A Practice of Anesthesia
for Infants and Children

A Practice of Anesthesia for Infants and Children

Fourth Edition

Charles J. Coté, MD, FAAP, MA(Hon)
Professor of Anaesthesia
Harvard Medical School
Director of Clinical Research, Division of Pediatric Anesthesia
MassGeneral Hospital for Children
Department of Anesthesia and Critical Care
Massachusetts General Hospital
Boston, Massachusetts

Jerrold Lerman, MD, FRCPC, FANZCA
Clinical Professor
Department of Anesthesia
Women and Children's Hospital of Buffalo
SUNY at Buffalo
Strong Memorial Hospital
University of Rochester
Rochester, New York

I. David Todres, MD
Professor of Pediatrics and Anaesthesia
Harvard Medical School
Chief, Ethics Unit
MassGeneral Hospital for Children
Department of Pediatrics
Massachusetts General Hospital
Boston, Massachusetts

SAUNDERS
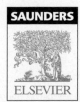
ELSEVIER

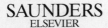

SAUNDERS
ELSEVIER

1600 John F. Kennedy Blvd.
Ste 1800
Philadelphia, PA 19103-2899

A Practice of Anesthesia for Infants and Children   ISBN: 978-1-4160-3134-5
Copyright © 2009 by Saunders, an imprint of Elsevier Inc.

Cover photo courtesy of Brian Smistek, Director of Medical Media, Women and
Children's Hospital of Buffalo, Buffalo, New York.

Notice

Knowledge and best practice in this field are constantly changing. As new research and experience
broaden our knowledge, changes in practice, treatment and drug therapy may become necessary or
appropriate. Readers are advised to check the most current information provided (i) on procedures
featured or (ii) by the manufacturer of each product to be administered, to verify the recommended
dose or formula, the method and duration of administration, and contraindications. It is the responsibility of the practitioner, relying on his or her own experience and knowledge of the patient, to make
diagnoses, to determine dosages and the best treatment for each individual patient, and to take all
appropriate safety precautions. To the fullest extent of the law, neither the publisher nor the editors
assume any liability for any injury and/or damage to persons or property arising out of or related to any
use of the material contained in this book.

The Publisher

Library of Congress Cataloging-in-Publication Data
A practice of anesthesia for infants and children / [edited by] Charles J. Coté, Jerrold Lerman, I. David
Todres.—4th ed.
    p. ; cm.
  Includes bibliographical references and index.
  ISBN 978-1-4160-3134-5 (alk. paper)
 1. Pediatric anesthesia.   I. Coté, Charles J.   II. Lerman, Jerrold.   III. Todres, I. David.
  [DNLM: 1. Anesthesia. 2. Child. 3. Infant.   WO 440 P895 2008]
  RD139.P73 2009
  617.9'6083—dc22   2008038001

Executive Publisher: Natasha Andjelkovic
Developmental Editor: Julie Mirra
Publishing Services Manager: Tina Rebane
Project Manager: Fran Gunning
Design Direction: Louis Forgione

Print in China

Last digit is the print number: 9   8   7   6   5   4   3   2   1

Working together to grow
libraries in developing countries

www.elsevier.com | www.bookaid.org | www.sabre.org

ELSEVIER   BOOK AID
            International   Sabre Foundation

Dedication

I wish to dedicate this edition of *A Practice of Anesthesia for Infants and Children* to my very wonderful friend, advisor, and mentor, David Todres, MD, who lost his battle with lymphoma on September 26, 2008. David was a unique individual who combined a wonderful sense of humor with his intelligence and dedication to making this world better and safer for children. In particular, he devoted much of his life in anesthesia and critical care medicine to challenging all of us on the ethics of our practices and on how to best protect the interests of our vulnerable young patients. David was a wonderful colleague who always looked at the bright side of every issue, including his own illness. He co-edited this text with me since its inception in 1982, an experience that profoundly impacted my life and career. We shared many nights at each other's homes reading aloud each chapter, realizing how effective it was to edit the material when the words were spoken rather than read. I believe that the success of the previous editions was due in no small part to this approach. Whenever we received a chapter that was not as well written as we had hoped, rather than sending it back to the author, David's approach was always "let's just rearrange the flowers to make it look better." These are wonderful words of advice that I shall always cherish.

Good-bye, David, we will all miss you. I hope to meet up with you "on the other side" so that together, we can once again "rearrange the flowers."

Charles J. Coté, MD

Contributors

Brian Anderson, PhD, FANZCA
Associate Professor
Department of Anaesthesiology
University of Auckland School of Medicine
Attending, Pediatric Anaesthesia and ICU
Starship Children's Hospital
Auckland, New Zealand
Orthopedic and Spine Surgery

Dean B. Andropoulos, MD, MHCM
Professor
Departments of Anesthesiology and Pediatrics
Baylor College of Medicine
Chief of Anesthesiology
Texas Children's Hospital
Houston, Texas
Cardiopulmonary Bypass and Management

Miriam Anixter, MD
Assistant Professor of Anesthesiology
University of Pittsburgh School of Medicine
Attending Anesthesiologist
Children's Hospital of Pittsburgh
University of Pittsburgh Medical Center
Pittsburgh, Pennsylvania
Organ Transplantation

M. A. Bender, MD, PhD
Associate Professor
Department of Pediatrics
Division of Hematology/Oncology
University of Washington School of Medicine
Director, Odessa Brown Sickle Cell Program
Odessa Brown Children's Clinic
Seattle, Washington
Essentials of Hematology

Charles Berde, MD, PhD
Professor of Anaesthesia (Pediatrics)
Harvard Medical School
Chief, Division of Pain Medicine
Department of Anesthesiology
Perioperative and Pain Medicine
Children's Hospital Boston
Boston, Massachusetts
Acute Pain

Frederic A. Berry, MD
Professor of Anesthesiology and Pediatrics
University of Virginia School of Medicine
Pediatric Anesthesiologist
University of Virginia Medical Center
Charlottesville, Virginia
Medicolegal Issues

Bruno Bissonnette, MD, FRCPC
Professor of Anesthesia
University of Toronto Faculty of Medicine
Toronto, Ontario, Canada
President and Founder
Children of the World Anesthesia Foundation
Thermal Regulation

Richard H. Blum, MD, MSE
Assistant Professor of Anaesthesia
Harvard Medical School
Senior Associate in Anesthesia and Medical Director
Post Anesthesia Care Unit
Children's Hospital Boston
Boston, Massachusetts
Pediatric Equipment

Adrian T. Bosenberg, MBChB, FFASA
Professor and Second Chair
Department of Anaesthesia
University Cape Town Faculty of Medicine
Chief Specialist Anaesthetist
Red Cross Children's War Memorial Hospital
Cape Town, South Africa
Pediatric Anesthesia in Developing Countries

Karen A. Brown, MD, FRCPC
Professor
Department of Anaesthesia
McGill University Faculty of Medicine
Staff Anesthesiologist
The Montreal Children's Hospital
Montreal, Quebec, Canada
Otorhinolaryngologic Procedures

Roland Brusseau, MD, FAAP
Instructor of Anaesthesia
Harvard Medical School
Assistant in Anesthesia
Children's Hospital Boston
Boston, Massachusetts
Fetal Intervention and the EXIT Procedure

James Cain, MD
Associate Professor
Department of Anesthesiology
University of Pittsburgh School of Medicine
Director of Trauma Anesthesiology
Children's Hospital of Pittsburgh
University of Pittsburgh Medical Center
Pittsburgh, Pennsylvania
Organ Transplantation

Anthony Chang, MD, MBA
Chief, Division of Cardiology
Medical Director, CHOC Heart Institute
Children's Hospital of Orange County
Orange, California
Cardiac Assist Devices

Carolyn I. Chi, MD
Fellow, Pediatric Endocrinology
Stanford University School of Medicine
Stanford, California
Essentials of Endocrinology

Franklyn Cladis, MD
Assistant Professor of Anesthesiology
University of Pittsburgh School of Medicine
Attending Anesthesiologist
Children's Hospital of Pittsburgh
University of Pittsburgh Medical Center
Pittsburgh, Pennsylvania
Organ Transplantation

Charles J. Coté, MD, FAAP, MA(Hon)
Professor of Anaesthesia
Harvard Medical School
Director of Clinical Research
Division of Pediatric Anesthesia
MassGeneral Hospital for Children
Department of Anesthesia and Critical Care
Massachusetts General Hospital
Boston, Massachusetts
The Practice of Pediatric Anesthesia; Preoperative Evaluation, Premedication, and Induction of Anesthesia; Pharmacokinetics and Pharmacology of Drugs Used in Children; Strategies for Blood Product Management and Reducing Transfusions; The Pediatric Airway; Burn Injuries; Regional Anesthesia; Sedation for Diagnostic and Therapeutic Procedures Outside the Operating Room; Procedures for Vascular Access; Pediatric Equipment

Joseph P. Cravero, MD
Professor of Anesthesiology and Pediatrics
Dartmouth Medical School, Hanover
Director of Pediatric Anesthesiology
Dartmouth Hitchcock Medical Center
Lebanon, New Hampshire
The Postanesthesia Care Unit and Beyond; Sedation for Diagnostic and Therapeutic Procedures Outside the Operating Room

Mark W. Crawford, MBBS, FRCPC
Associate Professor of Anesthesiology
University of Toronto Faculty of Medicine
Staff Anesthesiologist and Director of Research
The Hospital for Sick Children
Toronto, Ontario, Canada
Plastic and Reconstructive Surgery

Peter Crean, MBBCh, FRCA, FFARCS
Consultant Pediatric Anaesthetist
Royal Belfast Hospital for Sick Children
Belfast, United Kingdom
Essentials of Neurology and Neuromuscular Disease

Andrew J. Davidson, MBBS, MD, FANZCA
Clinical Associate Professor of Anaesthesiology
University of Melbourne Faculty of Medicine
Staff Anaesthetist
Royal Children's Hospital
Melbourne, Victoria, Australia
Interventional Cardiology

Peter J. Davis, MD, FAAP
Professor of Anesthesiology and Pediatrics
University of Pittsburgh School of Medicine
Anesthesiologist-in-Chief
Children's Hospital of Pittsburgh
University of Pittsburgh Medical Center
Pittsburgh, Pennsylvania
Essentials of Hepatology; Organ Transplantation

Hernando DeSoto, MD
Associate Professor, Department of Anesthesiology
University of Florida
College of Medicine–Jacksonville
Chief, Pediatric Anesthesia Division, and Medical Director,
   Operating Room
Shands Jacksonville Medical Center
Jacksonville, Florida
Trauma

Laura K. Diaz, MD
Assistant Professor of Anesthesiology and Critical Care Medicine
University of Pennsylvania School of Medicine
Staff Anesthesiology, Division of Cardiothoracic Anesthesia
The Cardiac Center at the Children's Hospital of Philadelphia
Philadelphia, Pennsylvania
Cardiac Assist Devices

Michael J. Eisses, MD
Assistant Professor, Department of Anesthesiology
University of Washington School of Medicine
Staff Anesthesiologist, Children's Hospital and Regional
   Medical Center
Seattle, Washington
Essentials of Hematology

Thomas Engelhardt, MD, PhD, FRCA
Honorary Senior Lecturer
University of Aberdeen Faculty of Medicine
Consultant Pediatric Anaesthetist
Department of Anaesthesia
Royal Aberdeen Children's Hospital
Aberdeen, United Kingdom
Plastic and Reconstructive Surgery

Lucinda L. Everett, MD, FAAP
Associate Professor of Anaesthesia
Harvard Medical School
Chief, Division of Pediatric Anesthesia
The MassGeneral Hospital for Children
Department of Anesthesia and Critical Care
Massachusetts General Hospital
Boston, Massachusetts
Pediatric Emergencies

Paul G. Firth, MBChB
Instructor in Anaesthesia
Harvard Medical School
Attending Anesthesiologist
Division of Pediatric Anesthesia
The MassGeneral Hospital for Children
Department of Anesthesia and Critical Care
Massachusetts General Hospital
Boston, Massachusetts
Essentials of Pulmonology

John Foreman, MD
Professor of Pediatrics
Duke University School of Medicine
Chief, Division of Pediatric Nephrology
Duke University Medical Center
Durham, North Carolina
Essentials of Nephrology

Gennadiy Fuzaylov, MD
Instructor in Anaesthesia
Harvard Medical School
Assistant in Anesthesia
Division of Pediatric Anesthesia
The MassGeneral Hospital for Children
Department of Anesthesia and Critical Care
Massachusetts General Hospital
Boston, Massachusetts
Pediatric Emergencies

Ralph Gertler, MD
Consultant Pediatric Cardiac Anesthesiologist
Institute of Anesthesiology
German Heart Centre of the State of Bavaria
Technical University Munich
Munich, Germany
Essentials of Cardiology; Cardiopulmonary Bypass and Management

Elizabeth A. Ghazal, MD
Assistant Professor of Anesthesiology
Loma Linda University School of Medicine
Loma Linda, California
Preoperative Evaluation, Premedication, and Induction of Anesthesia

Kenneth Goldschneider, MD
Associate Professor of Clinical Anesthesia and Pediatrics
University of Cincinnati College of Medicine
Director, Division of Pain Management
Cincinnati Children's Hospital Medical Center
Cincinnati, Ohio
Chronic Pain

Nishan Goudsouzian, MD, MS, MA(Hon)
Professor of Anaesthesia
Harvard Medical School
Pediatric Anesthetist
Division of Pediatric Anesthesia
The MassGeneral Hospital for Children
Department of Anesthesia and Critical Care
Massachusetts General Hospital
Boston, Massachusetts
Pharmacokinetics and Pharmacology of Drugs Used in Children

Eric F. Grabowski, MD
Associate Professor of Pediatrics
Harvard Medical School
Director, Cardiovascular Thrombosis Laboratory
Massachusetts General Hospital
Boston, Massachusetts
Strategies for Blood Product Management and Reducing Transfusions

Charles M. Haberkern, MD, MPH
Clinical Professor
Department of Anesthesiology
University of Washington School of Medicine
Staff Anesthesiologist
Children's Hospital and Regional Medical Center
Seattle, Washington
Essentials of Hematology

Gregory B. Hammer, MD
Professor of Anesthesia and Pediatrics
Stanford University School of Medicine, Stanford
Associate Director, Pediatric ICU
Director, Anesthesia Research
Lucile Packard Children's Hospital
Palo Alto, California
Anesthesia for Thoracic Surgery

Raafat S. Hannallah, MD
Professor of Anesthesiology and Pediatrics
The George Washington University Medical Center
School of Medicine and Health Sciences
Division of Anesthesiology
Children's National Medical Center
Washington, DC
Otorhinolaryngologic Procedures

Kenan E. Haver, MD
Assistant Professor of Pediatrics
Harvard Medical School
Associate Pediatrician
Massachusetts General Hospital
Boston, Massachusetts
Essentials of Pulmonology

Elaine Hicks, MA, MBBch, FRCPCH, MRCP(UK), DCH
Consultant Pediatric Neurologist
Royal Belfast Hospital for Sick Children
Belfast, United Kingdom
Essentials of Neurology and Neuromuscular Disease

Robert M. Insoft, MD
Assistant Professor of Pediatrics
Harvard Medical School
NICU Medical Director
Brigham and Women's Hospital
Boston, Massachusetts
Growth and Development

Andre Jaichenco, MD
Pediatric Anesthesiologist
Hospital Nacional de Pediatría S.Am.I.C.
Prof. Dr. Juan P. Garrahan
Buenos Aires, Argentina
Infectious Disease Considerations for the Operating Room

Zeev N. Kain, MD, MBA
Professor of Anesthesiology, Pediatrics, and Psychiatry
Chair, Department of Anesthesiology
Associate Dean of Clinical Research
University of California, Irvine, School of Medicine
Orange, California
Perioperative Behavior Stress in Children

Richard F. Kaplan, MD
Professor of Anesthesiology and Pain Medicine
The George Washington University Medical Center
School of Medicine and Health Sciences
Chief, Division of Anesthesiology and Pain Medicine
Children's National Medical Center
Washington, DC
Sedation for Diagnostic and Therapeutic Procedures Outside the Operating Room

Manoj K. Karmakar, MD, FRCA, DA(UK), FHKCA, FHKAM
Associate Professor and Director of Paediatric Anaethesia
Department of Anaesthesia and Intensive Care
The Chinese University of Hong Kong/Prince of Wales
  Hospital
Hong Kong, China
President Elect, Asian Society of Paediatric Anaesthesiologists
Ultrasound-Guided Regional Anesthesia

Babu V. Koka, MD
Assistant Professor of Anaesthesia
Harvard Medical School
Senior Associate in Anesthesia
Division Chief, Perioperative Anesthesia
Department of Anesthesiology
Children's Hospital Boston
Boston, Massachusetts
Anesthesia Outside the Operating Room

Elliot J. Krane, MD
Professor of Anesthesia and Pediatrics
Stanford University School of Medicine, Stanford
Director, Pain Management
Lucile Packard Children's Hospital
Palo Alto, California
Essentials of Endocrinology

C. Dean Kurth, MD
Professor of Anesthesia and Pediatrics
University of Cincinnati College of Medicine
Anesthesiologist-in-Chief
Department of Anesthesiology
Cincinnati Children's Hospital Medical Center
Cincinnati, Ohio
The Extremely Premature Infant (Micropremie)

Wing H. Kwok, MBChB, FANZCA, FHKCA, FHKAM
Adjunct Assistant Professor
Department of Anaesthesia and Intensive Care
The Chinese University of Hong Kong
Staff Specialist in Anaesthesia
Department of Anaesthesia and Intensive Care
Prince of Wales Hospital
Hong Kong, China
Ultrasound-Guided Regional Anesthesia

Geoffrey K. Lane, BPharm, MBBS, FRACP, FACC, FCSANZ
Staff Cardiologist
Lead Clinical Cardiac Catheterization Service
Royal Children's Hospital
Melbourne, Victoria, Australia
Interventional Cardiology

Jerrold Lerman, MD, FRCPC, FANZCA
Clinical Professor
Department of Anesthesia
Women and Children's Hospital of Buffalo
SUNY at Buffalo
Strong Memorial Hospital
University of Rochester
Rochester, New York
The Practice of Pediatric Anesthesia; Pharmacokinetics and Pharmacology of Drugs Used in Children; General Abdominal and Urologic Surgery; Plastic and Reconstructive Surgery; Malignant Hyerthermia

Steven Lichtenstein, MD
Clinical Associate Professor of Anesthesiology
University of Pittsburgh School of Medicine
Attending Anesthesiologist
Children's Hospital of Pittsburgh
University of Pittsburgh Medical Center
Pittsburgh, Pennsylvania
Organ Transplantation

Per-Arne Lönnqvist, MD, PhD, DEAA, FRCA
Professor of Paediatric Anaesthesia and Intensive Care
Department of Physiology and Pharmacology
Section of Anaesthesiology and Intensive Care
Karolinska Institute
Senior Consultant
Department of Paediatric Anaesthesia and Intensive Care
Astrid Lindgrens Children's Hospital
Karolinska University Hospital
Stockholm, Sweden
General Abdominal and Urologic Surgery

Igor Luginbuehl, MD
Assistant Professor of Anesthesiology
University of Toronto Faculty of Medicine
Staff Anesthesiologist
Department of Anesthesia
The Hospital for Sick Children
Toronto, Ontario, Canada
Thermal Regulation

Ralph A. Lugo, PharmD
Professor and Chair
Department of Pharmacy Practice
Bill Gatton College of Pharmacy
Adjunct Professor of Pediatrics
James H. Quillen College of Medicine
East Tennessee State University
Johnson City, Tennessee
Pharmacokinetics and Pharmacology of Drugs Used in Children

Jill MacLaren, PhD
Assistant Research Scientist
Department of Anesthesiology
University of California, Irvine, School of Medicine
Orange, California
Perioperative Behavior Stress in Children

Shobha Malviya, MD
Professor of Anesthesiology
University of Michigan
Ann Arbor, Michigan
Acute Pain

J. A. Jeevendra Martyn, MD
Professor of Anaesthesia
Harvard Medical School
Chief of Anesthesia, Shriners Burn Hospital
Attending Anesthesiologist
Massachusetts General Hospital
Boston, Massachusetts
Burn Injuries

Keira P. Mason, MD
Associate Professor of Anaesthesia (Radiology)
Harvard Medical School
Director, Radiology Anesthesia and Sedation
Children's Hospital Boston
Boston, Massachusetts
Anesthesia Outside the Operating Room

Linda J. Mason, MD
Professor of Anesthesiology and Pediatrics
Loma Linda University School of Medicine
Director of Pediatric Anesthesia
Loma Linda University Medical Center
Loma Linda, California
Preoperative Evaluation, Premedication, and Induction of Anesthesia

Linda C. Mayes, MD
Arnold Gesell Professor of Child Psychiatry, Pediatrics,
  and Psychology
Yale University School of Medicine
Staff Physician, Child Study Center
New Haven, Connecticut
Perioperative Behavior Stress in Children

Craig D. McClain, MD
Instructor in Anaesthesia
Harvard Medical School
Assistant in Perioperative Anesthesia
Children's Hospital Boston
Boston, Massachusetts
Fluid Management; Pediatric Neurosurgical Anesthesia

Angus McEwan, MBChB, FRCA
Honorary Senior Lecturer
Institute of Child Health, University College London
Consultant Anaesthetist
Great Ormond Street Hospital for Children
London, United Kingdom
Anesthesia for Children Undergoing Heart Surgery

Francis X. McGowan, Jr., MD
Professor of Anaesthesia (Pediatrics)
Harvard Medical School
Chief, Division of Cardiac Anesthesia
Director, Anesthesia/Critical Care Medicine Research
  Laboratory
Senior Associate in Cardiac Anesthesia
Children's Hospital Boston
Boston, Massachusetts
Cardiac Physiology and Pharmacology

Michael L. McManus, MD, MPH
Associate Professor of Anaesthesia
Harvard Medical School
Senior Associate in Critical Care Medicine and Perioperative
  Anesthesia
Children's Hospital Boston
Boston, Massachusetts
Fluid Management

Wanda C. Miller-Hance, MD
Associate Professor of Anesthesiology and Pediatrics
Baylor College of Medicine
Staff Physician
Texas Children's Hospital
Houston, Texas
*Essentials of Cardiology; Anesthesia for Noncardiac Surgery in
Children with Congenital Heart Disease*

Marilyn C. Morris, MD, MPH
Assistant Professor of Clinical Pediatrics
Columbia University College of Physicians and Surgeons
Attending, The Morgan Stanley Children's Hospital of
    New York
New York, New York
Cardiopulmonary Resuscitation

Neil S. Morton, MBChB, FRAC, FRCPCH, FFPmRCA
Senior Lecturer in Paediatric Anaesthesia and
    Pain Management
University of Glasgow
Consultant in Paediatric Anaesthesia and Pain Management
Royal Hospital for Sick Children
Glasgow, United Kingdom
Total Intravenous Anesthesia and Target-Controlled Infusion

Isabelle Murat, MD, PhD
Professor of Anesthesiology
Université Pierre et Marie Curie Paris VI
Chairman, Department of Anesthesia
Armand Trousseau Hospital
Paris, France
Pediatric Anesthesia in Developing Countries

Laura B. Myers, MD
Assistant Professor of Anaesthesia
Harvard Medical School
Associate in Anesthesia
Children's Hospital Boston
Boston, Massachusetts
Fetal Intervention and the EXIT Procedure

E. Kirk Neely, MD
Clinical Associate Professor of Pediatrics
Stanford University School of Medicine, Stanford
Lucile Packard Children's Hospital
Palo Alto, California
Essentials of Endocrinology

Jerome Parness, MD, PhD
Professor
Departments of Anesthesiology and Pharmacology
University of Pittsburgh School of Medicine
Staff Anesthesiologist
Children's Hospital of Pittsburgh
University of Pittsburgh Medical Center
Pittsburgh, Pennsylvania
Malignant Hyperthermia

David M. Polaner, MD, FAAP
Associate Professor of Anesthesiology
University of Colorado School of Medicine
Attending Pediatric Anesthesiologist
Chief, Acute Pain Service
The Children's Hospital Denver
Aurora, Colorado
Regional Anesthesia; Acute Pain

Erinn T. Rhodes, MD, MPH
Instructor in Pediatrics
Harvard Medical School
Director, Type 2 Diabetes Program
Physician in Medicine
Children's Hospital Boston
Boston, Massachusetts
Essentials of Endocrinology

Marcus R. Rivera, MD
Assistant Professor of Pediatrics
University of Pittsburgh School of Medicine
Attending, Department of Pediatrics
Division of Gastroenterology, Hepatology, and Nutrition
Children's Hospital of Pittsburgh
University of Pittsburgh Medical Center
Pittsburgh, Pennsylvania
Essentials of Hepatology

Jesse D. Roberts, Jr., MD, MS
Associate Professor of Anaesthesia (Pediatrics)
Harvard Medical School
Associate Pediatrician, Anesthetist, and Scientist
Division of Pediatric Anesthesia
The MassGeneral Hospital for Children
Department of Anesthesia and Critical Care
Massachusetts General Hospital
Boston, Massachusetts
Neonatal Emergencies

Mark A. Rockoff, MD, FAAP
Professor of Anaesthesia
Harvard Medical School
Associate Anesthesiologist-in-Chief
Children's Hospital Boston
Boston, Massachusetts
Pediatric Neurosurgical Anesthesia

Thomas M. Romanelli, MD
Instructor of Anaesthesia
Harvard Medical School
Assistant in Anesthesia
Division of Pediatric Anesthesia
The MassGeneral Hospital for Children
Department of Anesthesia and Critical Care
Massachusetts General Hospital
Boston, Massachusetts
Neonatal Emergencies

Allison Kinder Ross, MD
Associate Professor of Anesthesiology and Pediatrics
Duke University School of Medicine
Chief, Division of Pediatric Anesthesia
Duke University Medical Center
Durham, North Carolina
Essentials of Nephrology

Charles L. Schleien, MD
Professor of Pediatrics and Anesthesiology
Columbia University College of Physicians and Surgeons
Director of Pediatric Critical Care Medicine
The Morgan Stanley Children's Hospital of New York
New York, New York
Cardiopulmonary Resuscitation

Erik S. Shank, MD
Assistant Professor of Anaesthesia
Harvard Medical School
Associate Chief
Division of Pediatric Anesthesia
The MassGeneral Hospital for Children
Department of Anesthesia and Critical Care
Massachusetts General Hospital
Boston, Massachusetts
Burn Injuries

Robert L. Sheridan, MD
Associate Professor of Surgery
Harvard Medical School
Associate Chief of Staff and Attending Surgeon
Massachusetts General Hospital
Attending Surgeon, Shriners Burn Hospital
Department of Surgery
Boston, Massachusetts
Burn Injuries

Avinash C. Shukla, MBBS
Instructor in Anaesthesia
Harvard Medical School
Associate in Cardiac Anesthesia
Children's Hospital Boston
Boston, Massachusetts
Cardiac Physiology and Pharmacology

Adam Skinner, BSc(Hons), MBChB, MRCP(UK), FRCA
Consultant Paediatric Anaesthetist
Royal Children's Hospital
Melbourne, Victoria, Australia
Medications for Hemostasis; Interventional Cardiology

Timothy C. Slesnick, MD
Clinical Instructor in Pediatric Cardiology
Baylor College of Medicine
Staff Physician
Texas Children's Hospital
Houston, Texas
Essentials of Cardiology

Sulpicio G. Soriano, MD, FAAP
Associate Professor of Anaesthesia
Harvard Medical School
Senior Associate in Anesthesia
Children's Hospital Boston
Boston, Massachusetts
Pediatric Neurosurgical Anesthesia

James P. Spaeth, MD
Associate Professor of Anesthesia and Pediatrics
University of Cincinnati College of Medicine
Director of Cardiac Anesthesia
Department of Anesthesiology
Cincinnati Children's Hospital Medical Center
Cincinnati, Ohio
The Extremely Premature Infant (Micropremie)

Robert H. Squires, Jr., MD
Professor of Pediatrics
University of Pittsburgh School of Medicine
Clinical Director
Pediatric Gastroenterology, Hepatology, and Nutrition
Children's Hospital of Pittsburgh
University of Pittsburgh Medical Center
Pittsburgh, Pennsylvania
Essentials of Hepatology

James M. Steven, MD, SM
Associate Professor of Anesthesia and Pediatrics
University of Pennsylvania School of Medicine
Chief Medical Officer and Senior Anesthesiologist
The Children's Hospital of Philadelphïa
Philadelphia, Pennsylvania
Cardiac Physiology and Pharmacology

Robert C. Stough, MD
Associate Professor
Department of Anesthesiology
University of Pittsburgh School of Medicine
Staff Anesthesiologist and Director of Radiological
    Anesthesiology
Children's Hospital of Pittsburgh
University of Pittsburgh Medical Center
Pittsburgh, Pennsylvania
Malignant Hyperthermia

Christopher P. Stowell, MD, PhD
Assistant Professor of Pathology
Harvard Medical School
Director, Blood Transfusion Service
Massachusetts General Hospital
Boston, Massachusetts
Strategies for Blood Product Management and Reducing Transfusions

Santhanam Suresh, MD
Associate Professor of Anesthesia
Northwestern University Feinberg School of Medicine
Attending Anesthesiologist
Children's Memorial Hospital
Chicago, Illinois
Regional Anesthesia

Alexandra Szabova, MD
Assistant Professor of Clinical Anesthesia and Pediatrics
University of Cincinnati College of Medicine
Attending, Department of Anesthesia
Division of Pain Management
Cincinnati Children's Hospital Medical Center
Cincinnati, Ohio
Chronic Pain

Andreas Taenzer, MD, FAAP
Assistant Professor of Anesthesiology and Pediatrics
Dartmouth Medical School, Hanover
Co-Director, Pediatric Anesthesiology
Director, Pediatric Pain Service
Dartmouth Hitchcock Medical Center/Children's Hospital of
    Dartmouth
Lebanon, New Hampshire
The Postanesthesia Care Unit and Beyond

Joseph J. Tepas III, MD
Professor of Surgery and Pediatrics
University of Florida College of Medicine–Jacksonville
Chief, Division of Pediatric Surgery
Shands Jacksonville Medical Center
Jacksonville, Florida
Trauma

Joseph R. Tobin, MD
Professor of Anesthesiology and Pediatrics
Department of Anesthesiology
Wake Forest University School of Medicine
Winston-Salem, North Carolina
Ophthalmology

I. David Todres, MD
Professor of Pediatrics
Harvard Medical School
Chief, Ethics Unit
Division of Pediatric Anesthesia
The MassGeneral Hospital for Children
Department of Anesthesia and Critical Care
Massachusetts General Hospital
Boston, Massachusetts
The Practice of Pediatric Anesthesia; Growth and Development; Ethical Issues in Pediatric Anesthesiology; The Pediatric Airway; Neonatal Emergencies; Pediatric Emergencies; Cardiopulmonary Resuscitation

Robert D. Truog, MD
Professor of Medical Ethics and Anaesthesia (Pediatrics)
Director of Clinical Ethics
Harvard Medical School
Director, Institute for Professionalism and Ethical Practice
Senior Associate in Critical Care Medicine
Children's Hospital Boston
Boston, Massachusetts
Ethical Issues in Pediatric Anesthesiology

Susan T. Verghese, MD
Professor of Anesthesiology and Pediatrics
The George Washington University Medical Center School of Medicine and Health Sciences
Director of Cardiac Anesthesia
Department of Anesthesiology and Pain Medicine
Children's National Medical Center
Washington, DC
Otorhinolaryngologic Procedures

David B. Waisel, MD
Associate Professor of Anaesthesia
Harvard Medical School
Senior Associate in Anesthesia
Children's Hospital Boston
Boston, Massachusetts
Ethical Issues in Pediatric Anesthesiology

Samuel H. Wald, MD
Associate Clinical Professor
Department of Anesthesiology
David Geffen School of Medicine at UCLA
Los Angeles, California
Procedures for Vascular Access

Robert M. Ward, MD
Professor of Pediatrics
Director, Pediatric Pharmacology Program
University of Utah School of Medicine
Salt Lake City, Utah
Pharmacokinetics and Pharmacology of Drugs Used in Children

R. Grey Weaver, Jr., MD
Associate Professor
Department of Ophthalmology
Wake Forest University School of Medicine
Winston-Salem, North Carolina
Ophthalmology

Nicole E. Webel, MD
Acting Assistant Professor
Department of Anesthesiology
University of Washington School of Medicine
Staff Anesthesiologist
Children's Hospital and Regional Medical Center
Seattle, Washington
Essentials of Hematology

Rebecca W. West, JD
Assistant Professor of General Medicine
University of Virginia School of Medicine
CEO, Piedmont Liability Trust
Charlottesville, Virginia
Medicolegal Issues

Melissa Wheeler, MD
Chief of Anesthesiology
Shriners Hospitals for Children
Chicago, Illinois
The Pediatric Airway

Delbert R. Wigfall, MD
Associate Dean of Medical Education and Associate Professor of Pediatrics
Division of Pediatric Nephrology
Duke University School of Medicine
Durham, North Carolina
Essentials of Nephrology

Niall Wilton, MRCP, FRCA
Clinical Director
Paediatric Anaesthesia and Operating Rooms
Starship Children's Hospital
Auckland, New Zealand
Orthopedic and Spine Surgery

Andrew Wolf, MA, MBBCh, MD, FRCA
Honorary Professor of Anaesthesia
University of Bristol–Medicine
Consultant in Paediatric Anaesthesia and Intensive Care
Bristol Royal Hospital for Children
Bristol, United Kingdom
Medications for Hemostasis

Joseph I. Wolfsdorf, MB, BcH
Professor of Pediatrics
Harvard Medical School
Clinical Director and Associate Chief
Division of Endocrinology
Senior Associate in Medicine
Children's Hospital Boston
Boston, Massachusetts
Essentials of Endocrinology

Myron Yaster, MD
Richard J. Traystman Professor
Departments of Anesthesiology, Critical Care Medicine,
  and Pediatrics
Johns Hopkins University School of Medicine
Attending, Johns Hopkins Hospital
Baltimore, Maryland
*Sedation for Diagnostic and Therapeutic Procedures Outside the
Operating Room*

Preface

This fourth edition of *A Practice of Anesthesia for Infants and Children* has undergone a radical evolution from its original version published in 1985. Drs. Goudsouzian and Ryan have retired as editors, and Dr. Jerrold Lerman has joined Drs. Coté and Todres. Dr. Lerman brings a new, international perspective to the editorship. This book has blossomed from its humble beginnings as a synopsis of local practice to an international authoritative and evidence-based tome. In parallel with its growth, the contributorship has expanded beyond pediatric anesthesiologists to include pediatricians, internists, surgeons, a lawyer, and a pharmacologist. More than 20 of the pediatric anesthesiologists are also board-certified pediatricians, two with further subspecialty board certification (in cardiology and neonatology). The inclusion of 110 contributors from six continents represents a tribute to the global child-care network.

We have taken full advantage of advances in state-of-the-art publishing, including Internet access. This edition has a new feel and style to it; it is now divided into ten color-coded sections: Introduction, Drug and Fluid Therapy, The Chest, The Heart, The Brain and Glands, The Abdomen, Other Surgeries, Emergencies, Pain, and Special Topics. This color-coding format enables the reader to find chapters and topics of interest easily and quickly. In keeping with our mission to publish a comprehensive global text on pediatric anesthesia, we have expanded the number of chapters, as well as their content, to cover a wide range of anesthetic and pediatric subjects. To maintain a size similar to that of previous editions, we have shifted all but a few select references from each chapter to the accompanying website, with hypertext links to the original publications. Color has been added to the illustrations, photographs, and graphics to maximize clarity and to enhance visual appeal. In keeping with our mission to transform the book into a comprehensive text, we have included contributions from a number of pediatric specialists, who have shared their perspectives on and insights into basic pediatric physiology and the pathophysiologic implications of diseases in children. In each case, these specialists have been paired with a pediatric anesthesiologist to ensure a clinical anesthetic perspective.

The largest chapter of the book is that on pharmacology, with more than 1500 references; as in previous editions, this chapter benefits from the input of a neonatologist–pharmacologist and a clinical pharmacologist–pharmacist, with the addition of Dr.

Lerman as a coauthor for this edition. Throughout, this fourth edition maintains content on older medications, with the understanding that the book will be used by a wide variety of practitioners who work in very different environments. A separate chapter has been devoted to total intravenous anesthesia (TIVA) for children, an area of growing interest. The pediatric airway chapter now includes a discussion of the numerous supraglottic devices as well as emergency airway management strategies and equipment currently available for use in infants and children. The transfusion chapter has been updated with contributions from a pediatric hematologist (specializing in hemophilia) and the Director of the Blood Transfusion Service of the Massachusetts General Hospital. We also have added a variety of chapters dealing with such specialized issues as thoracic anesthesia, orthopedics, plastic surgery, general and urologic surgery, and the practice of anesthesia in medically disadvantaged countries. We have expanded the cardiac anesthesia section to include separate chapters on cardiopulmonary bypass, medications used for hemostasis, cardiac assist devices, and the cardiac catheterization laboratory. In the section on the abdomen, the chapter on organ transplantation remains a centerpiece. Other new chapters in this edition address medical-legal issues, infectious diseases, and the extremely premature infant, as well the ex-utero intrapartum treatment (EXIT) procedure. The trauma chapter is now coauthored by a pediatric trauma surgeon.

The increasing awareness of the importance of adequately treating children's pain is highlighted by chapters devoted to landmark- and ultrasound-guided regional anesthesia, chronic pain, and the management of acute postoperative pain. Various pain scoring systems for both normal and cognitively impaired children are discussed, to permit further insight into pain management strategies for these special children.

Finally, the accompanying website has enabled us to expand the audiovisual content of the book with a myriad of illustrations, pictures, video clips, and sample order forms. The addition of videos, in particular, affords the opportunity to view a hands-on approach to procedures such as ultrasound- and landmark-guided nerve blocks, catheter insertions, radiological investigations, ultrasound procedures, and echocardiograms, as well as various levels of sedation and analgesia. A pocket reference card is also provided that allows the reader to obtain general recommendations on doses of commonly used medications for a child of a given body weight.

Undertaking this revision has been quite a journey, oftentimes appearing to be a microcosm of the world and life. Many of our contributors have experienced a variety of life's challenges during the writing of their chapters. Nevertheless, they all have succeeded in crafting masterful chapters to create what we believe to be a state-of-the-art text on pediatric anesthesia.

The editors spent many days and nights "discussing" opposing viewpoints on many controversial issues in pediatric anesthesia before reaching common middle ground. It is our belief that these discussions, together with a global perspective on selection of our contributing authors, served to greatly strengthen the quality of the text and to infuse a truly international flavor.

We hope that *A Practice of Anesthesia for Infants and Children* will continue to provide a framework for students in our specialty, as well for the practicing clinician. We believe that the book is a truly practical resource for pediatric anesthesiologists and other pediatric care providers in clinical practice around the world.

Charles J. Coté, MD
Jerrold Lerman, MD
I. David Todres, MD

Acknowledgments

I wish to thank the Chairpersons of the Departments of Anesthesiology, Pediatrics, Surgery, and Internal Medicine around the world, who supported the academic endeavors of their staff and thus made it possible for them to contribute to this fourth edition of *A Practice of Anesthesia for Infants and Children*. In particular, I thank Dr. Richard J. Kitz, who originally had sufficient faith in a very junior attending to give me the time to be the initial engine in the development and growth of the first and second editions of this book while at the Massachusetts General Hospital. Later, Dr. Steven C. Hall provided similar support for the third edition while I was at the Children's Memorial Hospital in Chicago. Now I have returned to my roots and rejoined the staff at the Massachusetts General Hospital and the MassGeneral Hospital for Children. The wonderful support of Dr. Warren M. Zapol and recently Dr. Jeanine Wiener-Kronish has provided me the time to develop a totally new book. It has been a tremendous transition—from black and white to color, from 32 chapters to 53, from a national to a truly international text, with the addition of many multimedia bells and whistles, including our own website. Of most importance, I thank all of the wives, husbands, significant others, children, friends, secretaries, and staff members who lent their support to this wonderful international family of experts that has come together to produce the fourth edition.

Charles J. Coté, MD

Contents

Introduction

The Practice of Pediatric Anesthesia

CHAPTER 1

Charles J. Coté, Jerrold Lerman, and I. David Todres

Preoperative Evaluation and Management	Hearing
Parents and Child	Touch
The Anesthesiologist	**Airway and Ventilation**
Informed Consent	**Fluids and Perfusion**
Operating Room and Monitoring	**Conduct of Anesthesia Team**
Induction and Maintenance of Anesthesia	**Recovery Room**
Clinical Monitors	**Postoperative Visit**
Sight	**Summary**

IN THIS CHAPTER WE outline the basis of our collective practice of pediatric anesthesia. These basic principles of practice can be applied regardless of the circumstances; they provide the foundation for safe anesthesia.

Preoperative Evaluation and Management

Parents and Child

Anesthesiologists must assume an active role in the preoperative assessment of children. Ideally, the anesthesiologist performing the preoperative evaluation will also anesthetize the child. A complete medical and surgical history, family history, chart review, evaluation and review of laboratory, radiologic and other testing, and physical examination are performed on every patient to be anesthetized (see Chapter 4). When appropriate, the child should receive preoperative medical therapy to optimize his or her condition or conditions before receiving anesthesia (e.g., children with seizure disorders or reactive airway disease). In addition, the emotional state of the child and family must be considered and appropriate psychological and, if necessary, pharmacologic support provided. The anesthesia team, working in concert with surgical colleagues and nursing and child-life specialists, should find appropriate and creative techniques (e.g., videotapes, booklets, hospital tours, and trained paramedical personnel) to prepare the child and

family. The marked increase in outpatient surgical procedures has reduced the time available for interaction between the anesthesiologist and the family and child. Despite this reduced contact time, these support techniques should not be neglected.

Familiarity with a child's clinical and psychological status as well as the parental concerns is essential to delivering quality anesthesia care. To achieve the very best outcome for each child, it is essential to meet with the child and the parents together and establish rapport preoperatively. There are many developmental issues that surround the hospital experience: for example, teenagers fear loss of control, awareness, and pain; younger children fear mutilation from their surgery; and toddlers fear separation from their parents (see Chapter 3). However, for children who are old enough to understand (usually age 5 years and older), it is reasonable to explain in simple terms what anesthesia involves and what will transpire on entering the operating room. It is vital to speak directly to the child because he or she is the person having the surgery. Children at the age of reason have the same fears as adults. However, it is more difficult for them to articulate these fears to us and to their parents. It is important to explain that the sleep from anesthesia medicine is different from the sleep at home. Many children are fearful of not awakening. Children require reassurance that *they will not feel anything during surgery, that they will not wake up during the procedure, and that they will awaken at the conclusion.* The possibility of postoperative pain and the relief the child will receive in the form of nerve blocks and analgesics must be clearly presented to the parents and child. It is also important to explain to the child and the family what they can anticipate on entering the operating room and to explain the special monitoring you, as the anesthesiologist, will be providing for their child. A simple explanation of the monitors can be very reassuring to parents and interesting for many children: (1) the pulse oximeter (a Band-Aid–like device that lights up red and measures the oxygen in the bloodstream during anesthesia and recovery), (2) the blood pressure cuff (an *"arm hugger"* or *"muscle tester"*), (3) electrocardiogram leads (*"little sticky things that don't hurt so we can watch the heart beat"*), (4) we measure the oxygen you (your child) are (is) breathing; (5) we measure the concentration of the anesthesia medicines you (your child) are (is) breathing; (6) we measure the carbon dioxide you (your child) are (is) breathing so as to ensure that your (your child's) breathing is just right throughout the anesthesia. Sometimes asking teenagers if they have studied carbon dioxide in school science class helps them to better understand the monitors and provides reassurance as well as making it more interesting. The detail with which this is presented will vary from family to family and child to child as well as with the anesthesiologist's understanding of the needs of the child and family. By the end of the interview, however, the child and the parents should understand that you will be providing the quality of care that ensures their child's safety during anesthesia, thus reducing the parents' and child's anxiety. Explanation is also needed to describe the induction of anesthesia, and the degree of detail used will again depend on the developmental level of the child. For young children, one can present a plan to breathe "laughing gas" through a flavored mask, with a flavor that he or she can choose. Older children can be given the option of an intravenous induction, with nitrous oxide by mask to start the intravenous line relatively painlessly; or if they are needle phobic, they might be given the option of an inhalational induction. If parents are to be present during induction of anesthesia, it is essential to describe to them how they can assist in comforting their child and prepare them for what they might observe and experience to avoid any misconceptions. Parents should not be pressured into feeling that they must be present for induction of anesthesia. It must be clear that their presence during induction is for their child's benefit; and if at any time during the induction there is a new or additional risk to their child that they may be asked to leave and be escorted out of the operating room. Remind them that their presence at induction is for their child's benefit and a privilege, not a right. Thus, if there are issues with a difficult airway, the need for a rapid induction of anesthesia, or for the very young, then it would be inappropriate for the parents to be present and not in their child's best interest for physicians and nurses to be distracted at a time when everyone's attention needs to be focused on the child.

It is helpful and essential to explain to the parents specific changes in their child that might be observed at the time of anesthetic induction:

1. As anyone is anesthetized, the eyes may roll up: *"you might see your child's eyes roll up and this is completely normal and happens to all of us when we fall asleep; it is just that we are not looking for it."*
2. *"As people fall asleep they often make snoring noises and other noises from their throat; if your child does this it is completely normal."*
3. *"As the anesthetic reaches the brain the brain sometimes gets excited before it goes to sleep so it is common to see some children move their arms and legs or turn their head from side to side. This means the anesthetic is having its effect and even though your child appears to be partly awake he (or she) has received enough anesthesia to ensure that he (or she) does not remember this."*
4. *"If your child becomes frightened, we will increase the concentration of the anesthesia medicine rapidly and calm the child as quickly as possible."*
5. If the child is to have an intravenous induction, then informing the parents that their child might suddenly look pale and that the start of anesthesia will be very rapid is also helpful so as to avoid confusion about what the parents will observe.

These preemptive explanations are important to avoid unnecessarily making the parents anxious at a time when you need to focus on the child. It is common for parents to decline to be present during induction once they hear these explanations. Finally, reassure the parents that for surgeries in which nausea and vomiting are likely that appropriate prophylactic antiemetic therapy will be administered and that if pain is anticipated it will be aggressively managed in the operating room and recovery room. Anesthesiologists can provide valuable assistance in this respect because of their knowledge of the pharmacology of sedative and narcotic drugs (see Chapter 6), as well as their ability to perform neuroaxial and peripheral nerve blocks (see Chapters 42 to 44). The possible need for postoperative intensive care, including assisted ventilation, should be anticipated and fully discussed with the parents and child (if the child is of an appropriate age). If special monitoring is required in the operating room or postoperatively, this should be explained and the child assured that the intravenous catheters, airway devices, and all invasive monitoring devices will be placed after induction of anesthesia so as to avoid causing discomfort and will be removed as soon as the child's postoperative condition permits.

The anesthesiologist who sits down, who speaks slowly and clearly while answering questions, and who does not appear distracted and in a rush to leave presents a very different image from the anesthesiologist who stands tapping his or her toes, speaks quickly, and has one foot pointed toward the door. Details regarding the anesthetic should not be recited in a cold and technical manner but rather with communication that addresses the parents' and the child's questions and concerns. This dialogue is frequently given too little time, leaving the parents and child insecure and unnecessarily apprehensive. Body language is especially important during this preoperative interview. If the family speaks a different language than the anesthesiologist, then a medical interpreter should be sought.

The Anesthesiologist

Anesthesiologists must fully understand the proposed surgical or investigative procedure to facilitate the planning of an appropriate level of monitoring and selection of anesthetic drugs and technique. The anesthesiologist must anticipate the needs of the surgeon or proceduralist in terms of patient positioning for the procedure, the need for or avoidance of muscle relaxation, considerations regarding specific procedures (e.g., evoked motor and sensory potentials and anesthetic technique), intravenous fluid and blood product management (see Chapters 8 and 10), as well as the need for and strategies for perioperative pain and anxiety control (see Chapters 42–44). For complex cases, the anesthesiologist and surgeon should formulate a plan preoperatively and explain the plan to the parents and child. All important medical issues that require clarification should be investigated during the preoperative evaluation and planning process. It is useful to discuss your concerns with the appropriate medical consultants (e.g., the neurologist for the management of seizure medications in the perioperative period, the hematologist for the child with hemophilia, and others as indicated).

For the anesthesiologist to maximize the value from such consultations, it is important to focus the discussion with the medical specialist on the specific anesthetic or medical issue of concern. Consultant recommendations must be carefully reviewed and should reflect the consultant's understanding of the anesthesia process and what it is you need from him or her regarding management issues (see Chapters 11, 14, 22, 24, 26, and 28). Appropriate preoperative abstinence from food and fluid should always be ordered. Infants must receive special consideration; prolonged abstinence may lead to dehydration or hypoglycemia (see Chapters 4 and 8). Children may surreptitiously circumvent the preoperative fasting orders especially if the period of fasting is prolonged or other children in the vicinity are seen in the possession of food. One must always be prepared for the possibility of a full stomach and its sequelae. For example, the risk for pulmonary aspiration of gastric contents is increased in some children (e.g., those with obesity, previous esophageal surgery, difficult intubation, hiatal hernia). Management of the anesthetic in these children should be appropriately modified so as to minimize the risk of regurgitation and aspiration. Preoperative consideration must be given to proper psychological support, appropriate premedication, and the timing of the premedication (see Chapters 3 and 4). Premedication may be omitted because of the critical nature of a child's illness or because a child is especially cooperative. Psychological support of the child and parents must never be neglected, no matter how calm they might appear. Premedication may be administered on the ward or in the surgical waiting room. Once any medication is administered, a child must be observed for any compromise in cardiopulmonary function.

If the child is premedicated on the ward, transport to the operating room must be undertaken with caution and with appropriate monitoring. A critically ill child must be accompanied by skilled staff who will ensure continued infusion of vasoactive medications and who are skilled in the management of any emergencies that could arise during transport (see Chapter 39).

Informed Consent

The benefits and risks of the anesthetic procedure must be presented in clear, easily understood terms. At the same time, it is important not to present this in a manner that unduly frightens the child or parents. The details of such a presentation will depend, in part, on the severity of the underlying medical and surgical conditions and how these affect anesthetic management and the planned procedure. Thus, risk can be presented in general terms such as

- *"The risks of anesthesia are generally proportional to how healthy someone is. For example, if a child has a problem with*

the heart or lungs or kidneys, etc., then this would increase the risk from anesthesia. In your child's case these are our concerns" (and then elaborate the particular patient's issues, such as reactive airway disease, apnea of prematurity, etc.). *"Knowing these problems ahead of time makes it safer for your child because we can choose our anesthetic prescription according to your child's specific needs. However, there is always the possibility of allergic or unusual response to anesthetic medications that we cannot predict and that is why I will be observing your child very carefully with all the monitors that I described."*

We are designing our "anesthetic prescription" specifically for the specific needs of the child, and this notion should be described exactly this way to the parents; we are physicians and not technicians; and just as the pediatrician writes a prescription for antibiotics, anesthesiologists write the treatment prescription for anesthesia and administer it. If a child is critically ill or has a disease process that is an immediate threat to his or her life, then this must be explained to the family. If a parent asks about mortality risk, all one can say is that the mortality related to anesthesia varies from one in several hundred thousand for healthy children undergoing routine procedures to a much higher rate for children who are critically ill but that the mortality for any one child is never predictable.

Operating Room and Monitoring

For the anesthesiologist to successfully carry out a proposed anesthetic plan, the child's chart must be examined for pertinent information before induction of anesthesia; for children who have already been screened, the chart should be re-reviewed for new information that may have been added since the initial evaluation. It is most important that the child's identification bracelet be checked, especially if the anesthetizing team is different from the preoperative evaluation team. A "time out" for nurses, surgeon, and anesthesiologist to confirm the child's name, the planned surgical procedure, and the site of the surgical procedure (right or left side) is a vital part of the safety net we provide in the operating room. All equipment for induction and maintenance of anesthesia, including suction and all necessary monitoring devices, must be functioning and reliable (see Chapter 53). *Equipment must be checked by the anesthesia team taking care of the child.*

The degree of monitoring should be appropriate for the child's underlying clinical condition and the planned surgical procedure. In every situation, basic monitoring is essential; to this are added special monitoring devices as they become necessary. The basic monitors are the anesthesiologist's eyes, ears, and hands, which confer the ability to observe a child's color and chest movements, to listen for heart tones and breath sounds, and to palpate the arterial pulse and temperature of the skin. A precordial or esophageal stethoscope is a very useful and simple device that allows constant assessment of heart tones and the quality of breath sounds even when our attention is focused away from physiologic monitors. All children, except those undergoing the briefest noninvasive procedures, should have an intravenous line inserted to allow for fluid replacement and provide a route for rapid and predictable administration of drugs. If an intravenous line is already in place, it is vital to assure the adequacy of its function and size before anesthetic induction. Fluid replacement with balanced solution is particularly important in children who have undergone prolonged fasting or who have ongoing third space losses, although glucose-containing solutions may be preferable under specific circumstances (see Chapter 8). Continuous monitoring of the electrocardiogram, temperature, inspired oxygen concentration, oxygen saturation, expired carbon dioxide, and intermittent blood pressure determination are considered routine. Expired carbon dioxide monitors (especially those that display the waveform) and pulse oximetry are extremely important in the early detection of potential anesthetic-related events that, if undetected, could result in serious morbidity or mortality. Monitoring of the anesthetic agent is also helpful but not necessary. The role of wakefulness-monitoring devices in children is yet to be established, especially in children who are younger than 2 years of age.

Invasive cardiovascular monitoring (e.g., direct arterial blood pressure, central venous pressure, or very rarely pulmonary artery occlusion pressure) may be required for major surgery if extensive blood loss or major fluid shifts are anticipated or if a child is medically unstable. A urinary catheter provides indirect data reflecting intravascular volume status and organ perfusion in the presence of normal renal function. Monitoring urinary output is particularly useful for prolonged operations, for procedures involving major blood loss, when there is the potential for rapid or massive blood loss, when wide variations in blood pressure and fluid balance can be anticipated, or during induced hypotensive anesthesia. *In general terms, if a particular variable would be monitored in an adult, then the same approach should be adopted for a child.*

Invasive monitoring procedures are sometimes forsaken in a child because of the anesthesiologist's inexperience with pediatric techniques; the need for invasive monitoring is thus dismissed as being "excessive." These monitors, however, allow the accurate measurement of blood pressure, cardiac output, filling pressures, and cardiac and pulmonary function. In turn, they provide a safe mechanism for assessing the response to pharmacologic interventions, as well as the responses to administration of blood products, fluids, and vasoactive medications (see Chapter 49).

A cautionary note: With increased sophistication in monitoring, anesthesiologists have become more distanced than ever from their patients. Relying totally on mechanical monitoring devices to detect clinical abnormalities is dangerous. *The focus must always be on the child and the surgical field. Monitors may fail, and if the anesthesiologist focuses attention on the monitor in an effort to interpret it, rather than attending directly to the child, the child may suffer.* This is the reason that a precordial stethoscope is so useful; strong heart tones in the face of failed monitors provides assurance that the child is likely not in severe trouble. *Disabling monitor alarms for an extended period of time is a serious breech of safety and acceptable practice standards.* One of the editors knows of a child in whom all monitor alarms and sounds were disabled during the anesthetic, who was discovered dead at the conclusion of the procedure after an unrecognized, unintended tracheal extubation. Most importantly, the tone of the pulse oximeter should be audible by everyone in the operating room to detect decreasing oxygen saturation.

Induction and Maintenance of Anesthesia

Significant differences in the physiology and behavior of a child, especially a neonate, in comparison with an adult, mandate that the anesthesiologist not consider a child as merely a small adult. In an infant, the rate of uptake of inhalation anesthetic agents is more rapid than in an adult. An infant's response to most oral and intravenous medications is also different; therefore, changes made in concentration of an inspired inhalation agent should be more gradual and the doses of medication diluted and carefully titrated.

The approach to an anesthetic procedure in a child is in principle similar to that in an adult. In practice, however, it is often advisable to modify the sequence of application of monitoring devices. In a relatively stable child, anesthesia induction may proceed with a pulse oximeter and possibly a precordial stethoscope, with the remaining monitors applied after anesthesia is induced. This sequence often avoids a prolonged preparation phase during which a child may have more time to become anxious and distressed. In a critically ill child, however, while attempting always to approach a child in the least threatening way, establishing monitoring must not be compromised. Thus, therapeutic interventions in very sick children and adults proceed along similar pathways. Obviously in a struggling, upset child, some but not all monitors may be successfully applied. The pulse oximeter may not function in a struggling child until the finger or toe is relaxed.

Clinical Monitors

In children as in adults, monitoring begins with the basic observations of a child's general condition, the heart rate, blood pressure, respirations, and temperature. The most important aspect of basic monitoring consists of using the senses of sight, hearing, and touch to integrate all the data provided by patient observations and the monitors.

Sight
Constantly observing a child's chest excursions (depth and symmetry), the color of the nail beds, oral mucosa, and capillary refill provides vital information about the adequacy of ventilation and perfusion. Observation of the surgical field provides an immediate indication of the extent of fluid shifts and blood loss, the color of the blood in the surgical field, evidence of muscle relaxation, depth of anesthesia, and any physiologic problems that may be caused by the surgery (e.g., surgical retraction causing venous obstruction).

Hearing
Constantly listening to the pitch of the pulse oximeter as well as the heart tones and breath sounds through a precordial or esophageal stethoscope gives instant and continuous feedback about oxygenation (pulse oximeter), heart rate and rhythm, an impression of the cardiac output (changes in intensity of heart sounds), and the adequacy of ventilation (wheezing, stridor, laryngeal spasm, no air exchange). This information is particularly helpful in diagnosing arrhythmias, hypovolemia, anesthetic overdose, and airway obstruction. Listening to the sounds of

surgery may also be helpful, such as the sudden change in the noise of the suction device with rapid blood loss or the surgeon's comments regarding technical difficulties with the procedure.

Touch

Intermittently examining a child—especially palpating peripheral pulses and the skin—provides information that may confirm the auditory input about heart rate, cardiac output, blood pressure, perfusion, and temperature.

Airway and Ventilation

The most important consideration in the safe practice of pediatric anesthesia is attention to the adequacy of the airway. Obstruction occurs readily because of the unique characteristics of the infant and child airway (see Chapter 12). Thus, the anesthesiologist must maintain constant vigilance over the airway to ensure that it remains clear at all times. Airway obstruction may lead to hypoventilation, although the causes of hypoventilation may be central (narcotics or inhalation agents) or peripheral (muscle relaxants) in origin. Thus, anesthesiologists must always place emphasis and attention on constantly monitoring the adequacy of ventilation, particularly when administering anesthesia via a face mask; this is because the expired carbon dioxide tension may underestimate the true carbon dioxide tension as a result of a poor mask fit with air leaks and an obstructed airway. The capnogram is usually very accurate during mask anesthesia. Failure to detect an appropriate end-tidal carbon dioxide tension suggests inadequate ventilation or a mask leak or reduced pulmonary blood flow, with the result that the child's condition may deteriorate from lack of an adequate airway or dilution of anesthetic gas concentrations.

Although it is desirable to optimize ventilation by maintaining an arterial carbon dioxide pressure within the normal range (35 to 45 mm Hg), most healthy infants and children are not harmed by mild to moderate overventilation; however, severe underventilation has more serious implications.

Constant monitoring of inspired oxygen concentration, expired carbon dioxide concentration, and oxygen saturation is a valuable adjunct to the senses of sight, hearing, and touch. *Failure to ventilate adequately is probably the most important factor in the morbidity and mortality of children undergoing anesthesia.*

Fluids and Perfusion

Intraoperative fluid management is especially important in infants and children. Rapid development of hypovolemia with what may appear to be a trivial amount of blood loss or fluid shifts may occur in infants because they were fasted for a prolonged period preoperatively and because of their relatively small blood volume. Replacement of lost blood and basic fluid administration must be carefully titrated (using rate-limiting devices), because overhydration readily occurs. The anesthesiologist should have a clear plan for the type of fluid and the volume of fluid for perioperative administration. Preoperative calculation of maintenance, deficit, and potential third space losses helps in formulating this fluid management plan. A well-planned outline results in a rational and safe approach to correction of fluid deficit, maintenance, and losses (see Chapters 8 and 10).

Conduct of the Anesthesia Team

The anesthesiologist must maintain full concentration throughout the procedure; the child's safety is in his or her hands, and any inattention may place the child's life in jeopardy. Should members of the anesthesia team need to replace each other during the anesthetic procedure, it is essential that the "baton of responsibility" be passed in a smooth and coordinated manner. A clear dialogue between team members must be established about the nature of the surgery, the child's underlying conditions, anesthetic agents and other medications, fluid and blood product management, and any special problems. Drugs on the anesthesia machine must be clearly labeled by name and dosage; in infants, dilution of drugs and the use of tuberculin syringes further improve safety by limiting the amount of drug in each syringe and allowing more accurate dose administration.

Ongoing communication between the anesthesiologist and surgeon is important if the anesthesiologist is to anticipate potential changes in a child's physiologic status due to surgical manipulations and deal with them immediately, appropriately, and effectively.

The conclusion of an anesthetic procedure is fraught with potential problems. The anesthesiologist should not be left in the operating room without nurses or another physician or relax vigilance while a child is awakening and being transferred to the recovery room or intensive care unit. It is during this stage that airway obstruction, desaturation, vomiting, and excitement are likely to occur.

Records of an anesthetic procedure must be accurate and complete; however, anesthesiologists must avoid the compulsion to complete these during the procedure if a child's condition warrants special attention.

Recovery Room

The anesthesiologist's responsibility to a child continues into the recovery room. Transport to the recovery room must be carried out with appropriate monitoring, attention to a clear airway, and adequate ventilation, oxygenation, and perfusion. If necessary, battery-powered infusion pumps should be used to maintain accurate infusion of vasopressors. If there is need, oxygen should be administered and oxygen saturation monitored during transport. For children who are not yet fully awake, transport in the "tonsil position" (lateral decubitus position) rather than the common practice of supine is recommended so that—should regurgitation occur—it will flow away from the larynx and will be visualized immediately. In general, oxygen should be administered to children who have not yet awakened. The mask should be observed for condensation with each breath to assess the respiratory rate as well as gas movement with respiration. On arrival in the postanesthesia care unit (PACU), a clear summary of the medical and surgical problems of the child, important intraoperative events, timing of antibiotics, analgesics, local anesthetics or nerve blocks, and details of the anesthetic procedure are given to recovery room personnel. The PACU must be equipped with age- and size-appropriate resuscitation equipment. Vital signs (oxygen saturation, heart rate, blood pressure, respirations, and temperature) should be recorded on admission to the PACU and repeated at appropriate intervals thereafter (see Chapter 47). If appropriate, specific instructions should be given relating to fluid management, oxygen administration, drug therapy, analgesics, blood tests (e.g., hematocrit, blood gases, electrolytes, coagulation profile), and radiographs. Once the anesthesiologist is certain that the child is stable from a cardio-pulmonary standpoint and that all vital information has been provided to the PACU staff, then preferably the anesthesiologists or the PACU staff should inform the parents that their child has arrived safely in the PACU and then proceed to their next case.

Postoperative Visit

If the child has been admitted to the hospital for more than an overnight observation, it is good practice to visit the child and family postoperatively to assess the postanesthetic clinical course and discuss the child's reaction to the anesthetic procedure. A note documenting the visit should also be inserted into the child's record. All too often the anesthesiologist appears only preoperatively and is never seen again by the family, especially if there was a poor outcome. If the public is to understand and respect the profession of anesthesiology as a vital medical specialty, close interaction and trust among parents, child, and anesthesiologist are essential. A follow-up telephone call from the nursing staff is also useful in identifying and managing anesthesia-related postoperative issues.

Summary

This introductory chapter has outlined the fundamentals of safe pediatric anesthesia practice. The chapters that follow elaborate on these principles; our collective experience has been used to guide practicing anesthesiologists. We reiterate specific points throughout to emphasize their importance and to present several different perspectives on those issues.

Growth and Development

Robert M. Insoft and I. David Todres

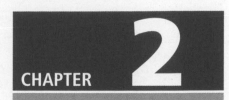

CHAPTER 2

AS AN INFANT GROWS and matures, vital changes occur that affect the child's response to disease, drugs, and the environment. Growth is an increase in physical size, and development is an increase in complexity and function. An overview of the subject is presented so that anesthesiologists can appreciate the uniqueness of developing children from both physical and psychological perspectives. We discuss the respiratory organ system in depth because of its primary considerations for anesthesiologists; however, it is necessary to integrate *all* organ systems so that a child is treated appropriately.

Normal and Abnormal Growth

Prenatal growth is the most important phase in development, comprising organogenesis in the first 8 weeks (embryonic growth), followed by the functional development of organ systems and maturation of the fetus to full term (fetal growth). Rapid growth occurs particularly in the second trimester; a major increase in weight from subcutaneous tissue and muscle mass occurs in the third trimester. The duration of gestation and the weight of an infant have an important relationship (Table 2-1); deviations from this relationship may be associated with (1) inadequate maternal nutrition (malnutrition or placental insufficiency); (2) significant maternal disease (pregnancy-induced hypertension, diabetes, collagen disorders); (3) maternal toxins (tobacco, alcohol, drugs); (4) fetal infections (toxoplasmosis, rubella, cytomegalovirus, syphilis); (5) genetic abnormalities (trisomy 21, 18, 13); and (6) fetal congenital malformations.

The term *prematurity* has conventionally been applied to infants weighing less than 2500 g at birth, but the designation *preterm infant* is more appropriate and is defined as one born before 37 completed weeks of gestation. A *term infant* is one born after 37 and before 42 completed weeks of gestation. *Post-term infant* refers to an infant born after 42 completed weeks of gestation.

Preterm infants are further classified according to their actual birth weight. A low birth weight infant (LBW) is one weighing less than 2500 g regardless of the duration of the pregnancy. A very low birth weight (VLBW) infant weighs less than 1500 g, and an extremely low birth weight infant weighs less than 1000 g. In addition, infants weighing less than 750 g are now

Table 2-1. The Relationship of Gestational Age to Weight

Gestation (weeks)	Mean Weight (grams)
28	1165 ± 109
32	1760 ± 128
36	2621 ± 274
40 (full term)	3351 ± 448

Data from Naeye RL, Dixon JB: Distortions in fetal growth. Pediatr Res 12:987, 1978

being called "micropremies"; there is very little published information regarding the anesthetic management of this vulnerable subpopulation of neonates (see Chapter 35).

An infant may also be classified as small for gestational age (SGA), large for gestational age (LGA), or appropriate for gestational age (AGA) depending on where the infant's birth weight plots out on a fetal growth curve. SGA infants (those whose weight is below the 10th percentile at any gestational age) have usually been affected by intrapartum factors that have led to intrauterine malnutrition, such as toxemia and placental insufficiency. Other known causes include intrauterine infections, chromosomal abnormalities, and congenital malformations.[1] SGA infants are particularly prone to hypoglycemia, hypocalcemia, polycythemia, hypothermia, and, potentially, mental and physical handicaps. Problems associated with length of gestation and body weight are summarized in Table 2-2.

Infants classified as LGA (those whose weight is above the 90th percentile at any gestational age) are usually born to mothers whose pregnancy has been complicated by diabetes. The increased weight is the result of organomegaly and excessive deposition of subcutaneous fat secondary to increased fetal insulin produced in response to maternal hyperglycemia. With improved control of maternal diabetes with home blood glucose monitoring, these infants are less likely to be LGA and therefore are at less risk for hypoglycemia, polycythemia, birth trauma, hyaline membrane disease, and congenital malformations.[2]

Gestational Age Assessment

The gestational age of an infant may be assessed in one of three ways. The most accurate means of assessing gestational age is by measuring the crown-rump length of the fetus during a first-trimester ultrasonographic examination. Another method involves calculating gestational age from the first day of the mother's last menstrual period, but this is commonly inaccurate, leading to errors in estimation. Finally, the Dubowitz scoring system is a well-accepted method combining neurologic and physical criteria of the infant to provide an accurate assessment of gestational age.[3,4] A summary of the more significant neurologic and physical signs of maturity is presented in Table 2-3.

Weight and Length

Assessment of growth is measured by changes in weight, length, and head circumference. Percentile charts are valuable for monitoring the child's growth and development. Deviation from growth within the same percentile for a child of any age is of greater significance than any single measurement (Figs. 2-1 and 2-2). Weight is a more sensitive index of well-being, illness, or poor nutrition than length or head circumference and is the most commonly used measurement of growth. Change in weight reflects changes in muscle mass, adipose tissue, skeleton, and

Table 2-2. Common Neonatal Problems with Respect to Weight and Gestation

Gestation	Relative Weight	Neonatal Problems at Increased Incidence
Preterm (<37 wk)	SGA	Respiratory distress syndrome Apnea Perinatal depression Hypoglycemia Polycythemia Hypocalcemia Hypomagnesemia Hyperbilirubinemia Viral infection Thrombocytopenia Congenital anomalies Maternal drug addiction Fetal alcohol syndrome
	AGA	Respiratory distress syndrome Apnea Hypoglycemia Hypocalcemia Hypomagnesemia Hyperbilirubinemia
	LGA	Respiratory distress syndrome Hypoglycemia: infant of a diabetic mother Apnea Hypocalcemia Hypomagnesemia Hyperbilirubinemia
Normal (37-42 wk)	SGA	Congenital anomalies Viral infection Thrombocytopenia Maternal drug addiction Perinatal depression Hypoglycemia
	AGA	–
	LGA	Birth trauma Hyperbilirubinemia Hypoglycemia: infant of a diabetic mother
Postmature (>42 wk)	SGA	Meconium aspiration syndrome Congenital anomalies Viral infection Thrombocytopenia Maternal drug addiction Perinatal depression Aspiration pneumonia Hypoglycemia
	AGA	–
	LGA	Birth trauma Hyperbilirubinemia Hypoglycemia: infant of a diabetic mother

AGA, appropriate for gestational age; LGA, large for gestational age; SGA, small for gestational age.

Table 2-3. Neurologic and External Physical Criteria to Assess Gestational Age

Physical Examination	Preterm (<37 wk)	Term (≥37 wk)
Ear	Shapeless, pliable	Firm, well formed
Skin	Edematous, thin skin	Thick skin
Sole of foot	Creases on anterior third	Whole foot creased
Breast tissue	Less than 1 mm diameter	More than 5 mm diameter
Genitalia		
Male	Scrotum poorly developed	Scrotum rugated
	Testes undescended	Testes descended
Female	Large clitoris, gaping labia majora	Labia majora developed
Limbs	Hypotonic	Tonic (flexed)
Grasp reflex	Weak grasp	Can be lifted by reflex grasp
Moro reflex	Complete but exhaustible (>32 wk)	Complete
Sucking reflex	Weak	Strong, synchronous with swallowing

Head Circumference

Head size reflects growth of the brain and correlates with intracranial volume and brain weight. Changing head circumference reflects head growth and is a part of the total body growth process; it may or may not indicate underlying involvement of the brain. The mean expected head circumference for preterm and full-term newborns is presented in Table 2-7. An abnormally large or small head may indicate abnormal brain development, which must alert the anesthesiologist to possible underlying neurologic problems. A large head may indicate a normal variation, familial feature, or pathologic condition (e.g., hydrocephalus or increased intracranial pressure), whereas a small head may indicate a normal variant, a familial feature, or pathologic condition such as craniosynostosis or abnormal brain development.

During the first year of life, head circumference normally increases 10 cm, and it increases 2.5 cm in the second year. By 9 months of age, head circumference reaches 50% of adult size, and by 2 years it is 75%. For the first 6 months of life, the circumference of the head is greater than that of the thorax. After 2 years of age, the head circumference increases much less

body water and thus is a nonspecific measure of growth. Measurement of length provides the best indicator of skeletal growth because it is not affected by changes in adipose tissue or water content.

Term infants may lose 5% to 10% of their body weight during the first 24 to 72 hours of life from loss of body water. Birth weight is usually regained in 7 to 10 days. A daily increase of 30 g (210 g/wk) is satisfactory for the first 3 months. Thereafter, weight gain slows so that at 10 to 12 months of age it is 70 g each week. For full-term infants, birth weight is expected to double at 6 months and triple by 1 year (Table 2-4).

Preterm infants may lose up to 15% of their body weight during the first 7 to 10 days of life. This significant weight loss is secondary to the fact that preterm infants have a higher percentage of total body water per unit weight than term infants do (Table 2-5). Regaining birth weight is very variable, depending on the infant's gestational age and medical problems. Although healthy LBW infants can regain birth weight in 10 to 14 days, VLBW and smaller infants may take as long as 3 to 4 weeks. Preterm infants gain weight more slowly than term infants (20 g/day) in general, but it is common for them to have significant growth spurts during the first year of life. *When plotting the weight of a premature infant on a growth chart, it is common to use the infant's corrected gestational age instead of his or her chronologic age during the first 2 years of the infant's life so as to correct for prematurity.*

Knowledge of the average weight at various ages is helpful in judging whether an infant possibly has a growth-limiting illness. Anesthesiologists should recognize an infant or child whose weight deviates from normal. Failure to thrive indicates that a serious underlying disorder that could significantly affect the anesthetic procedure may be present (Table 2-6).

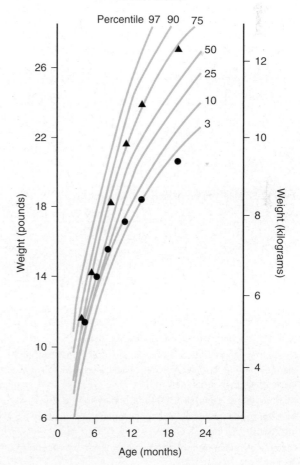

Figure 2-1. Postnatal growth curve (weight) for term male infants. This figure represents normal growth curves. *Triangles* indicate a normal child. *Circles* demonstrate failure to thrive in a child with severe renal failure.

LOW-BIRTH-WEIGHT INFANTS

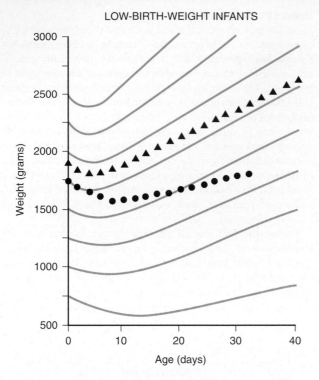

Figure 2-2. Postnatal growth curve (weight) for preterm infants. This figure represents normal growth curves for preterm infants. *Triangles* indicate a normal preterm infant. *Circles* demonstrate failure to thrive in an infant with bronchopulmonary dysplasia.

Table 2-4. Approximate Relationship of Age to Weight

Age (years)	Weight (kg)
1	10
3	15
5	19
7	23

Table 2-5. Relationship of Age to Total Body Water

Age	Body Water (percent)
Fetus	90
Preterm	80
Full-term	70
6-12 months	60

Table 2-6. Common Causes of Failure to Thrive

Genetic: parental size, chromosomal disorders

Nutritional: inadequate or inappropriate intake, malabsorption, diarrhea, vomiting, cystic fibrosis, celiac disease, carbohydrate intolerance, milk protein allergy

Malformations: especially cardiac or urinary tract

Infections: pulmonary, renal, hepatic, enteral, congenital infections

Metabolic/endocrine disorders: hypothyroidism, renal tubular acidosis

Preterm infants and those that are small for gestational age

Malignancy

Bronchopulmonary dysplasia

Table 2-7. Relationship of Head Circumference to Gestational Age

Gestation (weeks)	Head Circumference (cm)
28	25
32	29
36	32
40 (full term)	35

rapidly (i.e., 2 to 3 cm during the next 10 years). Head circumference is closely followed on standard percentile growth curves. As with weight, deviations of growth of the head within the same percentile are more significant than a single measurement; head circumference must be correlated with a child's body weight.

The anterior fontanelle should be palpated to assess whether it is sunken (dehydration) or bulging abnormally, which suggests increased intracranial pressure (hydrocephalus, infection, hemorrhage, increased $Paco_2$). If it is bulging, the sutures should be palpated for abnormal separation due to increased intracranial pressure. The anterior fontanelle closes between 9 and 18 months of age; the posterior fontanelle closes by about 4 months of age. Premature synostosis of sutures (craniosynostosis) can result in an abnormal head shape and may retard brain growth and development. The head may be abnormal in shape as a result of genetic and not necessarily pathologic causes. Cranial molding is seen particularly in LBW infants and is usually of no clinical importance.

Face

Although the cranial vault increases rapidly in size, the face and base of the skull develop at a slower rate. At birth, the mandible is small; but as a child develops, forward growth occurs, reducing the obliquity of the mandibular angle. Failure of prenatal development of the mandible may be associated with severe congenital defects (e.g., Pierre Robin, Treacher Collins, or Goldenhar syndromes). These syndromes often have other associated anomalies. After 2 years of age, although the cranial vault increases relatively little in size, a significant change in facial configuration occurs. The upper jaw grows rapidly to accommodate the developing teeth. In addition, the frontal sinuses develop by 2 to 6 years of age, and the maxillary, ethmoidal, and sphenoidal sinuses appear after 6 years of age.

Teeth

The first tooth, usually a lower incisor, erupts at approximately 6 months of age (deciduous dentition). Eruption of all deciduous teeth is usually complete by 28 months of age. Permanent teeth appear at 6 years, with the shedding of the deciduous teeth; this process takes place during the next 6 to 8 years. Poor nutrition and chronic illness may interfere with calcification of deciduous and permanent teeth. *Loose teeth should be sought in any child between the ages of 5 and 10 years* or when severe dental caries occur as a result of poor dental hygiene and infection. Care must be taken when placing an oral airway and performing laryngoscopy in children with loose teeth. Abnormally developed teeth occur with hereditary disturbances, Down syndrome, cerebral palsy, and nutritional defects. Premature infants may show severe enamel hypoplasia in their primary dentition.[5] Tetracycline administration during the period of calcification in children leads to permanent discoloration.

Body Composition

The more immature an infant, the greater the relative water content (see Table 2-5). Serial measurements of the extracellular volume of VLBW infants (<32 weeks of gestation) show a postnatal reduction of the extracellular volume with diuresis in the first 2 weeks of life. This represents a physiologic reduction of the expanded extracellular volume of a fetus. Hyponatremia occurring after the first 2 weeks of life may be an indication of excessive sodium loss and extracellular volume depletion.[6] Total body water decreases at the expense of the extracellular compartment, with adult levels attained at 1 year of age.[7,8] This finding has implications for drug dosage and distribution in the infant (see Chapter 6). Males have a higher percentage of water, whereas females have a slightly higher percentage of fat. The percentage decrease in extracellular volume is greater than the decrease in total body water because of the simultaneous increase in intracellular water.

Development of Organ Systems

Development of Airways and Lungs

Neonatal respiratory dysfunction is common because the process of lung development is protracted and differentiation of anatomic structures for gas exchange occurs late in gestation. The limit of viability is around the 24th week, when the lungs develop a gas-exchanging surface and surfactant production begins. Thereafter, survival increases markedly.

Laws of Lung Development

Normal lung growth is governed by three "laws" that describe the temporal development of the conducting airways, alveoli, and pulmonary vessels.[8]

1. *Airways:* The bronchial tree down to and including the terminal bronchioles forms by the 16th week of gestation. The acinus, consisting of all the airway structures distal to the terminal bronchiole and the entire gas-exchanging apparatus, develops throughout the remainder of gestation.
2. *Alveoli:* Alveoli develop mainly after birth, increasing in number until approximately 8 years of life and in size until growth of the chest wall ceases.
3. *Pulmonary vessels:* Arteries and veins accompanying the bronchial tree form by the 16th week of gestation. Those vessels lying within the acinus follow the development of the alveoli. The appearance and growth of arterial smooth muscle lags behind the sprouting of new vessels and is not completed until late adolescence.

Embryology of the Lungs

The lung bud appears as a diverticulum of the embryonic foregut around day 26 of gestation,[9] elongating to form the primordial trachea and branching to form the bronchial tree and the epithelial lining of the lungs, including the alveoli. By day 52, the segmental bronchi are present and the diaphragm is complete, marking the end of the embryonic phase of development, which is succeeded by three stages of fetal tissue differentiation (Fig. 2-3).[10]

1. The *glandular stage* (7-16 weeks) includes formation of intrasegmental airways and associated vessels. Differentiation of cartilage begins in the trachea and main-stem bronchi at 10 weeks, reaching the smallest bronchi at term.
2. The *canalicular stage* (16-24 weeks) involves growth of the liquid-filled airways, forming new branches that constitute the first vestiges of the acinus. By the end of this stage, two milestones are achieved: a viable gas-exchanging surface forms, and surfactant production begins.[11,12] At 24 weeks, the distance separating the capillaries from the potential air spaces is roughly two to three times the adult value, and the

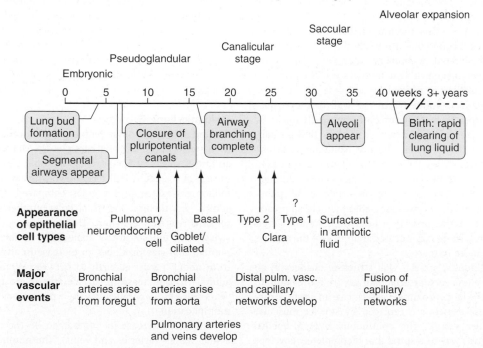

Figure 2-3. Timeline for fetal and postnatal lung development that incorporates salient events in the development of airway and alveolar and vascular components. (Reproduced and modified with permission from Jobe AH: Lung development and maturation. In Fanaroff AA, Martin RJ [eds]: Neonatal-Perinatal Medicine Diseases of the Fetus and Infant, 7th ed. 2002, p 975.)

type II pneumocytes begin producing surfactant.[13] Infants born at this gestational age may survive even though their lungs are very primitive and the surface area available for gas exchange is at an order of magnitude less than at term.[14]

3. The *terminal saccule* or *alveolar stage* (24 weeks to term) involves further intra-acinar branching of the airway epithelium, forming alveolar ducts and sacs.[15] The surface area available for gas exchange increases exponentially, and its thickness decreases.[14] From 30 to 36 weeks, surfactant secretion into the amniotic fluid increases, providing a clinically useful indicator of lung maturity.[16] The incidence of respiratory distress syndrome declines rapidly during this period and is very low after 35 to 36 weeks of gestation.

Development of the Pulmonary Vessels

The main pulmonary artery and veins develop with the heart and secondarily link up with the lungs. The main pulmonary artery, its first-degree branches, and the ductus arteriosus are derived from the right sixth branchial arch artery (its companion on the left side involutes). The four main pulmonary veins are derived from a vessel that sprouts from the left side of the embryonic atrium.

By the third week of gestation, the heart tube forms and connects with the arterial and venous systems at its cranial and caudal ends. Early in gestation, the heart is located ventrally in the pharyngeal region; it later moves into the thorax. The ventral aorta links with right and left dorsal aortas (which fuse caudally) via the paired branchial cleft arteries, which appear during the fifth week. The sixth arch arteries give off branches that connect with a preexisting vascular plexus in the lung bud. A few days later, the ventral aorta divides so that only blood from the right ventricle enters the lungs. Around this time, paired segmental branches of the dorsal aortas also supply the lungs. In normal development, these are lost; true bronchial arteries develop between weeks 9 and 12.

The main pulmonary veins develop a few days later than the pulmonary arteries. Venous blood initially drains into the systemic vessels of the foregut. A capillary outgrowth from the left side of the atrium connects with the lung vessels. The primitive pulmonary vein bifurcates several times, but the first two branches are later incorporated into the wall of the atrium, which is then perforated by four separate venous channels. By the seventh week, the typical fetal pattern of blood flow is established, that is, into the lungs via the main pulmonary artery, directly into the aorta via the larger ductus arteriosus, and from the lungs to the left atrium via the pulmonary veins.[9] Although intrapulmonary vessels develop at the same time as the epithelial elements with which they are associated (namely, all preacinar arteries form in the first 16 weeks of gestation), their branching pattern is more complicated than that of the airways because they are more numerous.[17,18]

In fetuses and adults, arterial wall structure changes in an orderly sequence along each arterial pathway from the hilum to the periphery.[19] The large proximal vessels have an elastic structure. Distally these vessels are replaced by smaller muscular arteries. In smaller vessels, the continuous layer of medial smooth muscle gives way to a spiral that incompletely envelops the arterial wall; these are called *partially muscular arteries*. The smallest vessels just proximal to the capillary bed lack a muscle layer and are called *nonmuscular arteries*.

Although the structural sequence is the same in fetuses and adults, important age-related differences are noted.[17] In a fetus, elastic tissue is less differentiated than in an adult, especially before 12 weeks, and mature smooth muscle is not present before 23 weeks. The zone of transition from the elastic to the muscular structure gradually extends peripherally during the first half of gestation, reaching the seventh generation (the same as in an adult) by the 19th week. The transition from muscular to partially muscular and from partially muscular to nonmuscular arteries occurs more proximally in a fetus than in an adult. At birth, no muscular arteries are found beyond the level of the terminal bronchiole, whereas in an adult, fully muscular arteries are found even in the walls of alveoli.[19] The fetal pulmonary circulation is less muscular than the adult circulation. However, fetal pulmonary arteries are more muscular; for muscularized vessels of a given external diameter, the muscle layer is thicker in a fetus than in an adult.[10]

Circulation of blood through the fetal pulmonary circuit is limited by vessel diameter, vessel number, and vasoconstriction.[20] In fetal lambs, during the second half of gestation, pulmonary blood flow increases from 3.5% to 10% of the combined output of the right and left ventricles, reflecting growth of the pulmonary vascular bed.[21] The increase in pulmonary blood flow occurring after birth is a consequence of rapid arterial dilation and the closure of extrapulmonary shunt pathways. Growth of the pulmonary vascular bed may be disturbed in many conditions, particularly those involving lung hypoplasia such as congenital diaphragmatic hernia (see Chapter 36). In cases of severe lung hypoplasia, the size and number of vessels may be so reduced that the pulmonary circulation cannot accommodate the cardiac output at normal pressure, even with maximal dilation.

The pattern of muscularization of pulmonary arteries may be disturbed prenatally, most strikingly in persistent pulmonary hypertension of the newborn. In this condition, muscularization of peripheral arteries is exaggerated; affected infants are born with smooth muscle down to the level of the alveolar wall, as found in adults.[22] Clinically, infants with persistent pulmonary hypertension of the newborn demonstrate increased pulmonary vascular reactivity, leading to episodic pulmonary hypertension and right-to-left shunting with resultant hypoxemia.[23]

Postnatal Lung Growth

Around birth, shallow indentations (primordial alveoli) appear in the walls of the terminal saccules.[24,25] Mature alveoli are seen around 5 weeks of age; alveolar multiplication continues until the age of 8 years.[8,25] Full-term newborns have approximately 20 million gas-exchanging saccules, compared with 300 million in adults.[25] For the first 3 years, alveolar numbers increase but size remains relatively constant. Thereafter, size increases progressively until full stature is achieved. The increase in alveolar number and size produces an increase in alveolar surface area from about $1.8 \, m^2$ at birth to between $40 \, m^2$ and $120 \, m^2$ in adults.[26] The increase in surface area is greatest in the first 5 years of life, paralleling the period of rapid alveolar multiplication.

As alveoli increase in number, so do the number of intra-acinar vessels (arteries and veins). The number of arteries per unit area of lung increases in the first 3 years of life but decreases after about 5 years as alveolar diameter increases.[25,27] Arterial structure also changes throughout childhood because there is a gradual peripheral extension of the smooth muscle layer.[8] There are no fully muscular arteries in the gas-exchanging region at birth. Fully muscular arteries are observed at the alveolar duct level by 10 years, but not until 19 years are they seen at the level of the alveolar wall. Postnatal proliferation and muscularization of the pulmonary vessels may be disturbed in any condition with abnormal pulmonary blood flow, most notably in association with congenital heart lesions with increased or decreased pulmonary blood flow (see Chapters 14, 15, 16, and 21).

Although airway number does not increase after the 16th week of gestation, growth in length and size continue throughout childhood. Comparisons of airway diameter at different levels and various ages indicate that growth is symmetrical in different parts of the bronchial tree, from the main-stem bronchi downward.[28]

Transition to Air Breathing

Fetal breathing movements have been detected as early as 11 weeks of gestational age; they are interspersed with long periods of apnea and produce little tidal movement of lung fluid.[29,30] The critical event in the change from placental to pulmonary gas exchange is the first inspiration, which initiates pulmonary ventilation, promotes the clearance of lung fluid, and triggers the change from the fetal to the neonatal pattern of circulation.

In late gestation, the volume of lung fluid approximates postnatal functional residual capacity (30 mL/kg).[31] During normal birth, a portion of this fluid is squeezed out through the upper airway as the thorax is compressed in the birth canal; elastic recoil of the chest wall helps to inflate the lungs. Fetal lung fluid is also resorbed by intrinsic lymphatic pathways leading from the lung. These events are not a necessary prelude to the first breath because most infants born by cesarean section have no difficulty clearing the fluid from their lungs.[32] The first breath is a gasp that generates a transpulmonary distending pressure of 40 to 80 cm H_2O.[33] This moves the tracheal fluid (100 times more viscous than air), overcomes surface forces that develop as the air/fluid interface reaches the small airways, and overcomes tissue resistance. As the lung fills with air, inspiration becomes less forceful. Lung fluid is expelled through the airway or absorbed into the lung interstitium, where it is drawn into the circulation by oncotic forces or carried away as increased lymph flow.[34] In some children, the removal of lung fluid may be delayed, producing the syndrome *transient tachypnea of the newborn*.[35] Tachypnea lasts for 24 to 72 hours and is associated with a characteristic chest radiographic appearance consisting of increased perihilar markings, fluid in the interlobar fissures, and streaky linear opacities in the parenchyma.

With the onset of pulmonary ventilation, pulmonary blood flow sharply increases. Decreased pulmonary vascular resistance (PVR) and increased peripheral systemic vascular resistance (loss of the umbilical circulation) are the two crucial events involved in the immediate transition from the fetal circulation to the normal postnatal pattern (see Chapters 14 and 16). The increase in systemic afterload causes an immediate closure of the flap valve mechanism of the foramen ovale and reverses the direction of shunt through the ductus arteriosus. Until these fetal shunt pathways close anatomically, the pattern of circulation is unstable. Increased pulmonary vascular reactivity in response to hypoxia and acidosis may precipitate a reversal to right-to-left shunting.

The decrease in PVR may be produced in part by mechanical stretching of small arteries or by the secretion of vasoactive substances triggered by lung inflation; however, the major factor is the sudden increase in oxygen in the pulmonary vessels with the onset of ventilation.[20,36] In addition to the immediate change in PVR that occurs in the first few hours of life, a slower increase occurs in the compliance of small muscular pulmonary arteries during the first few days of life, further contributing to a decline in pulmonary artery pressure and augmentation of pulmonary blood flow.[19]

In the first few minutes of life, a state of "normal" asphyxia exists as a result of impairment of placental blood flow during labor. The PaO_2 and pH are low, whereas the $PaCO_2$ is high immediately after birth, but these parameters change rapidly in the first hour of life. Extrapulmonary shunting through fetal channels and intrapulmonary shunting, probably through unexpanded regions of the lung, persist for some time after birth, so that in newborns the physiologic right-to-left shunt is about three times that in adults.[37]

Mechanics of Breathing

Chest Wall and Respiratory Muscles

The accessory muscles of inspiration are relatively ineffective in infants compared with those of adults because of an unfavorable anatomic rib configuration. In infancy, the ribs extend horizontally from the vertebral column, moving little with inspiration.[38] Furthermore, the chest wall is easily deformed, tending to move inward on inspiration. These factors increase the workload on the diaphragm. Consequently, and in contrast to an adult, thoracic cross-sectional area is fairly constant throughout the breathing cycle, and inspiration occurs almost entirely as a result of diaphragmatic descent. After assuming an upright posture, a young child gradually acquires the caudal slant and downward rotation of the ribs that are characteristic of an adult.

The chest wall of a newborn is floppy because it has a high content of cartilage, its musculature is poorly developed, and the ribs are incompletely calcified.[39] Intercostal muscle tone stabilizes the chest wall of a term neonate, who usually exhibits retractions only during rapid eye movement sleep when these muscles are inhibited.[40] Chest wall stiffness varies directly with gestational age; therefore, preterm infants have more severe retractions, which occur in all stages of the sleep-wake cycle.[41] Paradoxical chest wall movement commonly occurs in young children after infancy whenever there is an increase in respiratory effort. It frequently occurs under general anesthesia as a consequence of upper airway obstruction but may also be caused by depression of intercostal muscle tone. Inward movement of the rib cage opposes the inspiratory action of the diaphragm. As its severity increases, diaphragmatic displacement must also increase to maintain tidal volume. The increased workload may lead to diaphragmatic fatigue and respiratory failure or apnea, especially in preterm infants.[42,43]

The tendency to respiratory muscle fatigue is the result of the metabolic characteristics of the diaphragm, which has a low content of type I (slow twitch, high oxidative capacity) muscle fibers. Before 37 weeks of gestational age, fatigue-resistant fibers make up less than 10% of the total.[44] A high proportion of type I fibers confers fatigue resistance. Type I muscle fibers constitute about 50% of the fibers in an adult's diaphragm but only 25% of the diaphragm in a term infant (see Fig. 12-11).

Elastic Properties of the Lung

Changes in the static pressure-volume relationship of the lungs during growth are caused by increases in volume and changes in the elastic properties of lung tissue. Volume is the principal factor that determines lung compliance, which increases throughout childhood. To make comparisons that are less dependent on size, compliance is frequently indexed to some parameter of growth such as functional residual capacity (FRC) or total lung capacity (TLC). The resultant indexed value is called *specific compliance* to distinguish it from the raw value. Specific lung compliance remains relatively constant throughout childhood.[45] In contrast, specific compliance of the chest wall declines throughout childhood and adolescence, reflecting the progressive calcification of the ribs and the increasing bulk of the thoracic muscles. Specific compliance of the entire respiratory system also declines because of the changes in the chest wall.[46,47]

Elastic recoil pressure (the recoil pressure of the lung at a specified reference volume) increases throughout childhood, reaches a peak in late adolescence, and declines thereafter. Structural studies indicate that the period of increasing elastic recoil coincides with an increase in the pulmonary content of elastic fibers, whereas the phase of decreasing elastic recoil coincides with the gradual deterioration of these fibers with aging.[48,49] Elastic recoil is an important determinant of static lung volume.

Static Lung Volumes

Figure 2-4 summarizes the major differences in static lung volumes between infants and adults. TLC in relation to body weight is indicated for each, and other volumes are shown as fractions of TLC. More detailed information expressing static lung volumes on the basis of body weight are detailed in Table 2-8.

Total Lung Capacity

Adults have a markedly greater TLC than infants. This difference reflects the fact that TLC is an effort-dependent parameter, depending on the strength and efficiency of the inspiratory muscles, which can be estimated by the maximum inspiratory pressure at FRC. An adult can generate negative pressures in excess of 100 cm H_2O; negative inspiratory pressures as high as 70 cm H_2O have been recorded for neonates, a surprisingly high value in view of their underdeveloped musculature and highly compliant chest wall. This may be a consequence of the small radius of curvature of an infant's rib cage, which by the Laplace relationship converts a small tension into a large pressure difference.[48]

Functional Residual Capacity

Functional residual capacity is similar on a per-kilogram basis at all ages, but the mechanical factors on which it is based are different in infants and adults.[50] In adults, FRC is the same as the volume at which the elastic forces generated by the passive recoil of the chest wall are balanced by the recoil of the lung (Fig. 2-5); this is the volume attained at end-expiration with an open glottis.

In an infant, the elastic recoil of the chest is exceedingly small, and the recoil pressure of the lung is less than an adult's. An analysis of these forces reveals that if they are brought into equilibrium, a value for FRC around 10% of TLC is predicted instead of the observed value of slightly less than 40%.[51] Thus, the FRC in an infant is set by a cessation of exhalation at a lung volume in excess of its relaxation volume, so-called laryngeal braking, that is, prolongation of the expiratory time constant.[52]

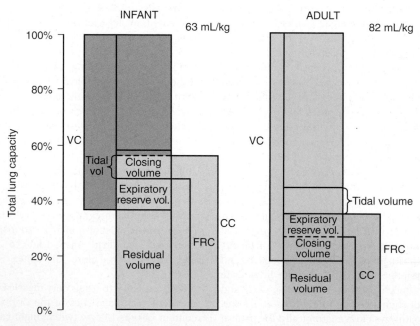

Figure 2-4. Total lung capacity in infants and adults. Note that, in infants, tidal volume breathing occurs at the same volume as closing volume. CC, closing capacity; FRC, functional residual capacity; VC, vital capacity. (Modified from Nelson NM: Respiration and circulation after birth. In Smith CA, Nelson NM [eds]: The Physiology of the Newborn Infant. Springfield, IL, Charles C Thomas, 1976, p 207.)

Table 2-8. Age-Dependent Respiratory Variables

	Newborn	6 months	12 months	3 years	5 years	12 years	Adult	Units
F	50 ± 1	30 ± 5	24 ± 6	24 ± 6	23 ± 5	18 ± 5	12 ± 3	Breaths per minute
TV	21	45	78	112	270	480	575	mL
	6-8						6-7	mL/kg
$\dot{V}_E$	1050	1350	1780	2460	5500	6200	6400	mL/min
	200-260						90	mL/kg/min
$\dot{V}_A$	665		1245	1760	1800	3000	3100	mL/min
	100-150						60	mL/kg/min
V_D/V_T	0.3						0.3	
V_{O_2}	6-8						3-4	mL/kg/min
VC	120			870	1160	3100	4000	mL
FRC	80			490	680	1970	3000	mL
	30						30	mL/kg
TLC	160			1100	1500	4000	6000	mL
	63						82	mL/kg
pH	7.3-7.4		7.35-7.45				7.35-7.45	
Pa_{O_2}	60-90		80-100				80-100	mm Hg
Pa_{CO_2}	30-35		30-40				37-42	mm Hg

F, frequency; FRC, functional residual capacity; Pa_{CO_2}, arterial carbon dioxide tension; Pa_{O_2}, arterial oxygen tension; TLC, total lung capacity; TV, tidal volume; $\dot{V}_A$, alveolar ventilation; V_D/V_T, dead space/tidal volume; $\dot{V}_E$, minute ventilation; VC, vital capacity; V_{O_2}, oxygen consumption.

Modified from O'Rourke PP, Crone RK: The respiratory system. In Gregory GA (ed): Pediatric Anesthesia, 2nd ed. New York, Churchill Livingstone, 1989.

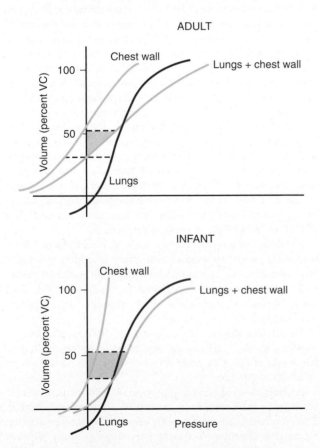

Figure 2-5. Lung volumes in infants and adults. (Modified and reproduced with permission from Pérez Fontán JJ, Haddad GG: Respiratory physiology. In Behrman RE, Kliegman RM, Jenson HB [eds]: Nelson Textbook of Pediatrics, 17th ed. Philadelphia, WB Saunders, 2003, p 1363.)

This observation is confirmed by the fact that apneic lung volume is less than FRC in an infant. This volume is close to the collapse volume of the lungs because intrapleural pressure is nearly equal to atmospheric pressure in an apneic infant whose chest wall elastic recoil pressure is so low. In fact, the major factor preventing complete collapse of the lungs is airway closure, which is directly related to lung elastic recoil.[48] It is unknown at what age FRC ceases to be determined by dynamic rather than passive factors.

An important clinical implication of the dynamic control of FRC is that an apneic infant has a disproportionately smaller store of intrapulmonary oxygen on which to draw than a similarly affected adult. This is one of the reasons hypoxemia develops rapidly if control of the airway is lost in an anesthetized infant.

Closing Capacity

As exhalation proceeds to completion, small airways in dependent regions of the lung close, leading to air trapping in the affected areas. Closing capacity is closely related to age, declining throughout childhood and adolescence and increasing thereafter throughout adult life. This pattern of change has been related to the development and deterioration of lung elastic tissue and its effect on recoil pressure. The latter is the principal determinant of transmural pressure and therefore patency of the smallest airways, which lack intrinsic stability because they contain no cartilage.

Closing volume is within the range of tidal breathing in some adults older than 40 years and some children younger than 10 years. It is not possible to measure closing volume in children younger than 5 years, but because elastic recoil pressure decreases to very low levels in infancy, it is likely that some airways remain closed throughout tidal breathing. This conclusion is supported by the finding that infants have a large "trapped gas volume" that is not in free communication with the conducting airways. Age-related changes in Pao_2, which parallel the changes in the difference between FRC and closing volume, may also be related to airway closure.[48]

Airway Dynamics

Resistance and Conductance
Airway resistance declines markedly with growth from 19 to 28 cm H_2O/L/sec in newborns to less than 2 cm H_2O/L/sec in adults.[50,53] Airway resistance is higher in preterm than in full-term infants. On the other hand, specific airways conductance (reciprocal of resistance) is higher in preterm infants, and it continues to decline throughout the first 5 years of life, probably reflecting disproportionate growth of the gas-exchanging region of the lungs.[54,55]

Distribution of Resistance
The distribution of airways resistance changes markedly around the age of 5 years. Airway resistance per gram of lung tissue is constant at all ages in the "central airways" (trachea to the 12th to 15th bronchial generation), whereas it decreases markedly around the age of 5 years in the "peripheral airways" (12th to 15th generation to the alveoli). These data explain why young children with inflammation of the small airways (bronchiolitis) suffer a severe impairment of respiratory function whereas older children and adults with similar pathology have a milder illness.[56]

Inspiratory and Expiratory Flow Limitation
Tracheal compliance in newborns is twice that of adults; it is even greater in preterm infants and appears to be a consequence of cartilaginous immaturity. The functional importance of this finding is that dynamic collapse of the trachea may occur with inspiration and expiration (see also Fig. 12-10).

Gas Exchange

Pulmonary gas exchange occurs by diffusion and has the same underlying mechanism for all ages. Of all the factors affecting pulmonary diffusing capacity, the one that changes most in childhood is the surface area of the alveolar-capillary membrane. Total diffusing capacity at term is similar to that of adults when referenced to oxygen consumption or alveolar ventilation, which has been interpreted to mean that gas exchange is flow limited rather than diffusion limited. This is not too surprising in view of the similarity of the thickness of the anatomic barrier to gas exchange in term infants and in adults. On the other hand, it must be borne in mind that the gas-exchanging surface area is smaller in relation to body size in infancy than in adulthood, suggesting that the physiologic reserve for diffusion is reduced in newborns.

Throughout growth and development, diffusing capacity increases linearly with height, which in turn is closely related to lung growth. The range of values at all ages is comparable to adult measurements when allowance is made for height. It is unknown whether diffusion limitation occurs in preterm infants, but the relationship of gestational age to both the thickness of the blood-gas barrier and its surface area suggests that the margin for diffusion limitation declines at earlier gestational ages. Despite the presumed absence of diffusion limitation, the alveolar-arterial oxygen difference $(A - aDo_2)$ is much higher in full-term neonates than in adults. Not surprisingly, it is even higher in preterm infants. The precise point in infancy at which adult values are reached is not known.

Venous admixture in infants is higher than in adults. The shunt fraction is estimated at 10% to 20% of cardiac output, with values at the upper end of the range occurring immediately postnatally, whereas the resting shunt fraction in adults is 2% to 5%. Intrapulmonary anatomic shunting, perhaps around the mouths of shallow developing alveoli, is a major cause of venous admixture. The nature of ventilation/perfusion imbalance in infants may be different from that in adults, arising from opening and closing of individual lung units rather than from decreased ventilation of open units.[37] Extrapulmonary right-to-left shunting contributes to $A - aDo_2$ in the first few hours of life but only episodically thereafter in association with transient reversal of the pressure gradient between the right and left atrium. Episodic shunting may continue up to the time of anatomic closure of the foramen ovale.

Regulation of Breathing
In neonates as in adults, Pao_2, $Paco_2$, and pH control pulmonary ventilation, with Pao_2 acting mainly through peripheral chemoreceptors in the carotid and aortic bodies and $Paco_2$ and pH acting on central chemoreceptors in the medulla. Infants respond to an increase in $Paco_2$ with an increase in alveolar ventilation just as adults; that is, they increase tidal volume and respiratory rate. The strength of the response is directly related to gestational and postnatal age, the principal change being an increase in the slope of the response rather than a change in the apneic threshold.[45,57] Unlike an adult, an infant's response to hypercapnia is not potentiated by hypoxia. In fact, hypoxia may depress the hypercapnic ventilatory response in term and preterm infants.[58]

High concentrations of oxygen depress the newborn's respiration, whereas low concentrations stimulate it. The hypoxic response is not sustained. However, sustained hypoxia leads first to a return to baseline ventilation and then to ventilatory depression. This pattern of response persists in normal term infants for the first week of life, after which the response to sustained hypoxia is replaced by a sustained increase in ventilation.[59] This pattern persists longer in preterm infants.

Relatively nonspecific factors such as blood glucose level, hematocrit, and temperature also affect breathing in infants. Hypoglycemia and anemia may limit substrate availability, especially in the presence of increased metabolic demand. Cold stress decreases ventilatory drive through an unknown mechanism.[60]

The Hering-Breuer reflex, consisting of induced apnea in response to lung inflation, appears to be operative in the first few weeks of life. This reflex does not appear to have a role in an adult's respiration.

Periodic breathing commonly occurs in newborns. It is characterized by recurrent pauses in ventilation lasting no more than 5 to 10 seconds, alternating with bursts of respiratory activity; Figure 2-6 illustrates a typical pneumogram study whereas Figure 2-7 illustrates a typical preterm infant with periodic breathing. Such episodes are not associated with any obvious physiologic impairment. This pattern of breathing is related to gestational age and to the sleep state. It is more common in preterm infants than in term infants and also occurs more

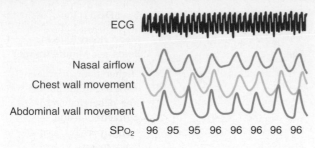

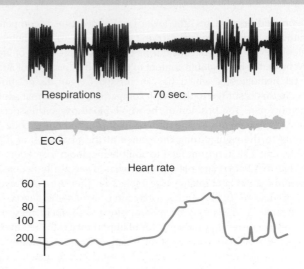

Figure 2-6. A typical respiratory sleep study in a normal newborn would include the electrocardiogram (ECG), nasal air flow (thermistor), chest wall and abdominal wall impedance, EEG, oxygen saturation, and other parameters. (Courtesy of Dr. Craig Canipari.)

Figure 2-8. Pneumogram of an abnormal preterm infant demonstrating apnea/bradycardia spells after general anesthesia. Note that severe bradycardia accompanies the apnea. (Courtesy of Dr. Dorothy Kelly.)

frequently during rapid-eye-movement sleep. Periodic breathing should be distinguished from clinical apnea, which occurs in as many as 25% of all preterm infants but especially in the most premature. Apnea of prematurity may be a life-threatening condition. Ventilatory pauses are prolonged and are associated with desaturation of arterial oxygen, bradycardia, and loss of muscle tone (Fig. 2-8). Apneic episodes may be terminated by tactile stimulation but in severe cases may require a resuscitative effort with bag-mask ventilation. Many factors have been implicated in the etiology of apnea of prematurity. These include brainstem immaturity, as reflected in decreased hypercarbic and hypoxic responses or in impulse conduction delays through the brainstem as assessed by auditory evoked potentials.[61] Respiratory fatigue precipitated by chest wall distortion has also been strongly implicated.[42] Treatment is directed at increasing the central drive to ventilation (theophylline or caffeine), stabilizing the chest wall (positive end-expiratory pressure), or providing stimulation by rocking and stroking.[62-67]

Prematurity is an important risk factor for life-threatening apnea in infants undergoing general anesthesia.[68] The risk of postanesthetic respiratory depression is inversely related to gestational age and postconceptual age at the time of anesthesia.[69] It has been stated that infants may be at risk up to 60 weeks' after conception[69-71]; however, the greatest risk is in infants 55 weeks or younger after conception. Infants considered at risk should be monitored in an environment where resuscitative equipment and trained personnel skilled in neonatal resuscitation are readily available (see Chapters 4, 35, and 36).

Normal Respiratory Parameters

The stimulus driving pulmonary ventilation is metabolic demand. The resting oxygen consumption of infants is twice that of adults (see Table 2-8), and this in turn leads to a doubling of alveolar ventilation on a per-kilogram basis.[72] Infants increase alveolar ventilation primarily by increasing respiratory rate rather than increasing tidal volume, the latter bearing a constant relationship to body size throughout life. It has been postulated that respiratory rate at different ages is set to minimize the sum of elastic and resistive work of breathing.

Static lung volume (including TLC, vital capacity, FRC, and residual volume) is linearly related to the logarithm of height. A divergence of lung growth between males and females begins in early childhood and produces persistent differences between the sexes in adult life.[73] Part of the increase in the so-called effort-dependent lung volumes (e.g., TLC, vital capacity) is related to the development and efficiency of the diaphragm and other inspiratory muscles. One measure of the role of muscle strength is the maximum inspiratory pressure at FRC. Maximum inspiratory pressure increases slightly throughout childhood and to a greater extent in adolescence, especially in males.

During the first few hours of life, Pao_2 and $Paco_2$ change rapidly as an infant recovers from the relative "asphyxia" associated with birth and a regular pattern of ventilation and stable lung volumes are established. Thereafter, these values remain fairly constant for the first week of life. Pao_2 continues to be

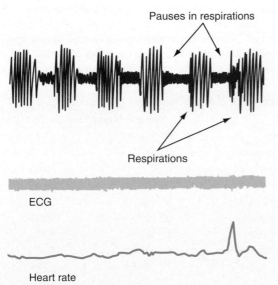

Figure 2-7. Pneumogram of a normal preterm infant, demonstrating the periodic type of respiratory pattern that is common in premature infants, that is, repetitive series of respirations followed by pauses. Note that there are no changes in the heart rate. (Courtesy of Dr. Dorothy Kelly.)

depressed in neonates. The lower PaO_2 of neonates is compensated by a higher oxygen-carrying capacity due to high hemoglobin levels, which decline during the first several weeks of life. At birth, the hemoglobin content of the blood is made up of 50% fetal hemoglobin, which has an in-vivo oxygen-dissociation curve that is shifted to the left in comparison with normal adult hemoglobin. The position of the whole-blood oxygen-dissociation curve depends on the ratio of adult to fetal hemoglobin. It shifts to the right during the course of the first week of life, reflecting a switch from fetal to adult hemoglobin formation.[45]

Normal $PaCO_2$ and pH are somewhat lower in the neonatal period than in later infancy (see Table 2-8). They are even lower in premature infants. Immediately after birth, some degree of metabolic acidosis may be present along with an increase in blood lactate level. Another factor of importance is the relatively large extracellular volume of an infant, leading to dilution of blood bicarbonate. The threshold for renal bicarbonate excretion is also reduced in premature infants.

The range of normal values for arterial pH, PaO_2, and $PaCO_2$ is stable from late infancy throughout adult life. However, average PaO_2 gradually increases throughout childhood, with a peak in late adolescence and a gradual decline thereafter throughout adult life. This pattern has been related to lung closing capacity, which is high in infancy, declines throughout childhood to late adolescence, and rises throughout adulthood. Newborns and older adults share the characteristic of closure of some airways during tidal ventilation.

Cardiovascular System

An understanding of cardiovascular development is important for anesthesiologists. This section briefly considers developmental changes in heart rate, blood pressure, cardiac output, and the electrocardiogram (ECG); a more detailed description is found in Chapter 16.

Heart Rate

Autonomic control of the heart in utero is mediated predominantly through the parasympathetic nervous system. It is only shortly after birth that sympathetic control appears. In newborns, the heart rate may have a wide variation that is within normal limits. In 50% of apparently healthy newborns, 24-hour ECG recordings have shown rhythm changes resembling complete, 2:1, or Wenckebach sinoatrial block.[74]

In older children, a significant number of arrhythmias and conduction abnormalities are also encountered, with marked fluctuations in heart rate due to variations in autonomic tone. The mean heart rate in newborns in the first 24 hours of life is 120 beats per minute. It increases to a mean of 160 beats per minute at 1 month, after which it gradually decreases to 75 beats per minute at adolescence (Table 2-9).[74]

Blood Pressure

Mean systolic blood pressure in neonates and infants rises from 65 mm Hg in the first 12 hours of life to 75 mm Hg at 4 days and 95 mm Hg at 6 weeks. There is little change in mean systolic pressure between 6 weeks and 1 year of age; between 1 year and 6 years, there is only a slight change, followed by a gradual rise.[75,76] These measurements apply to infants and children who are awake and quiet. The blood pressure of preterm infants in the first 12 hours is lower than in full-term infants; a gradual

Table 2-9. The Relationship of Age to Heart Rate*

Age	Mean Heart Rate in Beats per Minute (range)
Premature	120-170
0-3 months	100-150
3-6 months	90-120
6-12 months	80-120
1-3 years	70-110
3-6 years	65-110
6-12 years	60-95
>12 years	55-85

*Note that the heart rate will be lower during sleep.
Data from Mathers LH, Frankel LR: Pediatric emergencies and resuscitation. In Behrman RE, Kliegman RM, Jenson HB (eds): Nelson Textbook of Pediatrics, 17th ed. Philadelphia, WB Saunders, 2004.

rise in blood pressure occurs after birth—68/43 mm Hg on day 1 of life compared with 90/55 mm Hg on day 70 of life (Table 2-10).[77,78] It has also been noted that infants with birth asphyxia and those on ventilators have lower blood pressures.[79]

Cardiac Output

Myocardial performance may be seriously impaired in a critically ill infant or child. Measurement of cardiac output is a valuable indicator of myocardial contractility and may be superior to the traditional monitors of hemodynamic performance such as capillary refill, heart rate, blood pressure, and urine output. Determination of cardiac output and blood pressure allows calculation of systemic vascular resistance. It provides important information relating to the left ventricular afterload and allows rational application of pressor agents (vasoconstrictor, vasodilator) and inotropic drugs. Measurement of cardiac output may be carried out by the Fick method (using oxygen extraction) or thermodilution using a pulmonary artery flow-directed catheter. In neonates, the latter technique is rarely used because shunts at the atrial and ductal level introduce errors in interpreting the results.

Pulsed Doppler determinations of cardiac output appear to provide reasonable noninvasive estimates of cardiac output for clinical application in newborns. Cardiac output increases

Table 2-10. The Relationship of Age to Blood Pressure*

Age	Normal Blood Pressure (mm Hg)	
	Mean Systolic	Mean Diastolic
Premature	55-75	35-45
0-3 months	65-85	45-55
3-6 months	70-90	50-65
6-12 months	80-100	55-65
1-3 years	90-105	55-70
3-6 years	95-110	60-75
6-12 years	100-120	60-75
>12 years	110-135	65-85

*Note that the blood pressure will be lower during sleep or during anaesthesia.
Data from Mathers LH, Frankel LR: Pediatric emergencies and resuscitation. In Behrman RE, Kliegman RM, Jenson HB (eds): Nelson Textbook of Pediatrics, 17th ed. Philadelphia, WB Saunders, 2004.

linearly with increasing birth weight. An upper limit of 325 mL/min/kg and lower limit of 200 mL/min/kg are appropriate for clinical use.[80,81] This resting cardiac output is two to three times adult values. The relatively large cardiac output may reflect the higher metabolic rate and oxygen consumption compared with adults. This higher oxygen consumption may be related in part to the loss of body heat, which is relatively greater in newborns because of the larger surface area in relation to body mass. Pulsed Doppler estimation of cardiac output has been found helpful in assessing left ventricular myocardial dysfunction in neonates from perinatal asphyxia and acidosis and its response to therapy.[77,82,83]

Normal Electrocardiographic Findings from Infancy to Adolescence

Electrocardiographic findings undergo changes with age (see Chapter 14). Normal patterns in infants are distinctly abnormal if observed at a later stage of growth. The P wave reflects atrial depolarization and varies little with age. The PR interval increases with age (mean value for the first year is 0.10 second, increasing to 0.14 seconds at 12-16 years). The duration of the QRS complex increases with age, but prolongation greater than 0.10 seconds is abnormal at any age.

At birth, the QRS axis is right sided, reflecting the predominant right ventricular intrauterine development. It moves leftward in the first month as left ventricular muscle hypertrophies. Thereafter, the QRS follows a gradual change away from the initial marked right-sided axis.

In addition, T waves are upright in all chest leads. Within hours, they become isoelectric or inverted over the left chest; by the seventh day, the T waves are inverted in V_4R, V_1, and across to V_4; from then on, the T waves remain inverted over the right chest until adolescence, when they become upright over the right side of the chest again. Failure of T waves to become inverted in V_4R and V_1 to V_4 by 7 days may be the earliest ECG evidence of right ventricular hypertrophy.[84,85]

Studies of the ECG of preterm infants at 1 year of age show that for those without a history of bronchopulmonary dysplasia, the ECG findings are generally similar to the published norms for healthy 1-year olds. However, in those with residual lung disease, right ventricular hypertrophy is very prevalent. Thus, the ECG may be useful in the follow-up and assessment of infants with chronic residual lung disease.[86]

Renal System

In utero, the kidneys are active organs, producing a large volume of urine and helping to maintain amniotic fluid volume. Potter syndrome, characterized by a disfigured face, pulmonary hypoplasia, and skeletal deformities, is a result of lack of amniotic fluid secondary to renal agenesis. In utero, the fetus maintains its metabolic homeostasis through the placenta, and it is only after birth that the kidneys assume responsibility for metabolic function. More than 90% of newborns will have voided urine within the first 24 hours after birth. All normal infants should have voided within 48 hours after birth.[87]

At birth, glomerular filtration rate is 15% to 30% of normal adult values but reaches 50% of adult values on the 5th to 10th day and gradually attains adult values at the end of the first year of life.[88] Low glomerular filtration rate significantly affects the neonate's ability to excrete saline and water loads, as well as

drugs. Tubular function develops rapidly after 34 weeks of gestation.[89] An infant's immature kidneys respond to stress with changes in their capacity to function; however, a neonate's kidneys do not have the reserve to deal with the stress of serious illness.

The so-called physiologic acidemia of infancy is largely due to a diminished renal tubular threshold for bicarbonate.[90] An infant's kidneys concentrate urine to a maximum of 200 to 800 mOsm/L. This reflects some renal immaturity (fewer and shorter loops of Henle) but is in large part due to the low level of production and excretion of urea by a growing infant. An infant can dilute its urine (to a minimum of 50 mOsm/L) as can an older child; however, the rate of excretion of a water load is less. An infant's urea production is reduced as a result of growth, and thus "immature kidneys" are able to maintain a normal blood urea nitrogen level. *Elevated blood urea nitrogen, however, signifies renal failure, excessive dietary intake of protein (blood in the gastrointestinal tract, e.g., necrotizing enterocolitis), or interference with growth due to disease while intake of food has been maintained.*

Growth of renal length and cross-sectional area can be related to height or age. Capacity for growth extends into adulthood. For example, if one kidney is removed or destroyed, the remaining normal kidney hypertrophies; most compensatory growth occurs within 6 weeks and is usually complete within 6 months. Serious renal malfunctioning is usually associated with growth retardation. When this occurs, a child's rate of growth may be below the third percentile for chronologic age (see Fig. 2-1).

Hyperkalemia (defined as a serum potassium concentration of ≥6.8 mEq/L) has been noted in preterm infants weighing less than 1000 g and is associated with significant ECG dysrhythmias. Hyperkalemia appears to be partly related to immature distal tubule function and a relative hypoaldosteronism.[91]

Hepatic System

Development of the liver and bile ducts begins as an outgrowth of the foregut; by 10 weeks of gestation, the biliary tract has completed its development. The vitelline veins give rise to the portal and hepatic veins. Hepatic sinusoids form the ductus venosus, the bridge between the hepatic vein and the inferior vena cava. Most umbilical venous blood from the placenta passes through the ductus venosus to the inferior vena cava. The remainder passes via the portal vein through the liver to the hepatic veins. The portal venous drainage to the left lobe is less than to the right lobe, leading to a relative underdevelopment of the left lobe. The ductus venosus closes soon after birth.

At 12 weeks of gestation there is evidence of gluconeogenesis and protein synthesis; at 14 weeks, glycogen is found in liver cells. Although by late gestation liver cell morphology is similar to that of adults, the functional development of the liver is immature in newborns and more so in preterm infants. The liver has a major role in metabolism, controlling carbohydrate, protein, and lipid delivery to the tissues. Toward the end of pregnancy, large amounts of glycogen appear in the liver, and, as a result, preterm and SGA infants with smaller stores of glycogen may develop hypoglycemia. Bile acid secretion in newborns is depressed, and malabsorption of fat occurs.

The liver is the site for the synthesis of proteins; this process is active in fetal and neonatal life. In fetal life, the main serum protein is α-fetoprotein. This protein first appears at 6 weeks of gestation and reaches a peak at 13 weeks. Albumin synthesis starts at 3 to 4 months of gestation and approaches adult values at birth; in preterm infants, the level is lower. Proteins involved in clotting are also formed in the liver and are at a lower level than normal in preterm and full-term neonates for the first few days of life. Hematopoiesis occurs in the fetal liver, with peak activity at 7 months of gestation. After 6 weeks of age, hematopoiesis is confined to the bone marrow except under pathologic conditions, such as hemolytic anemia.

The capacity to enzymatically break down proteins is depressed at birth. This is particularly important in preterm infants, when high protein intake can lead to dangerous levels of serum amino acid concentrations. In the first weeks of life, drug metabolism is less efficient than in later life. In addition to less effective hepatic metabolism, altered drug binding by serum proteins and immature renal function contribute to the problem (see Chapter 6).

Physiologic Jaundice

Hyperbilirubinemia is an especially important problem in neonates. The mechanisms for producing jaundice are outlined in Table 2-11.[92,93] Increased concentrations of indirect bilirubin usually occur in the first few days of life. In term infants, bilirubin levels of 6 to 8 mg/dL are commonly seen within the first 3 days of life. In preterm infants, the peak level of 10 to 12 mg/dL occurs on the fifth to seventh day of life. After this period, levels gradually decrease to adult values of less than 2 mg/dL in 1 to 2 months for both term and preterm infants. The cause of nonhemolytic physiologic hyperbilirubinemia is excessive bilirubin production from breakdown of red blood cells and increased enterohepatic circulation of bilirubin with deficient hepatic conjugation due to depressed glucuronyl transferase activity. The relationship between breast feeding and hyperbilirubinemia has been well documented. It is usually delayed in onset (after the third day of life), its cause remains unclear, and it occurs in about 1% of breast-feeding infants. An earlier hypothesis ascribing it to inhibition of glucuronyl transferase by 3α, 20β-pregnanediol activity has not been substantiated.

Important pathologic causes of jaundice in newborns are presented in Table 2-12. Once the distinction between physiologic and hemolytic hyperbilirubinemia has been made, the underlying cause can then be treated and efforts can be directed at preventing bilirubin encephalopathy (kernicterus) by the use of phototherapy and, in selected cases, exchange transfusions. Sick preterm infants are especially at risk for kernicterus and are more aggressively treated at lower bilirubin levels than full-term infants.[94-99] Increasingly common is a form of cholestatic jaundice in LBW infants receiving prolonged hyperalimentation. Its mechanism is unclear, but it may be due to inhibition of bile flow by amino acids.[100-103] Future therapy for hyperbilirubinemia in LBW infants may include the use of tin-mesoporphyrin, which inhibits the production of bilirubin.[104,105]

Table 2-11. Causes of Jaundice in Neonates

Excess bilirubin production
Impaired uptake of bilirubin
Impaired conjugation of bilirubin
Defective bilirubin excretion
Increased enterohepatic circulation of bilirubin

Table 2-12. Pathologic Causes of Jaundice in Newborns

Antibody-induced hemolysis (Rh and ABO)
Hereditary red blood cell disorders (e.g., glucose-6-phosphate dehydrogenase deficiency, which gives rise to hemolysis from drugs or infection)
Infections (e.g., neonatal hepatitis, sepsis, severe urinary tract infections)
Hemorrhage into the body (e.g., intracerebral)
Biliary atresia
Metabolic (e.g., hypothyroidism, galactosemia)

Gastrointestinal Tract

In a fetus, the digestive tract consists of the developing foregut and hindgut. These rapidly elongate so that a loop of gut is forced into the yolk sac. At 5 to 7 weeks, this loop twists around the axis of the superior mesenteric artery and returns to the abdominal cavity. Maturation occurs gradually from the proximal to the distal end. Blood vessels and nerves (Auerbach and Meissner plexuses) are developed by 13 weeks of gestation, and peristalsis begins. Parotid, sublingual, and submandibular salivary glands arise from the oral mucosa. The pancreas arises from two outgrowths of the foregut; a diverticulum of the foregut gives rise to the liver.

Enzyme levels of enterokinase and lipase increase with gestational age but are lower at birth than in older children. Nevertheless, newborns and preterm infants are able to handle proteins reasonably well. Preterm infants, however, are unable to tolerate large protein loads. Fat digestion is limited, particularly in preterm infants, who absorb only 65% of adult levels. Neonatal duodenal motility undergoes marked maturational changes between 29 and 32 weeks of gestation. This is one factor limiting tolerance of enteral feeding before 29 to 30 weeks of gestation. Central nervous system abnormalities will delay these maturational changes.[106]

Anomalies arising from maldevelopment of the gut may be appreciated from an understanding of normal development.

- *Esophageal atresia and tracheoesophageal fistula.* This anomaly occurs when the respiratory tract fails to separate completely from the foregut at 4 weeks of gestation. Failure of separation may be seen as a laryngeal cleft. In its extreme form, the cleft may extend from the glottis to the carina (see Chapters 35 and 36).
- *Intestinal atresia and stenosis.* These anomalies are common causes of obstruction in newborns, particularly in the duodenal region; this lesion is frequently associated with Down syndrome. The cause may be a failure of recanalization in utero as a result of a vascular accident (intussusception, volvulus, or thrombosis).
- *Duplication and diverticulum.* These may be blind pouches or may communicate with the intestinal lumen. The mucosa frequently is gastric and may hemorrhage. Other complications include obstruction, perforation, and infection. Meckel diverticulum is relatively common and is due to persistence of the vitellointestinal duct.
- *Hirschsprung disease.* Hirschsprung disease is due to failure of development of the Meissner and Auerbach plexuses.

- *Peritoneal bands.* These bands, which cause obstruction, result from faulty rotation and fixation of the gut, most commonly at the duodenojejunal junction.
- *Omphalocele and gastroschisis.* In these conditions, intestine protrudes from the abdominal wall as a result of failure of closure of the rectus muscles (omphalocele) at 8 weeks of gestation or herniation of the intestine through a paraumbilical defect (gastroschisis) (see Chapter 36).

Swallowing

Swallowing is a complex procedure that is under central and peripheral control. The reflex is initiated in the medulla, through cranial nerves to the muscles that control the passage of food through the pharyngoesophageal sphincter. In the process, the tongue, soft palate, pharynx, and larynx all are smoothly coordinated. Any pathologic condition of these structures can interfere with normal swallowing. Neuromuscular incoordination, however, is more likely to be responsible for any dysfunction. This is particularly evident when the central nervous system has sustained damage either before or during delivery. With swallowing, pressure in the pharynx rises, the pharyngoesophageal sphincter opens, and peristaltic waves in the upper esophagus carry the bolus of food downward. Peristaltic waves are absent in the lower esophagus in infants, although present in adults. With the immaturity of the pharyngoesophageal sphincter, frequent regurgitation or "spitting" of gastric contents is observed even in healthy infants.

Gastroesophageal Reflux

Approximately 40% of newborns in the first few days of life regurgitate their food.[107] Lower esophageal pressures are diminished and take 3 to 6 weeks to achieve adult levels. Symptoms of reflux include persistent vomiting, failure to thrive, and, in severe cases, hematemesis and anemia, occasionally complicated by stricture formation. These symptoms are also found with hiatal hernia. Gastroesophageal reflux is one of a number of conditions associated with apnea and bradycardia in preterm infants.[108]

Meconium

Meconium is the material contained in the intestinal tract before birth. It consists of desquamated epithelial cells from the intestinal tract and bile, pancreatic and intestinal secretions, and water (70%). Meconium is usually passed in the first few hours after birth; virtually all term infants pass their first stool by 48 hours. However, passage of the first stool is usually delayed in LBW infants. Infants weighing less than 1500 g at birth may take up to 6 to 7 days, probably because of immaturity of the motility and lack of gut hormones due to delayed enteral feeding. This normal developmental delay should be appreciated, because late passage of the first stool raises the suspicion of a pathologic condition such as meconium ileus, meconium plug syndrome, or intestinal atresia.[109] Meconium ileus occurs in 10% of children with cystic fibrosis. The meconium is inspissated and causes intestinal obstruction. Newborns who fail to pass meconium may also be suffering from Hirschsprung disease; reduced colonic activity results in increased water absorption and inspissation of the meconium. Meconium in the amniotic fluid may indicate intrauterine asphyxia. Aspiration of meconium may have serious effects on pulmonary function, leading to pneumonia, pneumothorax, and persistent pulmonary hypertension (persistent fetal circulation).[110,111]

Pancreas

The placenta is impermeable to both insulin and glucagon. The islets of Langerhans in the fetal pancreas, however, secrete insulin from the 11th week of fetal life; the amount of insulin secretion increases with age. After birth, insulin response is related to gestational and postnatal age and is more mature in term infants.

Maternal hyperglycemia, particularly when uncontrolled, results in hypertrophy and hyperplasia of the fetal islets of Langerhans. This leads to increased levels of insulin in the fetus, affecting lipid metabolism and giving rise to a large, overweight infant characteristic of a mother with poorly controlled diabetes. Hyperglycemia alone is not instrumental in this effect; it may also be the result of an increase in serum amino acids found in diabetic mothers. Meticulous control of a mother's diabetes during pregnancy and delivery has led to a reduction in morbidity and mortality of the infants of diabetic mothers. Hyperinsulinemia of the fetus persists after birth and may lead to rapid development of serious hypoglycemia. In addition to severe hypoglycemia, these infants have an increased incidence of congenital anomalies.

Infants who are SGA are frequently hypoglycemic, and this may be the result of malnutrition in utero. Some of these infants secrete inappropriately large amounts of insulin in response to glucose and for this reason may suffer from serious hypoglycemia. In addition, hepatic glycogen stores are inadequate, and deficient gluconeogenesis exists. Preterm infants may be hypoglycemic without demonstrable symptoms, therefore necessitating close monitoring of blood glucose levels.

Full-term neonates undergo a metabolic adjustment after birth with regard to glucose. Studies have defined values for glucose levels below which there should be concern: plasma glucose levels less than 35 mg/dL in the first 3 hours of life; less than 40 mg/dL between 3 and 24 hours; and less than 45 mg/dL after 24 hours.[112] Others have defined hypoglycemia in full-term infants as a serum glucose concentration of less than 30 mg/dL in the first day of life or less than 40 mg/dL in the second day of life.[113] It is important to appreciate that infants, although showing no symptoms, may develop serious hypoglycemia leading to irreversible central nervous system damage. Other infants may present with convulsions, but signs may also be subtle (e.g., lethargy, somnolence, and jitteriness).

Hyperglycemia (plasma glucose ≥150 mg/dL) occurs in stressed neonates, particularly LBW infants infused with glucose-containing solutions. Hyperglycemia has been associated with infection as well as increased morbidity and mortality. Hyperglycemia commonly occurs in infants undergoing elective surgery under general anesthesia; infusion of glucose-containing solutions may aggravate the tendency to become hyperglycemic. Thus it is advisable that intraoperative glucose levels be monitored. Replacement of blood, "third space," and deficit fluid losses should be carried out with dextrose-free solutions. Maintenance fluid requirements may be replaced with glucose-containing solutions administered with a constant-infusion pump to avoid bolus glucose administration. A study in infants undergoing surgery under general anesthesia showed that postsurgical plasma glucose values were significantly higher than postinduction values; insulin changes were minimal.[114] The risk of hyperglycemia is considerably greater in infants weighing less than 1000 g compared with infants of 2000 g or more.[115] Hyperglycemia may be due to multiple causes, such as exogenous glucose solutions, lipid infusions, hypoxemia, sepsis, surgical procedures, and drugs such as theophylline. Hyperglycemia may also lead to osmotic diuresis and dehydration and has been associated with an increased incidence of intraventricular hemorrhage and handicap.

The mechanism of glucose intolerance in a neonate depends on the underlying cause. Hypoxemia stimulates α-adrenergic receptors and release of catecholamines while diminishing the insulin response.[116-118] Careful titration of glucose according to an infant's needs as measured by plasma blood glucose levels is required. Administration of 3 to 4 mg/kg/min dextrose in infants weighing less than 1000 g is a useful starting point.[119] Adjustments are made according to the infant's needs. Dextrose should be decreased in the infusate should plasma glucose levels exceed 150 mg/dL. If this maneuver is inadequate to achieve lower and safer blood glucose levels (i.e., levels are >250-300 mg/kg), a continuous insulin drip (0.05-0.2 units/kg/hr) can be administrated intravenously and titrated to achieve normoglycemia.[120]

Hematopoietic System

The blood volume of a full-term newborn is dependent on the time of cord clamping, which modifies the volume of placental transfusion. Blood volume is 93 mL/kg when cord clamping is delayed after delivery, compared with 82 mL/kg with immediate cord clamping.[121,122] Within the first 4 hours after delivery, however, fluid is lost from the blood and the plasma volume contracts by as much as 25%. The larger the placental transfusion, the larger this loss of fluid in the first few hours after birth, with resultant hemoconcentration. The blood volume in preterm infants is higher (90 to 105 mL/kg) than in full-term infants because of increased plasma volume.[121]

The normal hemoglobin range is between 14 g/dL and 20 g/dL. The site of sampling must be considered, however, when interpreting these values for the diagnosis of neonatal anemia or hyperviscosity syndrome. Capillary sampling (e.g., heel stick) gives higher values, as much as 6 g/dL, because of stasis in peripheral vessels leading to loss of plasma and hemoconcentration; thus a venipuncture is preferred. In 1% of infants, fetal-maternal transfusion occurs and may be responsible for some of the "lower normal" hemoglobin values reported.

Erythropoietic activity from the bone marrow decreases immediately after birth in both full-term and preterm infants. The cord blood reticulocyte count of 5% persists for a few days and declines below 1% by 1 week. This is followed by a slight increase to 1% to 2% by the 12th week, where it remains throughout childhood. Premature infants have higher reticulocyte counts (up to 10%) at birth. Abnormal reticulocyte values reflect hemorrhage or hemolysis.

In term infants, the hemoglobin concentration falls during the 9th to 12th week to reach a nadir of 10 to 11 g/dL (hematocrit 30% to 33%) and then rises. This decrease in hemoglobin concentration is due to a decrease in erythropoiesis and to some extent due to a shortened life span of the red blood cells. In preterm infants, the decrease in the hemoglobin level is greater and is directly related to the degree of prematurity; also, the nadir is reached earlier (4-8 weeks).[123] In infants weighing 800 to 1000 g, the decrement may reach a low of 8 g/dL. This "anemia" is a normal physiologic adjustment to extrauterine life. Despite the reduction in hemoglobin, the oxygen delivery to the tissues may not be compromised because of a shift of the oxygen-hemoglobin dissociation curve (to the right), secondary to an increase of 2,3-diphosphoglycerate.[124] In addition, fetal hemoglobin is replaced by adult-type hemoglobin, which also results in a shift in the same direction. In neonates, especially preterm infants, low hemoglobin levels may be associated with apnea and tachycardia.[125] Vitamin E administration does not prevent anemia of prematurity; no significant difference was noted between vitamin E-supplemented and unsupplemented groups in terms of hemoglobin concentration, reticulocyte and platelet counts, or erythrocyte morphology in infants at 6 weeks of age.[126] Infants with anemia of prematurity have been found to have an inadequate production of erythropoietin (the primary regulator in erythropoiesis). Some centers are now using recombinant human erythropoietin in VLBW infants to stimulate erythropoiesis and decrease the need for multiple transfusions.[127]

After the third month, the hemoglobin level stabilizes at 11.5 to 12.0 g/dL, until about 2 years of age. The hemoglobin values of full-term and preterm infants are comparable after the first year. Thereafter a gradual increase to mean levels at puberty of 14.0 g/dL for females and 15.5 g/dL for males is seen.

The white blood cell count may normally reach $21,000/mm^3$ in the first 24 hours of life and $12,000/mm^3$ at the end of the first week, with the number of neutrophils equaling the number of lymphocytes. It then decreases gradually, reaching adult levels at puberty. At birth, neutrophil granulocytes predominate but rapidly decrease in number so that during the first week of life and through 4 years of age the lymphocyte is the predominant cell. After the fourth year, the values approximate an adult's. Neonates have an increased susceptibility to bacterial infection, which is related in part to immaturity of leukocyte function. Sepsis may be associated with a minimal leukocyte response or even with leukopenia. Spurious increases in the white blood cell content may be due to drugs (e.g., epinephrine).

Thrombocytopenia occurs frequently in preterm infants suffering from hyaline membrane disease. Mechanical ventilation has been associated with a significant decrease in the platelet count in newborns.[128] There appears to be an inverse correlation between gestational age or birth weight and the severity of platelet reduction. A study of neonatal thrombocytopenia and its impact on hemostatic integrity showed that thrombocytopenic infants are at greater risk for bleeding than equally sick nonthrombocytopenic infants.[129]

Neonatal polycythemia (central hematocrit >65%) occurs in 3% to 5% of full-term newborns.[130] In studies of animals, hyperviscosity with a hematocrit exceeding 70% is associated with an increase in systemic and pulmonary vascular resistance and decreased cardiac output.[131] Using M-mode echocardiography, a study of neonates demonstrated an increase in PVR with hyperviscosity.[132] Partial exchange transfusion to lower the hematocrit and decrease the blood viscosity improves systemic and pulmonary blood flow and oxygen transport. The increased organ blood flow should prevent the cardiovascular and neurologic symptoms associated with the hyperviscosity syndrome.[133]

Coagulation in the Infant

At birth, vitamin K–dependent factors (i.e., II, VII, IX, and X) are at levels of 20% to 60% of adult values; in preterm infants, the values are even less. The result is prolonged prothrombin times, normally encountered in full-term and preterm infants. Synthesis of vitamin K–dependent factors occurs in the liver, which, being immature, leads to relatively lower levels of the coagulation factors, even with the administration of vitamin K. It takes several weeks for the levels of coagulation factors to reach adult values; the deficit is even more pronounced in preterm infants. Vitamin K prophylaxis has been reevaluated.[134] The findings show that the majority of cases of neonatal vitamin K deficiency occur in normal newborns. Thus, all newborns should receive prophylactic vitamin K soon after birth to prevent hemorrhagic disease of the newborn. Its omission could lead to serious and life-threatening consequences, especially if surgery is undertaken. Infants of mothers who have received anticonvulsant drugs during pregnancy may develop a serious coagulopathy similar to that encountered with vitamin K deficiency.[135] Vitamin K_1 administered to newborns usually reverses this bleeding tendency, but death has occurred despite therapy. Other risk factors include maternal use of drugs such as warfarin, rifampin, and isoniazid. Breast feeding may also be associated with severe vitamin K deficiency.

Neurologic Development

Reduction of perinatal mortality during the past decade has not resulted in the expected reduction in the prevalence of cerebral palsy. The strongest predictors of cerebral palsy appear to be congenital anomaly, LBW, low placental weight, or abnormal fetal position before labor and delivery and not perinatal complications such as perinatal asphyxia.[136]

An infant's normal mental development depends on maturation of the central nervous system. This development may be affected by physical illness or by inadequate psychosocial support. Delay in development in preterm infants, however, may be normal, depending on the degree of prematurity.

The rate of brain growth is different from the growth rate of other body systems. The brain has two growth spurts—neuronal cell multiplication between 15 and 20 weeks of gestation and glial cell multiplication—commencing at 25 weeks and extending into the second year of life. Myelination continues into the third year. Malnutrition during this phase of neural development may have profound handicapping effects. Knowledge of the normal pattern of a child's development allows one to evaluate the development of an individual child.

Normal brain development may be impaired by events leading to damage of the blood-brain barrier, particularly in an immature brain. The endothelial cells of the brain microvascular structure form tight junctions as a result of an interaction between the astrocytes of the brain and endothelial cells.[137] Plasma membrane transport selectively promotes the passage of essential substrates such as glucose, organic acids, and amino acids across the blood-brain barrier. Hypoxemia and ischemia may lead to a breakdown in this barrier, with resulting edema and increased intracranial pressure. Injury to the blood-brain barrier may be on the basis of abnormal entry of calcium or formation of free radicals. Further studies of the mechanism of this breakdown will lead to rational approaches to therapy. In preterm infants stressed by hypoxia, the blood-brain barrier may become particularly permeable to the water-soluble bilirubin, with possible damage to the brain.[138]

Normal newborns show various primitive reflexes, which include the Moro response and grasp reflex. Milestones of development are useful indicators of mental development and possible deviations from normal. It should be appreciated, however, that these milestones represent the *average,* and infants can vary in their rates of maturation of different body functions and still be within the normal range.[139] The Denver Developmental Screening Test is a useful scheme for assessing these milestones. The test focuses on four areas: (1) gross motor function, (2) fine motor and adaptive skills, (3) language, and (4) personal and social skills. Developing infants acquire motor skills. For effective movement, an infant needs postural control, which develops in a cephalocaudal direction. It starts with head control and progresses to sitting, standing, walking, and finally running (Table 2-13).

Adaptive skills are performed through well-coordinated fine motor movements (Table 2-14). Abnormal development may be reflected in a delay in appearance of a particular milestone or in its pathologic persistence with maturation in a child. For example, at 20 weeks, a child reaches and retrieves objects, frequently placing them in his or her mouth. As an infant matures, however, this behavior pattern usually ceases at 12 to 13 months of age; in infants with a mental abnormality, this practice may continue much longer.

Language development correlates closely with cognitive skills (Table 2-15). Personal and social skills are modified by environ-

Table 2-13. Relationship of Motor Milestones to Age

Motor Milestone	Age
Supports head	3 months
Sits alone	6 months
Stands alone	12 months
Balances on one foot	3 years

Table 2-14. Relationship of Fine Motor/Adaptive Milestones to Age

Fine Motor/Adaptive Milestones	Age
Grasps rattle	3 months
Passes cube hand to hand	6 months
Pincer grip	1 year
Imitates vertical line	2 years
Copies circle	3 years

Table 2-15. Relationship of Language Milestones to Age

Language Milestones	Age
Squeals	1.5-3.0 months
Turns to voice	6 months
Combines two words	1.5 years
Composes short sentences	2 years
Gives entire name	3 years

Table 2-16. Relationship of Personal-Social Milestones to Age

Personal-Social Milestones	Age
Smiles spontaneously	3 months
Feeds self crackers	6 months
Drinks from cup	1 year
Plays interactive games	2 years

Table 2-17. Causes of Developmental Delay

Infections (e.g., meningitis, encephalitis)
Head injury
Hypoxemia (e.g., near-drowning, carbon monoxide poisoning)
Metabolic (e.g., severe hypoglycemia, hypernatremia, hypothyroidism, phenylketonuria, chronic malnutrition)
Lead poisoning, addicting drugs
Degenerative disease of the nervous system
Cerebral tumor, vascular accident (intraventricular hemorrhage)
Congenital malformation
Prematurity

mental factors and cultural patterns (Table 2-16). Development of walking, speech, and sphincter control are most important. For appropriate evaluation consider familial patterns, level of intelligence, and physical illness. Deafness may cause delayed speech.

Developmental Issues

Children with developmental issues are delayed in *many* aspects of both cognitive and motor development. Smiling, vocalization, sitting, walking, speech, and sphincter control are delayed. When there is a delay in the eye following an object and the head turning in response to sound, blindness and deafness may erroneously be diagnosed. Drooling, common in young infants, is frequently prolonged for years in neurologically delayed children. Initially, a mentally handicapped infant appears to be inactive and may be seen as a "good child." The child later demonstrates constant and sometimes uncontrollable overactivity. In diagnosing a mental abnormality, anesthesiologists must be aware of possible pitfalls:

- Infants born prematurely will be delayed and should be assessed in terms of their conceptual age.
- Infants with cerebral palsy or sensory deficits (auditory and visual) may have normal mental development, but the handicap may interfere with assessment of mental status.
- The effects of drugs should be considered (e.g., barbiturates for epilepsy).

Developmental delay may be due to a wide range of causes, among which those listed in Table 2-17 should be considered.

Acknowledgment

We acknowledge the contributions of Ronald Gore, MD, from the second edition and Jonathan Cronin, MD, from the third edition.

Annotated References

Coté CJ, Zaslavsky A, Downes JJ, et al: Postoperative apnea in former preterm infants after inguinal herniorrhaphy: a combined analysis. Anesthesiology 1995; 82:809-822

Key reference describing risk factors for post-anesthesia apnea in former preterm neonates after surgical procedures.

DiFiore JM, Arko M, Whitehouse M, et al: Apnea is not prolonged by acid gastroesophageal reflux in preterm infants. Pediatrics 2005; 116:1059-1062

Recent reference detailing causes of apnea in preterm neonates.

Dubowitz LM, Dubowitz V, Goldberg C: Clinical assessment of gestational age in the newborn infant. J Pediatr 1970; 77:1-10

One of the first and most important references describing the physical examination of preterm infants.

Osborn D, Evans N, Kluckow M: Diagnosis and treatment of low systemic blood flow in preterm infants. NeoReviews.org 2004; 5: e109

Updated review on the most recent treatments for low blood pressure in preterm infants.

Reid L: 1976 Edward B. D. Neuhauser lecture. The lung: growth and remodeling in health and disease. AJR Am J Roentgenol 1977; 129:777-788

A key reference detailing the lung development of premature neonates.

References

Please see www.expertconsult.com

Perioperative Behavior Stress in Children

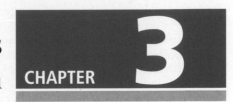

CHAPTER 3

Zeev N. Kain, Jill MacLaren, and Linda C. Mayes

Developmental Issues	**Pharmacologic Interventions versus Behavioral**
Cognitive Development and Understanding of Illness	**Interventions**
Attachment	**Postoperative Outcomes**
Temperament	Emergence Delirium
Preoperative Anxiety	Sleep Changes
Risk Factors	Other Behavioral Changes
Behavioral Interventions	Intraoperative Clinical Outcomes
Pharmacologic Interventions	**Summary**

INTEREST IN CHILDREN'S PERIOPERATIVE behavior has increased dramatically over the past 15 years. Specifically, there has been a recognition of the importance of developmental factors in perioperative research, resulting in a surge of investigation in this area. In this chapter, we discuss developmental considerations that are relevant to the child's perioperative experience (cognitive development, attachment and separation, temperament). We then offer a review and synthesis of recent data on preoperative anxiety and maladaptive behavioral and cognitive outcomes associated with surgery/anesthesia.

Developmental Issues

Cognitive Development and Understanding of Illness
The perioperative period is stressful for many individuals undergoing surgery, and this is especially true for children. Children's stress during the perioperative period results from multiple sources, one of which is a limited understanding of their illness and the need for surgery. Early developmental theories (e.g., those of Piaget[1,2]) suggest that a child's understanding of illness changes qualitatively as he or she matures cognitively. Although dated, Bibace and Walsh[3] described a model of the child's progressive understanding of illness that evolves from prelogical explanations such as phenomenism (e.g., magical thinking), to concrete-logical explanations such as contamination (e.g., eating bad food), to formal-logical explanations (e.g., physiologic causes). This is still currently the most widely cited model for the child's perspective of illness.

Although less theoretically developed, children's understanding of the treatments for illnesses is thought to follow a similar developmental pattern. In terms of understanding of surgery, a child's concepts are particularly underdeveloped. Young children have difficulty defining "an operation" suggesting that it is the same as being sick, going for a doctor's checkup, or taking a nap.[4] Given these developmental considerations, it is not surprising that young children are more likely to have misconceptions about hospitalization and surgery than older children and adults[5] and are at unique and disparate risk for perioperative stress when compared with adults.

Attachment
Another child-specific consideration during the perioperative period is his or her attachment style to the parent/caregiver and how the parent-child relationship influences the child's response to the separation associated with surgery/anesthesia. Although adults also undergo separation from family, the separation of children from their parents is particularly stressful.

Coping with separation is a lifelong challenge that is inevitable and necessary for a child's normal healthy development.[6] Separation experiences such as saying good-bye at the door of school or sleeping overnight at a friend's house facilitate normal childhood psychological growth and personality organization by mobilizing opportunities for learning and adaptation. Other separation experiences, especially those occurring in the context of loss, illness, or other stressors, can precipitate states of confusion, anger, and anxiety. Brief separations such as those associated with surgery are most stressful for infants, toddlers, and preschool-aged children. Indeed, for school-aged children, responses to separation may reflect, in part, response patterns established early in the preschool years.[6] For children with biologically based vulnerabilities, such as a sensitivity to novelty and transitions, even expected separations, may impose a greater degree of stress than for less sensitive children.[6] Similarly, for children with developmental delay, separations may be experienced with a degree of anxiety and developmental stress more like that experienced by a younger child.

One variable that is associated with children's response to separation is attachment. Attachment develops as a result of an infant's early experiences with the primary caregiver. Through interactions with the primary caregiver, an infant has the opportunity to develop a sense of trust and security in the reliability and predictability of his or her relationship and the world.[7] The style of attachment that an infant has developed is evident in the infant's responses to brief separations from the primary

25

caregiver. Children may be "securely attached," "insecurely attached," or "anxiously attached" to their parents.

Infants who are more "securely attached" to their parents deal more adaptively with the stress of brief separation and with the novelty of the hospital experience. These infants are more willing to explore their world and respond positively to their mother's return, using her as a secure, stable base from which to approach strangers and new situations.[8,9] In contrast, toddlers classified as "anxiously attached" to their mother tend to be distressed in unfamiliar situations, like those found in the perioperative environment, even when their mother is present. When their mother returns after brief separations, these infants tend to be angry and distressed and avoid physical contact. Another form of "insecure attachment" is avoidance. Avoidant children do not explore their surroundings as much as securely attached infants do and tend to ignore their mother. They rarely show distress on separation and avoid interactions with their mother when she returns. Conversely, "insecurely attached" infants are more easily distressed by even brief separations and spend more time trying to stay close to their parents. More anxious about novelty and separation, they are less likely to explore and less likely to adapt positively to new situations.

Temperament

Responses to the stress of the perioperative period in infancy and preschool years reflects in part the child's relationships with the parents *as well as* the child's temperament. Temperament refers to emotional responses that are characteristic of individual infants and young children. Clusters of related characteristics may constitute a temperament type. While conceptually related to personality, temperament characteristics in children are presumed to have primarily a genetic basis.[10] Later personality characteristics, such as adulthood characteristics, presumably reflect the interaction between temperament traits arising in early childhood and environmental influences. Some authors find that it is useful to classify infants with respect to three main dimensions: emotionality, activity, and sociability.[11] *Emotionality* refers to the ease with which an infant becomes aroused or anxious, especially in situations that might lead to fear, such as perioperative settings. *Activity* refers to the infant's customary level of energy and intensity of behavior. *Sociability* reflects the infant's tendency to approach or avoid others. These behavioral dimensions of temperament are also reflected in physiologic responses related to anxiety.[12] For example, measures of heart rate variability are closely related to infants' reactivity and lability in the first year of life.[13] Infants with less variability in heart rate (presumably reflecting increased sympathetic relative to parasympathetic influence on heart rate) are more labile and reactive to novelty. Infants who have a tendency to avoid novelty cry more easily and are less active in contrast to those who readily approach the unfamiliar. In long-term studies, infants who are inhibited in the face of novelty continue to be so through early school age.[14] Thus, temperament as a behavioral descriptor appears to characterize an enduring cluster of traits reflecting reactivity and anxiety regulation in the face of novelty.

In light of these issues, the child's developmental level is an important consideration in the perioperative period, especially on the child's perioperative behavior. The remainder of this chapter is a discussion of specific behavioral issues related to surgery in children. We focus on anxiety in the preoperative period, particularly at induction of anesthesia. We also present data on postoperative behavioral outcomes including emergence delirium, sleep, and other maladaptive behavioral changes.

Preoperative Anxiety

Anxiety in children undergoing anesthesia and surgery is characterized by feelings of tension, apprehension, and nervousness.[15] This response is attributed to separation from parents, loss of control, uncertainty about the anesthesia, and uncertainty about the surgery and its outcome.[15] It is estimated that between 40% and 60% of children develop significant fear and anxiety before their surgery.[16] Furthermore, separation from parents and induction of anesthesia have been found to be the most stressful times during the surgical/anesthesia experience. Some children verbalize their fears explicitly, whereas others express their anxiety only by changes in behavior. Children may appear scared or agitated, breathe deeply, tremble, stop talking or playing, and start to cry. Some may wet or soil themselves, display increased motor tone, and actively attempt to escape from medical personnel.[17] These behaviors may give children some sense of control in the situation and thereby diminish the damaging effects of a sense of helplessness.[15,17] In addition to the behavioral manifestations detailed here, several studies have documented that anxiety before surgery is associated with neuroendocrine changes, such as increased serum cortisol, epinephrine, growth hormone, and adrenocorticotropic hormone levels and increased natural killer cell activity.[18,19] Significant correlations between heart rate, blood pressure, and behavioral ratings of anxiety have also been reported.[20,21]

Risk Factors

Anxiety combined with distress before surgery is a clinically important phenomenon that should be treated as any other clinical phenomenon or disease. In epidemiologic terms, *all* diseases are characterized operationally by risk factors, interventions, and outcomes; preoperative anxiety is no exception. For the remainder of this chapter, we review the phenomenon of preoperative anxiety using the classic epidemiologic model of a disease (Fig. 3-1).

Identifying risk factors for preoperative anxiety is important because the routine use of pharmacologic and behavioral interventions may carry with them both advantages and disadvantages. Routine administration of sedative premedications, for example, may increase indirect pharmacy costs, increase the need for nursing staff, and increase appropriately monitored bed space in the preoperative holding area. Delayed discharge in children undergoing extremely short outpatient procedures may also occur. Similarly, behavioral preparation programs administered preoperatively are associated with increased hospital operational costs. Likewise, anxious children can utilize hospital resources that would be reduced with appropriate pharmacologic preparation. Thus, identifying children who are at a particularly high risk for developing extreme anxiety and distress before surgery would help guide the use of limited resources in the most beneficial directions.

Variation in children's behavioral responses to the perioperative experience has its origin in at least four domains:
- Age and developmental maturity
- Previous experience with medical procedures and illness

BEHAVIORAL PERIOPERATIVE STRESS

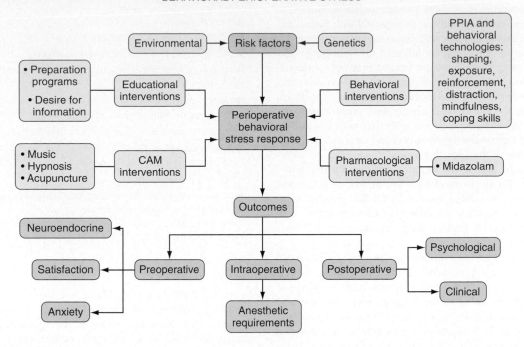

Figure 3-1. Operational overview of perioperative anxiety. PPIA, parental presence during induction of anesthesia. CAM, complimentary alternative medicine.

● Individual capacity for affect regulation and trait anxiety (baseline anxiety)

● Parental state (situational) and trait (baseline) anxiety

Previous studies that examined the behavioral responses to induction of anesthesia in children did so in terms of these four domains.[22-26] Children between the ages of 1 and 5 years are at greatest risk for developing extreme anxiety and distress. This is not surprising, because separation anxiety often does not peak until 1 year of age, and children older than the age of 5 years can more easily cope with new and unpredictable situations. A history of prior stressful medical encounters, such as in the pediatrician's office, the dentist's office, with previous surgery, or with previous hospitalization, affects how a child reacts to new medical encounters. These are each important risk factors for preoperative anxiety. Children who are shy and inhibited, as identified by temperament tests, are also at increased risk for developing anxiety and distress before surgery. In addition, children who lack good social adaptive abilities are likewise at risk.[26]

Parental characteristics also have a strong influence on a child's behavior during the perioperative experience. Children of parents who are more anxious, children of parents who use avoidance coping mechanisms, and children of separated or divorced parents all appear to be at high risk for developing preoperative anxiety.[27] Because children of anxious parents are more likely to experience high levels of preoperative anxiety, it is important to identify the predictors of increased *parental* preoperative anxiety. The gender of the parent (mothers are more anxious than fathers[28]), the child younger than 1 year of age, children with repeated hospital admissions, and baseline temperament of the child are predictors of increased parental preoperative anxiety.[27,29-31] Once one identifies those children and parents who are at the greatest risk for developing preopera-

tive anxiety and distress, one can then take steps to better treat this "at-risk" population.

Behavioral Interventions

Pharmacologic interventions (e.g., administration of premedications) and behavioral interventions (e.g., psychological preparation programs) are used to treat preoperative anxiety and distress in children and their parents.[16,32]

Preoperative Preparation Programs

Psychological preparation for children undergoing anesthesia and surgery has been widely advocated. These preparation programs may provide narrative information, an orientation tour of the operative facility, role rehearsal using dolls, modeling using videotapes or a puppet show, child-life preparation, or coping education and relaxation skills.[33-35]

Although there is general agreement in the medical community about the desirability of such programs, recommendations regarding the content of behavioral preoperative preparation programs differ widely. Preparation programs in the 1960s were information oriented and designed to facilitate emotional expression and trust between the medical staff, the child, and the parent.[36] Modeling techniques in which children and parents indirectly experienced anesthesia and surgery by viewing a video or a puppet show emerged in the 1970s.[37] This form of preparation was augmented in the late 1980s with child-life preparation and coping skills education.[34] Child-life specialists are trained individuals who facilitate development of coping skills and the adjustment of children and parents to the perioperative environment by providing play experiences, presenting information about events and procedures, and establishing supportive relationships with children and parents.[35] In making information accessible to children, child-life specialists incorporate descriptions of the sensations children will experience, provide opportunities to examine and manipulate equipment to be used in their care, and encourage rehearsal with dolls. Currently, development of coping skills is considered the most effective preoperative intervention, followed by modeling, play therapy, operating room tour, and printed material.[38] Interestingly, when development of coping skills preparation was compared with lower rated techniques, such as providing information and modeling, the highly rated coping skills preparation technique with child-life specialists was associated with less anxiety in the holding area on the day of surgery and on separation from parents on entry to the operating room.[39] In contrast, no differences were found among the various techniques during induction of anesthesia, in the recovery room period, or at 2 weeks postoperatively. Thus, from a cost-effectiveness point of view, one must decide whether the additional cost associated with child-life specialists is justified by reduction of anxiety *only* during the preoperative period.

It is important that these preparation programs are tailored to the individual, age-appropriate needs of each child. Several variables have been identified as influencing the response of children to preparation programs.[27] For example, children who are 6 years of age or older benefit most if they participate in a preparation program more than 5 days before the scheduled surgery and benefit least if the program is given only 1 day before surgery. In fact, older children prepared a week in advance showed an *increase* in anxiety level during and immediately after the preparation but demonstrated a gradual decrease in anxiety during the 5 days before the time of surgery.[40] To avoid increasing excessive anticipatory anxiety, older children should be given enough time to process the new information and to rehearse newly acquired coping skills. It is also important to realize that there may be a *negative* effect of a preparation program on children younger than 3 years of age. This may be a result of their inability to distinguish fantasy from reality.[1] A reality-based preparation program may do little to calm young children and may even exacerbate anxiety or sensitize the young child to the surgery. From age 3 to 6 years, children demonstrate an increasing ability to distinguish fantasy from reality; and by the age of 6 this distinction is usually accomplished.[1] The need to consider the age of the child who will most benefit from such programs thus relates to both the amount of anxiety such exposure might generate and the length of time over which the child can deal with knowing what will happen.

In addition to age and timing, previous experience in a hospital setting also influences the effectiveness of a preparation program. A child who was previously hospitalized is more likely to develop an exaggerated emotional response to a behavioral preoperative preparation program and the perioperative experience.[27,40-42] Information about what will occur as demonstrated by sensory expectation and doll play does *not* provide new information for these children. Furthermore, if the child has had a previous negative medical experience, the routine preparation may increase anxiety by triggering negative memories. In this case, alternative behavioral interventions, such as extensive individualized coping skills training combined with desensitization and actual practice, may be better suited and indicated.[41]

Because increased parental preoperative anxiety has been shown to result in increased preoperative anxiety in their children, preparation programs for surgery should also be directed at parents.[22] Although various interventions are routinely used

Table 3-1. The ADVANCE Preoperative Preparation Program

Anxiety reduction

Distraction on the day of surgery

Video modeling and education before surgery

Adding parents to the child's surgical experience and promoting family-centered care

No excessive reassurance—a suggestion made to parents for communication with children about surgery

Coaching of parents by researchers to help them succeed

Exposure/shaping of the child via induction mask practice (the mask placed over the child's nose and mouth to deliver anesthetic drugs)

Reproduced with permission from Kain ZN, Caldwell-Andrews AA, Mayes LC, et al: Family-centered preparation for surgery improves perioperative outcomes in children: a randomized controlled trial. Anesthesiology 2007; 106:65-74.

to reduce a child's anxiety, there is a paucity of information regarding interventions directed toward reducing parental anxiety.[43] One study demonstrated that parental preoperative anxiety decreased after viewing an educational videotape.[44] In conclusion, most studies to date suggest that preoperative preparation programs for children reduce preoperative anxiety and enhance coping.[34,40,45]

Parents whose child was undergoing immunization who were taught to be active in distracting their child through conversation and reading or in reassuring them through touch and eye contact were able to reduce their child's distress.[46] It may be that similarly effective methods of training and educating parents as to what to expect and how they can be most helpful to their child can be developed for enhancing the value of parental presence during induction of anesthesia. Indeed, this was the case in a randomized controlled trial evaluating a family-centered behavioral preparation program (ADVANCE) (Table 3-1).

Parents and children who received ADVANCE were less anxious before and during induction of anesthesia than parents and children who did not receive this program. In fact, ADVANCE was as successful as midazolam in managing children's compliance with and anxiety at induction of anesthesia (Table 3-2).[47] It is important to note that ADVANCE also decreased the time spent in the postanesthesia care unit and decreased the analgesic requirements during the postoperative period. A major disadvantage of ADVANCE, however, is its high cost and personnel requirements.

Finally, another study examined whether interactive music therapy is an effective intervention for preinduction anxiety in children undergoing outpatient surgery.[48] The investigators found no difference in anxiety during the induction of anesthesia between children in the music therapy group and those in the control group. An analysis controlling for therapist revealed that music therapy may be helpful on separation and entrance to the operating room, depending on the therapist. However, music therapy does not appear to relieve anxiety during the induction of anesthesia.

Parental Presence during Induction of Anesthesia

It is well established that most parents and children prefer to remain together during procedures such as immunization, bone

Table 3-2. Perioperative Outcomes of the ADVANCE Program

	Study Group					
	Control (n = 99)	Parental Presence (n = 94)	ADVANCE (n = 96)	Midazolam (n = 98)	P Value	Effect Size (95% CI)[¶]
Children's anxiety (mYPAS)						
Holding area	36 ± 16	35 ± 16	31 ± 12*	37 ± 17	.001	0.54 (0.78-0.30)
Introduction of mask at induction	52 ± 26	50 ± 26	43 ± 23[†]	40 ± 24	.018	0.33 (0.58-0.08)
Postanesthesia care unit						
Fentanyl consumption (μg/kg)	1.37 ± 2.00	0.81 ± 1.00	0.41 ±1.00[‡]	1.23 ± 2	.016	0.54 (0.75-0.24)
Time until discharge (min)	120 ± 48	122 ± 44	108 ± 46[§]	129 ± 44	.040	0.34 (0.60-0.09)

ADVANCE group anxiety scores:
*Significantly less than those in all other groups, $P < .01$.
[†]Significantly less than those in the control and parental presence groups, $P < .05$.
[‡]Significantly less than those in the control and midazolam groups, $P < .01$.
[§]Significantly less than those in the midazolam group, $P < .01$.
P values for parental presence and control groups = .07.
[¶]Cohen's d effect sizes were calculated for the intervention group vs. other groups combined.
CI, confidence interval; mYPAS, modified Yale Preoperative Anxiety Scale.
Reproduced with permission from Kain ZN, Caldwell-Andrews AA, Mayes LC, et al: Family-centered preparation for surgery improves perioperative outcomes in children: a randomized controlled trial. Anesthesiology 2007; 106:65-74.

marrow aspiration, and dental treatment.[49,50] Several survey studies have also indicated that most parents prefer to be present during induction of anesthesia regardless of the child's age or previous surgical experience.[51,52] This is even the case for those parents who have had previous experience with pharmacologic interventions. Indeed, one study reported that parents of children undergoing repeated surgery were likely to request parental presence regardless of their experience with prior parental presence or premedication of their child with midazolam.[53] That is, even if children were calm after midazolam during their first surgery, parents still preferred to be present during induction of anesthesia during the second surgery.

It is important to note, however, that parental presence during induction of anesthesia (PPIA) does not necessarily equate with appropriate choice of interventions. One study found that mothers who were most highly motivated to be present at induction of anesthesia also reported high levels of anxiety and their children were more distressed at induction.[54] That is, mothers who most want to be present during induction of anesthesia are the most anxious during induction and thus the anesthesiologist should consider carefully the option of permitting the very anxious mother to accompany her child to the operating room. Indeed, more than 90% of parents report some degree of anxiety during the anesthesia induction process.[55] The most upsetting factors are seeing the child go limp during induction and then having to leave their child.[55] This observation was confirmed by a study that examined heart rate, blood pressure, and skin conductance levels in mothers as they observed their child's induction of anesthesia.[56] The study found a moderate increase in heart rate and blood pressure among the mothers who were present during induction of anesthesia (Fig. 3-2). However, no cardiac arrhythmias or ischemic episodes were noted. Another study examined whether parental auricular acupuncture would reduce parental preoperative anxiety and thus allow children to benefit from parental presence during induction of anesthesia (Fig. 3-3).[57] A multivariate model also dem-

onstrated that children whose mothers had received the acupuncture intervention were significantly less anxious on entrance to the operating room and during placement of the anesthesia mask on their child's face. These investigators suggested that children of mothers who underwent acupuncture intervention benefitted from the reduction of maternal anxiety during the induction of anesthesia.[57]

There is also significant variability in the practice and attitudes about parental presence between anesthesiologists and surgeons from different parts of the world.[58-61] Survey studies reported that anesthesiologists from Great Britain support and allow parental presence during induction of anesthesia significantly more often than anesthesiologists from the United States. Although most Great Britain respondents (84%) allow parental presence in more than 75% of their cases, the majority of anesthesiologists in the United States (59%) *never* have parents present during induction. Twenty-three percent of United States anesthesiologists allow parents to be present during induction in less than 25% of routine cases, and only 10% of United States anesthesiologists have parents present during induction in more than 75% of cases. The reasons for these differences in practice between anesthesiologists from the United States and those from Great Britain may include the use of different induction techniques (mask induction in the United States versus intravenous induction in Great Britain), less concern about legal ramifications in Great Britain, and a stronger demand for parental presence in Great Britain. Within the United States, the prevalence of PPIA is becoming more common. One study comparing PPIA practices between 1995 and 2002 found that the overall prevalence of PPIA had increased, and geographic differences in PPIA use had decreased during the 7-year period (Fig. 3-4).[59,62]

Potential benefits from PPIA include minimizing the need for premedication and avoiding the screaming and struggling of the child that may result on separation from the parents. Other benefits, such as decreasing the child's anxiety during induction

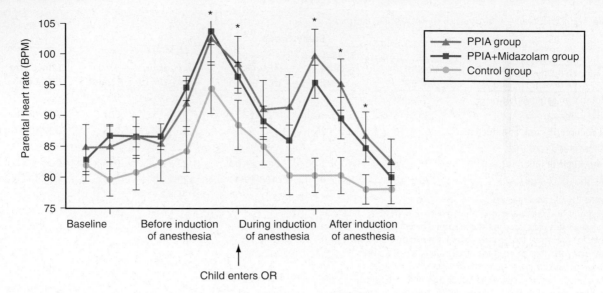

Figure 3-2. Changes in parental heart rate from baseline measurement until after induction of anesthesia. Data are reported as mean ± SE. *Asterisks* indicate time points at which differences between groups are statistically significant (*P* < .05). BPM, beats per minute; OR, operating room; PPIA, parental presence during induction of anesthesia. (From Kain ZN, Caldwell-Andrews AA, Mayes LC, et al: Parental presence during induction of anesthesia: physiological effects on parents. Anesthesiology 2003; 98:58-64.)

and potentially decreasing the long-term behavioral effects of surgery and anesthesia, remain controversial. Common objections to PPIA include concern about disruption of the operating room routine, compromising operative sterility, crowded operating rooms, and a possible adverse reaction of the parent. In

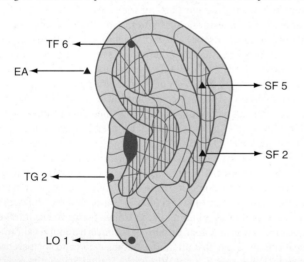

Figure 3-3. Location of acupuncture press needles in the ear for both the intervention and sham control groups. *Solid circles:* Intervention group (L01, lobe zone 1, master cerebral point; TF 6, triangular fossa zone 6, hypertension; TG 2, tragus zone 2 [tranquilizer point]). *Triangles:* Control group (EA, extraneous point; SF 2, scaphoid fossa zone 2, wrist; SF 5, scaphoid fossa zone 5, shoulder). (From Wang SM, Maranets I, Weinberg ME, et al: Parental auricular acupuncture as an adjunct for parental presence during induction of anesthesia. Anesthesiology 2004; 100:1399-1404.)

addition to its impacts on parents themselves, parental anxiety in the operating suite can result in increased child anxiety, prolonged induction, and additional stress on the anesthesiologist, especially if an anesthetic complication develops. For some children, their behavioral response to stress may be more negative when a parent is present than when the parent is absent.[63] In several reports PPIA resulted in disruptive behavior, parents failing to leave the room when requested, and even removal of a child from the operating room by a grandmother during the second stage of anesthesia.[64,65] However, one report has described a 4-year experience with 3086 children in a free-standing ambulatory surgery center in which no parent needed to be escorted from the operating room because of undue anxiety and only two parents developed syncope, with prompt recovery.[66]

The experimental evidence to date does not clearly support the routine use of PPIA.[58,67,68] Although early studies suggested reduced anxiety and increased cooperation if parents were present during induction,[69,70] later investigations indicate that routine PPIA may *not* always be beneficial.[58,67,68] One study demonstrated that only children who are older than 4 years of age, who also have a "calm" baseline personality or have a parent with a "calm" baseline personality, have been found to benefit from parental presence during induction of anesthesia.[58] When interpreting the results of these studies, however, several factors should be considered. First, the design of a randomized controlled study, while considered a gold standard in research, may *not* reflect the practice of *all* anesthesiologists. That is, although a randomized controlled study is applicable to centers that offer PPIA for *all* parents, it may not be applicable to centers in which each request for PPIA is considered individually based on personality characteristics of each child and parent. Such centers may have different results with PPIA than were demonstrated

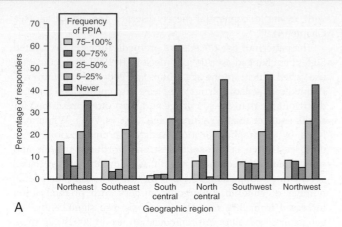

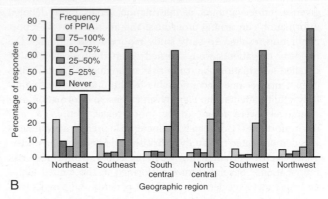

Figure 3-4. A, Frequency of parental presence during induction of anesthesia (PPIA) practice in the United States as of 2002. **B,** Frequency of PPIA practice in the United States as of 1995/1996. Data reported are medians (range, 0%-100%). (From Kain ZN, Caldwell-Andrews AA, Krivutza DM, et al: Trends in the practice of parental presence during induction of anesthesia and the use of preoperative sedative premedication in the United States, 1995-2002: Results of a follow-up national survey. Anesth Analg 2004; 98:1252-1259.)

in experimental studies. Second, allowing PPIA without adequate preparation of the parent may be counterproductive. Some parent behaviors, such as criticism, excessive reassurance, and commands, are associated with greater distress.[71]

Given the drawbacks just discussed, interests in this area have begun to shift toward an emphasis on individual factors in PPIA research. For example, several studies have evaluated child and parent predictors of benefit from PPIA. Older children, children with lower temperamental activity levels, parents with less state anxiety, and parents with lower external locus of control benefit most from PPIA.[29] The match between parent and child anxiety level also appears to be important. Calm children with anxious parents do more poorly during induction when compared with calm children with calm parents or anxious children with either calm or anxious parents.[29] Taking individual factors one step further, studies have begun to examine what parents actually do during induction of anesthesia, rather than simply comparing parental presence to absence. The development of a new tool for assessing child and adult behavior in the perioperative setting (The Perioperative Child-Adult Medical Procedure Interaction Scale [P-CAMPIS]) has been developed to facilitate such research (Fig. 3-5).[72] Preliminary validation of this measure indicates that parental behavior affects the child's anxiety during induction in a similar manner as it impacts a child's distress during immunizations.

At this point it is important to note the potential legal implications of parental presence during induction. One lawsuit has occurred in which a mother was invited by a nurse to accompany her son into an emergency treatment room.[73] According to the court, the mother fainted in the treatment room and suffered an injury to the head as a result of the fall. In its verdict, the Illinois Supreme Court stated that a hospital that *allows* a "non-patient" to accompany a patient during treatment does not have a duty to protect the non-patient from fainting. However, if the health care personnel *invite* the non-patient to participate in the treatment, then the hospital has a legal responsibility toward the non-patient. Because this is a unique individual state ruling, this concern may not apply in all situations or in all states. Each child must be considered individually regarding the

question of PPIA, and in certain states it may be important to document in the medical record that the parent requested that he or she be allowed to be present during anesthetic induction.

The Preoperative Interview

Although most anesthesiologists may not realize it, the preoperative interview is a behavioral intervention that is routinely administered to *all* patients undergoing anesthesia and surgery.[74] It is clear that anesthesiologists have an ethical and legal responsibility to disclose to children/parents detailed anesthetic risk information when obtaining informed consent, but how far this disclosure must extend remains controversial. A common reason given for not providing detailed anesthetic risk information is that it may increase the child's/parents' anxiety. Com-

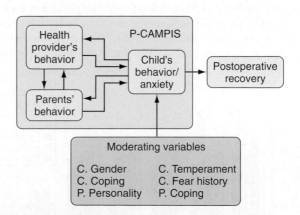

Figure 3-5. The conceptual framework that underlies the relation between a child's preoperative anxiety, parental behaviors, health care provider's behaviors, moderating variables, and postoperative recovery. C, child; P, parent; P-CAMPIS, Perioperative Child-Adult Medical Procedure Interaction Scale. (From Caldwell-Andrews AA, Blount RL, Mayes LC, Kain ZN: Behavioral interactions in the perioperative environment: a new conceptual framework and the development of the perioperative child-adult medical procedure interaction scale. Anesthesiology 2005; 103:1130-1135.)

parative studies investigating anxiety levels in adult patients given a limited amount of information versus more detailed information concerning procedural and anesthetic risks report conflicting results. An early study reported that although the majority of patients were satisfied when they received more detailed information about the risks of angiography, up to 35% of patients became uncomfortable by the information.[75] Similarly, adult patients who were given extensive information preoperatively were found to be more tense, depressed, and uncomfortable.[76] Conversely, no increase in preoperative anxiety was demonstrated in a study of British and Scottish men undergoing elective herniorrhaphy when presented with detailed risk information.[77] Several studies performed in the United States and Australia have demonstrated that patients and parents who received detailed information, including numerical estimates of anesthesia-related complications, were no more anxious than those given minimal information regarding risks.[78-80] Furthermore, parents have expressed their desire to have as much perioperative information about their child's surgery as possible.[79] Thus, the presentation of very detailed anesthetic information of what might go wrong should not increase parental or patient anxiety and has the advantage of allowing for fully informed choices. It should be emphasized, however, that anesthesiologists should note the particular coping style of the parent. Parents use different strategies to cope with or handle difficult, unclear, or unpleasant life experiences, such as a child undergoing surgery. Whereas some parents try to avoid information about unpleasant or unclear situations ("avoidance behavior"), others may seek any available information ("monitoring behavior").[81] While a "monitoring" parent will benefit from a large amount of perioperative information, an "avoiding" parent may react to the information with increased anxiety and distress. Thus, the amount of information provided should be tailored to the needs of the individual parent.

Pharmacologic Interventions

The primary goals of administering a premedication to children are to facilitate an anxiety-free separation from their parents and to facilitate a smooth, stress-free induction of anesthesia. Other effects that may be achieved by pharmacologic preparation of the child include amnesia, anxiolysis, prevention of physiologic stress, such as avoiding tachycardia in patients with cyanotic congenital heart disease, and analgesia (see Chapter 4).

The pattern of use of sedative premedications in the United States has changed over the past decade. In 1997, premedication use varied widely among age groups and geographic locations.[59] Premedicant sedative drugs were least often prescribed for children younger than 3 years of age and most often prescribed for adults younger than 65 years of age (25% vs. 75%). When analyzed by geographic location, sedative premedications were used least often in the southwest and northeast regions and most often in the southeast region. A follow-up study revealed several interesting changes (Fig. 3-6).[62] Most notably, the overall number of children undergoing surgery with premedication increased from 30% to 50%. There was also significantly less geographic variability in premedication use in 2002 than there was in 1997. In both years, the most commonly used sedative premedicant in the preoperative holding area was midazolam, followed by ketamine, transmucosal fentanyl, and meperidine. When data from several survey studies were reviewed, it was noted that anesthesiologists from the United States who allowed PPIA *least* frequently used sedative premedication *most frequently*, and vice versa.[59-61] Thus, most anesthesiologists in the United States use either parental presence or sedative premedication to treat preoperative anxiety in children.

Pharmacologic Interventions versus Behavioral Interventions

When pharmacologic interventions are directly compared with behavioral interventions, children receiving a sedative are less anxious and more compliant than those who are accompanied to the operating room by a parent.[68] Interestingly, parental anxiety is also less when the child receives a premedication. One study examined whether a combination of parental presence and sedative premedication is more effective than sedative premedication alone for reducing the anxiety of children and their parents and for improving parental satisfaction.[82] The investigators found that PPIA offers no additional anxiolysis for children who receive a sedative preoperatively. However, parents who accompany their sedated children into the operating rooms are themselves significantly less anxious and more satisfied both with the separation process and with the overall anesthetic, nursing, and surgical care provided. It is important to note that

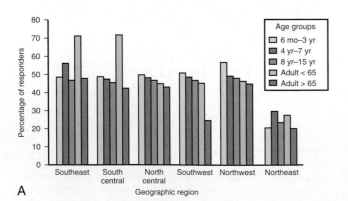
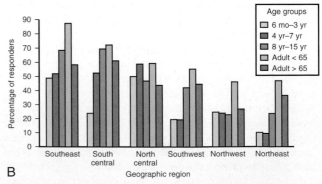

Figure 3-6. A, Frequency of sedative premedication practice in the United States as of 2002. **B,** Frequency of sedative premedication practice in the United States as of 1996. Data reported are medians (range, 0%-100%). (From Kain ZN, Caldwell-Andrews AA, Krivutza DM, et al: Trends in the practice of parental presence during induction of anesthesia and the use of preoperative sedative premedication in the United States, 1995-2002: Results of a follow-up national survey. Anesth Analg 2004; 98:1252-1259.)

these studies were conducted with parents who had no preparation for their presence at anesthesia induction. In a randomized controlled trial highlighted earlier,[47] premedication and an advanced behavioral preparation resulted in similar outcomes on child and parent anxiety at induction and child compliance with induction. Furthermore, children who received behavioral preparation evidenced significantly less emergence delirium and required less analgesia in the recovery room than children who received premedication.

In conclusion, although sedative premedications are effective for treatment of preoperative anxiety, they should *not* be used routinely in all children undergoing surgery. Their use should be directed to children who are at a significant risk for the development of preoperative anxiety. Variables such as age, duration of surgery, and potential recovery delays should also be considered. However, it is important to not withhold premedication if that premedication would likely be of benefit to a selected child. Even if the scheduled procedure is brief, if a particular child is very anxious, then that child will likely benefit from a premedication regardless of the negative effects on recovery and discharge.

Postoperative Outcomes

Four decades ago, it was proposed that moderate levels of preoperative anxiety in adult patients were associated with good postoperative behavioral recovery, whereas low and high levels of preoperative anxiety were associated with poor behavioral recovery.[83] Although this theory is intriguing, these studies were based on descriptive data from nonrandom, limited samples and retrospective reports of questionable validity. Subsequent studies have reported a linear rather than a curvilinear relationship between anxiety level and postoperative behavioral recovery.[84-87] In addition, increased preoperative anxiety in adult patients correlates with increased postoperative pain, increased postoperative analgesic requirements, prolonged recovery and hospital stay and behavioral changes after surgery.[22,88-91] A large-scale study that aimed to examine the question if preoperative anxiety is associated with adverse postoperative outcomes in children undergoing surgery found that anxious children experienced significantly more pain both during the hospital stay and over the first 3 days at home.[92] During home recovery, anxious children also consumed, on average, significantly more codeine and acetaminophen compared with the children who

were not anxious (Fig. 3-7). Anxious children also had a higher incidence of emergence delirium compared with those who were not anxious (9.7% vs. 1.5%) and had a greater incidence of postoperative anxiety and sleep problems. The investigators concluded that preoperative anxiety in young children undergoing surgery is associated with a more painful postoperative recovery and a greater incidence of sleep and other problems.[92]

The assumption that low preoperative anxiety is predictive of good postoperative outcomes underlies many interventions in which the aim is to reduce preoperative anxiety. To date, preoperative preparation studies in adult patients have used diverse postoperative outcome measures, including intensity of pain, analgesic requirements, postsurgical complications, length of hospital stay, patient satisfaction, blood cortisol levels, changes in blood pressure and heart rate, and behavioral indices of recovery.[86,93-100] Reviews of this research, while critical of the methodology, have concluded that psychologically prepared adult patients may have improved postoperative recovery.[89,93,96,101] In children, as indicated in the section describing preoperative preparation, a recent study reports that children who received the ADVANCE preoperative program experienced a lower incidence of emergence delirium, had a briefer stay in the recovery area, reported less postoperative pain, and required less analgesics as compared with a control group.[47]

Emergence Delirium

The first maladaptive behavioral change in children that may be evident after surgery is emergence delirium. This phenomenon is characterized by nonpurposeful restlessness and agitation, thrashing, crying or moaning, and disorientation. Published studies have reported up to 18% of all children undergoing surgery and anesthesia develop emergence delirium.[102] Factors such as young age, previous surgery, type of procedure, and type of anesthetic all affect the incidence of emergence delirium.[102,103] Preoperative anxiety has also been shown to be related to emergence delirium.[92,103] Furthermore, preoperative anxiety, emergence delirium, and postoperative maladaptive behavior changes have been shown to be closely related phenomena. One study found that the odds of experiencing marked symptoms of emergence delirium increased with increased anxiety scores and that the odds of the onset of new maladaptive behavioral changes also increased with the presence of emer-

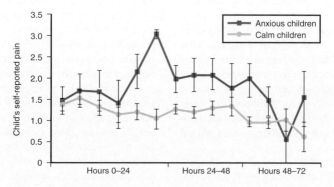

Figure 3-7. Children's self-reported postoperative pain as a function of preoperative anxiety. (From Kain ZN, Mayes LC, Caldwell-Andrews AA, et al: Preoperative anxiety, postoperative pain, and behavioral recovery in young children undergoing surgery. Pediatrics 2006; 118:651-658.)

gence delirium.[92] This finding is highly significant to practicing clinicians, who can now predict the development of adverse postoperative phenomena, such as emergence delirium and postoperative behavioral changes, based on levels of preoperative anxiety.

Sleep Changes

Changes in sleep patterns in the postoperative period have been well documented in adults and children. One study reported that 47% of children experienced sleep disturbances after anesthesia[104] and approximately 14% of children showed significant decreases in percentage of sleep after surgery. The most commonly identified predictor of sleep difficulties after surgery has been postoperative pain,[105] but psychological variables have also been shown to be important. Specifically, parental personality measures of anxiety and child measures of externalizing behavior have both been found to predict sleep efficiency in children after surgery.

Other Behavioral Changes

In addition to sleep, changes in daytime behavior in children after surgery/anesthesia have also been documented. A number of studies have indicated that up to 60% of children undergoing outpatient surgery may develop negative *postoperative* behavioral changes within 2 weeks after surgery.[106-108] These negative postoperative behaviors include sleep and eating disturbances, separation anxiety, apathy, withdrawal, and new-onset enuresis.[22,108] In fact, some children may develop long-lasting psychological effects that could have an impact on their responses to subsequent medical care. Interference with normal development has also been described.[109] A significant number of children demonstrate new negative behaviors postoperatively, such as new onset of general anxiety, night-time crying, enuresis, separation anxiety, temper tantrums, and sleep or eating disturbances. These behaviors may occur in up to 44% of children 2 weeks after surgery; about 20% of these children continue to demonstrate negative behaviors up to 6 months postoperatively.[22] The postoperative negative behavioral changes are likely the result of an interaction between the distress the child experiences during the perioperative period and the individual personality characteristics of the child. Previously, variables such as the age and temperament of the child and the state and trait anxiety of the parent have been identified as predictors for the occurrence of negative postoperative behavioral changes.[22] There is a paucity of data, however, regarding a possible association between the distress the child experiences during induction of anesthesia and the occurrence of these negative postoperative behavioral changes. One investigation concluded that extreme anxiety, such as with a "stormy induction" of anesthesia, was associated with an *increased* incidence of postoperative negative behavioral changes.[110] The investigators recommend that anesthesiologists advise parents of children who are anxious during induction of anesthesia of the increased likelihood that their children will develop postoperative negative behavioral changes, such as nightmares, separation anxiety, and aggression toward authority.[110]

Because the anxiety level of the child and mother in the preoperative holding area predicts the occurrence of negative postoperative behavioral problems,[22] it can be hypothesized that if sedative premedications reduce anxiety of the child and the parents in the preoperative holding area, they may also have an effect on negative postoperative behavioral outcomes.[71] One investigation of premedicated children found a significantly reduced incidence of negative behavioral changes during the first week after surgery.[111] This study suggests that reducing anxiety in the holding area had a beneficial effect on the preoperative behavior of the child as well as in the immediate postoperative period.[111]

Intraoperative Clinical Outcomes

It is commonly believed that increased anxiety before surgery is associated with increased intraoperative anesthetic requirements.[85,112] This belief, however, is based on early studies with questionable scientific validity,[113,114] many of which did not use validated scales to measure anxiety or control for potential confounding variables such as sedative premedication and the surgical procedure.[21] One investigation indicated that high baseline (i.e., trait) anxiety is associated with increased intraoperative anesthetic requirements. The investigators in that study controlled for the surgical procedure, used bispectral electroencephalographic analysis (the bispectral index [BIS]) monitoring to ensure the same anesthetic depth in all patients, and used a total intravenous anesthetic technique to ease the calculation of the anesthetics used.[115] As such, it does seem clear that a high baseline, or trait, anxiety is associated with increased intraoperative anesthetic requirements.

Although several review articles suggest that increased anxiety before surgery and anesthesia is associated with postoperative nausea and vomiting,[116] experimental data suggest that a child's anxiety in the preoperative holding area is not predictive of postoperative nausea and vomiting either in the postanesthesia care unit or at home.[117]

Summary

Approximately 3 million children undergo anesthesia and surgery in the United States every year. It is reported that 40% to 60% of these children develop behavioral stress before their surgery. Multiple interventions have been proposed to treat the preoperative behavioral stress response in children. Currently, however, there is a trend toward a *reduction* in both behavioral and pharmacologic preoperative interventions aimed at children. One possible reason for this trend may be that some physicians believe that reducing parental anxiety during the preoperative period is a surrogate outcome. Rather than evaluating the effects of various preoperative interventions on the transient preoperative behavior, some believe that we should concentrate on research directed at demonstrating that a reduction in preoperative anxiety can dramatically change postoperative outcomes. It is well established that low levels of preoperative anxiety are associated with good postoperative behavioral recovery, whereas moderate and high levels of preoperative anxiety are associated with poor postoperative behavioral recovery. A far more intriguing question is the possible association between preoperative anxiety and postoperative clinical recovery; quality research needs to be developed regarding the relationship between preoperative anxiety and postoperative recovery.

Annotated References

Kain ZN, Caldwell-Andrews AA, Mayes LC. Parental intervention choices for children undergoing repeated surgeries. Anesth Analg 2003; 96:970-5.

Children were assigned to parental presence at induction (PPIA), premedication with midazolam, PPIA + premedication, or no intervention at initial surgery. Children were then followed up at subsequent surgery and parental preference for intervention was assessed. Of parents whose children were assigned to PPIA, 70% would choose PPIA as intervention again. Of those assigned to premedication, only 23% would choose premedication again. Regardless of prior intervention, parents at subsequent surgery favored PPIA. Children's and parents' anxiety also affected parental preference for intervention.

Kain ZN, Caldwell-Andrews AA, Mayes LC, et al: Family-centered preparation for surgery improves perioperative outcomes in children: a randomized controlled trial. Anesthesiology 2007; 106:65-74.

This study evaluated the efficacy of a family-centered behavioral preparation program (ADVANCE) for children undergoing outpatient surgery (n = 408). Children were randomly assigned to no intervention, ADVANCE + PPIA, PPIA without advance, and midazolam premedication. Children in ADVANCE + PPIA displayed significantly less anxiety at induction than no intervention or PPIA alone. Anxiety and compliance in the ADVANCE + PPIA group were comparable to premedication. ADVANCE + PPIA was superior to all other groups on postoperative recovery variables.

Kain ZN, Hofstadter MB, Mayes LC, et al: Midazolam: Effects on amnesia and anxiety in children. Anesthesiology 2000; 93:676-684.

These researchers assessed children's memory at baseline and in four randomly assigned groups (5, 10, and 20 minutes post midazolam administration, and no midazolam [control]) of children (n = 118). Compared with controls, recall memory was impaired for children in the 10- and 20-minute post-midazolam groups. All midazolam groups demonstrated recognition deficits when compared with controls. In terms of perioperative anxiety, significant effects of midazolam were evidenced at approximately 15 minutes.

Kain ZN, Mayes LC, Caldwell-Andrews AA, et al: Preoperative anxiety and postoperative pain and behavioral recovery in young children undergoing surgery. Pediatrics 2006; 118:651-658.

This study assessed preoperative anxiety and postoperative pain and behavioral outcomes after surgery in 241 children. Children who displayed more preoperative anxiety were rated as having higher pain after surgery by their parents. Anxious children also consumed more analgesics at home after surgery and were more likely to experience emergence delirium and postoperative sleep disturbances.

Kain ZN, Mayes LC, Wang SM, et al: Parental presence during induction of anesthesia vs. sedative premedication: which intervention is more effective? Anesthesiology 1998; 89:1147-1156.

Eighty-eight children undergoing outpatient surgery were randomly assigned to parental presence at anesthesia induction, midazolam premedication, or no intervention. Children in the midazolam group exhibited significantly less perioperative anxiety than children in the parental presence or no intervention groups.

References

Please see www.expertconsult.com

Preoperative Evaluation, Premedication, and Induction of Anesthesia

CHAPTER 4

Elizabeth A. Ghazal, Linda J. Mason, and Charles J. Coté

Preparation of Children for Anesthesia

Fasting

Infants and children are fasted before sedation and anesthesia to minimize the risk of pulmonary aspiration of gastric contents. In a fasted child, only the basal secretions of gastric juice should be present in the stomach. In 1948, Digby Leigh recommended a 1-hour preoperative fast after clear fluids. Subsequently, Mendelson reported a number of maternal deaths that were attributed to aspiration at induction of anesthesia.[1] During the intervening 20 years, the fasting interval before elective surgery increased to 8 hours after all solids and liquids. In the late 1980s and early 1990s, an evidence-based approach to the effects of fasting intervals on the gastric fluid pH and volume proclaimed that fasting more than 2 hours after clear fluids neither increased nor decreased the risk of pneumonitis should aspiration occur.[2-10] The risk for pneumonitis had been predicated on two parameters: gastric fluid volume exceeding 0.4 mL/kg and pH less than 2.5 based on data that was never published in peer-reviewed literature.[1,11] In a monkey, 0.4 mL/kg of acid instilled endobronchially resulted in pneumonitis. The equivalent volume for tracheal aspiration that caused aspiration pneumonitis in rats was 0.8 mL/kg.[12] Using these corrected criteria for acute pneumonitis (gastric residual fluid volume 0.8 mL/kg and pH < 2.5), several fasting studies in children demonstrated no additional risk for pneumonitis when children were fasted for only 2 hours after clear fluids.[2-9]

The incidence of pulmonary aspiration in modern routine elective pediatric or adult cases without known risk factors is small.[13-16] Fasting for 3 hours instead of 2 hours after clear liquids in children provides flexibility in the operative schedule. The gastric residual volume half-life for clear liquids is approximately 15 minutes (Fig. 4-1). Clear liquids include water, fruit juices without pulp, carbonated beverages, clear tea, and black coffee. A scheduled operation on a preterm infant or neonate may occasionally be delayed, thus extending the period of fasting to a point that may be potentially dangerous (hypoglycemia or hypovolemia). In this circumstance it is recommended that appropriate fluids be administered via intravenous access before induction of anesthesia. Alternatively, if the period of delay is known, an infant is offered clear fluids until 2 hours before induction. The potential benefits of abbreviating

37

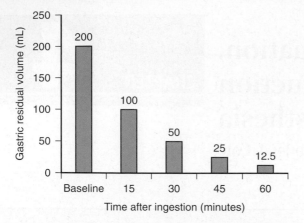

Figure 4-1. Clear liquids are rapidly absorbed from the stomach with a half-life of approximately 15 minutes. In this figure, for example, 200 mL of apple juice would be reduced to 12.5 mL after 60 minutes. (Data abstracted from Hunt JN, MacDonald M: The influence of volume on gastric emptying. J Physiol 1954; 126:459-474.)

the fasting interval to 2 hours includes a reduced risk of hypoglycemia, which is possible in debilitated, poorly nourished children, in children with metabolic dysfunction, and in (former) pre-term infants.[17-20] Additional benefits include decreased thirst, decreased hunger (and thus reduced risk the fasting child will "steal" another child's food), decreased risk for hypotension during induction, and improved child cooperation.[2,11,21]

Breast milk, which can cause significant pulmonary injury if aspirated,[22] has a very high and variable fat content (determined by maternal diet), which will delay gastric emptying.[21] *Breast milk should not be considered a clear liquid.*[23] Two studies estimated the gastric emptying times after clear fluids, breast milk, or formula in full-term and preterm neonates.[24,25] The results of these studies determined that the emptying times for breast milk in both age groups were substantively greater than after clear fluids. Moreover, the gastric emptying times for formula were substantively greater than those for breast milk. With half-life emptying times for breast milk of 50 minutes and for formula of 75 minutes, fasting intervals of 3.3 hours for breast milk and 5 hours for formula are required. More importantly perhaps was the large (15%) variability in gastric emptying times for breast milk and formula in full-term infants (Fig. 4-2, see website). Based in part on these data, the American Society of Anesthesiologists' Task Force on Fasting recommended the following guidelines: clear fluids, 2 hours; breast milk, 4 hours; formula, 6 hours; and solids, 8 hours (Table 4-1).[10]

Table 4-1. Preoperative Fasting Recommendations in Infants and Children

Clear liquids	2 hours
Breast milk	4 hours
Infant formula	6 hours*
Solids (fatty or fried foods)	8 hours

*Some centers now allow plain toast (no dairy products) up to 6 hours.[10]

Children who have been chewing gum must dispose of the gum by throwing it out, not swallowing it. Recent evidence suggests that chewing gum increases the gastric fluid volume but tends to increase fluid pH in children, leaving no clear evidence for an increased risk of regurgitation.[26] Consequently, we recommend that if the gum is discarded, then elective anesthesia can proceed without additional delay. If, however, the child swallows the gum, then surgery is cancelled because aspirated gum may be nearly impossible to extract from a bronchus or trachea.

Children can never be trusted to fast. Therefore, anesthesiologists must always be suspicious and question children just before induction if they have eaten or drunk anything (although the veracity of the answer is questionable). It is not unusual to find bubble gum, candy, or other food in a child's mouth. When the anesthesiologist suspects a full stomach, induction of anesthesia must be managed appropriately. The incidence of pulmonary aspiration of gastric contents during elective surgery in children ranges from 1 to 8.6 in 10,000, depending on the study.[13-15,27] In contrast, the frequency of pulmonary aspiration in children undergoing emergency procedures was more than 10-fold greater (1:373 or 1:4,544).[27] In both studies, serious respiratory morbidity and death did not occur. Risk factors for perianesthetic aspiration included neurologic or esophagogastric abnormality, emergency surgery (especially at night), American Society of Anesthesiologists' (ASA) physical status 3 to 5, intestinal obstruction, increased intracranial pressure, increased abdominal pressure, obesity, and the skill and experience of the anesthesiologist.[14]

The majority of aspirations in children occurred during induction of anesthesia, with only 13% occurring during emergence and extubation. In contrast, 30% of the aspirations in adults occur during emergence. In one study, bowel obstruction or ileus was present in the majority of infants and children who aspirated during the perioperative period.[27] The risk of aspiration was greater in children younger than 3 years of age.[27] A combination of factors may predispose the infant and young child to regurgitation and aspiration, including decreased competence of the lower esophageal sphincter, excessive air swallowing while crying during the preinduction period, strenuous diaphragmatic breathing, a shorter esophagus, and a smaller hydrostatic pressure gradient between the stomach and the larynx. In one study in children, nearly all cases of pulmonary aspiration occurred when they gagged or coughed during airway manipulation or during induction of anesthesia in which paralysis with muscle relaxants was not provided or given in insufficient doses so as to prevent a gag or cough.[27]

When aspiration does occur, morbidity and mortality are rare for elective surgical procedures and generally reflect their ASA physical status. The mortality rate reported was between 0.2:10,000 and zero.[13,14,27] Most ASA 1 or 2 patients who aspirate clear gastric contents generally have minimal or no sequelae.[13,27] Clinical signs of sequelae from aspiration are usually apparent in children within 2 hours of the regurgitation.[27]

Piercings

Body piercing is common practice in adolescents and young adults who require anesthesia and surgery. Piercings may appear anywhere on the body as a single piercing or be in many areas. To minimize the liability and risk of complications from these metal piercings, the managing principle is to remove them before surgery. Complications that may occur if piercings are left in situ are listed in Table 4-2 (see website).[28-30]

Psychological Preparation of Children for Surgery

The perioperative period is stressful and anxiety provoking for the child and family; many parents express more concern about the risks of anesthesia than those of the surgery. The factors that influence the ability of the child and family to cope with the stress of surgery include family dynamics, the child's developmental and behavioral status and cultural biases, as well as our ability to explain away misperceptions and misinformation. Because of logistics and today's practice constraints, there is limited time to evaluate family dynamics and establish rapport. It is therefore vital for the anesthesiologist to ensure that he or she interacts directly with the child in a manner consistent with the child's level of development. A specific child-oriented approach by the anesthesiologist, surgeon, nurses, and hospital staff is required. Preoperative evaluation is usually simplified once the basic concepts of how to evaluate a child are understood.

Although the preoperative evaluation and preparation of children are similar to those of adults from a physiologic standpoint, the psychologic preparation of infants and children is very different (see Chapter 3). Many hospitals have an open house or a brochure to describe the preoperative programs available to parents before the day of admission.[31] However, leaflets should not replace verbal communication with nursing and medical staff.[32] Anesthesiologists are encouraged to participate in the design of these programs so that they accurately reflect the anesthetic practice of the institution. The preoperative anesthetic experience begins at the time parents are first informed that their child is to have surgery or a procedure that requires general anesthesia. Parental satisfaction correlates with comfort of the environment and establishing trust between the anesthesiologist, the child, and parents.[33] If parental presence during induction is deemed to be in the child's best interest, a parental educational program that describes what the parent can expect to happen if he/she accompanies the child to the operating room can significantly decrease parental anxiety and increase their satisfaction.[34] The greater the understanding and amount of information that the parents have, the less their anxiety will be; this attitude, in turn, will be reflected in the child.[35,36]

Informed consent should include a detailed description of what the family can anticipate and our role to protect the welfare of their child. Before surgery, the anesthetic risks should be discussed in clear terms but in a reassuring manner by describing the measures that will be taken to carefully and closely monitor the safety of their child. Mentioning specific details and the purpose of the various monitoring devices may help diminish the parents' anxiety by demonstrating to them that their child will be anesthetized with the utmost safety and care. A blood pressure cuff will *"check the blood pressure,"* electrocardiographic monitors will *"watch the heartbeat,"* a stethoscope will help us *"to continuously listen to the heart sounds,"* a pulse oximeter will *"measure the oxygen in the bloodstream,"* a carbon dioxide analyzer will *"monitor the breathing,"* an anesthetic agent monitor will *"accurately measure the level of anesthesia,"* and an intravenous catheter will be placed *"to administer fluid and medications as needed."* Children who are capable and their parents should be given ample opportunity to ask questions preoperatively. Finally, they should be assured that our "anes-

thetic prescription" will be designed specifically for their child's needs, taking into account their child's underlying medical conditions and the needs of surgery to ensure optimal conditions for surgery, the safety of their child, and analgesia.

It has been shown that parents desire comprehensive perioperative information and that discussion of highly detailed anesthetic risk information does not increase parental anxiety level.[37] Inadequate preparation of children and their families may lead to a traumatic anesthetic induction and difficulty for both the child and the anesthesiologist, with the possibility of postoperative psychological disturbances.[38] Numerous preoperative educational programs for children and adults have evolved to alleviate some of these fears and anxiety. They include preoperative tours of the operating rooms, educational videos, play therapy, magical distractions, puppet shows, anesthesia consultations, and child life preparation.[39] The timing of the preoperative preparation is an important determinant of whether the intervention was effective. For example, children older than 6 years of age who participated in a preparation program more than 5 to 7 days before surgery are least anxious during separation from their parents, those who participated in no preoperative preparation were moderately anxious, and if they received the information 1 day before surgery they were the most anxious. The predictors of anxiety correlated also with the child's baseline temperament and history of previous hospitalizations.[40] Children of different ages vary in their response to the anesthetic experience (see Chapter 3).[41] Even more important may be the child's trait anxiety when confronted with a stressful medical procedure.[42]

Child Development and Behavior

Understanding age-appropriate behavior in response to external situations is essential (Table 4-3, see website). Infants younger than 10 months of age tolerate short periods of separation from their parents. Many do not object to an inhalation induction and frequently respond to the smell of the inhalation agents by sucking or licking the mask. These infants usually do not need to receive sedative premedication.

Children between 11 months and 6 years of age frequently cling to their parents. In an unfamiliar environment such as a hospital, preschool children tend to become very anxious, especially if the situation appears threatening. Their anxiety may be exacerbated if they sense that their parents are anxious. Efforts to educate the parents to allay their anxiety can reduce their child's anxiety.[31,43,44] A heightened anxiety response may lead to immediate postoperative maladaptive behavior, such as nightmares, eating disturbances, and new-onset enuresis. Compared with other patients, children 2 to 6 years of age are more likely to exhibit problematic behavior when separated from their parents (see Chapter 3).[41] Children who display one or more of the predictive risk factors would probably benefit from sedative premedication.[45-48] They are generally more content if their parents accompany them during induction of anesthesia or if they are sedated in the presence of their parent's in a nonthreatening environment before entering the operating room (see later).

Children older than age 6 years and those who attend preschool or kindergarten are more willing to accept brief periods of separation from their parents. They tend to be more independent than younger children because of their school experience. They are better able to communicate and have a greater understanding of their environment. Their sense of curiosity and interest in new things and their trust of adults can be used to elicit their cooperation for a mask induction of anesthesia without the need for premedication.

Children ages 4 to 10 years may exhibit psychological factors that are predictive of postoperative behavior (e.g., abnormal sleep patterns, parental anxiety, and aggressive behavior).[49,50] In addition, children who have pain on the day of the operation have behavioral problems that last longer than the duration of pain itself.[51] Therefore, preventing postoperative pain decreases and limits the duration of postoperative behavioral problems.

Special aspects of a child's perception of anesthesia should be anticipated; children often have the same fears as adults but are unable to articulate those fears. The reason and need for a surgical procedure should also be carefully explained to the child.

It is important to reassure children that anesthesia is a type of *deep sleep*, not the same as the usual nightly sleep but rather *a special type during which they will feel no pain from surgery and from which they will very definitely awaken*. Many children fear the possibility that they will wake up in the middle of the anesthetic and during surgery. They should be reassured that they will awaken *only* when the surgery is completed.

The words the anesthesiologist uses to describe to the child what can be anticipated must be carefully chosen, because children think concretely and tend to interpret the facts literally. Examples of this are presented by the following anecdotes:

A 4-year-old child was informed that in the morning she would receive a "shot" that would "put her to sleep." That night, a frantic call was received from the mother, describing a very upset child; the child thought she was going to be "put to sleep" like the veterinarian had permanently "put to sleep" her sick pet.

A 5-year-old child was admitted to the hospital for elective inguinal herniorrhaphy. He received heavy premedication and was sleeping on arrival in the operating room. After discharge, the parents frequently discovered him wandering about the house at night. On questioning, the child stated that he was "protecting" his family. He stated: "I don't want anyone sneaking up on you and operating while you are sleeping."

In the first example, the child's concrete thought processes misunderstood the anesthesiologist's choice of words. The second case represents a problem of communication: the child was never told he would have an operation.

The importance of proper psychological preparation for surgery should not be underestimated. Often, little has been explained to both patient and parents before the day of surgery. Anesthesiologists have a key role in alleviating fear of the unknown if they understand a child's age-related perception of anesthesia and surgery (see Chapter 3). They can convey their understanding by presenting a calm and friendly face (smiling, looking at the child and making eye contact), offering a warm introduction, touching the patient in a reassuring manner (holding a child's or parent's hand), and being completely honest. Children respond positively to an honest description of exactly what they can anticipate. This includes informing them of the slight discomfort of starting an intravenous line or giving an intramuscular premedication, the possible bitter taste of an oral premedication, or a mask induction for anesthesia.

The postoperative process, from the operating room to the recovery room, and the onset of postoperative pain should be described. Encourage the child and family to ask questions.

Strategies to maintain analgesia should be discussed including the use of long-acting local anesthetics; nerve blocks; neuraxial blocks; patient-controlled, nurse-controlled, or parent-controlled analgesia or epidural analgesia; or intermittent narcotics (see Chapters 42, 43, and 44).

As children age, they become more aware of their bodies and may develop a fear of mutilation. Adolescents frequently appear quite independent and self-confident, but, as a group, they have unique problems. In a moment their mood can change from an intelligent, mature adult to a very immature child who needs support and reassurance. Coping with a disability or illness is often very difficult for adolescents. Because they are often comparing their physical appearance with that of their peers, they may become especially anxious when they have a physical problem. In general, they want to know exactly what will transpire during the course of anesthesia. Adolescents are usually cooperative, preferring to be in control and unpremedicated preoperatively. The occasional overly anxious or rambunctious adolescent, however, may benefit from preanesthetic medication.

Monitoring the attitude and behavior of a child is very useful. A child who clings to the parents, avoids eye contact, and will not speak is very anxious. A self-assured, cocky child who "knows it all" may also be apprehensive or frightened. This "know it all" behavior may mask the child's true emotions, and he or she may decompensate just when his or her cooperation is most needed. In some cases, nonpharmacologic supportive measures may be effective. In the extremely anxious child, supportive measures alone may be insufficient to reduce anxiety and premedication is indicated.

Identifying a difficult parent or child preoperatively isn't always easy, especially if the anesthesiologist first meets the child or family just on the day of surgery and has limited time to assess the situation. Occasionally, we receive a warning regarding a difficult parent or child from the surgeon or nursing staff, based on their encounters with the family. With experience, some anesthesiologists will be able to identify difficult parents and children during the short preoperative assessment and make appropriate adjustments to the anesthetic plan.

The "veterans" or "frequent flyers" of anesthesia can also be difficult in the perioperative period. They have played the "anesthesia and surgical game" before and are not interested in participating again, especially if their previous experiences have been negative. These children may benefit the most from a relatively heavy premedication; reviewing previous responses to premedication will aid in the adjustment of the current planned premedication (e.g., adding ketamine and atropine to oral midazolam so as to achieve a greater depth of sedation).

It is important to observe the family dynamics to better understand the child and determine who is in control, the parent or the child. Families many times are in a state of stress, particularly if the child has a chronic illness; these parents are often angry, guilt ridden, or simply exhausted. Ultimately, the manner in which a family copes with an illness will largely determine how a child will cope.[52] The well-organized, open, and communicative family tends to be supportive and resourceful, whereas the disorganized, noncommunicative and dysfunctional family tends to be angry and frustrated. Dealing with a family and child from the latter category may be challenging. There is the occasional parent who is overbearing and demands total control of the situation. It is important to be empathetic and understanding but to set limits and clearly define the parents' role. They must be told that the anesthesiologist determines when the parent must leave the operating room; this is particularly true if an unexpected development occurs during the induction.

Parental Presence During Induction

One controversial area in pediatric anesthesia is parental presence during induction of anesthesia. Some anesthesiologists encourage parents to be present at induction, whereas others are uncomfortable with the process and do not allow parents to be present. Inviting the parent to accompany the child to the operating room has been interpreted by some courts as an implicit contract on the part of the caregiver who invited the parent to participate in the child's care; the institution was found to assume responsibility for a mother who suffered an injury when she fainted.[53] Each child and family must be evaluated individually—what is good for one child and family may not be good for the next (see Chapter 3).[54-57]

Studies have demonstrated that children older than age 4 years benefited from parental presence.[58,59] One study found that oral midazolam was more effective in reducing a child's anxiety than parental presence[60] and that parental presence combined with oral midazolam was no more beneficial in reducing a child's anxiety than oral midazolam alone.[61]

Do all parents who are present at induction of anesthesia of their children benefit? Events that upset them include seeing their child limp or upset during the induction and leaving their child after induction.[62,63] Studies have also shown that when mothers are present at induction of anesthesia their heart rates and skin conductance levels increase, although electrocardiographic abnormalities were not identified.[64] Finally, parents of children who have undergone repeated surgeries prefer to be present during induction of anesthesia.[65]

Over the past several years there have been significant increases in the number of anesthesiologists who use preoperative sedative premedication and/or parental presence for children undergoing surgery.[66] Anesthesiologists who practice in pediatric hospitals, more experienced anesthesiologists, and those who practice pediatric anesthesiology exclusively are more likely to favor parental presence.[67] Others believe they may be distracted or criticized by the parents, that it may impact resident education, or that it may have legal implications.[53,68,69] Each state has different legal implications regarding the health care worker inviting the parent to be present versus the parent requesting to be present.[53] If the practice of having parents present at induction is to work well, then the anesthesiologist must be comfortable with such an arrangement. No parent should ever be forced to be present for the induction of anesthesia, nor should any anesthesiologist be forced into a situation that compromises the quality of care he or she affords a child in need.

Parents must be informed about what to anticipate in terms of the operating room itself (equipment, surgical devices), in terms of what they may observe during induction (eyes rolling back, laryngeal noises, anesthetic monitor alarms, excitation), and when they will be asked to leave. They must also be instructed regarding their ability to assist during the induction process, such as by comforting their child and reassuring him or her to trust the anesthesiologist, distracting the child, and consoling the child. Personnel should be immediately available to escort parents back to the waiting area at the appropriate time. Someone should also be available to care for a parent who

wishes to leave the induction area or who becomes lightheaded or faints. An anesthesiologist's anxiety about parents' presence during induction decreases significantly with experience.[70]

Explaining what parents might see or hear is essential. We generally tell parents the following:

As you see your child fall asleep today there are several things you might observe that you are not used to seeing. First, when anyone falls asleep, the eyes roll up, but since we are sleeping we do not generally see it. You may see your child do that today, and I do not want you to be frightened by that—it is expected and normal. The second thing is that as children go to sleep from the anesthesia medications, the tone of the structures in the neck decreases so that some children will begin to snore or make vibrating noises. Again, I do not want you to be frightened or think that something is wrong. We expect this, and it is normal. The third thing you might see is what we call "excitement." As the brain begins to go to sleep it can actually get excited first. About 30 to 60 seconds after breathing the anesthesia medications, your child might suddenly look around or suddenly move his or her arms and legs. To you it appears that he is awakening from anesthesia or that he or she is upset. In reality, this is a good sign because it indicates to us that your child is falling asleep and that 15 to 30 seconds after that he or she will be completely anesthetized. Also you should know that even though your child appears to be awake to you, in reality he or she will not remember any of that. As soon as your child loses consciousness we will ask you to give your child a kiss and step out of the operating room.

This kind of careful preparation provides to the parents the confidence that the anesthesiologist really knows what he or she is talking about and it avoids frightening the parents. In general, the more information you can provide, the lower are the parental anxiety levels.

Occasionally the best efforts to relieve a child's anxiety by including parental presence and administration of a sedative premedication may not be successful and an anticipated smooth induction may not go as planned. There are three options that may be used depending on the age of the child: (1) re-negotiate, (2) hold the mask farther away from the face, or (3) suggest an intravenous or intramuscular induction, thus giving the child a choice and some control over the situation. Sedation can be considered if it was not already used (either intramuscular, oral, inhalational [nitrous oxide], or by another route). If an intramuscular shot or intravenous induction is proposed, the child will usually choose the mask. If the situation is totally out of control, either elective surgery can be rescheduled or intramuscular ketamine can be used if the parents choose to proceed. These situations are particularly difficult for the parents and the caregivers but must be handled on an individual basis.

History of Present Illness

The medical history of a child obtained during the preanesthetic visit allows the anesthesiologist to determine if the child is optimized for the planned surgery, to anticipate potential problems due to coexisting disease, to determine if appropriate laboratory or other tests are available or needed, to select optimal premedication, to formulate the appropriate anesthetic plan including perioperative monitoring, and to anticipate postoperative concerns including pain management and postoperative ventilatory needs. The history of the present illness is described to the physicians by the parents and verified by the referring or consultant surgeon's notes. If the child is old enough, it is helpful to obtain the child's input. The history should focus on the following aspects:

- A review of all organ systems (Table 4-4) with special emphasis on the organ system involved in the surgery
- Medications (over-the-counter and prescribed) related to and taken before the present illness, including herbals and vitamins
- Previous surgical and hospital experiences, including those related to the current problem
- The time of the last oral intake, time of last urination (wet diaper), or time of vomiting and diarrhea. It is essential to recognize that decreased gastrointestinal motility often occurs with an illness or injury.

In the case of a neonate, problems that may have been present during gestation and birth may still be relevant in the neonatal period and beyond (Table 4-5, see website). The maternal medical and pharmacologic history (therapeutic, drug abuse) may also provide valuable data for the management of a neonate requiring surgery.

Past/Other Medical History

The past medical history should include a history of all past medical illnesses with a review of organ systems, previous hospitalizations (medical or surgical), childhood syndromes with associated anomalies, medication list, herbal remedies, and any allergies, especially to antibiotics and latex. Whether the child was full-term or preterm at birth and, if preterm, any associated problems should be discerned, including admission to a neonatal intensive care unit (NICU), duration of tracheal intubation,

apnea/bradycardia history (including oxygen treatment and home apnea monitor and intraventricular hemorrhage), and congenital defects.

Examination of previous surgical and anesthetic records greatly assists in planning the anesthetic. Particular attention should be paid to any difficulties encountered with airway management, venous access, or emergence. The response to or need for premedication and the route of administration utilized should be noted.

Herbal Remedies

Increasing numbers of children who present for surgery have been ingesting herbal medicine products. During the preoperative interview, anesthesiologists should include specific inquiries regarding the use of these medications because of their potential adverse effects and drug interactions. Hospital surveys suggest that the use of herbal remedies ranges from 17% to 32%[71-73] of presurgical patients and 70% of these patients did not inform their anesthesiologist of such use.

A recent study from Hong Kong queried patients undergoing major elective surgery about their regular use of prepacked over-the-counter traditional Chinese herbal medicines (TCHMs) and TCHMs prescribed by a traditional Chinese medicine practitioner.[74] There was a high rate of recent TCHM (80% over-the-counter and 8% by prescription) use in this population. The TCHM-by-prescription users had a higher incidence of experiencing an adverse perioperative "event." In particular, this group

Table 4-4. Review of Systems: Anesthetic Implications

System	Questions to Ask	Possible Anesthetic Implications
Respiratory	Cough, asthma, recent cold	Irritable airway, bronchospasm, medication history, atelectasis, infiltrate
	Croup	Subglottic narrowing
	Apnea/bradycardia	Postoperative apnea/bradycardia
Cardiovascular	Murmur	Septal defect, avoid air bubbles in intravenous line
	Cyanosis	Right-to-left shunt
	History of squatting	Tetralogy of Fallot
	Hypertension	Coarctation, renal disease
	Rheumatic fever	Valvular heart disease
	Exercise intolerance	Congestive heart failure, cyanosis
Neurologic	Seizures	Medications, metabolic derangement
	Head trauma	Intracranial hypertension
	Swallowing incoordination	Aspiration, esophageal reflux, hiatus hernia
	Neuromuscular disease	Neuromuscular relaxant drug sensitivity, malignant hyperpyrexia
Gastrointestinal/hepatic	Vomiting, diarrhea	Electrolyte imbalance, dehydration, full stomach
	Malabsorption	Anemia
	Black stools	Anemia, hypovolemia
	Reflux	Possible need for full-stomach precautions
	Jaundice	Drug metabolism/hypoglycemia
Genitourinary	Frequency	Urinary tract infection, diabetes, hypercalcemia
	Time of last urination	State of hydration
	Frequent urinary tract infections	Evaluate renal function
Endocrine/metabolic	Abnormal development	Endocrinopathy, hypothyroid, diabetes
	Hypoglycemia, steroid therapy	Hypoglycemia, adrenal insufficiency
Hematologic	Anemia	Need for transfusion
	Bruising, excess bleeding	Coagulopathy, thrombocytopenia, thrombocytopathy
	Sickle cell disease	Hydration, possible exchange transfusion
Allergies	Medications	Possible drug interaction
Dental	Loose, carious teeth	Aspiration of loose teeth, subacute bacterial endocarditis prophylaxis

was twice as likely to have hypokalemia or impaired hemostasis (prolonged international normalized prothrombin ratio [INR] and activated partial thromboplastin time [aPTT]) than nonusers. However, there was no significant difference in the risk of perioperative events between self-prescribed TCHM users and nonusers. It is interesting to note that there is a difference between Western and oriental herbs. Western herbs are usually ingested as a single substance, whereas TCHMs consist of multiple herbs that are combined for their effects.[75]

The most commonly used herbal medications reported are garlic, ginseng, ginkgo biloba, St. John's wort, and echinacea.[76] The "g" herbals (together with feverfew [*Tanacetum parthenium*]) all increase the risk of bleeding. Although the dose of the active ingredient in each preparation may vary, the dose taken by the child may also vary and our ability to detect a change in platelet function and other subtle coagulation disturbances may be difficult. St. John's wort is the herb that most commonly interacts with anesthetic and other medications, usually via a change in drug metabolism. Evidence indicates that St. John's wort is a potent inducer of cytochrome P-450 enzymes and/or P-glycoprotein. A potentially fatal interaction between cyclosporine and St. John's wort has been well documented.[77-80] Heart, renal, or liver transplant recipients who were stabilized on a dose of cyclosporine showed decreased plasma levels and, in some cases, acute rejection episodes after taking St. John's wort. Herbal medicines are associated with cardiovascular instability, coagulation disturbances, prolongation of anesthesia, and immunosuppression.[81] A summary of the most commonly used herbal remedies and their potential perioperative complications is shown in Table 4-6 (see website).

To avoid potential perioperative complications, the ASA has encouraged the discontinuation of all herbal medicines 2 weeks before surgery,[82] although this recommendation is not evidence based. Indeed, some herbs such as valerian, used as a treatment of insomnia (*Valeriana officinalis*), should NOT be discontinued abruptly but tapered; otherwise they may result in a paradoxical and severe reaction.[83] Each herb should be carefully evaluated by using standard resource texts and a decision made regarding the timing of or need for discontinuation determined on a case-by-case basis.[84]

Anesthesia and Vaccination

Children may present for either emergency or elective surgery after having been recently immunized. The anesthesiologist and surgeon must then consider (1) if the immunomodulatory effects of anesthesia and surgery might affect the efficacy and safety of the vaccine and (2) if the inflammatory responses to the vaccine will alter the postoperative course.

How soon after a vaccine can children be anesthetized? A recent international survey[85] revealed that only about one third of responding anesthetists had the benefit of a hospital policy, ranging from a formal decision to delay surgery to an independent choice by the anesthesiologist. Sixty percent of respondents would anesthetize a child for elective surgery within 1 week of receiving a live attenuated vaccine (oral polio or measles, mumps, and rubella [MMR] vaccines), whereas 40% would not. The survey also revealed that 28% of anesthesiologists would delay immunization from 2 to 30 days after surgery.

A scientific review of the literature associating anesthesia and vaccination in children resulted in recommendations for immunizations in children.[86] The review demonstrated a brief and reversible influence on lymphoproliferative responses that generally returned to preoperative values within 2 days. Vaccine-driven adverse events (fever, pain, irritability) might occur but should not be confused with postoperative complications. Adverse events to inactivated vaccines such as diphtheria-tetanus-pertussis (DPT) become apparent from 2 days and to live attenuated vaccines such as MMR from 7 to 21 days after immunization.[86] Therefore, appropriate delays for the type of vaccine between immunization and anesthesia are recommended to avoid misinterpretation of vaccine-associated adverse events as postoperative complications. Because children remain at risk of contracting vaccine-preventable diseases, the minimum delay seems prudent, especially in the first year of life. Likewise, it seems reasonable to delay vaccination *after* surgery until the child is fully recovered. Other immunocompromised patients, such as human immunodeficiency virus (HIV)-positive children, cancer patients, or transplant recipients, have distinct underlying immune impairments, and the influence of anesthesia on vaccine responses has not been comprehensively investigated.

Family History

It is important to inquire about a family history, particularly focusing on a number of conditions, including malignant hyperthermia, prolonged paralysis associated with anesthesia (pseudocholinesterase deficiency), muscular dystrophy, sickle cell disease, bleeding (and bruising) tendencies, and drug addiction (drug withdrawal, HIV carrier).

Laboratory Data

The laboratory data obtained preoperatively in children should be appropriate to the history, illness, and surgical procedure. Routine hemoglobin testing or urinalysis is not indicated for most elective procedures in children; the value of these tests is questionable when the surgical procedure will not involve clinically significant blood loss.[87] There are insufficient data in the literature to make strict hemoglobin testing recommendations in healthy children. Most children's hospitals obtain a preoperative hemoglobin only for those who will undergo procedures with the potential for blood loss, those with specific risk factors for a hemoglobinopathy, former preterm infants, and those younger than 6 months of age. Coagulation studies (platelet count, INR, and partial thromboplastin time) may be indicated if major reconstructive surgery is contemplated, especially if warranted by the medical history, and in some centers before tonsillectomy. In addition, collection of a preoperative type-and-screen or type-and-crossmatch is indicated in preparation for potential blood transfusions depending on the nature of the planned surgery and the anticipated blood loss.

In general, routine chest radiography is not necessary; studies have confirmed that routine chest radiographs are not cost-effective in children.[88,89] The oxygen saturation of children who are breathing room air is very helpful. Baseline saturation of 95% or less suggests clinically important pulmonary or cardiac compromise and warrants further investigation.

Special laboratory tests, such as electrolyte and blood glucose determinations, renal function tests, blood gas analysis, blood concentrations of seizure medication and digoxin, electrocardiography, echocardiography, liver function tests, computed tomography, magnetic resonance imaging (MRI), or pulmonary function tests, should be performed when appropriate.

Pregnancy Testing

Pregnancy rates among teenagers in the United States are declining,[90] yet a small percentage of adolescent females may present for elective surgery with an unsuspected pregnancy. In 2003 the birth rate in girls aged 15 to 19 years was 41.6 births per 1,000 and for girls aged 10 to 14 years it was 0.6 per 1,000. However, routine preoperative pregnancy testing in adolescent females may present some ethical and legal dilemmas, including social and confidentiality concerns. This places the anesthesiologist in a predicament deciding whether to perform routine preoperative pregnancy screening.[90] Each hospital should adopt a policy regarding pregnancy testing to provide a consistent and comprehensive policy for all females who have reached menarche.

A survey of members of the Society for Pediatric Anesthesia practicing in North America revealed that pregnancy testing was routinely required by approximately 45% of the respondents regardless of the practice setting (teaching vs. non-teaching facilities).[87] A retrospective study reviewed the results of a 2-year study of mandatory pregnancy testing in 412 adolescent surgical patients[91]; the overall incidence of positive tests was 1.2%. Five of 207 patients aged 15 years and older tested positive, for an incidence of 2.4% in that group. Interestingly, none of the 205 patients younger than the age of 15 years had a positive pregnancy test.

The most recent ASA Task Force on Preanesthesia Evaluation[92] recognizes that a history and physical examination may not adequately identify early pregnancy and issued the following statement: *"The literature is insufficient to inform patients or physicians on whether anesthesia causes harmful effects on early pregnancy. Pregnancy testing may be offered to female patients of childbearing age and for whom the result would alter the patient's management."*[93] Because of exposure of the fetus to potential teratogens and radiation, and rodent evidence for anesthetic agent-associated apoptosis in the rapidly developing fetal brain, elective surgery with general anesthesia is not advised during early pregnancy. Therefore, if the situation is unclear and when indicated by medical history, it is best to perform a preoperative pregnancy test; and if the surgery is required, then a regional anesthetic is preferred.

Premedication and Induction Principles

General Principles

The major objectives of preanesthetic medication are to (1) allay anxiety, (2) block autonomic (vagal) reflexes, (3) reduce airway secretions, (4) produce amnesia, (5) provide prophylaxis against pulmonary aspiration of gastric contents, (6) facilitate the induction of anesthesia, and (7) if necessary, provide analgesia. Premedication may also decrease the stress response to anesthesia and prevent cardiac arrhythmias.[94] The goal of premedication for each child must be individualized. Light sedation, even though it may not eliminate anxiety, may adequately calm a child so that the induction of anesthesia will be smooth and a pleasant experience. In contrast, heavy sedation may be needed for the very anxious child.

Factors to consider when selecting a drug or a combination of drugs for premedication include the child's age, ideal body weight, drug history, and allergic status; underlying medical or surgical conditions and how they might affect the response to premedication or how the premedication might alter anesthetic induction; parent and child expectations; and the child's emotional maturity, personality, anxiety level, cooperation, and physiologic and psychological status. The anesthesiologist should also consider the proposed surgical procedure and the attitudes and wishes of the child and the parents.

The route of administration of premedicant drugs can be very important. Although a drug may be more effective and have a more reliable onset when given intravenously or intramuscularly, most pediatric anesthesiologists refrain from administering parenteral medication to children without intravenous access. Many children who are able to verbalize, report that receiving a needle puncture was their worst experience in the hospital.[95,96] In most cases, medication administered without a needle will be more pleasant for children, their parents, and the medical staff.

Drugs for premedication have been administered by many routes, including the oral, nasal, rectal, buccal, intravenous, and intramuscular routes. Previously, oral administration of drugs for premedication was thought to increase gastric residual volume and consequently increase the risk for pulmonary aspiration. However, unless a large volume of fluid is ingested, oral premedication does not increase the risk of aspiration pneumonia.[97] In general, the route of drug administration should depend on the drug, the desired drug effect, and the psychological impact of the route of administration. For example, a small dose of oral medication may be sufficient for a relatively calm child, whereas an intramuscular injection, such as ketamine, may be best for an uncooperative, combative, extremely anxious child. Intramuscular medication may be less traumatic for this type of child than forcing him or her to swallow a drug, giving a drug rectally, or forcefully holding an anesthesia mask on the face.[98]

Since Water's classic work in 1938 on premedication of children, numerous reports have addressed this subject.[99] Despite the wealth of studies, no single drug or combination of drugs has been found to be "ideal" for all children. Many drugs used for premedication have similar effects, and a specific drug may have various effects in different children or in the same child under different conditions.

Medications

Several categories of drugs are available for premedicating children before anesthesia (Table 4-7). Selection of drugs for premedication depends on the goal desired. Drug effects should be weighed against potential side effects, and drug interactions should be considered. Premedicant drugs include tranquilizers, sedatives, hypnotics, opioids, antihistamines, anticholinergics, H_2-receptor antagonists, antacids, and drugs that increase gastric motility. The most widely used premedication in both children and adults in North America is midazolam.[100]

Tranquilizers

The major effect of tranquilizers is to allay anxiety, but they also have the potential to produce sedation. This group of drugs includes the benzodiazepines, phenothiazines, and butyrophenones. Although benzodiazepines are widely used in children, phenothiazines and butyrophenones are not.

Benzodiazepines

Benzodiazepine derivatives are widely used for premedicating children. They are generally given to calm patients, allay anxiety, and diminish recall of perianesthetic events. At low doses,

Table 4-7. Doses of Drugs Commonly Administered for Premedication

Drug	Route	Dose (mg/kg)
Barbiturates		
Methohexital	Rectal	(10% solution) 20-40
	Intramuscular	(5% solution) 10
Thiopental	Rectal	(10% solution) 20-40
Benzodiazepines		
Diazepam	Oral	0.1-0.5
Midazolam	Oral	0.25-0.75
	Nasal	0.2
	Rectal	0.5-1.0
	Intramuscular	0.1-0.150
Phencyclidine		
Ketamine*	Oral	3-6
	Nasal	3
	Rectal	6-10
	Intramuscular	2-10
Alpha$_2$ Adrenergic Agonist		
Clonidine	Oral	0.004
Opioids		
Morphine	Intramuscular	0.1-0.2
Meperidine	Intramuscular	1.0-2.0
Fentanyl	Oral	0.010-0.015 (10-15 µg/kg)
Sufentanil	Nasal	0.01-0.003 (1-3 µg/kg)

*With atropine 0.02 mg/kg.

minimal drowsiness and cardiovascular or respiratory depression are produced.

Midazolam, a short-acting water-soluble benzodiazepine with an elimination half-life of about 2 hours, is the most widely used premedication for children.[66,100] The major advantage of midazolam over other drugs in its class is its rapid uptake and elimination.[101] It can be administered intravenously, intramuscularly, nasally, orally, and rectally with minimal irritation, although it leaves a bitter taste in the mouth or nasopharynx after oral and nasal administration, respectively.[102-108] Peak plasma concentrations of midazolam occur approximately 10 minutes after intranasal, 16 minutes after rectal, and 53 minutes after oral administration.[101,108,109] The bioavailability of midazolam after different routes of administration is a fraction of the bioavailability after intravenous administration, that is, about 0.9 after intramuscular injection and about 0.57 after intranasal, 0.4 to 0.5 after rectal, and about 0.3 after oral administration (see Chapter 6).[109,110] After oral and rectal administration there is incomplete absorption and extensive hepatic extraction of the drug during the first pass through the liver. Because of poor bioavailability of midazolam after oral and rectal administration, larger doses must be given via these routes than via parenteral routes to achieve the same effect. Most children are adequately sedated after receiving a midazolam dose of 0.025 to 0.1 mg/kg intravenously, 0.1 to 0.2 mg/kg intramuscularly, 0.25 to 0.75 mg/kg orally, 0.2 mg/kg nasally, or 1 mg/kg rectally.

Orally administered midazolam is effective in calming most children and does not increase gastric pH or residual volume.[111] Children who are premedicated with oral midazolam are calmer than those who are not premedicated, even when parents are present for the induction of anesthesia.[61] Initial studies of oral midazolam necessitated the institution to prepare a formulation by combining the intravenous formulation of midazolam with a variety of flavorings, syrups, or medications to mask the bitter taste. However, these have been replaced with a commercially prepared formulation in a concentration of 2 mg/mL. Two multicenter studies yielded different responses to the commercial preparation of oral midazolam in children.[112,113] In one study, 0.25, 0.5, and 1.0 mg/kg all provided satisfactory sedation and anxiolysis within 10 to 20 minutes,[113] whereas in the other study, 1.0 mg/kg provided greater anxiolysis and sedation than 0.25 and 0.5 mg/kg.[112] These differing results may be attributed to the older ages of children in the former study.[112]

Recent data suggest that the dose of midazolam increases as age decreases in children, similar to that for inhaled agents and intravenous agents. Thus, greater doses may be required in younger children to achieve a similar degree of sedation and anxiolysis. However, the formulation of the oral solution may also attenuate its effectiveness.[114,115] It should be noted, however, that a number of medications might affect the cytochrome oxidase system, thereby significantly affecting the first pass metabolism of midazolam. For example, grapefruit juice, erythromycin, protease inhibitors, and calcium-channel blockers depress CYP3A4 activity, resulting in unexpectedly greater blood concentrations of midazolam and prolonged sedation.[116-122] Conversely, anticonvulsants (phenytoin and carbamazepine), rifampin, St. John's wort, glucocorticoids, and barbiturates induce the 3A4 isoenzyme, thereby reducing the blood concentration of midazolam and its duration of action.* The dose of oral midazolam should be adjusted in children who are taking these medications.

Concerns have been raised about possible delayed discharge after premedication with oral midazolam. Oral midazolam, 0.5 mg/kg, administered to children 1 to 10 years of age did not affect awakening times, postanesthesia care unit or hospital discharge times, or time to extubation after sevoflurane anesthesia.[123] Similar results have been reported in children and adolescents after 20 mg of oral midazolam premedication. However, detectable preoperative sedation in this group of children was predictive of delayed emergence.[124] In children aged 1 to 3 years undergoing adenoidectomy as outpatients, premedication with oral midazolam, 0.5 mg/kg, delayed spontaneous eye opening by 4 minutes and discharge by 10 minutes as compared with placebo after 25 minutes of sevoflurane anesthesia; children who had been premedicated however, exhibited a more peaceful sleep at home on the night after surgery.[125]

What is the effect of oral midazolam on recovery from anesthesia? Oral midazolam decreased the infusion requirements of propofol by 33% during a propofol-based anesthetic, although the time to discharge readiness was delayed.[126] After oral midazolam premedication (0.5 mg/kg), induction of anesthesia with propofol, and maintenance with sevoflurane, emergence and early recovery were delayed by 6 and 14 minutes, respectively, in children 1 to 3 years of age undergoing ambulatory adenoidectomy compared with nonpremedicated children, although discharge times did not differ.[127] Increased postoperative sedation may be attributed to synergism between propofol and midazolam on γ-aminobutyric acid (GABA) receptors.[128]

One notable benefit of midazolam is anterograde amnesia; children who were amnestic about their initial dental

*See http://medicine.iupui.edu/flockhart/table.htm.

extractions tolerated further dental treatments better than those who were not amnestic.[129] It appears that memory becomes impaired within 10 minutes and anxiolytic effects are apparent as early as 15 minutes after oral midazolam.[130]

Although anxiolysis and a mild degree of sedation occur in most children after midazolam, a few will become agitated.[131] This can also occur with intravenous midazolam, 0.1 mg/kg. In the latter case, intravenous ketamine, 0.5 mg/kg, effectively reverses the agitation.[132] Adverse behavioral changes in the post-operative period have also been reported. In one study, oral midazolam resulted in less crying during the induction of anes-thesia but was associated with greater adverse behavioral changes (nightmares, night terrors, food rejection, anxiety, and negativism) up to 4 weeks postoperatively compared with the placebo-treated group.[133] This finding was not substantiated in another study.[45] One undesirable effect associated with mid-azolam, independent of the mode of administration (rectal, nasal, or oral), is hiccups; the etiology is unknown.

Anxiolysis and sedation usually occur within 10 minutes after intranasal midazolam.[134] It has been suggested that intranasal midazolam may be less effective in children with an upper respi-ratory tract infection (URI) and excessive nasal discharge.[108] Intranasal midazolam does not affect the time to recovery or the time to discharge a child from the hospital after surgical proce-dures at least 10 minutes in duration.[135,136] Although midazolam reduces negative behavior in children during parental separa-tion, nasal administration is not well accepted because it pro-duces irritation and discomfort that may outweigh the sedative effects.[137-139] A theoretical concern for the nasal route of admin-istration of midazolam is its potential to cause neurotoxicity via the cribriform plate.[108] There are direct connections between the nasal mucosa and the central nervous system (CNS) (Fig. 4-3, see website). Medications administered nasally reach high con-centrations in the cerebrospinal fluid very quickly.[140-142] Because midazolam with preservative has been shown to have neuro-toxic properties in an animal model, we do not recommend this route of administration unless it is with preservative-free midazolam.[143,144]

Sublingual administration of midazolam (0.2 mg/kg) has been reported to be as effective as, and better accepted than, intranasal midazolam.[145] Oral transmucosal midazolam given in three to five small allotments (0.2 mg/kg total dose) placed on a child's tongue at age 8 months to 6 years provides satisfactory acceptance and separation from parents in 95% of patients.[146]

There is another pharmacodynamic difference among benzo-diazepines that is important to consider when these drugs are administered intravenously. Entry into the CNS is directly related to fat solubility.[147,148] The greater the fat solubility, the more rapid the transit into the CNS. The time to peak CNS electroencephalographic effect in adults is 4.8 minutes for mid-azolam but only 1.6 minutes for diazepam (see Fig. 48-11). Therefore, when administering intravenous midazolam, one must wait an adequate interval between doses to avoid excessive medication and oversedation.

Diazepam is used to sedate older children but is rarely used in neonates, infants, and school-aged children. In infants and especially preterm neonates, the elimination half-life of diaze-pam is markedly prolonged because of immature hepatic function (see Chapter 6). In addition, the active metabolite (desmethyldiazepam) has pharmacologic activity equal to the parent compound and a half-life of up to 9 days in adults.[149] The most effective route of administration is intravenous, followed by oral and rectal. The intramuscular route is not recommended because it is painful and absorption is erratic.[150-154] A combina-tion of oral midazolam, 0.25 mg/kg, and oral diazepam, 0.25 mg/kg, was compared with oral midazolam, 0.5 mg/kg, alone in children undergoing adenotonsillectomy. The combination of oral midazolam and diazepam provided a more sedated child at the induction of anesthesia and less agitation during emer-gence.[155] The average oral dose for premedicating healthy chil-dren with diazepam ranges from 0.1 to 0.3 mg/kg; however, doses as large as 0.5 mg/kg have been used.[156] A rectal solution is more effective and reliable than rectally administered tablets or suppositories.[154,157] The recommended rectal dose of diaze-pam is 1 mg/kg, with serum concentrations peaking at approxi-mately 20 minutes.[157] However, when compared with rectal midazolam, rectal diazepam appeared to be less effective.[158]

Lorazepam (0.05 mg/kg) given orally or intravenously is used primarily in older children. The intravenous formulation is not used in neonates because it may be neurotoxic.[159,160] The advantages of lorazepam compared with diazepam are less tissue irritation and more reliable amnesia. It can be adminis-tered orally, intravenously, or intramuscularly and is metabo-lized by the liver to inactive metabolites. Compared with diazepam, the onset of action of lorazepam is slower and its duration of action is prolonged. These characteristics that may be appropriate for inpatients make it inappropriate for use in outpatients. When given the night before surgery in children undergoing reconstructive burn surgery, oral lorazepam, 0.025 mg/kg, significantly decreased preoperative anxiety.[161]

Butyrophenones

Droperidol is a major tranquilizer that is very rarely used for preanesthetic medication any longer. It is effective in preventing postoperative nausea and vomiting after strabismus surgery even in small doses (20 µg/kg).[162] However, most pediatric anes-thesiologists in the United States avoid its use after the Food and Drug Administration (FDA) issued a black box warning in 2001 regarding the association of droperidol with torsades de pointes and QTc interval prolongation.

Phenothiazines

Promethazine, a phenothiazine derivative, is occasionally admin-istered to control nausea and vomiting when opioids are used before anesthesia. It is more commonly used in combination with other medications by non-anesthesiologists for procedural sedation.[163] The recommended dose is 0.25 to 0.5 mg/kg intra-venously, intramuscularly, or orally. In addition to its sedative properties, promethazine is an H_1 blocker and has antiemetic, antihistaminic, anti–motion sickness, and anticholinergic effects. Its prolonged elimination half-life (8 to 12 hours) may make it inappropriate for children who are outpatients and who are at risk for postoperative airway compromise (e.g., children with obstructive sleep apnea), especially if other sedating/analgesic medications are needed. Dystonic reactions have also been reported.

Barbiturates

Barbiturates are among the oldest medications used for pre-medication in children but are infrequently used for this purpose any longer. The advantages of barbiturates include minimal respiratory or cardiovascular depression, anticonvulsant effects, and a very low incidence of nausea and vomiting. The major disadvantage of barbiturates is hyperalgesia. In some cases, a small dose administered to children with pain may intensify the pain and cause them to become uncooperative.

The relatively short-acting barbiturates *thiopental* and *methohexital* may be given rectally to premedicate young children who refuse other modes of sedation. These drugs are usually administered in the presence of the parents who may hold the child until the child becomes sedated.[164] The usual dose of rectal thiopental for children who have not received any other sedative is 30 mg/kg. This dose produces sleep in about two thirds of the children within 15 minutes.[165,166] Intravenous thiopental has an elimination half-life (9 ± 1.6 hours) that is longer than that of methohexital (3.9 ± 2.1 hours) owing to a slower rate of hepatic metabolism.[167] There are few data comparing the elimination kinetics of rectally administered barbiturates.

Methohexital is rarely used for premedication any longer, but when it was used rectally, a 10% solution was prepared in a dose of 20 to 30 mg/kg. With this dose, most children were sedated within 10 to 15 minutes.[168,169] The sedation may be profound, resulting in airway obstruction and laryngospasm. Hence, all children should be closely monitored with a source of oxygen, suction, and a means for providing ventilatory support; rectally administered methohexital has been reported to cause apnea in children with meningomyeloceles.[170,171] Children chronically treated with phenobarbital or phenytoin are more resistant to the effects of rectally administered methohexital, probably because of enzyme induction.[169,172]

Recovery after methohexital is relatively rapid because of the rapid redistribution and metabolism of the drug. A rectal dose of 25 mg/kg does not affect the discharge time from the hospital, but the time to return to full consciousness after a 30-minute or shorter surgical procedure is slightly prolonged in those children who are premedicated with methohexital rectally compared with those who receive 5 mg/kg of thiopental intravenously for the induction of anesthesia.[173]

Additional disadvantages of rectal methohexital include the unpredictable systemic absorption, defecation after administration, and hiccups. Older children (>6 years of age) may strenuously object to any rectal intervention while awake. The volume of methohexital is quite large in children who weigh more than 20 kg, thus increasing the risk of defecation and erratic absorption. Some children develop airway obstruction, apnea, seizure, or an allergic reaction.[171] Contraindications to methohexital include hypersensitivity, temporal lobe epilepsy, and latent or overt porphyria.[174-176] Rectal methohexital is also contraindicated in children with rectal mucosal tears or hemorrhoids because large quantities of the drug can be absorbed, resulting in respiratory or cardiac arrest.

Nonbarbiturate Sedatives

Chloral hydrate and *triclofos* are orally administered nonbarbiturate drugs that are used to sedate children; both have slow onset times and are relatively long acting. They are converted to trichloroethanol, which has an elimination half-life of 9 hours in toddlers (see Fig. 48-10).[177] Chloral hydrate is frequently used by non-anesthesiologists to sedate children.[178-180] It is rarely used by anesthesiologists because it is unreliable in producing sedation, it has a prolonged duration of action, it is unpleasant to taste, and it is irritating to the skin, mucous membranes, and gastrointestinal tract. An oral dose (50 to

100 mg/kg with a total maximum dose of 2 g) is most effective when administered $1\frac{1}{2}$ to 2 hours before anesthesia (see Chapters 6 and 48). Its use in neonates is not recommended because of impaired metabolism[181,182] nor is chronic administration recommended because of the theoretical possibility of carcinogenesis.[183,184] Children with hepatic failure may have prolonged action of chloral hydrate, and greater doses can produce significant respiratory depression in children with liver disease.

Opioids

Opioids may be useful to provide analgesia and sedation in children who have pain preoperatively. However, opioid use is associated with well-established side effects, including nausea, vomiting, respiratory depression, sedation, and dysphoria. Therefore, all children who receive an opioid premedication should be continuously observed and monitored with pulse oximetry.

Morphine sulfate may be given to children with preoperative pain, such as those with a limb fracture. The recommended dose for preanesthetic medication is 0.1 to 0.2 mg/kg intramuscularly 1 hour before the induction of anesthesia or 0.05 to 0.1 mg/kg intravenously. Morphine is also effective when given orally; rectal administration is not recommended owing to erratic absorption. Neonates are more sensitive to the respiratory depressant effects of morphine, and it is rarely used to premedicate that age group.[185]

Meperidine is a long-acting synthetic opioid with a slightly more rapid onset of action and reduced duration of action than morphine. The usual dose for premedication in children is 1 to 2 mg/kg intramuscularly 1 hour before induction. Meperidine may also be administered intravenously and orally. An oral dose of 1.5 mg/kg in combination with diazepam, 0.2 mg/kg, and atropine, 0.02 mg/kg, safely sedates patients before anesthesia.[97] Large doses or chronic administration of meperidine can cause CNS excitation (seizures, tremors, muscle twitches) owing to accumulation of the metabolite normeperidine.[186] Meperidine is not recommended for repeated use in children but is safe for short-term administration.[186] Currently, the primary indication for meperidine is to treat postoperative shivering.

Fentanyl may be administered by parenteral, transdermal, nasal, and oral routes. A "lollipop" delivery system, oral transmucosal fentanyl citrate (OTFC), is nonthreatening and more readily accepted by children than other routes as a premedicant and facilitates separation from parents.[187] Fentanyl is strongly lipophilic, and OTFC is readily absorbed from the buccal mucosa with an overall bioavailability of approximately 50%.[188,189] The optimal dose as a preanesthetic medication with minimal desaturation and preoperative nausea appears to be 10 to 15 µg/kg.[190,191] Children begin to show signs of sedation within 10 minutes after receiving this dose, although the blood levels of fentanyl continue to increase for up to 20 minutes after completion. Recovery from anesthesia after a premedication of 10 to 15 µg/kg of oral fentanyl is similar to that after 2 µg/kg intravenously.[190] Doses greater than 15 µg/kg are not recommended because of opioid side effects, particularly occasional respiratory depression. The incidence of the opioid-associated side effects is increased when the interval between completion of "lollipop" and induction of anesthesia is prolonged.[191-194] Ondansetron given after the induction of anesthesia does not decrease the incidence of opioid-related side effects such as nausea and vomiting.[195] OTFC is infrequently used as a premedicant today but rather is now primarily indicated for the treatment of breakthrough cancer pain. Fentanyl has also been administered nasally (1 to 2 µg/kg) but primarily after induction of anesthesia as a means of providing analgesia in children without intravenous access.[196]

Sufentanil is 10 times more potent than fentanyl. After a nasal dose of 1.5 to 3 µg/kg, children are usually calm and cooperative, and most separate with minimal distress from their parents.[134] However, several instances of reduced chest wall compliance have been reported in children after nasal sufentanil. In a study that compared the effects of nasally administered midazolam and sufentanil, midazolam caused more nasal irritation, whereas sufentanil caused more postoperative nausea and vomiting and reduced chest wall compliance. In addition, children in the sufentanil group were discharged approximately 40 minutes later than those in the midazolam group.[138] The potential side effects and prolonged hospital stay after nasal sufentanil makes it an unpopular choice for premedication.

Tramadol is a weak µ-opioid receptor agonist whose analgesic effect is mediated via inhibition of norepinephrine reuptake and stimulation of serotonin release. Tramadol is devoid of action on platelets and does not depress respirations in the clinical dose range.[197] Serum concentrations peak by 2 hours after oral dosing with clinical analgesia maintained for 6 to 9 hours. When oral tramadol (1.5 mg/kg) was given to children who had been premedicated with oral midazolam (0.5 mg/kg), it provided good analgesia after multiple dental extractions with no adverse respiratory or cardiovascular effects.[198] Intravenous tramadol (1.5 mg/kg) given before induction of general anesthesia has been compared with local infiltration of 0.5% bupivacaine (0.25 mL/kg) for ilioinguinal and iliohypogastric nerve blocks. Tramadol was as effective as the regional blocks in terms of pain control, although the incidence of nausea and vomiting was greater in the tramadol group. Time to discharge was similar in both groups.[199]

Butorphanol is a synthetic opioid agonist-antagonist with properties similar to those of morphine that can be administered nasally.[200] It is as effective as equipotent doses of intramuscular meperidine and morphine, with an onset of analgesic action in about 15 minutes and peak activity within 1 to 2 hours in adults. The most frequent side effect is sedation that resolves approximately 1 hour after administration. A dose of 0.025 mg/kg administered nasally immediately after the induction of anesthesia was shown to provide good analgesia after myringotomy and tube placement at the expense of increased incidence of emesis at home compared with children who received nonopioid analgesics such as acetaminophen.[201]

If opioids are used in combination with other sedatives such as benzodiazepines, the dose of each drug should be appropriately adjusted to avoid serious respiratory depression. For example, if fentanyl is indicated to control pain in a child who has already received midazolam, the fentanyl dose should be titrated in small increments (0.25 to 0.5 µg/kg) to prevent hypoxemia and hypopnea or apnea. When fentanyl or other opioids are combined with midazolam, they produce more respiratory depression than opioids or midazolam alone.[202]

Codeine is a commonly prescribed oral opioid that must undergo O-demethylation in the liver to produce morphine to provide effective analgesia. Five to 10 percent of children lack the cytochrome isoenzyme (CYP450 2D6) required for this conversion and therefore do not derive analgesic benefit. Codeine can be given orally or intramuscularly but should not be administered intravenously because of the risk of seizures. The usual oral dose of oral codeine is 0.5 to 1.5 mg/kg with an onset of action within 20 minutes and peak effects between 1 to 2 hours. Codeine has an elimination half-life of 2.5 to 3 hours. The combination of codeine with acetaminophen is effective in relieving mild to moderate pain. This combination was found to provide superior analgesia to acetaminophen alone after myringotomy and placement of pressure-equalizing tubes.[203,204] Codeine is associated with the unpleasant side effects of nausea and vomiting (see Chapter 6).

Ketamine

Ketamine is a phencyclidine derivative that produces dissociation of the cortex from the limbic system, producing reliable sedation and analgesia while preserving upper airway muscular tone and respiratory drive.[203] In infants younger than 3 months of age, the volume of distribution is similar to that in older infants but the elimination half-life is prolonged about threefold (185 vs. 65 minutes).[205] At equal doses on a milligram-per-kilogram basis, the dose of ketamine required to prevent gross movement in infants younger than 6 months of age is four times greater than in children 6 years of age.[206] Ketamine may be administered by intravenous, intramuscular, oral, nasal transmucosal, and rectal routes. The disadvantages of ketamine include increased oral secretions, nystagmus, an increased incidence in postoperative emesis, and possible undesirable psychological reactions, such as hallucinations, nightmares, and delirium. Concomitant administration of midazolam may eliminate or attenuate these emergence reactions.[207,208] The addition of atropine or glycopyrrolate is recommended to decrease the copious secretions that may lead to laryngospasm.[209]

Intramuscular ketamine is an effective means of sedating combative, apprehensive, or developmentally delayed children who are otherwise uncooperative and refuse oral medication. A low dose of 2 mg/kg is sufficient to adequately calm most uncooperative children in 3 to 5 minutes so that they will accept a mask for inhalation induction of anesthesia without prolonging the hospital discharge times even after brief surgical procedures.[98] However, the combination of intramuscular ketamine (2 mg/kg) and midazolam (0.1 to 0.2 mg/kg) significantly prolongs recovery and discharge times, making the ketamine/midazolam combination inappropriate for brief ambulatory procedures such as bilateral myringotomies and tube insertion.[210] A larger dose (4 to 5 mg/kg) sedates children within 2 to 4 minutes, and a dose of 10 mg/kg usually produces deep sedation that lasts from 12 to 25 minutes. Larger doses and repeated doses are associated with hallucinations, nightmares, vomiting, and unpleasant, as well as prolonged, recovery from anesthesia.[98,211] Concentrations of ketamine of 100 mg/mL are available in the United States and other countries for such purposes but they should be carefully labeled and stored to avoid mixing this concentration with formulations at reduced concentrations. The larger doses of intramuscular ketamine are particularly useful for the induction of anesthesia in children in whom there is a desire to maintain a stable blood pressure and in whom there is no venous access, such as those with congenital heart disease.

Oral ketamine alone and in combination with midazolam has been successfully used for premedication in both healthy children and those with congenital heart defects.[212] An oral ketamine dose of 5 to 6 mg/kg sedates most children within 12 minutes, and more than half of the children will be sedated sufficiently to permit establishing intravenous access.[210,213] A larger dose of 8 mg/kg has been shown to prolong recovery from anesthesia, although by 2 hours in the recovery room there was no difference compared with a smaller dose of oral ketamine (4 mg/kg).[214] The combination of oral midazolam and ketamine provides more effective preoperative sedation than either drug alone. This oral lytic cocktail is a good alternative for children who have had inadequate sedation with oral midazolam alone in the past. In one study, the combination of oral ketamine (3 mg/kg) and midazolam (0.5 mg/kg) did not prolong recovery time for surgical procedures that lasted more than 30 minutes.[215] Oral ketamine has also been used effectively to alleviate the distress of invasive procedures (bone marrow aspiration) in pediatric oncology patients.[216] Oral ketamine has not been associated with nightmares or emergence delirium.

Nasal transmucosal ketamine at a dose of 6 mg/kg is also effective in sedating children within 20 to 40 minutes before induction of anesthetia.[217] There is the potential that nasally administered ketamine could cause neural tissue damage if it reaches the cribriform plate. Because the preservative in ketamine is neurotoxic, preservative-free ketamine would appear to be safer to administer by the nasal route.[218] If ketamine is given by this route, we recommend the 100-mg/mL concentration to minimize the volume that must be instilled in the nose.

Rectal ketamine (5 mg/kg) produces good anxiolysis and sedation within 30 minutes of administration.[219] However, the rectal route does not provide reliable absorption.

α₂ Agonists

Clonidine, an α₂ agonist, causes dose-related sedation by its effect in the locus ceruleus through its inhibition of adenylate cyclase.[220] The plasma concentration peaks at 60 to 90 minutes after oral administration and at 50 minutes after rectal administration.[221] An oral dose of 3 µg/kg given 45 to 120 minutes before surgery produces comparable sedation to that of diazepam or midazolam.[222] Clonidine acts both centrally and peripherally to reduce blood pressure and therefore it attenuates the hemodynamic response to intubation.[223] It appears to be relatively free of respiratory depressant properties, even when administered in an overdose.[220] The sedative properties of clonidine reduce the dose of intravenous barbiturate required for induction of anesthesia.[223] Likewise, clonidine has been shown to reduce the minimal alveolar concentration (MAC) of sevoflurane for tracheal intubation[224] and the concentration of inhaled anesthetic, as judged by hemodynamic stability intraoperatively, for the maintenance of anesthesia.[225-227] The MAC for tracheal extubation (MAC-ex) with sevoflurane anesthesia in air and oxygen decreased by 36% and 60% with oral clonidine premedication (2 or 4 µg/kg, respectively). These doses did not prolong emergence from anesthesia or produce airway-related complications.[228] During the first 12 hours after surgery, oral clonidine (4 µg/kg) reduced the postoperative pain scores and the requirement for supplementary analgesics.[229,230] In children undergoing tonsillectomy, those who received oral clonidine, 4 µg/kg, exhibited more intense anxiety on separation and during induction than those who received midazolam (0.5 mg/kg). However, those who received clonidine had reduced mean intraoperative blood pressures, reduced duration of surgery,

anesthesia, and emergence, and decreased need for supplemental oxygen during recovery but greater postoperative opioid requirements, greater pain scores, and excitement. Parenthetically, these observations are not consistent with previously reported analgesic and anesthetic properties of clonidine. Even though discharge readiness, postoperative emesis, and 24-hour analgesic requirements were similar in both groups, midazolam was judged to be a better premedicant for children undergoing tonsillectomy.[231] Oral clonidine (4 µg/kg) reduces the incidence of vomiting after strabismus surgery compared with (1) a placebo, (2) clonidine (2 µg/kg), and (3) oral diazepam (0.4 mg/kg).[232] Oral clonidine combined with 0.15 mL/kg of apple juice 100 minutes before the induction of anesthesia does not affect the gastric fluid pH and volume in children.[233] An oral dose of 4 µg/kg attenuates the hyperglycemic response to a glucose infusion and the surgical stress in children undergoing minor surgery, possibly by inhibiting the surgical stress release of catecholamines and cortisol. Children who were involved in surgeries that lasted 1.7 hours did not develop hypoglycemia, but in the absence of intraoperative glucose infusions, there is a risk of hypoglycemia during operations of prolonged duration.[234] Although oral clonidine offers several desirable qualities as a premedication, particularly sedation and analgesia, the need to administer it 60 minutes before induction of anesthesia makes its use impractical in most clinical settings.[231]

Antihistamines

The popularity of antihistamines for premedication has declined because their sedative effects are variable. They are very rarely given to infants but may be occasionally indicated for older children, especially those who are hyperkinetic.

Hydroxyzine is mainly administered for its ataractic properties.[235,236] It also has antiemetic, antihistaminic, and antispasmodic effects with minimal respiratory and circulatory changes. It is usually administered with other classes of drugs as an intramuscular "cocktail" at a dose of 0.5 to 1.0 mg/kg.

Diphenhydramine is an H₁ blocker with mild sedative and antimuscarinic effects. The dosage for children is 2.5 to 5 mg/kg/day (maximum daily dose: 300 mg) in four divided doses orally, intravenously, or intramuscularly. Although the duration of action is 4 to 6 hours, it does not appear to interfere with recovery from anesthesia.[237] The combination of oral diphenhydramine (1.25 mg/kg) and oral midazolam (0.5 mg/kg) has been found to provide safe and effective sedation for healthy children undergoing MRI.[238] The combination was more effective than midazolam alone without a delay in discharge and recovery times.

Anticholinergic Drugs

Anticholinergic agents were commonly used in the past (1) to prevent the undesirable bradycardia associated with some anesthetic agents (halothane and succinylcholine), (2) to minimize the autonomic vagal reflexes manifested during surgical manipulations (e.g., laryngoscopy or strabismus repair), and (3) to reduce secretions. The most commonly used anticholinergic drugs are atropine, scopolamine, and glycopyrrolate. Undesirable effects of anticholinergics include tachycardia, dry mouth, skin erythema, and hyperthermia due to inhibition of sweating. Atropine and scopolamine cross the blood-brain barrier and with excessive doses may cause CNS excitation manifested as agitation, confusion, restlessness, ataxia, hallucinations, slurred speech, and memory loss.

Because most modern inhalational anesthetics are not associated with bradycardia, the routine use of an anticholinergic drug is not generally warranted. Most anesthesiologists administer these agents only when indicated, such as before intravenous succinylcholine, combined with ketamine, before laryngoscopy and intubation in neonates, and when surgery stimulates vagal reflexes, such as during strabismus repair. In the majority of cases, anticholinergics need not be given preoperatively but rather should be given after intravenous access is established.

The recommended doses of anticholinergics are *scopolamine*, 0.005 to 0.010 mg/kg, and *atropine*, 0.01 to 0.02 mg/kg. Atropine is more commonly used and blocks the vagus nerve more effectively than scopolamine, whereas scopolamine is a better sedative, antisialagogue, and amnestic. Infants who require atropine should receive it before heart rate decrease to avoid decreasing cardiac output because the onset time of the atropine is delayed with bradycardia.[239] Anticholinergic overdose may be treated with the centrally active anticholinesterase physostigmine (0.04 mg/kg).

Glycopyrrolate is a synthetic quaternary ammonium compound that does not cross the blood-brain barrier. It is twice as potent as atropine in decreasing the volume of oral secretions, and its duration of effect is three times greater. The recommended dose of glycopyrrolate (0.01 mg/kg) is one half that of atropine. The routine use of an anticholinergic drug for the sole purpose of drying secretions is probably unwarranted, because a dry mouth can be a source of extreme discomfort for a child. In one study, more adults who were premedicated with glycopyrrolate reported that they had a sore throat or hoarseness postoperatively than those who were not premedicated.[240] Therefore, it is best to reserve the use of glycopyrrolate for specific indications such as to limit sialorrhea associated with ketamine.

Topical Anesthetics

The child's exaggerated fear of the needle makes topical anesthetic creams an attractive alternative to intradermal infiltration. There are several needleless methods to minimize procedural pain, each with its own limitations.

EMLA cream (eutectic mixture of local anesthetic, Astra Zeneca, Wilmington, DE) is a mixture of two local anesthetics (2.5% lidocaine and 2.5% prilocaine). One-hour application of EMLA cream to intact skin with an occlusive dressing provides adequate topical anesthesia[241] for a variety of superficial procedures, including intravenous catheter insertion, lumbar puncture, vaccination, laser treatment of port-wine stains, and neonatal circumcision.[242-247] However, EMLA causes venoconstriction and skin blanching, both of which obscure superficial veins, making intravenous cannulation more difficult.[248] Methemoglobinemia, another limitation of EMLA cream, is the result of prilocaine.[249] However, a 1-hour application of EMLA cream and a maximum dose of 1 g did not induce methemoglobinemia when applied to intact skin of full-term neonates younger than 3 months of age.[250] Lidocaine toxicity from EMLA has been reported when applied to mucosal membranes, including the tongue, for extended periods of time.[251]

Ametop is a topical local anesthetic (4% tetracaine) that is available in the United Kingdom, Europe, and Canada (Smith and Nephew, Lachine, Quebec) but not in the United States. Its indications are identical to those of EMLA. Its characteristics include a 30- to 40-minute onset time, no venoconstriction or skin blanching, and no risk of methemoglobinemia.

ELA-Max (4% lidocaine) is another topical anesthetic cream that has been shown to decrease pain associated with dermatologic procedures,[252] including intravenous catheter insertion after only a 30-minute application.[253] In addition, ELA-Max blanches the skin to a lesser extent and dilates veins better than EMLA cream.[254] It includes no prilocaine, thus significantly eliminating the risk of methemoglobinemia.

A novel delivery device, the *S-Caine Patch* (ZARS, Inc., Salt Lake City, UT), is a eutectic mixture of lidocaine and tetracaine (70 mg of each per patch) that uses a controlled heating system to accelerate delivery and analgesic effect of the local anesthetic. An application time of 20 minutes lessens pain associated with venipuncture in children and is associated with only mild and transient local erythema and edema and no skin blanching.[255] A potential advantage over prilocaine-containing formulations is that methemoglobinemia has not been reported with tetracaine.

Other noninvasive topical anesthetic delivery systems are available, such as lidocaine iontophoresis using an impregnated electrode, current generator, and a return pad to carry ionized lidocaine through the stratum corneum.[256] This method has been shown to provide similar pain relief for insertion of intravenous catheters in children as EMLA cream but requires extra equipment and training for appropriate application.[257] Lidocaine iontophoresis also causes a stinging pain that some children experience during current application and potential skin burns from the electrodes.[258]

Nonopioid Analgesics

Acetaminophen is the most common nonopioid analgesic used for treatment of postoperative pain in children. It can be administered orally preoperatively, rectally immediately after the induction of anesthesia but before the start of surgery, or intravenously (where available) once an intravenous line has been established.

The oral doses of acetaminophen is 10 to 15 mg/kg recommended for the antipyretic effect are as effective as ketorolac (1 mg/kg)[259] at 10 or more minutes postoperatively for myringotomies with pressure-equalizing tube placement.[260] Oral acetaminophen is very rapidly absorbed with a bioavailability of 0.54.[260] Acetaminophen is also safe to use in neonates because the immature hepatic enzyme systems in neonates produce less toxic metabolites than in older children.[261-263] Other studies have shown that when acetaminophen is given preemptively, it has opioid-sparing properties that enhance analgesia in children after tonsillectomy.[264,265] Acetaminophen and codeine oral elixir given preoperatively provides superior analgesia to acetaminophen alone after myringotomy and placement of pressure-equalizing tubes.[204] However, in children undergoing tonsillectomy, the levels of pain control provided by acetaminophen with codeine or acetaminophen alone were similar and postoperative oral intake was significantly greater in children treated with acetaminophen alone.[266]

The pharmacokinetics of rectal acetaminophen (10, 20, and 30 mg/kg) yield peak blood concentrations between 60 and 180 minutes after administration, emphasizing the importance of administering the rectal acetaminophen immediately after induction of anesthesia to provide sufficient time to achieve therapeutic blood concentrations by the end of surgery.[267] With doses of 30 mg/kg rectal acetaminophen or less, children do not achieve peak or sustained serum concentrations that are associated with antipyresis (Fig. 4-4). Thus, based on these pharmacokinetics, the authors recommended that an initial dose of rectal acetaminophen of 40 mg/kg be followed by 20 mg/kg rectally every 6 hours; this dosing regimen was confirmed in a second study.[268] Several other single-dose rectal administration studies reported similar results.[269,270] For children undergoing tonsillectomy, a preoperative oral dose of 40 mg/kg plus 20 mg/kg rectally 2 hours later was associated with satisfactory pain scores for about 8 hours after administration.[260] At greater doses (40 to 60 mg/kg rectally) administered after induction of anesthesia but before surgery, children required less rescue morphine postoperatively and less analgesia at home than children who received either a placebo or 20 mg/kg of acetaminophen rectally.[265] In addition, the children who received larger doses of acetaminophen experienced less postoperative nausea and vomiting. However, until further safety data are developed, the initial dose of acetaminophen should not exceed 40 to 45 mg/kg with a total 24-hour dose of not more than 100 mg/kg in order to avoid hepatic toxicity. Acetaminophen administered rectally in a loading dose of 40 mg/kg and then 20 mg/kg either orally or rectally every 6 hours after elective craniofacial surgery yielded greater plasma concentrations and lower pain scores than those who received oral acetaminophen; this was in part related to some children vomiting the oral acetaminophen.[271]

A parenteral formulation of acetaminophen (*propacetamol*) may be administered in a dose of 30 mg/kg (15 mg/kg acetaminophen) every 6 hours to children 2 to 15 years of age. In a placebo-controlled trial in febrile children, this dose of propacetamol was superior to placebo.[272] Pharmacokinetic studies indicate that such a dose of propacetamol maintains therapeutic blood levels of acetaminophen of 10 μg/mL.[273] Pharmacokinetic data in infants indicate that 15 mg/kg of propacetamol four times daily is appropriate for neonates 10 days of age or younger but 30 mg/kg at the same frequency may be required in infants older than 10 days of age.[274] Hemostatic effects of large (60 mg/kg) doses of propacetamol have been studied in adult volunteers. The results indicate that this dose of propacetamol may transiently and reversibly inhibit platelet aggregation as well as decrease thromboxane activity, although less than ketorolac (0.4 mg/kg), but that the combination of the two may prolong this effect.[275]

Combinations of nonsteroidal inflammatory agents can be more effective in pain management than single-agent therapy. A combination of acetaminophen (10 mg/kg) and ibuprofen (10 mg/kg) alternating every 2 hours in children undergoing suboccipital craniotomy provided better pain scores and decreased narcotic and antiemetic requirements compared with those who received analgesic medications only when requested.[276] Hepatic failure in a 3-year-old child after acetaminophen and sevoflurane exposure for appendectomy underscores the necessity of avoiding toxic doses of acetaminophen. In the first 24 hours the child with hepatic failure had received 175 mg/kg of acetaminophen for an average dose of 100 mg/kg/day for 4 days. Fasting, a very large initial dose of acetaminophen, and sevoflurane may deplete glutathione stores and may have contributed to the problem. Fortunately, the child made a complete recovery after treatment with *N*-acetylcysteine.[277] *Because hepatic toxicity is a real and potentially fatal complication of an acetaminophen overdose, it is advised that a complete history of*

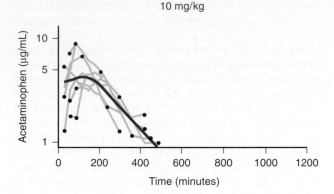

10 mg/kg

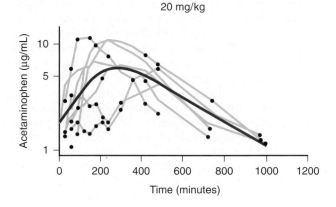

20 mg/kg

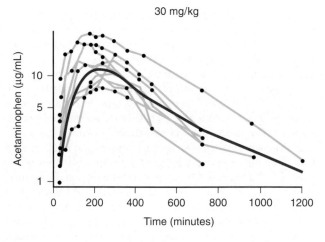

30 mg/kg

Figure 4-4. Levels of acetaminophen after rectal administration of 10, 20, or 30 mg/kg were recorded. Values for serum concentration of acetaminophen (*solid circles, teal lines*) are plotted against time for each child. Thick (*magenta*) lines indicate "average" values. Note that only children who received 30 mg/kg achieved the antipyretic threshold of 10 to 20 μg/mL but that even at this dose that range was not sustained. These data suggest the need to use a larger loading dose (~40 mg/kg) followed by subsequent doses of 20 mg/kg every 6 hours; see text for details. (From Birmingham PK, Tobin MJ, Henthorn TK, et al: Twenty-four-hour pharmacokinetics of rectal acetaminophen: an old drug with new recommendations. Anesthesiology 1997; 87:244-252.)

acetaminophen administration be taken before anesthesia and that a 100-mg/kg limit be placed on the 24-hour cumulative dosing.

Ibuprofen is a commonly used nonsteroidal anti-inflammatory drug. In children undergoing a variety of surgical procedures, rectal ibuprofen (40 mg/kg/day in divided doses) was given for up to 3 days. This was supplemented with intravenous or intramuscular morphine as clinically indicated; the need for additional morphine during the 3-day study period was less for those who received the rectal ibuprofen.[278] Children undergoing bilateral myringotomy who were given either oral ibuprofen (10 mg/kg) or acetaminophen (15 mg/kg) demonstrated similar blood concentrations.[279] Rectal ibuprofen alone is insufficient analgesia for children undergoing day-case adenoidectomy.[280] Acetaminophen/codeine combination has been shown to provide superior analgesia to ibuprofen after tonsillectomy. Furthermore, the ibuprofen-treated children demonstrated a significant increase in bleeding time.[281] However, in an unblinded study, ibuprofen was as effective as acetaminophen with codeine for postoperative pain control after tonsillectomy with less nausea and vomiting and no increase in bleeding.[282] The analgesic effectiveness of acetaminophen alone or combined with either ibuprofen or rofecoxib showed that the addition of ibuprofen but not rofecoxib to acetaminophen reduced the need for early analgesia in tonsillectomy patients by 50% as compared with acetaminophen alone.[283] Ibuprofen performs better than placebo and as well as acetaminophen in children undergoing dental procedures.[284] Ibuprofen should not be used in children with impaired renal function or in those who are hypovolemic owing to the increased risk of renal toxicity.[285,286]

Ketorolac is a nonsteroidal anti-inflammatory drug that can be administered parenterally and orally, intraoperatively, or postoperatively. It has an opioid-sparing effect, reducing the incidence of adverse effects of opioids such as respiratory depression, nausea, and vomiting. Features that may limit the usefulness of this drug include gastrointestinal irritation, the antiplatelet effects, and limited safety data. In children, small cohort pharmacokinetic studies failed to demonstrate any age-related differences in pharmacokinetics.[287] However, stereospecific pharmacokinetics of ketorolac in infants and toddlers aged 6 to 18 months showed differences in pharmacokinetics of the R(+) and S(−) isomers with more rapid elimination of the analgesic S(-) isomer. Thus, smaller dose intervals of 4 rather than 6 hours may be needed in infants older than 6 months to achieve serum concentrations at or above the adult effective concentration (EC_{50}) level.[288] Ketorolac has been shown to diminish emergence agitation and pain when given intravenously after induction for myringotomies with pressure-equalization tube insertion.[289] However, ketorolac (1 mg/kg) provided no better pain relief than rectal acetaminophen (35 mg/kg) in children undergoing tonsillectomy with or without adenoidectomy.[290] Ketorolac (1 mg/kg) intramuscularly or intravenously before tonsillectomy increased intraoperative and postoperative blood loss compared with children who received codeine (1.5 mg/kg) intramuscularly[291] or morphine (0.1 mg/kg) intravenously.[292,293] In the same study, there was no difference in the awakening time or readiness for discharge among the groups. In contrast, when ketorolac was given as a single dose at the end of tonsillectomy there was no increase in post-tonsillectomy hemorrhage, although duration of hospitalization and the likelihood of over-night admission decreased.[294] Ketorolac is a useful adjunct when given intravenously to supplement the local anesthesia infiltrated by the surgeon during inguinal herniorrhaphies.[295] Ketorolac (0.9 mg/kg) is an effective alternative to morphine (0.1 mg/kg), with less nausea and vomiting,[296] and decreases postoperative morphine requirements if continued at a dose of 0.5 mg/kg intravenously every 6 hours in infants and children.[297] This has also been confirmed in orthopedic surgery with the added benefit of decreasing the length of stay.[298] Single doses of ketorolac (0.8 mg/kg) are opioid sparing and decrease the frequency of urinary retention in orthopedic surgery when combined with patient-controlled analgesia with morphine.[299] In children undergoing strabismus surgery, ketorolac provided equivalent analgesia to fentanyl (1 µg/kg) or morphine (0.1 mg/kg) with less postoperative nausea and vomiting.[300,301] In children undergoing ureteral reimplantation, ketorolac decreases the incidence and severity of postoperative bladder spasms with no decrease in hematocrit or increase in serum creatinine.[302,303]

Because ketorolac can increase bleeding time, we recommend discussing its use with the surgeon and administration only after achieving hemostasis and completion of surgery. The safe use of this drug in infants younger than 6 months of age has been questioned, although a review of 53 infants who received ketorolac 48 hours after cardiac surgery and continuing for 3 days showed a minimal increase in serum creatinine and blood urea nitrogen at 48 hours after institution of the therapy but no increase in bleeding episodes.[304,305] This is a small sample size on which to base any conclusions regarding safety, and creatinine and blood urea nitrogen are not sufficiently sensitive indices of renal function. No data have been forthcoming to confirm the safety of ketorolac in any age group in children. Despite the varied doses described earlier, the recommended dose should be limited to 0.5 mg/kg with a maximal dose of 15 mg for children who weigh less than 50 kg and 0.5 mg/kg up to 30 mg every 6 hours for those who weigh more than 50 kg.

Rofecoxib, a nonsteroidal anti-inflammatory cyclooxygenase-2 (COX-2) inhibitor, offers the advantages of minimal effects on renal, gastrointestinal, and platelet function.[306-309] However, the use of COX-2 inhibitors is currently under reevaluation owing to increased metabolites reported among long-term users after large doses.[310]

Antiemetics

Antiemetic administration should be considered in children undergoing high-risk procedures such as tonsillectomy and strabismus repair as well as those who have a history of motion sickness or prior history of postanesthesia nausea and vomiting. The uses of these medications are presented elsewhere in the text (see Chapters 6, 31, 32, and 37).

Corticosteroids

Children who have been taking chronic corticosteroid therapy (e.g., for asthma, Crohn's disease, lupus, acute lymphocytic leukemia) or those who have discontinued chronic corticosteroid therapy in the last 6 months may suffer from suppression of the hypothalamic-pituitary-adrenal axis.[311] There is a paucity of evidence to support the need for supplemental corticosteroids in children receiving chronic corticosteroid therapy. In the past, the hypotension reported in those who were taking chronic corticosteroid therapy was likely the result of hypovolemia. Nonetheless, many endocrinologists continue to recommend a dose of supplemental corticosteroids before or shortly after induction of anesthesia for "stress" corticosteroid coverage. The usual recommended dose is 1 to 2 mg/kg of hydrocortisone (Solu-Cortef) intramuscularly or intravenously or an equivalent dose of dexamethasone (0.05 to 0.1 mg/kg) approximately 1 hour before the induction of anesthesia or as soon as intravenous access is established. For more complicated operations, the corticosteroid dose may have to be repeated every 6 hours for up to 72 hours (see Chapter 24).

Insulin

Optimal management of diabetic children undergoing surgery entails maintaining glucose homeostasis and avoiding hyperglycemia with resultant osmotic diuresis, impaired wound healing, and increased infection rate. Anesthesiologists should work together with each diabetic child's endocrinologist or primary care physician to carefully consider the child's specific diabetes treatment regimen, glycemic control, intended surgery, and anticipated postoperative care when devising the perioperative management plan. Diabetes mellitus is the most common endocrine problem encountered in children. The preoperative fasting time should be the same as that recommended for nondiabetic children. Every attempt should be made to schedule these children as the first case of the day to minimize the fasting period. Preoperative laboratory tests should include the hematocrit, serum electrolytes, and glucose levels; blood glucose concentrations should be measured at frequent intervals during the perianesthetic period. Several protocols have been crafted to control the blood sugar in children who are diabetic[312]; these are described in more detail in Chapter 24 (see also Figs. 24-1 to 24-8 that describe a variety of management strategies).

Antibiotics

Antibiotics are frequently administered to prevent or reduce infection in surgical patients. The appropriate timing of antibiotics is now a source of performance benchmarking for some insurance carriers, thus making communication with surgeons essential for the success of this anesthesiology-directed quality assessment measure. For prophylaxis against endocarditis in children with structural heart disease, antibiotics should ideally be administered either intravenously 30 to 60 minutes or orally 1 hour before the induction of anesthesia and surgery. In reality, in children these antibiotics are usually administered after induction of anesthesia and establishment of intravenous access (see also Tables 14-1 and 14-2).[313]

Antacids, H₂ Antagonists, and Gastrointestinal Motility Drugs

The risk of aspiration during induction of or emergence from anesthesia is increased in children who are developmentally delayed, have gastroesophageal reflux, experienced previous esophageal surgery, had a difficult airway, were obese, or had undergone a traumatic injury. Preanesthetic administration of drugs that reduce gastric fluid volume and acidity may decrease the risk of pulmonary acid aspiration syndrome (Table 4-8).[1,314] Gastric fluid pH may be increased by drinking a nonparticulate antacid such as sodium citrate; particulate antacids should be avoided because they can cause severe pneumonitis if aspirated.

Cimetidine and *ranitidine* are H₂-receptor antagonists that decrease gastric acid secretion, increase gastric fluid pH, and

Table 4-8. Doses of Antacids, H₂ Antagonists, and Gastrointestinal Motility Drugs

Drug	Dose
Antacids	
Bicitra	30 mL
Prokinetic	
Metoclopramide	0.1-0.15 mg/kg
H₂ Antagonists	
Cimetidine	5-10 mg/kg
Ranitidine	2.0-2.5 mg/kg
Famotidine	0.3-0.4 mg/kg

reduce gastric residual volume.[315,316] These drugs can be given orally, intravenously, or intramuscularly.

Metoclopramide is often administered with an H₂-receptor antagonist to increase lower esophageal sphincter tone, relax the pyloric sphincter and the duodenal bulb, and promote gastric emptying by increasing peristalsis of the duodenum and jejunum. The drug effect is apparent 30 to 60 minutes after oral administration and 1 to 2 minutes after intravenous administration.[317] Side effects such as extrapyramidal signs relate to its effect on the CNS through blockade of dopaminergic receptors.

Induction of Anesthesia

Preparation for Induction

Adequate preparation includes warming the operating room and ensuring that warming devices are properly functioning (e.g., heat lamps, warming blanket, forced air warmer) before the child's arrival, especially for young infants. The preinduction checklist should include a variety of sizes of masks, oral airways, laryngoscope blades, tracheal tubes (one size larger and one size smaller than the anticipated size), an appropriate size laryngeal mask airway, and functioning wall suction. The anesthesia machine and monitoring equipment should be prepared before the child's arrival in the operating room to ensure that all appropriate equipment is on hand and to minimize any last minute "commotion." One of the most essential monitors used during the induction of anesthesia is the precordial stethoscope. The bell from the stethoscope should have a double-stick adhesive attached ready for application before induction. A chair or stool for the child's parent to sit on helps avoid fainting episodes should the parent accompany the child. Ensuring a quiet, calm operating room environment, free of clanging instruments and loud conversations among the staff, allows for a smoother and less upsetting induction.

There are a variety of techniques for inducing general anesthesia. The technique used depends on a number of factors including the child's developmental age, understanding and ability to cooperate, and previous experiences, the presence of a parent and the interaction of these factors with the child's underlying medical or surgical conditions.

Inhalation Induction

The most common method of inducing anesthesia in children is inhalation by mask of the nonpungent volatile anesthetic agents sevoflurane or halothane. The anesthesiologist should be flexible and adapt an approach that suits the child, depending on age, degree of sedation, and cooperation.

If the child is already asleep on arrival in the operating room, it is possible to utilize the "steal induction" technique. The child is not touched or disturbed. After priming the breathing circuit with N$_2$O in O$_2$, the mask is gently placed near the child's face and gradually brought closer and closer until it is tightly applied to the face. After breathing N$_2$O for 1 to 2 minutes, sevoflurane is then gradually introduced up to its maximum (8%) concentration or halothane is administered in increasing concentrations as tolerated. Adequate monitoring must be instituted as soon as possible, and the child is then transferred to the operating table. This technique is atraumatic and avoids exposing the child to the "strange" operating room surroundings while awake. However, it is possible that the child may suffer psychological harm when he or she awakens to pain without realizing what has transpired.

When the child is reluctant to lie down on the operating table and insists on sitting up, induction should proceed with the child sitting on the operating room bed with his or her back supported by the anesthesiologist's chest. Some children may prefer to sit on the anesthesiologist's or their parent's lap (Fig. 4-5A, see website); they may be distracted by asking them to "blow up the balloon," where the balloon refers to the reservoir bag. If this approach is considered, it is advisable that this be undertaken only with children who are wearing diapers or sitting on a thick blanket to limit the spread of urine should the bladder be emptied during induction of anesthesia. The anesthesia machine should be within easy reach during such an induction, to allow control of the bag, pop-off valve, and vaporizer without interruption. An assistant should be at hand to help position and hold the child when needed. Other children can be distracted by allowing them to hold their favorite toy or security blanket during induction (Fig. 4-5B, see website).

If a parent wishes to accompany a young child to the operating room we generally allow the child to remain in the parent's lap for the induction. We request that the child be sitting facing forward in the parent's lap so there is free access to the child's face. It is vital to instruct the parent that he or she must have the arms tightly wrapped around the child (also holding the arms in such a way that the child cannot reach up to the face mask) and to warn him or her that as the child loses consciousness that the child will become limp. It is also important to have an experienced individual in front of the child and parent to hold onto the child as induction proceeds and help place the child on the operating room table after successful induction. At this point we ask the parent to kiss the child and step out of the operating room (Fig. 4-6, see website).

Some children refuse a mask or to have the face mask placed anywhere near their face. They may have an unknown fear of masks or have been traumatized previously with high concentrations of sevoflurane or halothane administered by face mask without nitrous oxide. The solution to this problem is to remove the mask, place the elbow of the breathing circuit between your fingers, and then cup your hands below the chin. Because nitrous oxide is heavier than air, cupped hands act like a reservoir. The hands are gradually brought closer and closer to the face until they gently cover the mouth. Once the child has an obvious effect from the N$_2$O, high concentrations of sevoflurane can be added. Younger infants who refuse a mask may be soothed by placing one's small finger ("pinky") in their mouth to suck on as the face mask is gently advanced to their nose and mouth for an inhalation induction (Fig. 4-7).

Inhalation with Sevoflurane

The traditional mask induction of anesthesia is accomplished by placing the mask lightly on the child's face and administering a mixture of N$_2$O in O$_2$ (2:1) for 1 or 2 minutes until the full effect of N$_2$O is achieved. Offering children the choice of a scented mask or "sleepy air," such as bubble gum or strawberry flavor (Lorann Oils, Lansing MI), applied to the inside of the face mask may disguise the odor of the plastic. Sevoflurane is then introduced and can be rapidly increased to 7% or 8%, without significant bradycardia or hypotension in otherwise healthy children, except in young infants (<6 months). After anesthesia is induced, the sevoflurane concentration should be maintained at the

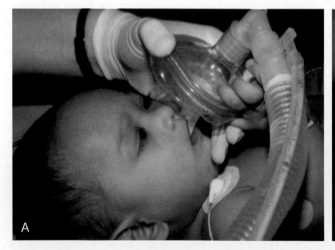
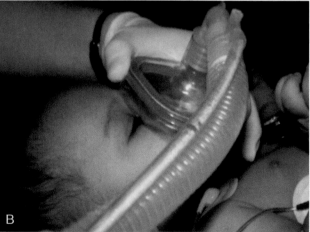

Figure 4-7. A, Infants 6 months of age or younger are often consoled during induction by placing a little finger ("pinky finger") of your hand in their mouth while you hold the face mask near their face with the rest of the hand. Generally they are so hungry that they will stop crying and eagerly suckle on your pinky finger. **B,** As the infant loses consciousness, the intensity of the suckling diminishes, the pinky finger is gently removed, and the face mask is fully applied.

maximum tolerable concentration until the intravenous line is established, but this concentration should be reduced if controlled ventilation is initiated so as to avoid overdose. The reason for maintaining delivery of a high concentration of sevoflurane is to minimize the risk of awareness during the early period of the induction sequence. Data from unpremedicated children (aged ≥ 3 years) indicate that sevoflurane is associated with small increases in heart rate, although heart rate does decrease to 80 to 100 beats per minute in some children after breathing sevoflurane for a period of time.[318] In contrast to halothane,[319] sevoflurane does not increase the myocardial sensitivity to epinephrine.[320] In a study of three techniques for delivering sevoflurane for induction of anesthesia, minimal differences were detected among the three: incremental increases in sevoflurane (2%, 4%, 6%, and 7%) in oxygen, a high concentration of sevoflurane (7%) in oxygen, and a high concentration of sevoflurane in a 1:1 mixture of N_2O and O_2.[321] When N_2O was added, there was a decreased time to loss of the eyelash reflex and a decreased incidence of excitement during the induction.

Agitation or excitement in early induction (shortly after loss of eyelash reflex) with sevoflurane has been observed. In addition, minor seizure-like activity characterized by muscular rigidity and uncoordinated movements of arms and legs occasionally occurs; the incidence varies among studies and appears to be related in part to the observer.[322,323] One study described minimal (minor) seizure-like activity in 80% of the children during sevoflurane induction (8% in O_2-N_2O, 1:1),[324] whereas another found none under similar conditions.[325] In our experience, rapid induction of anesthesia with nitrous oxide, oxygen, and sevoflurane 8% has not yielded instances of clinical seizure activity. No long-lasting neurologic or electroencephalographic sequelae due to the use of sevoflurane in children have been reported.

Inhalation Induction with Halothane

Halothane has largely been replaced by sevoflurane for inhalation induction of anesthesia because of halothane's slower wash-in and emergence and greater incidence of bradycardia, hypotension, and arrhythmias. When anesthesia is induced with halothane, the inspired concentration is gradually increased by 0.5% every two to three breaths up to 5%. Alternatively, a single-breath induction of anesthesia with 5% halothane can yield a rapid induction of anesthesia without triggering airway reflex responses.[326]

The inspired concentration of halothane should be decreased as soon as anesthesia is established to avoid heart rate slowing and myocardial depression. The child will autoregulate the depth of anesthesia as long as he or she is allowed to breath spontaneously; however, if respirations are controlled, then anesthetic overdose may easily occur (see Chapter 6).[327,328] Halothane sensitizes the heart to catecholamines, and ventricular arrhythmias may commonly be seen, especially during periods of hypercapnia or light anesthesia.[329]

If vital signs become abnormal during induction, the concentration of halothane should be reduced or discontinued and the circuit flushed with 100% oxygen. If bigeminy or short bursts of ventricular tachycardia occur, then the following strategies should be considered: (1) hyperventilation (to reduce the $Paco_2$) (2) deepening of the halothane anesthesia, or (3) change to an alternate potent inhalation agent.[329] There is no role for intravenous lidocaine to treat these arrhythmias.

During inhalation induction with either sevoflurane or halothane, if the oxygen saturation decreases (and there is no mechanical cause for the desaturation such as partial dislodgement of the oximeter probe, the patient clenching the fingers or toes, the blood pressure cuff inflating), 100% oxygen should be administered until the oxygen saturation returns to normal while addressing the cause of the desaturation. If the cause of the desaturation is not related to upper airway obstruction, then the most common cause of a desaturation in a healthy child is a ventilation/perfusion mismatch due to segmental atelectasis. The management is to recruit alveoli by applying a sustained inflation of the lungs to 30 cm H_2O for 30 seconds or as tolerated.[330] Alternately, mild to moderate upper airway obstruction from collapse of the hypopharyngeal structures or the development of mild laryngospasm causes hypoventilation and desaturation. Generally, this upper airway obstruction is readily relieved by gently applying a tight mask fit, closing the popoff valve sufficiently to generate 5 to 10 cm of positive end-expiratory pressure, and simply allowing the distending pressure of the bag to stent open the airway until the child is adequately anesthetized to tolerate the placement of an oral airway (see Figs. 12-10 and 37-2). Pressure should be applied to the superior pole of the condyle of the mandible to sublux the temporomandibular joint. This maneuver opens the mouth and may supplant the need for an oral airway.[331] Moreover, this maneuver translocates the mandible anteriorly and rotates the temporomandibular joint. The net effect is to pull the tongue off the posterior and nasopharyngeal walls, opening the laryngeal inlet (Video Clip 4-1, see website). It is very important to avoid applying digital pressure to the soft tissues of the submental region, leading to the tongue occluding the oropharynx and nasopharynx. If the child develops symptomatic bradycardia, then oxygenation and ventilation must first be established, followed by intravenous atropine (0.02 mg/kg) and, if necessary, chest compressions and intravenous epinephrine (see Chapter 40).

Inhalation Induction with Desflurane

Desflurane has a low blood gas partition coefficient (0.42) and has the fastest onset and offset of all potent volatile agents. However, it is very pungent and causes significant airway irritation, with inhalation induction attempts resulting in severe laryngospasm (49%), coughing, increased secretions, and hypoxemia.[332] Therefore, *desflurane is not recommended for inhalation induction in children* but may be used safely for maintenance of general anesthesia when the trachea has been intubated.

Hypnotic Induction

Hypnosis can reduce anxiety and pain in children with chronic medical problems and those undergoing painful procedures[333,334] as well as reduce preoperative anxiety. In a study in which hypnosis was compared with midazolam, 0.5 mg/kg, 30 minutes before surgery, hypnosis significantly reduced preoperative anxiety at the time of face mask application and the frequency of behavior disorders postoperatively compared with children who had received midazolam.[335] Hypnosis provided a relaxed state of well-being and enabled children to actively participate in anesthesia, thus leaving them with a pleasant memory. Unlike midazolam's anterograde amnesia, hypnosis may have the benefit of maintaining a pleasant memory to prevent fear during future anesthesia. Hypnosis is an altered state of consciousness with highly focused attention, based on the principle of dissociation.[336] Hypnosis results in a state of inner absorption that leads

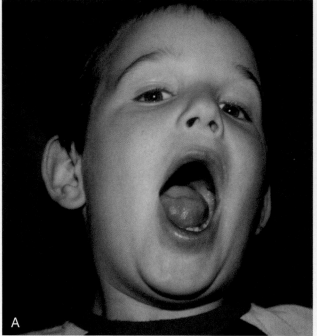

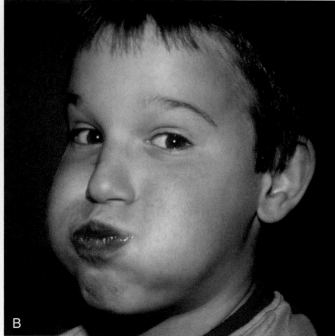

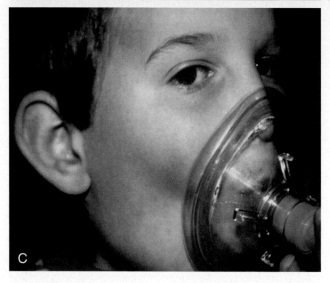

Figure 4-8. A single-breath induction is another useful method that is most appropriate for children 5 to 10 years of age. It is important to practice several times without the mask attached to the circuit prior to the actual induction (see text for details of preparing the circuit). This allows the child to become familiar with the feel of the mask as it is applied to the face and to properly time the sequence of events. **A,** Generally we ask the child to take "the biggest breath possible and hold it." **B,** Then we ask the child to "breathe all the way out until you have no more air in your lungs and hold it." **C,** Then we ask the child to take in "the biggest breath you have ever taken, hold it, then breath normally." If a full vital capacity breath is taken with a good mask seal around the mouth and nose, most children will lose their lid reflex within 30 to 45 seconds, which is similar to that produced by intravenous induction agents.

to a reduction in awareness of immediate physical surroundings and experiences. Children are more likely to be absorbed in fantasy with their natural power of playing making them more hypnotizable than adults.[337] Although an anesthesiologist may not have training in hypnosis, he or she can use hypnotic suggestions to help children even though an actual trance state is not induced. It may be helpful to engage children in age-appropriate scenarios, such as going to the zoo, a fancy tea party, a baseball game, or flying a jet. Words should be spoken slowly and rhythmically with descriptions of sights and sounds that are familiar to the child as well as repeated suggestions of "feeling good." The hypnotic suggestions distract the child so that the smell of anesthetic agent becomes the scent of the zoo animals, the tea brewing, the aviation fuel, and so on. Any number of stories can be told with the same result as long as one remembers to repeatedly say things that can be identified by the child and that fit with what the child is experiencing at the time of induction.

Modified Single-Breath Induction

The single-breath induction is especially appealing to children who desire to fall sleep "really fast" with a face mask because loss of consciousness is achieved much more rapidly than with a traditional escalating dose technique. It works best with older children, although some as young as 3 years old can be anesthetized with this technique if they are cooperative. Before beginning, the child should be coached through a mock induction by instructing him or her to "breathe in the biggest breath possible" and then "breathe all the way out until there is no more air in the lungs." Once this has been practiced once or twice, then a practice run is repeated with only the mask (no circuit) on the face.

Before induction, the circuit and reservoir bag are primed with 70% N_2O in O_2 and the maximum concentration of concentration of halothane or sevoflurane that is possible. This is achieved by running modest fresh gas flows through the circuit and intermittently emptying the reservoir bag manually into the scavenger system (i.e., with the circuit occluded). Once the circuit is primed with inhalation agent at high concentration, the distal end of the circuit is occluded (to avoid contaminating the operating room) and the child is instructed to take a deep breath of room air and to exhale all the air and hold expiration. The face mask is then placed securely over the child's mouth and nose while he or she is instructed to take in the "deepest breath ever" and "hold it, now just breathe normally." Loss of consciousness, as noted by loss of the eyelash reflex, results soon after this vital capacity breath (Fig. 4-8).[326,338]

Intravenous Induction

Intravenous induction is usually reserved for older children, those who request an intravenous induction, those with a previously established intravenous catheter, those with potential cardiovascular instability, and those who need a rapid-sequence induction because of a full stomach. There are many different options as far as medications that can be used for an intravenous induction in a child (Table 4-9). Ideally, all children should breathe 100% oxygen before intravenous induction of anesthesia. If the face mask is met with objections, oxygen may be insufflated without a mask by simply holding the Y-connector of the circuit between your fingers over or near the child's face.

Thiopental

Thiopental (sodium pentothal) has been the barbiturate most frequently used for induction of anesthesia in children, although more recently many clinicians have replaced it with propofol. The recommended induction dose of thiopental in healthy, nonpremedicated children is 5 to 6 mg/kg[339]; neonates require a smaller dose (3 to 4 mg/kg).[340] Debilitated or severely ill patients, those that are hypovolemic, and those that have been premedicated may also require a smaller dose for induction of anesthesia. The beta-elimination half-life of thiopental in neonates is twice that in their mothers (15 vs. 7 hours), so a single dose may produce excessively long effects in neonates.[341]

Methohexital

Methohexital is an ultra-short-acting oxybarbiturate that is infrequently used for induction of anesthesia today. The induction dose for children ranges from 1.0 to 2.5 mg/kg[342]; nonpremedicated children require the larger dose. Recovery from intravenous administration is more rapid than after thiopental.[343] Larger doses cause skeletal muscle hyperactivity and myoclonic movements. Pain at the injection site is common, necessitating pretreatment with intravenous lidocaine. Intravenous methohexital is also associated with hiccups.[342]

Propofol

Propofol is the most commonly used nonbarbiturate intravenous induction agent in children. The induction dose of propofol

varies with age: the ED_{50} for a satisfactory induction in healthy infants 1 to 6 months old is 3.0 ± 0.2 mg/kg, and in healthy children 10 to 16 years old it is 2.4 ± 0.1 mg/kg.[344] The ED_{95} in healthy unpremedicated children 3 to 12 years of age is 2.5 to 3.0 mg/kg.[345] The early distribution half-life is about 2 minutes, and the elimination half-life is about 30 minutes.[346] Clearance is very large (2.3 ± 0.6 L/min) and exceeds liver blood flow.[346] Advantages to using propofol for induction of anesthesia include a lower incidence of airway-related problems (e.g., laryngospasm), more rapid emergence,[347,348] and a lower incidence of nausea and vomiting.[349,350] The major disadvantage of propofol is pain at the site of injection, especially when administered in small veins.[344] The administration of lidocaine (0.5 to 1.0 mg/kg) while applying tourniquet pressure proximal to the injection site ("mini-Bier block") for 30 to 60 seconds before injecting the propofol effectively eliminates the pain. Other techniques reported to attenuate the pain include mixing lidocaine (0.5-1 mg/kg) with the propofol (but this should be done within 60 seconds of administration of the propofol), mixing thiopental with the propofol, refrigerating the propofol, pretreating with an opioid or ketamine, and diluting propofol to a 0.5% solution.[351-360]

In addition to its use as an induction agent, propofol can also be administered by infusion for total intravenous anesthesia (see Chapter 7) because of its relatively low context-sensitive half-time. It is especially useful for pediatric patients undergoing nonoperating room procedures such as computed tomography (CT), MRI, radiotherapy, bone marrow biopsy, upper and lower gastrointestinal endoscopy, and lumbar puncture.

Etomidate

Etomidate is a hypnotic induction agent that provides marked cardiovascular stability. It is indicated for the induction of anesthesia in children with cardiomyopathy or those who are hypovolemic after trauma. The recommended induction dose is 0.2 to 0.3 mg/kg depending on the cardiovascular status of the child. Myoclonic movements are associated with etomidate administration[361]; this agent can suppress adrenal steroid synthesis,[362] and it causes pain on injection.

Ketamine

Ketamine is a very useful induction agent for children with cardiovascular instability, especially in hypovolemic states, or for those who cannot tolerate a reduction in systemic vascular resistance, such as those with aortic stenosis or congenital heart disease in whom the balance between pulmonary and systemic blood flow is vital for maintaining cardiovascular homeostasis. Ketamine is a myocardial depressant that can result in systemic hypotension in children who already are maximally compensating with endogenous catecholamines.[363] The usual induction dose of ketamine is 2 mg/kg, which should be reduced in the presence of severe hypovolemia. Smaller doses of intravenous ketamine (0.25 to 0.5 mg/kg) have been used successfully for procedural sedation.

Ketamine is associated with increased oropharyngeal secretions, psychomimetic side effects (hallucinations, nightmares), and postoperative nausea and vomiting. The administration of an antisialagogue and midazolam is recommended to attenuate these side effects.

Intramuscular Induction

Although it is preferable to avoid intramuscular injections in children, there are occasions when this route may be indicated,

Table 4-9. Doses of Commonly Used Intravenous Induction Agents

Drug	Dose
Thiopental or thiamylal	5.0-8.0 mg/kg
Methohexital	1.0-2.5 mg/kg
Propofol	2.5-3.5 mg/kg
Etomidate	0.2-0.3 mg/kg
Ketamine	1.0-2.0 mg/kg

such as for the uncooperative child and adolescent who refuses all other routes of sedation (oral, intranasal, intravenous) and for those susceptible to malignant hyperthermia who have poor venous access. In infants, but especially in older children, intramuscular ketamine is a very useful drug because of the low volume of injectate (see earlier).[98] In infants and very small children, intramuscular methohexital (10 mg/kg of a 5% solution) produces a state of anesthesia within several minutes.

Rectal Induction

Rectal drug administration is ideally suited for an extremely frightened young child who rejects other forms of premedication and for those who are developmentally delayed. It is not desirable for older children and those who weigh more than 20 kg owing to volume limitations on the fluid injected and for concern over emotional consequences. Methohexital, thiopental, ketamine, and midazolam have all been studied for this use. For nonpremedicated children, the usual doses are thiopental (30 to 40 mg/kg), methohexital (20 to 25 mg/kg),[364] midazolam (1.0 mg/kg),[365] and ketamine (~5 mg/kg).

Disadvantages of rectal drug administration include failure of inducing anesthesia owing to poor bioavailability of the drug or defecation, as well as delayed recovery from anesthesia after brief procedures due to the variability of rectal drug absorption. Conversely, there can be a very rapid drug uptake leading to respiratory compromise.

Full Stomach and Rapid-Sequence Induction

A full stomach is one of the most common problems that pediatric anesthesiologists face. The preferred method to secure the airway in the presence of a full stomach is a rapid-sequence intravenous induction. Before this is undertaken, the anesthesiologist must ensure that the proper equipment is at hand: two functioning laryngoscope blades and handles (should a bulb or contact fail, a spare is available), two suctions (should the suction be blocked by vomitus or blood, a second is available), appropriate drugs, a leak-free anesthesia circuit, endotracheal tubes of appropriate sizes, and stylet. All monitors should be properly functioning, and, at a minimum, the pulse oximeter, blood pressure cuff, and precordial stethoscope applied (in a crying, struggling child the pulse oximeter may not function properly until after anesthetic induction). After intravenous access is established, the child is given atropine (0.02 mg/kg intravenously) and is denitrogenated with 100% oxygen ("preoxygenated") for several breaths. Studies of adult patients demonstrated that oxygen saturation remains greater than 95% for 6 minutes after only four vital capacity breaths of 100% oxygen.[366] Similar studies have not been performed in cooperative or uncooperative children; however, without preoxygenation, younger infants and children desaturate more rapidly after induction of anesthesia than older children and adults.[367,368] One study demonstrated a more rapid increase in the inspired oxygen concentrations in infants compared with older patients and that preoxygenation to an FEO_2 of 0.9 can be achieved in 100 seconds.[369] Even with a crying child, it is possible to increase the PaO_2 by enriching the immediate environment with high flows of oxygen. Preoxygenation should not be carried out in such a way that it upsets a child. Premedication (e.g., intravenous midazolam, 0.05 to 0.1 mg/kg) in divided doses may alleviate fear and anxiety before induction. It is important to preoxygenate children to avoid positive-pressure ventilation before intubation because positive-pressure ventilation might distend the already full stomach, leading to regurgitation and aspiration. After preoxygenation (and atropine), anesthesia is induced with intravenous thiopental (5 to 6 mg/kg),[339] propofol (3 to 4 mg/kg) intravenously,[370,371] ketamine (1 to 2 mg/kg), or etomidate (0.2 to 0.3 mg/kg), followed immediately by 2 mg/kg of succinylcholine. Succinylcholine is still the paralytic agent of choice for rapid onset and short duration. However, high-dose rocuronium may be used as an alternate muscle relaxant for a rapid-sequence induction should succinylcholine be contraindicated. One study demonstrated equivalent intubating conditions 30 seconds after rocuronium administration (1.2 mg/kg) or succinylcholine (1.5 mg/kg).[372] In that study, the mean time to return of 25% twitch was 46.3 ± 23.4 minutes (range, 30-72) for rocuronium compared with 5.8 ± 3.3 minutes (range, 1.5-8.25) for succinylcholine. However, if rocuronium is used with thiopental for induction, the thiopental must be cleared from the tubing before infusing rocuronium to prevent rocuronium from precipitating.[373] The availability of a new reversal agent (suggamadex) for rocuronium (and potentially vecuronium) may reduce concern about the prolonged duration of action of rocuronium and eliminate the need for intravenous succinylcholine (see Chapter 6).

Cricoid pressure (Sellick maneuver) should be applied as anesthesia is induced, and pressure should be maintained until the endotracheal tube is confirmed to be situated between the vocal cords and the lungs inflated.[374,375] Unfortunately, few apply cricoid pressure as originally described by Sellick. The neck is not hyperextended, and a hard neck rest is not placed beneath the cervical curve. By obliteration of the esophageal lumen, cricoid pressure is intended to prevent regurgitated material from reaching the pharynx. Before induction the cricoid ring is palpated between the thumb and the middle finger and, after the child has lost consciousness, pressure is steadily increased using the index finger. To prevent passive gastroesophageal reflux, a pressure of 30 to 40 Newtons (3 to 4 kg of force) must be applied to the upper esophagus (in adults), which creates an intraluminal pressure of approximately 50 cm H_2O in the upper esophagus.[376] However, active vomiting creates esophageal pressures greater than 60 cm H_2O that could overcome cricoid pressure, leading to regurgitation and pulmonary aspiration; or, if cricoid pressure is not relieved immediately, spontaneous rupture of the esophagus (Boerhaave's syndrome) may occur. Hence the contraindications to cricoid pressure should be carefully reviewed to avoid complications from this maneuver (see Table 37-1). Gastric insufflation is prevented in children with cricoid pressure during airway management via mask ventilation up to 40 cm H_2O peak airway pressure.[377] The Sellick maneuver should seal the esophagus in the presence of a nasogastric tube,[378] but removal of the nasogastric tube before intubation provides a better mask fit and exposure for intubation. If the nasogastric tube is left in place, leaving it open to atmospheric pressure will vent liquid and gas remaining in the stomach.

The results of surveys from the United Kingdom indicated that cricoid pressure was used in only 40% to 50% of children in whom it was indicated.[379,380] Reluctance to apply cricoid pressure may be attributed to a number of reasons, including the indications for its use and how often it is applied with the correct position and pressure.[381-383] In adults evaluated with MRI, the esophagus was situated lateral to the cricoid cartilage in more than 50% of patients without cricoid pressure and laterally displaced more than 90% of the time with cricoid pressure.[384] In addition, cricoid pressure may distort the anatomy of the upper airway, making laryngoscopy more difficult, and must sometimes be released to facilitate laryngoscopy and tracheal intubation, particularly in infants.[385] Cricoid pressure may also decrease upper and lower esophageal sphincter tone.[376,386] However, properly applied cricoid pressure can facilitate intubation with rapid-sequence induction and mask ventilation. Evidence suggests that the gastric residual volume in children undergoing emergency surgery is greater if a child is anesthetized within 4 hours of hospital admission (1.1 mL/kg).[387] If, on the other hand, surgery can be delayed for at least 4 hours, then the mean gastric residual volume is on average much less (0.51 mL/kg)[387]; this gastric residual volume is in fact similar to that observed in children who have fasted for routine surgical procedures (Fig. 4-9).[1] This does not imply that these children should not be regarded as having a full stomach; rather, the risk may be somewhat reduced if surgery can be delayed several hours. In addition, there is evidence to suggest that in emergency cases the size of the gastric residual volume (mL/kg) is in part dependent on the time interval between the last food ingestion and the timing of the injury. Children who last ate more than 4 hours before injury, as a group, have a gastric residual volume similar to those who fasted as if it were elective surgery (Fig. 4-10). *There is some comfort in these numbers, but one should never consider such children as not having a full stomach but rather as having a less full stomach.* Additionally, the possible value of H_2-blocking agents, metoclopramide, and clear antacids may be considered but their use in this regard is not evidence based. A modified rapid-sequence induction may be preferred in small infants who will likely develop oxyhemoglobin desaturation during brief periods of apnea and will therefore require assisted ventilation before intubating the trachea. Neonates may be intubated awake if indicated; this may provide a greater margin of safety because it preserves spontaneous ventilation as well as

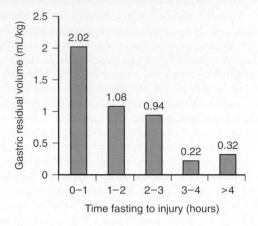

Figure 4-10. Mean gastric residual volume is plotted against time from last food ingestion to time of injury. These data suggest that the longer the time from ingestion to injury, the lower the risk for pulmonary aspiration of gastric contents. Also, if more than 4 hours has elapsed between the time of last food ingestion and time of injury, the risk is similar to that for patients with routine fasting. However, even with a 4-hour fasting time period, these patients must still be treated as though they have a full stomach. (Data abstracted from Bricker SRW, McLuckie A, Nightingale DA: Gastric aspirates after trauma in children. Anesthesia 1989; 44:721-724.)

laryngeal reflexes. Skillfully performed awake intubation in neonates is not generally associated with significant adverse cardiovascular responses and may be preferred in infants with hemodynamic instability.[388]

Special Problems

The Fearful Child

This is a difficult problem with no good solution. The child's fear is generally based on the unknowns of the hospital environment or the impending surgery. That is why it is so vital that as much information as possible is presented and queries as to why the child is afraid are so important. Frequently, just a few well-directed questions and honest answers will resolve many of the child's concerns. Often simply allowing a parent to hold a child during induction or allowing the child to hold the anesthetic mask themselves will stop the flow of tears. In other situations, one commonly practiced solution is to use intramuscular ketamine.

Anemia

The minimum hematocrit necessary to ensure adequate oxygen transport in children has not been well established. Preoperative hemoglobin testing, however, is of limited value in healthy children undergoing elective surgery when minimal blood loss is expected.[389] Children with chronic anemia, such as those with renal failure, do not require preoperative transfusion because of compensatory mechanisms, such as increased 2,3-diphosphoglycerate, increased oxygen extraction, and cardiac output. Elective surgery for children who are anemic should take into consideration the medical history, underlying diseases (hemoglobinopathies, von Willebrand, sickle cell, other factor deficiency), the nature of the surgery, and its urgency. Most pediatric anesthesiologists would recommend a hematocrit

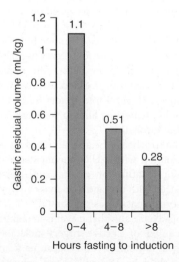

Figure 4-9. Mean gastric residual volume is plotted against hours of fasting before anesthetic induction in emergency pediatric cases. These data suggest that a 4-hour fast, if it does not compromise patient safety, may reduce gastric residual volume and therefore reduce (but not eliminate) risk for aspiration. (Data abstracted from Schurizek BA, Rybro L, Boggild-Madsen NB, Juhl B: Gastric volume and pH in children for emergency surgery. Acta Anaesthesiol Scand 1986; 30:404-408.)

greater than 25% before elective surgery in the absence of chronic disease. If significant blood loss is anticipated and the surgery is elective, then the cause of anemia should be investigated and treated and the surgery postponed until the hematocrit is restored to the normal range. *Healthy children scheduled for elective surgery that is not expected to cause substantive bleeding should not routinely receive a blood transfusion just to bring their hematocrit to 30%.*

Physiologic anemia of infancy occurs between 2 and 4 months of age. At this time there is an increased production of hemoglobin A and an increase in red cell 2,3-diphosphoglycerate, which contribute to a right shift of the oxygen-hemoglobin dissociation curve (see Chapter 9). Therefore, in infants 2 to 4 months of age, a reduced hemoglobin value is acceptable. Anemia, with a hematocrit of less than 30%, in former preterm infants represents a special category of patients who may have an increased incidence of postoperative apnea (see later), but transfusion is still not recommended.[390]

Upper Respiratory Tract Infection

Most anesthesiologists agree that the presence of an acute purulent URI, fever, change in mental state/behavior, or signs pertaining to a lower respiratory tract infection (i.e., wheezing and rales) are sufficient grounds to postpone elective surgery. However, the child with a nonpurulent active or recent URI (within 4 weeks) often presents a conundrum, even for the most experienced anesthesiologist.

It has been documented that 20% to 30% of all children have a runny nose during a significant part of the year. In the preanesthetic evaluation, we must rely on history, physical examination, and, rarely, laboratory data to decide whether to proceed with the anesthetic. A differential diagnosis of a child with a runny nose is presented in Table 4-10.

The perioperative and postoperative risks of anesthetizing children with URIs are incompletely understood. In part, this stems from study bias in that procedures for many children with symptomatic URIs are cancelled before the day of surgery, thus

Table 4-10. Differential Diagnosis of a Child with a Runny Nose

Noninfectious Causes
Allergic rhinitis: seasonal, perennial, clear nasal discharge no fever
Vasomotor rhinitis: emotional (crying), temperature changes
Infectious Causes
Viral infections
Nasopharyngitis (common cold)
Flu syndrome (upper and lower respiratory tract)
Laryngotracheal bronchitis (infectious croup)
Viral exanthems
Measles
Chickenpox
Acute bacterial infections
Acute epiglottitis
Meningitis
Streptococcal tonsillitis

precluding them from the studies. Another difficulty is the variable definition of a URI, which limits the external validity of these studies. Finally, study design flaws or inadequacies including retrospective studies, nonrandomized, and nonblinded studies have created inconsistencies among the published results.

A number of perioperative risks have been studied. The risk of postintubation croup was similar in children who had an active URI and those who did not. However, some children in that study had "tight-fitting" endotracheal tubes, which may have confounded the results.[391] Intraoperative complications including atelectasis and cyanosis were evaluated in a series of children with a history of a recent URI. Very severe complications were occasionally associated with the administration of anesthesia in those with recently infected airways. However, this study was retrospective in design and lacked a case/matched control population.[392] In another study, the incidence of intraoperative complications in children with a URI who were anesthetized was similar to that in children without a URI.[393] This study included children with an active URI at the time of anesthesia and some whose tracheas were intubated. However, they did report a greater incidence of respiratory complications in those who had recently had a URI. As in the previous study, this was a retrospective study. In a prospective cohort study of 489 children who were scheduled for myringotomy and tube placement, 50% underwent anesthesia and surgery for chronic ear infection and 50% were matched, nonanesthetized controls. There was no increased morbidity from face mask general anesthesia in this instance.[394] However, it is difficult to evaluate this study because bronchospasm would not be expected without endotracheal intubation.[395,396] Bronchospasm appears to occur more frequently in a child whose trachea is intubated and who has an active URI.[396] In a large study of 24,500 children, the incidence of bronchospasm in children with a URI (41:1000) was 10-fold greater than in those without a URI. Mechanical stimulation of the airway appeared to be an important contributory factor.[395] The incidence of laryngospasm in children with a URI (96:1000) is fivefold greater than it is in children without a URI (17:1000).[397] The incidence of minor but not major intraoperative hemoglobin desaturation events is greater in children with a URI than in those without a URI.[396] In another large study, the incidence of all respiratory-related adverse events combined in children with a URI was 9-fold greater than in those without a URI and 11-fold greater in children who had both a URI and required tracheal intubation.[398]

When the endotracheal tube and laryngeal mask airway were compared in children with a URI, the incidence of mild bronchospasm, major desaturation events, and overall respiratory events was reduced with the laryngeal mask airway although the incidence of laryngospasm was similar.[399,400]

Predictors of adverse anesthetic events in children with a URI who were scheduled for elective surgery included airway management (tracheal intubation > laryngeal mask airway), parent states that the child has a "cold," nasal congestion, snoring, passive smoking, induction agent (thiopental > halothane > sevoflurane ~ propofol), sputum production, and whether the neuromuscular agent was antagonized.[401] Propofol depresses laryngeal reflexes and may decrease airway responsiveness by relaxation of bronchial smooth muscle.[402,403] Several variables, including wheezing, fever, malaise, and age could not be excluded as predictors of adverse events because procedures in some children were deferred or cancelled after their preoperative visit.

A second study identified a similar set of predictors for adverse events in children with URI as those just mentioned.[404] Three children with a recent or active URI required unanticipated admission to hospital. Logistic regression determined that childhood risk factors associated with adverse outcomes included copious secretions ($P = .0001$), ex-premature infants ($P = .007$), nasal congestion ($P = .014$), passive (parental) smoking ($P = .018$), and reactive airway disease ($P = .028$). ASA status did not correlate with adverse outcomes. Age in the presence of a URI has not been an independent predictor of adverse events in most studies, although this study demonstrated that infants younger than 6 months old with active URIs had a greater incidence of bronchospasm (20.8 vs. 4.7%, $P = .08$) than older children.[404] This same study also demonstrated that the incidence of oxygen desaturation was greater in children younger than 2 years of age than older children (21.5 vs. 12.5%, $P = .023$). Endotracheal intubation in children younger than 5 years of age was an independent risk factor for postoperative respiratory adverse events ($P = .0002$).[404] Neither the duration of anesthesia nor the depth of anesthesia at the time of extubation (awake vs. deep) was identified as a risk factor. Children with active URIs who were anesthetized and maintained with sevoflurane had the smallest incidence of adverse events. The incidence of adverse respiratory events in children undergoing airway surgery was the greatest (e.g., tonsillectomy and adenoidectomy, direct laryngoscopy, and bronchoscopy). This study concluded that children with active and recent URIs (within 4 weeks) are at increased risk for adverse respiratory events, particularly if there was a history of reactive airway disease, of surgery that involved the airway, or of prematurity or passive smoke inhalation, nasal congestion or copious secretions, or requirement for an endotracheal tube.

In another study that examined the risk factors for adverse anesthetic events in children with URIs, adverse respiratory events were greater in children who were premedicated with midazolam, in children who were extubated while deeply anesthetized, or in children who had peak URI symptoms that occurred within the preceding 4 weeks. However, specific preoperative symptoms were not useful in predicting respiratory adverse events during emergence from anesthesia.[405]

Cancellation of cardiac surgery carries special import because of the risk that the child's heart will deteriorate or the disease process will progress (i.e., pulmonary hypertension) as well as the extensive time, materials, and personnel committed to a planned case. In a prospective study of children scheduled for cardiac surgery, the incidence of respiratory adverse events (29.2 vs. 17.3%, $P < .01$), multiple postoperative complications (25 vs. 10.3%, $P < .01$), and bacterial infection (5.2 vs. 1.0%, $P = .01$) were greater in those with a URI than in those without.[406] Logistic regression identified the presence of a URI as an independent risk factor for both postoperative infections and multiple postoperative complications. Although the duration of the ICU stay was greater for children with URIs (80 ± 90 vs. 60 ± 60 hours, $P < .01$), the duration of hospital stay was not (8.4 vs. 7.8 days, $P > .05$).

A national survey suggested that more experienced anesthesiologists are less likely to cancel surgery because of the presence of a URI.[407] In one survey, 40% of anesthesiologists with less than 10 years in practice reported "seldom" (1%-25% of time) cancel-

ing because of a URI compared with 27% of those with more than 10 years' experience. Cancellation may also impose emotional and economic burdens on the parents.[408,409] Factors that should be considered when deciding whether to proceed with elective surgery in a child with a URI are summarized in Table 4-11.

On the basis of the best evidence available at the present time, a child with a mild URI that is not of acute onset may be safely anesthetized for minor surgical procedures; if an endotracheal tube is required, then the risk of bronchospasm, laryngospasm, and desaturation events increases.[391,393-398,401,404] It is reassuring to note that most such adverse perioperative events are not associated with significant morbidity; that is, the severity of oxygen hemoglobin desaturation is similar in children with and without a URI.[396] Such children may also be more susceptible to mild episodes of oxygen desaturation in the recovery room. Once again, these episodes are readily treated with supplemental oxygen administration.[410]

Insofar as which techniques will help to prevent complications from a URI, pretreating healthy ASA I or II children with no lung disease having noncavity, nonairway surgery of less than 3 hours' duration with bronchodilators before anesthesia (either inhaled ipratropium or albuterol) provided no benefit. These children had either a URI within the preceding 6 weeks or an active URI. In addition there was no association between either a recent URI or an active URI and desaturation, wheezing, coughing, stridor, or laryngospasm causing desaturation in this select group.[411] Humidification, intravenous hydration, and anticholinergics may decrease complications,[407] although the results of at least one study suggested that glycopyrrolate did not reduce the incidence of perioperative adverse respiratory events when it was given after induction of anesthesia to children with URIs.[412]

It is prudent to consider postponing anesthesia in children with an active URI, which includes any one of the following: fever (>38.5°C), a recent onset of purulent nasal discharge, or "wet" cough, because this may represent a prodrome of a more serious or infectious illness (chickenpox, measles), systemic

Table 4-11. Factors Affecting Decision for Elective Surgery in Child with Upper Respiratory Tract Infection

Pro	Con
• Child has "just a runny nose," no other symptoms, "much better"	• Parents confirm symptoms: fever, malaise, cough, poor appetite, just developed symptoms last night
• Active and happy child	• Lethargic, ill-appearing
• Clear rhinorrhea	• Purulent nasal discharge
• Clear lungs	• Wheezing, rales
• Older child	• Child <1 year, ex-premie
• Social issues: hardship for parents to be away from work, insurance will run out	• Other factors: history of reactive airway disease, major operation, endotracheal tube required

Modified from Bailey AG, Badgwell JM: Common and uncommon coexisting diseases that complicate pediatric anesthesia. In Badgwell JM (ed): Clinical Pediatric Anesthesia. Philadelphia, Lippincott-Raven, 1997, p 383.

symptoms (not behaving normally, not eating), and those with lower respiratory tract symptoms (wheezing that does not clear with coughing). If a child is recovering from a URI, the child's physical examination should be near normal. If this is true, anesthesia can generally proceed without increasing the risks substantively. However, if the child with a URI requires prolonged endotracheal intubation, the clinician must use his or her judgment and experience together with consultation with the parents and surgeon to determine whether to proceed with or postpone anesthesia.[395-397,407,413]

If the decision is to postpone anesthesia, then how long should one wait before undertaking general anesthesia? Bronchial hyperreactivity, which is associated with URIs in children, shows spirometric changes in the lungs as late as 7 weeks after a URI.[413,414] Although these studies suggest that surgery should be postponed for at least 7 weeks after resolution of a URI, this plan is not practical because most children will be infected with a new URI by that time.

Postponing surgery until 2 weeks after resolution of the URI is a common but as yet unproven strategy. In fact, some data suggest that the incidence of adverse respiratory events is just as great in this population as it is in those who were anesthetized during the acute phase of the URI.[394,415] This 2-week waiting period may be acceptable in a child with uncomplicated nasopharyngitis.[416] Unfortunately, there is no consensus on the optimal time interval before surgery is rescheduled. In a survey of anesthesiologists, most wait 3 to 4 weeks before proceeding with surgery.[407] The rationale for this time period is that the risk of respiratory complications remains for 4 to 6 weeks.[404]

In conclusion, there is risk to anesthesia even in children without URIs. In children with a URI we must wait 4 to 6 weeks or longer to decrease these risks back to baseline. Therefore, in children who have had a URI we can tailor our anesthetic to further decrease these risks (propofol, laryngeal mask airway, or face mask instead of endotracheal tube) but the risk cannot be reduced to zero. Good judgment, common sense, clinical experience, and informed consent from the parents or guardians must be used when deciding whether to proceed or postpone the surgery. All of these deliberations and discussions including the risks and benefits should be documented in the chart (see Chapter 11 for additional discussion and perspectives).

Asymptomatic Cardiac Murmurs

The presence of a cardiac murmur is a common finding in children[417] and may have significant anesthetic implications. Never underestimate the potential implications of a newly diagnosed heart murmur. Generally, nonpathologic murmurs occur during systole and are soft and nonradiating with normal feel to peripheral pulses; there are normal blood pressures in both upper and lower extremities. However, if there is a harsh murmur that is not localized or if there are bounding pulses, then further evaluation is warranted. At least several times per year, children present with a previously unrecognized murmur and have a serious underlying structural heart defect. Sometimes even the experienced cardiologist cannot make a correct diagnosis by physical examination; an echocardiogram is required. Further history should be obtained to delineate the nature of the murmur. In the majority of cases, the parents may report that the murmur was previously detected by the child's pediatrician and determined to be an innocent flow murmur without any anatomic or physiologic abnormalities. If the murmur has not been previ-

Table 4-12. Grading of Heart Murmurs

Grade I	Heard only with intense concentration
Grade II	Faint, but heard immediately
Grade III	Easily heard, of intermediate intensity
Grade IV	Easily heard, palpable thrill/vibration on chest wall
Grade V	Very loud, thrill present, audible with only edge of stethoscope on chest wall
Grade VI	Audible with stethoscope off the chest wall

Modified from Emmanouilides GC, Allen HD, Riemenschneider TA, Gutgesell HP: Moss and Adams Heart Disease in Infants, Children, and Adolescents Including the Fetus and Young Adult, 5th ed. Baltimore, Williams & Wilkins, 1995.

ously detected, referral to a pediatric cardiologist is indicated or an echocardiogram by an experienced pediatric echocardiographer should be obtained before induction of anesthesia.[418] An innocent murmur is rarely louder than grade II/VI, and is not usually accompanied by other findings (Tables 4-12 and 4-13).[419] When a pediatric cardiologist confirms the classic clinical features of an innocent murmur, it has been suggested that the echocardiogram seldom reveals heart disease especially with older age at presentation.[420] However, even an experienced cardiologist can occasionally make a misdiagnosis; the only certain means to exclude a structural defect within the heart is with an echocardiogram.[421]

Fever

The presence of a low-grade fever before elective surgery poses a dilemma whether to proceed with anesthesia or to delay. In general, if a child has only 0.5°C to 1.0°C of fever and no other symptoms, this degree of fever is not a contraindication to general anesthesia. However, if the fever is associated with a recent onset of rhinitis, pharyngitis, otitis media, dehydration, or any other sign of impending illness, it is more prudent to postpone the procedure. If the planned surgery is of an urgent nature, every effort should be made to reduce the fever before induction of anesthesia, primarily to reduce oxygen demands. Reduction of the fever should not include aspirin, because it may interfere with platelet function and is associated with Reye syndrome. Ibuprofen may be associated with an increase in bleeding time[281] and should be avoided before surgery. On the

Table 4-13. Symptoms and Signs of Heart Disease

- Feeding difficulties: disinterest, fatigue, diaphoresis, tachypnea, dyspnea
- Poor exercise tolerance
- Tachypnea, dyspnea, grunting, nasal flaring, and intercostal, suprasternal, or subcostal retractions
- Frequent respiratory tract infections (a result of compression of airways by plethoric vessels leading to stasis of secretions and atelectasis)
- Central cyanosis (involving warm mucous membranes: tongue and buccal mucosa) or poor capillary refill
- Absent or abnormal peripheral pulses

Modified from Pelech AN: Evaluation of the pediatric patient with a cardiac murmur. Pediatr Clin North Am 1999; 46:167-188.

other hand, acetaminophen has no effect on platelet function and is an excellent antipyretic. It is rapidly absorbed when administered orally, producing adequate blood concentrations within several minutes. In contrast, rectal administration requires at least 60 minutes to achieve a significant blood concentration.[267,422] There is no evidence that an existing fever predisposes to a malignant hyperthermic reaction.[423]

Sickle Cell Disease

Whenever a child presents with either sickle cell disease (Hgb SS) or trait (Hgb Ss), the anesthetic and postanesthetic management must be modified (see Chapters 9 and 11).[424-445] It is important to obtain a complete family history and a sickle cell preparation if the child has not been previously tested. If the sickle cell preparation is positive and the surgery is elective, then a formal hemoglobin electrophoresis is indicated to more carefully delineate the nature of the hemoglobinopathy. It must be emphasized that the status of hydration and oxygenation is critical in all children with sickle cell disease or trait. Thus, a secure intravenous route with hydration of at least one and a half times maintenance is recommended well into the postoperative period, especially after procedures in which ileus may result (third-space losses). Meticulous attention to details to ensure a stable cardiovascular and ventilatory status establishes adequate oxygenation to prevent sickling. Pulse oximetry is of particular value in managing these children by providing an early warning of developing desaturation. Children with hemoglobin SC are especially at risk because they have a relatively normal hemoglobin level yet are extremely vulnerable to sickling and the complications of sickle cell crisis (see Chapter 9).[426,446]

Preoperative Transfusion

Because vaso-occlusive crises occur more frequently in the perioperative period, consideration should be given toward optimizing their care and anesthetic management. In a study of 54 children with sickle cell disease who were not transfused before 66 elective procedures, no intraoperative deaths occurred, although 26% had postoperative complications.[447] These data suggested that children who are scheduled for low-risk procedures do not require preoperative transfusions, whereas those who are scheduled for high-risk procedures (e.g., thoracotomy, laparotomy, or tonsillectomy and adenoidectomy) should be transfused preoperatively to a hemoglobin concentration of 10 g/dL. A large multi-institutional study reported that the incidence of sickle cell–related complications in children who were transfused to a hemoglobin value of 10 g/dL was reduced compared with those not transfused, although children in the transfusion group developed new antibodies. This could present difficulties for future crossmatching.[431,448] Single-unit transfusions or partial exchange transfusions appear to be as effective as full exchange transfusions.[434,448-450] Children with sickle cell disease should have a hematologic consultation preoperatively to assess the child's risk for perioperative complications and the need for transfusion (see Chapter 9).

Cognitively Impaired Children

Cognitively impaired children may be challenging to anesthetize because we often cannot explain the nature of the surgery and are unable to reassure them. A bad hospital experience can greatly magnify the difficulties of future admissions. Therefore, the care of these children requires the utmost in patience, understanding, preparation, and cooperation among the family, pediatrician, surgeon, anesthesiologist, and nursing staff. These children frequently have extensive medical and surgical histories and may be transported from a chronic care facility. Often they are wards of the state and require special consent for surgery and anesthesia; advanced planning is required if a caudal, epidural, or local block is planned for pain relief.

A complete history and a physical examination are essential before anesthetizing these children. Cognitive and communication problems may make this more difficult. Parents and caretakers are best to be involved during this period not only to gain information but also to allay the fears of the child. Postoperative analgesia is also important to discuss at this time because inadequate analgesia, anxiety, fear, and poor communication can lead to an increase in postoperative muscle spasms and pain. It is vital to obtain the medical records to become familiar with underlying present and past medical conditions; this can be particularly difficult if care has not been provided at a single institution.

Gastrointestinal reflux is common and may cause chronic respiratory problems. Salivary drooling due to pseudobulbar palsy with impaired swallowing may lead to aspiration. Medical treatment with anticholinergics may be indicated.

Respiratory disease is a common cause of death. Recurrent pneumonias, pulmonary aspiration, and chronic lung disease are aggravated by the inability to cough and poor nutritional state that decreases the immune response. Reactive airway disease may be present owing to chronic reflux, and many of these children will have a permanent tracheostomy. Scoliosis may compound the problem with a restrictive lung pattern. Noisy breathing may be indicative of upper airway obstruction that may worsen on induction or postoperatively. Patients may need frequent suctioning of the endotracheal tube to clear secretions.

Epilepsy occurs in 30% of children with cerebral palsy. Anticonvulsant therapy should be continued up to and including the day of surgery. Phenytoin, valproic acid, and phenobarbital may be given intravenously if needed (see Chapter 22).

Medical Therapy

Baclofen is a GABA receptor agonist with action in the dorsal horn of the spinal cord; it is commonly used to reduce the pain associated with muscle spasms and to delay development of contractures. It can be given intrathecally via an implantable pump, thus allowing a lower dose and fewer side effects, and should be continued during surgery. Baclofen is rarely implicated in delayed awakening, bradycardia, or hypotension during general anesthesia. Abrupt withdrawal can result in seizures, hallucinations, itching, and disorientation lasting up to 72 hours. Side effects such as urinary retention and hypotension may respond to reducing the dose.

Sedation may be valuable to decrease anxiety for both the parent and child, but children with poor pharyngeal coordination may need special precautions. Antacids, antiemetics, and drugs to reduce secretions may also be indicated. If premedication is chosen, oral midazolam, 0.25 to 0.5 mg/kg, or oral ketamine, 3 to 6 mg/kg, with atropine, 0.02 to 0.03 mg/kg, or glycopyrrolate, 0.02 mg/kg, may be considered.[451] Some anticonvulsants induce CYP450 3A4, thus reducing the effectiveness of the standard dosing of midazolam. Topical local anesthetics may be useful if an intravenous line will be started

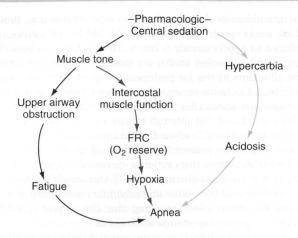

Figure 4-15. Pharmacologic interventions may result in several sequences of events leading to apnea. FRC, functional residual capacity.

techniques may offer an advantage, but apnea has also been associated with regional anesthesia techniques.[464,485,486] In a study comparing spinal and general anesthesia, the desaturation and bradycardia incidents but not apnea were reduced in the spinal group.[477] Another study of 55 preterm and former preterm infants with a mean postconceptual age of 43.3 weeks, half with coexisting disease, the incidence of postoperative apnea was 9.1%.[487] In a review of four studies that utilized regional (spinal, epidural, caudal) versus general anesthesia in former preterm infants undergoing inguinal herniorrhaphy in early infancy, there was no convincing evidence to support the use of spinal anesthesia as part of the standard practice in inguinal herniorrhaphy, although there was some evidence that spinal anesthesia reduced the incidence of postoperative apnea in an infant population who were not given additional sedation.[488] Spinal anesthesia is also associated with a significant failure rate or the need for multiple attempts to achieve accurate placement of the needle.[489,490] However, in an institution that routinely performs spinal anesthesia in infants, the success rate of placing a spinal block was 97.4% and an adequate level of spinal anesthesia was achieved in 95.4% of patients. Oxygen hemoglobin desaturation to less than 90% was noted in 0.6% and bradycardia (heart rate <100 beats per minute) in 1.6% of infants.[491] In addition, additives to prolong the duration of a spinal or caudal block such as clonidine have been associated with apnea.[492-495] In a study of 262 preterm infants (gestational age <37 weeks and postconceptual age <60 weeks) undergoing inguinal hernia repair with spinal anesthesia, the rate of perioperative apnea was 4.9%. All of these infants were inpatients undergoing therapy for apnea, with one third having supplemental anesthesia. Of the 103 infants who were managed on an outpatient basis after surgery (mean gestational age 33 weeks and mean postconceptual age <44.3 weeks), 39 had a history of apnea and none developed apnea postoperatively. The major flaw in this study is that none of the infants had apnea monitoring at home, so postoperative apneic episodes that could have resulted in hypoxic injury but not death could have gone undetected. In addition, the infants were not randomized to general or spinal anesthesia and the study was likely underpowered.[496] *In summary, these infants must not be anesthetized as outpatients even when a regional technique has been utilized; they still require postoperative monitoring for apnea.*

There is no consensus among anesthesiologists of the age beyond which the risk of perioperative apnea is zero in former preterm infants. This is a matter of balancing risks and benefits. The risk of developing perioperative apnea in former preterm infants who are not anemic (hemoglobin <10 g/dL) and who did not develop apnea in a postanesthesia care unit exceeds 1 in 200 (0.5%) until about 55 weeks' postconceptual age. Former preterm infants who have major organ surgery and/or preexisting major organ dysfunction (e.g., periventricular hemorrhage, bronchopulmonary dysplasia) may be at greater risk for developing perioperative apnea and therefore may benefit from extended postanesthesia monitoring. We recommend, and most institutions use, a criterion for admission of former preterm infants after surgery for infants who are younger than 60 weeks' postconceptual age.

With respect to full-term neonates, three reports have described infants who have developed apnea after an apparently uneventful general anesthetic procedure.[497-499] Thus, if a full-term infant who is younger than 44 weeks' postconceptual age demonstrates any abnormality of respiration after anesthesia, it is reasonable to admit the infant for further evaluation. The algorithms in Figure 4-16 can be used as a decision tree for outpatient surgery in the term and former preterm infant.

Bronchopulmonary Dysplasia

Bronchopulmonary dysplasia (BPD) is a form of chronic lung disease associated with prolonged mechanical ventilation and oxygen toxicity in the preterm neonate. Antenatal glucocorticosteroid, early surfactant therapy, and gentler modalities of ventilation currently utilized have minimized the severity of lung injury than was previously seen (see Chapters 11 and 36).

The clinical manifestations of BPD are tachypnea, dyspnea, and airway hyperactivity and oxygen dependence. These infants suffer from hypoxemia, hypercarbia, abnormal functional airway growth, tracheomalacia, bronchomalacia, subglottic stenosis, increased pulmonary vascular resistance, and congestive heart failure.[500-502] Pulmonary function abnormalities, including a reduced functional residual capacity, reduced diffusion capacity, airway obstruction, and reduced exercise tolerance may persist into the school-aged years. Many of these children also suffer neurodevelopmental problems and seizures due to intraventricular hemorrhage or hypoxic insults.[503-505] Some may have a cardiomyopathy due to corticosteroid therapy in the neonatal period or the combination of corticosteroid therapy and viral infections[506]; others may have systemic hypertension.[507] These children are often discharged home on oxygen therapy,[508] diuretics (pulmonary interstitial edema increases the possibility of respiratory failure),[509] and β_2 agonists. Hyperinflation and areas of increased density are often seen on chest radiographs.

Adequate preoperative preparation should focus on optimizing oxygenation, reducing airway hyperactivity, and correcting electrolyte abnormalities due to chronic diuretic therapy. These children require special attention to fluid balance with careful titration of intraoperative fluids. In addition, chronic air trapping should alert the anesthesiologist to the potential dangers of nitrous oxide. It is important to allow adequate expiratory time and to avoid excessive positive-pressure ventilation. Subglottic stenosis may be present owing to the prolonged

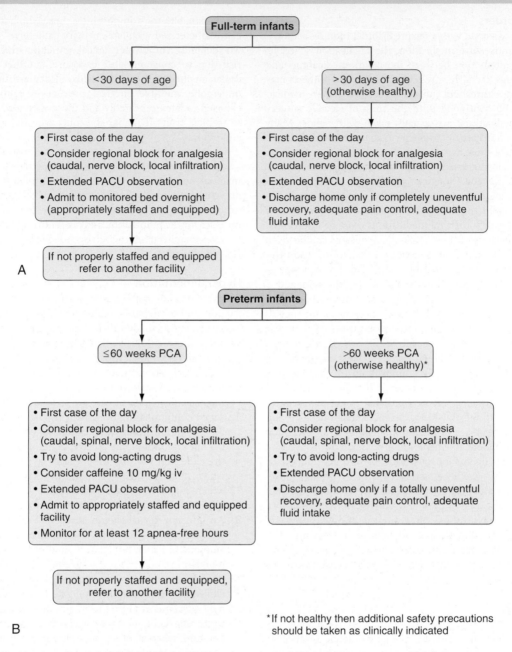

Figure 4-16. Algorithms used as a decision tree for outpatient surgery in term (**A**) and former preterm (**B**) infants.

intubation of these infants, potentially necessitating the use of a smaller endotracheal tube. The avoidance of tracheal intubation by using a laryngeal mask airway, when appropriate, may offer some advantage in reducing the incidence of coughing, wheezing, and hoarseness.[510] Spinal anesthesia for some procedures (e.g., inguinal hernia repair) may provide an acceptable alternative technique, avoiding the need for tracheal intubation. Chronic hypercarbia is often present.

Diabetes

Diabetes mellitus is the most common endocrine problem encountered in children. Preoperative assessment should include a thorough knowledge of the child's insulin schedule. The preoperative fasting time should be the same as that recommended for nondiabetics. Every attempt should be made to schedule a diabetic child as the first case of the day to minimize the fasting period (see earlier).

Several protocols have been advocated for glycemic control in diabetics. An intravenous infusion that contains 5% glucose at maintenance infusion rate should be started to avoid hypoglycemia. Half the normal insulin dosage is usually administered on the morning of surgery *after* the intravenous infusion is started: 5% glucose at the maintenance rate is continued throughout the surgical procedure. Serum glucose concentrations should be monitored both intraoperatively and postoperatively until the child is back on a routine schedule.[511] More detailed discussion of the perioperative management of the child with diabetes is addressed in Chapter 24.

Seizure Disorders

Management of a child with a seizure disorder requires a knowledge of the antiseizure medication, the medication schedule, and possible interaction between the child's medications and anesthetic drugs.[512-518] The stress of surgery and anesthesia may lower the seizure threshold and cause a seizure. Seizure medications should be continued until the time of elective surgery unless the medications are usually taken with solids. Many seizure medications are not available in an intravenous formulation. Fortunately, most have long therapeutic half-lives (24 to 36 hours) so that dosing usually can restart the night after surgery or the next day. Medications can also be given through a gastrointestinal tube, if present, unless the surgery involves the bowel. If the child requires strict pharmacologic control of a seizure disorder or if the oral medications must be interrupted for extended periods of time, oral anticonvulsants can be given intravenously (or equivalent substitute medications if intravenous formulations are not available). The adequacy of preoperative anticonvulsant blood levels should be assessed and a perioperative management plan developed with the child's neurologist (see Chapter 22). Blood concentrations of anticonvulsant drugs may need to be monitored postoperatively to ensure proper therapeutic effect, especially if the procedure has been associated with significant blood loss.[519-521] Most anesthetic and analgesic agents can be safely administered to children with seizure disorders. It is important to know the nature of the seizure disorder to avoid medications that might precipitate a seizure (e.g., methohexital can exacerbate temporal lobe epilepsy).[175] Multiple doses of meperidine could be an exception because its metabolite, normeperidine, possesses proconvulsant properties. Other agents, nitrous oxide, sevoflurane, etomidate, and some opioids have been associated with seizure-like movements in both healthy children and those with epilepsy, without serious sequelae. Some of these movements were more likely a benign form of myoclonus. Most anesthetic medications are anticonvulsant (sodium thiopental) or have little to no effect (propofol) on the seizure threshold. Virtually all general anesthetic agents are anticonvulsants in doses associated with loss of consciousness.

Latex Allergy

Latex is the most common cause of intraoperative anaphylactic reactions in children.[522] An IgE-mediated allergic reaction to latex may be severe and life threatening. The clinical manifestations of intraoperative reactions may differ from those of anaphylactic or anaphylactoid reactions outside of anesthesia; cutaneous manifestations are far less common. A delay in diagnosis may make treatment more difficult. In the preoperative history, it is crucial to inquire about previous exposure and sensitivity to latex but even in those without a history, it is important to ask whether the child can put a toy balloon to the lips or whether his or her tongue swells when the dentist places a rubber dam in the mouth. These simple queries may unexpectedly reveal a susceptibility to latex allergy. Those at risk for anaphylaxis to latex include children with neural tube defects (spina bifida, meningomyelocele), children with urinary tract anomalies who require frequent bladder catheterization, those with an immunologic predisposition (atopic individuals), those having undergone multiple surgeries, and health care workers who are exposed to latex.[523] Children with spina bifida have an increased risk if they have had more than six surgeries and/or

atopic skin, but, most importantly, those who have been chronically catheterized with latex urinary catheters.[524] Also, children who depend on home mechanical ventilation may be at increased risk due to constant latex exposure.[525] Other children who are at an increased risk for latex allergy are those who have undergone multiple surgical procedures and are therefore exposed to latex repeatedly and those with a history of allergy to tropical fruits (banana, chestnut, avocado, kiwi, pineapple, and others).[526-528]

It has been shown that pretreatment with antihistamines and corticosteroids successfully prevents reactions to radiocontrast material, but this same preventative treatment does not reliably prevent anaphylactic reactions to latex.[523,529] Avoidance of latex exposure (latex-free environment) is the most important measure for the preparation and prevention of latex anaphylaxis. If a latex anaphylactic reaction occurs, the treatment is epinephrine administration.

Hyperalimentation

Intravenous alimentation is frequently used as a means of life support and to prepare children for surgery. It is important for anesthesiologists to identify the composition and rate of administration of these fluids so that potential intraoperative complications can be avoided. Most of these solutions are hypertonic, have a high glucose content, and must be administered through a centrally placed intravenous route.

The basic principles of care are as follows:

1. Avoid contaminating the line. It is best not to puncture the line for administering medications or changing fluid.
2. Do not discontinue the glucose-containing solution because the child will then be in a relative hyperinsulinemic state, which might result in profound hypoglycemia, the signs of which might be masked by general anesthesia. Intralipid infusions should be discontinued before surgery.
3. An infusion device should be used at all times so that the rate of infusion is constant. Accidental rapid infusion of large amounts of hyperalimentation fluid may cause a hypertonic nonketotic coma.[530] There is no consensus on the intraoperative management of hyperalimentation solutions. Some clinicians reduce the infusion rate by 33% to 50% to avoid hyperglycemia resulting from a reduced metabolic rate due to the effects of anesthetic agents and a reduced body temperature, whereas others leave the infusion rate unchanged to avoid intraoperative hypoglycemia.
4. Perioperative and intraoperative monitoring of glucose, potassium, sodium, and calcium, as well as acid-base status, is important for long procedures.
5. Preoperative confirmation of correct intravascular line placement (radiograph or aspiration of blood) is important to avoid intraoperative complications such as hydrothorax or hemothorax.

Asthma and Reactive Airway Disease

Children with reactive airway disease or asthma who are scheduled for elective surgery should be free of wheezing.[531,532] Key considerations in the evaluation of the child with reactive airway disease include previous anesthetic history, allergies, cough or sputum production, medication regimen, hospital and emergency department visits (intubation or intravenous infusions), and level of activity. Physical examination should include attention to vital signs, wheezing, cough, type of breath sounds, use of accessory muscles, cyanosis, altered mental state, and level of hydration. Baseline measurements of the preoperative oxygen saturation in room air are useful particularly for the purposes of determining preexisting hypoxemia. Laboratory data may be unnecessary unless an acute infection is suspected. A baseline electrocardiogram and chest radiograph may be of value for a severely asthmatic child who may have chronic air trapping, pulmonary hypertension, pulmonary blebs, or pneumonitis. All medications should be maintained up to and including the morning of surgery so that the child is receiving optimal bronchodilator treatment.[533-536]

Preoperative preparation for mild asthma should include the administration of a nebulized β_2-adrenergic agonist 1 to 2 hours before surgery. For moderate asthma, additional optimization with any inhaled anti-inflammatory agent and regular use of nebulized β_2 agonists 1 week before surgery can be instituted. Severe asthmatics should visit their physician just before the scheduled surgery to optimize therapy; some children benefit from short-term oral corticosteroid therapy for several days before surgery.[533,537] Severe asthmatics may benefit from the addition of oral prednisone 3 to 5 days before surgery or oral dexamethasone for 2 days before surgery (see Chapter 11).[533,538]

Because the insertion of an endotracheal tube into the trachea is a common cause of bronchospasm, it may be prudent to avoid tracheal intubation and use a laryngeal mask airway in asthmatics. A laryngeal mask airway should not be used, however, if complete control of the airway is essential for the safe conduction of anesthesia and surgery. Having the child use a β_2-adrenergic agonist inhaler before the induction of anesthesia as well as establishing a deep plane of anesthesia before tracheal intubation may decrease the risk of bronchospasm that can occur with intubation.[539]

When elective or emergent surgery is required, a means for administering a bronchodilator through the endotracheal tube or laryngeal mask airway must be available. Specific adaptors allow the interface of metered-dose inhalers with the intact anesthesia circuit. These adapters are particularly helpful for timing delivery of drug during inspiration and much more effective in drug delivery than simply spraying the drug down an endotracheal tube but without the special adapter (see Figs. 11-10 and 37-11). However, delivered efficiency of albuterol by metered-dose inhaler through 3.0- to 6.0-mm tracheal tubes is poor (2.5%-12.3% of discharged dose) and can be dramatically increased by actuating the canister through a distally placed catheter.[540]

Emergency surgery may require general anesthesia despite the presence of continued bronchospasm (see Chapter 37). In this situation, the urgency of the operation must be balanced against the severity of the bronchospasm. Some control of bronchospasm should ideally be instituted before induction of anesthesia (oxygen administration, hydration, subcutaneous epinephrine, β_2-agonist therapy, corticosteroids, and antibiotics).

Acknowledgment

We wish to thank John F. Ryan, MD, Letty M. P. Liu, I. D. Todres, MD, Nishan G. Goudsouzian, MD, and Leila Mei Pang, MD, for their prior contributions to these topics.

Annotated References

Birmingham PK, Tobin MJ, Henthorn TK, et al: Twenty-four-hour pharmacokinetics of rectal acetaminophen in children: an old drug with new recommendations. Anesthesiology 1997; 87:244-252

The current recommended dose of rectal acetaminophen of 10 to 15 mg/kg yields peak serum concentration less than the antipyretic of 10 to 20 μg/mL. Based on the observed kinetics, the recommended initial dose should be approximately 40 mg/kg.

Craven PD, Badawi N, Henderson-Smart DJ, O'Brien M: Regional (spinal, epidural, caudal) versus general anaesthesia in preterm infants undergoing inguinal herniorrhaphy in early infancy [review]. Cochrane Database Syst Rev 2003; CD003669

The review found that there is not enough evidence from trials to show whether spinal block improves outcome for a preterm infant having surgery for inguinal hernia.

Henderson-Smart DJ, Steer P: Prophylactic caffeine to prevent postoperative apnea following general anesthesia in preterm infants [review]. Cochrane Database Syst Rev 2001; CD000048.

Caffeine can be used to prevent postoperative apnea/bradycardia and episodes of oxygen desaturation in growing preterm infants if clinically necessary. There is a need to determine with further studies which infants might benefit most by this treatment.

Holzman RS: Clinical management of latex-allergic children. Anesth Analg 1997; 85:529-533

Latex allergic children can be safely anesthetized if exposure to latex in the medical environment is avoided and administration of prophylactic medication to decrease the response is unnecessary.

Skinner CM, Rangasami J: Preoperative use of herbal medicines: a patient survey. Br J Anaesth 2002; 89:792-795

Self-administration of herbal medicine is common in patients presenting for anesthesia. Because of the potential for side effects and drug interactions, it is important for anesthesiologist to be aware of their use. This is a good overview of herbal medicines and potential perioperative complications with their use.

Warner MA, Warner ME, Warner DO, et al: Perioperative pulmonary aspiration in infants and children. Anesthesiology 1999; 90: 66-71

The frequency of perioperative pulmonary aspiration in children is quite low. Serious respiratory morbidity is rare, and there were no associated deaths in this review. Infants and children with clinically apparent pulmonary aspiration in whom symptoms did not develop within 2 hours did not have respiratory sequelae.

References

Please see www.expertconsult.com

Ethical Issues in Pediatric Anesthesiology

David B. Waisel, Robert D. Truog, and I. David Todres

ETHICAL DILEMMAS OCCUR IN the practice of pediatric anesthesiology. Can parents refuse resuscitation for their 2-year-old with terminal cancer? Should a hysterical 12-year-old be held down for an intramuscular injection of ketamine to subdue him for anesthesia? Can we practice intubation skills on deceased children? What factors matter in making these determinations? Bioethics is designed to help the motivated physician identify and resolve dilemmas such as these. This chapter seeks to provide a framework for thinking about these problems.

Informed Consent

The doctrine of informed consent centers on the belief that patients have a right to self-determination. Physicians facilitate this right by explaining to the patient the risks, benefits, and alternatives to the procedure and obtaining from the patient an active, voluntary, informed authorization to perform a specific plan.[1] Components of the informed consent process include competence and decision-making capacity, disclosure, and autonomy (Table 5-1).[2]

All adult patients are considered to be competent to make decisions unless ruled otherwise by a judge. Decision-making capacity, on the other hand, refers to the ability to participate in health care decisions and it may vary, depending on the patient's age, situation, and the level of risk in the decision. For example, a patient who normally has decision-making capacity may have a decrement in that capacity after sedation. The patient then may be capable of making decisions involving lesser risks but not greater risks. A patient gives evidence of decision-making capacity by being able to appreciate one's situation, to understand the proposed procedure and the alternatives, and to communicate a decision based on internally coherent reasoning.

It is often difficult to know what information to disclose to a patient. In the United States, the reasonable person standard requires disclosure to be to the level that would be desired by the hypothetical reasonable person. This approach, however, does not define exactly what information should be given. Some suggest that the subjective person standard may be more successful at fulfilling the spirit of informed consent.[1] This standard holds that informed consent should be matched to the wants and needs of the individual person giving consent. While this may be considered the ideal form of disclosure, its greater ambiguity makes it difficult to use as a legal standard.

One of the difficulties in assessing the literature that discusses patient's desires for information and participation in decision-making is that there is no standardized method for studying these variables or communicating measurements. Nonetheless, examining the literature does permit the drawing of general conclusions, particularly that patients differ to the extent they prefer to receive information and to participate in decision-making.[3-6] Studies focusing on the desire for information about anesthesia also indicate that patients vary in their desire to receive information and participate in decision-making. A study of Scots and Canadians found that for men younger than 50 years of age, 73% to 85% wanted to know more information overall and 10% to 19% wanted to know less.[7] In men aged 50 and older, 45% to 73% wanted to know more overall, and 16% to 21% wanted to know less. Even though individuals younger than the age of 50 as a group wanted to know more information, 18% of Scottish men and 11% of Canadian men younger than the age of 50 wanted to know less information, and in men older than 50, 45% of Scottish men wanted to know more and 73% of Canadian men wanted to know more.

A study of surgical outpatients in a hospital in the northeastern United States found that more than 85% of patients preferred extensive information in a wide variety of areas such as alternate anesthetic methods, preoperative medication, dangerous and common complications, and the postoperative expectations.[8] On the other hand, 10% did not want to know about alternative methods for anesthesia, 7% did not want to know

Table 5-1. Elements of Consent and Assent as Defined by the American Academy of Pediatrics Committee on Bioethics

Consent

1. Adequate provision of information including the nature of the ailment or condition, the nature of the proposed diagnostic steps or treatment, and the probability of their success; the existence and nature of the risks involved; and the existence, potential benefits, and risks of recommended alternative treatments (including the choice of no treatment)

2. Assessment of the patient's understanding of the above information

3. Assessment, if only tacit, of the capacity of the patient or surrogate to make the necessary decisions

4. Assurance, insofar as it is possible, that the patient has the freedom to choose among the medical alternatives without coercion or manipulation

Assent

1. Helping the patient achieve a developmentally appropriate awareness of the nature of his or her condition

2. Telling the patient what he or she can expect with tests and treatment

3. Making a clinical assessment of the patient's understanding of the situation and the factors influencing how he or she is responding (including whether there is inappropriate pressure to accept testing or therapy)

4. Soliciting an expression of the patient's willingness to accept the proposed care

From Committee on Bioethics, American Academy of Pediatrics: Informed consent, parental permission, and assent in pediatric practice. Pediatrics 1995; 95:314-317.

about preoperative medications, 11% did not want to know all possible complications, 10% did not want to know dangerous complications, and 7% did not want to know common complications. The study also found that women wanted more information than men, divorced subjects wanted more information than single or married subjects, and a history of previous surgery in a relative increased the desire for information.

In a two-part survey of parents of minors who had not spoken to anesthesiologists, 87% wanted to know the risk of death and 13% did not.[9] Seventy-four percent of respondents wanted to know all possible risks of anesthesia, whereas 24% wanted to know only those likely to occur and 2% wanted to know only those that may result in a significant injury. In the second part of the study, if the anesthesiologists mentioned or implied the risk of death, 88% responded that they wanted to know the risk of death whereas 11% did not. In the group that did not mention or imply the risk of death, 38% responded that they did not want the risk of death discussed and 47% wished it had been discussed. In a study of information preferences for parents, 96% of parents either "liked to know" or believed they had a "right to know" all possible complications, whereas 4% would "prefer not to know."[10] In some cases, parents with more advanced formal education desired more information.

In sum, patients vary in their desire for information and desire to participate in decision-making and it may be difficult to base informed consent practices on known but imperfect tendencies of sociodemographic variables such as age, ethnicity, gender, marital status, and history of previous surgery in a relative. In fact, several studies have concluded that only 15% to 20% of decision-making variability can be attributed to sociodemographic and acuity issues.[5] Furthermore, listing less relevant risks clutters the informed consent process and should be avoided unless specifically requested.[11] For that reason, one approach to informed consent can be to determine the available options and their associated risks. After that, perhaps the best way to determine the optimal extent of disclosure is to provide certain relevant information and then ask the patient if he or she wishes to know more.[7,9,12] The importance of personal interaction in the informed consent process is becoming increasingly recognized.[13]

The informed consent process should conclude with the autonomous authorization of the patient to have the specific procedure performed. This, in part, gives evidence that the patient freely chose to proceed. This desire to have the patient voluntarily pick the course of action does not preclude the anesthesiologist from offering suggestions. In fact, the communication of the anesthesiologist's opinion along with an explanation of the supporting reasons is a critical part of the informed consent process. With this information, the patient is better able to determine which anesthetic provides the most desired benefits. Persuasion, the act of using argument and reason to influence a patient's decision, is appropriate. Coercion, the outright use of a credible threat, or manipulation, the use of misleading information, is not. The freedom to choose may also be usurped by rushing the informed consent process, thereby limiting the time for patients to consider their options and formulate questions.

Two common misunderstandings exist in the process of obtaining of informed consent. The first is the belief that the requirements for informed consent must be achieved fully and perfectly for the consent to be valid. As a corollary, some clinicians believe that if an ideal quality of informed consent cannot be attained, then the entire concept is meaningless and should be abandoned. Mandating such an unobtainable level is unrealistic and destructive to the goals of informed consent.[14] Simply because the requirements cannot be totally achieved, however, does not mean that they cannot be successfully and sufficiently accomplished. Few, if any, can achieve the idealized requirements of informed consent. Many, however, can reach an adequate level to achieve substantial self-determination.

The second misunderstanding is the belief that an anesthesiologist successfully fulfills the obligation to obtain informed consent by completing the legal requirements. Informed consent has both a legal and ethical sense. The legal sense is defined by institutional policies, which may require completing a form or writing a progress note as defined by local statutes and hospital regulations. Fulfilling such policies does not necessarily achieve the goals of informed consent nor does it provide protection against liability. The anesthesiologist can best achieve both the legal and ethical senses of informed consent by making the patient a full partner in decision-making and actively seeking to fulfill the patient's informed consent needs.[15]

The Informed Consent Process for Pediatric Patients

Informed Permission

Parents have traditionally acted as the surrogate decision-makers for their children, and legally they or other appointed surrogates give consent for the child. But this consent does not fulfill the spirit of consent, which is based on obtaining a legally empowered individualized autonomous decision from the patient receiving the treatment. As such, the American Academy of Pediatrics has suggested that the proper role for the surrogate decision-maker is to provide *informed permission*.[2] Informed permission has the same requirements as informed consent, but it provides recognition that the doctrine of informed consent cannot apply. Throughout the discussion that follows, we will use the term *parent* to describe the individual who provides informed permission for the child. Whenever this term is used, however, it should be understood that parents may not always be the legal surrogate decision-maker (as when a child is in the custody of the state), and that the authority of the parents may be limited in older children and adolescents (as when an adolescent is legally judged to be "mature" or "emancipated").

Parents and physicians primarily use the concept of best interests to guide their decision-making about health care for minors. The *best interests standard* acknowledges that the cornerstone of informed consent, the right to self-determination, is not applicable when it is impossible to know or even surmise from previous interactions what a child's preference would be. Instead, this standard requires the decision-maker to select the care that is objectively the best. Using this standard, then, requires determining (1) who will make the decision and (2) what is the best care. The difficulties arise in assuming that there is always one best choice, because if there is it should not matter who makes the decision. However, in today's heterogeneous and multicultural society there is wide latitude of what constitutes acceptable decision-making, particularly in complex decisions about informed consent, end-of-life issues, and confidentiality. Traditionally, parents who are present and capable of participating in the decision-making process are well suited to be the primary decision-makers for their children. This is in part due to society's respect for the concept of the family and the assumption that parents care greatly for their children. And although we can never know what children would decide if they were capable of participating in the decision-making process, it is reasonable to assume that children will incorporate some of the parents' values as they grow and mature, making the values of the parents a good first approximation for the future values of the child.[16] For these reasons, parents have extensive leeway in determining what is in a child's best interests.

One way to decide what is in the best interests of the child is to define what choices fall outside the range of acceptable decision-making. Criteria to make this determination include the amount of harm to the child by the intervention or its absence, the likelihood of success, and the overall risk-to-benefit ratio.[17] In the classic Baby Doe case, a child was born with Down Syndrome and duodenal atresia and was permitted to die without intervention.[18] Public discussion ensued, and it was believed that not repairing a correctable lesion was outside the bounds of acceptable undertreatment. In fact, this spurred the "Baby Doe regulations," which defined what care must be given to certain infants.[19] In this effort to avoid unacceptable undertreatment,

some believe that such regulations cause unacceptable overtreatment of children, primarily because regulations are crude instruments for dissecting complex clinical situations.[20,21]

The continuum between unacceptable and acceptable treatment in the practice of anesthesiology provides clear extremes but an ambiguous gray zone. For example, it is nearly always considered unacceptable undertreatment for Jehovah's Witnesses to refuse a life-sustaining blood transfusion for their child. On the other hand, parents may decline to have an epidural placed in their child for postoperative pain management, depriving the child of an optimal source of pain control. This is not considered unacceptable undertreatment, in part because the harm is limited by other adequate methods of pain control.

In general, the anesthesiologist's sole responsibility is to the child. Parents and surrogates may not always make decisions that are in the child's best interests. Although anesthesiologists must respect the diversity of values in society and the relationship between the parent and the child, decision-making that imperils the health of a child needs to be challenged. Anesthesiologists who believe parents are choosing unacceptable treatments should determine the basis of this judgment, address those specific concerns, and involve other clinicians both to offer an assessment of the appropriateness of care and to engage the parent in discussion.[22] Charging parents of not acting in the child's best interests is serious and can have significant social, fiscal, and familial ramifications. If, however, after exhausting other options, anesthesiologists believe parents have chosen unacceptable treatments, they should report the situation to proper child welfare authorities for possible legal action.

The best interests standard may not be as singularly focused as it seems. Recent discussion has suggested that clinicians who care for children may legitimately consider family interests in decision-making about incompetent patients.[23] Although, one can imagine a range of roles for the family interests, family interests are likely to have more weight in decision-making when they are identified as likely important to the patient.[23] This reasoning is used, for example, to justify general anesthesia and bone marrow donation from a younger to an older sibling.

Assent

Although most children cannot legally consent to medical care (see exceptions later), children can and should share in decision-making to the extent their development permits (see Table 5-1). The participation of children should increase as they grow older and depends on both their maturity and the consequences involved in the decision.

Anesthesiologists should attempt to achieve both informed permission from the parent or surrogate and assent as appropriate from the child.[2,24] The "rule of sevens," a rule that comes from British Common Law and still has legal relevance, provides a useful way to approach the decision-making capacities of children. The "rule of sevens" views children younger than the age of 7 as incapable of decision-making capacity, children between the ages of 7 and 14 as unlikely to have decision-making capacity, and children older than age 14 as presumed to have decision-making capacity. In practice, then, it would need to be shown that children between ages 7 and 14 have decision-making capacity and that children older than 14 not have decision-making capacity.

Because infants and young children have no decision-making capacity, assent is not a viable option, and anesthesiologists should obtain informed permission from the parent.

School-aged children are developing decision-making capacity, so anesthesiologists should seek both informed permission from the parent and assent and participatory decision-making from the child. School-aged children are capable of using logic and reason and are able to define and relate multiple aspects of a situation. Younger children in this period tend to be more rigid and absolute in applying rules. For these children, "do's and don'ts" are very important, and breaking rules, even with good reason, can lead to harsh rebukes and loss of trust. Older school-aged children begin to develop the flexibility to understand motives and different situations. Such situations may include whether to sedate a 6-year old before an inhalation induction, to use an inhalation or intravenous induction of anesthesia in an 8-year old, and to place an epidural for postoperative analgesia in a 12-year old.

Some adolescents older than age 14 will have developed decision-making capacity and anesthesiologists should try to fulfill the ethical requirements of consent while obtaining assent. These adolescents have the ability to use abstract thought, apply complex reasoning, foresee outcomes, and understand concepts such as probability. The critical ability to simultaneously evaluate multiple options evolves at this time. Anesthesiologists should recognize that although some adolescents may have cognitive abilities similar to adults, these abilities do not necessarily translate into good decision-making skills, because adolescents may be hindered by other limitations, such as insufficient emotional development. Examples may include obtaining consents from a 14-year old for anesthesia for scoliosis surgery and from a 16-year old for an awake thoracic epidural placement for a pectus repair.

Pro forma solicitations of opinions are harmful. The American Academy of Pediatrics speaks directly to this point, emphasizing "no one should solicit a patient's views without intending to weigh them seriously. In situations in which the patient will have to receive medical care despite his or her objection, the patient should be told that fact and should not be deceived."[2]

Informed Refusal

The requirements to achieve an informed refusal of a procedure are similar to the requirements for informed consent in that decision-makers should be substantially well versed about the risks, benefits, and alternatives before declining. When parents refuse what clinicians believe is necessary care for a child who cannot participate in the decision-making process, clinicians may invoke the best interests standard as described earlier. This situation is more complicated when children express significant decision-making capacity and refuse nonemergent procedures. Anesthesiologists should respect the right of these children (typically those older than the age of 10 years) not to assent to a procedure and should go out of their way to avoid coercing or forcibly making the child have the procedure. Achieving the child's assent may necessitate further discussions with the child, parents, and other providers, and such discussions may best take place away from the operating room. In cases in which the parent and child disagree, clinicians should seek the assistance of others experienced in conflict resolution to help resolve the dispute with a minimum of rancor. For example, consider a 15-year old who arrives in the preoperative holding area for an elective knee arthroscopy. The day before she had given assent and her parents had given informed permission for anesthesia and surgery. In the holding area, she starts crying and refuses to cooperate. Rather than forcibly or surreptitiously sedating her, the anesthesiologist should try to discuss her concerns. If she is unable to discuss the issues, the anesthesiologist should consider physically removing her from the area and giving her time to regain composure before readdressing the situation. Often such simple actions will allow the situation to be resolved. If the withdrawal of assent was in part related to anxiety, she may assent to receiving ample premedication before returning to the holding area to permit her to receive the operation. It would be important to obtain her assent before administering the sedation, however, and not to simply assume that forceful or surreptitious administration is justified. These simple interventions can also be used in most urgent cases, when a trivial delay can often permit communication sufficient to obtain the child's assent.

Doctor, If This Were Your Child, What Would You Do?

In general, physicians should respond to this question by using medical facts to explain how certain values could be supported, so that decision-makers could choose the path that supports their values. This question, however, could be asked for a number of different reasons, forcing the physician to put the question into a broader context.[25,26]

A useful way to approach this question is to determine the sense in which the question is being asked. In one sense, for example, the parents may be overwhelmed by difficult-to-comprehend information. These parents are declaring that they cannot fully understand the choices and they need help making a reasonable decision. Perhaps they're actually asking what would give their child the best chance of getting better. In this situation, physicians should explain the reasons and values underlying their personal choice.

In the second situation, the parents are making a difficult choice and simply want support that they are making the right choice. Physicians should answer with their best judgment if they agree with the family. If they disagree with the family, physicians should lend support through comments such as "other parents in the same situation have made the same choice" or by acknowledging that it is normal to feel uncertain.[25] If the family persists in asking what they would do, physicians may wish to acknowledge that they may have chosen differently. Physicians should emphasize, however, that their decisions are guided by personal values and beliefs that are no more worthy than the parents' values and beliefs.

In the third situation, parents may be asking physicians for help in making a major life-altering decision. One way of approaching this question is to offer a process for answering the question (e.g., "My spouse and I would talk with the chaplain and with our parents to help arrive at a decision"). Physicians should feel comfortable admitting that they may not be able to determine what they would do if they were actually in that situation. Such honesty reinforces the difficulty of the decision for the parents.

Special Situations in Pediatric Informed Consent

Emancipated Minor Status and Mature Minor Doctrine

Some adolescents younger than age 18 have the legal right to consent to treatment.[27,28] The term *emancipated minor* refers to minors who have been given the global right to make their own health care decisions. This status is generally awarded to adolescents who are married, parents, in the military, and economically independent and may include adolescents who are pregnant. The mature minor doctrine holds that adolescents who have decision-making capacity are legally and ethically capable of giving informed consent in specific situations as determined by a court. Although particulars vary by state, the mature minor doctrine in general requires adolescents to be at least 14 years old and tends to permit decisions of lesser risk. The nearer the adolescent is to majority (usually an age of 18 years), the more likely the court is to grant the adolescent the ability to consent.[29]

Children of Jehovah's Witnesses

Jehovah's Witnesses interpret biblical scripture as prohibiting blood transfusions because blood holds the "life force" and that anyone who takes blood will be "cut off from his people" and not earn eternal salvation.[30,31] The courts have fairly consistently upheld the rights of nonpregnant adults who are not sole providers to refuse blood transfusions. The presumption is that they are making an informed decision about the risks and benefits of receiving blood. The courts, however, have uniformly intervened under the legal doctrine of *parens patriae*, the obligation of the state to protect the interests of incompetent patients, when Jehovah's Witnesses have refused blood transfusions on behalf of their children in both emergent and elective cases.[29,32,33]

Obtaining informed permission and assent for the care of a ward of a Jehovah's Witness should squarely address the transfusion issue. The child and family should be informed that attempts will be made to limit the need to give a blood transfusion and the anesthesiologist should clarify which interventions are acceptable. Deliberate hypotension, deliberate hypothermia, and hemodilution are often acceptable techniques. Synthetic colloid solutions, dextran, erythropoietin, desmopressin, and preoperative iron are usually acceptable. Some Jehovah's Witnesses will accept blood removed and returned in a continuous loop, such as cell saver blood. The family should know, however, that in a life-threatening situation, the anesthesiologist will seek a court order authorizing the administration of life-sustaining blood. Anesthesiologists should be familiar with the local mechanism (e.g., contacting hospital counsel) for obtaining a court order authorizing transfusion. In instances in which the likelihood of requiring blood is high, or the local judiciary is not that familiar with case law for Jehovah's Witnesses, the anesthesiologist may choose to obtain the court order before the operation.

A common concern is the sudden need for a transfusion in a healthy child having a low-risk procedure. For example, consider an otherwise healthy 7-year-old child of Jehovah's Witnesses having a tonsillectomy. The parents are told that the need for transfusion is unlikely and that a court order will be sought if transfusion becomes necessary. During the procedure, the carotid artery is punctured, leading to massive hemorrhage. In emergent situations such as these, based on the obligation to protect children, anesthesiologists should take the legally correct and ethically appropriate action of transfusing blood without the court order. Waiting for the court order may inappropriately result in functionally honoring the wishes of the parents while resulting in permanent harm to the child.

In elective procedures that may be safely delayed, the child and family may also consider postponing the procedure until the child is of sufficient age and maturity to decide about transfusion therapy. The problem lies in whether the delay may increase risk or decrease the likelihood of a good outcome. This decision requires the same balancing act as discussed in determining the best interests for a child. Questions that affect the decision include the quantitative change in risk or benefit, the quality of the risk or benefit, and the significance of it. For example, it may be easier to wait on a procedure that is purely cosmetic (although it would still be difficult) than to wait on a procedure that may lead to permanent injury and a shortened life.

Individual clinicians, perhaps with judicial support, may choose to honor the wishes of a mature minor. Particularly in a pediatric hospital, it is important to ensure the fidelity of the process, by ensuring that postoperative and on-call clinicians will honor the mature minor's wishes. Those arranging for the care of the mature minor should respect the values of clinicians by devising systems that do not put conscientious objectors in the untenable position of choosing between their principles and the promised care.

Confidentiality for Adolescents

The obligation to maintain confidentiality requires physicians to protect patient information from unauthorized and unnecessary disclosure. Confidentiality is necessary for the development of a patient-physician relationship that supports an open and uncensored flow of information and concerns. A trusting alliance is particularly important in the care of adolescents who are more likely to defer needed treatment because they are concerned about confidentiality.[34] Emancipated and mature minors have a right to complete confidentiality. For other adolescents, if maintaining confidentiality is of minimal harm, physicians should encourage adolescents to be forthright with parents but respect their decision not to be. On the other hand, if maintaining confidentiality may result in serious harm to the adolescent, physicians may be ethically justified in notifying the parents.[34] Possible exceptions to the principle of confidentiality are notifications required by law such as reporting statutes, parental notification, and when an adolescent makes a credible threat to harm another person.

The quality of the information obtained in the preoperative interview may be directly affected by the adolescent's trust of the anesthesiologist. The anesthesiologist can enhance this trust by interviewing the adolescent in private, acknowledging the adolescent's concerns about confidentiality, and following through on any promises made. Inadvertent breeches of confidentiality are as harmful as intentional ones, and anesthesiologists should be aware that many disclosures take place unwittingly in public spaces or social situations.[35]

Anesthesiologists may face confidentiality issues when an adolescent has a positive preanesthetic pregnancy test. Given the principles of confidentiality, in most cases it is likely to be ethically appropriate to inform only the adolescent of the positive pregnancy test.[36] In addition, adolescents in many locales have the legal right to keep this information private from their parents. Anesthesiologists must then share this information with the adolescent without letting the parents know. Because there are psychosocial and medical issues about adolescent pregnancy beyond the purview of most anesthesiologists, anesthesiologists should involve pediatricians, gynecologists, and social workers with expertise in adolescent issues in this discussion. Matters may become more complex if the surgeon, anesthesiologist, adolescent, and other advisors believe the case should be postponed and the adolescent chooses not to inform her parents about the results of the pregnancy test. Clinicians must be careful not to inadvertently inform the parents of the positive pregnancy test during these deliberations and the subsequent postponing of anesthesia and surgery.

The Adolescent and Abortion

Even though adolescents who are pregnant may be considered emancipated, many states require some form of parental involvement such as parental consent or notification before an elective abortion in an adolescent. If a state requires parental involvement, the ability of the adolescent to circumvent this regulation by seeking relief from a judge, known as judicial bypass, is available. Requirements and enforcement of statutes vary from state to state.[37] The need for parental involvement in adolescent abortions is not always legally straightforward, and it may be best to consult with hospital counsel in determining these issues. Although this is an area in which honorable people disagree, it is worth noting that both the American Academy of Pediatrics and the American Medical Association have issued statements affirming the rights of adolescents to confidentiality when an abortion is contemplated.[37,38]

Emergency Care

Children are frequently without their parents or surrogate decision-makers for a portion of each day. As such, it is likely that an anesthesiologist will at some point need to perform an emergent anesthetic for a minor who does not have a parent available to give legal consent or informed permission. In an emergency situation, the presumption is that necessary therapy is desirable and should be given.[39] It is reasonable to attempt to contact the parents or surrogate, but questions about reimbursement should not delay necessary treatment.[39] Emergencies include problems that could cause death, disability, and an increased risk of future complications.

This situation becomes more complex when an adolescent near majority refuses assent for emergency care that the parent desires. The right to refuse treatment turns on the adolescent's decision-making capacity and the resulting harm from the refusal of care.[2] If the harm is significant, and the adolescent's rationale is decidedly short term or filled with misunderstanding, it becomes necessary to consider whether the adolescent has sufficient decision-making capacity for this decision. In this situation, it may be appropriate to consider what is in the best interests of the adolescent. For example, a 15-year-old football player suffers a cervical fracture. He is brought to the preoperative holding area where he refuses emergency stabilization, stating that he does not want to live life without football. Most would hold that his conclusion implies less than full decision-making capacity, especially in light of the suddenness of the injury, and that he should receive emergency treatment. If, however, 12 months later he was quadriplegic and was continuing to refuse interventions to sustain life, then the clinicians caring for him would have to give serious weight to his requests.

The Impaired Parent

More than 11 million children live with parents who have substance abuse problems. These parents may have impaired judg-

ments and may be unable to fulfill surrogate responsibilities regarding informed permission, and they may be disruptive or dangerous. Clinicians should focus on the safety of the child, the impaired parent, and others, such as patients, parents, and employees in the area, and comply with reporting mandates and protect patient confidentiality.[40] As a general rule, clinicians should use the least restrictive means to decrease the risk from the impaired parent. If possible, caregivers may wish to postpone routine treatment until legal consent can be obtained from an unimpaired parent. Anesthesiologists will have to weigh the benefits of waiting with the risk that impaired parents may be less reliable and, for example, may not return for future visits. In this case, it may be wise to consider what is in the best interest of the child. It may be in the child's best interests to proceed with a routine procedure in the situation of an impaired parent unable to give legal consent. Anesthesiologists may wish to consult legal and risk management colleagues for guidance.

Forgoing Life-Sustaining Treatment

Do-Not-Resuscitate Orders

Do-not-resuscitate (DNR) orders are designed to permit children to forgo certain procedures because their likely benefits are not worth their likely burdens. DNR orders in children, as in adults, are not necessarily optimally done.[41] In one study of end-of-life care in children with cancer, discussions about possible limits on resuscitation were initiated too late, enacted too late, and used too infrequently.[42] Physicians may delay discussion of resuscitation status because they are unknowledgeable, untrained, or uncomfortable with having the discussion.[41,42] Changing care teams may also make it difficult to consummate plans over time. Parents may delay a timely DNR order because of delayed understanding or acceptance of the likely outcome, inappropriately equating withholding resuscitation to lack of care, concerns about betraying their child or because they consider such topics taboo.[41,42]

Do-Not-Resuscitate Orders in the Operating Room

DNR orders are predicated on the idea that patients may forgo certain procedures and their possible benefits because they choose not to undertake the associated burdens. The burdens may be related to either the resuscitation attempt itself or to the decrement in functional or cognitive capacity that would likely follow from even a successful attempt at resuscitation. This individualized weighing of the risk-to-benefit ratios of resuscitative procedures is as valid in the operating room as on the ward. For this reason, the American Academy of Pediatrics, the American Society of Anesthesiologists, and the American College of Surgeons recommend mandatory reevaluation of the DNR order before going to the operating room.[43-45]

Reevaluation of the DNR order requires clarifying the patient's goals for the proposed surgery and end-of-life care. For children, the anesthesiologist needs to involve the child, parents, and clinicians such as surgeons, intensivists, and pediatricians in determining appropriate goals for surgery. Although it is immensely difficult to define "benefit" and "burden," it is helpful to consider the guidelines set forth by the American Academy of Pediatrics. Benefits include prolongation of life under certain circumstances, improved quality of life (e.g., reduction of pain or the ability to leave the hospital), and increased enjoyment of life. Burdens may include intractable pain and suffering, disability, and events that cause a decrement in the quality of life, as viewed by the child and parents.[46] These guidelines may be helpful in considering short- and long-term goals and putting into appropriate context specific fears such as long-term ventilatory dependency, pain, and suffering. Decision-makers also should be educated about the differences between resuscitation on the ward and in the operating room. For example, anesthesia routinely brings about conditions such as apnea and hemodynamic instability that normally would require resuscitation when the child is on the ward. Surgical interventions may also increase the likelihood of needing resuscitation. Outcomes from a witnessed arrest such as one that would occur in the operating room, however, are likely to be better than from an unwitnessed arrest. By considering these issues, the anesthesiologist and appropriate parties can determine the desired extent of resuscitation by using either a goal-directed approach or procedure-directed approach.[44,47]

The goal-directed approach permits decision-makers to guide therapy by prioritizing outcomes rather than procedures. After defining desirable outcomes, decision-makers have clinicians use clinical judgment to determine how specific interventions will affect achieving the goals. Predictions about the success of interventions that are made by the anesthesiologist at the time of the resuscitation are likely to be more accurate than predictions made preoperatively, when the quality and nature of the problems are not known. Therapy may be guided by goals rather than specific procedures because during the perioperative period children are cared for by dedicated clinicians for a short period of time. This allows these clinicians to have the necessary discussions with the decision-makers to be able to understand and therefore implement the specific plans. It is helpful to define a goal-directed approach by discussing with children and parents, as appropriate, the burdens they are willing to accept, the benefits they want, and the likelihood of distinct outcomes. For example, some may wish to undertake a significant burden of resuscitation if the likelihood of leaving the hospital is high but not if it is low. Others may choose to accept only minor burdens in the form of pain and suffering and only if the likelihood of returning to their preoperative function is very high. In our experience, most decision-makers choose a goal-directed approach such that they would desire therapy if the interventions and burdens were temporary and reversible; in other words, if they could return to their current state without suffering too much.

Although a goal-directed approach provides a necessary degree of flexibility, some individuals prefer the control of the procedure-directed approach. The procedure-directed approach replicates successful mechanisms used to document DNR orders on the ward. A checklist of specific interventions is presented, and the decision-makers choose which interventions may be used. Anesthesiologists can advise children and parents based on the benefit and burden of each intervention, as well as the likelihood of that intervention achieving the desired goals. Interventions frequently on such lists include tracheal intubation or other airway management, postoperative ventilation, chest compressions, defibrillation, use of vasoactive drugs, and invasive monitoring.[44,47] The strength of the procedure-directed approach is that it is unambiguous and clearly defines which procedures are desired. This important feature is necessary for ward medicine, where a child may have multiple clinicians throughout his or her stay. The procedure-directed approach,

however, does not allow for clinical subtleties that may be difficult to precisely document and define.[48,49] The procedure-directed approach may also place anesthesiologists into challenging ethical situations, such as when the anesthesiologist has agreed not to perform a procedure (e.g., tracheal intubation) for a complication that was unanticipated and entirely reversible (e.g., inadvertent morphine overdose).

In practice, both methods may be used to facilitate discussion before completing documentation in accordance with institutional policies. An important part of the reevaluation is determining postoperative plans. A patient may want therapy continued for a limited time before withdrawing it. This expresses the patient's belief that a burden (a few days of ventilatory support) may be worth a benefit (extubation of the trachea) but at some point the increasing burden may not be worth the decreasing likelihood of the benefit. Indeed, it is well accepted that withholding and withdrawing life-sustaining treatments are conceptually equivalent actions (although emotionally different) and the considerations in making the decisions should be the same.[50] Some physicians may feel uncomfortable in withdrawing care after its initiation, mistakenly believing that starting a treatment requires them to continue it or that withdrawing implies that they have failed in their duties. By recasting the purpose of postoperative ventilation as a trial of therapy to achieve a specific goal, physicians may be psychologically more comfortable with withdrawing care.

In pediatrics there is less importance placed on determining postoperative plans ahead of time, because parents usually are available in the postoperative period to make decisions regarding therapy. In that case, it is not unreasonable to favor a trial of therapy.

The American Academy of Pediatrics suggests that legitimate procedures for a child with a DNR order would include procedures that will decrease pain, provide vascular access, enable the child to be able to be discharged from hospital (e.g., gastrostomy tube), treat an urgent problem unrelated to the primary problem (e.g., appendicitis), or treat a problem that may be related but is not considered a terminal event (e.g., bowel obstruction). Specific information that is useful to give children and parents is listed in Table 5-2.[45]

Readers should not misinterpret the focus of this discussion on maintaining some form of perioperative DNR order to mean

---

Table 5-2. Components of a Pediatric DNR Discussion

- Planned procedure and anticipated benefit to child
- Likelihood of requiring resuscitation
- Reversibility of likely causes
- Description of potential interventions and their consequences
- Chances of success
- Ranges of outcomes with and without resuscitation
- Intended and possible venues and types of postoperative care
- Establishment of an agreement through a goal-oriented approach, a procedure-oriented approach, or a revocation of the DNR order for the perioperative period
- Documentation

From Fallat ME, Deshpande JK. Do-not-resuscitate orders for pediatric patients who require anesthesia and surgery. Pediatrics 2004; 114:1686-1692.

that it is inappropriate to revoke the DNR order. In many cases, perioperative revocation is likely to be preferred. Children and families do not have to worry if a certain intervention is considered to be resuscitative, and they do not have to worry about limiting potentially therapeutic anesthetic or surgical interventions. As such, the chance of quality survival after an arrest in the operating room is greater than after an arrest elsewhere. When perioperative revocation of DNR status is desired, however, physicians should discuss and document the timing and process of reinitiating the DNR status, the identity and roles of surrogate decision-makers, and the desired extent of postoperative care. This is particularly critical if there is no surrogate decision-maker available postoperatively.

Barriers to Honoring Preferences for Resuscitation

Perhaps the most significant barrier to acceptance and implementation of perioperative DNR orders is the bias physicians have against understanding why children and parents of patients may choose to refuse resuscitation.[51] In an extensive study of end-of-life care, physicians believed that 46% of patients' requests to forgo cardiopulmonary resuscitation (CPR) were appropriate whereas they believed that 86% of decisions to receive it were appropriate.[52] Patients place more emphasis and value on their functional status and how they perform the activities of daily living than do physicians, who tend to focus more on diagnosis and life expectancy.[53]

There are other reasons why children and parents are "encouraged" to accept resuscitation in the operating room. Anesthesiologists may believe that consent for anesthesia is inconsistent with refusal of resuscitation. Although it is true that anesthetic practice consists of a spectrum of interventions that are broadly considered to be resuscitation, it is certainly possible to provide both regional and general anesthetic treatments to children while agreeing to withhold resuscitative treatments such as chest compressions and cardioversion. In addition, a desire to receive surgical therapy may be considered inconsistent with the wish to limit resuscitation. However, it is clear that children and parents may want the benefits of the placement of an indwelling venous access or repair of a painful broken bone, for example, only when certain burdens are not foisted upon them, such as an extensive postoperative stay in the intensive care unit or the loss of certain faculties.[54]

The closely linked environment of the operating room, in which cause and effect is attributed to a specific physician and action, may influence physicians' attitudes toward perioperative DNR orders. Physicians may believe that while it is acceptable to honor a refusal for medical treatments that might delay death caused by disease, it may be somewhat less acceptable to honor a refusal of treatment that might delay death caused by an iatrogenic event. Indeed, some physicians would perform CPR in opposition to declared preferences in cases in which iatrogenic problems caused or contributed to the child's arrest.[55,56] To children and parents, however, it is likely to be wholly irrelevant whether the cardiac arrest was iatrogenic; what is relevant are the factors they considered in requesting limited resuscitation, including, for example, their physical and mental status after the arrest.[54] The benefits of continued therapy after certain types of iatrogenic arrests should be addressed as part of the perioperative DNR interview to help children and parents arrive at an informed decision.[56]

System problems may affect the ability for anesthesiologists to adequately reevaluate DNR orders for the perioperative period. Production pressure to do a high volume of cases in the operating room makes it difficult to address any problem that requires time to investigate and resolve. The ability of anesthesiologists to reevaluate the DNR order may be hindered by insufficient physician knowledge and a lack of standardized procedures for addressing perioperative DNR orders.[57]

Another barrier may be fear of being sued. Specific statutory provisions often address requirements for DNR orders, including explicit immunity provisions. Clinicians who act in accordance with statutory requirements are often protected from liability when they honor a child's or family's refusal of resuscitation.[51] Some statutes confer immunity on clinicians who resuscitate a patient who has a DNR order, provided they have a good-faith belief that no order exists. Given the well-established right of children and parents to refuse medical treatment and the paucity of cases finding physicians liable for honoring DNR requests, the risk of liability for honoring an appropriately entered perioperative DNR order is not great and is likely to be less than the risk of not honoring the order.[51]

Concepts of Inadvisable Care and Futility

The concept of futile care has undergone a number of changes over the past decade.[58] Previously, attempts were made to define futile care based on a specific percent likelihood of achieving a certain outcome (e.g., CPR is futile when the likelihood of a child with this disease being discharged from the hospital is less than 1% with 95% confidence). This approach failed, in large part because it was difficult to know with any certainty the likelihood of success in the individual child. Policies based on this approach inappropriately de-emphasized the importance of individual values and preferences, such as the willingness to atypically undertake extensive burdens for relatively minor or highly unlikely benefits.[59]

A clearer way to think about futility is to separate those treatments that will not accomplish their intended goals from treatments that have a very low likelihood of accomplishing their goals. Therapy may be labeled "futile" when it cannot accomplish its intended specific goal, such as, for example, successfully resuscitating an infant who has been asystolic and has not responded to CPR for 30 minutes. In this sense, then, because questions about futile care arise rarely, futility policies are less important.

However, having policies to help resolve differences of opinions about applying treatments with low likelihoods of success is important. For example, continuing substantial cardiopulmonary support in a neonate with a grade IV intraventricular hemorrhage, necrotizing enterocolitis, complex heart disease, and trisomy 13 is probably not futile, although it may be inadvisable, because it may be in the infant's interest to discontinue extensive support. Treatments with low likelihoods of success may be considered inadvisable because of burden to the child, cost, or uncertain benefit, but they are not futile. Good policies are procedure-based, public, reflect the moral values of the community, and include processes for identifying stake holders, for initiating and conducting the policy, for commencing appellate mechanisms, and for determining relevant information.[58] Discussions about inadvisable treatment should bear in mind qualitative and quantitative considerations. The qualitative aspects define the goals of the treatment, and the quantitative aspects state the likelihood of achieving a defined result. When offering likelihoods of a result, physicians should be clear whether the information used to form the estimation is based on intuition or clinical experience or from rigorous scientific studies. Scoring systems useful for population predictions in determining potentially inadvisable care should be considered as contributory but not determinative for decision-making for individuals. In Texas, a legislative approach was adopted for resolving disputes about medical futility, empowering physicians to unilaterally withhold or withdraw treatments they regard as futile provided they obtain the agreement of the hospital ethics committee. The impact of this legislation is being closely monitored, and until more data are available this will remain a controversial strategy for conflict resolution.[60-62]

Decision-making for a child near the end of life should be based on the best interests of the child. Given improvement in medicine, clinicians should be aware that it is often hard to predict success in very young children. Furthermore, parents tend to be very involved in the care of their children and pediatric doctors may feel a need to "protect" their patients. When both parents and clinicians are invested in the child's well being, there is a greater possibility of disagreements causing conflict. A useful approach to resolving conflicts has been proposed by the President's Commission for the Study of Ethical Problems in Medicine and Biomedical and Behavioral Research (Table 5-3).[16] In short, only if a therapy is clearly beneficial (as in blood transfusion for anemia) may clinicians override parental preferences and even then, out of respect, the appropriateness of the treatment and the process of decision-making should undergo an external review, which will often be medical, ethical, or legal. Because pediatric anesthesiologists are providing care for increasingly younger children, anesthesiologists should be aware of the improving outcomes for the most preterm infants. The best information suggests that for those infants at the threshold of viability (22-25 weeks), survival increases with each week of gestation but the rate of moderate or worse disability does not improve and remains at 30% to 50%.[63]

Table 5-3. Suggested Approach for Resolving Disputes about Appropriate Care

	Parents Prefer to *Accept* Treatment	Parents Prefer to *Forgo* Treatment
• Physicians consider treatment *clearly beneficial*	Treat	Provide treatment during review process
• Physicians consider treatment to be of *ambiguous or uncertain benefit*	Treat	Forgo
• Physicians consider treatment to be *inadvisable*	Provide treatment during review process	Forgo
• Physicians consider treatment to be *futile*	Review	Forgo

From President's Commission for the Study of Ethical Problems in Medicine and Biomedical and Behavioral Research: Deciding to Forgo Life-Sustaining Treatment: Ethical, Medical and Legal Issues in Treatment Decisions. Washington, DC, U.S. Government Printing Office, 1983.

Withdrawing Therapy

When therapy is being withdrawn, particularly when a child is disconnected from mechanical ventilation, family members may request that the child receive sedation. The criteria of benefits to burdens should be applied when determining the appropriateness of sedation. In most cases, the benefit of administering sedation is to minimize discomfort and suffering whereas the only burden associated with giving sedation is the decreased likelihood of a remote possibility of survival. Physicians may indeed feel uncomfortable that they are causing death. When faced with this problem, some appeal to the *doctrine of double effect*, which assesses the rightness of the action based on its intent, which is to minimize pain and suffering, rather than on its foreseeable but unintended side effect (double effect), which is to hasten the child's death. Others criticize the doctrine of double effect because it oversimplifies the concept of intentionality and justifies the action through the physician's intent, rather than the patient's authorization. If anesthesiologists are uncomfortable providing analgesia and sedation in these circumstances, they should decline to provide care and consider finding a suitable replacement.[64]

Clinicians should realize the complexity in skillfully withdrawing therapy and providing good end-of-life care.[65,66] Specifically, anesthesiologists should not use paralytic agents to minimize potentially upsetting patient movements during the withdrawal of therapy.[67] Paralytic agents hide signs of discomfort and distress that physicians should use as indicators to provide additional sedation and analgesia. Explaining this to family members may help them tolerate otherwise upsetting movements or events.

Commonly limited interventions are CPR and hemodialysis; less invasive therapies are often not limited, most likely because they involve a lesser burden. In one study, the most common reasons for limiting treatments were an incomparable benefit-burden ratio, prior poor quality of life, and the likelihood that therapy would not leave the child with an acceptable quality of life.[68]

Improving Communication in Pediatric Intensive Care Units

Many of the 55,000 annual pediatric deaths in the United States occur in pediatric intensive care units.[66] To support these children and their families, pediatric intensivists should emphasize interdisciplinary communication, tailor communication style to parents, and maximize meaningful parental participation in care.[66] The goal is to be an empathic professional who establishes compassionate relationships with family by managing emotional, informational, and care needs.[69] In nearly all conversations, clinicians should explain the meaning of the conversation in terms of overall care.[70] Table 5-4 lists parental desires in terms of end of care in the intensive care unit.

Communication is not solely about transfer of information. Parents respond and benefit from the relational aspects of compassion, mercy, authenticity, and integrity.[71] More colloquially, the relational aspect is referred to as "being there," interacting with the parents as a caring person with feelings and emotions.[72] For example, although some clinicians may believe it is inappropriate to show emotion, parents appreciate compassion and some level of distress at the sharing of bad news, rather than cold, hard professionalism.[70]

Table 5-4. Parent's Desires for Communication in the Intensive Care Unit

1. **Honest and complete information** tailored to the parent's needs and information-receiving preferences. Comprehension of the child's potential trajectories permits better participation in care and a greater chance of appropriate end-of-life care.

2. **Ready access to staff**, to include periodic scheduled informal visits to the bedside and the availability of email interactions. The goal is to provide the parents with easy and frequent opportunities to have their questions answered, with sufficient repetition and clarification of the "big picture."

3. To maximize successful **communication**, clinicians should actively assess the parent's preferences for communication and decision-making. This includes considering how to relate information to parents when clinicians have different management opinions. Parents frequently recognize that there are differences of options, and some prefer to hear the range of options whereas others prefer to hear only the recommended option.

4. **Emotional expression and support by staff** is critical to parents. To do this successfully, clinicians should adapt their style to patient preferences. Most clinicians should adopt practices that give parents more room to control the conversation, including talking less, listening more, and tolerating silence as parents gather themselves to continue communicating.

5. **Preservation of the integrity of the parent-child relationship** means enabling parents to continue in their self-identified and prominent role as decision-maker and protector. Loss of this role harms parents and may impair their ability to participate in decision-making for the child.

6. **Faith and spiritual matters** are highly personal, and parents may feel uncomfortable expressing their faith in an institutional setting. Spiritual matters should be accepted and integrated into the intensive care unit practice to benefit those who benefit from spiritual support.

Modified from Meyer EC, Ritholz MD, Burns JP, Truog RD: Improving the quality of end-of-life care in the pediatric intensive care unit: parents' priorities and recommendations. Pediatrics 2006; 117:649-657.

Difficult discussions merit thoughtful accommodations. A quiet, private room with sufficient space, atmosphere, and seating facilitates communication. The family should be able to stay in the room for private reflection after the discussion. Proper personal self-care is necessary to enable clinicians to focus on the family's needs and desires. Clinicians should ensure they have an unsoiled professional appearance and that personal needs are met before beginning the discussion with the family. It is helpful to have more than one clinician enter into the meeting, both to provide support to the other clinician and to provide another opportunity for the family members to "connect" with the clinical staff. In pediatrics, this second person may be the primary nurse, intensive care unit social worker, or chaplain. Parent's lifelong views of these events are profoundly colored by their vivid memories and strong feelings of these seminal discussions. How difficult discussions are handled often becomes the basis for the family's intensive care unit narrative.

Palliative Care

Anesthesiologists, in their role as pain management specialists, intensive care unit doctors, or in the operating room, may participate in pediatric palliative care. Palliative care emphasizes relationship-centered care and should be available to children with a wide variety of diseases (Table 5-5).[73]

Euthanasia

Although euthanasia has been permitted in the Netherlands for some time, only recently have there been reports of euthanasia for children. Sixteen-year olds may now request euthanasia, and 12- to 15-year olds may request euthanasia with their parent's approval. On reflection, it is reasonable for teenagers to want to minimize suffering and pain at the end of life. Similar to euthanasia in the adult patient, the adolescent must have decision-making capacity; must clearly, voluntarily, and repeatedly request to die; must have an incurable condition associated with severe, unrelenting, and intolerable suffering; and should not be making the request due to inadequate comfort care. Consultation with other experts should be made to review and verify the facts about prognosis and current comfort management.[74]

However, there is a concern that there is a "slippery slope" extending to euthanasia in children younger than 12 years and to those unable to formulate requests. In the Netherlands, approximately 1% of neonatal and infant deaths are related to decisions to actively end the life of infants not dependent on life-sustaining technology.[75] In children older than 1 year, 36% of all deaths are preceded by an end-of-life decision and 2.7% are preceded by the use of drugs explicitly intended to hasten death. In those cases, 0.7% of the time the decision was made at the child's request and 2% of the time the decision was made at the family's request. In a survey of Dutch pediatricians, approximately half of the pediatricians were willing to use lethal drugs at the child's request when the parents agree, more than one third are willing to end the life of an unconscious child based on the parents recommendation, and some respondents were willing to provide euthanasia for a child even when the parents did not agree with the child's request for euthanasia.[76]

Donation after Cardiac Death

In organ procurement after the declaration of death through neurologic criteria (i.e., brain death), the child is declared dead before being brought to the operating room and the organs are then retrieved while body homeostasis is maintained through mechanical ventilation, pharmacologic therapy, and other standard resuscitative techniques.[77] Recent controversies in the ethics of organ recovery center on non–heart-beating cadaver organ donation, now known as donation after cardiac death (DCD).[78] In DCD, the child is not declared dead before being brought to the operating room for organ retrieval. In this case, it is determined that the child has no significant likelihood of survival after the withdrawal of life support and that, given the benefits and burdens of the situation, it is appropriate to withdraw life-sustaining therapy. If the child dies after life-sustaining therapy is withdrawn, the child is declared dead by cardiac criteria and the organs are retrieved.

Pediatric DCD protocols offer the potential of increasing the number of organs available for donation from 3% to 10%.[79,80]

Table 5-5. Palliative Care

WHO	• All children suffering from chronic, life-threatening, and terminal illnesses are eligible, including those with:
	    Diseases in which curative therapy may fail (e.g., malignancies with poor prognoses)
	    Diseases that require long periods of hospitalizations to prolong life (e.g., severe epidermolysis bullosa or immunodeficiencies)
	    Progressive diseases in which treatment is palliative (e.g., severe osteogenesis imperfecta)
	    Severe nonprogressive disabilities that are at risk for coexisting diseases
	• Do not resuscitate orders should not be required
	• Prognosis for short-term survival is not required

WHAT	• Child-focused, family-oriented, and relationship-centered care that focuses on relief of suffering and enhancing quality of life • Prioritization of participation of the child and family in decision-making • Caring for the child as a unique individual • Caring for the family as a functional unit • Care is not directed at shortening life
HOW	• An interdisciplinary team is always available to families to provide continuity • Facilitation and documentation of communication are critical tasks of the team
WHY	• Respite care and support are essential for families
WHERE & WHEN	• Care is coordinated across all sites of care delivery • Care is incorporated into mainstream medical care • Bereavement care should be provided for as long as needed

From Himelstein BP: Palliative care for infants, children, adolescents, and their families. J Palliat Med 2006; 9:163-181.

There are a number of ethical issues regarding DCD protocols (Table 5-6). Core arguments center on whether protocols seriously alter the dying process by shifting decision-making away from the best interests of the dying child and by interfering with the family's ability to be with their dying child. Pediatric DCD has additional issues. There is a greater risk of premature withdrawal of therapy because neurologic prognoses are more uncertain in children. In addition, in many cases the surrogate is not fulfilling a previous wish of the child because the child has not formally or informally expressed interest in donating organs. Because donating organs cannot be in the best interests of such a child, the decision for pediatric DCD is often made because the family believes donation is what the child would have wanted or because donation benefits the family by ameliorating the pain of the child's death.

Table 5-6. Decided and Undecided Ethical Issues Surrounding Donation after Cardiac Death

Should interventions be permitted prior to withdrawal of care?	The burdens from the interventions are not in the best interests of the child. On the other hand, the burdens of the interventions are mostly theoretical and may improve the quality of the transplanted organs.
Should withdrawal of therapy occur in the intensive care unit or in the operating room?	Withdrawing therapy in the operating room may increase the quality of the organs transplanted. Withdrawing therapy in the ICU is likely to be less upsetting to the family and more consistent with the premise of withdrawing therapy for the child's benefit. In addition, it may remove some of the awkwardness if the child does not die within the defined interval.
Who should withdraw therapy?	To be consistent with the premises of withdrawal of therapy, it should be the same person who would normally withdraw therapy from the child. Even if the decision is made to withdraw therapy in the operating room, an anesthesiologist who has not been caring for the child should not be asked to withdraw therapy because of the physical location of the event.
How long should there be cessation of cardiac function for a child to be declared dead?	Proposed times may be based on the premises of how long it would take to autoresuscitate as compared with how long it would take to be resuscitated through medical care.
Contents of a good donation after cardiac death policy	• Acceptable interventions before withdrawing therapy • Acceptable locations of withdrawing therapy • Amount of time to wait until death before forgoing procurement • Which individual should withdraw therapy • What to do if family will not leave after death is declared

Pediatric Issues in Clinical Anesthesia Practice

Special Requirements for Pediatric Research

The anesthesiologist Henry K. Beecher was one of the first to propose different requirements for pediatric research as compared with adult research.[81] Because children may be incapable of understanding and consenting to experiments and because they are vulnerable to abuse and at risk for long-term harm, most proposed pediatric research is closely examined.[81] Federal guidelines give four categories of pediatric research with each ascending category requiring greater scrutiny of the risk-to-benefit ratio, especially in research without therapeutic benefit for the subject (Table 5-7). Whereas obtaining the assent of the child whenever possible is important for therapeutic medical procedures, it is absolutely essential in the context of research, along with the informed permission of the parents.

Informed consent and assent for research requires the decision-makers to be fully educated about the risks, benefits, and alternatives of the proposed research. In addition, subjects and parents, as appropriate, must be informed that they are free to withdraw from the study at any time without prejudice. Other ethical requirements of research hold. A study must provide quality care for the subject and legitimate options for the nonparticipant. The investigator should have good reason to believe the study will sufficiently benefit the subject or science as a whole with respect to the incurred risk. A poorly conducted study wastes resources and puts subjects at risk and, if published, may affect treatment decisions and harm other children. Institutional review boards help ensure that these principles are met by monitoring and safeguarding the quality of the research as well as the informed consent processes.

Some states allow children to assent to minor risk research without parental permission, but most states do not have explicit provisions. Most states honor the mature minor and emancipated minor conditions. Assent should be sought whenever a child has sufficient capacity. Assent is not necessary for proceeding if the child is incapable of assent or if the prospect of direct benefit which is important to the child's health, is available only in the context of the clinical investigation. Assent can be waived when it involves no more than minimal risk to the subjects, will not adversely affect the rights of the subjects, or could not practically be carried out without the waiver.[82] Parental permission may be waived when it would be unreasonable, such as in matters of child abuse.[83]

Minimal Risk

Minimal risks are defined as those risks that are not greater in and of themselves than those ordinarily encountered in daily life or during the performance of routine physical or psychological examinations. Most interpret this to mean the risks encountered in daily life by healthy children, such as running in the back yard, playing sports, and riding in a car.[84,85] A less-favored relative interpretation uses as a benchmark those risks encountered in the daily life of children who will be enrolled in the research. In other words, if a child were to live in a manner that exposed the child to risk, such as repeated general anesthetics, then it would be acceptable to expose a child to that risk in a study.

Individuals are poor at estimating the risk level of activity and often correlate risk to familiarity, control of activity, and reversibility of the potential harms.[85] Institutional review boards may reject low-risk studies because they involve unfamiliar matters while approving studies that have excessive risks. While there is variation by age, some broad strokes about risks encountered in daily life are possible.[85] In car trips for children younger than 15, the risk of mortality is 1 in 16,666,666 trips and the risk of hospitalization is 1 in 1 to 3 million trips. Combining the upper end of risk for roundtrip car travel, bathing, and playing, it is estimated that cumulative daily risk of mortality for children younger than 15 is 1 in 666,666.[85]

Minor Increase over Minimal Risk

The category "greater than minimal risk and no prospect of direct benefit to individual subjects, but likely to yield generalizable knowledge about the subject's disorder or condition . . . which is of vital importance" is based on the idea that it is acceptable to expose a child to a "minor increase over minimal risk" under certain conditions.[82] Parsing the regulation may help clarify this somewhat unhelpful definition. One suggestion has been that minor increase means that the pain, discomfort, or stress must be transient, reversible, and not severe.[84] Condition should be used to mean a set of characteristics "that an established body of scientific or clinical evidence has shown

---

Table 5-7. Federal Classifications for Pediatric Research

1. Research not involving greater than minimal risk
   a. IRB determines minimal risk.
   b. IRB finds and documents that adequate provisions are made for soliciting assent from children and permission from their parents or guardians.

2. Research involving greater than minimal risk but presenting the prospect of direct benefit to the individual subjects
   a. IRB justifies the risk by the anticipated benefit to the subjects.
   b. The relation of the anticipated benefit to the risk is at least as favorable as that presented by available alternative approaches.
   c. Adequate provisions for assent and permission

3. Research involving greater than minimal risk and no prospect of direct benefit to individual subjects but likely to yield generalizable knowledge about the subject's disorder or condition
   a. IRB determines the risk represents a minor increase over minimal risk.
   b. The intervention or procedure presents experiences to subjects that are reasonably commensurate with those inherent in their actual or expected medical, dental, psychological, social, or educational situations.
   c. The intervention or procedure is likely to yield generalizable knowledge . . . which is of vital importance for the understanding or amelioration of subject's disorder or condition.
   d. Adequate provisions for assent and permission

4. Research not otherwise approvable that presents an opportunity to understand, prevent, or alleviate a serious problem affecting the health or welfare of children

IRB, institutional review board.
From U.S. Department of Health and Human Services 45CFR46 Subpart D. Additional protection for children involved as subjects in research. 1991.

to negatively affect children's health and well-being or to increase the risk of developing a health problem in the future."[84] Interpreting "condition" to include having the potential to have the condition permits otherwise healthy children to participate in research for diseases that they may develop, such as cellulitis. The words "vital importance" imply that the evidence supporting the relevance of the study should require a higher order of proof.

Imperative for Pharmacologic Research

Through the mid 1990s, more than 70% of new molecular entities were without pediatric drug labeling. Inadequate information exposed children to age-specific adverse reactions, ineffective treatment due to inappropriate dosing, and lack of access to new drugs because physicians tended to prescribe less effective known medications. Inadequate research into pediatric drugs forced physicians to prescribe drugs in nonstandard ways, such as sprinkled or crushed tablets. Even when there is some pediatric labeling, there is very little labeling for children younger than the age of 2 years.

The U.S. Food and Drug Administration (FDA) has been trying to address this problem. The following selective history highlights the overall intent: (1) to ensure that children get the same benefits of pharmacologic advances as adults and (2) to ensure that research is performed in the youngest children, infants, and neonates, so that they benefit, too. Advocates should also learn from this history that implementing regulatory changes to benefit children may require a number of attempts to have the desired effect. For example, in 1979, an FDA requirement to include specific pediatric information on the label actually led to less pediatric labeling because of the expense of getting this information. In 1994, the FDA began requiring sponsors to explain why pediatric labeling cannot occur but did not require sponsors to perform pediatric studies. The 1997 FDA Modernization Act and the 1998 Final Rule: Pediatric Studies required more data on pediatric studies in exchange for the benefit of an additional 6 months of exclusivity. With these requirements, the FDA required studies if a new drug may be used in a substantial number of children or may provide a meaningful therapeutic benefit or if inadequate labeling could pose significant risks. The pharmaceutical industry responded vigorously to the additional 6 months of exclusivity. Medications approved during this process included over-the-counter ibuprofen for younger children, a new oral formulation of midazolam, and use of ranitidine in the neonatal population.

However, the exclusivity provision was not a panacea. Sponsors did not study generic drugs or drugs with insufficient sales. Furthermore, there was no incentive to do sequential pediatric studies. In other words, once exclusivity was credited for older pediatric age groups there was no incentive to conduct studies in younger groups. In 2002, the Best Pharmaceuticals for Children Act created the Office of Pediatric Therapeutics to coordinate activities within the FDA that affect children and a Foundation of the National Institutes of Health for the study of drugs in children. It reauthorized the extended patent exclusivity. It increased the amount of public safety reporting, but reporting remained voluntary.

In December 2003, the Pediatric Research Equity Act was enacted. It *required* studies of drugs and biological products that have a new indication, new dosage form, new routes, new dosing regimen, or new active ingredient. Studies could be waived if studies are impracticable, if therapy would be ineffective or unsafe in pediatric patients, or if there would be no meaningful therapeutic benefit over existing therapies and the moiety would not be likely to be used in a substantial number of children. Some labeling changes that arose out of these efforts include warnings about using propofol for long-term sedation, rare cases of seizures with the use of sevoflurane, and dosing of midazolam in children with congenital heart diseases and pulmonary hypertension.

Advocacy and Good Citizenship

One of the obligations of pediatric clinicians is advocacy. Obligations of physicians arise from an implicit social contract. Society supports medical students, interns and residents, and physicians by providing opportunities to train, to perform research, and, perhaps most importantly, to learn from and with patients.[86] In return, society expects physicians to manage matters in their spheres of influence; society expects anesthesiologists to "manage all things anesthesia."

An additional implicit obligation is to manage those issues that "directly influence individuals' health" in the practitioner's community.[87] The idea of "community" suggests that there are some specific individuals other than patients to whom physicians have obligations. These may be individuals in the same physical location as the physician or patients to whom the physician has a special obligation, such as children. The obligation to be involved is more relevant when the harm clearly and straightforwardly affects health (e.g., childhood obesity). Physicians should participate in activities that improve community health that are consistent with the individual's "expertise, interests, and situations."[87] Table 5-8 lists potential areas of advocacy for pediatric anesthesiologists and methods for participation.

Pain Management

For years it was thought that neonates had immature neurologic pathways that did not respond to pain and that if they did have pain, they did not remember.[88,89] Indeed, myths like these led to the Liverpool technique in which neonates received muscle relaxants and minimal anesthesia for surgery.

Table 5-8. Examples of Advocacy and Participation

- Raising public awareness about a health or social issue
- Writing a letter, signing a petition, or participating in another form of public advocacy and lobbying
- Working informally with others to solve a health problem in the community
- Encouraging a medical society to act on an issue that concerns the public health
- Serving in a local organization, political interest group, or political organization
- Topics of particular relevance to pediatric anesthesiologists
  - Pediatric obesity
  - Pediatric sedation in hospitals
  - Child abuse
  - Health care access
  - Role of subspecialty training in improving care for children

From Gruen RL, Pearson SD, Brennan TA: Physician-citizens—public roles and professional obligations. JAMA 2004; 291:94-98.

Older children also have had their pain undertreated due to limited training and knowledge about pediatric pain, the difficulty in doing pain research on children, and the mistaken belief that children are more prone to addiction and respiratory depression. Perhaps the most important factor in whether pain is adequately treated is the ability of the child to verbalize discomfort.[90]

Aside from the humanitarian imperative to control pain, children do in fact have a physiologic response to pain and adequate pain control may lead to less morbidity and mortality (see Chapters 44 and 45).[91] Comfortable children are more capable of achieving the goals of assent and are more cooperative with care. The obligation to provide postoperative pain management requires anesthesiologists to minimize pain in the least objectionable ways. Limitations to achieving successful analgesia after surgery include inadequate postoperative care facilities, inexperience, and no designated pain service.[92]

Components of pain management include analgesia and elimination of fear, which often includes obliteration of awareness, anxiolysis, and perhaps amnesia. Amnesia and anxiolysis without adequate pain control, particularly for a procedure that will be repeated such as sampling bone marrow, does not wholly fulfill the humanitarian and physiologic goals and should not be confused with adequate pain management. Similarly, control of pain without sufficient management of awareness and fear is not desirable care.

The concept of suffering deserves special note. Suffering is an intensely personal feeling that can be defined as "the state of severe distress associated with events that threaten the intactness of the person."[93] Suffering should be considered when evaluating pain control, and adequate steps should be taken to find and alleviate sources of suffering. Factors that may contribute to a child's suffering include not knowing the origin or meaning of the pain, inability to influence important aspects of care such as pain management, and a belief that the pain will never be relieved.[93] This is especially true in children, where pain is often interpreted as punishment for something that the child has done wrong. Anesthesiologists can help minimize suffering by clearly communicating about these issues with parents and children and affording children as much control of their care as possible.

Medical Error

Medical error may be the result of human mistakes or system flaws or, most commonly, both.[94] Anesthesiologists have an obligation to work to reduce system flaws, including participating in quality improvement activities such as data collection, following policies meant to improve care in high-risk situations (e.g., nosocomial infections), and actively engaging in policies designed to reduce medical errors (e.g., universal standards of patient identification). Although many anesthesiologists may not understand or appreciate why they are being asked to do "extra" steps, it is vital for anesthesiologists (as well as all physicians) to subsume personal preferences for the good of "the team" and willingly participate in those activities to further the common good. Similar to the blind men describing an elephant by the parts of the elephant's body they are holding, it is difficult for individual anesthesiologists to appreciate the big picture sufficiently to understand the purposes of policies.[95] When anesthesiologists believe that policies are harmful or unnecessary, they are obligated to raise these questions through appropriate channels. Surreptitiously circumventing policies may harm patients, does not permit remediation of the policy, and weakens the fidelity of the entire system, encouraging others to "make their own rules."

Production Pressure

Anesthesiologists are prone to production pressure, which has been defined as "the internal or external pressure on the anesthetist to keep the operating room schedule moving along speedily."[96] Indeed, nearly half of surveyed anesthesiologists reported seeing what they considered unsafe anesthetic practices in response to this production pressure.[97] As a consequence, anesthesiologists may not want to take the time to allow a child to ask questions about the anesthetic, to adequately premedicate an anxious child, or to engage the parents in a lengthy discussion about postponing the surgery because their child has a mild upper respiratory infection. Anesthesiologists should also be cognizant of their level of skill in providing anesthesia. For example, the "routine" tonsillectomy may be beyond some anesthesiologists' ability in the child with multiple congenital deficits. Anesthesiologists have an obligation to the patient and themselves to only provide care within their skills and to recognize when economic and administrative pressures may induce them to do otherwise.

Another source of production pressure may be from managed care organizations. The concept of managed care is neither good nor bad. At its best, managed care can encourage preventative care, continuing patient-physician relationships, collaborative relationships among primary care clinicians and specialists, and good performance improvement programs. At its worst, managed care can result in a mercurial bureaucratic system that prioritizes short-term cost-containment and seeks a young and predominantly healthy customer population to avoid paying for expensive care.[98] Managed care organizations accomplish these goals by "managing" or controlling physician and patient behavior through the use of case managers to coordinate care, financial and administrative incentives to encourage physicians to conserve resources, gatekeeping devices to control access to specialty care, and practice guidelines to limit imaging tests, expensive drugs, and longer hospital stays. Physicians have the obligation to participate in managed care to ensure it is performed well and should participate in legislative initiatives to curb potential abuses, work with managed care organizations to design systems that minimize conflicts of interest, and actively fight abuses on an individual level. Anesthesiologists need to closely examine any managed care organization contract for inherent problems, that may include compensation through financial incentives, plans that do not have a reasonable or responsive appeals process, and policies that have an undefined physician termination procedure.[99,100]

Suspicion of Child Abuse

Each year, 2% to 3% of children are abused. Child abuse includes acts of physical abuse, sexual abuse, emotional abuse, and neglect. Anesthesiologists are in a unique position to recognize some forms of physical abuse given their more than usual attention to patients' hands, arms, ankles, and faces. Anesthesiologists should be particularly sensitive to bruises or burns in the shape of objects, injuries to soft tissue areas such as upper arms, unexplained mouth and dental injuries, fractures in infants, and height and weight less than the 5th percentile (see Chapter 39 and Fig. 39-10).[101-104] Children who have physical or mental handicaps are particularly prone to abuse.[105] Stunningly, child abuse occurs in the hospital and even while a child is undergoing diagnostic or therapeutic care.[106] Anesthesiologists, as all physicians, are legally required to report the suspicion of child abuse or neglect to appropriate authorities. Indeed, in most jurisdictions, a physician can be criminally prosecuted if found liable for failing to report suspected child abuse.[17,101]

To help clinicians recognize possible child abuse, the American Academy of Pediatrics has suggested that "child abuse should be considered as the most likely explanations for inflicted skin injuries if they are non-accidental and there is any injury beyond temporary reddening of the skin."[107] Other markers of concern are injuries that do not appear accidental, injuries that fit a biomechanical model (e.g., a handprint), and injuries that are not developmentally appropriate, would not occur naturally, and are not explained by the offered history (see Chapter 39).[107]

Complementary Medicine

Anesthesiologists may meet families who prefer to use complementary and alternative medicine for their child. Complementary and alternative approaches include acupuncture, manual therapies, herbal therapies and nutritional supplements, mind/body therapies, and energy medicine such as Reiki.[108] Complementary and alternative approaches have been shown to have a range of benefits.[109] Among other reasons, parents may choose complementary and alternative medicine because it provides an opportunity to actively help their child fight illness. While it is important to honor the parent's desires, it is also important to ensure that children are not hurt either by the addition of potentially harmful therapies or by the forgoing of useful mainstream therapies (see Chapter 6).[109] Anesthesiologists should be careful to avoid derogating complementary and alternative approaches chosen. If one is chosen, anesthesiologists should be willing to help in monitoring and evaluating complementary and alternative medicine approaches.

Practicing Procedures on Deceased Children

Practicing procedures in newly deceased children may allow junior clinicians an opportunity to gain valuable experiences under controlled circumstances without exposing children to risk.[110] Such procedures, however, should be undertaken with respect. Physicians should obtain permission to practice procedures, just as they would obtain permission for autopsies or the procurement of organs. Although each institution has to determine appropriate policy, we believe that consent is best obtained and documented by oral discussion with the parents and by a written note in the medical record. An additional paper form for this rare event seems cumbersome and unnecessarily stressful to the parents and adding a statement about the procedure to forms discussing autopsy seems like an inappropriate combination of activities. Procedures should be nonmutilating, such as tracheal intubation. Only those clinicians who have a legitimate need to learn should be permitted to perform the technique. This group is not necessarily limited to physicians, because others, such as emergency medical technicians, may need this skill. The procedure should be performed under supervision and after proper preparation. This groundwork legitimizes the exercise as an educational experience while fulfilling the obligation to treat the body and its donation with respect.

Molecular Genetic Testing

Genetic testing can be used to confirm a diagnosis or determine carrier status or for asymptomatic testing for disorders of late onset.[111] Benefits of testing include an elimination of uncertainty and the initiation of appropriate surveillance and care. On the other hand, because people share genes, people may learn about their own genetic predisposition without giving consent or receiving appropriate pretesting counseling. Family secrets may be unwittingly exposed. Minors, of course, present with additional informed consent issues. Determining genetic predisposition in a child keeps the child from choosing in the future whether to obtain that knowledge. To that end, the American Academy of Pediatrics recommends that testing should be offered only when there are immediate medical benefits and when there is a benefit to another family member and no expected harm to the child. Other testing should be deferred until the child is able to appreciate the social, psychological, and economic consequences of genetic testing.[111] Disorders that are diagnosable by mutation analysis include types of neurofibromatosis, types of muscular dystrophies, hemophilia A, cystic fibrosis, and craniofacial anomalies.[111]

The Fetus

One of the more perplexing aspects of caring for the fetus is the view of the maternal-fetal relationship. It is instructive to examine the positions of the American Academy of Pediatrics and the American College of Obstetricians and Gynecologists (Table 5-9).[112-114] The statements of these organizations are similar, but there are some important, subtle differences when the interests of the mother and fetus diverge, such as when the mother wishes to refuse a likely beneficial treatment for the fetus. Broadly, the American Academy of Pediatrics advocates more for the fetus, particularly when there is an effective intervention to an irreversible harm and the intervention poses only a small risk to the mother. The American College of Obstetricians and Gynecologists is more concerned about the complex issues of overriding maternal autonomy, such as the criminalization of not complying with medical recommendations.

The Ethics Consultation Service

The ethical dilemmas that occur in the practice of anesthesiology may be difficult for the practitioner to resolve alone. Ethics committees and their consulting services act in an advisory role to help clinicians, patients, and families amicably resolve ethical dilemmas.[115] Anesthesiologists may find ethics consultation helpful with questions about informed consent, decision-making capacity, resuscitation decisions, and resolving disagreements among patients, families, and clinicians.[115-117]

A survey of ethics consultation services conducted in 2000 gives insight into what clinicians can expect from an ethics consult.[118] Although most ethics consultation services use a small group (typically around three people) to perform consults, some use the entire committee and some use a single individual. Physicians, nurses, social workers, chaplains, administrators, and lay people serve on ethics committees and perform consults. Common characteristics of ethics consultations services are that they permit anyone to request an ethics consultation; require notification (not permission) of the child, parents, and attending physician before performing the consult; and recognize that choosing to follow the recommendations is wholly voluntary.

Table 5-9. Positions of the American Academy of Pediatrics and the American College of Obstetricians and Gynecologists on Ethical Considerations and Maternal Choices in Fetal Therapy

	American Academy of Pediatrics	American College of Obstetricians and Gynecologists
Priority	Respect for principle of maternal autonomy Fetal concerns may trump maternal autonomy	Respect for principle of maternal autonomy Fetal concerns may not trump maternal autonomy
Type of Medical Treatment Worthy of Judicial or Physical Intervention	If the intervention has been demonstrated to be effective If nonintervention will lead to significant and irreversible harm If there is minimal maternal risk from the intervention	If there is a high probability of serious harm to the fetus If there is a high probability of significant benefit to the fetus If there is a relatively small risk to the pregnant woman If no comparably effective less invasive options are available Intervention only under extraordinary circumstances of conflict
Use of Physical Intervention	Physical intervention may be acceptable if judicial authorization has been obtained	Physical intervention is never acceptable
Psychosocial Aspects	Psychosocial aspects of overriding a woman's autonomy is not addressed	Significant concern about overriding maternal autonomy, including: • criminalization of noncompliance with medical recommendations • loss of trust in the health care system • social costs of compromising liberty
Conflict Resolution	Does not ask physicians to consider subordinating their view Does not suggest it is reasonable to transfer the patient's care	Physicians should make reasonable attempts to explain recommended treatments and to persuade the woman to comply Physicians should subordinate their values if necessary, because it is the woman's decision Suggests it may be reasonable to transfer care

Data from references 112 to 114.

After consultations, clinicians feel greater satisfaction in managing cases with ethical conflicts, not only because of their heightened awareness of the expert consulting services available but also because of their increased knowledge and comfort in dealing with these issues. Ethics committees are also available to consult on policy development and to organize continuing educational programs.

Summary

Ethical issues in the care of children tend to center on questions about decision-making capacity. Infants and children are often incapable of successfully "speaking for themselves" and may be in need of supervision and protection. This protection is generally well executed by the parents, but at times is not, and the state, through clinicians and the legal system, must sometimes seek to ensure proper care for children by balancing the "natural rights" of the parents with the obligation of the state to protect the child. Those caring for adolescents need to incorporate the increasingly accepted concept of children as active participants in determining their care. Many anesthesiologists who are uncomfortable with this approach become even more threatened when they realize that there are different categories of decision-making that require considerations of the child and the situation. Finally, there is the problem of defining what criteria should be used to determine what is in the best interests of the minor. Decisions such as these may appear difficult at best and insurmountable at worst. Anesthesiologists can help themselves and their patients by utilizing available resources such as ethics consultation services for guidance and conflict resolution.

Annotated References

Committee on Bioethics, American Academy of Pediatrics: Informed consent, parental permission, and assent in pediatric practice. Pediatrics 1995; 95:314-317
This article is the fundamental explanation of informed consent for children. Pay particular attention to the introduction, in which Dr. William Bartholome (in absentia) exhorts clinicians to respect "the experience, perspective and power of children."

Consensus statement of the Society of Critical Care Medicine's Ethics Committee regarding futile and other possibly inadvisable treatments. Crit Care Med 1997; 25:887-891
This article explains the importance of recognizing the ethical and clinical differences between futile treatment and other inadvisable treatments and expands on the classifications used in this chapter.

Gruen RL, Pearson SD, Brennan TA: Physician-citizens—public roles and professional obligations. JAMA 2004; 291:94-98
This article provides a thoughtful perspective on obligations of physicians.

Kon AA: Answering the question: "Doctor, if this were your child, what would you do?" Pediatrics 2006; 118:393-397
This article helps anesthesiologists understand and answer this deceptively simple question.

Fallat ME, Deshpande JK: Do-not-resuscitate orders for pediatric patients who require anesthesia and surgery. Pediatrics 2004; 114:1686-1692
This article is a complete explanation of perioperative do-not-resuscitate orders for children.

References

Please see www.expertconsult.com

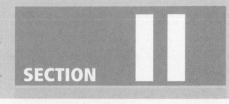

Drug and Fluid Therapy

SECTION **II**

Pharmacokinetics and Pharmacology of Drugs Used in Children

CHAPTER **6**

Charles J. Coté, Jerrold Lerman, Robert M. Ward,
Ralph A. Lugo, and Nishan Goudsouzian

Codeine	**Antiemetics**
Tramadol	Metoclopramide
Nonsteroidal Anti-inflammatory Agents	5-Hydroxytryptamine Type 3 Receptor (5-HT₃) Antagonists
Ketorolac	
Acetaminophen	**Anticholinergics**
Sedatives	Atropine and Scopolamine
Diazepam	Glycopyrrolate
Midazolam	**Antagonists**
Dexmedetomidine	Naloxone
Chloral Hydrate	Naltrexone
Antihistamines	Methylnaltrexone
Diphenhydramine	Flumazenil
Cimetidine, Ranitidine, and Famotidine	Physostigmine

THE **PHARMACOKINETICS AND PHARMACODYNAMICS** of most medications, when used in children, especially neonates, differ from those in adults.[1-11] Children exhibit different pharmacokinetics from adults because of their altered protein binding, larger volume of distribution (Vd), smaller proportion of fat and muscle stores, and immature renal and hepatic function.[2,3,12-19] These factors and individual differences in drug metabolic enzymes may reduce a drug's metabolism and/or delay elimination and, in some cases, may increase metabolism.[7,20-22] This necessitates modification of the dose and the interval between doses to achieve the desired clinical response and avoid toxicity.[7] In addition, some medications may displace bilirubin from its protein binding sites and possibly predispose an infant to kernicterus.[23-28] The capacity of the end organ, such as the heart or bronchial smooth muscle, to respond to medications may also differ in children compared with adults. In this chapter we discuss basic pharmacologic principles as they relate to drugs commonly used by anesthesiologists.

Drug Distribution

Protein Binding

The degree of protein binding is usually less in preterm and term infants than in older children and adults. This may be attributed in part to the lower concentrations of total protein and albumin (Fig. 6-1).[29] Many drugs that are highly protein bound in adults have less of an affinity for protein in neonates (Fig. 6-2, see website).[29-33] Lower protein binding results in a greater free fraction of medications, thus providing more free medication and greater pharmacologic effect.[2,3,12,14,17] This effect is particularly important for medications that are highly protein bound because the reduced protein binding increases the free fraction of the medication. For example, phenytoin is 85% protein bound in healthy infants but only 80% in those who are jaundiced. This equates to a 33% increase in the free fraction of phenytoin when jaundice occurs (Fig. 6-3, see website). Differences in protein binding may have considerable influence on the response to medications that are acidic and are, therefore, highly protein bound (e.g., phenytoin, salicylate, bupivacaine, barbiturates,

antibiotics, theophylline, and diazepam).[17] In addition, some medications, such as phenytoin, salicylate, sulfisoxazole, caffeine, ceftriaxone, diatrizoate (Hypaque), and sodium benzoate, compete with bilirubin for binding to albumin (see Fig. 6-3 on website). If large amounts of bilirubin are displaced, particularly in the presence of hypoxemia and acidosis, which open the blood/brain barrier, kernicterus may result.[24,25,30,33-35] Because these metabolic derangements often occur in sick neonates coming to surgery, special care must be taken when selecting

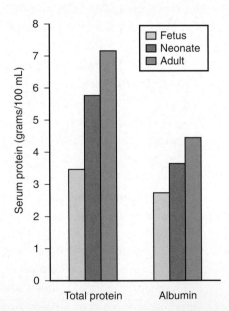

Figure 6-1. The changes in total serum protein and albumin values with maturation. Note that total protein and albumin are less in preterm than term infants and less in term infants than adults. The result may be altered pharmacokinetics and pharmacodynamics for drugs with a high degree of protein binding because less drug is protein bound and more is available for clinical effect. (Data from Ehrnebo M, Agurell S, Jalling B, et al: Age differences in drug binding by plasma proteins: studies on human fetuses, neonates and adults. Eur J Clin Pharmacol 1971; 3:189-193.)

medications for the anesthetic.[35] Medications that are basic (e.g., lidocaine or alfentanil) are generally bound to plasma α_1-acid glycoprotein; α_1-acid glycoprotein concentrations in preterm and term infants are less than in older children and adults. Therefore, for a given dose, the free fraction of a drug is greater in preterm and term infants.[36-38]

Body Composition

Volume of Distribution

Preterm and term infants have a much greater proportion of body weight in the form of water than older children and adults (Fig. 6-4).[19] The net effect on water-soluble medications is a greater Vd in infants, which in turn increases the initial (loading) dose, based on weight, to achieve the desired serum level and clinical response.[2,3,14,39,40] Term neonates often require a greater initial loading dose (milligrams per kilogram) for some medications (e.g., digoxin, succinylcholine, and antibiotics), than older children.[39-43] However, neonates also tend to be sensitive to the respiratory, neurologic, and circulatory effects of many medications and therefore tend to be more responsive to these effects at reduced blood concentrations than are children and adults. Preterm infants are usually more sensitive than term neonates and in general require even lower blood concentrations.[2] On the other hand, dopamine may increase blood pressure and urine output in term neonates only at doses as large as 50 μg/kg/min. This dose, which would induce intense vasoconstriction in adults, suggests that neonates are less sensitive in their cardiovascular responsiveness.[3,41,44-47] *It is important to carefully titrate*

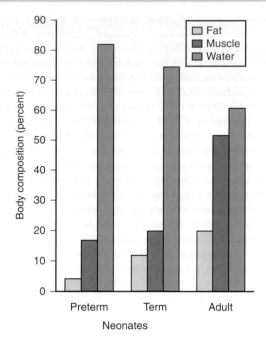

Figure 6-5. Changes in body content for fat, muscle, and water that occur with maturation. Note the small fat and muscle mass in preterm and term infants. These factors may greatly influence the pharmacokinetics and pharmacodynamics of medications that redistribute into fat (e.g., barbiturates) and muscle (e.g., fentanyl) because there is less tissue mass into which the drug may redistribute. (Data from Friis-Hansen B: Body composition during growth: in-vivo measurements and biochemical data correlated to differential anatomical growth. Pediatrics 1971; 47:264-274.)

the doses of all medications that are administered to preterm and term infants to the desired response.

Fat and Muscle Content

Compared with children and adolescents, preterm and full-term neonates have a smaller proportion of body weight in the form of fat and muscle mass; with growth, the proportion of body weight composed of these tissues increases (Fig. 6-5).[2-4,19,45,46,48,49] Therefore, medications that depend on their redistribution into muscle and fat for termination of their clinical effects likely have a large initial peak blood concentration. These medications may also have a more sustained blood concentration because neonates have less tissue for redistribution of these medications. An incorrect dose may result in prolonged undesirable clinical effects (e.g. barbiturates and opioids may cause prolonged sedation and respiratory depression). The possible influence of small muscle mass on the response to muscle relaxants is exemplified by achieving neuromuscular blockade at lower serum concentrations in infants.[41]

Metabolism and Excretion

Hepatic Blood Flow

The liver is one of the most important organs involved in drug metabolism. Hepatic enzymatic drug metabolism usually converts the medication from a less polar state (lipid soluble) to a more polar, water-soluble compound (see later). Although no categorical statement applies to all drugs and enzymes, the

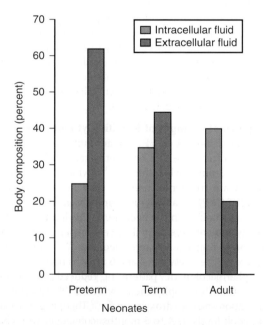

Figure 6-4. Changes in the intracellular and extracellular compartments that occur with maturation. Note the large proportion of extracellular water in preterm and term infants. This large water compartment creates an increased volume of distribution for highly water-soluble medications (e.g., succinylcholine, antibiotics) and may account for the large initial "loading" dose (mg/kg) required for some medications to achieve a satisfactory clinical response. (Data from Friis-Hansen B: Body composition during growth: in-vivo measurements and biochemical data correlated to differential anatomical growth. Pediatrics 1971; 47:264-274.)

Table 6-2. Developmental Patterns for Important Conjugation (Phase II) Reactions in the Neonate

Enzymes	Selected Substrates	Developmental Patterns
Uridine diphosphoglucuronyltransferase (UDP-GT)	Chloramphenicol, morphine, acetaminophen, valproic acid, lorazepam	Ontogeny is isoform specific. In general, adult activity is achieved by 6-18 months of age. May be induced by cigarette smoke and phenobarbital.
Sulfotransferase	Bile acids, acetaminophen, cholesterol, polyethylene, glycols, dopamine, chloramphenicol	Ontogeny seems to be more rapid than UDP-GT; however, it is substrate specific. Activity for some isoforms may exceed adult values during infancy and childhood, e.g., that responsible for acetaminophen metabolism.
N-Acetyltransferase 2	Hydralazine, procainamide, clonazepam, caffeine, sulfamethoxazole	Some fetal activity present by 16 weeks. Virtually 100% of infants between birth and 2 months of age exhibit the slow metabolizer phenotype. Adult activity present by 1-3 years of age.

Adapted from Leeder JS, Kearns GL: Pharmacogenetics in pediatrics: implications for practice. Pediatr Clin North Am 1997; 44:55-77.

understanding the immaturity of UDP-GT and its role in the elimination of chloramphenicol. Infants accumulated high concentrations of chloramphenicol and developed fatal circulatory collapse, a condition known as the gray baby syndrome.[116-118] Although the clearance of chloramphenicol is low during the neonatal period, appropriate dosage adjustments and monitoring allow safe treatment of preterm- and full-term infants with chloramphenicol.[119]

Morphine, acetaminophen, and lorazepam also undergo glucuronidation. The major steps in the metabolic disposition of morphine in children and adults is glucuronidation in the 3- and 6-position.[63,120] The limited ability of neonates to glucuronidate morphine necessitates dosage adjustment.[121-123] Detailed studies have shown that morphine clearance,[122,124] in particular 3- and 6-glucuronide formation, is limited at birth and increases with birth weight,[123] gestational age,[83] and postnatal age.[120,121] In some studies, morphine clearance approaches adult values by 1 month,[121,125] although others reported that the clearance does not reach adult values until at least 5 to 6 months.[122,126] Overall, the maturation of glucuronosyltransferase enzymes varies among isoforms, but, in general, adult activity is reached by 6 to 18 months of age.[94]

In contrast to glucuronosyltransferase, the sulfotransferase enzyme system is well developed in the neonate, and for some compounds it may compensate for limited glucuronidation. In adults, the primary pathway for acetaminophen metabolism is glucuronidation, yet its half-life is only moderately prolonged in neonates compared with older infants and adults.[127-129] This occurs because the neonate forms more sulfate than glucuronide conjugate, leading to a greater percent of the dose excreted as the acetaminophen-sulfate conjugate.[128,129] This metabolic pattern of preferential sulfation of acetaminophen persists into childhood.[128,130]

Alterations in Biotransformation

Many biotransformation reactions, especially those involving certain forms of cytochrome P-450, are inducible before birth through maternal exposure to drugs, cigarette smoke, or other inducing agents. Postnatally, biotransformation reactions may be induced through drug exposure (see Tables 6-1 and 6-2) and may be slowed by hypoxia/asphyxia, organ damage, and/or

illness. Postnatal changes in hepatic blood flow, protein binding, and/or biliary function may also alter drug elimination. Further studies of drug metabolism in preterm and term infants will lead to safer and more effective pharmacotherapeutic regimens.

Genotypic Variations in Drug Metabolism

Single nucleotide changes or polymorphisms (SNPs) in the DNA sequence in CYP enzymes usually decrease but may increase metabolic activity for a specific drug substrate.[131] Much of the explanation for variations in drug responses within large populations that are described as "biologic variation" likely relates to genetic differences in drug metabolism, receptor binding, and intracellular coupling to effector mechanisms. Following the recognition that certain individuals had exaggerated hypotensive responses to debrisoquine, the enzyme responsible for its metabolism, CYP2D6 became one of the first drug-metabolizing enzymes identified.[132-134] Earlier studies had shown that individuals might possess normal or reduced metabolic activity (poor metabolizers) for debrisoquine and sparteine.[133,135] The frequency of poor metabolizers varied among ethnic groups, occurring in approximately 7% of whites[136] and 0% to 1% of Chinese and Japanese.[137]

Codeine, is primarily a pro-drug that undergoes metabolic activation by CYP2D6 O-demethylation to morphine.[138] Without O-demethylation, codeine confers a small fraction of the analgesic molar potency of morphine, and much of its analgesic effect is likely contributed by a metabolite, codeine 6-glucuronide.[139] For the 2% to 10% of the population who are CYP2D6 poor metabolizers, codeine causes limited opioid effects.[140,141] For other drugs, ranging from propranolol to warfarin to methotrexate, reduced metabolism through genetic polymorphisms of other enzymes leads to exaggerated effects when administered in conventional doses.[131] Similar variations in activity have been reported for many of the CYPs involved in drug metabolism in humans.[142] Genotyping has become a routine part of the evaluation before treatment with methotrexate for detection of reduced activity of thiopurine methyltransferase that may be lethal with treatment with conventional dosages.[143,144] Genotyping has been proposed before drug treatment and as a guide to drug selection when specific SNPs have been correlated with adverse drug reactions or clinically significant alterations in metabolism.[92] Although hundreds of possible SNPs have been identified that account for much of the variation in drug effects among individuals, Andersson and associates have discussed which specific SNPs of CYP2C9, CYP2C19, CYP2D6, CYP3A, and uridine diphosphate-glucuronosyltransferase 1A1 (UGT1A1) account for a sufficient number of adverse pharmacologic outcomes to warrant clinical testing when it becomes feasible.[92] Until genotyping for many more abnormalities in drug metabolizing enzymes, receptors, and channels becomes a routine part of drug treatment, careful attention to a history of adverse drug reactions in the child and first-degree relatives and careful attention to recording current reactions are the best guides to detect clinically important variations in drug metabolism.

Renal Excretion

The renal function in preterm and term infants is less efficient than in adults even after adjusting for the differences in body weight. This reduced efficiency is related to the combination of incomplete glomerular development, low perfusion pressure, and inadequate osmotic load to produce full countercurrent effects.[145-150] Preterm and term neonates have immature glomerular filtration and tubular function; both develop rapidly during the first few months of life. Healthy term neonates have relatively normal renal drug clearance by 3 to 4 weeks of age. Glomerular filtration and tubular function are nearly mature by 20 weeks of age and fully mature by 2 years of age (Fig. 6-7).[146-150] For these reasons, *drugs that are excreted primarily through glomerular filtration or tubular secretion, such as aminoglycoside and cephalosporin antibiotics, have a prolonged elimination half-life in neonates* (Fig. 6-8, see website).[151-153]

In the presence of renal failure, one or two doses of drugs that are excreted via the kidneys often achieve and maintain prolonged therapeutic drug levels if there is no alternate pathway of excretion. The first dose may be removed from the circulation by distribution and tissue binding. *Whenever administering a medication to a preterm or term infant, one must consider the contribution of renal function in the termination of its action.*

The pharmacokinetics and pharmacodynamics of the old muscle relaxant, curare, exemplify the complex interaction of increased Vd, smaller muscle mass, and decreased rate of excretion due to immaturity of glomerular filtration. The initial dose of curare needed to achieve neuromuscular blockade is similar in infants and adults.[41] In infants, however, this blockade is achieved at reduced serum concentrations compared with older children or adults, corresponding to differences in muscle mass. A larger Vd (total body water) accounts for the equivalent dose for each kilogram of body weight, and the reduced glomerular function in infants compared with older children or adults accounts in part for the longer duration of action.[41] As in the case of drugs excreted by the liver, there is a triphasic developmental response to drugs excreted by the kidneys: a prolonged half-life in neonates (immature renal function), a shortened half-life in young children (maturation of the kidneys and increased renal perfusion delivering more drug to the kidneys), and a greater elimination half-life in adolescents and adults (decreased renal function and decreased proportional renal blood flow). Reduced protein binding in neonates and preterm infants increases the free fraction of drugs delivered to the kidneys and liver for metabolism; however, this also increases the fraction of drugs available to cross biologic membranes. This greater unbound fraction causes more drug to be available to have effect or a greater potential for toxicity.[2,3,16,17]

Pharmacokinetic Principles and Calculations

Changes in drug concentrations within the body over time are referred to as pharmacokinetics. The principles and equations that describe these changes can be used to adjust drug doses rationally to achieve more effective drug concentrations at the site of action.[80,81,154-156] The equations in this section are intended for general and practical use, whereas the more rigorous mathematical intricacies of pharmacokinetics are covered elsewhere.[157-160]

Within the body, a drug may diffuse between several body fluids and tissues at different rates, yet the consistent change in its circulating concentration may be used to characterize its kinetics and to guide dosages. The rate of removal of drug from the circulation usually fits either first-order or zero-order exponential equations. The difference between these two types of rates has important implications for drug treatment.

First-Order Kinetics

Most drugs are cleared from the body with first-order exponential rates in which a constant fraction or constant proportion of drug is removed per unit of time. Because the proportion of drug cleared remains constant, the higher the concentration, the greater the amount of drug removed from the body. Such rates can be described by exponential equations that fit the following form:

$$C = C_0 e^{-kt} \quad \text{(Eq. 1)}$$

where C is the concentration at time t, C_0 is the starting concentration (a constant determined by the dose and distribution

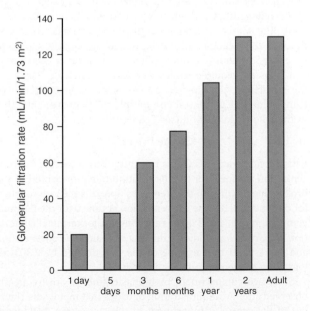

Figure 6-7. Changes in glomerular filtration rate (GFR) versus age. Note the rapid development of glomerular function during the first year of life. Abnormal as well as immature renal function may delay drug excretion. (Data from Chantler C: Clinical Pediatric Nephrology. Philadelphia, JB Lippincott, 1976.)

volume), and k is the elimination rate constant with units of time^{-1}. First-order indicates that the exponent is raised to the first power ($-kt$ in Equation 1). Second-order equations are those that are raised to the second power, such as $e^{(z)2}$. First-order exponential equations, such as Equation 1, may be converted to the form of the equation of a straight line ($y = mx + b$) by taking the natural logarithm of both sides, after which they may be solved by linear regression.

$$\ln C = \ln C_0 + (-kt) \qquad \text{(Eq. 2)}$$

If ln (i.e., natural logarithm) C is graphed versus time, the slope is $-k$, and the intercept is $\ln C_0$. If log (i.e., common logarithm) C is graphed versus time, the slope is $-k/2.303$, because ln x equals $2.303 \log x$. When graphed on linear-linear axes, exponential rates are curvilinear and on semilogarithmic axes, they produce a straight line.

Half-Life

Half-life, the time for a drug concentration to decrease by one half, is a familiar exponential rate used to describe the kinetics of many drugs. *Half-life is a first-order kinetic process, because the same proportion or fraction of the drug is removed during equal periods of time.* As described earlier, the greater the concentration, the greater the amount of drug removed during each half-life.

Half-life can be determined by several methods. If concentration is converted to the natural logarithm of concentration and graphed versus time, as described in Equation 2, the slope of this graph is the elimination rate constant, k. For both accuracy and precision, at least three concentration-time points should be used to determine the slope, and they should be obtained over an interval during which the concentration decreases at least in half. In clinical practice, for infants and small children, however, k is often estimated from just two concentrations obtained during the terminal elimination phase. With multiple data points, the slope of ln C versus time may be calculated easily by least-squares linear regression analysis. Half-life ($T^1/_2$) may be calculated from the elimination rate constant, k (time^{-1}), as follows:

$$T^1/_2 = \frac{\text{Natural logarithm (2)}}{k} = \frac{0.0693}{k} \qquad \text{(Eq. 3)}$$

Graphic techniques may be used to determine half-life from a series of timed measurements of drug concentration. The concentration-time points should be graphed on semilogarithmic axes and used to determine the best fitting line either visually or by linear regression analysis. This approach is illustrated in Figure 6-9, in which the best-fitting line has been drawn to the concentration-points and crosses a concentration of 20 at 100 minutes and a concentration of 10 at 200 minutes. The concentration has decreased by one half in 100 minutes so the half-life is 100 minutes. The elimination rate constant is 0.693/100 min^{-1} or 0.00693 min^{-1}.

First-Order Single-Compartment Kinetics

The number of exponential equations required to describe the change in concentration determines the number of compartments. Although a drug may be diffusing among several tissues and body fluids, its clearance often fits first-order, single-compartment kinetics if it quickly distributes homogeneously

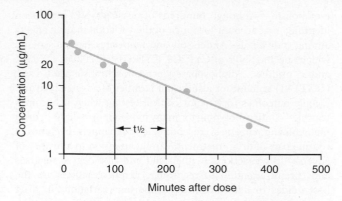

Figure 6-9. Graphic determination of half-life. Half-life can be determined from a series of concentration-time points on a semi-logarithmic graph, if the kinetics are exponential. The concentrations are plotted on semi-logarithmic axes; the best-fit line is drawn to the points; convenient concentrations are chosen that decrease in half, such as 20 and 10, as illustrated; and the interval between those concentrations is the half-life, which is 100 minutes in the illustration.

within the circulation and is removed rapidly from the circulation through metabolism or excretion. This may be judged visually, if a semilogarithmic graph of the change in drug concentration fits a single straight line. Kinetics may appear to be single-compartment, when they are really multiple compartments, if drug concentrations are not measured soon enough after IV administration to detect the initial distribution phase (α phase).

First-Order Multiple-Compartment Kinetics

If drug concentrations are measured several times within the first 15 to 30 minutes after IV administration as well as during a more prolonged period, more than one rate of clearance is often present. This can be observed as a marked change in slope of a semilogarithmic graph of concentration versus time (Fig. 6-10). The number and nature of the compartments required to describe the clearance of a drug do not necessarily represent specific body fluids or tissues. When two first-order exponential equations are required to describe the clearance of drug from the circulation, the kinetics are described as first-order, two-compartment (e.g., central and peripheral compartments) that fit the following equation (see Fig. 6-10)[154]:

$$C = Ae^{-\alpha t} + Be^{-\beta t} \qquad \text{(Eq. 4)}$$

where concentration is C, t is time after the dose, A is the concentration at time 0 for the distribution rate represented by the broken line graph with the steepest slope, α is the rate constant for distribution, B is the concentration at time 0 for the terminal elimination rate, and β is the rate constant for terminal elimination. Rate constants indicate the rate of change in concentration and correspond to the slope of the line divided by 2.303 for logarithm concentration versus time.

Such two compartment or biphasic kinetics are frequently observed after IV administration of drugs that rapidly distribute out of the central compartment of the circulation to undergo hepatic metabolism or renal excretion.[154] In such situations, the initial rapid decrease in concentration is referred to as the α distribution phase and represents distribution to the peripheral (tissue) compartments in addition to drug elimination. The

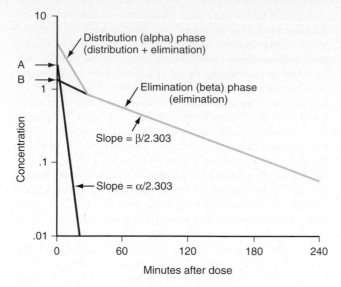

Figure 6-10. Two compartment kinetics in a semi-logarithmic graph. The initial rapid decrease in serum concentration reflects distribution and elimination followed by a slower decrease due to elimination. Subtraction of the initial decrease in concentration due to elimination using the concentrations from the elimination line extrapolated back to time 0 at B produces the lower line with a steep slope = α(distribution rate constant)/2.303. The terminal elimination phase has a slope = β(elimination rate constant)/2.303.

terminal (β) phase begins after the inflection point in the line when elimination starts to account for most of the change in drug concentration. To determine the initial change in concentration due to distribution (see Fig. 6-10), the change in concentration due to elimination must be subtracted from the total change in concentration. The slope of the line representing the difference between these two rates is the rate constant for distribution. A more detailed mathematical discussion may be found elsewhere.[154,157]

Although many drugs demonstrate multiple-compartment kinetics, many studies of kinetics in neonates do not include enough samples immediately after dosing to determine both compartments. For clinical estimates of dose and dosing intervals, it is often not necessary to use multiple-compartment kinetics. To minimize cost, limit blood loss, and simplify pharmacokinetic calculations, dose adjustments are often based on only two plasma concentrations (peak and trough) and assume linear, single-compartment kinetics (e.g., gentamicin and vancomycin). Because the elimination rate constant should be determined from the terminal elimination phase, it is important that peak concentrations of multiple-compartment drugs not be drawn prematurely, that is, during the initial distribution phase. If drawn too early, the concentrations will be greater than those during the terminal elimination phase (see Fig. 6-10), which will overestimate the slope and the terminal elimination rate constant.

Zero-Order Kinetics

The elimination of some drugs occurs with loss of a *constant amount per time, rather than a constant fraction per time*. Such rates are termed zero-order, and because $e^0 = 1$, the change in the amount of drug in the body fits the following equation[157]:

$$-dA/dt = k_0 \qquad \text{(Eq. 5)}$$

where dA is the change in the amount of drug in the body (mg), dt is the change in time, and k_0 is the elimination rate constant with units of amount/time. After solving this equation, it has the following form:

$$A = A_0 - k_0t \qquad \text{(Eq. 6)}$$

where A_0 is the initial amount of drug in the body and A is the amount of drug in the body (in milligrams) at time t.

Zero-order kinetics may be designated saturation kinetics, because such processes occur when excess amounts of drug saturate the capacity of metabolic enzymes or transport systems. In this situation, only a constant amount of drug is metabolized or transported per unit of time. If kinetics are zero order, a graph of serum concentration versus time is linear on linear-linear axes and is curved when graphed on linear-logarithmic (i.e., semilogarithmic) axes. Clinically, first-order elimination may become zero order after administration of excessive doses or prolonged infusions or during dysfunction of the organ of elimination. Certain drugs administered to neonates exhibit zero-order kinetics at therapeutic doses and may accumulate to excessive concentrations, including caffeine, chloramphenicol, diazepam, furosemide, indomethacin, and phenytoin.[161] Some drugs (e.g., phenytoin) may exhibit Michaelis-Menten kinetics (i.e., first order at low concentrations and zero order after enzymes are saturated at higher concentrations). For these drugs, a small increment in dose may cause disproportionately large increments in serum concentrations (Fig. 6-11).

Apparent Volume of Distribution

The apparent Vd is a mathematical term that relates the dose to the circulating concentration observed immediately after administration. It might be viewed as the volume of dilution that can be used to predict the change in concentration after a dose is diluted within the body. Vd does not necessarily correspond to

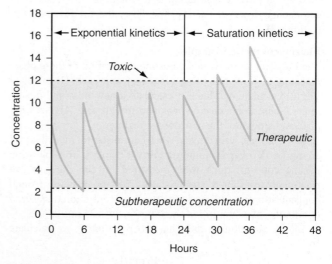

Figure 6-11. Transition from exponential to saturation kinetics. During every-6-hour dosing, concentrations during the first 24 hours reflect exponential kinetics with a half-life of 3 hours (k = 0.231/hr) followed by a change to saturation kinetics at 24 hours with elimination of 1.0 mg/hr, leading to drug accumulation to toxic concentrations.

a physiologic body fluid or tissue volume, hence the designation "apparent." For drugs that distribute out of the circulation or bind to tissues such as digoxin, Vd may reach 10 L/kg, a physical impossibility for a fluid compartment in the body. This illustrates the mathematical nature of Vd. The units used to express concentration are amount/volume and may help to remind the reader of the following equation that expresses the relation between dose in amount per kilograms and the Vd in volume per kilograms that dilutes the dose to produce the concentration:

$$\text{Concentration change (mg/L)} = \frac{\text{Dose (mg/kg)}}{\text{Vd (L/kg)}} \quad \text{(Eq. 7)}$$

If concentration is expressed with the unconventional units of milligrams per liter rather than micrograms per milliliter (which is equivalent), it is easier to balance the equation. This equation serves as the basis for most of the pharmacokinetic calculations because it is easily rearranged to solve for Vd and dose. It is also important to note that this equation represents the change in concentration after a rapidly administered IV dose of a drug whose elimination is long compared with the time for distribution. After a mini-infusion (e.g., vancomycin or gentamicin), a more complex exponential equation may be required to account for drug elimination during the time of infusion.[157] For neonates in whom drug elimination is relatively slow, only a small fraction of drug is eliminated during the time of infusion, and such adjustments can be omitted, whereas more complex equations may be needed in older children.

Knowledge of the apparent Vd is essential for dosage adjustments. Vd may be calculated by rearranging Equation 7.

$$\text{Vd (L/kg)} = \frac{\text{Dose (mg/kg)}}{\text{C (post dose)} - \text{C (pre dose) (mg/L)}} \quad \text{(Eq. 8)}$$

The concentration after a drug infusion, C (post dose), must be measured after the distribution phase to avoid overestimating the peak concentration that would, in turn, lead to an erroneously low Vd. For the first dose, the predose concentration is 0.

Pharmacokinetic Example

The following example illustrates the application of these pharmacokinetic principles using a four-step approach: (1) calculate Vd; (2) calculate half-life; (3) calculate a new dose and dosing interval based on a desired peak and trough; and (4) check the peak and trough of the new dosage regimen.

For example, vancomycin was administered in a dose of 15 mg/kg IV over 60 minutes every 12 hours. The following plasma concentrations were measured on the third day of treatment (presumed steady-state). The predose or trough concentration was 12 mg/L; the peak concentration, measured 60 minutes after the *end* of the infusion, was 32 mg/L.

Step 1: Substituting the data into Equation 8, we calculate Vd.

$$\text{Vd (L/kg)} = \frac{15\,\text{mg/kg}}{32\,\text{mg/L} - 12\,\text{mg/L}}$$

$$= \frac{15\,\text{mg/kg}}{20\,\text{mg/L}}$$

$$= 0.75\,\text{L/kg}.$$

Step 2: At steady-state, peak and trough concentrations reach the same levels after each dose. The time between the peak and trough concentrations is 10 hours, that is, 12 hours minus 1 hour infusion minus 1 hour to peak concentration. Half-life may be solved by rearranging Equation 2 to solve for k (elimination rate constant) and substituting the calculated k into Equation 3. In this case, the calculated elimination rate constant is 0.098 hours^{-1} and the corresponding half-life is 7.1 hours. However, a practical and clinically applicable "bedside" approach may be used without need for logarithmic calculations. For example, the plasma concentration decreased from 32 to 16 mg/L in one half-life and then from 16 to 12 mg/L in a fraction of the second half-life. At the end of the second half-life, the concentration would have decreased to 8 mg/L. Because 12 mg/L is the midpoint between the first and second half-lives, 1.5 half-lives have elapsed during the 10 hours between the peak and trough. Thus, if one assumes a linear decline, the half-life may be estimated as 6.67 hours (10 hours ÷ 1.5 half-lives). Note that the error between the actual half-life of 7.1 hours and the estimated half-life (6.67 hours) is a result of the linear assumptions of this calculation between half-lives. In fact, first-order elimination is a nonlinear process and concentration will actually decline from 32 mg/L to 22.6 mg/L during the first 50% of the first half-life rather than from 32 mg/L to 24 mg/L using this linear approach. The same occurs during subsequent half-lives. However, the small error associated with this method is often acceptable for rapid bedside estimates of pharmacokinetic parameters.

Step 3: A new dosage regimen must be calculated if the concentrations are unsatisfactory. Accordingly, one must decide on a desired peak and trough concentration. If, for example, the desired vancomycin peak and trough concentrations were 32 mg/L (20-40 mg/L) and 8 mg/L (5-10 mg/L), respectively, then Equation 8 may be rearranged to solve for the new dose.

$$\text{Dose (mg/kg)} = \text{Vd (L/kg)} \times [\text{C (peak desired)} - \text{C (post desired) (mg/L)}] \quad \text{(Eq. 9)}$$

$$\text{Dose (mg/kg)} = 0.75\,\text{L/kg} \times (32\,\text{mg/L} - 8\,\text{mg/L})$$

$$\text{Dose (mg/kg)} = 18\,\text{mg/kg}$$

The current dose produces a peak of 32 mg/L that is in the recommended therapeutic range, and lengthening the dosing interval to 2 half-lives (13⅓ hours) after the peak is reached (2 hours after beginning the dose infusion) will produce a trough concentration of 8 mg/L. The dose interval should be increased to 16 hours and the dose increased to 18 mg/kg.

Step 4: Estimating peak and trough concentrations with the new regimen provides a good double check against a mathematical error. Sixteen hours after the 15 mg/kg dose is administered (or approximately 2 half-lives after the measured peak), the trough should be approximately 8 mg/L. At this time, administration of 18 mg/kg will raise the concentration by 24 mg/L (assuming a Vd of 0.75 L/kg) to a peak concentration of 32 mg/L.

Repetitive Dosing and Drug Accumulation

When multiple doses are administered, the dose is usually repeated before complete elimination of the previous one. In this situation, peak and trough concentrations increase until a steady-state concentration (C_{ss}) is reached (see Fig. 6-11). The average C_{ss} can be calculated as follows:[155]

$$AvgC_{ss} = \frac{1}{Clearance} \times \frac{f \times D}{\tau} \qquad \text{(Eq. 10)}$$

$$= \frac{1}{k \times Vd_{(area)}} \times \frac{f \times D}{\tau}$$

$$= \frac{1.44 \times T^{1/2}}{Vd_{(area)}} \times \frac{f \times D}{\tau} \qquad \text{(Eq. 11)}$$

In Equations 10 and 11, f is the fraction of the dose that is absorbed, D is the dose, τ is the dosing interval in the same units of time as the elimination half-life, k is the elimination rate constant, and 1.44 equals 1/0.693 (see Equation 3). The magnitude of the average C_{ss} is directly proportional to a ratio of $T^{1/2}/\tau$ and D.[155]

Steady State

Steady state occurs when the amount of drug removed from the body between doses equals the amount of the dose.[156,160] Five half-lives are usually required for drug elimination and distribution among tissue and fluid compartments to reach equilibrium. When all tissues are at equilibrium (i.e., steady state), the peak and trough concentrations are the same after each dose. However, before this time, constant peak and trough concentrations after intermittent doses, or constant concentrations during drug infusions, do not prove that a steady state has been achieved because drug may still be entering and leaving deep tissue compartments. During continuous infusion, the fraction of steady-state concentration that has been reached can be calculated in terms of multiples of the drug's half-life.[155] After three half-lives, the concentration is 88% of that at steady state. When changing doses during chronic drug therapy, the concentration should usually not be rechecked until several half-lives have elapsed, unless elimination is impaired or signs of toxicity occur. Drug concentrations may not need to be checked if symptoms improve.

Loading Dose

If the time to reach a constant concentration by continuous or intermittent dosing is too long, a loading dose may be used to reach a greater constant concentration more quickly. This frequently is applied to initial treatment with digoxin, which has a 35- to 69-hour half-life in term neonates and an even longer half-life in preterm infants.[162] Use of a loading dose produces a greater circulating drug concentration earlier in the therapeutic course, but the equilibration to reach a true steady state still requires treatment for five or more half-lives. Loading doses must be used cautiously, because they increase the likelihood of drug toxicity, as has been observed with loading doses of digoxin.[3,16,17,162]

Central Nervous System Effects

Laboratory data have demonstrated the lethal dose in 50% of animals (LD_{50}) for many medications to be significantly less in neonates than in adult animals.[163,164] The sensitivity of human neonates to most of the sedatives, hypnotics, and narcotics is clinically well known and may in part be related to increased brain permeability (immature blood-brain barrier or damage to the blood-brain barrier) for some medications.[165-171] Laboratory studies have demonstrated greater brain concentrations of mor-

phine and amobarbital in infant than in adult animals.[172] Incomplete myelination in infants may make it easier for drugs that are not particularly lipid soluble to enter the brain at a greater rate than if the blood-brain barrier were intact.[165,166,172,173] A study that examined morphine requirements and the plasma concentrations of morphine that were required to provide analgesia in postoperative infants and children from neonates to 3 years of age found the greatest plasma analgesic concentrations and the fewest adjustments for additional morphine in neonates from birth to 4 weeks of age compared with older infants and children.[174] When considering the use of any centrally acting medication in children younger than 1 year of age and particularly those younger than 48 weeks' postconceptual age, one must balance the potential risks and benefits. Dosage must be carefully calculated and titrated to allow the lowest dose that provides the required patient response. Careful monitoring of vital signs is important because prolonged effects or adverse clinical responses may occur in children of any age but particularly in infants in whom maturation of the central nervous system (CNS) may be incomplete.

The Drug Approval Process, the Package Insert, and Drug Labeling

One area of concern has been the general lack of approval of many medications for populations of pediatric patients. This is particularly ironic because most of the changes in legislation pertaining to pharmaceuticals have been a result of adverse events in infants and children. The 1938 Federal Food, Drug, and Cosmetic Act[175] replaced the original Federal Food and Drugs Act of 1906 (Wiley Act)[176] because nearly 100 individuals, mostly children, were poisoned by diethylene glycol (an antifreeze analogue for vehicles) that had been added to an elixir of sulfanilimide. This new legislation prohibited the addition of poisonous substances (unless they were demonstrated to be safe in low concentrations) and instituted other measures to protect the consumer. The next major piece of legislation was the Kefauver-Harris Amendments, which were passed in 1962 as a result of the thalidomide catastrophe.[177] This legislation strengthened the safety standards by requiring the drug company to demonstrate effectiveness before marketing. The U.S. Food and Drug Administration (FDA) then allowed drugs to be marketed to adults as "safe and effective," but now the drug label was required to indicate that "safety and effectiveness had not been established in children" because no pediatric trials had been carried out. As a result, this had an enormous negative impact on drug development for children and led Shirkey to coin the now common expression "therapeutic orphans" when referring to drug development for children.[178] Until the late 1990s, nearly 80% of approved medications contained language within the drug label (package insert) that excluded children of varying ages. The majority of the drugs that we use in the operating room and the intensive care unit today have similar language.[179] Common examples of disclaimers for drugs used in our daily practice include that for bupivacaine ("Until further experience is gained in children younger than 12 years, administration of Sensorcaine [bupivacaine HCl] injection is not recommended.")[180] and for fentanyl ("It should not be administered to children 2 years of age or younger because safety in this age group has not yet been established.").[181] Such disclaimers are

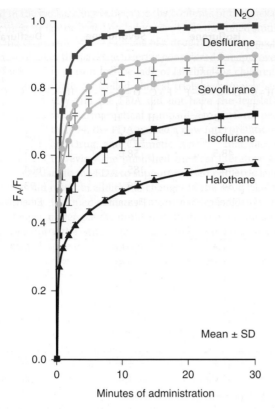

Figure 6-12. Wash-in (or FA/FI) of N$_2$O, desflurane, sevoflurane, isoflurane, and halothane in adults. The order of wash-in (N$_2$O > desflurane > sevoflurane > isoflurane > halothane) is inversely related to their solubilities in blood. (Redrawn from Yasuda N, Lockhart SH, Eger EI 2nd, et al: Comparison of kinetics of sevoflurane and isoflurane in humans. Anesth Analg 1991; 72:316-324.)

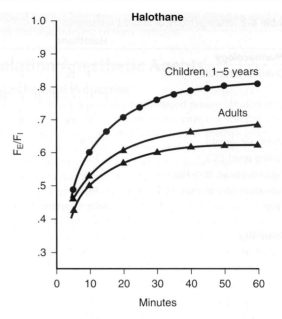

Figure 6-13. Rate of rise of expired to inspired partial pressures (FE/FI) of halothane in children and adults. (Redrawn from Salanitre E, Rackow H: The pulmonary exchange of nitrous oxide and halothane in infants and children. Anesthesiology 1969; 30:388-394.)

to the threefold greater metabolic rate and, therefore, threefold greater alveolar ventilation in neonates compared with adults. This is true for both spontaneous and controlled ventilation, depending on the settings used during controlled ventilation.

Uptake of anesthetic from the lungs (into blood) is the product of the cardiac output, tissue/blood solubility, and alveolar to venous partial pressure gradient. If any one of these factors diminishes or approaches zero, uptake decreases. The net effect is discussed next.

Factors Affecting the Uptake (Removal) of Anesthetics from the Lungs

Cardiac Output

The rate of increase in FA/FI is inversely related to changes in cardiac output: that is, the smaller the cardiac output, the more rapid the increase in FA/FI and vice versa (Fig. 6-15, see website).

Table 6-5. Determinants of the Rapid Wash-In of Inhalational Agents in Infants

- Greater alveolar ventilation to functional residual capacity ratio
- Greater fraction of the cardiac output distributed to the vessel-rich group
- Reduced tissue/blood solubility
- Reduced blood/gas solubility

As cardiac output diminishes, removal of anesthetic from the lungs diminishes and the rate of equilibration of FA/FI increases. Thus, a child in heart failure who receives an inhalational induction may reach greater anesthetic concentrations in the lungs than expected more rapidly than one with a normal cardiac output, a very serious problem if the "overpressure" technique has been used because this may result in an acute anesthetic-induced myocardial depression and decompensation of cardiac output. Conversely, in a high cardiac output state (as in the case of anxiety), the greater blood flow through the lungs removes anesthetic from the alveoli, thus reducing the alveolar partial pressure of anesthetic, which slows the rate of equilibration of FA/FI. The impact of changes in cardiac output on FA/FI depends, in part, on the solubility of the anesthetic: the more soluble the anesthetic (e.g., halothane), the greater the effect of changes in cardiac output on FA/FI and the less soluble the anesthetic (sevoflurane and desflurane), the less the effect.[194] This is another safety feature of the less soluble anesthetics.

Paradoxically, the greater cardiac index in neonates actually speeds the increase in FA/FI. This has been attributed to the preferential distribution of the cardiac output to the vessel-rich group (VRG) of tissues (brain, heart, kidney, splanchnic organs, and endocrine glands) in neonates. The VRG receives a greater proportion of the cardiac output in neonates compared with adults because it comprises 18% of the body weight in the former compared with only 8% in the latter. As a result of the increased blood flow to the VRG, the partial pressures of anesthetics in the VRG equilibrate with those in the alveoli more rapidly in neonates than in adults. Because the uptake of anesthetic by tissues other than those in the VRG in neonates is small, the rapid increase in FA/FI in the VRG and blood suggests that the partial pressure of anesthetic in venous blood returning to the lungs rapidly approaches the partial pressure in the alveoli. Uptake of anesthetic from the lungs then diminishes, as discussed later. The net effect of the greater cardiac output in neonates is paradoxical in that it speeds the equilibration of anesthetic partial pressures in the VRG and thus speeds the equilibration of FA/FI. This also accounts for part of the "downward spiral" that occurs when an excessive concentration of inhaled agent (particularly the soluble anesthetic halothane) is administered to a neonate or infant during controlled ventilation, as discussed later.

Solubility

Inhalational agents partition into two compartments in body fluids and tissues: (1) an aqueous phase and (2) a protein/lipid phase. This partitioning is analogous to the distribution of gases such as oxygen in blood between the aqueous phase (dissolved fraction) and hemoglobin (bound fraction). Because inhaled anesthetics move along partial pressure gradients and not concentration gradients within and between fluids and tissues, the rate of increase of FA/FI and, therefore, the anesthetic partial pressure in blood determines how rapidly anesthetics move into and out of tissues and affect organ function (e.g., central nervous and cardiac systems).

The rate of increase of FA/FI of inhalational anesthetics, which varies inversely with the solubility of the anesthetic in blood, follows the order: nitrous oxide > desflurane > sevoflurane > isoflurane > enflurane > halothane > methoxyflurane (see Table 6-3 and Fig. 6-12).[194,195] Although the solubilities of nitrous oxide and desflurane are similar, the rate of increase in FA/FI of nitrous oxide is more rapid than that after desflurane because of the concentration effect from administering 70% nitrous oxide. After a stepwise change in the inspired partial pressure of less soluble anesthetics, the alveolar partial pressure equilibrates rapidly with the new inspired partial pressure. Because the wash-out of these anesthetics is equally rapid (see later), the inspired partial pressure can be adjusted to previous values rapidly by decreasing the inspired partial pressure. Thus, anesthetic depth can be controlled more rapidly with a less soluble (i.e., desflurane or sevoflurane) than with a more soluble inhalational anesthetic (i.e., halothane).

The blood solubility of xenon is one-third that of nitrous oxide and desflurane (see Table 6-3). Although the tissue solubility of xenon has not been determined, its low blood solubility would lead us to speculate that its wash-in is the most rapid of the inhalational anesthetics currently in use.

Age is an important determinant of the solubility of inhalational anesthetics in blood. The blood solubilities of halothane, isoflurane, enflurane, and methoxyflurane are 18% less in neonates than they are in adults (Fig. 6-16, see website; see Table 6-3).[203] Serum cholesterol and proteins (including albumin) account for these age-related differences in blood solubilities of anesthetics.[203,204] In contrast, the blood solubility of the less soluble anesthetic sevoflurane is similar in neonates and adults.[204] Factors that do not appear to significantly affect the blood solubility of most anesthetics include age-related differences in hemoglobin, serum concentration of α_1-acid glycoprotein, and prematurity.[203,204]

The tissue/gas solubilities of the inhalational anesthetics in the VRG in neonates are approximately one-half those in adults (Fig. 6-17, see website).[205] The reduced tissue solubilities of halothane, isoflurane, enflurane, and methoxyflurane in neonates are attributable to two differences in the composition of tissues: (1) greater water content and (2) decreased protein and lipid con-

centrations. In terms of the uptake and distribution of anesthetics in tissues, the tissue/blood solubilities determine the speed of equilibration of anesthetics in tissues. The reduced tissue solubilities of inhalational anesthetics decrease the time for partial pressure equilibration of anesthetics (see time constant, later). Although the partial pressures of inhalational agents in tissues cannot easily be measured in vivo, they may be estimated by their concentrations in the exhaled or alveolar gases. The solubilities of the inhalational anesthetics in the brain of adults vary approximately 50% from desflurane to halothane (see Table 6-3). In the case of neonates, the reduced tissue solubilities of inhalational anesthetics speed the rate of increase in FA/FI compared with the rates in adults. In the cases of sevoflurane and desflurane, their respectively low but similar blood solubilities and likely similar tissues solubilities in neonates and adults offer a safety factor in neonates compared with adults because tissue equilibration of these insoluble inhalational anesthetics should be similar in both age groups. In contrast, the reduced tissue solubility of halothane in neonates likely results in a more rapid and unexpected anesthetic effect compared with the time course in adults.

We can estimate the time to equilibration of anesthetic partial pressures in tissues, such as the brain, by calculating the time constant for equilibration in brain tissue. The time constant (tau τ) for equilibration of anesthetic partial pressure in the brain is based on the expression:

$$\tau_{brain} = \frac{\text{Volume of the brain (mL)} \times \text{Brain/blood solubility}}{\text{Brain blood flow (mL/min)}}$$

where one time constant is the time for 63% equilibration of brain to blood anesthetic partial pressures. If the blood flow to the brain is approximately 50 mL/min/100 g of brain tissue and the brain/blood solubility for a particular inhalational anesthetic is 2.0 (assuming the density of brain tissue is 1 g/mL, then the time constant is:

$$\tau_{brain} = \frac{100\,\text{mL} \times 2}{50\,\text{mL/min}} = 4\,\text{minutes}$$

Knowing that two time constants achieves 86% equilibration, three time constants achieves 95%, and four time constants achieves 98%, then the time to 86% equilibration of anesthetic partial pressures in this example is 8 minutes, 95% equilibration is 12 minutes, and 98% equilibration is 16 minutes. If the brain/blood solubility were halved to 1.0, as it might be in the case of the neonate, then the time to 95% equilibration would decrease by 50% to 8 minutes. *Thus, the time to equilibration of anesthetic partial pressure within the brain of the neonate would be approximately one half that of the adult but still requires 8 minutes!* This holds true for the more soluble anesthetics such as halothane, whose tissue solubility in neonates is diminished compared with adults[205] but not for the less soluble anesthetics such as desflurane and sevofluran, whose tissue solubilities may be similar in neonates and adults.

Whereas the pharmacokinetics of inhalational anesthetics during the first 15 to 20 minutes depend primarily on the characteristics of the VRG, the pharmacokinetics during the subsequent 20 to 200 minutes depend primarily on those of the muscle group.[194] The solubility of inhalational anesthetics in skeletal muscle varies directly with age in a logarithmic relationship.[205] Thus, the lower solubility of inhalational anesthetics in the muscle of neonates and the smaller muscle mass speed the increase in Fa/Fi during this period compared with that in adults. This effect of age on the solubility of anesthetics in muscle has been attributed to age-dependent increases in protein concentration (i.e., muscle bulk) during the first 5 decades of life and in fat content during the subsequent 3 decades of life.[205] Overall, the reduced solubility combined with the reduced muscle mass in neonates (and infants) decreases uptake by the muscle group, leaving the Fa/Fi to equilibrate more rapidly in neonates compared with adults.

The net effect of these differences between neonates and adults is to speed the equilibration of anesthetic partial pressures in alveoli and tissues and thereby speed the rate of increase in Fa/Fi in neonates compared with adults.[197,198] This is particularly true for the more soluble anesthetics such as halothane. However, the difference in the rate of wash-in of less soluble anesthetics such as sevoflurane and desflurane between neonates and adults may be diminished.

Alveolar to Venous Partial Pressure Gradient

The difference in the anesthetic partial pressures between the alveolus and venous blood returning to the heart is a measure of the driving force of inhalational anesthetics from the alveoli into the bloodstream. As the anesthetic partial pressures in the VRG, muscle group, and others approach equilibration and less anesthetic is taken up by those tissues, the anesthetic partial pressure in the blood returning to the heart is similar to that when it left the alveoli. Thus, the driving force for anesthetics to move along a partial pressure gradient from the alveoli to the blood is diminished. This reduces the partial pressure gradient and diminishes the uptake of anesthetic from the alveoli.

Second Gas Effect

When two anesthetics are administered simultaneously, the wash-in of the anesthetic administered in a small concentration may be increased if the uptake of the second anesthetic is relatively large.[194] Nitrous oxide is the only anesthetic for which the uptake may be relatively large compared with that of the potent inhalational anesthetics as described earlier. Recent evidence, however, has cast doubt on the clinical relevance of the second gas effect.[206,207] These new data suggest that the concentrating effect, if it exists in humans at all, is a small and weak effect.

Induction

The more rapid increase in Fa/Fi of insoluble anesthetics compared with soluble anesthetics is generally thought to result in a more rapid induction of anesthesia. However, this is not necessarily true. Whereas the wash-in of inhalational anesthetics is determined by the pharmacokinetics of the agents, the speed of induction of anesthesia depends not only on the wash-in but also on (1) the solubility of the agent, (2) the rate of increase of the inspired concentration, (3) the maximal inspired concentration, and (4) respirations (including airway irritability and the mode of ventilation [spontaneous or controlled]). It is the combination of these four factors that determines the relative rate of induction of anesthesia.

The rate of wash-in of inhalational anesthetics into the lungs varies inversely with their solubilities in blood. Although anesthetics that are less soluble (e.g., sevoflurane and desflurane) wash in to the lungs more rapidly than more soluble anesthetics (e.g., halothane), the more rapid increase in Fa/Fi of less soluble

anesthetics is offset by their greater minimum alveolar concentration (MAC) (see Table 6-3). To ensure that induction of anesthesia is as rapid with less soluble anesthetics as it is with more soluble anesthetics, two criteria must be satisfied. First, the inspired concentration of the less soluble anesthetic must be increased in greater increments (based on the relative MAC values and wash-in profile, where MAC is defined as the minimum alveolar (or end-tidal or end-expiratory) anesthetic concentration at which 50% of subjects do not move in response to a noxious stimulus) than the more soluble anesthetic and, second, the maximum inspired concentration of the less soluble anesthetic must provide an alveolar concentration that is equipotent with that of the more soluble anesthetic. Theoretically, the overpressure technique should provide rapid and similar rates of induction of anesthesia with anesthetics of differing solubilities. However, if the maximum inspired anesthetic concentrations from the vaporizers preclude the delivery of equipotent concentrations or if airway irritability (as in the case of coughing and breath holding) interrupts the smooth delivery of anesthetic, induction of anesthesia will not be comparable.

To illustrate this, we contrast the rate of equilibration of Fa/Fi for sevoflurane and halothane during the first few minutes of induction of anesthesia (see Fig. 6-12). For this discussion, we rely on the wash-in of inhalational anesthetics in adults because comparable data for children are not available. In adults, Fa/Fi for halothane reaches 0.35 in the first few minutes of anesthesia. Given the previous data from Salanitre and Rackow,[197] Fa/Fi in children should increase more rapidly than that in adults, reaching perhaps 0.45 in the same time frame. For the maximum inspired concentration of halothane of 5%, the alveolar or end-tidal concentration achieved in the first few minutes in a child is 0.45 × 5% = 2.25%. With a MAC for halothane in children of 1.0%, this is equivalent to 2.25%/1% or 2.25 MAC multiples. Contrast this to the wash-in of sevoflurane during the same time frame. The Fa/Fi for sevoflurane reaches 0.5. Because of its low blood solubility, the Fa/Fi for sevoflurane in children is likely to be similar to that in adults in the same time frame. With a vaporizer that delivers a maximum inspired concentration of sevoflurane of 8%, the alveolar or end-tidal concentration in children achieved in the first few minutes is 0.5 × 8% = 4%. Given that the MAC for sevoflurane in children is 2.5%, 4% sevoflurane is equivalent to 4%/2.5% or 1.6 MAC multiples. This number of MAC multiples for sevoflurane is approximately 25% less than that achieved with halothane. This model will result in even greater differences between halothane and sevoflurane if the sevoflurane vaporizer is limited to 5% or 7%, as it is in some countries.

A similar but more clinically important case can be made for neonates (with a MAC for halothane of 0.87%) in whom the Fa/Fi for halothane reaches 0.5 in the first few minutes of anesthesia, resulting in an alveolar concentration of 5% × 0.5/0.87% or 2.9 MAC multiples. Although the Fa/Fi for sevoflurane in neonates (with a MAC for sevoflurane of 3.3%) also reaches 0.5 in the first few minutes of anesthesia, the alveolar concentration reaches 8% × 0.5/3.3% or only 1.2 MAC multiples. In this case, the MAC multiples of sevoflurane are approximately 40% those of halothane! Thus it is difficult to rapidly induce a deep level of anesthesia with sevoflurane in neonates and infants, as it was with halothane in the past. More importantly, however, an anesthetic overdose during induction with sevoflurane is much less likely to occur, than it was with halothane.

These two examples illustrate several extremely important features of the pharmacology of sevoflurane that distinguishes it from halothane. First, it may be difficult to rapidly achieve a deep level of anesthesia with sevoflurane in children (as was previously done with halothane) when sevoflurane is the sole anesthetic. Hence, inserting an IV catheter or performing laryngoscopy or bronchoscopy immediately after induction of anesthesia with sevoflurane may result in a physiologic or motor (withdrawal) response, even if the inspired concentration remains at 8%. We caution against decreasing the inspired concentration of sevoflurane (and nitrous oxide) as soon as the eyelash reflex is lost or the child appears to have lost consciousness because a deep level of anesthesia has not been achieved. In such cases, supplemental IV anesthetics may be required to rapidly deepen the level of anesthesia. Second, these examples illustrate an important safety feature of sevoflurane. With the current vaporizer design, excessive concentrations of sevoflurane cannot be administered to neonates and infants because their large MAC values more than offset their reduced solubilities. These insights contribute to the cardiovascular safety profile of sevoflurane and may help to explain why the morbidity and mortality associated with sevoflurane in children appear to be less than with halothane.[208]

Control of Anesthetic Depth

Two feedback responses modulate the depth of anesthesia during inhalational anesthesia: (1) a negative-feedback respiratory response and (2) a positive-feedback cardiovascular response. The feedback responses refer to the relationships between the inspired concentration of anesthetic and depth of anesthesia. After an increase in the inspired concentration, a negative feedback response refers to a decrease in the depth of anesthesia, whereas a positive-feedback system refers to an increase in the depth of anesthesia. Two examples that follow are used to illustrate the importance of these responses in clinical pediatric anesthesia practice.

During spontaneous respirations, as the partial pressure of inhaled anesthetics increases, alveolar ventilation decreases, thereby limiting both the wash-in of anesthetics and the depth of anesthesia achieved (Fig. 6-18A, see website).[209] This negative-feedback response is a protective mechanism that permits the safe use of inspired concentrations of inhalational anesthetics that are severalfold greater than MAC (overpressure technique) during spontaneous respirations. Excessive depth of anesthesia cannot normally be achieved during spontaneous respirations (irrespective of the inspired concentrations of anesthetics, even if multiple anesthetics are administered simultaneously), because of the negative-feedback effect such anesthetic concentrations have to depress minute ventilation. As alveolar ventilation decreases and the wash-in of anesthetics slows, the uptake of anesthetic by blood slows and the delivery of anesthetics to the VRG slows. When the partial pressure of anesthetics in the VRG exceeds that in blood, anesthetics move along their partial pressure gradients from the VRG into blood and other tissues, thus decreasing the depth of anesthesia. As the depth of anesthesia decreases, alveolar ventilation again increases and uptake of anesthetic from the alveoli resumes. *Thus, spontaneous ventilation protects against an anesthetic overdose by its negative feedback effect on respirations.*

In contrast to the negative-feedback effect of spontaneous ventilation, the positive-feedback effect of controlled ventilation relentlessly delivers inhaled anesthetic to the alveoli, increasing F_A/F_I but at the same time diminishing cardiac output (Fig. 6-18B, see website).[209] The decrease in cardiac output limits the uptake of anesthetic from the alveoli, further increasing F_A/F_I. Hence, as cardiac output decreases, F_A/F_I increases and the depth of anesthesia increases, thereby further decreasing cardiac output. For a given minute ventilation, the speed at which cardiovascular collapse can occur in a neonate is reflected in part in the maximum MAC-multiples the vaporizers can deliver (Table 6-6). This is a positive-feedback response. This response creates a downward spiral that may result in death if it is not interrupted.

In a model of uptake and distribution, dogs who breathed spontaneously received up to 6% inspired concentrations of halothane[209]; the anesthetic was tolerated without cardiovascular collapse because the negative feedback response of respiratory depression prevented excessive concentrations of anesthetic from depressing the VRG. In contrast, when ventilation was controlled, cardiovascular collapse occurred at inspired concentrations $\geq 4\%$ and some dogs succumbed. High concentrations of inhalational anesthetics (i.e., as those used in the overpressure technique) are commonly administered during inhalational inductions either as stepwise increases in inspired concentrations or as a single-breath high concentration. *These high concentrations are tolerated provided that spontaneous respiration is maintained. If, however, ventilation is controlled, then cardiovascular collapse becomes a substantive risk.* This is of particular concern in neonates and small infants who are more susceptible to the cardiodepressant effects of inhaled agents.[194]

Shunts

Two types of shunts exist in the lungs and heart: left-to-right or right-to-left. Left-to-right shunts refer to conditions in which blood recirculates through the lungs (usually via an intracardiac defect such as a ventricular septal defect). Right-to-left shunts refer to conditions in which venous blood returning to the heart bypasses the lungs as in an intracardiac shunt (cyanotic heart disease) or intrapulmonary shunt (pneumonia or an endobronchial intubation). The effects of shunts on the rate of increase in F_A/F_I are poorly understood. In general, left-to-right shunts do not significantly affect the pharmacokinetics of inhalational anesthetics (they may affect IV medications), provided cardiac output remains unchanged. In contrast, right-to-left shunts can significantly delay the equilibration of F_A/F_I of inhalational anesthetics. The magnitude of the delay with a right-to-left shunt depends on the solubility of the anesthetic: the wash-in of less soluble anesthetics is delayed to a greater extent than that of the more soluble anesthetics.[194] These effects are independent of the location of the shunt: intracardiac or intrapulmonary.

Table 6-6. Maximal Alveolar Concentration (MAC) Multiples for a Neonate Allowed by Current Vaporizers

Agent	Maximum Vaporizer Output (%)	MAC (%)	Maximum Possible MAC Multiples
Halothane	5	0.87	5.75
Isoflurane	5	1.20	4.2
Sevoflurane	8	3.3	2.42
Desflurane	18	9.16	1.96

See text for further discussion.

To understand the effects of a right-to-left shunt on the pharmacokinetics of inhalational anesthetics, it is useful to consider a simplified model of a right-to-left shunt using the lung to mimic the shunt. In this model, each lung is represented by one alveolus and each lung is perfused by one pulmonary artery (Fig. 6-19). When a tracheal tube is positioned with its tip at the mid-trachea level (Fig. 6-19A), ventilation is divided equally between both lungs, thereby yielding equal anesthetic partial pressures in both pulmonary veins (PV = 1). However, if the tip of the tracheal tube is advanced into the right main-stem bronchus (equivalent to a right-to-left shunt) (Fig. 6-19B), all of the ventilation is delivered to one lung, that is, the ventilation to that lung is doubled, whereas ventilation to the nonventilated lung is zero. Under these conditions, ventilation remains unchanged. For the remainder of this discussion, it is important to recognize that with a right-to-left shunt, the end-tidal and blood partial pressures may differ, the magnitude of which will depend on the solubility of the anesthetic.

When a more soluble anesthetic (e.g., halothane) is administered through a tracheal tube that is positioned in the right main-stem bronchus (to model a right-to-left shunt), the increased ventilation to that lung speeds the increases in FA/FI (as described earlier) such that it compensates, for the most part, for the absence of ventilation to the contralateral lung (Fig. 6-19B).[194] The more soluble the anesthetic, the closer the partial pressure of anesthetic in the combined pulmonary vein that drains both the ventilated and nonventilated lungs approximates the partial pressure from delivering the anesthetic through a tube in the trachea. The net effect of a right-to-left shunt on the FA/FI of a more soluble inhalational anesthetic is thus negligible.

In contrast, when a less soluble anesthetic (e.g., sevoflurane or desflurane) is administered in the presence of such a right-to-left shunt, the increase in ventilation to the lung minimally increases the FA/FI, because increasing ventilation has a diminishing effect to speed FA/FI as the solubility of the anesthetic decreases (see earlier) (Fig. 6-19C).[194] Consequently, the increase in FA/FI in the ventilated lung is insufficient to offset the absence of anesthetic in the blood draining the nonventilated lung. The *net effect is to almost halve* the anesthetic partial pressure in the combined pulmonary vein. The less soluble the anesthetic, the greater the discrepancy between the anesthetic partial pressure in the pulmonary vein that drains the ventilated and nonventilated lungs and the partial pressure when the tube is in the trachea. The overall effect is to slow induction of anesthesia or even limit the depth of anesthesia that can be achieved.[210,211]

Few studies have documented the clinical importance of such a shunt.[210,211] Clinical situations that have posed challenges with these shunts include children with right-to-left cardiac shunts and infants with chronic lung disease. In the past, very soluble anesthetics such as methoxyflurane (blood/gas solubility of 12) would have been unaffected by a right-to-left shunt. In the case of halothane, the most soluble anesthetic currently available, anesthesia remained quite effective in children with right-to-left shunts even though the ratio of arterial to inspired partial pressures lagged behind the ratio when the shunt was closed.[211] The most likely explanation was the 5% inspired concentration of halothane from the vaporizer, which permitted a 5 × MAC overpressure effect. Although the ratios of the arterial to inspired partial pressures of sevoflurane and desflurane have not been measured in children with right-to-left shunts, we expect they will pose even greater difficulties than halothane, particularly with their limited overpressure effect (i.e., the maximal inspired concentrations of the vaporizers are limited to 3 MAC or less [see Table 6-6]). Our experience suggests that when we use these less soluble anesthetics in such circumstances (e.g., bronchoscopy for a bronchial foreign body), IV anesthetics are needed to deepen the level of anesthesia in infants and younger children.

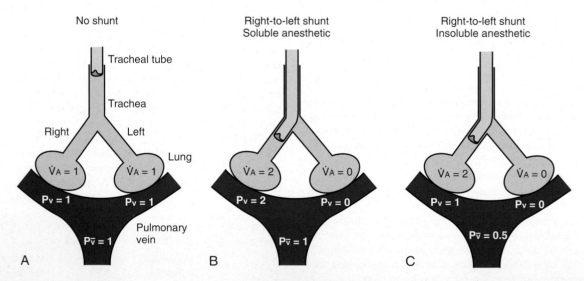

Figure 6-19. Effect of shunt on the rate of increase of anesthetic partial pressure in blood using a model. **A,** Normal situation with no shunt, equal ventilation to both lungs, and normocapnia. **B,** The effect of a right-to-left shunt (via an endobronchial intubation) with a more soluble anesthetic (i.e., halothane). Ventilation and therefore normocapnia are maintained, and hypoxic pulmonary vasoconstriction is negligible. In this case, the increased ventilation to the ventilated lung speeds the increase in FA/FI and offsets the effect of the shunt. Results in terms of the mixed pulmonary venous partial pressure of the anesthetic (P$\bar{v}$ = 1) are similar to those in **A. C,** The effect of shunt with a less-soluble anesthetic (i.e., desflurane or sevoflurane). Because the increase in alveolar ventilation does not increase FA/FI in the ventilated lung, the shunted blood has a dramatic effect to reduce the anesthetic partial pressure in the blood (P$\bar{v}$ = 0.5). (Redrawn from Lerman J: Pharmacology of inhalational anaesthetics in infants and children. Paediatr Anaesth 1992; 2:191-203.)

Wash-out and Emergence

The wash-out of inhalational anesthetics follows an exponential decay (the inverse of the wash-in curves, see Fig. 6-12).[195] The order of the wash-out of the anesthetics parallels their blood solubilities, that is, anesthetics that wash out first are those that are least soluble in blood (see Table 6-3).[195] Halothane is the one exception to this order; its wash-out is as rapid as that of isoflurane, likely because its metabolism is 15- to 20-fold greater than that of isoflurane (see later). The order of the wash-out of anesthetics in children should be similar to that in adults. However, the rate of wash-out of inhalational anesthetics in neonates and infants is likely to be more rapid than that in adults for the same reasons the rate of wash-in is more rapid (see Table 6-5). Further studies are required to substantiate this notion.

A more sophisticated approach to the wash-out of inhalational anesthetics is to use the context-sensitive half-time, which is a measure of the time to decrease the anesthetic partial pressure, by 50%. Using a computer model and pharmacokinetic data from adults, the context-sensitive half-times of the potent inhalational anesthetics enflurane, isoflurane, sevoflurane, and desflurane were similar (<5 minutes) and were unaffected by the duration of the anesthetic.[212] The 80% decrement times were similar for desflurane and sevoflurane (<8 minutes) whereas those for isoflurane and enflurane were greater (30 and 35 minutes). However, after 6 hours of simulated anesthesia, the 90% decrement times differed substantially: 14 minutes for desflurane, 65 minutes for sevoflurane, 86 minutes for isoflurane, and 100 minutes for enflurane. These data suggest that the early recovery (up to 80% decrement in partial pressure) after inhalational anesthesia is similar among these four anesthetics (although sevoflurane and desflurane are more rapid) but after 6 hours (i.e., prolonged anesthesia) 90% decrement is achieved much more rapidly with desflurane than with the remainder.

Switching from one anesthetic to another, less soluble anesthetic, to facilitate a rapid emergence from anesthesia is a common practice in pediatric anesthesia. Few data exist to substantiate such a practice (see later).

In animal models, recovery of motor function (an indicator of more complete recovery than simple measurement of expired anesthetic concentrations) parallels the wash-out of inhalational anesthetics from fastest to slowest: desflurane < sevoflurane < isoflurane < halothane.[213] Notably, the time to recovery increases in parallel with the duration of anesthesia.[213] In pediatric studies in which the recovery times after two or more anesthetics were compared, the end-tidal concentrations of the anesthetics were maintained at approximately 1 MAC until the conclusion of surgery after which the anesthetics were abruptly discontinued.[214-216] In this paradigm, it is not surprising that the rates of recovery paralleled the rates of wash-out, which in turn paralleled the solubilities of the inhalational anesthetics, including xenon and desflurane.[217] In clinical practice, however, anesthetic concentrations are gradually tapered as the end of surgery approaches. This practice may attenuate the differences in the rates of recovery among inhalational anesthetics.

Pharmacodynamics of Inhaled Anesthetics

Minimum Alveolar Concentration

Minimal alveolar concentration is defined as the minimum alveolar (or end-tidal or end-expiratory) anesthetic concentration at which 50% of patients do not move in response to a noxious stimulus. The classic stimulus for MAC is skin incision;

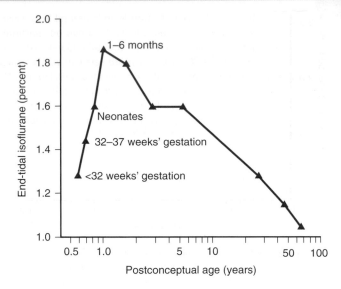

Figure 6-20. MAC of isoflurane in preterm and full term neonates, infants and children. MAC increased with gestational age in infants younger than 32 weeks' gestation (1.3%), reaching a zenith in infants 1 to 6 months of age of 1.87% and decreased thereafter with increasing age to adulthood. Postconceptual age is the sum of the gestational age and postnatal age in years. (Data from Cameron CB, Robinson S, Gregory GA: The minimum anesthetic concentration of isoflurane in children. Anesth. Analg. 1984; 63:418-420 and LeDez KM, Lerman J: The minimum alveolar concentration (MAC) of isoflurane in preterm neonates. Anesthesiology 1987; 67:301-307)

throughout the remainder of this chapter, MAC will refer to this stimulus. MAC has also been determined in response to other stimuli, including tracheal intubation, insertion of a laryngeal mask airway, tracheal extubation, and awake responsiveness. The difference in the potency (or MAC) of inhalational anesthetics varies inversely with the lipid solubility of these anesthetics; that is, as the lipid solubility decreases, the potency decreases in parallel (i.e., MAC increases) (see Table 6-3).

In children, MAC varies significantly with age. For example, the MAC of halothane increases as age decreases, reaching a maximal value in infants 1 to 6 months of age (1.20 ± 0.06%) and then decreases by about 30% to (0.87 ± 0.03%) in full-term neonates.[218,219] Similar relationships hold true for isoflurane and desflurane (Figs. 6-20 and 6-21, see website for Fig. 6-21).[220,221] However, the relationship for sevoflurane differs from that of the other inhalational anesthetics in that the MAC of sevoflurane does not increase steadily as age decreases (Fig. 6-22).[222] In fact, the MAC of sevoflurane in neonates and infants younger than 6 months of age is 3.3%, whereas in older infants and children it is 2.5%.[222-225] The explanation for this different relationship for sevoflurane remains unclear.

The MAC of inhalational anesthetics in preterm neonates has been determined for isoflurane (Fig. 6-20). The (mean ± SD) MAC of isoflurane in preterm neonates younger than 32 weeks' gestation (1.28 ± 0.17%) is 10% less than it is in neonates of 32 to 37 weeks' gestational age (1.41 ± 0.18%), which in turn is 12% less than it is in full-term neonates (1.60 ± 0.03%).[226]

The etiology of these age-dependent changes in MAC remains elusive. Several possible causes have been proposed, including maturational changes in the CNS and neurohumoral factors, but none has been confirmed.

Cardiovascular System

Inhalational anesthetics (with the exception of xenon) affect the cardiovascular system either directly (by depressing myocardial contractility, altering the conduction system, or by dilating the peripheral vasculature) or indirectly (by affecting the balance of parasympathetic and sympathetic nervous systems and neuro-humoral, renal, or reflex responses). The cardiovascular responses to inhalational anesthetics in children are further complicated by maturational changes in the cardiovascular system and its responsiveness to these anesthetics. When all of these developmental changes are taken into consideration there is a reduced margin of safety between adequate anesthesia and severe cardiopulmonary depression in infants and children compared with adults. The salient features of the immature cardiovascular system in infants and children at both the macroscopic and microscopic levels have been reviewed.[286]

Assessment of cardiovascular variables in infants and children presents a challenge for clinicians. Although blood pressure and electrocardiography are standard monitors of hemodynamics in infants and children of all ages, measures of cardiac output and myocardial contractility are much more difficult to quantitate accurately. Two-dimensional echocardiography and impedance cardiometry have been used to estimate cardiac output and myocardial contractility in infants and children,[287-290] although the echocardiographic measurements are subject to variability depending on the preload and afterload. Load-independent derived echocardiographic variables (stress-velocity and stress-shortening indices) have improved the accuracy of echocardiographic estimates of myocardial function and are used with increasing frequency.[291] Transesophageal echocardiography is used much more frequently in children, although its use is limited to children with congenital heart disease undergoing cardiac surgery.

In children, several factors determine the blood pressure responses to inhalational anesthetics, including the particular anesthetic studied, the dose, the presence of a premedication, the level of preoperative anxiety, and the systemic pressure measured: systolic, diastolic, or mean. Most studies demonstrate modest, dose-dependent decreases in blood pressure with all of the inhalational anesthetics, although the magnitude of the changes varies. In a direct comparison of sevoflurane and halothane, systolic blood pressure decreased 7.5% at 1 MAC sevoflurane and 12.5% at 1 MAC halothane but returned to awake values at 1.5 MAC with both anesthetics.[291] In children older than 1 year of age, systolic blood pressure decreased 0% to 11% at 1 MAC sevoflurane and 22% to 28% at 1 MAC desflurane compared with awake values.[221,222] At 1 MAC, mean blood pressure in children decreased 15% to 25% with isoflurane and sevoflurane.[288,290] All of the inhalational anesthetics (in concentrations up to 1.5 MAC) modestly depress the systemic blood pressure in children.

Myocardial contractility decreases to a greater extent during halothane (up to 1.5 MAC) than during isoflurane or sevoflurane anesthesia, as evidenced by decreases in cardiac output and ejection fraction in healthy children.[289,290,292] Cardiac index decreased to similar extents with halothane and sevoflurane at 1 and 2 MAC: 10% at 1 MAC and 20% to 35% at 2 MAC.[290] Ejection fraction decreased 30% at 0.5 and 1.5 MAC halothane compared with awake values but is unchanged at equipotent concentrations of isoflurane.[288] The addition of nitrous oxide to halothane or isoflurane in infants and small children depresses myocardial function to a similar extent as equipotent anesthetic concentrations of halothane or isoflurane in oxygen.[292] In children, halothane decreases myocardial contractility in a dose-dependent manner and to a greater extent than the ether anesthetics. Isoflurane and sevoflurane decrease myocardial contractility to a lesser extent than halothane and are preferred for children with limited cardiovascular reserves. Intravenous atropine restores the decrease in myocardial function in part, associated with halothane anesthesia,[292-295] whereas IV balanced salt solution restores the decrease in myocardial function associated with isoflurane anesthesia.[289]

The mechanism by which inhalational anesthetics depress myocardial function remains controversial. Studies in both animal and human myocardial cells suggest that halothane, isoflurane, and sevoflurane directly depress myocardial contractility by decreasing intracellular Ca^{2+} flux. Inhalational anesthetics decrease the Ca^{2+} flux by their action on the calcium channels themselves, ion exchange pumps, and the sarcoplasmic reticulum.[286] Evidence suggests that inhalational anesthetics attenuate contractility of ventricular myocytes via voltage-dependent L-type calcium channels (which are responsible for release of large amounts of calcium from the sarcoplasmic reticulum).[296,297]

That neonates and infants are more sensitive to the depressant actions of inhalational anesthetics than are older children is supported by experimental evidence of maturational differences between neonatal and adult rat, rabbit, and feline myocardium.[297,297-300] Structural differences that may account in part for the changes in myocardial sensitivity to inhalational anesthetics with age include a reduction in contractile elements, immature sarcoplasmic reticulum, and functional differences in calcium sensitivity of the contractile elements, calcium channels, and the sodium-calcium pump in the neonatal myocardium.[286,296-298,300-303] The determinants of Ca^{2+} homeostasis in neonatal ventricular myocardial cells depend on trans-sarcolemmal Ca^{2+} flux to a far greater extent than on the sarcoplasmic reticulum.[286] This is based on a growing body of experimental evidence that includes the finding that the concentration of the Na^+-Ca^{2+} exchange protein in the neonatal myocardium, a protein that regulates trans-sarcolemmal flux of Ca^{2+}, exceeds that in adult cells by 2.5-fold and that its concentration decreases with age as the concentration of L-type voltage-dependent calcium channel increases.[298] Furthermore, halothane reversibly inhibits the Na^+-Ca^{2+} exchange protein in immature myocardial cells.[298] The sarcoplasmic reticulum is poorly developed in neonatal myocardial cells, and this finding weighs heavily against the sarcoplasmic reticulum being the major source of Ca^{2+} required for myocardial contractility. Further research is required before the contribution of each aspect of Ca^{2+} homeostasis to myocardial contractility in the neonate can be confirmed.

Ever since the introduction of halothane into clinical practice, clinicians have been aware of a greater incidence of hypotension and bradycardia in neonates who were anesthetized with halothane than in adults. However, this was not the case when *equipotent* concentrations (~1 MAC) of halothane[219,294] were administered to neonates and older infants 1 to 6 months of age. Subsequent studies demonstrated that isoflurane,[304] sevoflurane,[222] and desflurane[221] all decreased systolic pressure in neonates to similar extents as in older infants 1 to 6 months of age. Interestingly, systolic blood pressure decreased 30% in response to 1 MAC sevoflurane in neonates and infants 1 to 6 months of age, which was substantively greater than the 5% decrease in older infants and children up to 12 years of age.[222] In the case of desflurane, systolic blood pressure decreased 30% in response to 1 MAC desflurane across all age groups.[221] These data suggest that systolic blood pressure decreases up to 30% in response to 1 MAC of all inhalational anesthetics in infants and children and that caution should be exercised when administering these anesthetics to infants and children who are at risk for hemodynamic instability or in whom greater concentrations of inhaled anesthetics are required. On the basis of echocardiographic determinations, cardiac output and ejection fraction decrease in a dose-dependent fashion from awake to 1.5 MAC halothane and isoflurane in neonates and infants.[287] In a comparison of sevoflurane and halothane up to 1.5 MAC in infants, sevoflurane maintained cardiac index but decreased blood pressure and systemic vascular resistance.[305] Myocardial contractility decreased in a dose-dependent manner with halothane as well as with sevoflurane, although the decrease with the former exceeded that with the latter.

The baroreflex response is also depressed in infants with both halothane[306] and isoflurane,[307] albeit to a greater extent with halothane. In view of the greater incidence of hypotension in neonates and infants than older children, an intact baroreflex could offset in part, the cardiovascular consequences. However, inhalational anesthetics blunt this response, leaving the infant vulnerable to the direct cardiodepressant actions of the anesthetics. Prophylactic anticholinergics augment the cardiac output by increasing the heart rate.

Two studies evaluated the effects of inhalational anesthesia on the hemodynamics of children with congenital heart disease undergoing cardiac surgery.[308,309] The key findings were that sevoflurane maintained cardiac index and heart rate with less hypotension and negative inotropic effect than halothane. Isoflurane maintained cardiac index and ejection fraction, increased heart rate, and caused less depression of mean arterial pressure than halothane.[308] Sevoflurane was also associated with fewer episodes of severe hypotension and reduced need for vasopressors and chronotropes during emergence than halothane.[309]

Inhalational anesthetics also vary in their effect on cardiac rhythm. Halothane slows the heart rate, in some cases leading to junctional rhythms, bradycardia, and asystole. This response is dose dependent. Three mechanisms have been proposed to explain the genesis of halothane-associated dysrhythmias: a direct effect on the sinoatrial node, a vagal effect, or an imbalance in the parasympathetic/sympathetic tone. It has also been suggested that the etiology of the bradycardia during halothane anesthesia may be a withdrawal of sympathetic tone. Bradycardia is particularly marked in the neonate, presumably because parasympathetic influences predominate over the sparse sympathetic innervation of the myocardium in this age group. Junctional rhythms are also common during halothane anesthesia. Atrial or ventricular ectopic beats are rare except in the presence of hypercapnia.[310] In infants and children anesthetized with halothane, 10 μg/kg atropine increases heart rate greater than or equal to 50% and promotes sinus rhythm.[311] This dose of atropine also increases blood pressure in infants ≥2 years of age and children.

Halothane also sensitizes the myocardium to catecholamines, particularly in the presence of hypercapnia and "light anesthesia."[310] Halothane decreases the threshold for ventricular extrasystoles during epinephrine administration threefold.[312-314] In contrast, isoflurane, desflurane, and sevoflurane maintain or increase heart rate during the early induction period of anesthesia,[216,221,222,288,290,304,305,315-317] although a slowing of the heart rate has been reported during sevoflurane anesthesia. When bradycardia occurs in an anesthetized child, hypoxia must be considered first before other causes such as a direct drug effect (i.e., high concentration of halothane). Isoflurane, desflurane, and sevoflurane do not sensitize the myocardium to catecholamines to the same extent as halothane, and ventricular arrhythmias are rare.[312,313,318] The mechanism by which the sinus node controls automaticity is incompletely understood but may include K^+ currents, hyperpolarization-activated current, and T and L forms of Ca^{2+} currents.[286] Moreover, developmental changes in these channels likely account, in part, for the differential effects of inhalational anesthetics on heart rate with age.[301]

Recent concerns of a relationship between inhalational anesthetics and prolonged QT interval that progressed to induce cardiac arrest or torsades de pointes have emerged. Although the ether inhalational anesthetics prolong the QTc interval,[319,320] this alone appears to be insufficient to induce torsades de pointes. Torsades de pointes depends on the transmural dispersion of repolarization across the myocardial wall, which is defined as the interval between the peak and end of the T wave on an electrocardiogram. Recent evidence has demonstrated that the risk of torsades de pointes during sevoflurane anesthesia is minimal because transmural dispersion of repolarization is limited.[321]

Paroxysmal increases in blood pressure (both systolic and diastolic pressures) and heart rate have been reported in adults after a rapid increase in the inspired concentration of isoflurane or desflurane.[322] This occurs as a result of a massive sympathetic response, mediated by norepinephrine and/or epinephrine, that culminates in tachycardia and hypertension.[323,324] Further increases in the inspired concentration of the inciting anesthetic while attempting to attenuate the tachycardia and hypertension are ineffective and may perpetuate or augment the response. In order to restore vital signs to normal, the inciting anesthetic should be discontinued and replaced with another anesthetic. Repetitive small increases (1%) in the inspired concentration of the putative anesthetic produces transient but attenuated catecholamine bursts and cardiovascular responses compared with larger increases in concentration.[325,326] Fentanyl (2 μg/kg), esmolol, and clonidine have all been shown to be effective in preventing, attenuating, or eliminating these responses.[327-329] The origin of these responses is unknown, although the rapidity of the response points to the lung.[330] Others, however, dispute this notion, contending that two sites must be responsible for triggering the sympathetic discharge; the lung and the VRG,[331] with the latter mediating the greater response.[331,332] Neuroexcitatory responses have not been reported in children with isoflurane, desflurane, or sevoflurane.[333]

Xenon offers an immense advantage over the ether-based inhalational anesthetics in that it maintains circulatory stability. This anesthetic may have a niche role when anesthetizing infants and children with congenital and acquired heart disease. However, the effects of xenon on the hearts in children have not been studied.

Respiratory System

During spontaneous ventilation, both tidal volume and respiratory rate vary with the specific anesthetic, depth of anesthesia,

A recent concern has been the potential for fire and explosions in the operating room when sevoflurane was administered in the presence of desiccated Baralyme.[483,484] This has not been reported with the other anesthetics.[484] The exothermic reaction that occurred caused parts of the anesthetic machine to melt beyond use (see Chapter 53, Fig. 53-10). The putative flammable products have been attributed to the degradation of sevoflurane at high temperatures in the presence of desiccated Baralyme. Evidence suggests that sufficient hydrogen may be produced in the presence of 8% sevoflurane and at temperatures in excess of 300°C to ignite and cause an explosion.[485] Although exceedingly rare, this catastrophic response resulted in the withdrawal of Baralyme production in August 2004.

Nitrous Oxide

Nitrous oxide confers several properties that differ substantively from the potent inhalational anesthetics that merit consideration. Because nitrous oxide is 34 times more soluble in blood than nitrogen ($\lambda_{blood/gas}$ for nitrous oxide is 0.47 vs. $\lambda_{blood/gas}$ for nitrogen 0.014), nitrous oxide diffuses into gas cavities that are filled with nitrogen more rapidly than nitrogen egresses. Consequently, the volume of the cavity expands. However, the magnitude of the increase in the volume of the cavity depends, in part, on the concentration of nitrous oxide administered, as determined by the formula $100/(100 - \%N_2O)$. The rate at which the cavity expands also depends on the source of the blood supply: those cavities in which the blood supply decreases as the volume of the cavity increases (e.g., a loop of obstructed bowel) will expand slower and to a smaller overall volume than a cavity in which the blood supply is independent of the cavity volume (e.g., a pneumothorax). By using a model of these conditions the time to double the volume of a loop of obstructed bowel with nitrous oxide was estimated to be 120 minutes, whereas the time to double the volume of a pneumothorax was one tenth, or 12 minutes.[486] Any gas-filled cavities within the body are vulnerable for expansion if nitrous oxide is administered, including obstructed bowel,[486] pneumothorax, gas cavities within the eye, endotracheal tube cuffs,[487] laryngeal mask airways,[488,489] bubbles in veins,[490] and a pneumoencephalogram.[491] Theoretically, nitrous oxide should be avoided during laparoscopic surgery to avoid expanding CO_2 bubbles that reach the venous circulation.

Inhalational anesthetics confer a very low risk for postoperative nausea and vomiting. In contrast, nitrous oxide is considered to be an emetogenic anesthetic. In a large meta-analysis of the impact of nitrous oxide on the incidence of postoperative nausea and vomiting in adults, the authors determined that for emetogenic surgery, eliminating nitrous oxide was salutary (number needed to treat of six) whereas for nonemetogenic surgery there was no benefit from omitting nitrous oxide.[492] Hence, avoiding nitrous oxide in surgery that is emetogenic is reasonable. However, the authors also reported that the number needed to harm in the form of intraoperative awareness when nitrous oxide was omitted from the anesthetic was 46, or more than 2%! Hence, omitting nitrous oxide from the anesthetic prescription requires very careful consideration, assessment, and monitoring for awareness.

A number of studies investigated the contribution of nitrous oxide to postoperative vomiting in children. Although there is some evidence that avoiding nitrous oxide reduces the incidence of postoperative vomiting in children,[493] the preponderance of evidence shows no benefit.[494-498] In part, this may be attributed to the multiplicity of factors that contribute to postoperative vomiting, as well as the salutary effects of other factors such as the use of propofol and/or antiemetics. In none of the studies in which nitrous oxide was omitted in children was awareness reported.

Environmental Impact

Currently, the National Institute of Occupational Safety and Health (NIOSH) recommendations limit the chronic exposure to nitrous oxide to 25 ppm and to inhalational anesthetics to 10 ppm. The basis for these recommendations is uncertain but may be attributed to the risk of teratogenicity and end-organ dysfunction. In pediatric anesthesia, mask anesthesia and/or uncuffed tracheal tubes and laryngeal mask airways in children leak inhalational anesthetics into the environment. As a result there is local exposure to inhaled anesthetics during anesthesia in children that should be considered.

Concern over the pollution of the stratosphere and ozone layer depletion by polyhalogenated anesthetics has raised further questions for the long-term use of these agents and the need to fully recycle or adsorb the waste gases.[499] The polyhalogenated compounds are produced in extremely low concentrations; and although they have a high molecular weight, atmospheric winds likely facilitate their transfer to the stratosphere to do harm to the ozone layer. However, the most compelling data of their limited impact on the environment relate to their half-lives. The half-lives of these polyhalogenated anesthetics in the stratosphere are approximately 5 years. Contrast these to nitrous oxide, a compound with a very small molecular weight (in comparison with potent inhalational anesthetics), which is administered in high concentrations (50%-70%) and which has a half-life in the stratosphere of 120 years! Nitrous oxide is a known greenhouse gas and depletes the ozone layer. The case for banning the polyhalogenated anesthetics pales in comparison with the enormous potential environmental impact of nitrous oxide. Although nitrous oxide is a serious greenhouse pollutant, medical sources account for less than 5% of the volume pumped into the atmosphere. Industrial sources account for the remaining 95%. Highly efficient scrubbers and absorbers are being developed to prevent atmospheric pollution and recycle expensive anesthetics (e.g., xenon) but their use remains experimental at this time. We should all limit the fresh gas flow and concentration of polyhalogenated anesthetics in our practice to preserve the ozone layer.

Oxygen

The appropriate concentration of oxygen to be delivered for each anesthetic is carefully titrated to an individual's needs. Requirements are monitored by inspired oxygen concentration measurement, oxygen/hemoglobin saturation (pulse oximetry), and arterial blood gas determinations. Oxygen is often liberally administered in excess of a patient's metabolic needs. However, potential dangers in this excess should be noted, particularly in two areas: (1) Pulmonary oxygen toxicity is well documented; despite the fact that it develops slowly, general recommendations are to use an air/oxygen combination for prolonged procedures when nitrous oxide is contraindicated.[500] (2) Of additional concern is the remote possibility of adverse effects on the immature neonatal retina leading to retinopathy of prematurity (ROP).[501-508] When using portable oxygen tanks a good rule of thumb to determine the capacity of an E-cylinder is as follows: pounds of pressure × 0.3 divided by gas flow = minutes of oxygen delivery left in the tank.

Several cases of ROP have been reported in infants whose only known exposure to supplemental oxygen occurred in the operating room; it should be noted that no new cases related to operating room management have been reported since 1981![509,510] In the earlier cases of ROP, cardiovascular instability related to the disorder requiring surgery may have been the major factor predisposing to ROP along with prematurity. Many factors contribute to the development of ROP; it has been reported in children with cyanotic congenital heart disease, infants not exposed to exogenous oxygen, and even in stillborn infants.[511,512] A possible relationship of the development of ROP to arterial carbon dioxide variations, hypercarbia, hypotension, candida sepsis, red blood cell transfusions, corticosteroid therapy, duration of ventilation, elevated blood glucose values, a deficiency of insulin-like growth factor, and vascular endothelial growth factor, as well as hypoxemia and fluctuating levels of oxygen, have all been suggested.[513-528] Other factors such as exogenous bright light, maternal diabetes, and maternal antihistamine use within 2 weeks of delivery have been found to be risk factors; the evidence for vitamin E deficiency is less convincing.[529-531] Recently, the possibility of a genetic predisposition, that is, a genetic polymorphism altering control of neovascularization, has been proposed.[527,532-534] The use of continuous transcutaneous oxygen tension monitoring was not found to reduce the risk of ROP in infants weighing less than 1000 g compared with controls.[535] It appears the major risk factor for developing ROP is extreme prematurity; *oxygen therapy represents only part of this complex problem*.[503,504,506] The incidence of ROP is predominantly limited to infants weighing 1000 g or less, but it is a concern in infants with a birth weight less than 1500 g born at less than 28 weeks' gestation.[536-538]

The embryonal development of the retina involves the progressive increase in vascularization of retinal vessels in a nasal to temporal direction. Exposure to high blood oxygen concentrations results in vasoconstriction of retinal vessels, probable occlusion of these vessels by thrombi, development of new vessels (neovascularization), formation of arteriovenous anastomoses, vascularization of the vitreous, and, in some cases, fibrous degeneration and retraction of the scar (i.e., cicatrization and retinal detachment).[504,506] This sequence of events apparently does not occur when vascularization of the retina is complete (at about 44 weeks' postconceptual age).[539,540]

The evidence implicating hyperoxia as contributing to the development of ROP must be recognized but placed in proper perspective. Although it was thought that tight control of oxygen saturation and minimizing exposure to exogenous oxygen would reduce the incidence of ROP,[541] a multicenter study, the Supplemental Therapeutic Oxygen Prethreshold Retinopathy of Prematurity study (STOP-ROP), failed to support that hypothesis.[542] In fact, the conclusion reached stated, "Although the relative risk/benefit of supplemental oxygen for each infant must be individually considered, clinicians need no longer be concerned that supplemental oxygen, as used in this study, will exacerbate active prethreshold ROP."[543] This study suggests that anesthesiologists should take practical precautions to protect an infant's retinas from hyperoxemia without unnecessarily endangering the infant. One possibility is to discuss with the surgeon post-

ponement of elective surgery on a neonate younger than 44 weeks' postconceptual age to allow for further retinal maturation. Obviously, a life-threatening surgical problem must be corrected promptly. Once the decision has been made to proceed with surgery, an ophthalmologic assessment to document possible preexisting ROP is desirable but often not practical. No comprehensive epidemiologic studies have yet examined anesthetic risk factors, but, given the many cofactors that are associated with this entity, it appears that anesthesia management, although very important, is a small piece of this puzzle.

Bearing in mind the possible role of hyperoxia and hypercarbia, intraoperative management must include careful monitoring of inspired oxygen and expired carbon dioxide concentrations. Pulse oximetry allows an anesthesiologist to adjust the inspired concentration of oxygen. Maintaining the oxygen saturation at 93% to 95% results in a PaO$_2$ of approximately 70 mm Hg.[505,544] Unfortunately, individual oximeters may vary considerably in terms of their accuracy, so practitioners must be familiar with their equipment.[545] Most anesthesia machines are equipped with flow ratio valves that prevent the delivery of less than 25% oxygen. The use of air blended with oxygen can be used to further reduce the inspired oxygen concentration. A transport system equipped with an air/oxygen blender is desirable to continue the titration of oxygen therapy from the operating room to the intensive care unit. While avoiding hyperoxia, one must never lose sight of the importance of *avoiding hypoxemia; hypoxemia is life-threatening whereas hyperoxia is not*. One cannot be faulted if ROP should occur, provided a reasonable and safe approach to oxygen administration and ventilation has been made.

Intravenous Anesthetic Agents

The anesthetic effects of IV agents are primarily reflected by brain concentrations; to achieve anesthesia, it is necessary to obtain an adequate cerebral blood level. Each drug administered is rapidly redistributed from vessel-rich well perfused areas (brain, heart, lung, liver, and kidneys) to muscle, and finally to vessel-poor less well perfused areas (bone, fat). Thus, termination of the effect of a single drug dose is primarily determined by redistribution. Protein binding, Vd, body composition, cardiac output, distribution of cardiac output, metabolism, and excretion all alter the pharmacokinetics and pharmacodynamics of IV drugs. Anesthetic depth may be altered if a constant cerebral blood level is not maintained. The changes in body composition and the blood-brain barrier that occur during maturation may also greatly affect the duration of action of IV drugs, especially in neonates.

Barbiturates

Methohexital
Methohexital (Brevital) is a short-acting barbiturate for the IV induction of anesthesia (1 to 2 mg/kg). Administered intravenously as a 1% solution (10 mg/mL), it produces pain at the injection site; hiccups, apnea, and seizure-like activity may also be occasionally observed.[546,547] Methohexital has minimal effects on cardiovascular function (increased heart rate) in children.[548,549] Methohexital may be contraindicated in children with temporal lobe epilepsy.[546] Slow IV titration averts apnea. A possible advantage of methohexital over thiopental is that its

rate of metabolism is greater, suggesting a more rapid recovery when large doses have been administered.[550-552]

Rectal methohexital in a 10% solution (20 to 30 mg/kg) is a safe and atraumatic method of induction with an acceptable incidence of undesired side effects (hiccups 13%, defecation 10%).[553] It is an excellent sedation technique for brief radiologic procedures such as computed tomographic (CT) scans, when a single rectal administration of a 10% solution (100 mg/mL given through a well-lubricated catheter) is often sufficient for the 10- to 30-minute procedure.[554,555] Absorption by this route is quite variable and may account for an occasional child with prolonged or rapid onset of sedation.[550,556] This technique and dosage have been used safely in children from 3 months to 6 years of age. It is a useful adjunct to induction of anesthesia in older mentally handicapped children or in children who are excessively fearful of the anesthesia mask or an IV needle. It is also an alternative for children who are still in diapers and who are not candidates for other premedicants such as midazolam (e.g., a child taking erythromycin).[557,558]

Oxygen desaturation after sedation with rectal methohexital occurs in approximately 4% of cases and is usually related to airway obstruction; this is generally readily corrected by repositioning the head.[553,559] Although methohexital is an exceedingly safe medication, it should be administered only under the supervision of a physician trained in airway management to ensure adequacy of the airway and ventilation. Blood pressure monitoring and equipment for airway management and ventilation should be readily available because airway obstruction, seizures, or apnea may rarely occur.[560] *Children must not be left unobserved after administration.*

Thiopental

The induction of anesthesia in healthy, unpremedicated children with IV thiopental (2.5%) is achieved with a dose of 5 to 6 mg/kg.[561-563] The duration of the clinical effect of thiopental depends primarily on redistribution rather than metabolism (10%/hr). As a result, repeated doses of thiopental may accumulate, causing prolonged sedation. Children 5 months to 13 years of age, however, metabolize thiopental almost twice as rapidly as adults (Fig. 6-23, see website).[564-566] The elimination half-life of thiopental in neonates is greater than that in adults and children[567,568] because of the reduced clearance in neonates. Acute tolerance to thiopental, well demonstrated in adults, may also occur in children.[569] A total IV dose of 10 mg/kg is generally the upper limit; however, with this dose, it is common to have a prolonged period of sedation after brief surgical procedures. Thiopental is a weak vasodilator and a direct myocardial depressant; both of these effects may cause significant systemic hypotension in the *hypovolemic* state (e.g., dehydration due to prolonged fasting or trauma).[570]

Thiopental in a 10% solution (20 to 30 mg/kg) may also be used for induction of anesthesia by rectal instillation when methohexital is contraindicated (temporal lobe epilepsy).[546] The period of sedation may be longer for thiopental than for methohexital, partly because of the reduced rate of metabolism of thiopental.[571]

Thiopental has also been used in the pediatric critical care setting as a continuous high-dose infusion (approximately 2 to 4 mg/kg/hr) to control intracranial hypertension. Monitoring the blood concentration of thiopental may be useful during such therapy to avoid depressing myocardial function. The elimination half-life of thiopental after a continuous infusion may be markedly prolonged compared with that after a single bolus (11.7 vs. 6.1 hours).[565,566] These findings may in part be attributed to the underlying illness, intercurrent drug treatment, and delayed metabolism (i.e., converting the kinetics from first to second order).[572]

Propofol

Propofol (Deprivan) is a sedative-hypnotic agent useful for both the induction and maintenance of anesthesia.[573] Because of its limited solubility in water, it was initially formulated in a Cremophor EL solvent. However, severe anaphylactoid reactions[574,575] led to a new solvent, 10% intralipid. Diprivan is formulated with 1% propofol, 10% soybean oil, 1.25% egg yoke phosphatide (ovolecithin), 2.25% glycerol, EDTA (ethylenediamine tetraacetic acid), and sodium hydroxide to maintain a pH of 7.0 to 8.5. This formulation of propofol has a white milky appearance because it is a lipid macroemulsion with average droplet size of 0.15 to 0.3 μM (where 5 to 7 μM is required to pass through capillaries).[576] These droplets remain distinct in suspension owing to the negative surface charges on the phosphate moieties in the ovolecithin phospholipids in the aqueous outer layer. These droplets may coalesce if the negative surface charges on the emulsion droplets dissipate, which is a slow naturally-occurring process but which may also be precipitated by physical maneuvers (freeze-thawing, high temperatures, and agitation) and by changes in the chemical composition of the emulsion, such as by decreasing pH or the addition of electrolytes (i.e., sodium, potassium, calcium, and magnesium) and medications (i.e., lidocaine [see later]).[576] Soybean oil is composed of long-chain triglycerides (LCT), defined by the 12-22 carbon atoms in their skeletons: linoleic acid (54%), oleic acids (26%), linolenic acid (7.8%), and stearic acid (2.6%). EDTA was introduced into Diprivan after 1998 as an antimicrobial agent. Generic formulations of propofol are also available; these contain sulfites or metabisulfite as the antimicrobial agent.

Propofol is a highly lipophilic drug that is rapidly distributed into vessel-rich organs, accounting for its rapid onset and usefulness as an induction agent. Termination of this effect is effected by the combination of rapid redistribution and rapid hepatic and extrahepatic clearance.[577-579] The rapidity of the redistribution from vessel-rich organs accounts for its brief action and the need for repeated small boluses or a constant infusion to maintain a stable plane of anesthesia/sedation. Pharmacokinetic studies demonstrated a larger Vd at steady state (Vd_{ss}) (9.7 L/kg) in children compared with adults and more rapid redistribution but a clearance (34 mL/min/kg) that is similar to or greater than that reported in adults.[574,580-582] Clearance of propofol in neonates is 66% less than that in children and adults.[583-585] Although interindividual variability in the pharmacokinetics in neonates is large, the reduced clearance suggests that recovery after propofol in neonates may be prolonged and that repeat doses may not be required as frequently as in older children and adults. Propofol is conjugated to a water-soluble glucuronide in the liver and excreted in the urine.[574] Propofol also undergoes extensive extrahepatic metabolism (lung, kidney), as evidenced by the similar pharmacokinetics in infants with biliary atresia and healthy controls.[586] However, variability in the pharmacokinetics of propofol in the literature likely reflects differences in sampling time, pharmacokinetic modeling, and duration of sampling among the studies.[582]

Although measuring the concentration of propofol in blood has been the sole means to assess its disposition in vivo, alternate noninvasive techniques have been sought to provide online measurements. Mass spectrometry of the exhaled breath from adults and children,[587,588] a technique that is similar to end-tidal gas monitoring of inhalational anesthetics, has proven to provide stable estimates of the concentration of propofol in blood. Further refinement will be required before a commercially viable monitor is available for clinical use.

In unpremedicated children, the dose of propofol required for loss of the eyelash reflex generally increases with decreasing age.[589-593] The ED_{50} for loss of the eyelash reflex in infants (1-6 months) is 3 ± 0.2 mg/kg, which decreases in children (1-12 years) to 1.3 to 1.6 mg/kg and increases in older children (10-16 years) to 2.4 ± 0.1 mg/kg. A more linear decrease in propofol dosing with increasing age between infants and children 12 years of age was determined in Chinese children.[592] They noted a 10% decrease in the propofol dose for the ED_{95} between younger than age 2 years, 2 to 5 years, and 6 to 12 years. ED_{90-95} for loss of eyelash reflex for all age groups is 50% to 75% greater than the ED_{50}.[589,591] Larger doses may be required for acceptance of the face mask.[589,594] The dose of propofol in neonates has not been clearly established. In one study, a dose of 2.5 mg/kg permitted tracheal intubation in the majority of neonates, although the exact dose used was not specified.[595] Successful insertion of a laryngeal mask airway in unpremedicated children requires an even larger dose of propofol (5.4 mg/kg [4.7-6.8 mg/kg, 95% confidence interval]).[596] After induction of anesthesia with sevoflurane and nitrous oxide, preliminary evidence suggests that satisfactory conditions for tracheal intubation without prolonged apnea was achieved with 1.4 mg/kg in children undergoing tonsillectomy and adenoidectomy.[597]

Propofol is widely used as a continuous infusion or in intermittent doses in children undergoing brief procedures in radiology such as MRI, CT, and interventional radiology; during medical procedures such as oncology and gastroenterology; and for children with MH.[598-602] Although early evidence suggested that 100 µg/kg/min propofol was required after a halothane induction to maintain immobility during MRI,[598] subsequent studies showed that much larger doses are required in unpremedicated children or after sevoflurane inductions.[599] Specifically, initial infusion rates of propofol of 200 to 250 µg/kg/min (12-15 mg/kg/hr) or even greater may be required. This initial rate may be greater or less depending on the age of the child, that is, the younger the child and the presence of cognitive impairment increase the infusion dose requirements to prevent movement. Midazolam premedication may reduce the propofol requirements, but it delays emergence after brief procedures. Some advocate intermittent boluses of propofol for some procedures (upper endoscopy and oncologic medical procedures), whereas others advocate continuous infusions. In one study, systolic blood pressure decreased more and the total dose of propofol was greater when continuous infusions were used compared with intermittent boluses.[602] If minor movement can be tolerated (i.e., medical procedures), then intermittent boluses may be preferred for brief procedures, whereas if immobility is required (radiation oncology and radiologic procedures), then infusions are preferred. In some clinical scenarios, such as radiation oncology, burns, and oncology procedures, repeated sedation with propofol over a prolonged period is required. There is no evidence that tolerance to propofol develops.[603]

Propofol affects a number of organ system responses in vivo. Systolic blood pressure decreases approximately 15% in children,[580,594,604,605] which is similar to what occurs in adults.[606] Most studies reported similar decreases in blood pressure after propofol and thiopental.[605,607] The incidence of apnea after an induction bolus of either propofol or thiopental is similar.[594,604,605,607] The major clinical disadvantage of propofol in children is pain with IV injection. This pain can be diminished by using any one of a number of strategies, including injecting propofol into a large vein; pretreatment with IV lidocaine (0.5 mg/kg), meperidine, nitrous oxide, metoprolol, and tramadol; and combining a small dose of lidocaine (0.5 to 1.0 mg/kg) with the propofol.[580,589,594,605,607-612] Perhaps the most effective method of diminishing pain is to use lidocaine (0.5-1.0 mg/kg) pretreatment as a "manual" Bier block applied proximal to the IV site for about 30 seconds before the propofol is injected (Fig. 6-24, see website). The number needed to treat to prevent pain with such a maneuver in adults is less than two, indicating that this technique is extremely effective.[611] A recent call for the use of lidocaine to attenuate the pain associated with IV injection of propofol should make this routine.[613] Parenthetically, any parenteral form of lidocaine, including those that contain preservative, may be administered intravenously combined with or before propofol without triggering an anaphylactoid reaction.

The mechanism by which IV propofol causes pain has been attributed to the nociceptive effects of trace concentrations of this sterically hindered phenolic compound in the outer aqueous layer of the Diprivan micelles. When the concentration of propofol in the aqueous outer layer coating the micelles is reduced (i.e., by increasing the concentration of medium-chain triglycerides in the formulation) irritation of the endothelial nociceptive nerve endings and the severity of the pain during injection are attenuated.[614]

Indicators for recovery from anesthesia such as time to eye opening and time to extubation are more rapid in children induced with propofol when compared with thiopental and maintained with propofol.[615-620] Recovery of psychomotor function is more rapid after a propofol induction and maintenance of anesthesia compared with thiopental/isoflurane anesthesia.[621] Recovery room stay and time to hospital discharge are reduced with propofol.[616,617] Emergence delirium rarely occurs after propofol anesthesia in children.[424,622-624]

Propofol reduces the incidence of nausea and vomiting when used as an induction agent or when used for the maintenance of anesthesia.[616,625-631] However, there have been conflicting results for particular procedures such as strabismus repair and tonsillectomy and when the drug is combined with opioids.[632-635] Nausea and vomiting may be considered surrogate endpoints for serious adverse outcomes after surgery in children. No studies have demonstrated clinically important abbreviated times to discharge or decrease in overnight admission rate for vomiting and/or dehydration in children treated with propofol. Short-term infusions of propofol for surgical or medical procedures have shown that the depth of sedation is easily controlled by adjusting the infusion rate while still ensuring rapid and complete recovery.[636-640] Propofol infusions are particularly well suited for minor radiologic and medical procedures such as oncology. Compared with thiopental, propofol is less irritating to the airway, which translates into a reduced incidence of laryngospasm.[607,641-643] Insertion of a laryngeal mask airway is substantively easier and more successful after a propofol induction compared with thiopental.[578,596,644,645]

Propofol compromises airway patency and respiration in children. The upper airway narrows during propofol infusion in children particularly in the hypopharyngeal region, but it does remain patent.[646] If airway obstruction occurs, the chin lift maneuver augments the patency of the upper airway.[647,648] Theoretically, collapse of the upper airway increases in parallel with the dose of propofol by direct inhibition of genioglossus muscle activity as well as an inhibition of centrally mediated airway dilatation and airway reflexes.[649] All of these upper airway changes are reversed on emergence from anesthesia.[650] When propofol is given as an IV bolus, transient apnea may occur.[592,597,605] Concerns over atelectasis and airway obstruction have prompted some to insert a tracheal tube or laryngeal mask airway in children sedated with propofol during medical procedures. However, recent evidence suggests that the incidence of atelectasis in children who are breathing spontaneously with an unprotected airway is less than in those whose tracheas are intubated.[651]

Diprivan and the current lipid-based generic formulations of propofol must be handled with aseptic techniques because the lipid is a culture medium.[652] Propofol 1% can support the growth of at least four well-known organisms: *Staphylococcus aureus*, *Pseudomonas aeruginosa*, *Escherichia coli*, and *Candida albicans*.[653-655] When Diprivan was first introduced, it was prepared (as are all lipid emulsions) under strict aseptic conditions, with a layer of nitrogen above the liquid emulsion in each vial.[576] Once opened, external contamination of the vials, however, resulted in severe sepsis and several deaths before antimicrobial agents were mandated to be added to the propofol formulations to prevent or retard bacterial growth. In very small concentrations, EDTA inhibits bacterial growth by chelating vital trace metals without affecting the emulsion droplet size or stability. Other formulations of propofol contain sulfite or metabisulfites, which release sulfur dioxide that prevents bacterial growth. Sulfites are more effective at reduced pH values, but there is a limit to how acidic the emulsion can become because this destabilizes the emulsion droplets. To further prevent any risk of bacterial contamination, all opened vials of propofol should be discarded after 6 hours. These strategies have eliminated concerns of bacterial contamination of propofol and episodes of sepsis in patients.

Long-term propofol infusions were used extensively for sedation in intensive care units after recognizing that its favorable pharmacokinetics will facilitate a rapid wake-up.[577] However, a report of five deaths in infants and children (4 weeks to 6 years of age) who were sedated with Diprivan raised serious doubts about the safety of such a practice.[656] The syndrome, now known as propofol infusion syndrome (PRIS), occurs primarily but not exclusively in children who are sedated for prolonged periods in intensive care units.[656-660] The most common prescription for developing PRIS is prolonged sedation at a rate of more than 5 mg/kg/hr (70 μg/kg/min) for more than 48 hours. Manifestations of PRIS include the insidious onset of lipemia, metabolic acidosis, hyperkalemia, and rhabdomyolysis that may precipitously transform into profound myocardial instability and cardiovascular collapse that is refractory to all resuscitative efforts. Manifesting signs may be subtle, with the sudden onset of bradycardia that is refractory to the usual interventions. Of greater concern is a recent case in which a brief 6-hour infusion

of propofol resulted in an unexplained metabolic acidosis in a 5-year old undergoing an arteriovenous malformation resection.[661] Suspicion was raised that this may have been PRIS in evolution. Propofol was discontinued, and the signs of PRIS abated. In an adult neurosurgical intensive care unit where propofol sedation was used, 5 deaths prompted a review of 12 deaths.[662] It was determined that for every 1 mg/kg/hr that the propofol infusion exceeded 5 mg/kg/hr, the odds ratio of death was 1.93. After a total to date of at least 28 deaths in children and 14 adults, the FDA cautioned against the use of propofol for long-term sedation. Predisposing risk factors include concomitant catecholamine/inotrope infusions or high-dose corticosteroids and sepsis. Mortality currently exceeds 80%, although early institution of hemodialysis may improve survival.

Unraveling PRIS has proven to be difficult. Early investigations noted that during PRIS, the blood concentrations of malonylcarnitine and C5-acylcarnitine increased. These compounds are known to inhibit carnitine palmoyl transferase and the transfer of LCT into mitochondria.[663,664] Propofol may also directly inhibit carnitine palmoyl transferase to impede flux of LCT into the mitochondria. Within the mitochondria, propofol uncouples β spiral oxidation at complex II in the respiratory chain, which, in turn, inhibits transmembrane flux of LCT into mitochondria, strangling the mitochondria from a much needed source of energy. To reduce the risk of PRIS, new formulations of propofol are being developed that contain less or no LCT. Medium-chain triglycerides (MCTs) are replacing LCTs in propofol. The clinical importance of these developments requires further investigations with multicenter studies.[665]

There are no commercially available alternate lipid formulations of propofol currently on the market, although four are under investigation: SAZN 1% and 6%, Propofol-Lipopuro, IDD-D (insoluble drug delivery microdroplet), and Ampofol. SAZN 6% is formulated with MCT/LCT and has a similar pharmacology to Diprivan but with a much reduced incidence of pain on injection. Lipopuro is also similar in properties to Diprivan, although the 2% propofol concentration produced a similar incidence of pain as Diprivan. Propofol IDD-D (insoluble drug delivery-microdroplet) is another formulation that is based on a microdrop delivery system in which 2% propofol is combined with the 4% non-Soya MCTs without preservatives. It needs no antimicrobial protection. The pharmacology of IDD-D is similar to that of Diprivan and produces severe/moderate pain in less than one third of those who received Diprivan. One of the metabolites of this formulation, octanoate, can in theory produce neurologic complications, although the concentrations are likely subtoxic.[666] The final preparation is Ampofol, which is a 1% propofol infusion in 5% soybean oil and 0.6% lecithin.[667] The major detraction of Ampofol is the fourfold greater incidence of moderate pain on injection compared with Diprivan.

The safety of propofol in the neonatal period has raised concerns with some practitioners after at least four unexpected but profound episodes of cardiorespiratory collapse in neonates.[668,669] In these cases, precipitous and severe decreases in systolic blood pressure, heart rate, and oxygenation were observed after a single induction dose of propofol (1-7 mg/kg) in neonates without evidence of congenital heart defects or cardiomyopathy. Resuscitation was extremely difficult in all cases despite intervention with both inotropic and chronotropic agents. A myriad of causes of bradycardia associated with propofol administration have been proposed.[670] In a comprehensive review of bradycardia after propofol in children and adults, the authors concluded that "propofol carries a finite risk for bradycardia with potential for major harm."[671] Whether these responses reflect acute right-to-left shunting, a return to fetal circulation, or some as yet unclear cause has not been confirmed; readers should exercise caution when propofol is used to induce anesthesia in neonates.

Although anaphylactoid reactions have been reported after propofol administration in children, specific causes for the allergic reaction have not been identified.[672] In some instances, the "reactions" were primarily respiratory and attributed to preservatives such as metabisulfites.[673] However, 13 of 14 adults who developed anaphylactoid reactions after receiving a single dose of propofol displayed a hypersensitivity response to propofol during immunologic testing.[674] Similar testing in children has not been reported. When Diprivan was first introduced, clinicians were advised to avoid it in children (and adults) with "egg allergy." However, in the past 2 decades, the absence of any reports of anaphylactoid reactions to Diprivan when given to children with egg allergy has led to a relaxation of that concern. The egg proteins present in Diprivan are derived from ovolecithin, which is from egg white. Because the precise egg proteins against which children are allergic are never determined and given the wide array of proteins present in eggs, the probability of developing a cross-reaction with Diprivan is considered exceedingly unlikely. Hence, egg allergy is no longer considered a contraindication to Diprivan.

In an effort to divest propofol of its lipid carrier and pain during IV administration, aqueous-based formulations of propofol are under development for parenteral use. The first two formulations, propofol phosphate and Aquavan, undergo enzymatic hydrolysis in blood to remove the phosphate moieties yielding the active form of propofol.[675,676] Because this enzymatic process takes several minutes to release propofol, this formulation may be inadequate for a rapid induction of anesthesia but rather may render it useful for sedation and for procedures when the time of onset of anesthesia is not crucial. Neither formulation is associated with pain when injected into a vein. Even more interesting is the absence of a risk of microbial infection because this preparation does not include any lipid carrier. Pharmacokinetic data in adults indicate a delay to peak blood concentration after parenteral administration compared with Diprivan and an increased context-sensitive half-life. The most recent development is a liquid microemulsion formulation of propofol that contains two polyethylene glycol-based compounds to stabilize the microemulsion known as Aquafol (Daewon Pharmaceutical Co, Ltd, Seoul, Korea).[677] The pharmacodynamics and safety of Aquafol were similar to those of Diprivan in adults, although differences were noted in the pharmacokinetics. There are no data in children.

Ketamine

Ketamine (Ketalar) is a derivative of phencyclidine that similarly antagonizes the N-methyl-D-aspartate (NMDA) receptor.[678] Its action is related to central dissociation of the cerebral cortex, and it also causes cerebral excitation. The latter property may be responsible for precipitating seizures in susceptible children and the reason that processed EEG monitoring devices do not work with ketamine sedation/anesthesia.[679-683] Ketamine is an excellent analgesic and amnestic; the recommended dose for induction of anesthesia is 1 to 3 mg/kg intravenously or 5 to 10 mg/kg intramuscularly.[684,685] The duration of action of a single IV dose is 5 to 8 minutes with an α-elimination half-life of 11 minutes and a β-elimination half-life of 2.5 to 3.0 hours.[686,687] Further supplementary doses of 0.5 to 1.0 mg/kg are administered when clinically indicated. Atropine or another antisialagogue should usually accompany the initial dose to diminish the production of copious secretions that occur with ketamine.[688,689] Ketamine may also be administered in very low doses intravenously (0.25-0.5 mg/kg) or intramuscularly (1-2 mg/kg) either alone or in combination with low-dose midazolam (0.05 mg/kg [50 µg/kg]) along with atropine (0.02 mg/kg) for sedation for a variety of procedures such as oncology evaluations, suture of lacerations, or radiologic interventions.[684,685,690-695] Bioavailability after intramuscular (IM) administration is approximately 93% in adults and even greater in children.[696-698] If an antisialagogue is not administered, there is a greater risk for laryngospasm.[699] Larger doses of ketamine will produce a state of general anesthesia.[700-702] Even after small doses there is potential for apnea or airway obstruction, particularly when combined with other sedating medications.[700,703,704] Ketamine has also been administered orally, nasally, and rectally both as a premedication before general anesthesia and for procedural sedation.[549,705-720] Oral ketamine administered as a premedicant has also been reported to reduce emergence delirium; there is conflicting evidence regarding the efficacy of ketamine to reduce pain scores after tonsillectomy.[721-723]

The bioavailability of ketamine is approximately 93% after IM administration, 50% after nasal administration, 25% after rectal administration, and 17% after oral administration (Table 6-14).[698,724] There are concerns regarding both rectal and nasal drug administration. Rectal ketamine administration can result in very irregular and less predictable times of onset and peak sedation just as with rectal barbiturates. Nasal drug administration can result in drug entering directly into the CNS by tracking along neurovascular tissue of the nasal mucosa.[725-729] Because the preservative in ketamine has been shown to be neurotoxic, there is the theoretic possibility of CNS toxicity because of the preservative.[730,731] Until better safety information is available, this route of drug administration is not recommended unless preservative-free ketamine is used. Ketamine has also been administered as a means of providing epidural analgesia.[685,732-736] The same admonition regarding neuraxial administration of ketamine applies here even more importantly; *epidural ketamine must not be administered unless it is preservative free.* The use of ketamine is also increasing for postoperative pain management when administered in small doses as an opioid-sparing drug.[684,685,737-740] A new indication that requires further investiga-

Table 6-14. Ketamine Equivalency by Route of Administration*

Route	Dose (mg/kg)	Approximate Bioequivalence (mg/kg)
Intravenous	2	2
Intramuscular	2	2.15
Nasal	2	4
Rectal	2	8
Oral	2	11.75

*Note that these are estimates and that there is extreme patient-to-patient variability.
Extrapolated from data from references 696 to 698.

tion in children is the topical application for the treatment of mucositis and other painful conditions.[190,741-746]

Ketamine increases heart rate, cardiac index, and systemic blood pressure; it also increases pulmonary artery pressure in adults but has a small effect on respiration.[747,748] In children, there is apparently no effect on pulmonary artery pressure provided that ventilation is controlled.[749] If a child is sedated with ketamine but allowed to breathe spontaneously, increases in end-tidal CO_2 could increase pulmonary artery pressures.[750] Ketamine sedation has been shown to maintain peripheral vascular resistance, thus affecting intracardiac shunting less than propofol in children sedated for cardiac catheterization.[751] However, the combination of ketamine and propofol might be superior to either drug alone in this circumstance.[752,753] Ketamine has negative inotropic effects in those who depend on vasopressors.[754] The effect of ketamine on the musculature of the upper airway differs from that of midazolam; in adults, ketamine does not cause airway obstruction, whereas midazolam does.[755] Ketamine has one of the best safety profiles of any anesthetic agent. After unintended overdoses as great as 56 mg/kg IM and 15 mg/kg IV,[756] the duration of sedation lasted between 3 and 24 hours; respiratory depression occurred in four children, whereas tracheal intubation was required in two. Provided the children who received an overdose are monitored and airway patency is maintained, recovery will occur without incident. This report combined with the minimal effect of ketamine on airway patency may explain in part the successful widespread use of this anesthetic by nonanesthesiologists. However, there remains a small but consistent incidence of adverse airway-related events such as laryngospasm, apnea, and airway obstruction associated with ketamine use, underscoring the need to ensure that the personnel responsible for administering ketamine are trained in advanced airway management. Ketamine also relaxes the smooth musculature of the airway stimulated by histamine[757]; treatment of acute asthma with subanesthetic doses has yielded mixed results.[758-760]

The onset of anesthesia after IV ketamine is approximately 30 seconds. This is usually heralded by horizontal or vertical nystagmus.[748,761] Studies separating equi-anesthetic doses of ketamine isomers identified a reduced incidence of side effects, more potent analgesia, and fewer cardiovascular effects with the dextro-isomer rather than the levo-isomer of ketamine.[684,748,762-764] Acute tolerance to ketamine has been reported.[765] Children require greater doses of ketamine (milligrams per kilogram) than adults because of more rapid degradation; however, there is considerable patient-to-patient variability.[697,748,762]

The most common adverse reaction to ketamine is postoperative vomiting, which occurs in 33% of children.[761] Intraoperative and postoperative dreaming and hallucinations occur more commonly in older than in younger children.[761] The incidence of these latter adverse effects may be reduced to approximately 4% when ketamine is supplemented with a benzodiazepine.[766,767] One clinical report described two children, each 3 years of age, who had recurrent nightmares and abnormal behavior persisting for 10 months after a single ketamine administration.[768] A soporific environment may reduce the incidence of emergence phenomena.[769]

Indications

Ketamine is useful for children who are developmentally delayed or those who are too frightened to come to the operating room and become combative. Ketamine can be used in very low doses (0.25-0.5 mg/kg) for short-term procedures such as diagnostic spinal punctures and bone marrow aspiration and in larger doses for radiotherapy, angiography, and cardiac catheterization. Ketamine may be particularly valuable for burn dressing changes, suture removal, induction of anesthesia in hypovolemic children, children in whom application of a face mask may prove hazardous, such as with epidermolysis bullosa, and children who require invasive monitoring before induction of general anesthesia.[748,762,770-772] Ketamine has been successfully used even in neonates with less apparent cardiovascular depression than with halothane or isoflurane.[771]

Contraindications

Ketamine may produce increases in intracranial pressure (ICP) as a result of cerebral vasodilation; it also increases $CMRo_2$. Ketamine may be contraindicated in children with intracranial hypertension.[773,774] This concern regarding ICP has been recently challenged[775,776]; adult patients whose lungs were mechanically ventilated and who were sedated with a ketamine infusion demonstrated a decrease in ICP after bolus doses of 1.5, 3.0, and 5.0 mg/kg.[777] The caveat is that the tracheas were already intubated, ventilation was controlled, and they were sedated. Until further studies re-examine the role of ketamine when it is combined with medications that are known to reduce ICP, it is still generally not indicated for emergency airway management of children with a head injury. There may be a use for ketamine sedation in the intensive care unit where there is meticulous attention to airway management and control of ventilation.[776]

A 30% increase in IOP has been noted; thus, ketamine may be potentially dangerous in the presence of a corneal laceration.[778] In children with active upper respiratory tract infections, copious secretions produced by ketamine may well exacerbate an already irritable airway and result in laryngospasm.[688,699] Ketamine may cause an incompetent gag reflex and thus should not be administered in anesthetic/induction doses to children with a full stomach without appropriate airway management. Ketamine may not be useful as the sole anesthetic agent in any surgical procedure in which total control of the child's position is necessary because purposeless movements frequently occur. Ketamine may be inappropriate in any child with a history of psychiatric or seizure disorder because of its psychotropic and epileptogenic effects.[679,748,779] In addition, studies in mice and rats have correlated ketamine treatment with increased neuronal apoptosis during rapid synaptogenesis after birth.[678,780-782] In neonatal rhesus monkeys, up to 3 mg/kg ketamine failed to yield evidence of apoptosis.[783] At this time, the clinical importance of these findings to humans is unclear because apoptosis has been studied only in laboratory animals. It is unclear whether these data can be extrapolated from animals to developing humans. Similar observations in rodents have been made with isoflurane, nitrous oxide, benzodiazepines, and other medications commonly used to provide sedation/analgesia and anesthesia to infants. However, current anesthetic practice should not change until rigorous scientific investigations are carried out.[784]

Although the administration of ketamine appears simple, its side effects are potentially dangerous. *Ketamine must be administered only by physicians experienced with managing a compromised airway.* We urge that it not be used as a premedication unless given in the presence of continuous supervision by properly trained personnel.

Etomidate

Etomidate (Amidate) is a steroid-based hypnotic induction agent. As in the case of propofol, etomidate is painful when administered intravenously. However, concerns regarding the risks of anaphylactoid reactions and suppression of adrenal function have resulted in most anesthesiologists avoiding this induction agent in routine cases.[785] Etomidate is very useful in children with head injury and those with an unstable cardiovascular status such as children with a cardiomyopathy because of the virtual absence of adverse effects on the hemodynamics or cardiac function.[786,787] It is often used by emergency department physicians for management of the airway.[788-790] Commonly used doses include 0.2 to 0.3 mg/kg before administration of a low-dose opioid and a muscle relaxant. Etomidate is often used to facilitate endotracheal intubation in critically ill children, that is, those in whom it would seem to offer the most advantage. Because a very large proportion of critically ill children, particularly those resistant to vasopressors, suffer from relative adrenal insufficiency, corticosteroid supplementation may be indicated in such patients in whom etomidate is deemed necessary for their safe airway management.[791,792]

Muscle Relaxants

The measurement of evoked responses after an electrical stimulus is the standard method for evaluating neuromuscular function. This method allows nearly instantaneous evaluation of the degree of neuromuscular blockade in the unconscious individual. The force of contraction of the thumb, the accelerometer, or the electromyogram may be used to make this assessment.[793] Twitch tension measurements use the force of contraction of the adductor pollicis. This muscle is the only thumb muscle supplied by the ulnar nerve; measurements therefore approach the single-muscle precision of the experimental nerve muscle preparation.[437] The evoked tension of the adductor pollicis in response to stimulation of the ulnar nerve can be recorded by a force displacement transducer (Fig. 6-25A, see website). With the electromyogram, the compound muscle action potential is recorded by surface or needle electrodes applied to any muscle, usually the adductor pollicis brevis, the abductor digiti minimi, or the first dorsal interosseous muscle of the hand (see Fig. 6-25B). To achieve reproducibility and to ensure full activation of all stimulated nerve and muscle fibers, the stimuli should be supramaximal in intensity, square wave in nature, and no longer than 0.2 msec in duration.

Clinically, three types of stimulation are used (Fig. 6-26, see website):

1. Single twitch (0.1 to 0.25 Hz [cycles/second])
2. Train-of-four (2 Hz for 2 seconds)
3. Tetanus (50 Hz, usually for 5 seconds)

Single-twitch rates are useful whenever there is an observable control response. By comparing the percentage change of twitch tension before and after administration of the neuromuscular blocking agent, one can assess the degree of paralysis. Single stimuli detect relatively high degrees of neuromuscular blockade. In fact, depression of the twitch response can be observed only if more than three fourths of the postsynaptic receptors are blocked.[794]

The *train-of-four* is the most commonly used method for assessing nondepolarizing neuromuscular blockade. It consists of four supramaximal stimuli applied to the ulnar nerve at a frequency of 2 cycles/second. The ratio of the amplitude of the fourth twitch to the first is an indicator of the degree of neuromuscular blockade. The main advantage of the train-of-four is that it does not require a control measurement. Furthermore, the train-of-four technique can be repeated every 10 seconds, thus allowing rapid changes in neuromuscular blockade to be closely monitored.[437] In general, when the train-of-four is zero, the conditions for tracheal intubation are satisfactory (excellent or good).[795] Preterm infants younger than 32 weeks' postconceptual age have reduced train-of-four values (83 ± 2%) than more mature neonates (Fig. 6-27, see website).[796] In full-term infants younger than 1 month of age, the height of the fourth evoked response of the train is about 95%.[797] The change to the greater value during the first month of life probably indicates maturation of the myoneural junction. In children 2 months of age and older, all components of the train-of-four are nearly equal (100%).[796]

Tetanic stimulation is usually obtained by supramaximally stimulating the nerve for 5 seconds or more. During tetanic stimulation synthesis of acetylcholine increases; however, this increase is limited. If the duration of stimulation is too prolonged or the frequency of stimulation is too great, fade occurs; that is, a decrement in the height of tetanus is noted. The usual explanation for the occurrence of fade is that during repetitive stimulation, the acetylcholine output per impulse wanes. Under normal circumstances, the diminution of acetylcholine output does not affect transmission because of the continuing excess of both acetylcholine and receptors at the myoneural junction (safety factor). During partial receptor blockade with a nondepolarizing relaxant, the progressive diminution of acetylcholine output eventually results in a decreased number of stimulated receptors and a consequent decrease in the amplitude of contraction. An alternative notion holds that fade is not simply the consequence of a spontaneously occurring decrease in the transmitter action but is in fact due to a different and separate action of the drug. This suggests that the relaxant has a prejunctional effect.[798] In infants and children anesthetized with halothane, the percent of fade during tetanic stimulation for 5 seconds at 20 cycles/second is 5% and at 50 cycles/second it is 9%.[797] These values are comparable to those for adults.[799] If the duration of stimulation is prolonged, an even greater degree of fade may be noted. In small infants, a more than 50% decrement in the height of tetanus has been observed during 15 seconds of tetanic stimulation; this decrement is even more marked in preterm infants.[800,801] These findings suggest that small infants can indeed sustain short periods of tetanic stimulation, but their musculature becomes fatigued more quickly than that of older children.

The integrity of the myoneural junction can also be analyzed by evaluation of post-tetanic facilitation. The increased synthesis and release of acetylcholine that occur during tetanic stimulation continue for a short interval after the stimulation has stopped. This increased production normally does not result in facilitation because all the muscle fibers are excited by the stimulus. In the presence of nondepolarizing (competitive) neuromuscular blockade, however, the increased post-tetanic acetylcholine release stimulates a greater number of muscle fibers, producing the characteristic post-tetanic facilitation.[799]

The post-tetanic count has been used to evaluate intense neuromuscular blockade in children.[802,803] This is a measure obtained by applying a 50-cycle/second tetanic stimulus to the ulnar nerve for 5 seconds, followed by single-twitch stimulation at 1 cycle/second; the number of twitches observed in the post-tetanic period is known as the post-tetanic count (Fig 6-28, see website). Because tetanus and post-tetanic responses are indicators of deep neuromuscular blockade, they can usually be elicited during recovery before the reappearance of the train-of-four. At very deep levels of blockade, no tetanus or post-tetanic effect can be seen; as the patient recovers, a single post-tetanic response eventually manifests itself. The number of post-tetanic counts increases as recovery proceeds until, at post-tetanic counts of six to seven, the first twitch of the train-of-four reappears. It has been shown that during recovery, the first post-tetanic response precedes the first response of the train-of-four by 5 to 10 minutes with intermediate relaxants and by 20 to 30 minutes with long-acting relaxants.[802,803]

In a clinical situation in which neuromuscular recording instruments are not available, the number of contractions during train-of-four are counted. This technique depends on the fact that the number of twitches in the train-of-four usually correlates well with the degree of blockade. When the height of the first twitch is about 21% of control, three contractions are usually detected during train-of-four stimulation; at a single-twitch height of 14% of control, two contractions are in evidence, and when the single-twitch height is about 7%, only one contraction is detected.[804] During procedures in which a child's hand is covered by surgical drapes, palpating the number of contractions provides a satisfactory alternative. The number of contractions during train-of-four stimulation thus yields a practical assessment of neuromuscular blockade. For more profound blockade, the post-tetanic counts can be used intermittently. However, repeated tetanic stimulation is not ideal because it is painful and can lead to post-tetanic exhaustion.

Although twitch monitoring is the standard method of evaluating neuromuscular blockade, the neuromuscular blockade in one group of muscles can differ substantively from that in another. For example, 1.7 times more relaxant is required to block the diaphragm and the vocal cords than the adductor pollicis.[805,806] Nonetheless, recovery of the twitch response is also approximately 50% more rapid in these central muscles. Accordingly, it is conceivable that children could cough or react during intubation in the absence of the twitch response when it is measured peripherally. Perhaps more importantly, when the peripheral twitch response has recovered at the end of the procedure, it is a clear indication that the diaphragm and the vocal cords are in a more advanced stage of recovery. Monitoring the orbicularis oculi contraction (as an estimate of the relaxation of central muscles) to predict whether the conditions for tracheal intubation are suitable is preferred because it occurs before the twitch response of the adductor muscle of the thumb.[807]

Succinylcholine

Succinylcholine is the only depolarizing relaxant used in children. Infants are more resistant to its neuromuscular effects than adults.[808] Early studies demonstrated that the degree of neuromuscular blockade achieved by 1 mg/kg IV in infants is about equal to that produced by 0.5 mg/kg in older children.[809] The increase in dose requirement in younger children is thought to result from the drug's rapid distribution into the infant's large extracellular fluid volume (Tables 6-15 [on website] and 6-16).

As in adults, administration of a continuous infusion of succinylcholine in infants and children results in tachyphylaxis

Table 6-16. Suggested Standard Intubating Doses of Commonly Used Relaxants in Infants and Children

	Infants		Children	
	mg/kg	µg/kg	mg/kg	µg/kg
Succinylcholine	3	3000	1.5-2	1500-2000
Cisatracurium	0.1	100	0.1-0.2	100-200
Atracurium	0.5	500	0.5	500
Rocuronium*	0.25-0.5	250-500	0.6-1.2	600-1200
Pancuronium	0.1	100	0.1	100
Vecuronium	0.07-0.1	70-100	0.1	100

*Low-dose rocuronium (0.3 mg/kg) allows tracheal intubation after 3 minutes during inhalational anesthesia in children but then is easily antagonized in about 20 minutes. Large-dose rocuronium (1.2 mg/kg) may be used as a substitute for succinylcholine for rapid intubation in children.

(increased requirement). In addition, phase II block may be produced, as evidenced by a train-of-four less than 50% (blockade similar to that produced by nondepolarizing muscle relaxants). In children, tachyphylaxis generally develops after administration of about 3 mg/kg of succinylcholine and phase II block develops during tachyphylaxis after 4 mg/kg.[810,811]

Succinylcholine is effective when administered by the IM route; in this instance, complete paralysis is achieved in 3 to 4 minutes. Evidence of relaxation of the respiratory muscles, as manifest by decreased positive pressure required to ventilate by face mask, can be detected before the abolishment of the twitch response. A dose of 2 mg/kg IM does not achieve satisfactory relaxation in all children, whereas the higher dose of 3 mg/kg IM produces a mean twitch depression of 85%; 4 mg/kg produces profound relaxation in all children, but its effects may last up to 20 minutes.[812] In infants younger than 6 months of age, a dose of 5 mg/kg IM is required to achieve profound relaxation; maximal twitch depression occurred a mean of 3.3 ± 0.4 minutes.[813] Recovery from the neuromuscular effect of IM succinylcholine is faster in infants than in children. Changes in the heart rate after IM succinylcholine are not pronounced. Consequently, routine IM administration of atropine with IM succinylcholine is not generally indicated.[814] Succinylcholine has also been administered intralingually.[815,816] One study examined the time to clinical apnea in 60 children younger than 10 years of age. Succinylcholine (1.1 mg/kg) resulted in apnea in 75 ± 4 seconds when administered intralingually, in 35 ± 1 seconds when administered intravenously, and in 210 ± 17 seconds when administered intramuscularly.[816] In that study, 8 of 10 children who did not receive concomitant atropine developed an arrhythmia (primarily bradycardia). A second study limited to only 15 children examined the time to maximal twitch response after succinylcholine (3 mg/kg) when administered by the submental route into the base of the tongue.[815] Five children received the drug into the quadriceps femoris, five intralingually without tongue massage, and five intralingually with tongue massage; the time to maximal twitch depression was 265 ± 63 seconds intralingually without massage, 133 ± 12 seconds intralingually with massage, and 295 ± 43 seconds when injected into the quadriceps femoris. Thus, there are limited data regarding alternate routes of administration of succinylcholine that might speed the onset of relaxation during an emergency when an IV line is not in place. These limited data suggest that the time of onset of succinylcholine after intralingual administration is more rapid than it is after IM injection. Caution should be exercised, however, when administering sublingual or intralingual medications. To preclude an intralingual hematoma, it is advised that a 25-gauge needle be used and the blood vessels on the undersurface of the tongue identified to minimize the risk of puncture. Sublingual succinylcholine is an alternative to the IV route, but it should be preceded by a vagolytic agent to avoid arrhythmias. The submental approach would seem to avoid the potential for causing bleeding from the tongue.

Cholinesterase Deficiency

Plasma cholinesterase is a circulating glycoprotein that metabolizes succinylcholine into succinylmonocholine. Activity of plasma cholinesterase may decrease as a result of a congenital enzyme variant or an acquired cause. This enzyme codes at the E1 locus of the long arm of chromosome 3. Ninety-six percent of the population is homozygote for the "usual" cholinesterase enzyme (E^u) and 4% are homozygous or heterozygous for the variant alleles.[817] Five alleles code for the majority of cholinesterase enzyme: (1) normal cholinesterase enzyme which is designated by "usual" (E^u); (2) decreased cholinesterase activity or quantity which is designated as atypical (E^a) (homozygote in 1:3000 to 1:10,000); (3) fluoride resistant allele (E^f) (homozygote in 1:150,000); (4) silent allele (E^s) (homozygote 1:10,000); and (5) the Cynthiana (C_5) or Neitlich variant which is associated with an increase in (or rapid) cholinesterase activity.[818] Variations on the silent gene have been detected in Eskimo populations with three variants labeled: S for silent, T for trace, and R for residual. The duration of succinylcholine in children who are homozygous for the silent gene is 3 to 4 hours. Additional genetic variants of pseudocholinesterase have been identified, including types H, J, and K, which represent a 60%, 66%, and 30% reduction in enzyme activity, respectively.

Heterozygote atypical (E^uE^a), which occurs in 1:30 of the population, may prolong neuromuscular blockade by only a few minutes and may go undetected. In contrast, homozygote atypical (E^aE^a), which occurs in approximately 1:3000 population, may cause paralysis for up to 1 hour after a single dose of succinylcholine.[26] Of the genetic variants of cholinesterase, silent gene (E^s) confers the least pseudocholinesterase activity and therefore the most prolonged duration of paralysis. Homozygote (E^sE^s) occurs in 1:100,000 population and may result in 8 hours of paralysis. Plasma cholinesterase activity is more often diminished when a genetic variant is present, but a number of clinical conditions may also reduce its activity. These include severe liver disease, malnutrition, organophosphate poisoning, severe burns, renal failure, plasmapheresis, and medications (cyclophosphamide, echothiophate iodide, oral contraceptives).[817,819,820] Several conditions are associated with increase in plasma cholinesterase activity, including thyroid disease, obesity, and nephrotic syndrome, and cognitively challenged children are also affected.[817,821-823]

Plasma cholinesterase activity is determined by the percent inhibition of benzyl choline degradation by the amide local anesthetic dibucaine when it is incubated with a sample of plasma. With the homozygous normal allele (E^uE^u), dibucaine profoundly inhibits pseudocholinesterase activity (approximately 80%), whereas with the homozygous atypical allele (E^aE^a),

it inhibits the activity by only 20%. When fluoride is added to the plasma, fluoride inhibits E^uE^u 60% but inhibits E^fE^f only 36%. Thus, a low dibucaine number indicates a deficiency of pseudocholinesterase.

Side Effects of Succinylcholine

Temporomandibular Joint Stiffness

Intravenous succinylcholine is infrequently associated with an increase in masseter muscle tone that limits mouth opening (trismus), particularly when given during halothane anesthesia. The incidence of isolated trismus when IV succinylcholine is administered during halothane anesthesia, 0.3% to 1%, is severalfold greater than that after IV thiopentone and succinylcholine, 0/4457 (upper 95% confidence of 7/10,000).[824,825] The increase in masseter muscle tone after succinylcholine is transient, lasting for only a few minutes and occurring despite abolition of the evoked twitch response in the masseter and peripheral muscles. The increase in masseter muscle tone is usually mild and can be overcome by manually distracting the mandible.[826] However, on rare occasions, the increase in muscle tone may be so severe that extreme and sustained force is required to open the mouth, thus interfering with the smooth endotracheal intubation. Whether this increased tone is related to the "trismus" (so-called "jaws of steel") (see Fig. 41-2) encountered in children with MH remains a matter of debate.[827] Prospective studies designed to evaluate masseter muscle tone have failed to demonstrate a child with a marked increase in masseter tone who later developed evidence of MH.[828,829] In several retrospective reports, however, a number of children experienced trismus and did develop or have a positive test response for MH.[830-832] These studies failed to clarify how best to proceed when trismus occurs. Some advocate canceling the surgical procedure, treating the child as susceptible to MH, and recommending a muscle biopsy.[832,833] This recommendation is based on a 50% incidence of positive muscle biopsies for MH in children who developed trismus after succinylcholine. Others advocate continuing the procedure, avoiding further exposure to triggering agents by changing the anesthetic technique to one that is free of triggers, observing for signs of MH (e.g., increased CO_2 production or tachycardia) and, if indicated, initiating arterial and central venous blood gas sampling as well as early treatment.[834,835] Finally, others have advocated continuing with the original triggering anesthetic while monitoring for signs of MH.[824] For the most part, this entire issue has become moot since sevoflurane has supplanted halothane as the primary inhaled anesthetic in children and the FDA issued a "black box" warning regarding the routine use of succinylcholine for tracheal intubation in children. Curiously, the now widespread use of nondepolarizing relaxants has generated several purported reports of masseter muscle rigidity after use of these agents. Whether these cases actually represent nondepolarizing relaxant-induced masseter spasm or a combination of light anesthesia and incomplete muscle relaxation is unclear at this time.[836-838]

Arrhythmias

Changes in heart rate are frequently observed after the administration of succinylcholine. Heart rate usually increases transiently after succinylcholine, and this response appears to be more pronounced in the presence of sevoflurane than halothane.[839] Succinylcholine-associated arrhythmias are rarely due to ventricular irritability. Prior IV administration of an anticho-

of adults.[883-886] However, on rare occasions there may be resistance to vecuronium in neonates.[887]

Muscle relaxants are often administered to critically ill children. Vecuronium has been popular because of the absence of cardiovascular side effects and because its metabolites do not seem to have CNS effects. However, adult and pediatric patients in intensive care units have had residual weakness after the discontinuation of vecuronium.[888-890] In one study in which the rate of infusion was adjusted by accelerometry, all children recovered within 1 hour. Of note in these children, the requirements of neonates and small infants was 45% less than those of older children.[891] In this respect, cisatracurium seems to offer an advantage because its recovery from prolonged infusion in children is faster than that of vecuronium.[892]

Rocuronium

Rocuronium (Zemuron) is a monoquaternary steroidal muscle relaxant similar to vecuronium. It has the fastest onset of action of the intermediate-acting nondepolarizing relaxants because of its low potency and greater dose requirements.[893] The onset of action of rocuronium is 20 to 70 seconds faster than vecuronium, although its duration of action is similar.[894] Rocuronium is eliminated primarily by the liver; the kidney excretes about 10%.[895-900] Renal failure does not affect the onset of rocuronium-induced neuromuscular blockade in adults or children. However, it may prolong the duration of action of rocuronium in adults, a finding not shared by children older than 1 year of age.[895,897,900]

Rocuronium has an ED_{95} of 303 µg/kg in children during halothane anesthesia[901] with slightly greater doses required during $N_2O : O_2$ opioid anesthesia.[902-904] After the administration of 600 µg/kg rocuronium, two times ED_{95}, 90% and 100% neuromuscular block occurred in 0.8 and 1.3 minutes (see Tables 6-15 [on website] and 6-16). At this dose, heart rate increased by approximately 15 beats per minute in children. The mean time to recover to 25% of control was approximately 28 minutes and for recovery to 90% it was 46 minutes.[904]

For brief cases in which the children are anesthetized with 8% inspired sevoflurane, 0.3 mg/kg rocuronium yields satisfactory intubating conditions in children within 2 to 3 minutes.[905] This dose of rocuronium can be antagonized within approximately 20 minutes of administration.[900] The intubating conditions after rocuronium (600 µg/kg) have been compared with those after vecuronium (100 µg/kg), atracurium (500 µg/kg), and succinylcholine (1 mg/kg). The authors found that tracheal intubation could be performed within 60 seconds in all the children who had received rocuronium or succinylcholine but not until 120 seconds after vecuronium and 180 seconds after atracurium.[906,907] The intubating conditions at 60 seconds are improved by increasing the dose[908]; by increasing the dose to 1.2 mg/kg (three to four times ED_{95}), the intubating conditions are similar to those after succinylcholine.[863,904] At the higher doses, heart rate increases transiently while systolic and diastolic pressures are unchanged.[901,909] It is unclear whether this increase in heart rate after rocuronium is due to pain on injection or an inherent chronotropic effect.[910] Dosing studies in infants 2 to 11 months of age demonstrated a slightly faster onset of neuromuscular blockade than in older children with the same dose (600 µg/kg). The times to 90% and 100% twitch depression were 37 and 64 seconds, respectively. In infants, the rate of onset of neuromuscular blockade 60 seconds after rocuronium is comparable to that after succinylcholine.[901,911]

Neonates appear to be more sensitive to rocuronium than older infants.[912] In neonates, the duration of action of 600 µg/kg is approximately 90 minutes and there is marked patient to patient variability. Consequently, 450 µg/kg rocuronium provides adequate intubating conditions with a duration of action of approximately 1 hour.[912]

In a pharmacokinetic study, the clearance of rocuronium in infants was less than in children (4 vs. 7 mL/kg/min), whereas the Vd was greater in infants. The mean residence time was 56 minutes in infants versus 26 minutes in children, thus explaining the prolonged duration of action of rocuronium in infants compared with children. In a steady-state target-controlled infusion study, the potency of rocuronium was greatest in infants, least in children, and intermediate in adults.[913] The greater plasma clearance and smaller Vd of rocuronium in children compared with infants and adults result in a markedly smaller mean residence time and a decreased duration of neuromuscular blockade.[914] Consistent with the dose-response effects of curare and vecuronium in infants, smaller plasma concentrations of rocuronium are required in the effect compartment in infants than in children to produce the same degree of neuromuscular blockade.[41] Sevoflurane markedly potentiates the effects of rocuronium.[915]

If an IV route is unavailable, the IM route for rocuronium is a reasonable alternative. IM rocuronium (1.8 mg/kg, three times the IV intubating dose) provided poor intubating conditions 4 minutes after administration in most children. Neuromuscular blockade (>98%) was achieved in 6 to 8 minutes.[916] The bioavailability of IM rocuronium at these doses is approximately 80%[917]; IM rocuronium appears to be a viable alternative to IM succinylcholine although the time of onset of neuromuscular blockade is very slow and may not be appropriate for emergent situations. The duration of IM rocuronium (~80 ± 22 minutes) is much greater than that after IM administration of succinylcholine.[916]

Clinical Implications When Using Short- and Intermediate-Acting Relaxants

Short- and intermediate-acting relaxants have great utility in infants and children because of the large number of brief surgical procedures performed. Because of their short duration of action, these drugs can be given in one intubating dose (atracurium [500 µg/kg]; cisatracurium [200 µg/kg]; vecuronium [100 µg/kg]; rocuronium [600 µg/kg]) and a light anesthetic level maintained throughout the procedure. If more than 45 minutes elapse since the last dose of one of these relaxant drugs, one may reasonably assume that neuromuscular function has nearly recovered, but safe practice would recommend confirming *recovery of neuromuscular integrity by clinical signs or by assessment with a neuromuscular blockade monitor. We recommend antagonism in all infants despite clinical signs of recovery.*

The benzylisoquinoloniums and organosteroidal neuromuscular blocking drugs are acidic compounds (pH 3 to 4) that can precipitate thiopental (pH 10 to 11) if admixed.[918] Consequently, when these drugs are administered in tandem, the IV tubing should be thoroughly flushed between the thiopentone and these relaxants. Vecuronium and rocuronium are painful when administered intravenously in a small vein during the light stages of anesthetic. This pain is usually demonstrated by withdrawal of the hand. Pain can be attenuated by deepening the level of anesthesia or pretreating with fentanyl, lidocaine, or ketamine.[919,920]

Long-Acting Nondepolarizing Relaxants

For almost half a century the mainstay of muscle relaxants was curare (*d*-tubocurarine). After the development of intermediate relaxants, its use diminished because its duration of action was too great for most surgeries and large doses released histamine. Curare is no longer available. Because curare is considered the quintessential muscle relaxant, it was the basis of the majority of early studies of muscle relaxants in children. These studies demonstrated that the Vd was greater and plasma concentrations less in small infants and neonates than in older children and adults at the same degree of neuromuscular blockade. In addition, the reduced plasma clearance, which was attributed to immaturity of renal function, prolonged the duration of neuromuscular blockade.

Following curare, several long-acting relaxants with minimal adverse side effect were developed. These included metocurine, pipecuronium, and doxacurium, which are two, four, and ten times as potent as curare, respectively. The only long-acting relaxant that is still used in some institutions is pancuronium.

Pancuronium

Pancuronium bromide (Pavulon) is a bisquaternary ammonium steroidal compound with nondepolarizing neuromuscular blocking properties. It is more potent than curare, metocurine, and gallamine with a slightly shorter duration of action.[921] It induces mild tachycardia (increased cardiac output in infants) but has no histamine-releasing properties. As a result, systolic blood pressure tends to increase.[922] Pancuronium (100 μg/kg) provides satisfactory conditions for tracheal intubation in 70% to 90% of infants and children within 150 seconds of administration. Increasing the initial dose to 150 μg/kg provides satisfactory intubating conditions in all children within 80 seconds (see Tables 6-15 [on website] and 6-16).[866,923]

Pancuronium is frequently advocated for cardiac surgery and other high-risk procedures in infants and children. The anesthetic technique of high-dose opioid with air-oxygen-pancuronium is well tolerated by infants from a cardiovascular perspective. The vagolytic effect (tachycardia) of pancuronium counteracts the vagotonic effect (bradycardia) of potent opioids, and its relaxant properties counteract opioid-induced chest wall and glottic rigidity.[924] Pancuronium has been used to facilitate ventilation in preterm infants in neonatal intensive care units.[925] Because pancuronium increases the heart rate, blood pressure, and plasma epinephrine and norepinephrine levels in neonates, there is some concern that it may contribute to the risk of an intracerebral hemorrhage.[926] Accordingly, it would seem prudent to administer pancuronium with either general anesthesia or with adequate sedation, to blunt adverse cardiovascular responses. Vecuronium may offer an advantage over pancuronium because it does not significantly increase the blood pressure.[927-931] Nasotracheal intubation or intratracheal suctioning in neonates who are paralyzed with pancuronium results in smaller increases in intracranial pressure than in neonates who are not paralyzed.[931,932] By abolishing fluctuations in cerebral blood flow through the use of muscle relaxants, the incidence and severity of intraventricular hemorrhages should theoretically be reduced.

Antagonism of Muscle Relaxants

General Principles

In children and especially infants, oxygen consumption is greater than it is in adults. Therefore, a slight diminution in respiratory muscle power may lead to hypoxemia and CO_2 retention. Consequently, it is very important that neuromuscular function is returned to normal at the end of the surgical procedure. Neonates are at greater risk for residual neuromuscular blockade than adults for several reasons, including (1) immaturity of the neuromuscular system, as evidenced by the reduced train-of-four, post-tetanic facilitation, tetanus:twitch ratios, and the marked fade during prolonged tetanic stimulation; (2) greater elimination half-life of relaxants; (3) the reduced number of type I muscle fibers in the ventilatory musculature (thus being more susceptible to fatigue [see Chapter 12, Fig. 12-11])[933]; and (4) the closing lung volume of a neonate overlaps with the tidal volume (i.e., airway closure occurs at the end of expiration).[934] If respiration is mildly impaired as a result of residual muscle paralysis, even more alveoli will collapse. The result may be hypoxemia as well as hypercarbia and acidosis, which may potentiate and prolong the duration of action of the muscle relaxant, thus creating a vicious cycle.

When monitoring neuromuscular blockade in infants and children, train-of-four monitoring of the adductor pollicis overestimates the degree of neuromuscular blockade in the diaphragm.[806] Larger doses of muscle relaxants are required to block the diaphragm than the adductor pollicis train-of-four would suggest. Therefore, if the train-of-four of the adductor has fully recovered, one can assume that the diaphragm has fully recovered.

Clinical evaluation of the adequacy of antagonism in infants is more difficult than in children or adults. Neither grip strength nor voluntary head lifting can be elicited; rather, it is important when working with infants to observe the clinical conditions preoperatively (muscle tone, depth of respiration, vigor of crying) and to aim for a comparable level of activity in the post-antagonism period. Useful clinical signs that the neuromuscular blockade has been antagonized include the ability to flex the hips, flex the arm, and lift the legs and the return of abdominal muscle tone.[935] Inspiratory force may be measured; a negative force of −25 cm H_2O or greater indicates adequate antagonism.[936] A crying vital capacity greater than 15 mL/kg indicates an adequate respiratory reserve. The train-of-four is a valuable aid because it can be used in the smallest of infants in whom the force of contraction can easily be palpated (four equal contractions indicating adequate antagonism).

The dose requirement of anticholinesterase agents to antagonize neuromuscular blockade in children is less than adults.[937] However, the speed of antagonism depends on the extent of neuromuscular blockade at the time of the antagonism as well as the type and dose of antagonizing agent.[137-139] In the presence of four train-of-four responses with fade, 20 μg/kg of neostigmine preceded by 10 to 20 μg/kg of atropine or 5 to 10 μg/kg of glycopyrrolate is sufficient to achieve full recovery of muscle strength. This dose of neostigmine can be repeated if required (up to 70 μg/kg). Doses of neostigmine in excess of 100 μg/kg may induce a paradoxical weakness from excessive acetylcholine at the neuromuscular junction. Edrophonium has a theoretical advantage over neostigmine because its onset is 2 to 3 minutes faster than that of neostigmine. Whether this difference is clinically important is debatable. The dose of edrophonium for children is greater than it is for adults; at least 0.3 mg/kg is needed, but 0.5 to 1.0 mg/kg is most common.[938-942]

Some have suggested that it is not necessary to antagonize intermediate-acting relaxants, particularly if a lengthy time interval has elapsed since the last dose. With the advent of reliable neuromuscular monitors and their use in conjunction with clinical observations and measurements of respiratory adequacy, clinicians are more confident that antagonism was not always required. This may be particularly appropriate for the short- and intermediate-acting relaxants, particularly atracurium or cis-atracurium, which are hydrolyzed in plasma. Children have the additional advantage of recovering from neuromuscular blockade more rapidly than adults.[941,942] In infants, the elimination of all muscle relaxants might be delayed, necessitating antagonism of any neuromuscular blockade. Most importantly, if there is any concern that some degree of neuromuscular blockade persists, then the blockade must be antagonized.

Hypothermia potentiates the action of most nondepolarizing muscle relaxants and delays their elimination.[943] This effect can create a special problem at the end of a surgical procedure when the children attempt to resume spontaneous ventilation. Shivering increases oxygen consumption and augments the load on the respiratory system. If the respiratory muscles are unable to match this increased load, hypoxemia and CO_2 retention may occur, which, in turn, may lead to acidosis, which again may potentiate the relaxant. To avoid the extra cardiorespiratory load in a postsurgical infant, it is reasonable to warm the infant if his or her temperature is less than 35° C (95° F). Once the core temperature is above this level, antagonism of neuromuscular blockade may be attempted if appropriate.

All antibiotics theoretically have neuromuscular depressing properties when administered in association with relaxants.[944] Among the antibiotics, aminoglycoside derivatives such as gentamicin, tobramycin, and neomycin have the greatest effect. A single clinical dose of antibiotic will likely have minimal effect on the neuromuscular blockade.[945] This factor alone does not rule out the possibility that large concentrations of antibiotics, especially in the presence of other potentiating factors, may augment the neuromuscular blockade. The clinical importance of the interaction of antibiotics with muscle relaxants to prolong neuromuscular blockade has diminished with the introduction of intermediate-acting neuromuscular blocking agents.

Suggamadex

Recent research into the pharmacology of antagonizing muscle relaxants more rapidly and more effectively has yielded a new approach involving a "donut"-shaped molecule that reversibly encapsulates steroidal muscle relaxants.[946] Suggamadex (ORG 25969) is composed of cyclic oligosaccharides that are cyclodextrin compounds with hydrophobic molecules within the center (Fig. 6-29).[947,948] This compound encapsulates rocuronium, forms a stable complex, and prevents further action of the rocuronium. The complex is then excreted unchanged by the kidneys. The chemical encapsulation decreases the plasma concentration of rocuronium, thus promoting the dissociation of rocuronium from the acetylcholine receptor, speeding recovery of muscle strength. As more rocuronium dissociates, it, too, is encapsulated, thus reversing even very intense neuromuscular blockade from rocuronium. Three minutes after 0.6 mg/kg rocuronium produced profound neuromuscular block in adult volunteers, a single dose of suggamadex, 2 mg/kg or greater, reversed the neuromuscular block within 2 minutes.[949] If further clinical trials confirm the safety and efficacy of this new concept and studies in children demonstrate safety and efficacy, then suggamadex may be effective in antagonizing large doses of rocuronium rapidly, efficiently, and soon after the onset of neuromuscular blockade.[950-954] Under these circumstances, rocuronium might then supplant succinylcholine in most circumstances, including rapid-sequence intubations for brief procedures in children.

Relaxants in Special Situations

Of the many drug combinations possible, that of succinylcholine after a halothane induction seems to be most likely to trigger MH[955] (see Chapter 41). The use of depolarizing neuromuscular blocking agents in combination with halogenated agents should be avoided in children at risk for this syndrome.[956] The safest general anesthetic technique for children at risk for MH is an opioid/N_2O/O_2 combination with benzodiazepines, propofol, and a nondepolarizing relaxant. Nondepolarizing agents devoid of cardiovascular side effects may offer an advantage in not causing tachycardia, an early sign of MH.[957] Currently, there is some concern of the potential association between mitochondrial disease and MH. A major review, along with evidence from pathology specimens from patients who either had or had a

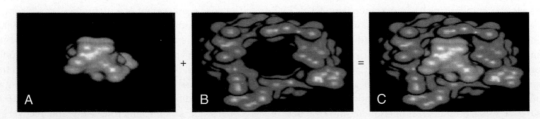

Figure 6-29. X-ray crystallography of the rocuronium molecule (shown in *blue*) (**A**) and suggamadex (*green ring*) (**B**). The 3-D conformation of the rocuronium molecule complements the conformation of the inner ring of suggamadex (**C**). The rocuronium/suggamadex complex (**C**) is stable, without a dissociation constant and is excreted unchanged via the kidneys. (Redrawn from Gijsenbergh F, Ramael S, Houwing N, van IT: First human exposure of Org 25969, a novel agent to reverse the action of rocuronium bromide. Anesthesiology 2005; 103:695-703.)

family member with MH, suggest that this is not at all clear and may be a case of "fortuitous association."[958] Because many of these children are bedridden, it would seem prudent to avoid succinylcholine, although there are "inadequate data to support the recommendation . . . that the anesthetic plan for patients with mitochondrial disease should routinely include MH precautions."[959]

The use of muscle relaxants in children with neuromuscular and mitochondrial diseases has been the subject of debate. Rhabdomyolysis has been reported after succinylcholine in children with Duchenne muscular dystrophy (see Chapters 22 and 41). It is prudent to avoid succinylcholine in any child with a suspicious neuromuscular or mitochondrial disease (see earlier). The response of children with neuromuscular disease to nondepolarizing relaxants is variable. Most are relatively sensitive to the relaxant, particularly those with muscular dystrophy, because of muscle wasting. The duration of neuromuscular blockade is often prolonged. Rarely, resistance may be evident as a result of chronic immobilization. Of all the nondepolarizing relaxants, we recommend cisatracurium because of its multiple sites of degradation that are independent of organ function.[960-962] The dose requirement of atracurium in children with Duchenne muscular dystrophy is similar to that in unaffected children, although the duration of action may be prolonged.[960] The dose response of rocuronium in children with Duchenne muscular dystrophy shows marked prolongation of both the onset and recovery times (two to three times normal).[963] Thus, relaxants should be administered with caution in children with severe preexisting respiratory dysfunction, because even a small dose of muscle relaxant may cause profound muscle weakness and the need for ventilatory support. Similarly, it is important to antagonize any residual neuromuscular blockade at the end of surgery. *If there is any doubt about the competence of the neuromuscular junction, the trachea should remain intubated until muscle strength has recovered.*

Succinylcholine can cause hyperkalemia in children with burns, which may cause a cardiac arrest.[964] The more extensive the burn, the more likely and the greater the hyperkalemic response. An 8% burn is the smallest burn that has been associated with hyperkalemia. Although most instances of cardiac arrest have occurred 20 to 50 days after the burn injury, exaggerated increases in the plasma concentration of potassium after succinylcholine can occur within a few days of the burn. However, hyperkalemia after succinylcholine has not been reported in the first 24 to 48 hours after a burn. Hyperkalemia is thought to result from the upregulation of acetylcholine receptors along the surface of the muscle membrane in the postburn phase (see Chapter 34).[965]

Children with burns may require two to three times the usual IV dose of nondepolarizing relaxants. This resistance peaks about 2 weeks after the burn, persists for many months in those with major burns, and decreases gradually as the burns heal. The degree of resistance appears to correlate with both the extent of the burn and the period of healing. The resistance can be explained, in part, by an increase in the Vd of the relaxant (including binding to an increased plasma concentration of α_1-acid glycoprotein) and an increase in number, sensitivity, and type of extrajunctional acetylcholine receptors (see Chapter 34).

Opioids

Morphine

Morphine is the most frequently used opioid to treat postoperative pain in children and is the standard against which all other opioids are compared. It may be administered by intermittent bolus, continuous infusion, or patient-controlled analgesia (see Chapter 44).[966-968] The usual initial IV dose is 0.05 to 0.2 mg/kg. A reduced dose may be indicated in children who are critically ill, are receiving supplemental analgesics, and/or have obstructive sleep apnea.[969-971]

A number of studies have examined the kinetics of IV morphine in children.[124,125,174,972-979] The clearance of IV morphine, which ranges from 79 to 133 minutes, is more rapid in children than in adults.[973,978] However, if the children require pressor support, the elimination half-life is prolonged (to ~400 minutes).[974,980] Studies of morphine pharmacokinetics in term and preterm infants demonstrate reduced clearance and a variable and markedly prolonged elimination half-life.[121,124,125,174,972,975,976,981,982] Morphine clearance increases with age, reaching adult values by about 3 months after birth in children with normal hearts and by about 6 months in those with heart disease (Fig. 6-30).[122,972,979]

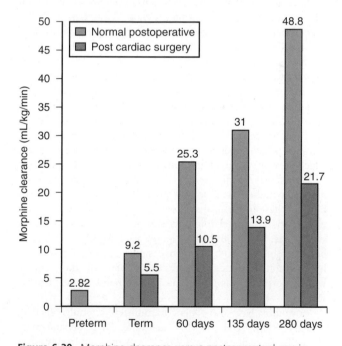

Figure 6-30. Morphine clearance versus postconceptual age in normal postoperative infants and infants undergoing cardiac surgery. Note that there is a rapid increase in an infant's ability to metabolize morphine in the first several weeks of life and that some infants achieve adult values by 1 month of age. Also note that after cardiac surgery infants have a marked impairment of morphine metabolism, which may reflect the use of vasopressors and/or decreased cardiac output to the liver. There is extreme patient-to-patient variability at all ages; preterm infants have the lowest clearance of any age group. (Data from Lynn A, Nespeca MK, Bratton SL, et al: Clearance of morphine in postoperative infants during intravenous infusion: the influence of age and surgery. Anesth Analg 1998; 86:958-963; and Mikkelsen S, Feilberg VL, Christensen CB, Lundstrom KE: Morphine pharmacokinetics in preterm and mature newborn infants. Acta Paediatr 1994; 83:1025-1028.)

Morphine is glucuronidated in neonates and infants to morphine-3 and morphine-6 glucuronide, with morphine-3 glucuronide accounting for a greater fraction of the clearance (85% vs. 55%).[972,975] These developmental factors for morphine metabolism explain in part the prolonged duration of action of morphine in neonates. It also suggests that some infants older than 1 month are able to equal or exceed the reported clearance of morphine in adults.

The major risk associated with opioid use in infants and children is respiratory depression.[983,984] Morphine infusion rates of 10 to 30 µg/kg/hr provide adequate postoperative analgesia without respiratory depression.[977] Postoperative analgesia is achieved at reduced infusion rates in infants greater than or equal to 4 weeks of age (~5 µg/kg/hr for neonates, ~8.5 µg/kg/hr at 1 month, ~13.5 µg/kg/hr at 3 months, ~18 µg/kg/hr at 1 year, and slightly less than ~16 µg/kg/hr for 1 to 3 year olds).[174] When respiratory depression from morphine occurs, it results from diminished tidal volume and respiratory rate. Whether morphine causes a parallel shift in the CO_2 response curve or a change in the slope as well as a parallel shift has not been clearly established. Morphine appears to depress respiration in neonates to a greater extent than meperidine.[985] In neonatal rats, the brain uptake of morphine is two to three times that in adult rats, in part owing to the immature blood-brain barrier.[165] This may explain the fivefold reduced LD_{50} of morphine in neonatal versus adult animals.[163-165] This immaturity of the blood-brain barrier may account in part for the increased sensitivity of the neonate to morphine compared with meperidine or fentanyl; because of their lipophilicity, the latter two opioids rapidly cross an adult's or infant's blood-brain barrier, that is, there is essentially no blood-brain barrier.[174,986,987] Alternatively, altered pharmacokinetics could lead to drug accumulation in some infants.[125] Another possibility is a maturation of the pharmacodynamic effects on respiration rather than altered pharmacokinetics, that is, a maturation of the sensitivity of the respiratory center to morphine rather than brain equilibrium.[988] Whether one or more of these mechanisms is relevant, morphine must be used with caution in preterm infants and in infants younger than 1 year of age. Significant histamine release may follow a rapid IV bolus of morphine and, on rare occasions, may result in systemic hypotension.[989] Urticaria over the course of the vein in which morphine was infused is a local, not systemic, allergic reaction.

Morphine has also been administered orally, rectally, transtracheally, and in the epidural and subarachnoid spaces (see Chapters 42 and 44).[990-999] Rectal administration is generally not recommended because of extremely irregular absorption (6%-93% bioavailability)[1000] and the potential for delayed respiratory depression.[1001] Table 6-17 summarizes the relative doses of opioids administered via the parenteral and oral routes.

Meperidine

The principal role of meperidine (Demerol) in children is to stop shivering. Although its onset time is more rapid than morphine, the risk of seizures after repeated dosing in children has all but removed it from clinical use. The impression that meperidine causes less histamine release than morphine has been questioned.[1002] The purported benefits of substituting meperidine for morphine in children who are hypovolemic or asthmatic are questionable.

Table 6-17. Relative Comparison of Commonly Used Oral and Parenteral Opioids

Drug	Parenteral Dose (mg)	Oral Dose (mg)	Half-Life (hr)
Morphine	10	30-40	2.0-3.5
Hydromorphone	1.5-2.0	6.0-7.5	2-4
Oxycodone		15-30	2-4
Methadone	7.5-10.0	15	22-25
Meperidine	75-100	300	3-5
Codeine	120-130	200	3
Fentanyl	0.1	0.1	0.5

Adapted from Lugo RA, Kern SE: Clinical pharmacokinetics of morphine. J Pain Palliat Care Pharmacother 2002; 16:5-18.

The dose of meperidine is 1 to 2 mg/kg, although reduced doses should be used in critically ill children (see Table 6-17). Peak plasma values after IV, IM, and rectal administration are 5 ± 1 minutes, 10 ± 2 minutes, and 60 ± 10 minutes, respectively.[1003,1004] Rectal administration of meperidine in children results in wide variations in systemic blood values (32% to 81% of administered dose) and is not recommended.[1005] The elimination half-life of meperidine in children after IV administration is approximately 3 ± 0.5 hours[1005] with a variable half-life in neonates between 3.3 and 59.4 hours.[1006]

Respiratory depression in infants after meperidine appears to be less than after morphine.[985] The LD_{50} of meperidine in the neonatal animal is only 20% less than in the adult animal, corresponding with the human clinical response.[163] This is consistent with the reduced respiratory depression with meperidine compared with the equivalent dose of morphine. This difference between morphine and meperidine, however, may be related in part to differences in their relative ability to cross the blood-brain barrier, that is, their relative fat solubility. Studies in neonatal rats have shown greater brain concentrations of morphine compared with mature rats,[1007] whereas the brain concentrations of meperidine in the same two groups are similar.[165] Because morphine is less fat soluble than meperidine, more morphine likely crosses the immature blood-brain barrier in the neonate than in the more mature child.[174] As with any opioid, the use of meperidine in very young infants must be accompanied by careful observation for respiratory depression and airway obstruction because the pharmacokinetics vary considerably.[1006] Because repeated doses of meperidine may result in the accumulation of normeperidine, which itself may cause seizures,[1008,1009] this drug has been removed from the formulary in most children's hospitals. We do not recommend the use of this opioid other than for a single dose administration.

Hydromorphone

Hydromorphone (Dilaudid) is commonly used when prolonged analgesia is required.[1010-1013] Morphine is often changed to hydromorphone to reduce the side effects or because of concern of accumulation of morphine metabolites, particularly in the presence of renal failure.[1014] Hydromorphone is five times more potent than oral morphine and 5 to 7.5 times more potent than the IV formulation.[1015] Hydromorphone is commonly administered IV, orally, in the epidural space, and more recently through the nasal mucosa.[1010,1011,1014,1016-1019] Its bioavailability is about 55% after nasal and oral administration and about 35% after rectal administration (not recommended).[1020-1022] The pharmacokinetics of hydromorphone are similar in children and adults with a half-life of 2.5 ± 0.9 hours.[1020,1023] Table 6-17 summarizes the relative doses of opioids administered via the parenteral and oral routes.

Oxycodone

Oxycodone (OxyContin) is another long-acting opioid that is usually administered orally and is available in a controlled-release formulation.[1024-1026] The bioavailability is 60% to 86% in adults.[1027-1030] Oxycodone may also be administered rectally, with a similar bioavailability, although absorption can be prolonged.[1029] The IV formulation of oxycodone significantly depresses respiration.[1031,1032] As with many medications, interindividual variability in the elimination half-life of oxycodone in the neonate is extreme.[1033,1034] In children, the elimination half-life after IV, buccal, IM, or orogastric administration is 2 to 3 hours.[1035] The bioavailability after various routes is IM, 68%; buccal, 55%; and orogastric, 37%.[1035,1036] This opioid is commonly used to transition from patient-controlled analgesia and to treat chronic painful conditions (see Chapters 44 and 45). Table 6-17 summarizes the relative doses of opioids administered via the parenteral and oral routes.

Methadone

The primary indication for methadone in children is to wean from long-term opioid infusions to prevent withdrawal and to provide analgesia when other opioids have failed or have been associated with intolerable side effects.[1024,1037-1043] In adults, the mean elimination half-life after oral administration is prolonged, 33 to 46 hours. Interindividual variability in the elimination of methadone in children is marked.[1044,1045] Table 6-17 summarizes the relative doses of opioids administered via the parenteral and oral routes.

Fentanyl

Fentanyl (Sublimaze) is the most commonly used opioid during general anesthesia in infants and children. It is particularly effective in the care of high-risk preterm and term neonates as well as in infants and children during cardiac surgical procedures. High doses of fentanyl (10 to 100 µg/kg) are often administered to maintain cardiovascular homeostasis.[924,1046-1056] Fentanyl may be administered intravenously, intramuscularly, as a supplement to epidural analgesia, orally (transoral mucosal absorption), and transdermally—both passively and by iontophoresis.[1057-1062]

The pharmacokinetics and pharmacodynamics of fentanyl vary substantively among neonates, infants, and children. Compared with term neonates, the clearance of fentanyl in preterm infants is extremely variable and markedly prolonged (mean elimination half-life is 17.7 ± 9.3 hours). Respiratory depression is also prolonged in preterm infants.[1046,1063,1064] Compared with older infants, the clearance of fentanyl is reduced in term neonates (elimination half-life is prolonged).[1047,1063,1064] Seventy-seven percent of fentanyl is bound to α_1-acid glycoprotein in preterm infants and 70% in term infants.[36] The clearance of fentanyl in older infants (>3 months of age) and children is greater than in adults (30.6 mL/kg/min vs. 17.9 mL/kg/min, respectively) resulting in a reduced elimination half-life (68 minutes vs. 121 minutes, respectively).[1046,1049,1063-1065] Several

factors are particularly important in the clearance of fentanyl: hepatic blood flow, hepatic function, and age-dependent changes in Vd.[1047,1050,1051,1066] Factors that decrease hepatic blood flow decrease the delivery and therefore metabolism of fentanyl in the liver. In infants undergoing abdominal surgery that is associated with an increase in intra-abdominal pressure (e.g., repair of omphalocele) the clearance of fentanyl may be markedly reduced.[1047,1050,1051] This has been attributed to a decrease in hepatic blood flow.[1067,1068] However, in neonatal lambs, the hepatic extraction ratio of fentanyl was noted to be much less than in adults, an effect that would decrease the contribution of liver blood flow to drug metabolism. When the intra-abdominal pressure was increased in these lambs, the hepatic extraction ratio decreased further. In this model, the decreased clearance of fentanyl was attributed not to a decrease in the hepatic blood flow but rather to the immature cytochrome enzyme system in the neonate and to a maldistribution of blood away from regions of concentrated cytochrome enzyme activity.[1069]

One additional concern in neonates is an apparent interaction between fentanyl and midazolam. Profound hypotension has been reported after a bolus of midazolam in neonates in whom fentanyl was infused and vice versa.[1070]

The pharmacokinetics of fentanyl are also variable in children undergoing cardiac surgery. This may be attributed in part to the nature of the cardiac surgical defect, the effect of the defect on hepatic blood flow, the Vd, the use of vasopressors, and the child's age.[1048,1066] Hypothermia has also been shown to significantly alter fentanyl kinetics.[1071] The pharmacokinetics of fentanyl in critically ill children receiving long-term infusions is also quite variable with a mean terminal elimination half-life of 21 hours and a range of 11 to 36 hours.[1072] The infusion rates of fentanyl that are required to achieve a similar level of sedation/analgesia may vary as much as 10-fold.[1072] This variability in pharmacokinetics and pharmacodynamics strongly reinforces the need to titrate the dose to effect and to be prepared to provide postoperative ventilatory support as needed. Children who receive a chronic infusion of fentanyl are at risk of rapidly developing tolerance to the opioid. On discontinuance of the infusion, these children may demonstrate signs of withdrawal. All long-term infusions should be tapered slowly over days rather than abruptly discontinuing the infusion.[1064,1073,1074]

With low-dose fentanyl, the termination of action is primarily a combination of redistribution and rapid clearance by the liver.[1064,1075] High-dose fentanyl, on the other hand, accumulates in muscle and fat and is therefore released (recirculated) more slowly, thus accounting in part for the prolonged respiratory depression after high doses. There is no evidence of dose-dependent kinetics, that is, there is no tissue or enzyme saturation in the clinically used ranges.[1075] In some respects, the pharmacology of opioids is very similar to thiopental: at low doses their clinical effect is terminated by redistribution, whereas at high doses their clinical effect is terminated by metabolism.[1076-1080]

The usual initial dose of fentanyl is 1 to 3 µg/kg, a dose that may be supplemented as clinically indicated. Fentanyl is highly lipid soluble and rapidly crosses the blood-brain barrier. This characteristic may in part explain why the LD_{50} for fentanyl in neonatal animals is 90% of that in adult animals; the maturation of the blood-brain barrier offers little resistance to the entry of fentanyl (unlike morphine) into brain tissue.[987,1078] Little research has addressed the relationship between blood fentanyl concentrations and ventilatory depression in children. Some data suggest that neonates are no more sensitive to this opioid than are adults, because the blood-brain barrier should have little effect on the ability of fentanyl to enter the CNS.[1047,1079] In animals, there is little developmental change in fentanyl-induced respiratory depression, an effect very different from that of morphine.[988] Other data suggest that older infants (>3 months) are less sensitive to fentanyl-induced respiratory depression than are adults.[1067,1079] Continuous intraoperative and postoperative infusions of fentanyl are common in children of all ages.[1048,1080,1081] However, the context-sensitive half-life of fentanyl increases dramatically as the duration of the infusion increases (beyond 2 hours) (Fig. 6-31).[1082] Fentanyl is also used to provide patient-controlled analgesia (see Chapter 44).[1083,1084]

Chest wall and glottic rigidity have been reported after IV administration of opioids, although most often after fentanyl. The reason for this is not clear.[1085-1090] Glottic rigidity may account for the inability to ventilate by bag and mask after IV fentanyl.[1088] This adverse response can be minimized by administering the opioid slowly, and it can be reversed by administering either a muscle relaxant or naloxone. One other concern is the rare association of increased vagal tone with bolus administration; bradycardia may have profound effects on the cardiac output of neonates. Additionally, fentanyl markedly depresses the baroreceptor reflex control of heart rate in neonates.[1091] It is for these reasons that the combination of pancuronium and fentanyl became popular.

Oral transmucosal fentanyl (Fentanyl Oralet; Anesta/Abbott Laboratories) was one of only several medications approved by the FDA for premedication of children, although this formulation is no longer marketed. A new formulation (Actiq; Cephalon, Inc.) has been approved for adults and currently under investigation in children for the treatment of breakthrough pain.[1092,1093] Fentanyl is rapidly absorbed through the oral mucosa, which bypasses the liver.[634,1058,1059,1094-1098] Nonetheless, approximately half the absorption is gastrointestinal. The bioavailability of this formulation in children (33%) is less than that in adults (50%).[1058,1059] Uptake continues for a period of time after consumption, which potentially can provide analgesia for several hours.[634,1058,1059] The main concerns with preoperative fentanyl administration were the apparent high incidence of desaturation and vomiting before induction of anesthesia.[1096,1097] Subsequent studies and personal experience suggest that administration of doses less than or equal to 15 μg/kg and induction of anesthesia within a short time of completion (10-20 minutes) markedly reduces or eliminates these potential complications.[634,1058,1059] The use of this formulation is likely going to be limited to the treatment of breakthrough pain.

The fentanyl patch was developed to provide an extended release of fentanyl similar to that provided with a continuous IV infusion.[1057,1099-1108] *This formulation was not designed to be administered to treat postsurgical pain but rather for those who require opioids chronically.* In adults, uptake of fentanyl begins within 1 hour and achieves therapeutic levels within 6 to 8 hours and peak levels at 24 hours.[1105,1108,1109] In children, the peak occurs earlier, at about 18 hours.[1110] The skin acts as a reservoir and even after removal of the patch, uptake continues for several hours with an elimination half-life of 14.5 ± 6 hours.[1110] Fentanyl uptake is markedly affected by skin blood flow, skin thickness, location of the patch, and adherence to the skin.[1111-1114] Alterations in skin blood flow may increase absorption (e.g., fever).[1115] The use of this medication should be limited to pain specialists who have familiarity with the unusual pharmacokinetics of this drug delivery system.[1116] Children may be particularly vulnerable to the rapid drug absorption compared with adults because they have thinner skin and better skin blood flow.[725] One study suggests that the pharmacokinetics of fentanyl by this route in children and adult patients are similar.[1110] A multicenter study in children 2 to 16 years of age reported satisfactory chronic analgesia. However, it should be noted that the data submitted to the FDA revealed plasma concentrations of fentanyl in children 1.5 to 5 years of age that were twice those in adults.[1117] These data are consistent with another study that found a negative correlation between fentanyl concentrations and age, that is, greater concentrations in younger children.[1110] Accordingly, it seems prudent to begin with the smallest size patch and gradually increase as indicated (see Chapters 44 and 45). Finally, all patches, including those that have already been used, still contain large amounts of fentanyl that may cause a fatal intoxication if accidentally ingested by a child.[1118,1119] Proper disposal of these opioid-containing patches is required. Table 6-17 summarizes the relative doses of opioids administered via the parenteral and oral routes.

Alfentanil

Alfentanil (Alfenta) is a fentanyl analogue whose main advantage is its reduced lipid solubility and smaller Vd compared with fentanyl.[1120] Studies indicate that brain concentrations of alfentanil are sevenfold to ninefold less, the Vd is four times less, and protein binding is greater than fentanyl.[1121] Alfentanil is more rapidly eliminated from the body than fentanyl, resulting in more frequent dosing. The pharmacokinetics of alfentanil in children and adults are independent of the dose, thus providing a wide margin of safety, that is, *the larger the dose, the greater*

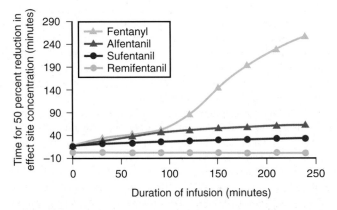

Figure 6-31. This figure is a simulation of the time required for a 50% reduction in the effective site concentration of remifentanil (*yellow circles*), sufentanil (*purple circles*), alfentanil (*brown triangles*), and fentanyl (*blue triangles*) after an infusion (duration of 0 to 240 minutes) designed to maintain a constant effect site concentration. Note that there is a completely flat curve for remifentanil, suggesting that a plateau effect is rapidly reached with remifentanil compared with the other opioids such that even after a long infusion, the time to 50% reduction in effect concentration is still under 4 minutes. (Redrawn and modified with permission from Westmoreland CL, Hole JF, Sebel PS, et al: Pharmacokinetics of remifentanil (GI87084B) and its major metabolite (GI90291) in patients undergoing elective inpatient surgery. Anesthesiology 1993; 79:893-903.)

the amount of drug metabolized.[1121-1125] The Vd in children and adults are similar, although clearance is greater in children (11.1 ± 3.9 mL/kg/min vs. 5.9 ± 1.6 mL/kg/min). As a result, the elimination half-life in children is less (63 ± 24 vs. 95 ± 20 minutes).[1122-1125] The Vd and elimination half-life in infants 3 to 12 months of age and older children are similar.[1124] Because clearance is markedly diminished in children with hepatic disease, clinical effects are prolonged in those with reduced hepatic blood flow (e.g., preterm infants, children with increased intra-abdominal pressure, children receiving vasopressors, and those with some forms of congenital heart disease).[1120,1126,1127] Compared with older children, the Vd in preterm infants is larger (1.0 ± 0.39 vs. 0.48 ± 0.19 L/kg), clearance is less (2.2 ± 2.4 vs. 5.6 ± 2.4 mL/min/kg), and the elimination half-life (525 ± 305 vs. 60 ± 11 minutes) is markedly prolonged.[1128,1129] Renal failure has little effect on its elimination.[1130] Because less alfentanil is bound to α_1-acid glycoprotein in preterm infants (65%) than in term infants (79%), an increased fraction of alfentanil is available for biologic effect in the former.[36]

The pharmacokinetics and pharmacodynamics of alfentanil suggest potential applications for the rapid control of analgesia and awakening from anesthesia. Alfentanil (10 µg/kg) has been combined with propofol (2.5 mg/kg) for tracheal intubation without a muscle relaxant.[1131] High-dose alfentanil is also used for cardiac procedures.

Sufentanil

Sufentanil (Sufenta) is a potent synthetic narcotic that in many respects is similar to fentanyl and alfentanil. The elimination of sufentanil is unaffected by renal failure but markedly altered by factors that influence hepatic blood flow; cirrhosis apparently has little effect on its elimination.[1120,1132,1133] The majority of studies of IV sufentanil in children have focused on those undergoing cardiac surgery. Evidence has shown age-dependent pharmacokinetics in which neonates have a larger Vd_{ss}, reduced clearance, and a greater and more variable elimination half-life than older children and adults (Fig. 6-32, see website).[1134-1136] Significant differences have been found between neonates from birth to 7 days of age and those studied a second time at 20 to 28 days of age, suggesting a marked improvement in hepatic blood flow, increased cardiac output, and rapid development of hepatic metabolic pathways.[1134] Because the three infants studied over time all had evidence of congestive heart failure and hepatic dysfunction, we cannot be certain which factor is more important. However, hepatic blood flow is most likely the major factor that influences drug elimination. Elimination may be more rapid in infants without congenital heart disease, as has been described with morphine and alfentanil.[977,979,1120,1127]

In general, children clear most drugs more rapidly from the bloodstream than do infants and adults. Bradycardia and asystole have been observed after a bolus administration of sufentanil, suggesting that the simultaneous administration of a vagolytic agent (atropine, glycopyrrolate, or pancuronium bromide) may be efficacious with rapid administration.[1137,1138] Transmucosal drug administration via the nasal mucosa has been investigated, with an ever-present risk of respiratory depression.[1139-1141] Several studies demonstrated that children are more likely to accept nasal sufentanil compared with nasal midazolam, although there was a greater incidence of vomiting after sufentanil and several children experienced decreased chest wall compliance after or during induction of anesthesia.

The dose of sufentanil that is most efficacious when administered intranasally is 2 to 3 µg/kg.[1140,1141]

Remifentanil

Remifentanil (Ultiva) is the newest in the family of synthetic opioids.[1142,1143] This opioid is unique because an ester linkage in the molecule allows rapid degradation to a carboxylic acid metabolite by blood and tissue esterases.[1144] This implies that metabolism would be unaffected by hepatic or renal function.[1145] The active metabolite of remifentanil that is eliminated by the kidneys, has approximately 1/300th to 1/1000th the opioid activity of the parent compound and, theoretically, could accumulate and cause clinical manifestations in children with impaired renal function.[1146] One study in adults failed to demonstrate any residual opioid effects after a 12-hour infusion in patients with renal failure.[1147] Perhaps the most important characteristic of remifentanil is its very brief half-life and the associated rapid recovery within about 10 minutes. Clearance is three to four times hepatic blood flow and dose dependent, that is, clearance increases as more drug is administered.[1146] Unlike all other opioids administered by infusion, the duration of effect is independent of both the dose administered and the duration of the infusion: the context-sensitive half-life, or the time required for a 50% reduction in drug effect, is constant (see Fig. 6-31).[1146] For example, when the infusions of remifentanil studied differed as much as 20-fold, the time to return to spontaneous respirations varied by only 1 to 3 minutes.[1145,1148] For opioids, its effect on respiration is an excellent reflection of its pharmacodynamic effects.[1149] After 3-hour infusions of alfentanil and remifentanil in adults, the elimination half-lives were 47.3 ± 12 minutes for alfentanil compared with 3.2 ± 0.9 minutes for remifentanil. The time to recover 50% of the minute ventilation, a pharmacodynamic effect of opioid, was 54.0 ± 48.1 minutes for alfentanil compared with 5.4 ± 1.8 minutes for remifentanil.[1149]

One theoretical concern that is associated with the long-term administration of remifentanil is the development of acute tolerance. In a study of adult volunteers, the analgesic threshold was one fourth of the peak values within 3 hours.[1150] A study of adolescents undergoing spinal instrumentation for scoliosis has also demonstrated acute tolerance.[1151] These data suggest that the infusion rates should be modified during the infusion of remifentanil to maintain a stable level of analgesia.

Remifentanil has an important role in providing safe analgesia to children of all ages, but in particular very sick infants and children.[1152-1155] Its main advantage is the ability to provide an intense opioid effect during the procedure with cardiovascular stability and then transition to a less intense opioid effect, allowing for early extubation.[1152,1156] A pharmacokinetic study after a bolus of 5 µg/kg found age-related differences with a larger Vd, a reduced maximal concentration (Cmax), an equivalent half-life and a greater clearance in infants younger than age 2 years than in older children and adults (Table 6-18, see website).[1157] *Remifentanil is the only drug for which there is a greater rather than a reduced clearance in neonates*, and the reason that it is so valuable in this age group.[1158-1165] These pharmacologic effects have important clinical implications because they translate into rapid titratability of the opioid effect, without regard for prolonged sedation. *This opioid should be administered only by continuous infusion. If an IV line becomes interrupted, kinked, or disconnected, the opioid effect will rapidly dissipate and the child will show evidence of pain.* Therefore, this drug should be "piggy backed" into a continuous infusion carrier as close to the IV as possible to provide smooth constant drug delivery. This also means that at the end of a procedure the anesthetic plan must include a transition to some other form of analgesia, including another opioid or a regional block.[1166]

Remifentanil is administered as a loading dose, 0.1 to 0.25 µg/kg and followed by an infusion of 0.25 to 0.5 µg/kg/min. The infusion may be titrated to effect with little fear of producing an "overdose" because of the very favorable pharmacokinetics. As with many synthetic opioids, severe bradycardia and hypotension may occur after bolus administration, especially large doses.[1157,1167] Remifentanil may have a direct negative chronotropic effect; therefore, the concomitant use of a vagolytic or pancuronium may prevent this adverse cardiac response.[1168,1169] However, because the plasma half-life is so brief there is rarely a need for a bolus because a steady-state opioid concentration occurs within three to five half-lives. Conversely, this negative chronotropic effect and the concomitant reduction in blood pressure can be used to induce controlled hypotension.[1170,1171] Remifentanil would seem to be the ideal opioid to provide a deep analgesic effect that allows spinal cord–evoked motor and sensory monitoring.[1172] Nonetheless, anesthesia is not produced by opioids alone. An anxiolytic must be administered to ensure that amnesia occurs. The half-lives of all anxiolytics exceed that of remifentanil, and this needs to be considered during recovery. Remifentanil complements propofol for short-term analgesia during total IV anesthesia for a variety of surgical and nonsurgical procedures as well as analgesia/sedation in the intensive care unit.[1081,1161,1162,1169,1173-1178] We have commonly used a fixed combination of remifentanil (5 µg/mL) in propofol (10 mg/mL), starting at a propofol infusion rate of 150 µg/kg/min for upper and lower gastrointestinal endoscopic procedures. For upper endoscopy, topicalizing the tongue and pharynx with lidocaine helps blunt responses to passing the endoscope through the oropharynx. The infusion rate is adjusted according to the child's responses.

Remifentanil has also been used to supplement propofol to facilitate endotracheal intubation without the use of a muscle relaxant. Two dose-response studies found that about 3 µg/kg of remifentanil combined with 4 mg/kg propofol provided the best intubating conditions. Intubating conditions were the same as with mivacurium or succinylcholine. Resumption of spontaneous respiration after a remifentanil/propofol combination was similar to that after succinylcholine.[1179,1180] It would seem that this combination is a reasonable alternative to succinylcholine to facilitate endotracheal intubation in children in whom succinylcholine is contraindicated, when the duration of intubation is anticipated to be brief, or when spontaneous ventilation is desired.

Butorphanol and Nalbuphine

Butorphanol (Stadol) and nalbuphine (Nubain) are synthetic narcotic agonist-antagonist analgesics that are apparently equianalgesic.[1181-1184] Both drugs seem to induce sedation as a common side effect, which can be used to advantage.[1181,1185] The mean elimination half-life of nalbuphine in adults is 2.2 to 2.6 hours[1186-1188] but is shorter in children (0.9 hour).[1189] The half-life of butorphanol is similar to that of nalbuphine at about 3 hours in adults.[1184,1190,1191] Both of these drugs can be administered orally with bioavailability in young adults of 12% to 17%, but this

dramatically increases to about 80% when administered to the nasal mucosa.[1187,1191-1193] The claimed advantage of this family of drugs is adequate analgesia with a ceiling on respiratory depression[1181,1182,1194-1196]; thus, there is some popularity for use in children.[1189,1197-1202] The administration of butorphanol by the nasal route may offer particular advantage for children without IV access.[1197,1203,1204,1204-1206] One report suggests a lower rate of postoperative vomiting after butorphanol compared with morphine.[1198] Another describes the use of rectal administration; as expected the authors found irregular absorption but peak blood levels were relatively rapidly achieved (25 ± 11 minutes) and the elimination half-life was 2.7 ± 0.7 hours.[1207] What must be remembered is that these agents may reverse µ receptor–mediated analgesic effects of the more potent opioids and should therefore be used as the initial or the sole opioid. This family of drugs has had mixed results in reversing or preventing opioid-induced pruritus.[1208,1209] Another appealing pharmacodynamic effect is sedation, particularly when compared with midazolam.[1181,1184,1185,1185,1210,1211] Butorphanol has also been administered by the caudal epidural route (25 µg/kg).[1212,1213]

Codeine

Codeine, also known as methylmorphine, is a naturally occurring weak mu-receptor prodrug with a potency that is approximately one tenth that of morphine. It is a mild to moderate opioid analgesic that is used to treat mild to moderate postoperative and nonoperative pain. The primary routes for delivery of codeine are the oral and IM routes, although the rectal route has been advocated.[1214] The dose of codeine by all three routes is similar, 0.5 to 1.5 mg/kg. Intravenous codeine was used in the past, but serious life-threatening side effects including transient but severe cardiorespiratory depression[1215-1217] and seizures[1218] led to proscription of this route of delivery.

Codeine's popularity as a perioperative analgesic in children is based in part on its favorable pharmacokinetics. When given orally, it is rapidly and completely absorbed, with 50% undergoing first-pass hepatic metabolism. Bioavailability after oral codeine is 90%, although after surgery the bioavailability may be quite variable (12%-84%).[1219,1220] Blood levels after oral codeine peak by 1 hour. Its terminal elimination half-life is 3 to 3.5 hours. When given by the IM and rectal routes, peak blood levels are achieved rapidly, within 0.5 hour, with the blood levels after the rectal route being less than after the IM route. The duration of action after these two routes of administration is 1 to 2 hours. The elimination half-life after rectal administration in children is approximately 2.6 hours in children but 4.6 hours in infants,[1221] suggesting the need for a much greater interval between subsequent doses in infants.

In vivo, 5% to 15% of codeine is excreted unchanged in the urine. The remaining 85% to 95% undergoes metabolism in the liver by one of three routes: glucuronidation (principal route), *O*-demethylation, and *N*-demethylation.[1219] Five to 15% of codeine undergoes *O*-demethylation to morphine. This metabolic pathway depends on CYP2D6, an enzyme responsible for the metabolism of more than 20% of prescribed medications. The *N*-demethylation pathway depends on the CYP 3A enzyme system.

CYP2D6 activity in fetal liver microsomes is either absent or less than 1% of adults values.[1221] *O*-demethylation begins postnatally with rapid maturation of this enzyme system irrespective of the gestational age at birth, although activity may remain less than 25% of adult values at 5 years of age. Interestingly, CYP2D6 is a noninducible enzyme whose activity, however, may vary with certain disease states, including malignancy, cigarette smoking, and some chronic inflammatory diseases (rheumatoid arthritis).[1219] Glucuronidation is immature at birth but develops throughout infancy, whereas N-demethylation is fully mature at birth.

Variability in the clinical response to codeine prompted investigations into genetic variants or polymorphisms of CYP2D6. This enzyme is mapped to chromosome 22 at 22q13.1. Fifty-five polymorphisms of CYP2D6 have been described to date with a frequency that exceeds 1% of the population.[1222] These include both functional and nonfunctional polymorphisms as well as gene duplication. The polymorphisms are numbered with *1 being the normal or wild allele (the * denotes an allele). The mutant alleles, *3, *4, *5, *6, and *9, for example, confer no CYP2D6 activity.[1219,1222,1223] The latter polymorphisms account for more than 90% of the poor metabolizers (see later). Variants *2, *10, and 17 have modestly reduced activity and are referred as intermediate metabolizers.[1219] To further complicate the genetic pattern, multiple copies of the same genes[1223] may be present in some individuals, resulting in bizarre phenotypes. The wide array of CYP2D6 polymorphisms of codeine may be summarized into three broad categories: poor metabolizers (negligible morphine produced [PM]), extensive metabolizers (normals [EM]) and ultra-extensive metabolizers (rapid and large amounts of morphine [UM]). Up to 10% of whites and 30% of Hong Kong Chinese are PM, rendering codeine an ineffective analgesic for these children.[1219] Alternately, 29% of the Ethiopian and 1% of Swedish, German, and Chinese populations are UM.[1219] Recent evidence suggested that the frequency of CYP2D6 polymorphisms, particularly children who are PM, may be more common and more varied than previously thought. Children with these polymorphisms who also have upregulated opioid receptors as a result of chronic intermittent nocturnal hypoxia may be particularly vulnerable to a mishap after a usual or subclinical dose of codeine.[1224] Consequently, the wide clinical response to a standard (or less than standard) dose of codeine necessitates careful monitoring in those with compromised cardiorespiratory status.

Codeine may be effective for pain control, although its limited conversion to morphine likely makes it suitable for only mild and moderate forms of pain. The limited conversion to morphine and fewer side effects of codeine has made it popular for infants and young children, particularly when a single dose is involved. There is some evidence that codeine is associated with less nausea and vomiting than morphine.[1225] Evidence from children who are PM suggested that codeine is a less reliable analgesic than morphine and that the analgesia did not correlate with the phenotype or morphine blood concentration.[1219]

Tramadol

Tramadol (Ultram) is a relatively new medication that is a weak opioid with minimal effects on respiration and that causes monoaminergic spinal cord inhibition of pain.[1226-1229] This formulation is structurally related to morphine and codeine.[1229] Two enantiomers provide analgesia; one is a mu opioid receptor agonist, and the other inhibits neuronal reuptake of serotonin and inhibits norepinephrine uptake, thus producing "multimodal antinociception."[1229] When administered orally to children, the elimination half-life is 3.6 ± 1.1 hours and when

administered intravenously the half-life is 6.4 ± 2.7 hours.[1230-1232] Tramadol has been shown to have extensive polymorphism regarding the cytochrome system with about 95% of patients showing rapid metabolism but 5% showing slow metabolism.[1229] An elegant study of preterm infants has demonstrated that clearance of tramadol is low in 25-week gestation infants (4.32 mL/min/kg) but that it rapidly matures to adult values by 60 weeks' postconceptual age (9.32 mL/min/kg).[1233] Clearance in children is similar to that in adults.[1230] Tramadol has been shown to be effective for moderate to severe pain in a variety of pediatric populations and may offer some advantage for the treatment of pain after tonsillectomy in children with obstructive sleep apnea.[1234-1242] Tramadol (1.5-2 mg/kg) has been administered rectally with peak plasma concentrations occurring at approximately 2 hours.[1243] Tramadol has also been administered in the caudal epidural space[1013] with longer-lasting analgesia than when administered intravenously.[1244] Caudal epidural tramadol (5%, 2 mg/kg) was also compared with caudal epidural bupivacaine (0.25%, 2 mg/kg) and found to provide superior analgesia.[1245] *Caudal administration is not recommended until further clarification of potential neurotoxicity.*[1234,1246] Tramadol has also been very useful as a transition to oral analgesics after IV therapy (see Chapter 44).

Nonsteroidal Anti-inflammatory Agents

Ketorolac

Ketorolac (Toradol) is an NSAID with very potent analgesic properties.[1247-1251] It is an important adjuvant to the treatment of postoperative pain, especially for children who require prolonged pain management.[1252] It is particularly useful for the transition from IV to oral therapy. The pharmacokinetics after a single dose are similar in adults and children. The terminal elimination half-life in children 4 to 8 years of age is approximately 6 hours according to one study but the range was 3.5 to 10 hours.[1253] Another study found a considerably shorter β-elimination half-life (2.26 ± 1.35 hours) for children 3 to 8 years of age.[1254] An additional study found a β-elimination half-life of 3.3 ± 1.9 hours for children 1 to 16 years of age but with a Vd smaller than that reported by other investigators.[1253-1255] These differences in pharmacokinetics may reflect differences in the duration of sampling times. The analgesic properties of ketorolac are similar to those of low-dose morphine for post-tonsillectomy analgesia.[1251,1256] The major use in pediatrics is as an adjuvant to opioid analgesia or for treatment of mild to moderate pain where there is a desire to reduce the potential for respiratory depression or for nausea and vomiting.[1249,1257-1262]

One of the major concerns with ketorolac is the inhibition of platelet function through inhibition of cyclooxygenase and the potential for post-surgical bleeding. Ketorolac has been shown to have minimal effect on prothrombin and partial thromboplastin times but has been shown to cause modest increases in the bleeding time.[1249,1263-1266] The effects of ketorolac on platelet function are different than those of aspirin. With aspirin, the antiplatelet effect lasts for several days after a single administration because of the irreversible acetylation of platelet cyclooxygenase. However, with ketorolac, this effect is reversible and therefore the effect is dependent on the presence of ketorolac within the body.[1267] Therefore, the antiplatelet effects of ketorolac are gone when the drug has been excreted. This effect on platelet function has been of most concern in children undergoing adenotonsillectomy.[1268-1271] In the studies reporting posttonsillectomy bleeding, most involved administration of the ketorolac during or at the beginning of the surgical procedure before hemostasis was achieved. In addition, the increased incidence of bleeding appears to be primarily during the first 24 hours, which corresponds to the several half-lives it would take to eliminate ketorolac from the body. The incidence of bleeding after the first 24 hours does not appear to be different.[1272] It would therefore be reasonable to not administer this medication until the end of surgery after hemostasis is achieved. Some practitioners eschew this issue altogether and only administer ketorolac when the potential for a life-threatening hemorrhage is less.[1205] Concerns regarding the possibility of postoperative hemorrhage appear to be valid, but the true frequency of life-threatening bleeding due exclusively to ketorolac is quite small.[1261,1273-1276] Many clinicians discuss the possible use of ketorolac with the surgeon before administering it and document the conversation in the anesthesia record. Ketorolac has been safely used to provide analgesia for preterm and term infants, but the pharmacokinetics in this age group have not been described.[1277]

Another concern is the potential for adverse effects on bone healing, particularly spinal fusion.[1278,1279] Evidence suggests that nonunion of the spine is associated only with large dose and not low-dose ketorolac. Ketorolac has been used safely to provide analgesia for other types of orthopedic conditions as well.[1280,1281] One other concern is the report of sudden and profound bradycardia after rapid IV administration of ketorolac.[1282] Although the mechanism of this response is unclear, ketorolac should be administered slowly when given intravenously.

Acetaminophen

Acetaminophen (Tylenol) is useful as an adjunct to spare opioids.[1283-1290] Acetaminophen can be administered orally before induction of anesthesia to achieve a therapeutic blood concentration at the time of emergence even after brief surgery such as myringotomy and tube insertion. Oral acetaminophen is rapidly absorbed with a measurable blood concentration within minutes of ingestion.[1291,1292] An oral dose of 10 to 20 mg/kg provides a blood concentration within the therapeutic antipyretic range of 10 to 20 µg/mL. The blood concentration required for analgesia has not been established. For procedures of greater duration, rectal administration of acetaminophen at the beginning of surgery provides therapeutic blood concentrations at the time of emergence and before the child would be likely to tolerate oral medications. Rectal administration of acetaminophen, however, is associated with very irregular absorption with peak blood levels achieved 60 to 180 minutes after administration.[1291,1293-1295] It is for this reason that it must be administered at the beginning rather than the conclusion of surgery. Several studies have shown that larger (up to 45 mg/kg) than the recommended doses (10-15 mg/kg) are required to achieve therapeutic blood concentrations for antipyresis.[1283,1289,1293,1296] Another study suggested that an initial rectal dose of 40 mg/kg with subsequent six hourly doses of 20 mg/kg produce the desired blood concentration (Feverall, Upsher-Smith, Minneapolis, MN).[1297] However, this study was limited to 24 hours and did not examine other brands of rectal acetaminophen. Therefore, no recommendations can be made regarding continued rectal dosing beyond 24 hours or dosing of

other brands of acetaminophen. Large doses of acetaminophen (40-60 mg/kg) have been shown to have morphine-sparing effects. Further studies are required before doses greater than 40 mg/kg can be recommended because of the risk of hepatotoxicity.[1290,1298,1299] The current maximum 24 hour dosing of acetaminophen is 90 to 100 mg/kg/day. Acetaminophen has been used extensively in preterm and term neonates. Neonates have a larger Vd and smaller clearance that is related to postconceptual age compared with older children.[1284,1285,1291,1295,1300,1301] An IV formulation of acetaminophen (proparacetamol) is available in some countries. This formulation allows for more predictable dosing and a means of providing mild analgesia to children undergoing brief operative procedures such as tonsillectomy.[1294,1302-1305]

Sedatives

Diazepam

Diazepam (Valium) is rapidly absorbed after oral administration, with peak plasma levels at 30 to 90 minutes; the absorption rate has been found to be more rapid in children than in adults.[1306,1307] Oral diazepam is administered in a dose of 0.2 to 0.3 mg/kg. It has been used extensively as a premedication, as an adjunct to balanced anesthesia, and for sedation, amnesia, and control of seizures. Intramuscular administration is painful and results in irregular absorption; plasma levels are only 60% of those obtained with a similar oral dose.[1308-1310] The recommended IV dose is 0.1 to 0.2 mg/kg. Diazepam has been administered rectally to children in doses ranging from 0.3 to 1.0 mg/kg with satisfactory results.[1311-1314] One study found a more rapid uptake during the first 2 hours after administration when administered in liquid rather than suppository form.[1311]

Diazepam is highly plasma bound, with a serum half-life varying from 20 to 80 hours. Its half-life is reduced in younger adults and children (approximately 18 hours).[1311] This latter observation may reflect the greater hepatic blood flow that facilitates hepatic metabolism in younger compared with older children.[96,1315] Hepatic disease may also decrease the elimination of diazepam.[1315] Studies in neonates who received diazepam transplacentally just before delivery demonstrate prolonged drug effects and serum half-lives (40-100 hours), probably as a result of immature hepatic excretory mechanisms and reduced hepatic blood flow (Fig. 6-33, see website).[96,1306,1316] Diazepam is broken down to active metabolites (desmethyldiazepam) with similar potency to the parent compound and with half-lives as long or longer than the parent compound, thus emphasizing the importance of not administering this benzodiazepine to neonates.[1306,1317,1318] The preservative benzyl alcohol is present in many formulations of diazepam. This preservative should be avoided in neonates because it is difficult to metabolize, is associated with kernicterus, and can cause a metabolic acidosis.[1319] The amount of benzyl alcohol that accompanies a usual dose of diazepam would likely be insufficient to cause harm to the neonate.[1320] Diazepam has respiratory depressant effects that are quite variable, especially when combined with opioids.[1321]

Diazepam is useful as an oral premedication, although midazolam has overshadowed this role. Its main disadvantage when given intravenously is pain. Administering IV lidocaine before the diazepam and administering the valium slowly through a rapidly flowing IV catheter minimizes this pain. Diazepam is avoided in neonates and infants because of its prolonged half-life. Finally, diazepam should not be administered intramuscularly because of the pain and erratic absorption.

Midazolam

Midazolam (Versed) is a water-soluble benzodiazepine that offers significant clinical advantages over diazepam. It is not painful when administered intravenously or intramuscularly. Midazolam is only one of a few medications that are approved as premedicants in children and is the only benzodiazepine approved by the FDA for use in neonates. Its clearance in adults (1.8-6.4 hours) is reduced compared with children (1.4-4.0 hours).[1322-1326] Its clearance is even further reduced in neonates and preterm infants when compared with toddlers and older children (6-12 hours) (see Fig. 6-33, see website).[1327,1328] The elimination half-life is still less in preterm infants less than 32 weeks' gestational age.[1064,1327,1328] The recommended infusion rate of midazolam is 0.5 µg/kg/min for preterm infants less than 32 weeks' gestational age and 1.0 µg/kg/min for infants more than 32 weeks' gestational age. Any factor that impairs hepatic blood flow (e.g., cardiac surgery with bypass compared with cardiac surgery without bypass) may decrease its elimination, although cirrhosis only minimally affects its elimination in adults.[1329,1330] The elimination half-life is also prolonged in hypovolemic states and in children receiving vasopressors.[1330,1331] Midazolam offers the best pharmacokinetic profile for neonates because the active metabolite has a half-life similar to the parent compound but with minimal clinical activity.[1064] *Bolus administration to preterm and term neonates has been associated with profound hypotension; the likelihood seems to be greater if the patient is receiving fentanyl.[1070] Likewise, a neonate receiving a midazolam infusion is more likely to suffer profound hypotension with a bolus of fentanyl.* Rapid IV and nasal administration have also been associated with seizure-like activity, although it appears that this is myoclonic rather than true seizure activity.[1332] Midazolam has been administered as a continuous infusion both in the operating room as an adjunct to general anesthesia and in the intensive care unit.[1333-1336] The plasma concentrations of midazolam correlate reasonably with the depth of sedation.[1337,1338] Prolonged administration does lead to tolerance, dependency, and benzodiazepine withdrawal.[1339,1340] Long-term infusions, particularly in neonates, should be tapered over days while carefully monitoring for signs of withdrawal (vomiting, agitation, sweating, bowel distention, seizures, change in neurologic status).[1074,1341,1342] A theoretical concern associated with midazolam is benzyl alcohol toxicity with the development of metabolic acidosis and gasping respirations.[1343,1344] The 24-hour dose of benzoyl alcohol in midazolam when administered according to recommended dosing guidelines should not cause toxicity.

Midazolam is the most commonly used benzodiazepine in pediatric anesthesia.[1345] It is administered orally, nasally, and rectally as well as intravenously and intramuscularly.[712,1139,1323,1330,1346-1359] The desired clinical effects include antegrade amnesia (approximately 50%)[1360-1362] as well as sedation and anxiolysis before induction of anesthesia or a medical procedure.[712,1346,1347,1350-1352,1355,1356] One study suggested that its amnestic properties may be superior to those of diazepam.[1363] The clinical endpoint with midazolam may differ somewhat when compared with diazepam. Midazolam produces a general calming effect with minimal sedation and little effect on speech. In contrast, diazepam frequently causes obvious sedation and

Table 6-19. Dosing and Onset Times of Midazolam in Infants and Children (Not Neonates)

Route	Dose (mg/kg)	Time of Onset (min)	Time to Peak Effect (min)
Intravenous	0.05-0.15	Immediate	3-5
Intramuscular	0.1-0.2	3-5	10-20
Oral	0.25-0.75	5-30	10-30
Nasal	0.1-0.2	3-5	10-15
Rectal	0.75-1.0	5-10	10-30

slurring of speech. It is important to appreciate the subtle difference between these medications to avoid relative overdose, particularly when using midazolam in combination with other potent CNS depressants.

When midazolam was first introduced, a number of deaths were attributed to respiratory depression. These deaths were probably the result of combining large doses of midazolam with other medications, particularly opioids. An important pharmacologic difference between the benzodiazepines is that the time to achieve peak CNS effect with midazolam, 4.8 minutes, is almost threefold greater than with diazepam, 1.5 minutes (see Fig. 4-4, see website).[1364,1365] This is due to the greater fat solubility of diazepam and therefore a more rapid transit into the CNS.[1366] Accordingly, we must wait sufficient time between doses of midazolam (3-5 minutes) to achieve the peak CNS effects before considering supplemental doses or other medications.[1367] In general, the dose of midazolam is one-third to one-fifth that of diazepam, especially when combined with a potent opioid such as fentanyl. Whenever midazolam is administered either alone or in combination with other medications, it is vital that the child be constantly monitored for respiratory depression because midazolam depresses the hypoxic ventilatory response and has been associated with respiratory arrest.[1368,1369] Midazolam increases upper airway obstruction, particularly in those with obstructive sleep apnea, by reducing pharyngeal muscle tone.[1370] In addition, midazolam and nitrous oxide together cause significant upper airway obstruction.[1371] Interestingly, a study of dental patients suggested that mouth opening further increases upper airway collapse, thus increasing the airway obstruction.[1372] One final concern relates to the administration of drugs that interfere with the cytochrome isoforms that metabolize midazolam (CYP 4503A 4). Examples of such drugs/foods are grapefruit juice, erythromycin, calcium channel blockers, and protease inhibitors.[57,557,558,1373-1376] The net effect is to prolong the duration of action of midazolam.

Midazolam has been used as an induction agent but is not as satisfactory as other agents.[1323] One author (CJC) has administered as much as 1.0 mg/kg intravenously to a child without producing unconsciousness. The same dose given orally produces sedation and hallucinations (JL). Commonly used doses and routes of administration are presented in Table 6-19. The nasal route has some proponents,[1346] although there is a direct connection with the CNS at that level (see Fig. 4-3, see website).[725] Because midazolam is neurotoxic when applied directly to neural tissue,[731] there is the theoretical risk of CNS toxicity.[725] In addition, 85% of children who receive nasal midazolam cry and complain of the bitter aftertaste that lasts for days.[1139,1348] It would seem prudent to avoid this route of administration because the oral route appears to be equally effective and without risk.

Table 7-1. Manual Infusion Schemes

Drug	Loading Dose	Maintenance Infusion	Notes
Propofol[23]	1 mg/kg	10 mg/kg/hr for 10 min, then 8 mg/kg/hr for 10 min, then 6 mg/kg/hr thereafter	Adult regimen to achieve blood concentration of 3 µg/mL Underdelivers to children and achieves lower blood concentration of 2 µg/mL
Propofol[22]	1 mg/kg	13 mg/kg/hr for 10 min, then 11-mg/kg/hr for 10 min, then 9 mg/kg/hr thereafter	Concurrently with alfentanil infusion
Alfentanil[29]	10-50 µg/kg	1-5 µg/kg/min	Results in blood concentration of 50-200 ng/mL
Remifentanil[1]	0.5 µg/kg/min for 3 min	0.25 µg/kg/min	Produces blood concentrations of 6-9 ng/mL
Remifentanil[1]	0.5-1.0 µg/kg over 1 min	0.1-0.5 µg/kg/min	Produces blood concentrations of 5-10 ng/mL
Sufentanil[1,30]	0.1-0.5 µg/kg	0.005-0.01 µg/kg/min	Results in blood concentration of 0.2 ng/mL for sedation and analgesia
Sufentanil[1,30]	1-5 µg/kg	0.01-0.05 µg/kg/min	Results in blood concentrations of 0.6-3.0 ng/mL for anesthesia
Fentanyl[29]	1-10 µg/kg	0.1-0.2 µg/kg/min	
Ketamine[29]	1-2 mg/kg	0.1-2.5 mg/kg/hr	Lower dose and infusion rate for analgesia and sedation. Higher dose and infusion rate for anesthesia titrated to effect
Midazolam[29]	0.05-0.1 mg/kg	0.1-0.3 mg/kg/hr	

For a fixed infusion rate, it takes five half-lives to reach a steady-state concentration (98% of the target) in the blood (Fig. 7-1). To more rapidly achieve steady-state conditions, a bolus dose or loading infusion may be administered. This rapidly fills the volume of distribution, after which a new rate of infusion is calculated to maintain the blood concentration (Fig. 7-2).

To understand the disposition of drugs after an intravenous dose, it is useful to consider a three-compartment model. The drug is delivered and eliminated from a central compartment V1 (which includes the blood) but also distributes to and redistributes from two peripheral compartments, one representing well-perfused organs and tissues (fast compartment, V2) and the other representing more poorly perfused tissues such as fat (slow compartment, V3) (Table 7-2). The transfer of the drug between the central compartment (V1) and the two peripheral compartments (V2, V3) and also the elimination of the drug from the central compartment is described by a series of rate constants indicating the distribution back and forth between paired compartments, such as V1 to V2 and then V2 back to V1 = k_{12} and k_{21} (k_{12}, k_{21}, k_{13}, k_{31}, k_{10}). The target organ that intravenous anesthetic agents affect is the brain. Therefore, a fourth rate constant is added to describe the equilibration between the central compartment and the effect site in the brain (k_{e0}). This compartment is not represented by a volume but rather by the time required to equilibrate. Consequently, there is a time lag before changes in the blood concentration are reflected in the effect site (see Figs. 7-1 and 7-2).

A hydraulic model is useful for understanding these concepts. The central compartment is connected to the peripheral compartments and effect site by a series of pipes of different diame-

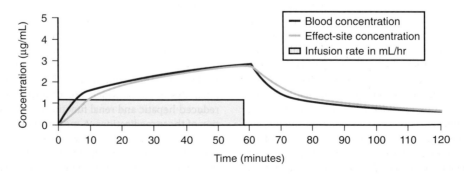

Figure 7-1. Fixed rate infusion of propofol at 10 mg/kg/hr with no bolus dose in a healthy 10-kg, 1-year-old infant. Steady state is not reached after 1 hour. There is a lag of effect-site concentration behind blood concentration both during infusion and after stopping infusion. Effect-site concentration reaches blood concentration at about 1 hour. Context-sensitive half-time = 9 minutes.

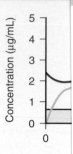

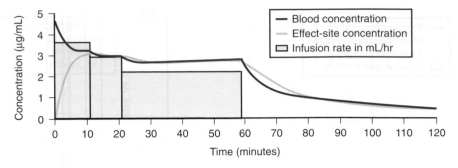

Figure 7-2. Manual infusion in a healthy 70-kg 40-year-old. Diprifusor pharmacokinetic data set. Bolus dose was 1 mg/kg, then 10 mg/kg/hr for 10 minutes, 8 mg/kg/hr for 10 minutes, then 6 mg/kg/hr thereafter until 60 minutes when infusion is discontinued. Maximum blood concentration is 4.5 μg/mL. Effect-site concentration reaches 3 μg/mL after around 10 minutes but drifts down to around 2.6 μg/mL and then very gradually rises. Context-sensitive half-time after 1 hour = 7 minutes.

Figure 7-4. Manual infusion of propo 8 mg/kg/hr for 10 minutes, then 6 mg dose not equilibrate until 11 minutes. a sufficient depth of anesthesia for sur

therefore is related to the duration of (except remifentanil [see later]). T *sensitive half-time (CSHT)* where th the infusion. For an individual dru context-sensitive half-times can be the elimination half-lives against th (Fig. 7-6). The context-sensitive half become parallel to the time (*x*) axis has become context *in*sensitive. Th nearly all intravenous anesthetics. Th whose half-time becomes context i ately after initiation of the infusion rapid and complete. The capacity of system is enormous, suggesting that constant rate, regardless of the dura 7-3, see Fig. 7-6). The relevant pharr remifentanil, alfentanil, and sufentan 7-4.[1] The differences in context-ser trated in Table 7-3 and Figure 7-6. Fe sensitive half-time when given by in this dramatically increases as the increases. Alfentanil's context-sensiti stant after approximately 90 minutes fentanil, alfentanil, and sufentanil ar young infants due to immaturity or a enzyme systems, whereas clearance age independent because tissue throughout the body and fully matu

ters and also a drainage pipe to represent elimination (Fig. 7-3). The height of the columns of fluid (which represents concentration of drug) illustrate the gradient down which drug travels between the central and peripheral compartments, and this can be animated over time to show filling and emptying of compartments relative to each other. The diameter of the interconnecting pipes between the central and peripheral compartments represents the intercompartment clearances, and size of the drainage channel represents elimination. This hydraulic analogy is used in the TIVA Trainer simulation program.[19]

Fixed Infusion Rate and a Three-Compartment Model
When a fixed infusion rate is started (see Fig. 7-1), the blood concentration will increase but, almost simultaneously, distribu-

Table 7-2. Nomenclature for TCI Systems		
Term	**Meaning**	**Units**
TCI	Target-controlled infusion	
Vc or V1	Central compartment volume	L
V2	Fast compartment volume (vessel rich group) = V1 × k_{12}/k_{21}	L
V3	Slow compartment volume (vessel poor group) = V3 × k_{13}/k_{31}	L
Cl 1	Elimination clearance = V1 × k_{10}	L/hr
Cl 2	Clearance between V1 and V2 = V2 × k_{21}	L/hr
Cl 3	Clearance between V1 and V3 = V3 × k_{31}	L/hr
Cp	Blood concentration	
Ce	Effect-site concentration	
T	Target concentration	
CALC	Concentration calculated by TCI software	
MEAS	Concentration measured	
k_{10}	Elimination rate constant	/min
k_{e0}	Rate constant for equilibration between blood and effect-site	/min
k_{12}, k_{21}	Rate constants for movement between V1 and V2	/min
k_{13}, k_{31}	Rate constants for movement between V1 and V3	/min

tion of drug to the fast compartment and elimination both begin. Distribution of drugs throughout the body contributes more to the removal of drug from blood than elimination for most medications. The one important exception to this is remifentanil, where extremely rapid tissue esterase clearance dominates. As the concentrations within each compartment equilibrate, the concentration gradient between compartments lessens (slowing drug transfer between compartments) but distribution to the slow compartment continues along with elimination. The net effect is that the blood concentration continues to increase, albeit at a slower rate. As the blood concentration increases toward equilibrium, elimination becomes relatively more important. Note how far behind the effect-site concentration lags (see Fig. 7-1). Eventually, after several hours (or in some cases, days), a steady state is reached where infusion rate equals elimination rate.

Bolus and Variable Rate Infusion in a Three-Compartment Model
A bolus dose can start to fill the central compartment, but then the rate of infusion should decrease in a stepwise manner to maintain a constant effect-site concentration until a steady state is reached. As drug is delivered into the central compartment, it continuously distributes into the peripheral compartments to the effect site all the while it is continuously being eliminated. The infusion rate must vary because it has to match the changes in the contribution of distribution and elimination as the infusion continues (Figs. 7-4 and 7-5). When the infusion is stopped, then elimination will continue to drain the central compartment, and drug will continue to distribute to V2 and V3 along concentration gradients from V1 for some time. Equilibrium may be reached, but the drug now begins to move back from the peripheral compartments into the central compartment, maintaining the central compartment drug concentration for a period of time. This can continue for a protracted interval, particularly for highly lipid soluble drugs that have a very large slow compartment V3 and a reservoir or depot effect (see Fig. 7-3F). Eventually the central compartment concentration will decrease. For most anesthetics, the longer the duration of an infusion, the more the drug has distributed into the peripheral compartments and the larger the reservoir of drug to be redistributed back into the central compartment and eliminated once the infusion ceases. The half-time of the decrease in drug concentration

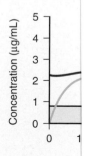

Figure 7-5. Manual infusion of propof 11 mg/kg/hr for 10 minutes, then 9 mg dose not equilibrate until 20 minutes. B hour to 2.6 μg/mL.

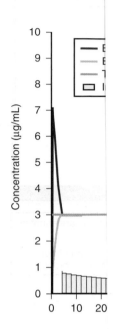

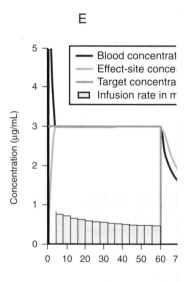

E

F

Figure 7-3 (continued). E, Or
maintenance effect-site concen
of the concentration of C1 and
although blood and effect-site
antiemetic and anxiolytic effect

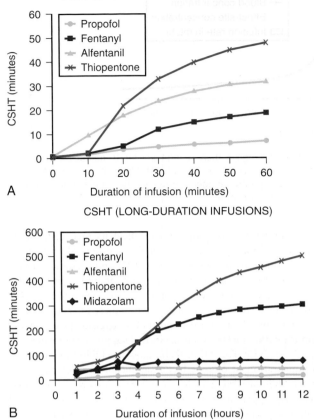

A

B

Figure 7-6. A, Context-sensitive half-times after short duration infusions. **B,** Context-sensitive half-times after longer duration infusions. For very lipid soluble drugs such as fentanyl and propofol, V3 is very large compared with V1. Intercompartmental clearance between V1 and V3 is given by the equation $V1 \times k_{13} = V3 \times k_{31}$, which implies that if V1 is much smaller than V3, rapid distribution from V1 to V3 is associated with very slow redistribution from V3 to V1. This is indeed seen with propofol and fentanyl, which have slow offset of effects after prolonged infusion. Propofol has a context-sensitive half-time that varies between around 3 minutes for a short duration infusion to 18 minutes after a 12-hour infusion. This is because elimination is quite rapid compared with the rate of redistribution from V3. For alfentanil, the concentration of the un-ionized form is 100 times greater than that of fentanyl (pKa alfentanil 6.4, fentanyl 8.5). Alfentanil therefore has a more rapid onset time and shorter half-life k_{e0}, a smaller V1, lower volume of distribution at steady-state, and lower clearance than fentanyl. Fentanyl does, however, have a shorter context-sensitive half-time than alfentanil after a short duration infusion lasting less than 2 hours (**A**); but for longer duration infusions, alfentanil reaches a maximum context-sensitive half-time after about 90 minutes, whereas for fentanyl the context-sensitive half-time continues to increase after 12 hours (**B**). This is because fentanyl has a huge V3, and redistribution back to V1 maintains the blood concentration when the infusion stops. CSHT, context-sensitive half-time.

tion once the block becomes established. Nitrous oxide and low doses of volatile agents also act synergistically with propofol and opioids.

Manual Infusion Schemes

Propofol

A simple scheme was devised by Roberts and associates[23] to maintain a blood concentration of propofol in healthy adults of 3 µg/mL. A bolus dose of 1 mg/kg is followed by a continuous infusion of 10 mg/kg/hr for 10 minutes, then 8 mg/kg/hr for 10 minutes, then 6 mg/kg/hr thereafter. When this "10, 8, 6" regimen is modeled and verified using the Marsh model[3] for an adult patient, the estimated blood concentration slightly exceeds 3 µg/mL but remains reasonably stable. This simple dosing regimen is every effective in adults (see Fig. 7-2). However, when the same regimen is modeled using the "Paedfusor" pharmacokinetic data set for a child 1 year old and weighing 10 kg, the blood concentration achieved is approximately 2 µg/mL but decreases slowly over time. Thus, this regimen delivers a sub-

Table 7-4. Pharmacokinetic Parameters for Short-Acting Opioids

	Remifentanil[31,32]	Alfentanil[33]	Sufentanil[34]
V1	$5.1-0.0201 \times (age - 40) + 0.072 \times (LBM - 55)$	Male: $0.111 \times$ weight Female: $1.15 \times 0.111 \times$ weight	$0.164 \times$ weight
V2	$9.82-0.0811 \times (age - 40) + 0.108 \times (LBM - 55)$	12.0	$0.359 \times$ weight
V3	5.42	10.5	$1.263 \times$ weight
k_{10}	$2.6-0.0162 \times (age - 40) + 0.0191 \times (LBM - 55)/V1$	0.356/V1	0.089
k_{12}	$2.05-0.0301 \times (age - 40)/V1$	0.104	0.35
k_{21}	$2.05-0.0301 \times (age - 40)/V2$	0.067	0.16
k_{13}	$0.076-0.00113 \times (age - 40)/V1$	0.017	0.077
k_{31}	$0.076-0.00113 \times (age - 40)/5.42$	0.0126	0.01
k_{e0}	$0.595-0.007 \times (age - 40)$	0.77	0.12

Age in years; weight in kilograms; LBM, lean body mass.
From Absalom A, Struys MMRF: An Overview of TCI and TIVA. Ghent, Belgium, Academia Press, 2005.

Table 7-5. Differences between Adult and Pediatric Pharmacokinetic Parameters

Age	Vd (mL/kg)	Elimination Half-life (min)	Clearance (mL/min/kg)
1-3 yr	9500	188	53
3-11 yr	9700	398	34
Adult	4700	312	28

Notes: The apparent volume of distribution of propofol in the child is twice that of adults. The clearance of propofol in young children is twice that of adults and elimination is much more rapid.

therapeutic blood concentration of propofol in children. The subtherapeutic concentrations of propofol occurred because of a larger central compartment and an increased clearance of propofol in children compared with adults (see Fig. 7-4, Table 7-5). When the "Paedfusor" is used to calculate the dose of propofol that is required to achieve a blood concentration of 3 µg/mL, the bolus dose needed is 50% greater than in adults (1.5 mg/kg) and the infusion rates needed are approximately "19, 15, 12" each for 10 minutes. In addition, it takes approximately 15 minutes for the effect-site concentration to reach 3 µg/mL (Fig. 7-7). These data from the "Paedfusor" support the notion that the dosing of propofol infusion in young children is approximately twice that in adults.

Opioids

Simple manual infusion regimens can be used for the opioids fentanyl, alfentanil, remifentanil, and sufentanil. The manual infusion regimens for these opioids in children are summarized in Table 7-1. Transitioning to maintenance analgesia after infusions of these opioids is a significant issue, and it is important to ensure either adequate regional or local anesthesia techniques are established or that adequate doses of systemic analgesia are given well before the infusion is discontinued. Transitioning is somewhat smoother after sufentanil than after alfentanil or remifentanil in children. The problem of acute tolerance to ultra-short-acting opioids has been noted after use of remifentanil in surgery for pediatric scoliosis.[24]

Ketamine

Ketamine can be used in a simple basic manual regimen as a loading dose of 1-2 mg/kg and a maintenance infusion of 0.1-2.5 mg/kg/hr depending on whether the target state is for analgesia, sedation or anesthesia (see Table 7-1).

Midazolam

Slow bolus dosing of up to 0.1 mg/kg followed by an infusion rate of 0.1 mg/kg/hr provides baseline sedation with adjustments and additional bolus doses often needed. Caution is required, with bolus dosing in neonates and infants and in the critically ill because hypotension may occur and the depth of sedation achieved with midazolam is tremendously variable (see Table 7-1).

Target-Controlled Infusion

A target-controlled infusion (TCI) is controlled by a computer that performs rapid sequential calculations every 8 to 10 seconds to determine the infusion rate required to produce a user-defined drug concentration in the central compartment (which includes the blood) or at the effect site of action of the drug in the brain.[1] *Thus, TCI may be blood targeted or effect-site targeted.* The standard nomenclature for TCI systems is listed in Table 7-2. Modern TCI systems are computer-controlled syringe drivers capable of infusion rates up to 1200 mL/hr with a precision of 0.1 mL/hr. They incorporate a user interface and display and a range of safety alarms, monitoring functions, and warning systems. For most programs, the user has to choose a drug and its concentration from a menu and one must also select a pharmacokinetic model. The models suitable for use in children are quite limited, and some models are not suitable for all age groups. Others may be suitable but have not been validated in younger children; neonatal and infant models are quite rare. Experience with the various models may be gained by running the simulation programs such as TIVA Trainer (http://eurosiva.org/), Rugloop (http://www.demed.be/rugloop.htm), and Stelpump and Stanpump (http://anesthesia.stanford.edu/pkpd/HTML%20Web%20pages/) on a personal computer. TIVA Trainer v8.5 (2006)[19] now allows uploading of new models via a central website and server and contains details and simulations of pediatric models for propofol and neonatal and pediatric models for sufentanil, in addition to a wide range of adult models for propofol, alfentanil, remifentanil, fentanyl, ketamine, and midazolam. The simulation shows animated graphs of blood and

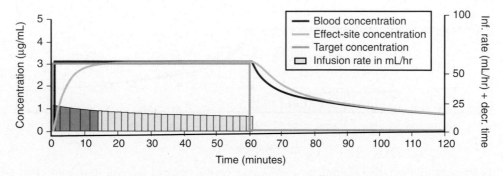

Figure 7-7. TCI. Paedfusor PK data set. Blood-targeted infusion of propofol in healthy 1-year-old, 10-kg child. Blood target = 3 µg/mL. Infusion stopped at 60 minutes (i.e., blood target = 0 µg/mL). Bolus dose of 1.4 mg/kg delivered, then stepwise-reducing infusion of from 19.1 mg/kg/hr to 9.5 mg/kg/hr at 1 hour. Effect-site concentration does not reach 3 µg/mL until 15 minutes 44 seconds. Total dose of propofol = 13.6 mg/kg. Context-sensitive half-time = 10 minutes.

Table 7-6. "Paedfusor" Pharmacokinetic Data Set

1-12 yr	$V1 = 0.4584 \times weight$; $V2 = V1 \times k_{12}/k_{21}$; $V3 = V1 \times k_{13}/k_{31}$
	$k_{10} = 0.1527 \times weight^{-0.3}$
	$k_{12} = 0.114$; $k_{21} = 0.055$
	$k_{13} = 0.0419$; $k_{31} = 0.0033$
	$k_{e0} = 0.26$
13 yr	$V1 = 0.400 \times weight$
	$k_{10} = 0.0678$
	(other constants as above)
14 yr	$V1 = 0.342 \times weight$
	$k_{10} = 0.0792$
	(other constants as above)
15 yr	$V1 = 0.284 \times weight$
	$k_{10} = 0.0954$
	(other constants as above)
16 yr	$V1 = 0.22857 \times weight$
	$k_{10} = 0.119$
	(other constants as above)

Note: The k_{10} value in the age group 1-12 years is a negative power function of weight that reflects the increasing clearance values in younger children.
Data from references 3, 25, 26, and 35.

Table 7-7. Comparison between "Paedfusor" and Kataria Models for Propofol in Children

	"Paedfusor"[3,25,26,35]	Kataria[27]
V1	$0.458 \times weight$	$0.41 \times weight$
V2	$0.95 \times weight$	$0.78 \times weight + 3.1 \times age$
V3	$5.82 \times weight$	$6.9 \times weight$
k_{10}	$0.1527 \times weight^{-0.3}$	0.085
k_{12}	0.114	0.188
k_{21}	0.055	0.102
k_{13}	0.0419	0.063
k_{31}	0.0033	0.0038
k_{e0}	0.26*	N/A*

*This is the value for adults, but Munoz and colleagues[28] have studied these two models to define a more accurate k_{e0} for children age 3-11 years, and the values are 0.91 for "Paedfusor"[3,25,26,35] and 0.41 for Kataria.[27]

effect-site concentrations against time, infusion rates, volumes, compartment sizes, and many other features.

The models within TCI systems are derived from studies of small numbers of healthy patients and are only a guide to drug administration for an individual patient. The accuracy of TCI propofol was assessed by Marsh and associates[2,3] in children.

The model was found to perform well in a small prospective series of healthy children. In children undergoing cardiac surgery, the model performed significantly better than the adult model in adults.[25,26] TCI propofol has been incorporated into a modified version of the commercial "Diprifusor" device and is known as the "Paedfusor,"[26] which has been evaluated clinically and performs well[2-5] (Table 7-6). Another pediatric propofol model that has been reasonably well validated is that of Kataria and coworkers[27] (Table 7-7). Experience shows that the models may need to be adapted and that clinicians need to learn how to use the model to optimize levels of anesthesia, ensure stability

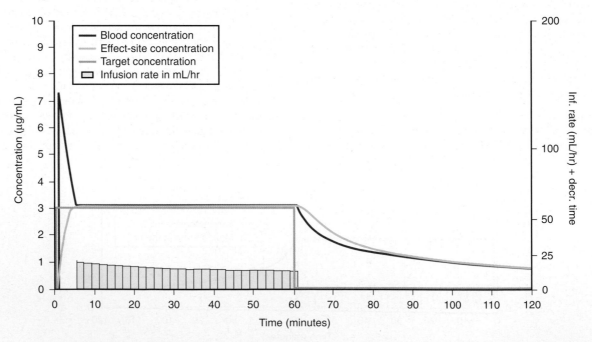

Figure 7-8. TCI. Paedfusor PK data set. Effect-site-targeted infusion of propofol in healthy 1-year-old, 10-kg child. Effect-site target = 3 µg/mL. Infusion stopped at 60 minutes (i.e., effect-site target = 0 µg/mL). Bolus dose of 3.4 mg/kg delivered at 45.5 mL/hr to accentuate the gradient from blood to effect site. Then infusion switches off for 4 minutes. Peak blood concentration after bolus dose = 7.1 µg/mL. Stepwise-reducing infusion of from 15.7 mg/kg/hr to 9.5 mg/kg/hr at 1 hour done. Effect-site concentration reaches 3 µg/mL at 3 minutes 39 seconds. Total dose of propofol = 14 mg/kg. Context-sensitive half-time = 10 minutes 37 seconds.

Table 7-8. Example of Target-Controlled Infusion (5 μg/mL) Based on Calculated Blood-Concentration Targeting Compared with Calculated Effect-Site Concentration Targeting for a Healthy 1-Year-Old (Weight 10 kg), using the "Paedfusor" Pharmacokinetic Data Set

	Blood Concentration Targeting	Effect-Site Concentration Targeting
Loading dose	1.7 mg/kg	5.7 mg/kg*
Maximum blood target reached	5 μg/kg	12 μg/kg*
Total propofol infused after 60 minutes	23.2 mg/kg	23.3 mg/kg
Time to achieve effect site target of 5 μg/mL	17.5 min	4.5 min†

*Potential for hemodynamic changes due to high peak blood concentration from larger bolus dose.
†Very much shorter time to achieve effect-site target.

during induction and maintenance phases, and enhance recovery speed and quality. The "Paedfusor" model makes an allowance for the steady increase in elimination clearance in younger children, particularly those below 30 kg in weight (see Tables 7-6 and 7-7, Fig. 7-8). The lower age and weight limits for each model also differ with age 1 year and 5 kg for the "Paedfusor" system and 3 years and 15 kg for the Kataria system. In the "Paedfusor" program, the adult value for k_{e0} of 0.26 is used but there is no value for this parameter in the Kataria model (see Tables 7-6 and 7-7). Thus, effect-site targeting is only possible with the "Paedfusor" (Table 7-8), although it may not be particularly accurate. Munoz and associates attempted to define a more accurate k_{e0} for children in an ingenious study using auditory evoked responses and both the "Paedfusor" and Kataria models.[28] They found that the time to peak effect after a bolus dose was greater in children than adults and the median k_{e0} values for the "Paedfusor" and Kataria models for children age 3 to 11 years were 0.91 min^{-1} and 0.41 min^{-1}. This should allow more accurate effect-site targeting using propofol in the future.

References

Please see www.expertconsult.com

Fluid Management

Craig D. McClain and Michael L. McManus

ELECTROLYTE DISTURBANCES ARE COMMON in children because of their small size, large surface area to volume ratio, and immature homeostatic mechanisms. As a result, fluid management can be challenging. On the ward, in the operating room, or in the intensive care unit, additional difficulties may result when fluid management is not tailored to the individual or when therapeutic decisions are based on extrapolations from adult data. To better understand the former and to limit the latter, in this chapter we review the basic mechanisms underlying fluid and electrolyte regulation, the developmental anatomy and physiology of fluid compartments, and the management of selected pediatric disease states relevant to anesthesia and critical care.

Regulatory Mechanisms: Fluid Volume, Osmolality, and Arterial Pressure

Water is in thermodynamic equilibrium across cell membranes and moves only in response to the movement of solutes (Fig. 8-1, see website). Movement of water is described by the Starling equation:

$$Q_f = K_f[(P_c - P_i) - \sigma(\pi_c - \pi_i)]$$

where Q_f is fluid flow; K_f is the membrane fluid filtration coefficient; P_c, P_i, π_c, and π_i are hydrostatic and osmotic pressures on either side of the membrane; and σ is the reflection coefficient for the solute and membrane of interest. The reflection coefficient gives a measure of a solute's permeability and, therefore, its contribution to osmotic force after equilibration. Across the blood-brain barrier, for example, σ for sodium approaches 1.0,[1] whereas in muscle and other cell membranes, σ is on the order of 0.15 to 0.3.[2] Thus, when isotonic sodium-containing solutions are given intravenously, usually only 15% to 30% of administered salt and water remains in the intravascular space while the remainder accumulates as interstitial edema.[3,4] In contrast, hypertonic solutions permit greater expansion of circulating blood volume with lower fluid loads and less edema.[5-7]

Both the amount and concentration of solute are tightly regulated to maintain the volumes of intravascular and intracellular compartments. Because sodium is the primary extracellular solute, this ion is the focus of homeostatic mechanisms concerned with maintenance of intravascular volume. When osmolality is held constant, water movement follows sodium movement. As a result, total body sodium (although not necessarily serum Na^+) and total body water generally parallel one another. Because sodium "leak" across membranes limits its contribution to the support of intravascular volume, this compartment is also critically dependent on large, impermeable molecules such as proteins. In contrast to sodium, albumin molecules, for example, follow the Starling equilibrium with a reflection coefficient in excess of 0.8.[8] Soluble proteins create the so-called *colloid oncotic pressure*, approximately 80% of which is contributed by albumin.

Although the presence of albumin supports intravascular volume, protein leak into the interstitium (and consequent water movement) may limit its effectiveness. It has been observed, for example, that the reflection coefficient for albumin decreases by as much as one third after mechanical trauma.[9] Furthermore, because of ongoing leakage, a slow continuous infusion of albumen is superior to bolus administration for increasing the serum albumen concentration in critically ill individuals.[10]

Potassium is the primary intracellular solute, with approximately one third of cellular energy metabolism devoted to Na^+/K^+ exchange. Sodium continuously leaks into cells along its concentration gradient, yet is rapidly extruded in exchange for potassium. As the cell is exposed to varying osmolarity, water movement occurs, causing cell swelling or shrinkage. Because stable cell volume is critical for survival, complex regulatory mechanisms have evolved to ensure that stability is maintained.[11,12] The processes by which swollen cells return to normal size are collectively termed *regulatory volume decrease* processes, and those returning a shrunken cell to normal are termed *regulatory volume increase* processes (Fig. 8-2). With sudden, brief changes in osmolality, regulatory volume increase or decrease processes are activated after small (1%-2%) changes in cell volume, returning cell volume to normal primarily through transport of electrolytes. If anisosmotic conditions persist, chronic compensation occurs through the accumulation or loss of small organic molecules termed *osmolytes* (e.g., polyols, sorbitol, myoinositol), amino acids and their derivatives (e.g., taurine, alanine, proline), and methylamines (e.g., betaine and glycerylphosphorylcholine).

Like intracellular volume, circulating blood (intravascular) volume is also tightly controlled. Increases in intravascular volume result from increases in sodium and water retention, whereas decreases in intravascular volume result from increases in excretion of sodium and water. As noted earlier, serum osmo-lality must be maintained within a very narrow range if serum sodium is to be an effective focus of intravascular volume control. Thus, serum osmolality is usually maintained between 280 and 300 mOsm/L. Changes in osmolality as small as 1% begin to elicit regulatory mechanisms.

Serum osmolality is primarily regulated by antidiuretic hormone (ADH), thirst, and renal concentrating ability. Because the indirect aim of osmolar control is actually volume control, these same osmoregulatory mechanisms are also influenced by factors such as blood pressure, cardiac output, and vascular capacitance.[13,14] In pathologic conditions such as ascites or hemorrhage, intravascular volume preservation takes precedence over osmolality and osmoregulatory mechanisms operate to restore intravascular volume, even at the expense of disrupting physiologic solute balance.

For example, ADH is released from neurons of the supraoptic and paraventricular nuclei in response to osmolar fluctuations in cell size. Solutes that readily permeate cell membranes, such as urea, raise serum osmolality without eliciting ADH release. Infusion of solutes with high actual or effective σ's at the cell membrane (e.g., sodium and mannitol) elicits a robust ADH release. ADH release begins when serum osmolality reaches a threshold of approximately 280 mOsm/L. Rapid increases in osmolality lead to more vigorous release of ADH than do slow increases. Hypovolemia and hypotension diminish the threshold for ADH release and increase the "gain" of the system by exaggerating the rate of rise of serum ADH levels (Fig. 8-3, see website). Thus, in a volume-depleted or hypotensive child, brisk ADH release occurs in response to plasma osmolalities as low as 260 to 270 mOsm/L. It has been hypothesized that different populations of vasopressin-secreting cells are responsive to osmotic and baroreceptor-mediated information.

Intravascular fluid volume, salt and water intake, electrolyte balance, and cardiovascular status are joined at many levels.[15] For example, as vascular fullness and systemic blood pressure increases, ADH release ceases and both *pressure diuresis* and *natriuresis* occur.[16] The resulting relationship of urinary output versus arterial pressure is termed the *renal function curve* and its intersection with salt and water intake determines the *equilibrium point* at which arterial blood pressure ultimately

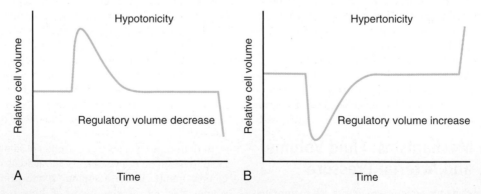

Figure 8-2. Activation of mechanisms regulating cell volume in response to volume perturbations. Volume-regulatory losses and gains of solutes are termed *regulatory volume decrease* (**A**) and *regulatory volume increase* (**B**), respectively. The course of these decreases and increases varies with the type of cell and experimental conditions. Typically, however, a regulatory volume increase mediated by the uptake of electrolytes and a regulatory volume decrease mediated by the loss of electrolytes and organic osmolytes occur over a period of minutes. When cells that have undergone a regulatory volume decrease (**A**) or increase (**B**) are returned to normotonic conditions, they swell above or shrink below their resting volume. This is due to volume-regulatory accumulation or loss of solutes, which effectively makes the cytoplasm hypertonic or hypotonic, respectively, as compared with normotonic extracellular fluid. (From McManus ML, Churchwell KB, Strange K: Regulation of cell volume in health and disease. N Engl J Med 1995; 333:1260-1266. ® Massachusetts Medical Society.)

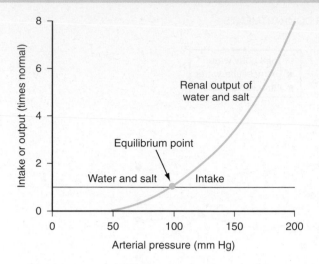

Figure 8-4. Analysis of arterial pressure regulation by equating the renal output curve with the salt and water intake curve. The equilibrium point describes the level to which the arterial pressure will be regulated. (That portion of the salt and water intake that is lost from the body through nonrenal routes is ignored in this figure.) (From Guyton AC, Hall JC [eds]: Textbook of Medical Physiology. Philadelphia, WB Saunders, 1996, pp 221-237.)

and complement the more immediate activity of the sympathetic nervous system. In addition to high pressure sensors, such as aortic arch and carotid sinus baroreceptors, intravascular volume information is provided by low pressure thoracic sensors. For this reason, effective increases or decreases in intrathoracic blood volume may mimic changes in whole-body volume status and produce natriuresis, diuresis, or fluid retention. Intravascular volume may also be sensed as the stretch of atrial muscle fibers leading to release of atrial natriuretic peptide.[17] Although its complete physiologic role is uncertain, atrial natriuretic peptide may serve to "fine tune" volume status by causing modest vasodilation, gently increasing glomerular filtration rate (GFR) and decreasing reabsorption of sodium. The combination of complex autoregulatory mechanisms with complementary actions operating on varying time scales, all responding to different, yet interrelated, effector stimuli yields an elegant system by which the mature individual may maintain circulation amid a variety of challenges. In this context, it is interesting to observe that successful heart transplant recipients, despite general cardiovascular stability, typically manifest fundamental derangements in body fluid homeostasis.[18]

Maturation of Fluid Compartments and Homeostatic Mechanisms

Body Water and Electrolyte Distribution

Much of our understanding of the development of body water compartments is derived from deuterium oxide dilution studies performed in the 1950s.[19] In a series of 21 neonates, total body water (TBW) was 78 ± ~5% of the body weight. Subsequent measurements in fewer subjects showed that TBW decreased to approximately 60% in the second 6 months of life with most of the loss being extracellular. A smaller decrease (to about 57%) is observed late in childhood (Fig. 8-6). When TBW is expressed in terms of surface area rather than weight, it decreases briefly during the first postnatal month and then increases steadily to adulthood. This "increase" reflects growth and the steady decrease of surface area to volume ratio. After 3 postnatal months, extracellular water and plasma volume, expressed as functions of surface area and ideal body weight, remain constant. Using these data, formulas such as $TBW = 0.135 \times W^{0.666} \times H^{0.535}$ (SD = 8.7%) and $TBW = 0.843 \times W^{0.891}$ (SD = 9.2%) have been generated and nomograms constructed (W, weight; H, height).

rests (Fig. 8-4). Equilibrium (chronic) blood pressure is influenced only by shifts of the renal function or fluid intake curves. Transient changes in arterial pressure secondary to peripheral resistance changes are always resolved by opposing changes in total body salt and water.

In response to a decreasing arterial pressure, the renin-angiotensin system is mobilized. With decreased renal perfusion, juxtaglomerular cells release renin, which, in turn, converts renin substrate (angiotensinogen) to angiotensin I. Angiotensin I is then rapidly converted to angiotensin II by angiotensin-converting enzyme present in lung endothelium. Angiotensin II supports arterial pressure in three ways: (1) direct vasoconstriction, (2) increased salt and water retention (via renal vasoconstriction and decreased glomerular filtration), and (3) stimulation of aldosterone secretion (Fig. 8-5).

Antidiuretic hormone, pressure diuresis, and the renin-angiotensin system permit wide ranges in salt and water intake without large fluctuations in blood pressure or volume status. All serve to support the systemic circulation when threatened

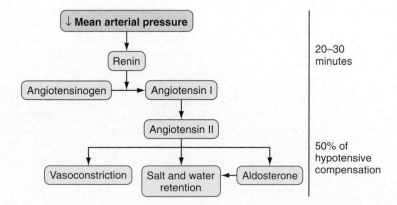

Figure 8-5. Physiologic responses to hypotension.

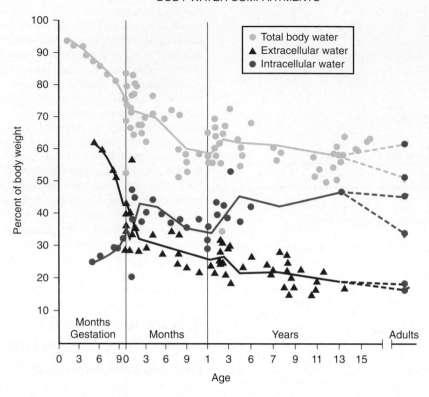

Figure 8-6. Total body water (*blue circles*), extracellular water (*purple triangles*), and intracellular water (*orange circles*) as percentages of body weight in infants and children, compared with corresponding values for the fetus and adults. (From Friis-Hansen B: Body water compartments in children: changes during growth and related changes in body composition. Pediatrics 1961; 28:169-181.)

The importance of the extracellular compartment, its relationship to the intracellular space, and much of the chemical anatomy of both were first described by Gamble in educational monographs issued during the first part of the 20th century (Fig. 8-7, see website).[20,21] The chemical compositions of mature body fluid compartments are provided in Table 8-1.

Circulating Blood Volume

Circulating blood volume in infants and children has been studied extensively using a variety of methods. By using the iodine 121-labeled human serum albumin technique, the blood volume in neonates was 82 ± 9 mL/kg, although substantial variability may result from the degree of placental-fetal transfusion.[22] In low birth weight, preterm, or critically ill infants, values as great as 100 mL/kg have been measured.[23] Blood volume then increases slightly during the first few months of life, reaching its zenith at 2 months of age (~86 mL/kg), returning to near 80 mL/kg in the second year of life, and then stabilizing between 75 and 80 mL/kg until adolescence. In general, the blood volume to weight ratio decreases with growth. The most accurate basis for prediction of blood volume is lean body mass, the consideration of which removes any male to female variation even into adulthood.[24] An estimate of the circulating blood volume is presented in Table 8-2.

Table 8-1. Composition of Body Fluid Compartments

	Extracellular Fluid	Intracellular Fluid
Osmolality (mOsm)	290-310	290-310
Cations (mEq/L)	155	155
Na^+	138-142	10
K^+	4.0-4.5	110
Ca^{2+}	4.5-5.0	–
Mg^{2+}	3	40
Anions (mEq/L)	155	155
Cl^-	103	–
HCO_3^-	27	–
HPO_4^{2-}	–	10
SO_4^{2-}	–	110
PO_4^{2-}	3	–
Organic acids	6	–
Protein	16	40

Table 8-2. Estimate of Circulating Blood Volume

Age	Estimated Blood Volume (mL/kg)
Preterm infant	100
Full-term neonate	90
Infant	80
School age	75
Adults	70

Maturation of Homeostatic Mechanisms

Renal development begins at approximately 5 weeks' gestation and continues in a centrifugal pattern until the full complement of nephrons is in place by around the 38th week. In the outermost regions of the renal cortex, postnatal nephron differentiation may continue for several weeks to months. In the early stages of gestation, renal blood flow is approximately one fifth of normal. Initially this is related to structural immaturity, and later it is due to increased renovascular resistance. By 38 weeks' gestation, renal blood flow is approximately one third of normal. High renovascular resistance protects the developing nephron from both pressure and volume overload. Resulting renal contribution to metabolic homeostasis in utero is limited.

As with the pulmonary bed, vascular resistance in the kidney decreases after birth, leading to abrupt increases in renal blood flow and GFR. In utero, despite a low GFR, urine output is brisk, owing to poor reabsorption of salt and water. Plasma renin activity is increased in utero, decreases immediately after birth, and then increases again as excess extracellular water is mobilized and excreted. Aldosterone levels are increased in cord blood and are maintained at this level for the first 3 days of life. The increased aldosterone may be necessary for sodium retention during periods of increased anabolism early in life.

Intrarenal gradients of NaCl and urea are less steep in the immature kidney, and full nephron length has yet to be achieved. Consequently, urine concentrating ability is limited in neonates, with maximum urine osmolality being about half that of the adult (700-800 mEq/L vs. 1300-1400 Eq/L). In part, this also relates to low circulating ADH levels and decreased renal responsiveness to ADH. Although overall ADH production is not impaired, excessive secretion may occur in some disease states. Limited urine-concentrating ability necessitates large urine volumes for elimination of large solute loads.

In the first year of life, renal plasma flow and GFR are approximately one half the adult values of 350 and 70 mL/min/m^2, respectively.[25] Consequently, serum creatinine is increased in term and preterm infants yet normalizes in the second month of life. Fractional excretion of sodium (FE_{NA}) is markedly increased in preterm, decreases somewhat by term, and stabilizes at adult levels by the second month of life. Although the adult kidney may easily achieve FE_{NA} values as low as 0.5%, the 34-week infant is limited to no less than 2%.

These maturational features make it very difficult for the preterm or young infant to handle fluctuations in fluid and solute loads. Both sodium conservation and regulation of extracellular fluid volume are impaired relative to the older child and adult. Limited GFR makes excretion of a fluid challenge difficult. Excessive urinary sodium loss leads to increased maintenance requirements. Hyponatremia is common. Conversely, diminished concentrating ability increases free water losses during excretion of a solute load, whereas high surface area to volume ratios produce increased evaporative water loss. Consequently, fluid requirements are relatively high and dehydration is common. Errors in medical management are poorly tolerated. Fortunately, the most severe impairment exists in preterm infants and the majority of homeostatic mechanisms are fully developed after the first year of life.

Fluid and Electrolyte Requirements

Holliday summarized the evolution of contemporary hydration therapy.[20] In 1832, Latta first reported the use of intravenous fluids in the resuscitation of patients dehydrated by cholera.[26] In 1918, growing information on the subject permitted Blackfan and Maxcy to successfully treat nine infants by intraperitoneal injection.[27] In 1923, Gamble detailed the anatomy of fluid and electrolyte compartments, introducing the use of milliequivalents to clinical practice.[21] This paved the way for the development of the "deficit therapy" regimen of Darrow.[28]

In subsequent decades, various recipes for replacement of extracellular and intracellular fluid losses were suggested. For the most part, these failed because of excessive potassium and insufficient sodium content. Hyponatremia was common. When repletion of extracellular losses became the focus, rapid restoration of extracellular fluid using solutions high in sodium became commonplace. This, along with oral rehydration, is the preferred method of treatment today.

The concept of "maintenance fluids" is a complex subject. Although water and salt are required to sustain life, it is fair to say that for an individual child at any particular time, the precise amounts necessary are unknown (and perhaps unknowable). In the context of individual variability, complex homeostatic mechanisms, and changing requirements, the "dose" of salt and water required for "maintenance" cannot be calculated precisely. Instead, fluids and electrolytes, like anesthetics, are titrated to effect with general guideposts provided by clinical assessment, basic physiologic principles, and limited published data. The term *maintenance fluids* is often more limiting than helpful and in all cases is less precise than other terms familiar to anesthesiologists such as *minimal alveolar concentration* (MAC) or *effective dose 50%* (ED_{50}).

Calculations for a first approximation of "the maintenance need for water in parenteral fluid therapy" were provided by Holliday and Segar in 1957.[29] Integrating the relevant known physiology to date, these authors observed that "insensible loss of water and urinary water loss roughly parallel energy metabolism and do not parallel weight." However, because water utilization parallels energy metabolism, energy metabolism follows surface area, and surface area follows weight, it should be possible to "estimate" water requirement (in a nonlinear fashion) from weight alone. The authors then proceeded under a series of assumptions to extrapolate from limited data to a "relationship between weight and energy expenditure that might easily be remembered."

Assuming energy requirements of "hospitalized patients" to be "roughly midway between basal and normal levels," a curve of caloric requirement versus weight was constructed. Such a curve could be seen as composed of three linear sections: 0-10 kg, 10-20 kg, and 20-70 kg (Fig. 8-8). Viewed in this manner, the authors reasoned that "fortuitously, the average needs for water, expressed in milliliters, equals energy expenditure in calories": 100 mL/kg/day for weights to 10 kg, an additional 50 mL/kg/day for each kilogram from 11 to 20 kg, and 20 mL/kg/day more for each kilogram beyond 20 kg. In anesthetic practice, this has been further simplified (Table 8-3) (see later).

Estimation of pediatric electrolyte needs was difficult and required use of less precise data. Assuming that human milk contained the minimal electrolyte requirement for infants and

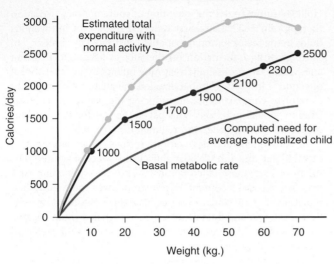

COMPARISON OF ENERGY EXPENDITURE
IN BASAL AND IDEAL STATE

Figure 8-8. The upper and lower curves were plotted from data from the study by Talbot.[107] Weights at the 50th percentile level were selected for converting calories at various ages to calories related to weight. The computed line for the average hospitalized child was derived from the following equations:
1. 0-10 kg: 100 kcal/kg.
2. 10-20 kg: 1000 kcal + 50 kcal/kg for each kg over 10 kg.
3. 20 kg and up: 1500 kcal + 20 kcal/kg for each kg over 20 kg.
(From Holliday MA, Segar WE: The maintenance need for water in parenteral fluid therapy. Pediatrics 1957; 19:823-832.)

coupling this observation with Darrow's work,[30] Holliday and Segar concluded that "maintenance requirements for sodium, chloride, and potassium were 3.0, 2.0, and 2.0 mEq/100 calories/day, respectively."

The simplicity and elegance of the Holliday and Segar formula have made it a great service to all physicians as the starting point for fluid management in healthy children. In the operating room, the formula is particularly useful in estimating deficits after a period of NPO status. However, its blind application to all situations is unwarranted and its uncritical use was unintended. As the authors cautioned, "understanding of the limitations and of exceptions to the system are required. Even more essential is the clinical judgment to modify the system as circumstances dictate." General water losses for infants and children are summarized in Table 8-4.

Neonatal Fluid Management

In the first few days of life, isotonic losses of salt and water cause the normal neonate to lose 5% to 15% of its body weight.

Although GFR rises rapidly, urine output is initially low and renal losses are modest. Day 1 fluid requirements of the wrapped neonate, therefore, are relatively low. Over the first few days of life, losses and requirements increase. In the poorly feeding infant, progression to hypernatremia and dehydration are common. When intake is appropriate, the term infant will regain body weight in the first week of life.

Three distinct phases of fluid and electrolyte homeostasis have been described in low[31] and very low birth weight[32] infants. In the first day of life, there is minimal urine output and body weight is stable despite low fluid intake. In the second phase, days 2 and 3 of life, diuresis occurs irrespective of the amount of fluid administered. By the fourth and fifth days of life, urine output begins to vary with changes in fluid intake and state of health.

Prematurity increases neonatal fluid requirements significantly. Fluid requirements are therefore estimated and then titrated to the infant's changing weight, urine output, and serum sodium. Sodium levels are routinely measured every 6 to 8 hours until equilibrium is established around 150 mEq/L.

No less important is glucose homeostasis. In the ninth month of gestation, the fetus begins to form glycogen stores at a rate of over 100 kcal/day. Thus, in the unstressed, term infant, hepatic glycogen stores are 5% of body weight. Immediately after birth, glycogenolysis depletes most of these stores within the first 24 to 48 hours. Gluconeogenesis must then proceed to yield glucose at a rate of around 4 mg/kg/min.

At birth, fetal serum glucose is 60% to 70% of maternal levels. Levels may decrease within the first hours of life before recovering but should exceed 45 mg/dL to avoid neurologic injury. Symptoms of hypoglycemia may include jitteriness, lethargy, temperature instability, and convulsions. Ten percent dextrose in water ($D_{10}W$) may be given as a bolus of 2 to 4 mL/kg followed by a continuous infusion providing 4 to 6 mg/kg/min. The serum glucose concentration is then followed every 30 minutes and the infusion titrated upward as necessary. It is important that the amount of glucose being provided is calculated in milligrams per kilograms per minute to avoid errors during fluid changes and to facilitate the diagnosis of persistent hypoglycemia.

Typical *day 1* infant fluid orders call for 70 to 80 mL/kg of $D_{10}W$. Because $D_{10}W$ contains 10 g glucose/dL, this provides

$$10 \text{ g/dL} \times 70\text{-}80 \text{ mL/kg/day}$$
$$= 7\text{-}8 \text{ g/kg/day}$$
$$= 0.333 \text{ g/kg/hr}$$
$$= \text{approximately 5 mg/kg/min.}$$

On *day 2*, fluids are routinely increased to at least 100 mL/kg/day and sodium is added at 2 to 3 mEq/dL. When urine

Table 8-3. Relationship between Weight and Hourly or Daily Maintenance Fluid Requirements of Children

Weight (kg)	Maintenance Fluid Requirements	
	Hour	Day
<10	4 mL/kg	100 mL/kg
10-20	40 mL + 2 mL/kg for every kg >10 kg	1000 mL + 50 mL/kg for every kg >10
>20	60 mL + 1 mL/kg for every kg >20 kg	1500 mL + 20 mL/kg for every kg > 20

Table 8-4. Normal Water Losses for Infants and Children

Cause of Loss	Volume of Loss (mL/100 kcal)
Output	
Urine	70
Insensible loss	
Skin	30
Respiratory tract	15
"Hidden intake" (from burning 100 calories)	15
Total	100

output is established, potassium is added at 1 to 2 mEq/dL. The final solution, containing 30 mEq Na⁺ and 10 to 20 mEq K⁺/L, approximates the 0.2 normal saline (NS) "maintenance" solution commonly used in older children.

In the neonatal intensive care unit, fluid management focuses on provision of adequate nutrition, maintenance of electrolyte balance, and limitation of fluid overload. The last factor is of particular concern because plasma oncotic pressure is lowered in preterm infants and the whole-body protein reflection coefficient is below adult values.[33] Very low birth weight infants are at particular risk for fluid and electrolyte imbalances.[34] Even modest fluid overload, therefore, may exacerbate pulmonary edema, prolong ductal patency, and more readily produce congestive heart failure. This perspective typically accompanies the infant to the operating room, where the primary considerations are routinely quite the opposite: restoration of circulating blood volume after third space accumulation, maintenance of intravascular volume amid ongoing blood loss, replacement of potentially massive evaporative losses, and maintenance of blood pressure despite anesthetic-induced vasodilation and increased venous capacitance. During surgery, these concerns must take precedence; yet unnecessary administration of fluid is best avoided.

Intraoperative Fluid Management

Intravenous Access and Fluid Administration Devices

In pediatrics, the first step toward intraoperative fluid management is often the most challenging, that is, gaining intravenous access. In general, simple procedures in healthy children are successfully approached using a single peripheral intravenous line. Although preferences vary among anesthesiologists, establishing intravenous access is most easily accomplished after induction of anesthesia. In young children, anesthesia is often induced by inhalation and a catheter is inserted by an assistant into a hand or foot vein. In older children, or when intravenous access is desirable before anesthesia is induced, intravenous access may be facilitated by the use of topical anesthesia (e.g., EMLA cream, amethocaine, lidocaine infiltration) or sedation or both.

Complex surgeries in sicker children usually require at least two large-bore catheters. In pediatrics, however, "large bore" is a relative term, with 22-gauge catheters typically providing sufficient access in infants. Preferred sites for larger catheters include antecubital and saphenous veins. In cases in which access to the central circulation is required (as for pressure monitoring, infusion of vasoactive medications, or prolonged access), longer catheters may be placed via the femoral, subclavian, or internal jugular veins (the latter usually via a high, anterior approach).[35] Although secure access may also be obtained via the external jugular vein, it is often difficult to negotiate the J wire or catheter tip into the central circulation.[36]

In selecting the appropriate intravenous catheter, it is useful to consider the relative effects of catheter length and diameter on solution flow rates. Longer catheters produce more resistance to flow and are therefore not preferred over shorter catheters when rapid infusion of large volumes of fluids is required (see Figs. 53-1 and 53-2). In vitro, catheters that were designed for peripheral venous access had 18% to 164% greater flow rates when compared with the same-gauge catheters designed for central venous use. Under pressure, as might be employed during emergent volume resuscitation, rates differed up to 17-fold.[37] Although this seems to suggest that short peripheral catheters should be preferred, in-vivo data are more complex. In animal models, it seems that overall catheter flow rates are below in-vitro rates and that central access presents somewhat less resistance to flow than peripheral access.[38] Finally, when weighing the risks and benefits of central versus peripheral access, it is also interesting to consider that central administration of resuscitation medications may provide little practical advantage over peripheral administration.[39]

Intraosseous devices are now commonly used in the initial resuscitation of critically ill or injured children (see Fig. 49-6).[40,41] Flow rates via these devices seem to be less dependent on needle diameter than on resistance in the marrow compartment.[42] In the operating room, the intraosseous route has been used for both induction and maintenance of anesthesia.[43-45] However, onset of drug effect is less predictable and they are more easily dislodged than intravenous catheters. Potential complications include compartment syndrome[46-48] and, very rarely, damage to the growth plate.[41,49] Thus, such devices are probably best considered an emergency or last-resort option.[44]

To prevent accidental volume overload, the amount of intravenous fluid available to administer to a child at any one time should not exceed the child's calculated hourly requirement. Particularly in infants, a volumetric chamber should be used to limit the amount of fluid available for infusion. Similarly, a microdrip infusion set limits the rate of fluid administration and permits much greater control. Although a fluid infusion pump provides the most precise mode of regulating the rate of fluid administration (and is therefore very useful in providing supplemental fluids or medications), such devices are impractical on primary access lines because they hinder the ability to administer drugs or fluids rapidly. In addition, the clinician should be mindful that pumps may continue to infuse through dislodged catheters and may give inappropriate reassurance of adequate intravenous access and fluid administration.

In neonates and small infants, when rapid infusion of resuscitation solutions or blood products is anticipated, many practitioners find it helpful to include a stopcock manifold in-line. Additional fluids may then be drawn up into 60-mL syringes and warmed separately. During periods of sudden blood loss, stored syringes may then be inserted into the manifold and a known volume rapidly infused.

Finally, in prolonged surgeries, or when volume replacement is great, it is imperative that all intravenous infusions be adequately warmed. Also, in younger infants and children in whom communication exists between the right and left sides of the circulation (e.g., patency of the foramen ovale), an in-line "bubble" filter is desirable.

Choice and Composition of Intravenous Fluids

In the early 1960s,[50] simultaneous measurements of plasma and extracellular fluid volumes demonstrated that, during surgery, plasma volume is supported at the expense of the extravascular space. At the same time, isotonic fluid is, to varying extents, redistributed from the extracellular and intravascular spaces to a third, nonfunctional space. Because of the differences in fluid distribution and renal function in infants compared with older children, it was at first unclear that these findings could be extended to infancy. Thus, fluid restriction remained the

Table 8-5. Composition of Extracellular Fluid and Common Intravenous Solutions

	Cations (mEq/L)				Anions (mEq/L)			
	Na^+	K^+	Ca^{2+}	Mg^{2+}	NH_4^+	Cl^-	HCO_3^-	HPO_4^-
Extracellular fluid	142	4	5	3	0.3	103	27	3
Lactated Ringer's solution	130	4	3			109	28	
0.45 NaCl	77					77		
0.9% NaCl (normal saline)	154					154		
3% NaCl	590					590		

standard of care until careful studies specifically demonstrated that fluid and electrolyte requirements are often extremely large in neonates who are undergoing major surgical procedures.[51-53]

Although hypotonic fluids are selected for maintenance hydration throughout the hospital (according to the reasoning outlined previously), isotonic solutions are preferred intraoperatively for several reasons. First, most ongoing volume losses are isotonic, consisting of shed blood and interstitial fluids. Second, large volumes of hypotonic solutions may rapidly diminish serum osmolality, producing very low concentrations of electrolytes (in particular, sodium) and undesirable fluid shifts. Indeed, even large volumes of "isotonic" fluids have been shown to significantly decrease serum osmolality in adult volunteers.[54] Third, as discussed earlier, the plasma volume expansion necessary in response to diminished vascular tone under anesthesia is difficult to achieve even with isotonic fluids. Finally, increases in ADH and other elements of intraoperative physiology result in free water retention in excess of sodium if inadequate amounts of the latter are provided.

The compositions of commonly used intravenous solutions are presented in Table 8-5. Assuming normal plasma osmolality of 275 to 290 mOsm/L, it is noteworthy that 0.9% NS is slightly hypertonic to plasma and that lactated Ringer's solution is isotonic, although slightly hyponatremic. For dextrose-containing solutions, added osmolality is rapidly dissipated as sugar is metabolized, resulting in increased volumes of free water. Thus, administration of 5% dextrose in water is ultimately equivalent to administration of free water.

The routine intraoperative use of glucose-containing solutions has been a subject of debate. As a rule, operative stress evokes physiologic responses that increase serum glucose. In practice, therefore, hypoglycemia is seldom a problem in healthy children when glucose is omitted from intravenous fluids.[55,56] Indeed, the risk should be particularly small if the period of fasting is limited to less than 10 hours.[56] At the same time, rapid administration of dextrose solutions may certainly produce acute hyperglycemia and hyperosmolality.[55,56] Thus, glucose-containing solutions should not be used to replace fluid deficits, third space losses, or blood losses. Some populations, such as debilitated infants,[57] children who are malnourished, or those undergoing cardiac surgery, have been shown, however, to be at risk for intraoperative hypoglycemia.[58,59] Thus, use of glucose-containing solutions, along with intraoperative glucose monitoring, may be useful in these children.

Hyperalimentation

It is now nearly routine practice that critically ill children arrive in the operating room with hyperalimentation solutions infusing. Common contents of hyperalimentation solutions are shown in Table 8-6. In general, children require 0.5 to 3.0 mg/kg/day of protein. Children receiving parenteral nutrition preoperatively should continue to receive those infusions separately, and a corresponding volume should be deducted from isotonic operative fluids. Common infusions of hyperalimentation include an infusion of Intralipid and another of a high concentration of a glucose solution. It is prudent to discontinue the Intralipid solution during surgery; but if that is not possible, then every effort should be made to avoid accessing any ports in the line to reduce the risk of contaminating the Intralipid. Conversely, the concentrated glucose solution should be continued at the same rate (since circulating insulin concentrations would be increased in response to the glucose concentration). Because of hyperglycemic responses to the stress of surgery, some practitioners routinely decrease hyperalimentation infusion rates by one third to one half. If this practice is followed, clinicians should consider checking serum glucose levels at regular intervals to avoid intraoperative hypoglycemia. If the glucose infusion is reduced, we recommend ad hoc testing for serum glucose concentrations. Under no circumstances should

Table 8-6. Common Contents of Parenteral Nutrition Solutions*

Carbohydrates

10%, 12.5%, 20%, 25%, 30% Dextrose

Limited to D_{10} or $D_{12.5}$ if through a peripheral catheter

Protein

In the form of amino acids

0.5, 1.0, 1.5, 2.0, 2.5, or 3.0 g/kg/day

Lipids

10%, 20% Lipids

Standard Additives (all per 1000 mL of solution)

Sodium: 30 mEq

Potassium: 20 mEq

Calcium: 15 mEq

Magnesium: 10 mEq

Phosphorus: 10 mM

Heparin

*Common contents of parenteral nutrition solutions containing dextrose, protein, lipids, and standard additives such as electrolytes. *These values represent standard starting points that may be modified based on individual patient needs.*

concentrated glucose solutions (such as D_{10} or D_{20}) be abruptly discontinued because the increased levels of circulating insulin could theoretically cause precipitous decreases in the serum glucose concentration.

When necessary, glucose-containing solutions are best administered as a separate "piggyback" infusion using an infusion pump or other rate- or volume-limiting device so as to avoid accidental bolus administration.

Fasting Recommendations and Deficit Replacement

Fasting recommendations have evolved significantly. The goal of fasting is to minimize the volume of gastric contents and thereby lessen the risk of vomiting and aspiration during induction of anesthesia. In children as opposed to adults, this is of particular concern because, in many institutions, induction is more often accomplished by inhalation than intravenous anesthesia and the period of vulnerability to regurgitation is potentially protracted compared with an intravenous induction.

At issue are the effectiveness of fasting in lowering a child's gastric volume and the benefits of this when weighed against the added discomfort and risk of dehydration. It seems unlikely, for example, that a hungry, thirsty, and agitated child who has been NPO since bedtime the previous evening is at an overall decreased anesthetic risk when compared with the child who has been permitted clear liquids 2 to 3 hours before surgery. Nonetheless, until recently, long periods of preoperative fasting was the rule. Fortunately, numerous studies of gastric volume and pH have convincingly demonstrated that clear liquids are rapidly emptied from the stomach and the stimulated peristalsis actually serves to decrease gastric volume and acidity. Taking this together with the benefits of improved hydration and mental status, it is clear that prolonged NPO status is unwarranted. The specific NPO guidelines currently in use in many institutions are included in Table 8-7.[59a]

With briefer NPO periods, replacement of the fasting deficit becomes less critical. Typically, in calculating maintenance requirements and deficits, anesthesiologists have reduced the work of Holliday and Segar to the following shorthand:

Hourly maintenance fluid rate = 4 mL/kg/hr for the first 10 kg
= 40 mL/hr + 2 mL/kg/hr for the second 10 kg (11-20 kg)
= 60 mL/hr + 1 mL/kg/hr for each kilogram >20 kg thereafter

Thus, fluid requirements for a 30-kg child would be 40 + 20 + 10 = 70 mL/kg/hr. Traditionally, the estimated deficit is calculated as the above hourly requirement multiplied by the number of NPO hours. However, such calculations tend to overestimate the true requirements because they neglect physiologic conser-

vation of water with increasing dehydration. Thus, complete replacement of the calculated deficit is frequently unnecessary. Conversely, as discussed earlier, factors such as fever, prematurity, and renal concentrating ability may significantly increase real fluid requirements above these estimates.

In practice, there is considerable variability in the speed and extent to which estimated deficits are replaced. As a general principle, however, deficits are usually replaced by 50% in the first hour and the remainder over the subsequent 2 hours. In procedures that are brief, such as tonsillectomy where the risk of postoperative nausea and vomiting is increased, more rapid replacement may be warranted.

Assessment of Intravascular Volume

Once the child is anesthetized, many clinical clues to volume status are lost or confounded by operative events. For example, although a fairly reliable indicator of volume status in the quietly resting preoperative child, tachycardia may result from any number of factors besides intravascular volume status during surgery. It is the challenge of the anesthesiologist to view the entire clinical picture, consider the possibilities, integrate them into a hypothesis, and then test the hypothesis.

Assessment of intravascular volume begins with knowledge of age-related norms for heart rate and blood pressure (see Tables 2-9 and 2-10). Is the heart rate persistently increased or does it vary with surgical stimulation? Is the pulse pressure narrow or, more ominously, is the blood pressure reduced for age? Does it vary with positive-pressure breaths? Are the extremities warm? Is capillary refill brisk? What is the urine output? Are these variables changing? What is the rate of the change? When hypovolemia is suspected, observing the response to a 10- to 20-mL/kg bolus of isotonic crystalloid or colloid may test the hypothesis.

Measurement and continuous monitoring of central venous pressure are often helpful in assessing the status of circulating volume (see Figs. 49-2 to 49-5). In addition to traditional central lines introduced into the superior vena cava or left atrium, animal[60] and limited clinical[61] data suggest that femoral lines that terminate in the abdominal vena cava may also be useful. In one study of 20 infants and children, comparison of right atrial and inferior vena caval pressures found close agreement with average end-expiratory pressure differences of less than 1 mm Hg.[61] Assessment of changes in the contour of the arterial waveform may also be helpful in assessing volume status and the response to volume administration (see Fig. 10-11).

Ongoing Losses and Third Spacing

During all surgical procedures, fluid loss from the vascular space is primarily the result of three simultaneous physiologic processes. First, whole blood is shed at various rates and must be replaced. Second, capillary leak and surgical trauma result in extravasation of isotonic, protein-containing fluid into nonfunctional compartments (the so-called third space). Third, anesthetic-induced relaxation of sympathetic tone produces vasodilatation and relative hypovolemia (a "virtual" loss). In very small patients, a fourth source of losses must also be carefully considered: direct evaporation. These ongoing losses are often difficult to quantitate (or even estimate). Although these losses occur in children of all sizes, the small circulating blood volume of an infant (e.g., for a 5 kg infant = 80 mL/kg × 5 kg = 400 mL) leaves little room for error. Faced with uncertainty, the prudent

Table 8-7. Preoperative Fasting Recommendations in Infants and Children

Clear liquids	2 hours
Breast milk	4 hours
Infant formula	6 hours*
Solids (fatty or fried foods)	8 hours

*Some centers now allow plain toast (no dairy products) up to 6 hours.[59a]

response is constant vigilance and reliance on general principles.

As a rule, just as in adults, shed blood is replaced 1 mL for 1 mL of blood loss with colloid (5% albumin or blood) or 3 mL for 1 mL of blood loss with isotonic crystalloid, such as lactated Ringer's solution. Isotonic crystalloid is also used to replenish third space losses. Surgical procedures involving only mild tissue trauma may entail third space losses of 3 to 4 mL/kg/hr. More extensive surgical procedures involving moderate trauma may require replacement equivalent to 5 to 7 mL/kg/hr to adequately support intravascular volume. In small infants undergoing very large abdominal procedures, the losses may approach 10 mL/kg/hr or more.[51,53] These "losses" are lost from the vascular compartment and include both evaporation and redistribution of fluid. The latter must be most carefully considered, because, for reasons outlined previously, such redistribution is exacerbated by continued fluid administration.

Although necessary intraoperatively, third space accumulation represents whole-body salt and water overload that will need to be mobilized postoperatively. The price of unchecked fluid administration is generalized anasarca, pulmonary edema, bowel swelling, and laryngotracheal edema. In the healthy child, this relative fluid overload is well tolerated, with most excess fluid excreted over the first 2 postoperative days. In children with impaired pulmonary, cardiac, or renal function, however, such fluid excess may result in clinically important postoperative morbidity.

Postoperative Fluid Management

General Approach
Well-planned postoperative fluid management complements the intraoperative plan and accounts for evolving physiology as the child recovers. Replacement of fluid deficits is completed. Ongoing losses are replaced. The child is repeatedly reassessed and intake is adjusted until normal fluid and electrolyte homeostasis has returned. To aid in decision-making, trends in vital signs are identified, all sources of fluid intake and output are quantitated, urine-specific gravity is followed, daily weights are obtained, and serum electrolytes are measured.

In simple outpatient surgeries, discharge is possible when fluid deficits are replaced. In complex children, replacement fluids may require hourly readjustment that is based on the prior hour's intake and output. Rather than reacting to single pieces

of data, such as low urine output, overall patterns must be discerned. High urine output and low urine specific gravity may indicate overhydration or diabetes insipidus. Oliguria may suggest hypovolemia when accompanied by high urine specific gravity and clinical signs of dehydration or low cardiac output when accompanied by signs of poor perfusion. In the well-hydrated patient, oliguria may represent renal failure if the urine specific gravity is normal (or dilute) or the syndrome of inappropriate antidiuretic hormone secretion (SIADH) if the urine is concentrated. A careful physical examination is necessary; in many cases, certainty in diagnosis requires simultaneous measurement of serum and urine electrolytes.

Frequently, losses via surgical or gastric drains may be large in both real and relative terms. For example, a neonate with a nasogastric tube may lose more than 100 mL/kg/day (normally 20-40 mL/kg/day) in gastric fluid. Therefore, in determining the volume and composition of replacement fluids, it is sometimes helpful to consider the electrolyte content of various losses (Table 8-8).

Postoperative Physiology and Hyponatremia
For a variety of reasons, children retain salt and water postoperatively. Contributing factors include neuroendocrine activation by stress, continued capillary leak with third space accumulation, and hypovolemic stimulation of ADH or renin secretion. As outlined earlier, intravascular volume depletion is a potent nonosmotic signal for fluid retention and may override osmotic signals under a variety of clinical circumstances.

At the same time, ongoing fluid and electrolyte losses after surgery may be large. Chest tubes, nasogastric suction, weeping incisions, and even continued slow bleeding can account for significant losses in children. Postoperatively children are often entirely dependent on intravenous fluids for replacement of these and other losses.

Thus, unless isotonic, sodium-containing fluids are provided, postoperative children are universally at risk for developing hyponatremia. In a retrospective review of 24,412 surgical admissions to a large children's hospital, the incidence of significant postoperative hyponatremia was found to be 0.34% and mortality in these previously healthy children was high (8.4%).[62] This measured incidence, 340 cases and 29 deaths per 100,000, would suggest 7,448 cases of postoperative hyponatremia and 626 associated childhood deaths per year in the United States alone from an entirely avoidable cause.

Table 8-8. Composition of Body Fluids

Source	Na$^+$ (mEq/L)	K$^+$ (mEq/L)	Cl$^-$ (mEq/L)	HCO$_3^-$ (mEq/L)	pH	Osmolality (mOsm/L)
Gastric	50	10-15	150	0	1	300
Pancreas	140	5	0-100	100	9	300
Bile	130	5	100	40	8	300
Ileostomy	130	15-20	120	25-30	8	300
Diarrhea	50	35	40	50		
Sweat	50	5	55	0	Alkaline	
Blood	140	4-5	100	25	7.4	285-295
Urine	0-100*	20-100*	70-100*	0	4.5-8.5*	50-1400*

*Varies considerably with fluid intake.
From Herrin J: Fluid and electrolytes. In Graef JW (ed): Manual of Pediatric Therapeutics, 6th ed. Philadelphia, Lippincott-Raven, 1997, pp 63-75.

In reviewing the etiology of hyponatremia, two factors stand out: extensive extrarenal loss of electrolyte-containing fluid and intravenous replacement with hypotonic fluids.[62] In addition, delay in recognition often plays a major role in associated morbidity. The solution seems a simple one: (1) administration of hypotonic fluids without a specific indication should be minimized postoperatively, (2) ongoing losses should be replaced in a timely fashion, and (3) serum electrolytes should be measured in children exhibiting potential symptoms of hyponatremia (see subsequent discussion).

Postoperative Pulmonary Edema

Children who receive large volumes of fluid intraoperatively are at risk for developing pulmonary edema as third space fluids are mobilized. Usually, fluid mobilization begins to occur on the second postoperative day and continues through days 3 or 4. Although this is less common in children than in the elderly, it occurs occasionally in children with burn injuries[63] or pediatric patients receiving large amounts of fluid during resuscitation from trauma or sepsis. In one review,[64] 13 patients (11 adults and 2 children) were identified who developed postoperative pulmonary edema. All began to exhibit symptoms within 36 hours after surgery, and all received perioperative fluids in excess of 67 mL/kg.

Pathophysiologic States and Their Management

Fluid Overload and Edema

Edema is essentially a "sodium disease," representing sodium and water overload, with excessive fluid residing in the extracellular space. Although intracellular volume changes can sometimes be substantial, prolonged cell swelling represents failure of essential volume regulatory functions and is likely a preter-minal event. In fluid-overload states, plasma volume is generally elevated unless the balance of Starling forces is disturbed, as in nephrotic syndrome or lymphatic obstruction. Edema formation is opposed by (1) low compliance of the interstitial compartment, (2) increased lymphatic flow, (3) osmotic washout of interstitial proteins, and (4) impedance and elasticity of the proteoglycan gel. The differential diagnosis of fluid overload and edema formation is presented in Table 8-9. Principles of therapy for fluid overload states include the following:

- Fluid restriction
- Salt restriction
- Diuresis, dialysis
- Salt-poor albumin for diminished plasma volume

Dehydration States

For reasons outlined earlier, dehydration states are common in children. The extent of dehydration is best assessed by weight because clinical signs such as tachycardia, capillary refill, and skin elasticity,[65] although often reliable, may be influenced by factors other than hydration status. Capillary refill time of 1.5 to 3.0 seconds, for example, suggests a fluid deficit of between 50 and 100 mL/kg, yet this sign is extremely dependent on ambient temperature.[66] Similarly, poor skin elasticity reflects significant volume loss, yet elasticity may be well preserved in children with hypernatremic dehydration.[65] Clinical signs associated with varying levels of dehydration are presented in Table 8-10.

As a first approximation, correction of most dehydration states in older children is most readily achieved with administration of a simple bolus of 0.9 or 0.45 NS. In mild-to-moderate acute dehydration states, 0.33 NS in 20-mL/kg boluses has also been applied with good results.[67] When caring for infants or children with unusual, prolonged, or severe dehydration, however, management must be more precise. Kallen has

Table 8-9. Differential Diagnosis of Fluid Overload and Edema Formation

Condition	Differential Diagnosis
Imbalance of intake and output	Salt poisoning
	Formula dilution errors
	Intravenous infusion errors
	Drugs given as sodium salts
Steroid excess with normal sodium intake	Congenital adrenal hyperplasia
	Exogenous steroids
Perceived decreases in effective plasma volume	↓ MAP → baroreceptors → ↑ sympathetic tone, ADH, renin, aldosterone
	Vasodilators
	Congestive heart failure
	Cirrhosis
	Nephrotic syndrome
Impaired sodium excretion	Chronic renal failure
	Acute glomerular disease (↓ GFR with normal tubular function)
	Nonsteroidal anti-inflammatory drugs (↓ PGE_2 and RBF)
Water excess	SIADH
	Hypotonic infusion
	Stress (↑ ADH)

ADH, antidiuretic hormone; GFR, glomerular filtration rate; MAP, mean arterial pressure; PGE_2, prostaglandin E_2; RBF, renal blood flow; SIADH, syndrome of inappropriate antidiuretic hormone secretion.

Table 8-10. Clinical Signs and Symptoms for Estimation of Severity of Dehydration in Infants

| Clinical Signs | Degree of Dehydration | | |
	Mild	Moderate	Severe
Weight loss (%)	5	10	15
Behavior	Normal	Irritable	Hyperirritable to lethargic
Thirst	Slight	Moderate	Intense
Mucous membranes	May be normal	Dry	Parched
Tears	Present	±	Absent
Anterior fontanelle	Flat	±	Sunken
Skin turgor	Normal	±	Increased

Modified from Herrin J: Fluid and electrolytes. In Graef J (ed): Manual of Pediatric Therapeutics, 6th ed. Philadelphia, Lippincott-Raven, 1997, pp 63-75.

proposed a framework for approaching the dehydrated child that, although intended for the pediatrician, may be used by the anesthesiologist when facing a complex condition.[68] This approach uses a five-point assessment that calls attention to the following questions:

1. *Does a volume deficit exist and, if so, how great is it?*

   As noted previously, assessment of this is best made by weight, yet ballpark estimates of 3% (mild), 6% (moderate), and 9% (severe) may be made in older children based on clinical signs (see Table 8-10). Infants must be managed by weight only.

2. *Does an osmolar disturbance exist? Is it acute or chronic?*

   Identification of osmolar imbalance is made through measurement of serum sodium. The majority of clinically encountered dehydration states (~80%) are isotonic ($Na^+ = 130\text{-}150$ mEq/L). These patients have experienced isotonic losses and are easily managed by almost any strategy.

   Approximately 15% of dehydrated children present with hypertonic dehydration ($Na^+ > 150$ mEq/L). These children are at greatest risk and have usually experienced the greatest fluid losses for a given set of clinical signs.[69] If the condition is chronic, they may require extensive, slow rehydration over much longer periods.[70]

   Five percent of children may present with hypotonic dehydration and serum sodium levels below 130 mEq/L. For a given fluid deficit, these individuals are often more symptomatic than others and their requirement for sodium replacement is greatest. Surprisingly, rapid improvement in clinical condition often results from the first fluid bolus.

   In general, chronic dehydration states must be repaired slowly and acute dehydration states (<24 hours) may be corrected more rapidly. This is because cell volume equilibration occurs acutely through gain or loss of electrolytes (which may be moved rapidly) whereas cell volume equilibration occurs chronically through gain or loss of osmolytes (which are moved more slowly).[11] Re-equilibration of brain cell volume during correction of hypertonicity is often very slow, mandating patience in correction of chronic fluid deficits. Similarly, rapid correction of hyponatremic disturbances can be hazardous,[62] even when seemingly "safe" isotonic solutions are employed.[71]

3. *Does an acid-base abnormality exist?*

   Quantitation of the child's acid-base status gives useful, although limited, information as to the severity of dehydration. When evaluating acid-base status, it is important to recall that bicarbonate reabsorption and urine acidification are limited in preterm and young infants, leaving even the normal infant in a state of mild metabolic acidosis (pH, 7.3; Tco_2 20-21 mEq/L [normal 22-26 mEq/L]). Although slow spontaneous correction of acid-base status is typically observed on rehydration, rapid fluid boluses in poorly perfused children may result in a transient "reperfusion acidosis" as returning circulation washes the products of anaerobic metabolism out of the tissues. In this setting, or when renal insufficiency exists, blood-buffering capacity is such that children with serum bicarbonate concentrations below 8 mEq/L or pH less than 7.2 may benefit from administration of supplemental base (sodium bicarbonate) (Fig. 8-9).[68]

   Rapid bedside evaluation of acid-base status utilizes the following general relationships: a pH decrease of 0.1 unit accompanies a base excess (BE) of approximately 6 mEq/L or an increase in Pco_2 of 10 to 12 mm Hg. The total replacement base required is then determined by the following equation:

   $$\text{Dose (mEq)} = 0.3 \times \text{Wt (kg)} \times \text{BE (mEq/L)}$$

   Clinically, a smaller sodium bicarbonate dose (1-2 mEq/kg) is given initially, the response is verified by blood gas analysis, and the remaining doses are titrated to effect.

4. *Is renal function impaired?*

   Initial evaluation includes information as to last urine void and recent urine output, measurement of urine specific gravity, and serum levels of blood urea nitrogen and creatinine. If uncertainty persists, measurement of serum and urine electrolytes for comparison and calculation of the FE_{Na} is indicated (see Chapter 26).

   FE_{Na} values less than 1% imply prerenal conditions causing renal dysfunction, whereas FE_{Na} values greater than 2% to 3% suggest renal insufficiency. In prematurity, however, values as high as 9% may be seen in otherwise normal infants.

5. *What is the state of potassium balance?*

   Potassium homeostasis is critical to life, and serum potassium levels are generally maintained within a very narrow range. Nonetheless, serum potassium levels do not reflect whole-body stores and substantial potassium depletion may exist in the presence of modest changes in serum potassium concentration (K^+_{serum}). Gastrointestinal losses or metabolic acidosis is usually accompanied by a potassium deficit, whereas other dehydration states are not. Rapid fluid boluses or pH correction, or both, may acutely reduce K^+_{serum},[72] and

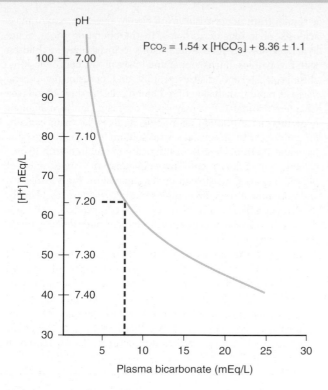

Figure 8-9. This figure, based on data from children with metabolic acidosis,[108] depicts the displacement of pH as serum bicarbonate declines. The zone of rapid pH displacement (pH < 7.20) has a slope that is several times greater than the zone of gradual pH displacement (pH 7.20 or higher). As the pH moves through the zone of rapid pH displacement, a further decline of serum bicarbonate, of as little as 1 or 2 mEq/L, produces a highly leveraged further decrease of pH. (From Kallen RJ: The management of diarrheal dehydration in infants using parenteral fluids. Pediatr Clin North Am 1990; 37:265-286.)

In the graph: $P_{CO_2} = 1.54 \times [HCO_3^-] + 8.36 \pm 1.1$

refractory hypokalemia may occur in children deficient in magnesium.[73] In all cases, adequate renal function should be present before administration of potassium and complete repletion should be accomplished over 48 to 72 hours.

Once the nature and severity of dehydration have been determined, the clinician may proceed using any one of a variety of correction strategies. In one approach, moderate to severe dehydration deficits may be estimated, as in Table 8-10. Fluid and electrolyte repair may then proceed according to a three-phase approach wherein circulating plasma volume, perfusion, and urine output are restored rapidly using isotonic crystalloid or colloid solution and remaining deficits are corrected over 24 hours as outlined[74]:

- *Emergency Phase:* 20-30 mL/kg isotonic crystalloid/colloid bolus
- *Repletion Phase 1:* 25-50 mL/kg (or half of deficit) over 6 to 8 hours. Anions: Cl⁻ 75%, acetate 25%
- *Repletion Phase 2:* remainder of deficit over 24 hours (isotonic) or 48 hours (hypertonic). Include calcium replacement as necessary.

Hypernatremia and Hyponatremia

As previously detailed, disorders of sodium equilibrium are primarily marked by disturbances of fluid balance and are corrected according to the principles outlined earlier.

Serious hypernatremia or hyponatremia is accompanied by neurologic symptoms whose severity is determined by the degree and rate of change of serum sodium concentration (Na^+_{serum}).

Hypernatremia

Unlike in adults, *acute hypernatremia* is common in children. A mortality rate of greater than 40% for the acute disorder and 10% for the chronic disorder has been quoted for hypernatremia (serum sodium >160 mEq/L). Mortality and permanent neurologic injury are even more common in infants. Depending on degree and duration, neurologic findings include irritability and coma. Seizures may be a presenting symptom, yet are more commonly encountered after the start of therapy. Children with acute conditions are usually symptomatic, whereas those with chronic conditions (acclimated individuals) may be asymptomatic. General principles for treatment of hypernatremia are as follows:

- In the setting of circulatory collapse, colloid or NS bolus should be administered. Although debatable, colloid bolus provides the theoretical benefit of sustained hemodynamic support with lower fluid load. Saline, in contrast, rapidly re-equilibrates, necessitating repeated boluses while adding to the total salt burden.
- On the basis of the principles outlined earlier, fluid deficit should be assessed as accurately as possible and corrected over 48 hours. Free water excess will be required. Continued reassessment of serum sodium and osmolality should be made, aiming for correction of no more than 1 to 2 mOsm/L/hr. Because of possible associated hypoglycemia, some solutions should be glucose-containing and serum glucose levels should be monitored.
- Vigilance for seizures, apnea, and cardiovascular compromise should be maintained, because such complicating factors can be the primary determinates of successful outcome.

Hyponatremia

Hyponatremia is also common in infants and children. Increasing prevalence due to erroneous formula dilution has intermittently been reported.[75,76] In the practice of anesthesiology, mild hyponatremia is a common postoperative condition after surgery of any severity[77]; in neurosurgical patients, hyponatremia may represent cerebral salt wasting or SIADH.[78] In general, symptomatic patients are acutely hyponatremic and asymptomatic individuals are chronically hyponatremic.[79] After surgery, acutely hyponatremic children may present with nonspecific symptoms that are often erroneously attributed to other causes. Early central nervous system symptoms include headache, nausea, weakness, and anorexia. Advancing symptoms include mental status changes, confusion, irritability, progressive obtundation, and seizures. Respiratory arrest (or irregularity) is a common manifestation of advanced hyponatremia.

When approaching the correction of hyponatremia, symptomatic children must be considered a medical emergency, whereas asymptomatic children do not require rapid intervention. Correction of chronic hyponatremia must be slow and limited to no more than 0.5 mEq/L/hr so as to avoid neurologic complications.[80] The best treatment for acute hyponatremia is early recognition and intervention. Because hypoxia will exacerbate neurologic injury, the simple ABCs of resuscitation are attended to first and the airway is secured in the child with seizures or respiratory irregularity. Hyponatremic seizures may be quieted by relatively modest (3-6 mEq/L) increases of serum sodium.[81] In several series,[76,82,83] such limited, rapid correction of symptomatic hyponatremia with hypertonic saline (514 mEq/L NaCl) was found to be well tolerated. It should be emphasized, however, that complete correction is unnecessary and unwise.[84] Initial therapy is aimed at raising serum sodium no more than is necessary to stop seizure activity (usually 3-5 mEq/L). Further correction is carried out over several days. Hypertonic saline may be used for correction until the serum sodium increases to greater than 120 mEq/L. Total sodium deficit is estimated as follows:

Sodium change (mEq/L) × fraction TBW (L/kg) × weight (kg) = mEq sodium

$(\text{Desired } [Na^+]_{serum} - \text{Observed } [Na^+]_{serum}) \times 0.6^* \times \text{weight (kg)}$ = mEq sodium required

In the 25-kg child with a serum sodium of 110 mEq/L, to correct to 125 mEq/L using hypertonic saline (514 mEq/L), infuse

(125 mEq/L − 110 mEq/L) × 0.6 × 25 = 225 mEq total

or

225 mEq/514 mEq/L = 0.44 L over 48 hours = 9 mL/hr

Because such calculations involve estimates, frequent measurement of serum sodium values is necessary during correction. As with hypernatremia, much of the morbidity and mortality associated with hyponatremia relates to complicating factors such as seizures and hypoxia that may occur during therapy. Thus, children undergoing therapy should be cared for in a monitored setting. When overzealous correction has occurred (seizures), there may be value in acutely re-lowering Na^+_{serum} using hypotonic fluids,[79] although such therapy is not without its own hazards.

General principles for treatment of hyponatremia are as follows:

- Asymptomatic hyponatremia in and of itself need not be rapidly corrected. Associated cardiovascular compromise due to volume depletion may be addressed by colloid bolus or administration of isotonic saline (1 L/m²/day). Provision of sodium is accompanied by free water restriction.
- Symptomatic hyponatremia is a medical emergency and may sometimes reflect irreversible neurologic injury. Correction should be rapid, yet limited, as discussed previously. A dose of 3 mL/kg of 3% saline (514 mEq/L) may be administered over 20 to 30 minutes to halt seizures.
- Subsequent correction is accomplished through calculation of sodium deficit and provision of sodium so as to slowly correct at a rate not to exceed 0.5 mEq/L/hr or 25 mEq/L (total) in 24 to 48 hours.
- If attendant fluid load is excessive or if oliguria is present, diuretics may be useful.

Disorders of Potassium Homeostasis

Hyperkalemia
Hyperkalemia is occasionally the presenting finding in conditions such as congenital adrenal hyperplasia. More commonly,

*As discussed earlier, TBW may range from 75% in infancy to 60% or less in older children.

it results from acute renal insufficiency, massive tissue injury, acidosis, or iatrogenic mishaps. In the operating room, acute hyperkalemia may follow the use of succinylcholine in children with myopathies, burns, upper and lower motor neuron lesions, chronic sepsis and disuse atrophy, and occasionally during massive, rapid transfusion of red blood cells or whole blood (see Chapters 6 and 10).[85] It may occur as a late sign in malignant hyperthermia. Although neurologic status is the main concern for children with abnormal serum sodium levels, cardiac status (rate and rhythm) determines the care of children with hyperkalemia. In children with hyperkalemia, the appearance of peaked T waves is followed by lengthening of the PR interval and widening of the QRS complex until P waves are lost. Finally, the QRS complex merges with its T wave to produce a sinusoidal pattern (Fig. 8-10). Successful treatment traditionally utilizes the following approach:

- Emergent therapy is first directed toward antagonism of potassium's cardiac effects by administration of calcium (calcium chloride 0.1 to 0.3 mL/kg of a 10% solution or calcium gluconate 0.3 to 1.0 mL/kg of a 10% solution over 3 to 5 minutes). (*Note:* Calcium does not decrease the serum potassium concentration but rather reestablishes the gradient between the resting membrane potential [increased in

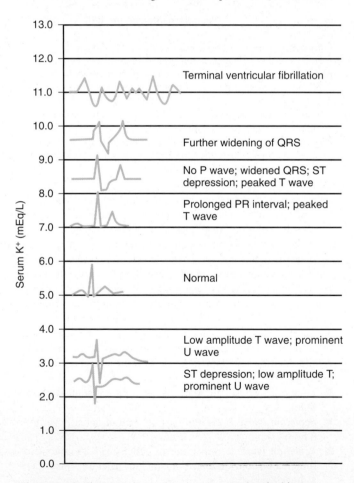

Figure 8-10. Electrocardiographic changes associated with hyperkalemia. (From Williams GS, Klenk EL, Winters RW: Acute renal failure in pediatrics. In Winters RW [ed]: The Body Fluids in Pediatrics: Medical, Surgical, and Neonatal Disorders of Acid-Base Status, Hydration, and Oxygenation. Boston, Little, Brown, 1973, pp 523-557.)

the presence of hyperkalemia] and the threshold potential [determined by the calcium concentration] as well as increases the refractory period of the action potential, the net effect being the prevention of spontaneous depolarization).

■ Serum potassium is then reduced by returning potassium to the intracellular space by correcting acidosis through administration of sodium bicarbonate (1-2 mEq/kg), mild to moderate hyperventilation, and administration of a β agonist.

■ To maintain potassium in the intracellular space, glucose and insulin are administered by infusion (0.5-1 g/kg glucose with 0.1 U/kg insulin over 30-60 minutes).

■ After stabilization, attention is directed toward removal of the whole-body potassium burden (Kayexalate, dialysis) and correction of the underlying cause (Fig. 8-11).

The knowledge that β-adrenergic stimulation modulates the translocation of potassium into the intracellular space[86,87] has prompted the consideration of β agonists in the treatment of acute hyperkalemia.[88-91] In children, a single infusion of salbutamol (5 μg/kg over 15 minutes) has been shown to effectively lower serum potassium concentrations within 30 minutes. The rapidity, efficacy, and safety observed with this therapy in a study of 15 children led its authors to conclude that salbutamol is a reasonable first-choice treatment for hyperkalemia.[88] In addition

to intravenous therapy, both salbutamol[92] and albuterol[91] have been found to be effective when given by inhalation.

This route has the significant advantages of being readily available in emergency departments and not requiring intravenous access. However, the observation that a paradoxical exacerbation of hyperkalemia sometimes occurs on initiation of treatment,[92] together with concerns regarding the possibility of associated arrhythmias,[93] suggests that more experience is required before such therapy can be considered the standard of care. Inhalation of albuterol during such an event in the operating room may speed the reduction in serum potassium while instituting other methods of treatment.

Hypokalemia

Hypokalemia is most common in children as a complication of diarrhea or persistent vomiting associated with gastroenteritis. In the operating room or intensive care unit, hypokalemia may also accompany a wide variety of other conditions, including diabetes, hyperaldosteronism, pyloric stenosis, starvation, renal tubular disease, chronic steroid or diuretic use, and β-agonist therapy. Severe hypokalemia is accompanied by electrocardiographic changes, including QT prolongation, diminution of the T wave, and appearance of U waves (see Fig. 8-10).

TREATMENT ALGORITHM FOR HYPERKALEMIA

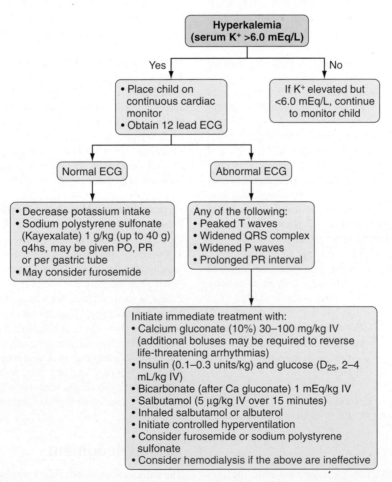

Figure 8-11. After stabilization, attention is directed toward removal of the whole-body potassium burden (Kayexalate, dialysis) and correction of the underlying cause.

As noted previously, serum potassium levels do not accurately reflect total potassium homeostasis and low serum levels may or may not be associated with significant total body potassium depletion. Indeed, the extracellular fraction of potassium is only a tiny proportion (approximately 3%) of the entire body store. The precise point to begin replacement therapy, therefore, is controversial, and total replacement requirements are impossible to calculate. In general practice, serum potassium values (K^+_{serum}) between 2.0 and 2.5 mEq/L are corrected before surgery on the assumption that further decreases may predispose the child to arrhythmias and hemodynamic instability.

Potassium replacement is best accomplished orally over an extended period while the underlying cause is evaluated and treated. When intravenous correction is required, concentrations up to 40 mEq/L may be given slowly (*not to exceed 1 mEq/ kg/hr*) in a monitored setting. Because such solutions often cause phlebitis, large-bore or central catheters are preferred. In the setting of hypochloremic hypokalemia, chloride deficits must first be replaced, usually via administration of normal saline.

Syndrome of Inappropriate Antidiuretic Hormone Secretion

The many factors capable of stimulating ADH release make the syndrome of inappropriate ADH release common (see Chapter 26). As detailed earlier, intravascular depletion is the most potent stimulus for vasopressin release, yet the term *inappropriate* generally refers to control of osmolality. Pain, surgical stress, critical illness, sepsis, pulmonary disease, central nervous system injury, and a variety of drugs may all stimulate ADH release above and beyond that necessary to maintain osmolar balance.

SIADH is common in children yet often overlooked. Minor head trauma, for example, may elicit spikes in ADH levels, although infrequently to the point of producing serious hyponatremia and seizures.[94] Urine output in postoperative spinal fusion patients is often reduced by elevated ADH levels and routinely returns within 24 hours without specific therapy.[95] Infants with bronchiolitis and hyperinflated lungs frequently possess markedly elevated plasma ADH levels and exhibit fluid retention, weight gain, urinary concentration, and plasma hypo-osmolality until their illness begins to resolve.[96] Hyponatremia to the point of seizures, however, is only occasionally observed.

The diagnosis of SIADH rests on the identification of impaired urinary dilution in the setting of plasma hypo-osmolality. Hyponatremia ($Na^+ < 135$ mEq/L), serum osmolality less than 280 mOsm/L, and urine osmolality greater than 100 mOsm/L in the absence of volume depletion, cardiac failure, nephropathy, adrenal insufficiency, or cirrhosis are generally considered sufficient for diagnosis. Therapeutic principles are similar to those of hyponatremia and rest on the following:
- Free water restriction
- Repletion of sodium deficits (if present)
- Countering of vasopressin effects with judicious use of diuretics

Diabetes Insipidus

In the operating room and the intensive care unit, diabetes insipidus is most commonly associated with the care of neurosurgical patients.[97-99] Diabetes insipidus is also caused by neuroendocrine failure in brain death, and management may be necessary if organ donation is requested.[100,101] Diabetes insipidus results from decreased secretion of, or renal insensitivity to, vasopressin (see Chapter 26). Manifestations include massive polyuria, volume contraction, dehydration, and plasma hyperosmolality. Dilute polyuria (<250 mOsm, >2 mL/kg/hr) in the presence of hypernatremia ($Na^+ > 145$ mEq/L) with hyperosmolality (>300 mOsm/L) is the hallmark. In central diabetes insipidus, administration of desmopressin produces urine concentration yet water deprivation does not. Postoperative diabetes insipidus may initially be difficult to distinguish from mobilization of operative fluids.

Children with craniopharyngiomas or a similarly situated pathologic lesion may not manifest vasopressin deficiency early in the disease but become symptomatic preoperatively after steroid administration or intraoperatively on surgical manipulation. Postoperative diabetes insipidus typically begins the evening after surgery and may resolve in 3 to 5 days if osmoregulatory structures have not been permanently injured. An often-confusing triphasic response may also occur wherein postoperative diabetes insipidus appears to resolve, fluid status normalizes, or SIADH appears and then vasopressin secretion ceases and diabetes insipidus returns. It is hypothesized that this pattern reflects nonspecific vasopressin release from a degenerating pituitary gland.

Attempts have been made to develop protocols for perioperative management of diabetes insipidus.[102] Because vasopressin is difficult to titrate to urine output, our practice involves maximal antidiuresis and fluid restriction. In this setting, volume status must be monitored closely because urine output is no longer a marker of renal perfusion. Children who need close perioperative monitoring for the development of diabetes insipidus include those with preexisting diabetes insipidus as well as those who will undergo procedures that may increase the risk of development of diabetes insipidus. Children who undergo resection of craniopharyngiomas, pituitary lesions, or other procedures that involve resection/manipulation of the pituitary stalk are at particular risk.[103]

Hyperchloremic Metabolic Acidosis

Administration of large amounts of 0.9% NaCl (NS) can lead to excess serum chloride.[104] The chloride content of NS is 154 mEq/L. This excess of chloride ions can subsequently lead to a hyperchloremic acidosis, which has been categorized as a "strong-ion acidosis."[105,106] This type of acidosis results from an excess of strong anions (e.g., lactate, ketoacids, sulfates) relative to the strong cations. Thus, as the strong ion difference increases, acidosis occurs. The magnitude of the acidosis is related to the amount of 0.9% NaCl administered as well as the rate of administration. Scheingraber and associates demonstrated that infusions of NS of 35 mL/kg over 2 hours in healthy patients undergoing gynecologic surgery resulted in acidosis. Acidosis did not occur with similar infusions of lactated Ringer's solution.[104]

Acknowledgment

The authors acknowledge the contributions of Letty M. P. Liu to previous editions of this chapter.

Annotated References

Arieff AI, Ayus JC, Fraser CL: Hyponatraemia and death or permanent brain damage in healthy children. BMJ 1992; 304:1218-1222

Much concern has been displayed in recent years to iatrogenic hyponatremia caused by administration of hypotonic solutions. This study highlights the grave consequences of such errors.

Constable PD: Hyperchloremic acidosis: the classic example of strong ion acidosis. Anesth Analg 2003; 96:919-922

This review is an excellent description of alternative methods of evaluating acid-base status. The focus of this paper is in the physiology behind the acidosis created by large, rapid administration of normal saline.

Friis-Hansen B: Body water compartments in children: changes during growth and related changes in body composition. Pediatrics 1961; 28:169-181

This classic paper is important because it describes the developmental aspects of fluid compartments in children from infants to teenagers.

Holliday MA, Segar WE: The maintenance need for water in parenteral fluid therapy. Pediatrics 1957; 19:823-832

This classic paper represents the background for contemporary fluid management in pediatrics. This article discusses the fluid requirements in healthy children and provides a basis for calculation of fluid deficits during the perioperative period. The figures quoted in this study may not represent intraoperative fluid requirements in children with varying disease states.

Shires T, Williams J, Brown F: Acute change in extracellular fluids associated with major surgical procedures. Ann Surg 1961; 154:803-810

This classic study from 1961 describes the phenomenon of fluid movement throughout the various compartments during surgical procedures. Specifically, it showed that, during surgery, plasma volume is supported at the expense of extravascular volume. The concept of "third spacing" of isotonic fluids is also described.

References

Please see www.expertconsult.com

Essentials of Hematology

Charles M. Haberkern, Nicole E. Webel, Michael J. Eisses, and M. A. Bender

CHAPTER 9

| The Basics |
| Laboratory Values and Diagnostic Tests |
| Guidelines for Transfusion |
| **Hemolytic Anemias** |
| Hereditary Spherocytosis |
| Glucose-6-Phosphate Dehydrogenase Deficiency |
| Hemoglobinopathies |
| **Thrombocytopenia** |
| Idiopathic Thrombocytopenia Purpura |
| **Coagulation Disorders** |
| Screening |
| von Willebrand Disease |
| Hemophilia |
| **Cancer and Hematopoietic Stem Cell Transplantation** |
| Cancer |
| Hematopoietic Stem Cell Transplantation |

HEMATOLOGIC DISEASES IN CHILDHOOD may present to the anesthesiologist in many different ways. They may be the primary cause for a surgical procedure, such as hereditary spherocytosis in a child undergoing splenectomy, or a factor complicating a surgical procedure, such as sickle cell disease in a child undergoing tonsillectomy. In addition, questions related to such hematologic problems as anemia, thrombocytopenia, coagulopathy, childhood cancer, and hematopoietic stem cell transplantation are often raised in the perioperative setting.

In this chapter we address the hematologic considerations and disease entities of significant interest to pediatric anesthesiologists in the perioperative period. We shall highlight issues of importance to the hematologist that the anesthesiologist should incorporate into the care of a child.

The Basics

Laboratory Values and Diagnostic Tests

What is a "normal" hematocrit or platelet count for an infant or child who comes to the operating room? Red blood cell, white blood cell, platelet, and coagulation indices evolve in varying ways through late gestation, the neonatal period, infancy, and childhood (Table 9-1).

The full-term neonate has a relative polycythemia, reticulocytosis, and leukocytosis compared with the child. The term neonate has prolongation of both prothrombin time (PT) and activated partial thromboplastin time (aPTT) owing to a relative deficiency in vitamin K–dependent factors. In addition, the neonate has decreased plasma concentrations of proteins C and S, a condition that increases the likelihood of thrombosis.[1] The hematologic indices of the preterm neonate are closer to those of the child except for PT and aPTT, both of which are prolonged in the preterm neonate. This has been attributed to deficiencies in vitamin K–dependent factors, as well as an approximate 10% reduction in the plasma concentration of fibrinogen. The international normalized ratio (INR), a normalized PT, has an average value of 1.0 through all age groups.

After the immediate neonatal period, preterm and full-term infants experience "physiologic anemia," presumably due to the downregulating effect of increased oxygen supply in extrauterine life on erythropoiesis and to the dilutional effect of a rapidly increasing blood volume. Preterm infants reach their nadir hemoglobin of 7 to 9 g/dL at 3 to 6 postnatal weeks, and full-term infants reach their nadir hemoglobin level of 9 to 11 g/dL at 8 to 12 postnatal weeks. Most hematologic values reach adult norms by the end of infancy, although some continue to change gradually into the second decade. All of these changes underscore the importance of laboratory reports with age-adjusted standards.

There is no ideal single screening test to assess the *bleeding risk* of a child in the perioperative period. What about bleeding time and the thromboelastogram (TEG)?

Bleeding time appears to be greater in the infant and child (and less in the neonate) than it is in the adult, but the range of values is wide and overlapping (see Table 9-1). Although this test is potentially helpful in predicting post-tonsillectomy and adenoidectomy hemorrhage,[2] as well as hemorrhage after percutaneous renal[3] and liver[4] biopsy, there is little evidence to support its use as a screening test to predict bleeding in the presence of a careful, inclusive clinical history.[5,6]

The TEG has been utilized to evaluate and investigate coagulation status in children undergoing spinal fusion,[7] neurosurgical procedures,[8] and cardiopulmonary bypass for cardiothoracic procedures.[9] Although the TEG may provide useful information in the surgical setting to evaluate fibrinolysis, hypercoagulability, and other coagulation perturbations, its use is usually limited to clinical scenarios with dynamic coagulation changes, such as open-heart surgery with cardiopulmonary bypass and liver transplantation. The platelet function analyzer (PFA-100) analysis is an additional test increasingly utilized for the assessment

Table 9-7. Agents That May Precipitate Hemolysis In G6PD Deficiency

Antibiotics
Sulfonamides

Co-trimoxazole (Bactrim, Septrin)

Dapsone

Chloramphenicol

Nitrofurantoin

Nalidixic acid

Antimalarials
Chloroquine

Hydroxychloroquine

Primaquine

Quinine

Mepacrine

Other Medications
Aspirin

Phenacetin

Sulfasalazine

Methyldopa

Vitamin C (large doses)

Hydralazine

Procainamide

Quinidine

Chemicals
Moth balls (naphthalene)

Methylene blue

Food
Fava ("broad") beans

Table 9-8. Perioperative Considerations and Concerns in G6PD Deficiency

Preoperative
History of hemolysis and precipitating factors

Hemoglobin, reticulocyte count

Intraoperative
Avoidance of triggering agents

Caution in use of high doses of agents that increase methemoglobin, especially in infants

Hemoglobin and urine output in high-risk settings (e.g., cardiopulmonary bypass)

Postoperative
Hemoglobin, reticulocyte count, urine output if hemolysis

particularly susceptible to both symptomatic methemoglobinemia (owing to their low NADH dehydrogenase activity) and to methemoglobin-induced hemolysis if G6PD deficient. Furthermore, *treatment of methemoglobinemia with methylene blue is contraindicated in these infants because the agent itself may precipitate hemolysis.*[39] It should also be noted that hemolysis has occurred during cardiopulmonary bypass in G6PD-deficient children.[41,42]

Hemoglobinopathies

Sickle Cell Disease
First identified by Herrick about 100 years ago, sickle cell disease is a group of inherited hemoglobinopathies with a widely varying worldwide prevalence. The disease affects about 1 : 375 African American births[43] and includes the following: sickle cell anemia (HbSS), which accounts for about 70% of the American sickle cell disease population; sickle cell/hemoglobin C disease (HbSC), about 20% of the sickle population; sickle cell/β-thalassemia (HbSβ disease), about 10%; and a host of other, uncommon sickle variants.[44] Both HbSC and sickle cell/hemoglobin D disease (HbSD) have the potential for significant clinical sickling. Sickle cell trait (HbAS), in which approximately 40% of

hemoglobin is hemoglobin S, occurs in about 8% of African Americans and in a much smaller percentage of Hispanic and other American subpopulations. The sickle gene is found commonly in Africa, Mediterranean areas, southwestern Asia, and other areas where malaria has been historically endemic and for which the gene is protective. Sickle hemoglobinopathies have many implications for perioperative care, and they increase perioperative morbidity and mortality.

Pathophysiology
Hemoglobin A is composed of two α- and two β-globin chains. Hemoglobin S is caused by a mutant β-globin gene on chromosome 11 leading to a single amino acid substitution (valine for glutamate at position 6). Replacement of negatively charged and hydrophilic glutamate by noncharged and hydrophobic valine leads to instability of the hemoglobin molecule and decreased solubility of the molecule when deoxygenated. Hemoglobin polymers form, generating long helical strands and inducing a process that leads to hemoglobin precipitation and hemolysis.[45]

Classically, the pathophysiology and clinical complications of sickle cell disease were thought to be related primarily to accumulation in the microvasculature of sickled erythrocytes in the setting of factors that promote hemoglobin deoxygenation (i.e., hypoxia, acidosis, hyperthermia) and interfere with peripheral perfusion (i.e., dehydration and hypothermia). This accumulation of sickled cells compromises microcirculation, produces ischemia, and thereby generates further red cell sickling and end organ compromise.

It is now appreciated that the pathophysiologic process in sickle cell disease is much more complex.[45-47] Interactions among red cells, endothelial cells, and such plasma constituents as thrombin contribute to microvascular occlusion.[48] Inflammation, vascular endothelial adhesion abnormalities, platelets, and coagulation cascade activation all contribute to vaso-occlusive related complications. The sickle red cell membrane, exposed to the destructive oxidant effects of intracellular iron, develops altered transmembrane ion transport pathways, which lead to altered permeability to sodium, potassium, and calcium, thereby producing cellular dehydration and irreversible sickling.[49] Membrane abnormalities of phospholipid content also contribute to its deformability, and exposure of phosphatidyl serine facilitates activation of the clotting cascade. These and other factors then lead to entrapment of irreversibly sickled red cells in the microcirculation, activation of coagulation and inflammatory pathways, ischemia, and infarction of tissue. At the same time, chronic intravascular hemolysis decreases production of nitric oxide (NO), while increased scavenging decreases its bioavailability. The resulting deficiency of NO contributes to endothelial dysfunction and such disease com-plications as pulmonary hypertension, priapism, and skin ulceration.[49,50]

Clinical and Laboratory Features and Treatment

Sickle cell disease is a multisystem process involving potentially most organs of the body and often necessitating surgical intervention. Based on data collected in the early 1990s, approximately one third of patients with HbSS disease have a progressive disease with organ dysfunction and death; about half have significant but less devastating disease; and the remainder have a reasonably stable, slowly progressive clinical course.[51] Therapeutic interventions and genetic factors account in large part for the differences in outcome. Children with persistence of hemoglobin F (which itself protects against the effects of deoxygenation on red cells) and those with HbSC or HbSβ$^+$ (as compared with HbSS or HbSβ$^\circ$), have fewer complications (see later).

Early diagnosis and treatment of sickle cell disease have been remarkably facilitated over the past decades by the widespread institution of neonatal screening, first utilized by the state of New York in 1975. The majority of screening programs use isoelectric focusing of an eluate from dried blood spot samples also used to screen for other disorders. Because a small percentage of children with sickle cell disease are non–African American (i.e., Native American, Hispanic, and even Caucasian),[43] selective screening may not detect all affected infants. As of 2006, all 50 states and the District of Columbia screen all neonates for sickle hemoglobinopathies. Families of infants diagnosed with sickle trait (HbAS) on neonatal screening may not be made aware of the diagnosis, but fortunately these infants rarely develop significant clinical problems in the perioperative period.

Affected children born within the United States before universal neonatal screening and those born outside the United States and not receiving regular health care may not have received diagnosis and appropriate care before a surgical procedure. Notwithstanding controversy over the utility of nonselective preoperative screening,[52] children at risk whose hemoglobin status is not known preoperatively should be tested with a sickle screening test, followed by a hemoglobin electrophoretic evaluation if screening is positive. However, infants younger than 6 months of age may have a false-negative screening test because of presence of fetal hemoglobin, although electrophoresis should be diagnostic. Children older than age 10 years with a normal hemoglobin value *and* unremarkable clinical history are probably at a reduced risk for clinically significant hemoglobinopathy.[53]

Common clinical symptoms of sickle cell disease in children include chronic hemolytic anemia, recurrent episodes of vaso-occlusive pain crisis (VOC), acute chest syndrome (ACS), infection, renal insufficiency, osteonecrosis, and cholelithiasis. Chronic pulmonary and neurologic disease (e.g., stroke) are additional causes of significant morbidity and mortality.[44] In the perioperative period, the most common complications in sickle cell children include acute chest syndrome (about 10%), fever or infection (about 7%), VOC (about 5%), and transfusion-related events (about 10%).[54]

Chronic hemolytic anemia is a hallmark of HbSS disease and is characterized by a baseline hemoglobin value of 5 to 9 g/dL (often >9 g/dL in HbSC disease), reticulocytosis (5%-10%), and a distinctive red cell morphology on peripheral smear.[47] Chronic hemolysis is associated with increased red cell turnover and a propensity to form biliary stones. It may be complicated by other anemic events: acute splenic sequestration, typically in infants and young children following a viral illness; acute aplastic anemia, typically in association with parvovirus B19 infection. For some children, chronic and acute severe anemia is managed with red cell transfusions, although these children are prone to develop alloantibodies to red cell antigens. Most children are maintained on chronic folic acid therapy to prevent megaloblastic erythropoiesis that can accompany increased requirements for red cell production.

VOC in sickle cell disease occurs as a result of episodic microvasculature occlusions at one or more sites. The occlusive process occurs most commonly in phalanges (dactylitis, or "hand-foot syndrome"), long bones, ribs, sternum, spine and the pelvis; it also can occur in the mesenteric microvasculature, thereby producing abdominal pain that may mimic a surgical acute abdomen. These crises are managed with hydration, warmth, acute and chronic pain management (including opioids, anti-inflammatory agents, and complementary modalities), and often in-hospital care. It is essential to foster an ideal environment for pain control (e.g., calm, pleasant distractions as well as supportive personnel and objects). For children who have frequent and/or severe crises, oral hydroxyurea therapy has been shown to be effective in decreasing the frequency of events through a number of mechanisms, including the following: inhibiting hemoglobin precipitation by increasing fetal hemoglobin concentrations; reducing the white blood cell count; modifying inflammatory response; and facilitating NO metabolism.[50,55,56] Inhaled NO itself may prove to be effective therapy for VOC.[57]

ACS is characterized by development of acute respiratory symptoms concurrent with a new infiltrate evident on chest radiography, usually defined as involvement of at least one complete lung segment.[58] ACS frequently occurs with VOC, and its clinical presentation is quite variable, including fever, tachypnea, cough, and hypoxemia. The process may be self-limited over a period of a few days, or it may progress to respiratory failure (15%) and even death. The variable presentation is in part due to the complex and variable pathogenesis of ACS. An episode may be due to single or multiple causes, including infection (bacterial [often *Chlamydia* or *Mycoplasma*], viral and mixed flora), pulmonary fat embolism, pulmonary infarction, and pulmonary hemorrhage.[59] Acute management includes supportive care and oxygen, antibiotics to cover encapsulated and atypical organisms, bronchodilators, pain control, ventilatory support as needed and, often, transfusion. Incentive spirometry or continuous positive airway pressure can also be helpful, especially in the perioperative setting. Hydroxyurea therapy and chronic transfusion therapy have been shown to decrease ACS frequency, whereas inhaled NO has been shown to ameliorate the process acutely.[50,60-62] Children with sickle cell disease have also been shown to commonly have increased airway reactivity, which may be due in part to NO deficiency and which is responsive to bronchodilator therapy.[63,64] In later life children with sickle cell disease may develop restrictive lung disease and pulmonary hypertension, the development of which

can be effective in managing of VOS as well as providing perioperative anesthetic care.[103] Hyperventilation should be avoided because of its potential to reduce cerebral perfusion in children at an increased risk of stroke.[104] The use of a tourniquet in HbSS and HbAS diseases has been questioned.[105-107] However, tourniquets have been applied intraoperatively for up to 2 hours without complication, and the predominance of evidence supports their safe use as long as they are used carefully and selectively in combination with general guidelines of perioperative care.[108-111] Intraoperative blood salvage via cell saver devices has also been used safely in sickle cell patients,[112] although there is some evidence that the salvage device itself may produce sickling in the processed blood.[113] Cardiopulmonary bypass would seem to be an optimal setting in which to induce sickling, given the cold, hypoxic, acidotic, and stagnant environment created therein. Although there are reports of bypass surgery conducted in children with both HbSS and HbAS with standard bypass procedures without transfusion,[114-116] these children are generally managed with aggressive exchange transfusion before or during bypass.

Thalassemias

The thalassemia disorders are among the most common genetic disorders worldwide, and they are characterized by a perturbation of the normal 1:1 ratio of α to β polypeptide chains, usually due to reduced synthesis of one polypeptide. The clinical severity of the disease in a child is a function of the degree of alteration of the synthetic ratio, ranging from an asymptomatic carrier state to chronic symptomatic hemolytic anemia to fetal death due to hydrops fetalis. α-Thalassemias commonly affect children of Southeast Asian descent and also occur in those of African and Mediterranean descent; β-thalassemias also affect primarily children of Mediterranean, African, and Southeast Asian descent. Whereas state neonatal assays screening for HbS can often detect many forms of α-thalassemia, these tests can detect only profound forms of β-thalassemia because of the small levels of adult β chains in the neonate. The concomitant presence of qualitatively abnormal hemoglobins (e.g., HgS or HgE) affects the clinical course of the disease. Both the primary hemolytic anemia and therapy utilized in the treatment of the disease may affect perioperative care.

Pathophysiology

Anemia in thalassemia is the result of both hemolysis and ineffective erythropoiesis, the latter the result of accelerated cell apoptosis triggered by excess deposition of unpaired globin chains in erythroid precursors.[117] Unpaired globin subunits are oxidized and form hemichromes, whose rate of formation determines rate of hemolysis. Because unpaired α chains undergo this process more readily than do β chains, β-thalassemia tends to be more severe than α-thalassemia. Precipitation of hemichromes leads to a complex process that includes release of toxic agents and formation of reactive oxygen species; alteration of red cell membranes (causing cells to become rigid, aggregate, and disintegrate); and, finally, activation of the coagulation process. As a result of chronic anemia and ineffective erythropoiesis, bone expansion and extramedullary hematopoiesis may develop in the liver and spleen, and marrow space expansion at sites such as the cranium and paravertebral areas can lead to disfiguring bony changes.

Clinical and Laboratory Features and Treatment

The disease picture in α-thalassemia is due to complete loss of expression of one to four α-globin genes. As a four-gene globin deletion, it is characterized by hydrops and in-utero or perinatal death; as a three-gene deletion, or hemoglobin H (HgH), it is characterized by chronic hemolytic anemia, which may be exacerbated by exposure to stress and oxidants and which may necessitate intermittent transfusion therapy[118]; as a two-gene deletion, it is characterized by mild, clinically insignificant microcytic anemia; and as a one-gene deletion, it is characterized by a "silent" carrier with no anemia or microcytosis.

The clinical picture in β-thalassemia is due to partial or complete loss of expression of two β-globin genes. The broad spectrum of disease is due to both the number of genes affected and the degree to which each is affected. Where only one β-globin gene is affected (β-thalassemia trait), mild microcytic anemia is the primary clinical manifestation. Where both β-globin genes are affected, the clinical picture may be mild to moderate (thalassemia intermedia) or severe, requiring chronic transfusions (thalassemia major, or "Cooley anemia"). Children with HgE-β-thalassemia have symptoms ranging from very mild to severe, depending on the level of expression of the mutant β-globin gene.

In thalassemia, clinical problems result from complications of the anemia, transfusions required to maintain hemoglobin over 9 g/dL, resultant iron overload, and chelation therapy. These complications include transfusion-associated alloimmunization and infection, splenomegaly, bone abnormalities (secondary to extramedullary hematopoiesis, chelation therapy, and other factors), endocrine dysfunction (including hypogonadism, hypopituitarism, and diabetes mellitus), short stature, pulmonary hypertension, venous thrombosis and thromboembolism, and cardiomyopathy (primarily due to iron overload). Thalassemia patients have been noted to be hypercoagulable,[119] a condition that may be exaggerated after splenectomy.[119,120] Routine therapies currently utilized for the treatment of severe disease and prevention of complications include phenotypic matching and leukocyte reduction of transfused blood, chelation therapy, and hormone and vitamin D therapy. When an appropriate donor is available, hematopoietic stem cell transplantation is recommended before severe liver damage occurs because it provides a potential cure for thalassemia. To ameliorate the course of the disease, other therapies are under investigation, including administration of erythropoietin, fetal hemoglobin modifiers (e.g., hydroxyurea), antioxidants, and gene therapy.

Perioperative Considerations

Children with moderate or severe thalassemia may require cholecystectomy, splenectomy, and vascular access placement for frequent transfusions or other therapies.[121] In addition, demineralized long bones may be prone to fracture and older children may require osteotomies for bony deformities. Bony abnormalities of the maxillofacial area may render securing the airway challenging.[122] Laparoscopic techniques for cholecystectomy[123] and splenectomy have been used successively in children with thalassemia, although it has been noted that perioperative hypertension may be a common problem in laparoscopic splenectomy.[124,125] Open-heart surgery requiring cardiopulmonary bypass with judicious use of sodium nitroprusside therapy has been successively performed in a patient with HgH disease.[126] Perioperative considerations and concerns for children with

Table 9-10. Perioperative Considerations and Concerns in Thalassemia

Preoperative

Hemoglobin

Transfusion crossmatch if appropriate (antibody-matched, leukocyte reduced for frequently transfused children)

Evaluation for endocrine dysfunction (e.g., diabetes mellitus, hypopituitarism)

Cardiac function, including echocardiogram (when appropriate)

Hepatic function, awareness of risk of cirrhosis and iron or viral-induced damage

Airway evaluation

Pre-splenectomy antibiotics and immunizations (when appropriate)

Intraoperative

Preparation for possible difficult airway

Careful positioning of demineralized extremities

Attention to cardiovascular function, including post-splenectomy hypertension

Physiologic effects of laparoscopy on circulatory and respiratory function

Prophylaxis for thromboembolism

Postoperative

Monitoring of cardiac function

Prophylaxis for thromboembolism

---

thalassemia, especially for those with thalassemia major, are listed in Table 9-10.

Thrombocytopenia

Platelets are an essential component in the coagulation cascade. Their lifespan is normally 7 to 10 days, and they are distributed between the bloodstream (two thirds) and spleen (one third). In children, platelets may decrease in number due to a decrease in production or increase in consumption, or they may be abnormal in their function. Bleeding typical of platelet disorders often involves skin and mucous membranes. Although there are many causes of thrombocytopenia in infants and children, both primary and secondary, the focus of this discussion is on idiopathic thrombocytopenic purpura.

Idiopathic Thrombocytopenic Purpura

Idiopathic thrombocytopenic purpura (ITP) is the most common cause of acute-onset thrombocytopenia in the otherwise healthy child, and it commonly presents in the operative setting. ITP has an estimated incidence of about 4 per 100,000 children, and it is usually a benign, self-limited disorder affecting children between the ages of 2 and 10.[27] Diagnosis is by exclusion, and the differential list is extensive.

Pathophysiology

This disorder is characterized by thrombocytopenia (platelet count <100,000/mm^3), shortened platelet survival, presence of antiplatelet antibody in the plasma, and increased megakaryocytes in the bone marrow. Platelet autoantibodies may exist

alone or as part of immune complexes, and they are usually IgG in type; they often show specificity for platelet membrane glycoproteins IIb/IIIa and Ib/IX.[127] Thrombocytopenia develops when the reticuloendothelial system, typically the spleen, destroys the antibody-covered platelets.

Clinical and Laboratory Features and Treatment

Typically, ITP in children is a benign process after a viral illness or immunization that presents as petechiae of mucosal surfaces or purpura over bony prominences. This process resolves within weeks or months regardless of therapy. Chronic ITP is ITP that persists for more than 6 months. Rarely, hospitalization is required, although treatment is indicated when platelet counts are less than 10,000 to 20,000/mm^3, especially when surgery is required or life-threatening emergencies such as intracranial hemorrhage (0.1%-0.9% incidence) occur.[127] Medical treatment options include the following: corticosteroids, which inhibit phagocytosis of antibody-coated platelets in the spleen and inhibit antibody production; antimetabolites, notably vincristine; intravenous immunoglobulin (IVIg), which may block reticuloendothelial Fc-receptors; and, in Rh-positive patients, anti-D immunoglobulin, which may block Fc receptors and thereby render them unavailable to antibody-covered platelets. Platelet transfusions are generally recommended only in the setting of life-threatening emergencies. Splenectomy removes a major site of platelet destruction and is recommended as an option only in chronic, symptomatic ITP or acute life-threatening ITP unresponsive to medical treatment.[128,129] This procedure, commonly performed laparoscopically, has a success rate of about 75%.[130-132]

Perioperative Considerations

In view of the clinical and laboratory features of ITP, the anesthesiologist providing care for the child with ITP who is undergoing splenectomy or incidental surgery should give consideration to concerns listed in Table 9-11. A hematologist should be consulted to assess the need for medical therapy, including platelet transfusion, before surgery.

Coagulation Disorders

Children may present for surgery with a personal or family history suggestive or indicative of a bleeding disorder. The anesthesiologist must decide expeditiously whether to postpone surgery to further evaluate and/or treat the child. A careful history, physical examination, and family history, followed by laboratory evaluation in consultation with a hematologist, are all important elements in screening for, diagnosing, and treating a bleeding disorder in the perioperative setting.

Screening

The clinical history of the child and family is the most essential screening tool. Important in the family history are family members who have been labeled as "bleeders," who have required blood transfusion unexpectedly during surgery, or who returned to surgery for unexpected postoperative bleeding; a history of maternal menorrhagia may also be significant. Suggestive signs and symptoms in a child's personal history are "easy bruising," mucosal bleeding, and in older girls menorrhagia. Although diagnosing "easy bruising" is subjective, one should suspect bleeding tendencies if skin bruising occurs in nontraumatized

to morbidity and mortality are related to infection, regimen-related toxicity, and alloreactivity.[160]

Host defenses, both immunologic and physical, are impaired throughout the transplantation process. Children are vulnerable to a wide range of routine and opportunistic pathogens, including bacteria, fungi, and viruses.

Regimen-related toxicity can involve literally every organ of the body through the direct and indirect effects of radiation and chemotherapy (see Table 9-16). Mucositis is common and can place children at increased risk of aspiration and airway compromise.[161] Sinusoidal obstruction syndrome (SOS, previously called veno-occlusive disease [VOD]) occurs in 10% to 60% of children and is characterized by hepatomegaly, jaundice, and weight gain; its presence requires careful attention to fluid balance as sodium administration must be minimized.[162,163] Other gastrointestinal complications include hemorrhage,[164] infection, and opiate-induced abdominal pain and distention (narcotic bowel syndrome). Pulmonary complications occur in about half of HSCT patients[165,166] and include infection, hemorrhage, edema, acute respiratory distress syndrome (ARDS), and idiopathic pneumonia syndrome (IPS), a noninfectious inflammatory lung process.[167] Cardiac complications occur in 5% to 10% of patients, including toxicity from anthracyclines or cyclophosphamide (in doses exceeding 200 mg/kg)[168] and hypertension from cyclosporine or glucocorticoids. Acute renal failure occurs in 30% to 50% of children[169] and warrants judicious use of fluids in these patients[170]; hemorrhagic cystitis is also common.[171] A process of thrombotic microangiopathy similar to hemolytic uremic syndrome may occur in children receiving cyclosporine or the calcineurin inhibitor, tacrolimus.[172] Central nervous system complications include infection, hemorrhage, and both encephalopathy and peripheral neuropathy secondary to metabolic and chemotherapeutic effects.[173-177]

Graft-versus-host disease (GVHD) is the clinical manifestation of the recognition of recipient alloantigens by donor T cells. Acute GVHD is a common event (incidence depending on histocompatibility of donor and recipient) occurring before day 100 post transplant, and it is characterized by inflammatory dermatitis, enteritis, and/or hepatitis. Chronic GVHD occurs in 30% to 60% of patients,[178] typically after day 100 post transplant, and has many features of autoimmune diseases (e.g., sclerodermatous changes; dry mouth and conjunctivae; esophagitis; pulmonary dysfunction, including bronchiolitis obliterans; contractures of extremities and soft tissue; alopecia; and thrombocytopenia). Opportunistic infections are common during chronic GVHD. Biopsy is often indicated to distinguish acute and chronic GVHD from other causes for specific complications in order to guide therapy. Hemolysis is an additional manifestation of alloantigenicity, the result of major and minor blood group incompatibilities between donor and recipient.

Perioperative Considerations

Surgical and procedural interventions are common throughout the transplant process and are similar to those described earlier for children with cancer. An additional surgical procedure that is an integral component of HSCT is harvesting of hematopoietic stem cells, whether from the recipient or another individual. Harvesting of bone marrow in children generally requires general anesthesia, although the procedure can be performed under spinal anesthesia with equivalent safety.[179] The donor is usually placed in a prone position to extract approximately 10 mL/kg (recipient weight) of marrow from the posterior iliac crests. When stem cells are obtained from peripheral blood, placement of vascular access in children usually requires sedation or general anesthesia. There is little evidence to support the avoidance of nitrous oxide for harvesting procedures, a concern raised in the past due to the ability of nitrous oxide to affect methionine synthase activity and, thereby, DNA synthesis.[180]

In view of the wide range of complications occurring in children undergoing HSCT, there are many issues to consider, as enumerated earlier for children with cancer (see Table 9-17). Of note, radiation, glucocorticoids, mucositis, and chronic GVHD may all contribute to an airway that is friable, prone to dental injury, and difficult to properly position for endotracheal intubation. Chemotherapy and GVHD may affect the skin and make venous access difficult. Chronic GVHD can lead to both sclerodermatous changes, which can profoundly restrict range of motion, and sicca, which may necessitate use of artificial tears. GVHD may alter gut motility and delay gastric emptying. Immune compromise increases the risk of infection from vascular access lines and, therefore, mandates meticulous technique at all times. Chemotherapy may compromise cardiac and pulmonary function, alter hepatic metabolism of medications, and limit renal handling of fluid challenges. Immune compromise and modifications resulting from a transplant require special processing of blood components, as recommended by hematology and blood bank consultants (see Tables 9-3, 9-4, and 9-5). In general, only irradiated, leukocyte-reduced, cytomegalovirus-negative (where the recipient is cytomegalovirus negative) blood components should be administered, and blood typing is dependent on engraftment of donor antigens. It is critical to coordinate the choice of blood products with the transplant service because often blood type changes from that of recipient to that of donor.

References

Please see www.expertconsult.com

Strategies for Blood Product Management and Reducing Transfusions

Charles J. Coté, Eric F. Grabowski, and Christopher P. Stowell

DESPITE ADVANCES IN PEDIATRIC surgery, the number of infants and children sustaining major operative blood loss remains high. Little information has been gathered about when to expect coagulation defects in the pediatric age group. Advances in blood banking, use of component therapy, and the use of various alternatives to allogeneic transfusion have altered the problems associated with blood replacement. Most studies of massive blood transfusion have involved adult patients whose blood replacement has been with either whole blood or modified whole blood. The majority of recommendations regarding the use of fresh frozen plasma (FFP) and platelets are based on these studies and not on large series of patients whose blood replacement has been made exclusively with component therapy.[1]

The judicious use of blood transfusion is imperative both because the supply is limited and because transfusions can incur various complications. The risk of these complications varies around the world. In countries with sophisticated health care systems, the most common serious hazards of transfusion are hemolytic transfusion reactions due to ABO incompatibility (usually as a result of mistransfusion), bacterial infection, and transfusion-related acute lung injury. In developing countries the risk of infectious disease transmission may be high owing to the presence of endemic infections in the population and the technical or logistic limitations of donor screening.

Perhaps nothing has changed the use of blood products by surgeons and anesthesiologists more than the threat of the acquired immunodeficiency syndrome (AIDS).[2-4] Although infection with human immunodeficiency virus (HIV) is now by no means the most common disease associated with blood transfusion, it has been the most publicized in the lay press and is still feared in the public mind. The implementation of donor education programs, improved health history screening, new tests, and new test technologies (Table 10-1) have markedly altered the spectrum of transfusion-transmitted infectious agents in the developed world. The risks of some of the infectious and noninfectious hazards of transfusion are summarized in Table 10-2.

Despite marked reduction of the transmission of HIV, hepatitis C virus, and hepatitis B virus, transfusions can incur other deleterious effects.[5,6] Therefore, it is still vital that there be clear medical justification for every blood transfusion. The benefits of each transfusion must be weighed against the potential infectious, immunologic, and metabolic risks.[7] It is in the child's best interest to transfuse with a clear clinical goal and in the anesthesiologist's best interest to document the reason for each

Table 10-4. Composition of RBC-Containing Components

Parameter	CPDA-1 Whole Blood*	CPDA-1 RBC*	Additive Solution RBC†
Storage time (days)	35	42	42
Volume RBC (mL)‡	203	203	203
Residual plasma (mL)§	248	50	30
Hematocrit (%)‡	40	72	53
pH	6.98	6.71	6.6
Adenosine triphosphate (% of day 1)	56	45	60
2,3-DPG (% of day 1)	<10	<10	<10
Plasma [K⁺] (mEq/L)¶	27.3	78.5	50

*At 35 days outdate.
†At 42 days outdate.
‡Based on collection of 450 mL of whole blood at hematocrit of 45%.
§Note that the concentration of factors V and VIII is reduced to 20% to 50% of normal levels (0.2-0.5 units/mL). The other clotting factors are quite stable.
¶Although the K⁺ concentration varies considerably, the total amount of extracellular K⁺ is 5 to 7 mEq per unit for all of these RBC components. This is because the volume of residual plasma plus anticoagulant preservative is much different, as reflected in the final hematocrit of the units.

Table 10-7. Common Initial Doses of Blood Components and Expected Effect

Component	Dose	Effect
PRBCs	10-15 mL/kg	Increase hemoglobin by 2-3 g/dL
Platelets	5-10 mL/kg	Increase platelet count by 50,000 to 100,000/mm³
Fresh frozen plasma	10-15 mL/kg	Factor levels increase by 15%-20%
Cryoprecipitate	1-2 units/kg	Increase fibrinogen by 60-100 mg/dL

RBCs bear glycoconjugate antigens of the ABH Histo-Blood Group System. During the first year of life, infants begin to elaborate alloantibodies to whichever A or B antigens they lack. These isoagglutinins are invariably present after a few months of age and constitute a formidable immunologic obstacle to transfusion or transplantation across this ABO barrier. Therefore, RBC for transfusion must be compatible with the ABO isoagglutinins of the intended transfusion recipient. By the same token, components with a large volume of plasma (e.g., whole blood, FFP, apheresis platelets) must be selected to be compatible with the A and/or B antigens expressed on the recipient's RBCs. Therefore, PRBCs must be ABO *compatible* with the recipient, whereas whole blood must be ABO *identical*; Table 10-5 summarizes the permissible combinations. Note that only RBCs express the Rh(D) antigen. Rh(D)-positive patients may receive either Rh(D)-positive or Rh(D)-negative RBCs. Rh(D)-negative patients are routinely given Rh(D)-negative RBCs for any elective transfusions, but in the setting of massive transfusion it may be necessary to switch to Rh(D)-positive RBCs to preserve the supply of Rh(D)-negative RBCs. The blood bank will generally determine when to make this switch based on the inventory and will do so more quickly for a patient who is either a male or a postmenopausal female (Table 10-6). The object is to avoid exposing a female with child-bearing potential to Rh(D)-positive RBCs and eliciting the formation of the anti-D alloantibody that is responsible for the most severe forms of hemolytic disease of the newborn. Table 10-7 presents a common initial volume of PRBCs to increase the hemoglobin by 2 to 3 g/dL.

Platelets

Platelets may either be obtained from a whole blood donation or collected by apheresis. Whole blood–derived platelets are

Table 10-5. ABO Compatibility of Blood Components

Recipient ABO Group	Acceptable Component ABO Groups (Second Choice)			
	Whole Blood	PRBC	FFP/Cryo	Platelets
O	O	O	O (A, B, AB)	O (A, B, AB)
A	A	A (O)	A (AB)	A (AB)*
B	B	B (O)	B (AB)	B (AB)*
AB	AB	AB (A, B, O)	AB	AB*

*Can give out of group apheresis platelets (or whole blood–derived platelets for small child) if plasma is removed or replaced.

Table 10-6. Rh(D) Compatibility of Blood Components

Recipient Rh(D) Type	Acceptable Component Rh(D) Types (Second Choice)			
	Whole Blood or PRBCs	FFP/Cryo	Apheresis Platelets	Whole Blood–Derived Platelets
Rh(D) positive	Rh positive (Rh negative)	Any	Any	Rh positive (Rh negative)
Rh(D) negative	Rh negative (Rh positive)*	Any	Any	Rh negative (Rh positive)*†

*Depending on inventory, blood bank may switch to Rh(D) positive, particularly for male patients or postmenopausal females.
†Consider Rh immune globulin for females of child-bearing potential receiving whole blood–derived platelets from Rh(D) positive donors.
Cryo, cryoprecipitate; FFP, fresh frozen plasma.

separated by centrifugation and suspended in 40 to 60 mL of plasma at a concentration that is two to four times greater than in the circulation. Each unit contains a minimum of 5.5×10^{10} platelets and is stored at 20°-24°C with gentle continuous agitation for a maximum of 5 days. One unit of whole blood–derived platelets would be expected to increase the platelet count of a 70-kg adult by 5,000 to 10,000/mm^3 and increase the count in an 18-kg child by 15,000/mm^3.[18,19] A unit of platelets obtained by apheresis contains at least 3×10^{11} platelets in 200 to 400 mL of plasma, or the equivalent of approximately 6 units of whole blood–derived platelets. A common dose for pediatric patients is 0.1 to 0.3 unit/kg of body weight, or 10 to 15 mL/kg (see Table 10-7); this dose usually produces an increment of 30,000 to 90,000/mm^3. In the setting of dilutional thrombocytopenia with ongoing losses, or a consumptive coagulopathy (e.g., disseminated intravascular coagulation), larger doses (0.3 unit/kg or more) may be required to boost the platelet count above 50,000/mm^3. Because platelets are suspended in plasma that contains the anti-A and anti-B isoagglutinins, they should be ABO compatible with the recipient's RBCs. Some donors have high titer isoagglutinins that can produce hemolysis in transfusion recipients if a large enough volume of plasma is given.[20] The transfusion of plasma-incompatible, whole blood–derived platelets to adult recipients does not produce clinically significant hemolysis because the volume of plasma is so small. However, apheresis platelets (and whole blood–derived platelets for small children) should be ABO compatible with the recipient's RBCs. Because platelets do not express Rh antigens, matching for Rh(D) antigen is not necessary for apheresis platelets that contain virtually no RBCs. Whole blood–derived platelets may contain enough RBCs to provoke Rh alloimmunization so platelets from Rh(D)-negative donors are given preferentially to Rh(D)-negative recipients with child-bearing potential. Should a premenopausal female receive whole blood–derived platelets from an Rh(D) positive donor, Rh immune globulin can be administered within 72 hours to prevent alloimmunization. Note that platelets should never be withheld in an emergency situation because of Rh(D) incompatibility.

Platelets are essential to hemostasis associated with the vascular injury of surgery and thus are necessary for the control of surgical bleeding. Platelets are also required for the maintenance of an intact endothelial barrier to spontaneous blood loss. The number of platelets required to provide adequate hemostasis in the surgical setting is much greater than the level needed to provide prophylaxis against spontaneous hemorrhage. A platelet count of 10,000/mm^3 is generally considered to be adequate to prevent either spontaneous bleeding or bleeding from minor invasive procedures (e.g., lumbar puncture, line placement) in an otherwise stable child. If overt signs of bleeding are present or a more significant hemostatic challenge in the form of a surgical procedure is imminent, then a level of 30,000 to 50,000/mm^3 may be required.[21-25] A target level of 50,000/mm^3 is also appropriate in the setting of massive transfusion.[22,26-28] Platelets may also be required for children with adequate counts but in whom platelet function is impaired. Many medications (e.g., aspirin, nonsteroidal anti-inflammatory agents, Plavix, glycoprotein IIa/IIIb receptor inhibitors such as abciximab) and some conditions (e.g., renal failure with blood urea nitrogen levels >60 mg/dL) cause abnormal platelet function, which may interfere with surgical hemostasis, in which case it may be necessary to maintain the platelet count at a somewhat greater level, at

least until the effect of the medication wears off or the child's platelets are largely replaced by banked platelets.[29,30] There are a few settings in which even greater levels (100,000/mm^3) are sought such as intracranial, ophthalmic, and otologic surgery.

There is no clear-cut threshold regarding platelet count and clinical bleeding in the perioperative period; each child must be individually assessed by constantly observing the surgical field for evidence of abnormal bleeding.[31] Unfortunately, we are currently lacking a well-validated bedside tool to assess platelet function. The utility of the thromboelastogram and other devices to measure platelet function under controlled flow conditions, such as the platelet function analyzer (PFA), are under investigation. The standard technique for diagnosis and evaluation of thrombocytopathies remains Born-O'Brien platelet aggregometry but it is not useful in the intraoperative setting.[32] In any event, it is thrombocytopenia rather than a newly acquired platelet function defect that most commonly occurs in the operative setting and massive transfusion.

A child occasionally presents for surgery with a previously characterized platelet dysfunction that may be associated with bleeding. If the child has a normal platelet count, it is a reasonable practice to be sure that the blood bank has an adequate platelet supply available for the operating room but to withhold transfusion until the child demonstrates pathologic bleeding.

Several additional points should be considered[33]:

1. Not all hospitals have platelets in the inventory. Unless the need is anticipated before surgery, platelets may not be available when required.

2. For children who are thrombocytopenic before surgery, it is recommended that platelets be infused just before the surgical procedure to ensure the greatest levels during the time of peak demand.

3. Platelets should be filtered only by large-pore filters ($\geq$150 μm) or leukocyte-reduction filters (if indicated); micropore filters may adsorb large numbers of platelets and therefore diminish the effectiveness of a platelet transfusion.

4. Platelets are suspended in plasma, which may help to replenish coagulation factors other than factors V and VIII, which are labile.

Platelets should not be refrigerated or placed in a cooler with ice before administration because they will be rapidly cleared from the circulation.

Special Processing of Cellular Blood Components

Leukocytes (WBCs) collected with whole blood donations partition into both the platelet and PRBC components; few intact WBCs can be found in FFP. Passenger WBCs are responsible for most febrile, nonhemolytic transfusion reactions, HLA alloimmunization, and transmission of cytomegalovirus (CMV). To prevent these complications of transfusion, WBCs can be very effectively removed (2-3$_{\log}$ reduction) by passage through leukocyte-reduction filters that may be done shortly after collection or at the bedside. Note that leukocyte reduction by filtration is a superior technique to washing or freezing-deglycerolizing, which was used in the past. Table 10-8 lists children who may benefit from receiving leukocyte-reduced cellular components (i.e., RBCs or platelets).

CMV transmission can also be reduced by screening donors for CMV exposure (testing for antibody to CMV), although leukocyte reduction is the more widely used approach. Although primary CMV infection is benign in children with intact immune

declines below 15%, subendocardial myocardial ischemia may develop.[481,487,489,492] It is at this extreme level of anemia that dissolved oxygen begins to assume a more important role.[485] There are a number of reports of extreme acute normovolemic hemodilution with successful outcome (hemoglobin as low as 2 g/dL) without the production of lactic acid.[481,493]

Control of the child's metabolic rate is very important during extreme hemodilution should a rapid hemorrhage occur without adequate blood products to replace losses. Therefore, inducing a slight degree of hypothermia (33°-34°C), controlled ventilation to maintain a constant carbon dioxide value, and a high inspired oxygen tension (and therefore an increased dissolved oxygen value) have allowed the survival of patients with hematocrits as low as 4%.[493] These extreme levels of hemodilution cannot be recommended as an elective effort to reduce blood transfusions. However, these reports[481,493] do indicate how well healthy patients tolerate such low oxygen-carrying capacity provided that they are under the effects of anesthesia, they are normovolemic, they are slightly hypothermic, and they are on 100% oxygen.

A right shift in the oxygen-hemoglobin dissociation curve secondary to increased erythrocyte 2,3-DPG improves oxygen release to tissues. This compensatory mechanism occurs primarily during chronic anemia and becomes important when the hematocrit falls below 20%; this compensatory mechanism is less important during the development of acute anemia.[448,467,468,487] It is our practice never to allow the hematocrit to fall below 15%, and we prefer to maintain it closer to 20%.

Lung Water

Pulmonary interstitial water increases with hemodilution; this amount is quantitatively greater with crystalloid than colloid replacement. However, there is no clinical difference as measured by arterial blood gases.[494-496] There appears to be no clinical advantage of colloid over crystalloid hemodilution, and the cost of the latter is much less.

Effects on Muscle Relaxants

Several studies have demonstrated a prolonged duration of action and an increased potency of many muscle relaxants (succinylcholine, pancuronium, curare, rocuronium, and vecuronium).[497-501] It is unclear why the potency of muscle relaxants is increased. These effects may relate to a number of factors, including alterations in protein binding, volume of distribution, alterations in distribution of blood flow to organs that metabolize or excrete these medications, and acute changes in electrolytes, ionized calcium, and blood flow to tissues.[497] A more important consideration is that the use of muscle relaxants prevents shivering. Because shivering increases oxygen consumption, such increases in oxygen consumption are not desirable during isovolemic hemodilution because the ability to compensate for the increased oxygen demand may be compromised.[502]

Technique and Key Concepts

We allow blood to run directly from an arterial line into sterile blood collection bags with the appropriate anticoagulant. Each bag is weighed before any blood is transferred to determine precisely the volume that has been removed. The bag is placed on a scale below the level of the child to accurately measure the amount of blood withdrawn. The bag is frequently but gently agitated to ensure even distribution of the anticoagulant.

The volume of blood to be withdrawn should be calculated preoperatively to reduce the hematocrit to the 20% to 25% range. Care must be taken to replace the blood removed with either 5% albumin milliliter for milliliter or 2 to 3 mL of lactated Ringer's solution for each milliliter of blood removed. Sometimes an even greater volume of replacement fluid is needed.[463] A reasonable estimate of the adequacy of replacement is to obtain a baseline CVP and then maintain the same CVP as blood is withdrawn and substituted with colloid or crystalloid. It is preferable to hemodilute before the surgical incision, although this can also be done during the initial phases of surgery. The major concern is to maintain a normal circulating blood volume and provide adequate oxygen-carrying capacity. It is therefore important to make an educated guess about how much blood loss is anticipated so that the autologous blood can be reinfused in place of homologous blood. It is important to remember that a small-pore filter (20 μm) traps many of the platelets that a large-pore filter (≥150 μm) allows to pass.

Indications

Hemodilution may be indicated in any procedure in which blood loss is expected to exceed one half the child's blood volume.

Contraindications

Hemodilution is contraindicated in children with sickle cell disease, septicemia, or compromised function of any major organ that may be significantly affected by changes in perfusion and oxygenation. *We do not recommend combining extreme hemodilution (hematocrit <25%) with controlled hypotensive anesthesia.* Therefore, children with moderate anemia are not good candidates because not enough units can be removed to make the technique effective.

Complications

The major complications of hemodilution relate to blood volume status, hemoglobin content (removing too much blood), and coagulopathy (dilution of clotting factors). Anesthesiologists must pay meticulous attention to blood volume replacement. As long as normovolemia is maintained and the hematocrit exceeds 15% (preferably around 20%), problems with organ perfusion or oxygenation should not occur. Sepsis is a theoretical concern if strict sterile techniques were not followed during the collection process.

Advantages

The benefits of this technique are that the units collected at the beginning of the procedure pose no risk of infection (unless contaminated by bacteria in the collection process) or mistransfusion (if they are not removed from the operating room). It yields a net saving in loss of red blood cell mass because the surgical losses occur at a hematocrit of 15% to 20% compared with 30% to 45%. The net use of banked RBCs is reduced if 2 or 3 units can be removed at the beginning of the procedure. Obviously this technique can be used only in teenagers and the most frequent population to which this technique is applied is spine instrumentation.

The Jehovah's Witness Patient

This subpopulation of children presents a particular medical/legal dilemma.[503,504] Transfusion management of anyone with a religious objection to transfusion will depend in part on the urgency of the surgical procedure and underlying medical condition of the child. If not an emergent situation, a meeting with the patient (or the parents or guardian if a minor), the patient's spiritual advisor (if the child so chooses), and representatives of the team that will be caring for the patient should be held to allow the child to clearly articulate his or her wishes with respect to the refusal of transfusion and its consequences and to discuss possible alternatives including the use of erythropoietin, iron therapy, acute normovolemic hemodilution, intraoperative cell recovery/reinfusion, and the use of antifibrinolytic medications.[474,475,505-507] In addition, specific inquiries should be made for each child's beliefs regarding the use of albumin and intraoperative cell recovery/reinfusion if the circuit is not continuously connected to the child and, in particular, what the child's response would be if a life-threatening event occurred while he or she was under anesthesia.[465,508] All of these discussions need to be carefully documented in the child's record and informed consent signed beforehand. Not all hospitals or physicians are willing to participate with these kinds of manipulations, in which case arrangements should be made to transfer the child to the care of institutions or physicians who are willing to work with these constraints. Note that the courts have consistently ruled that the adult patient or emancipated minor has a right to refuse transfusion.[466,509] Physicians have the moral (and legal) obligation to respect those beliefs if an adult or teenager has made a completely informed decision understanding that he or she might die or suffer permanent injury without a transfusion should a life-threatening situation occur. However, in the case of a minor child, the courts have ruled that the fate of the minor child cannot be determined by the parents' religious convictions. The most important issue is full and open discussion including the fact that every effort will be made to respect the person's religious beliefs. It should also be recalled that for children a court order can generally be obtained to save the child's life; parents should be informed of this possibility beforehand.[510] For a more complete ethical discussion regarding this issue, see Chapter 5.

Acknowledgment

The authors wish to thank Richard M. Dsida for his prior contributions to this chapter.

Annotated References

Dzik WH, Stowell CP. Transfusion and coagulation issues in trauma. In Sheridan RL (ed): The Trauma Handbook of the Massachusetts General Hospital. Philadelphia, Lippincott Williams & Wilkins, 2004, pp 128-147

This chapter discusses the issues and complications of massive transfusion, and provides a practical guide for management of this difficult clinical situation.

Lacroix J, Hébert PC, Hutchinson JS, et al. Transfusion strategies for patients in pediatric intensive care units. N Engl J Med 2007; 356:1709-1719

This landmark, multicenter, clinical trial compared outcomes in pediatric patients randomized to RBC transfusion thresholds of 9.5 g/dL or 7 g/dl. There were no differences with respect to new or progressive multiple-organ failure, mortality, or other clinical outcomes between the two groups which highlights the capacity of even acute ill pediatric patients to tolerate anemia.

Ness PM, Cushing MM. Oxygen therapeutics: Pursuit of an alternative to the donor red blood cell. Arch Pathol Lab Med 2007; 131:734-741

This review provides a comprehensive and balanced summary of the development of synthetic oxygen carriers and the current challenges they face making the transition from the laboratory to the clinic.

References

Please see www.expertconsult.com

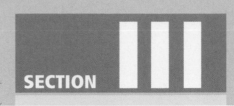

The Chest

Essentials of Pulmonology

Paul G. Firth and Kenan E. Haver

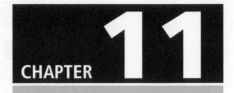

Respiratory Physiology	Lower Airway Disease
Preoperative Assessment	Cystic Fibrosis
Pulmonary Function Tests	Sickle Cell Disease
Perioperative Etiology and Epidemiology	**Summary**
Upper Respiratory Tract Infection	

MAINTENANCE OF ADEQUATE GAS exchange and delivery is a fundamental goal of anesthesia. Although the lungs play an important role in acid-base balance, temperature regulation, metabolism, and endocrine signaling, the preservation of oxygen and carbon dioxide (CO_2) equilibrium is the principal pulmonary function of immediate concern to the anesthesiologist. Respiratory problems are common in children and are frequently encountered by anesthesiologists during perioperative consultations, intraoperatively, or in intensive care units. Problems range from mild acute respiratory tract infections to chronic lung disease with end-stage respiratory failure. In this chapter we discuss the basics of respiratory physiology, assessment of pulmonary function, and practical anesthetic management of specific pulmonary problems. Airway and thoracic aspects pertinent to ventilation are discussed in Chapters 12 and 13, whereas pulmonary issues specific to neonates, intensive care, or other disease states are addressed in the relevant chapters.

Respiratory Physiology

The morphologic development of the lung begins several weeks into the embryonic period and continues into the first decade and beyond postnatal life.[1] Intrauterine gas exchange occurs via the placenta, but the respiratory system develops in preparation for extrauterine life when gas exchange transfers abruptly to the lungs. The respiratory system is an outgrowth of the ventral wall of the foregut. During the embryonic period of development of the first few postconceptual weeks, lung buds form as a projection of the endodermal tissue. During the pseudoglandular period, extending to the 17th week of life, rapid lung growth is accompanied by formation of the bronchi and branching of the

airways down to the terminal bronchioli. Further development of bronchioli and vascularization of the airways occurs during the canalicular stage of the second trimester. The saccular stage begins at approximately 24 weeks, when terminal air sacs begin to form. Proliferation of capillary networks surrounding these air spaces become sufficient for pulmonary gas exchange by 26 to 28 weeks, when extrauterine survival of premature neonates becomes possible. Formation of alveoli occurs by lengthening of the saccules and thinning of the saccular walls and has begun by the 36th postconceptual week in most human fetuses (Fig. 11-1). The vast majority of alveolar formation occurs after birth, however, typically continuing to as late as 8 to 10 years postnatally. The neonatal lung at birth commonly has 10 to 20 million terminal air sacs (many of which are saccules rather than alveoli), which is one tenth of the number in the mature adult lung. Growth of the lungs after birth is primarily due to an increase in the number of respiratory bronchioles and alveoli and not due to an increase in the size of the alveoli.

Respiratory rhythmogenesis, as seen by rhythmic thoracic movement, begins well before birth and may be necessary for normal anatomic and physiologic lung development. At birth, interruption of umbilical blood flow initiates rhythmic breathing. Amniotic fluid is expelled from the lungs via the upper airways with the first few breaths, with residual fluid draining through the lymphatic and pulmonary channels in the first days of life. Changes in Po_2, Pco_2, and pH cause an acute decrease in pulmonary vascular resistance and a consequent increase in pulmonary blood flow. Increased left atrial and decreased right atrial pressure reverse the pressure gradient across the foramen ovale, causing functional closure of this left-to-right one-way flap valve. Expansion of the lungs combined with increased pulmonary blood flow initiates the abrupt transition to

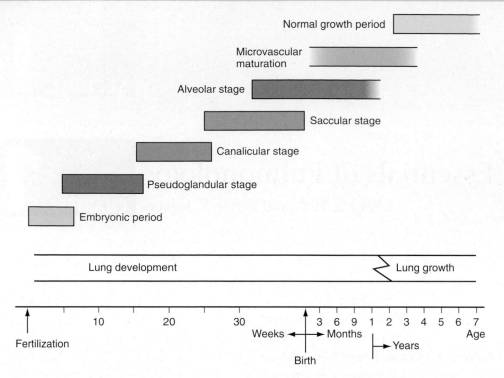

Figure 11-1. Timetable for lung development. (Reproduced and modified with permission from Guttentag S, Ballard PL: Lung development: embryology, growth, maturation, and developmental biology. In Tausch HW, Ballard RA, Gleason CA [eds]: Avery's Diseases of the Newborn, 8th ed. Philadelphia, WB Saunders, 2004, p 602.)

extrauterine gas exchange. Continuous increased arterial oxygen levels following birth, in comparison with intrauterine levels, augment and maintain ventilatory rhythm.

Breathing is controlled by a complex interaction of input from sensors, integration by a central control system, and subsequent output to effector muscles.[2] Afferent signaling is provided by peripheral arterial chemoreceptors, central brainstem chemoreceptors, upper airway and intrapulmonary receptors, and chest wall and muscle mechanoreceptors. The peripheral arterial chemoreceptors consist of the carotid and aortic bodies, with the carotid bodies playing the greater role in arterial chemical sensing in humans. The carotid bodies sense both Pao_2 and hydrogen ion concentration. The central chemoreceptors are responsive to $Paco_2$ and hydrogen ion concentration and are thought to be located at or near the ventral surface of the medulla. The nose, pharynx, and larynx have a wide variety of pressure, chemical, temperature, and flow receptors that can cause apnea, coughing, or changes in ventilatory pattern. Pulmonary receptors lie in the airways and lung parenchyma. The airway receptors are subdivided into the slowly adapting receptors, or pulmonary stretch receptors, and the rapidly adapting receptors. The stretch receptors, found in the airway smooth muscle, are thought to be involved in the balance of inspiration and expiration. The rapidly adapting receptors lie between the airway epithelial cells and are triggered by noxious stimuli such as smoke, dust, and histamine. Parenchymal receptors, or juxtacapillary receptors, are located adjacent to the alveolar blood vessels; they respond to hyperinflation of the lungs, to various chemical stimuli in the pulmonary circulation, and possibly to interstitial congestion. Chest wall receptors include mechanoreceptors and joint proprioceptors. Mechanoreceptors in the

muscle spindle endings and tendons of respiratory muscles sense changes in length, tension, and movement.

Central control of respiration is maintained by the brainstem (involuntary) and cortical (voluntary) centers. Although the precise mechanism of the neural ventilatory rhythmogenesis is unknown, the pre-Bötzinger complex and retrotrapezoid nucleus/parafacial respiratory group, neural circuits in the ventrolateral medulla, are thought to be the respiratory rhythm generators.[3] These neuron groups fire in an oscillating pattern, an inherent rhythm that is moderated by inputs from other respiratory centers. Involuntary integration of sensory input occurs in various respiratory nuclei and neural complexes in the pons and medulla, which modify the baseline pacemaker firing of the respiratory rhythm generators. The cerebral cortex also affects breathing rhythm and influences or overrides involuntary rhythm generation in response to conscious or subconscious activity, such as emotion, arousal, pain, speech, breath holding, and other activities.[2]

The effectors of ventilation include the neural efferent pathways, the muscles of respiration, the bones and cartilage of the chest wall and airway, and elastic connective tissue. Upper airway patency is maintained by connective tissue and by sustained and cyclical contraction of the pharyngeal dilator muscles. The diaphragm produces the majority of tidal volume during quiet inspiration, with the intercostal, abdominal, and accessory muscles (sternocleidomastoid and neck muscles) providing additional negative pressure. The elastic recoil of the lungs and thorax produces expiration, with inspiration an active, and expiration a passive action in normal lungs during quiet breathing. During vigorous breathing or with airway obstruction, both inspiration and expiration become active processes.

Preoperative Assessment

The preoperative assessment of the respiratory system in a child is based on history, physical examination, and evaluation of vital signs. Further investigations, such as laboratory, radiographic, and pulmonary function studies, may be indicated if there is doubt as to the diagnosis or severity of the pulmonary disease. Because ventilation is a complex process involving many systems beyond the lung, preoperative pulmonary appraisal must include airway, musculoskeletal, and neurologic assessment that might impact gas exchange under anesthesia or in the postoperative period. The potential impact of esophageal reflux, cardiac, hepatic, renal, or hematologic disease on gas exchange and pulmonary function should also be considered. The child's reaction to the presence and approach of medical staff may determine the order and even the position of the history and examination.

The history should establish the current respiratory status, the presence of chronic and present status of pulmonary disease. Because children may be unwilling or unable to give a reliable history, parents or caregivers are often the sole or an important supplemental source of information. Respiratory issues especially pertinent to the pediatric population include upper respiratory tract infections (URIs), reactive airway disease/asthma, ventilatory problems relating to prematurity, and congenital diseases. Viral URIs are common in children, and the time, frequency, and severity of infection should be established. Reactive airway disease is also widespread in the pediatric population, and the precipitants, frequency, severity, and relieving factors should be determined. Chronic pulmonary diseases often have a variable clinical course, and a history of acute exacerbations of chronic problems should be elicited. The conceptual age at birth, the current postconceptual age, neonatal respiratory difficulties, and prolonged intubation in the neonatal period are particularly important to ascertain in the younger child because subglottic stenosis and/or tracheomalacia are common sequelae. Whereas congenital lesions may manifest at birth, symptoms of airway obstruction may only become evident later in life.

Physical examination begins when you enter the room. Particularly with young children, your best opportunity to observe them before they react to your presence is from across the room, and inspection from a distance can provide useful information. Respiratory rate is a sensitive marker of pulmonary problems, and scrutiny before a young child becomes agitated and hyperventilates is an important means of assessment. Pulse oximetry, the "fifth vital sign," is a useful baseline indicator of oxygenation. Nasal flaring, intercostal retractions, and the marked use of accessory respiratory muscles are all signs of respiratory distress. General appearance is also important. Apathy, anxiety, agitation, or persistent adoption of a fixed posture may indicate profound respiratory or airway difficulties, whereas intense cyanosis can also be detected from a distance. Weight may relate to pulmonary function: patients with chronic severe pulmonary disease are often underweight owing to retarded growth or malnourishment, whereas severe obesity can produce airway obstruction and sleep apnea. Inspection of the chest contour may reveal hyperinflation or thoracic wall deformities.

Closer physical examination adds further information. Auscultation may reveal wheezes, rales, fine or coarse crepitus, transmitted breath sounds from the upper airway, altered breath sounds, or cardiac murmurs. Chest percussion can provide an estimate of the position of the diaphragm and serve as a useful marker of hyperinflation. Patience, a gentle approach, and warm hands will improve diagnostic yield and patient satisfaction.

Pulmonary Function Tests

Further investigations of pulmonary function include chest radiography, measurement of hematocrit, arterial blood gas analysis, pulmonary function tests, and sleep studies. Special investigations are not routinely indicated preoperatively and should be reserved for times when the diagnosis is unclear, the progression or treatment of a disease needs to be established, or the severity of impairment is not evident. In most cases, a comprehensive history and careful physical examination will be adequate to establish an appropriate anesthetic plan. Before requesting a new investigation, the clinician should have a clear idea of what question is being asked and how the answer will modify anesthetic management and outcome.

Pulmonary function tests enable clinicians to (1) establish mechanical dysfunction in children with respiratory symptoms, (2) quantify the degree of dysfunction, and (3) define the nature of the dysfunction as obstructive, restrictive, or mixed obstructive and restrictive.[4] Figure 11-2 illustrates a normal pulmonary function test (normal flow-volume loop and spirometry parameters). Pulmonary function studies include dynamic studies, measurement of static lung volumes, and diffusing capacity. The

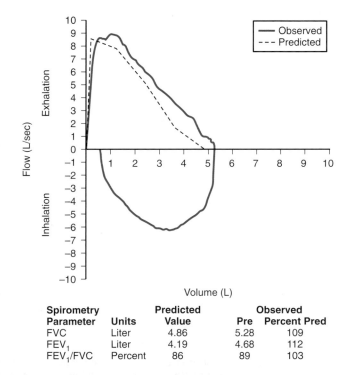

Spirometry Parameter	Units	Predicted Value	Pre	Observed Percent Pred
FVC	Liter	4.86	5.28	109
FEV$_1$	Liter	4.19	4.68	112
FEV$_1$/FVC	Percent	86	89	103

Figure 11-2. Normal pulmonary function test (*broken line, predicted curve, solid line, measured curve*). The normal flow-volume curve obtained during forced expiration rapidly ascends to the peak expiratory flow. Shortly after reaching the peak expiratory flow (highest point on curve), the curve descends with decreasing volume following a reproducible shape that is independent of effort. In this normal flow-volume curve, the FEV$_1$/FVC, FEV$_1$, and FVC are all within the normal range for this child's age, height, gender and race. The shapes of both the inspiratory and expiratory limbs are normal as well. Pre, prebronchodilator; Pred, predicted.

and 6 years from a cohort of 1246 neonates. By the age of 6 years, 48.5% of the children had experienced at least one documented episode of wheezing and were categorized into three groups. "Transient wheezers" are children who wheeze only in response to viral infections, typically during the first 3 years of life. "Non-atopic wheezers" are children who wheeze beyond the first few years of life, often in response to viral infections, but who are less likely to persistently wheeze in later childhood. "Atopy-associated wheezers" are children with a reversible wheeze together with a tendency toward IgE-mediated hypersensitivity; they have the greatest risk of persistent symptoms into late childhood and adulthood.[29]

The development of asthma is a complex process that probably involves the interaction of two crucial elements: host factors (specifically genetic modifiers of inflammation) and environmental exposures (e.g., viral infections, environmental allergens, and pollution) that occur during a crucial time in the development of the immune system.[27] The population of young children who wheeze, therefore, includes a spectrum of disorders rather than one specific pathologic process.

Asthma must be differentiated from other distinct causes that produce similar symptoms (Table 11-5). Tracheomalacia or bronchomalacia may produce wheezing, but this tends to be present from birth, which is unusual for asthma. The wheezing is commonly of a single pitch and is heard loudest in the central airways, as opposed to asthma, which typically produces polyphonic sounds from the lung periphery. Breathing difficulties due to chronic aspiration are often related to feeding times. Unremitting wheeze or stridor is often due to a fixed obstruction or foreign body. Chronic cough is the most common manifestation of asthma in children. Many children who cough may never be heard to wheeze and still have asthma. A cough with or without wheeze may be due to a viral infection, whereas a persistent productive cough may suggest suppurative lung disease such as cystic fibrosis. The response of the cough to asthma medication suggests the diagnosis of asthma.

The exact incidence of perioperative complications in the pediatric asthma population is difficult to ascertain, owing to variations in the definition of asthma, the definition and detec-

Table 11-5. Causes of Wheezing in Children

Acute	
Asthma	Pneumothorax
Foreign body	Endobronchial intubation
Bronchiolitis	Herniated ETT cuff
Inhalation injury	

Recurrent or Persistent	
Asthma	Mediastinal mass
Foreign body	Tracheomalacia/bronchomalacia
Bronchiolitis	Vascular ring
Cardiac failure	Tracheal web/stenosis
Cystic fibrosis	Bronchial stenosis
Sickle cell disease	Roundworm infestation
Recurrent aspiration	

tion of complications, the presence of coexisting diseases, overlap with adult populations, and changing anesthetic management techniques. A retrospective review of 706 adult and pediatric patients with a rigorous definition of asthma found an incidence of documented bronchospasm of 1.7% and no pneumonia, pneumothorax, or death.[32] Of 211 children younger than age 12 years, none developed bronchospasm at the time of surgery. A retrospective review of over 136,000 computer-based anesthetic records found an incidence of 0.8% of bronchospasm in patients with asthma.[33] By contrast, older studies from the 1960s noted incidences of wheezing of 7% to 8% in asthmatic patients.[34,35] A blinded, prospective study of 59 asthmatic patients detected transient wheezing after intubation in 25% of cases; however, most events were brief and self-limited.[36] An editorial review of the subject of asthma and anesthesia concluded that, although the true incidence of major complications is low, severe adverse outcomes do result from bronchospasm and patients with asthma are at heightened risk for severe morbidity.[37]

Both the severity and the control of asthma must be established preoperatively. The two aspects of the current disease state should be clearly differentiated.[38] For example, severe asthma may be well controlled, whereas mild asthma may be poorly controlled, but both situations may have heightened potential for perioperative complications because even the child with intermittent asthma can have a severe exacerbation. Severity and control may be assessed by the frequency of symptoms, medication use, emergency department attendance, hospitalizations, and need for ventilatory support. Maintenance treatment of asthma is based on a stepwise approach; the type of therapy is, therefore, often an indication of severity. An approach to assessment of severity and control in children aged 5 to 11 years is outlined in Tables 11-6 and 11-7 (see website). Short-acting inhaled β agonists are first-line therapy, with inhaled corticosteroids for those with persistent symptoms poorly managed by bronchodilators as the preferred second step. Alternative treatments at this step include a leukotriene receptor antagonist, a mast cell stabilizer such as cromolyn sodium or nedocromil, and a methylxanthine bronchodilator such as theophylline. The third step in therapy involves increasing the dose of inhaled corticosteroid or the addition of an alternative treatment to a lower dose of corticosteroid; a long-acting β agonist, a leukotriene-receptor antagonist, or theophylline may be considered. Step 4 involves a medium dose of corticosteroid together with a long-acting β agonist. The final steps of therapy include a high dose of inhaled corticosteroid or commencing an oral corticosteroid (Fig. 11-9, see website).

Most children with asthma have disease that is intermittent or persistent but mild and will be treated with inhaled short-acting β agonists on an as-needed basis, alone or in combination with low-dose inhaled corticosteroids or an adjunctive therapy. Poor control may relate to poor compliance with medication, inadequate inhaler technique, or incorrect diagnosis. Severe asthma is diagnosed when symptom control is poor despite high doses of corticosteroids (steps 5 or 6 in Fig. 11-9 [see website]). A small group of children have "brittle asthma" that is difficult to control despite optimal therapy and may lead to life-threatening respiratory compromise. A history of severe attacks or admission to intensive care is particularly ominous.

Special investigations are not routinely indicated but may be useful in specific circumstances. A chest radiograph is not usually helpful to assess the severity of asthma but can help diagnose a superimposed infection, pneumothorax, or pneumomediastinum during an acute exacerbation. Pulmonary function tests are important in following long-term response to therapy but are of little use in the immediate routine preoperative workup of cases at a stable clinical baseline. The measurements of nitric oxide and various inflammatory markers are primarily of use as research tools at present but their role in asthma management is evolving.

Although an assessment of disease severity is essential, an important caveat is that many asthma deaths in the community setting occur not in those with severe disease but in those with what was thought to be mild or moderate disease. Asthma is often undertreated,[38] so the sensitivity of medication prescription as a marker of disease activity must be viewed with some caution. Some studies of asthma have found a poor correlation between assessment of disease sensitivity and the occurrence of perioperative bronchospasm. Disease *activity*, as noted by recent asthma symptoms, use of medications for symptom treatment, and recent therapy in a medical facility for asthma, was significantly associated with perioperative bronchospasm in one study.[32]

Children should continue their regular medications before anesthesia. Midazolam has been reported to be a safe premedication for asthmatics.[39] Corticosteroids may help prevent perioperative bronchospasm, although controlled clinical data to substantiate this practice are lacking.[40] Inhaled β agonists before or shortly after induction of anesthesia attenuate the increases in airway resistance associated with tracheal intubation.[41,42] Ketamine is the traditional choice of intravenous induction agent in patients with severe asthma, although this has not been substantiated in clinical trials.[43,44] Propofol is typically preferred over thiopentone because it causes less bronchoconstriction.[36,45] Both halothane and sevoflurane are used extensively as inhalation induction agents.

Airway manipulation is a potent stimulus for bronchospasm. In children with URIs, when the airways may be acutely hyperactive, the avoidance of intubation is associated with a reduced incidence of pulmonary complications.[19] There are inadequate clinical outcome data on the perioperative management of asthma to make definitive recommendations about airway management. Nevertheless, avoidance of airway stimulation when possible seems a sensible approach. For short cases, a face mask may be adequate; a laryngeal mask airway similarly is less of an irritant than an ETT. If endotracheal intubation is mandatory, a deep plane of anesthesia blunts airway hyperreactivity. Similarly, unless contraindicated by other factors, deep extubation may be preferable for the same reason. Surgical stimulation is another trigger of bronchospasm, and anesthetic depth and analgesia should be adequate to prevent this response.

Intraoperative bronchospasm is characterized variously by polyphonic expiratory wheeze, prolonged expiration, active expiration with increased respiratory effort, increased airway pressures, a slow upslope on the end-tidal CO_2 monitor, raised end-tidal CO_2, and hypoxemia (see also Fig. 37-9A-B). Other causes of wheezing must be excluded, such as partial ETT obstruction (secretions or herniation of the cuff causing obstruction), mainstem intubation (deep endobronchial intubation), aspiration, pneumothorax, or pulmonary edema. Mechanical obstruction of the circuit or ETT must also be excluded. First-line responses to bronchospasm involve removing the triggering

stimulus if possible, deepening anesthesia, increasing FIO_2 if appropriate, and increasing expiratory time to minimize alveolar air trapping. In severe status asthmaticus, ventilation strategy should focus primarily on achieving adequate oxygenation, rather than attempting to normalize $PaCO_2$ at the potential cost of inducing pulmonary barotrauma. Inhaled β agonists can be delivered by nebulizer or by a metered-dose inhaler down the airway device with specially designed adaptors (see also Fig. 37-10). Alternatively, a 60-mL syringe can be used to deliver doses of the nebulizer into the breathing circuit (Fig. 11-10). All children who experience anything more than minor bronchospasm should also receive corticosteroids if they have not already done so.

The anesthesiologist may be involved in the management of bronchospasm when consulted to assist a child in the emergency department or on the wards. A drowsy, silent child with a quiet chest on auscultation is in imminent danger of respiratory arrest and requires emergent intubation by an experienced practitioner. Signs and symptoms to assess the severity of an asthma exacerbation are outlined in Table 11-8, and an algorithm for management issued by the American National Heart, Lung and Blood Institute is presented in Figure 11-11 (see website). Oxygen is recommended for most children to maintain the hemoglobin saturation greater than 90%. Repetitive or continuous administration of short-acting β agonists is first-line therapy for all children and is the most effective way of reversing airflow obstruction. The addition of ipratropium to a β agonist may produce additional bronchodilation and have a modest effect to improve outcome. Systemic corticosteroids should be given to those who do not respond completely and promptly to β agonists. For severe exacerbations unresponsive to the treatment listed earlier, intravenous magnesium may decrease the likelihood of intubation, although the evidence is limited. Current recommended drug dosages are listed in Table 11-9 (see website). Methylxanthines such as theophylline are not recommended as treatment for acute exacerbations because they produce no added benefit but expose the child to the complications from toxicity. Antibiotics are not recommended except for comorbid conditions. Aggressive hydration is not recommended for adults or older children, although it may be indicated in younger children who become dehydrated as a result

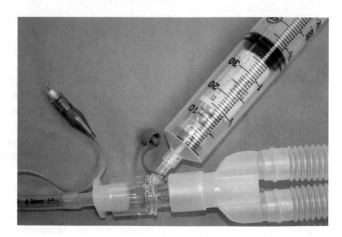

Figure 11-10. A 60-mL syringe may be attached to a port in the circuit to administer aerosolized drugs such as albuterol.

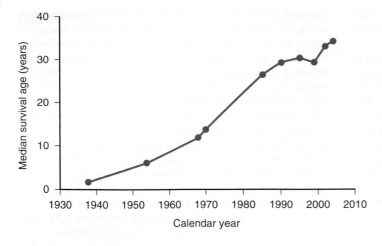

Figure 11-12. Median survival for patients with cystic fibrosis at various times since the first description of the disease. Data before 1970 are gleaned from the then-current literature. Data since 1985 are from the Cystic Fibrosis Foundation Data Registry and represent projections of median survival age for a child born in that year with cystic fibrosis. (Reproduced from Davis PB: Cystic fibrosis since 1938. Am J Respir Crit Care Med 2006; 173:475-482.)

disorders is the next most common procedural category that requires anesthesia in the CF population. Other indications for anesthesia include bronchoscopy and pulmonary lavage, gastrointestinal endoscopy, sclerosing injection of varices due to portal hypertension, insertion of venous access devices, and incidental surgical problems.[52-54] The pediatric anesthesiologist may be involved in the care of adult patients because of the perception that CF remains a "pediatric disease." Surgical procedures typically include treatment of recurrent pneumothorax, cholecystectomy, and lung or cardiac transplantation. Consultation may also be requested for obstetric cases as increasing numbers of patients survive to adulthood.

Pulmonary disease is the predominant concern when planning an anesthetic. Historically, morbidity and mortality from pulmonary complications were high. A retrospective 18-year review of 133 anesthetics in 93 patients, published in 1964, noted perioperative mortality of 27%, with pulmonary complications occurring in 42% of cases.[55] A retrospective 11-year review of 144 anesthetics, published in 1972, reported a perioperative mortality of 4%.[51] More recent studies record better outcomes. A 1985 study of 126 anesthetics found no mortality and a CF-specific complication rate, predominantly pulmonary, of 9%.[52] A 1984 study of 18 patients for pleural surgery concluded that, although the risks for this procedure were great, the anesthetic hazards of CF could be minimized with careful management.[56] A study of 11 patients undergoing anesthesia for injection of esophageal varices found no serious anesthetic complications

but detected significant deterioration in pulmonary function tests shortly after anesthesia[57]; it was unclear if these changes persisted past the immediate postoperative period. A larger study found no difference between pulmonary function tests measured 3 months before and 3 months after surgery.[52] A recent study of 199 anesthetics in 53 patients for ear/nose/throat surgery found a 5% incidence of minor pulmonary problems and no deaths.[58] These limited data suggest that although pulmonary complications are a problem, they can be successfully anticipated and preempted by modern anesthetic management techniques.

An assessment of the severity, current state and progression of pulmonary disease should guide anesthetic planning. Fitness is a positive predictor of survival,[46] and exercise tolerance is a useful marker of pulmonary function. The quality and quantity of secretions, recent and chronic infections, the use and effectiveness of bronchodilators, and number of hospitalizations are also important points to elucidate on history. Examination of the cardiopulmonary systems should aim to detect compromise of cardiac, pulmonary, and hepatic function. Special investigations are not routinely indicated but may quantify organ dysfunction in end stages of the disease. Arterial blood gas analysis, chest radiography, pulmonary function tests, electrocardiography, echocardiography, and liver function tests may assist the planning of anesthetic technique in selected children.[54] Pulmonary function should be optimized preoperatively, with chest physiotherapy, bronchodilators, and humidified nebulizers to improve clearance of secretions.

Children are often emotionally vulnerable, not simply owing to the usual preoperative anxieties but secondary to the psychological consequences of progression of an ultimately fatal disease. A preoperative visit should aim to allay distress; oral benzodiazepines have been successfully used as anxiolytics.[52,58] Prophylactic use of osmotic laxatives may be indicated if opioid-induced ileus is anticipated.[54] Although aspiration has not been reported as a complication in the literature, the incidence of gastroesophageal reflux is high and antacid premedication may be considered.[59]

Inhalation induction may be prolonged due to large FRC, small tidal volumes, and ventilation/perfusion mismatch. Common intraoperative problems include obstruction by inspissated secretions, airway hyperreactivity, and hypoxemia.

Table 11-10. The Most Frequent Indications for Anesthesia in Cystic Fibrosis

Neonates	Children/Teenagers	Adults
Meconium ileus	Nasal polypectomy	Esophageal varices
Meconium peritonitis	Intravenous access	Recurrent pneumothorax
Intestinal atresia	Ear/nose/throat surgery	Cholecystectomy
		Lung (liver) transplantation

Reproduced from Della Rocca G: Anaesthesia in patients with cystic fibrosis. Curr Opin Anaesthesiol 2002; 15:95-101.

Pneumothorax, consequent on high ventilatory pressures and rupture of bullae, is a less common complication. Postoperative tribulations include impaired clearance of secretions, atelectasis, pneumonia, and respiratory failure. Anesthesia should be deep enough to prevent bronchospasm or increased shunting during surgical stimulation or airway suctioning but ideally should not compromise postoperative respiratory function. Regional anesthesia is an ideal option if not contraindicated by coagulopathy or patient refusal. For general anesthesia, short-acting agents are preferred to minimize postoperative respiratory compromise. A cuffed ETT is often required, owing to the great airway pressures needed for adequate ventilation.

Because dehydration of secretions is a central pulmonary issue in CF, general anesthesia poses specific problems. During spontaneous ventilation under normal conditions, inspired gases are warmed to body temperature and saturated with water vapor, reaching this state at a point just below the carina.[60] This region is known as the isothermic saturation point and ensures that the lower airways are kept moist and warm.[61] The alveolar environment in optimal circumstances has a saturated water vapor pressure of 47.1 mm Hg and an absolute humidity of 43.4 g/m^{-3} at 37°C. The inspiration of cold, desiccated anesthetic gases and vapors can impair the warming and humidification of the airways. The use of any airway device—oropharyngeal airway, laryngeal mask, or ETT—bypasses the nasal and oropharyngeal passages and delivers cold, dry gas to a varying extent farther down the airway.[62] This shifts the isothermic saturation point distally, forcing bronchi that normally function in optimal conditions to take part in heat and gas exchange.[61] These parts of the airway are less adapted to moisture exchange and tend to dehydrate more rapidly, thereby impairing the mucociliary escalator and predisposing to impaction of secretions.[63,64] Direct impairment of mucociliary motion by anesthetic medications, as well as blunting of the cough response and ventilatory drive, can contribute further to the problem. Particular attention should, therefore, be directed to hydrating the airway in the perioperative period, to minimize the exacerbation of the primary pathologic pulmonary process of CF. Inhalation of hypertonic saline (7% sodium chloride) accelerates mucus clearance and improves lung function[65-67] and is now part of the routine maintenance management of CF. Nebulized saline treatments should be continued up to the start of anesthesia and recommenced after the procedure is complete. Inhaled gases should be humidified or an artificial "nose" inserted into the circuit to conserve airway moisture and minimize inspissation of secretions. Bronchial washing and suction can be used to clear secretions for more prolonged procedures, under a depth of anesthesia adequate to prevent bronchospasm.

At the conclusion of surgery, complete reversal of neuromuscular blockade should be confirmed. Whenever possible, the child should be extubated and encouraged to breathe spontaneously. A 30- to 40-degree head-up position assists movement of the diaphragm and ventilation. Postoperatively, physiotherapy, airway humidification, close attention to analgesia, and early mobilization should aim to enhance clearance of secretions and minimize atelectasis. The use of regional or local anesthesia, plus non-opioid analgesics, is useful to avoid respiratory depression. Ambulatory surgery is optimal, if feasible, because it minimizes disruption to the patient's schedule and decreases exposure to nosocomial infection.

Sickle Cell Disease

Sickle cell disease (SCD) is an inherited hemoglobinopathy resulting from a point mutation on chromosome 11. The mutant gene codes for the production of hemoglobin S, a mutant variant of the normal hemoglobin A. This leads to widespread and progressive vascular damage.[68,69] Clinical features of the disease include acute episodes of pain, acute and chronic pulmonary disease, hemorrhagic and occlusive stroke, renal insufficiency, and splenic infarction, with mean life expectancy shortened to just over 3 decades.[70] Perioperative problems and management are covered in more detail in Chapter 9, and this discussion will be limited to a brief review of the pulmonary pathology of SCD.

The acute chest syndrome (ACS) is an acute lung injury caused by SCD. Diagnostic criteria include a new pulmonary infiltrate involving at least one lung segment on the radiograph (excluding atelectasis), combined with one or more symptoms or signs of chest pain, pyrexia greater than 38.5°C (101.3°F), tachypnea, wheezing, and cough.[71-73] Precipitants include infection, fat embolism after bone marrow infarction, pulmonary infarction, and surgical procedures.[73-75] Potential risk factors for the development and severity of perioperative ACS include a history of lung disease, recent clustering of acute pulmonary complications, pregnancy, increased age, and the invasiveness of the surgical procedure.[68] However, a study of 60 laparoscopic surgeries noted an association between younger age and ACS, which the authors suggested may be related to reduced temperatures and greater relative blood loss as a proportion of total blood volume in smaller children.[76]

Minor procedures such as inguinal hernia repair or distal extremity surgery have a low risk of pulmonary complications (none to 5%), whereas intra-abdominal or major joint surgery has an ACS rate of 10% to 15%.[75,77,78] Although overall perioperative mortality specifically from SCD appears to be quite small, slightly under 1%,[75] ACS can lead to prolonged postoperative hospitalization, respiratory failure, and death. One study of 604 patients noted that ACS typically developed 3 days postoperatively and persisted for 8 days; 2 patients died in approximately 60 episodes.[74]

SCD also causes chronic lung damage, known as sickle cell lung disease (SCLD).[79] Because lung function has not yet been assessed longitudinally in a cohort from early childhood to adulthood, the precise pathology of and relationship between the obstructive and restrictive patterns of lung disease is unclear.[80] Children appear to have a predominantly obstructive pattern,[81] whereas adults have more restrictive pulmonary findings.[79,82,83] The later stages of lung damage involve decreased vital and total lung capacities, impaired gas diffusion, pulmonary fibrosis, pulmonary artery hypertension, right-sided cardiomyopathy, and progressive hypoxemia.[79,83] The development of pulmonary artery hypertension, which can precede clinically apparent lung damage, is a particularly ominous sign of disease progression and is associated with heightened risk of sudden death.[82] Recurrent ACS is an independent risk factor for the development of end-stage SCLD, but subtle evidence of parenchymal and vascular damage commonly precedes clustered episodes of ACS.[79]

Assessment of lung function should include a history of the occurrence, frequency, severity, and known precipitants of ACS and a search for progression of chronic lung damage. A recent chest radiograph will serve as a baseline for comparison if postoperative radiographs are needed and can also delineate lung pathology. Early features of lung damage include decreased distal pulmonary vascularity and diffuse interstitial fibrosis, whereas later stages are characterized by pulmonary fibrosis and right ventricular hypertrophy.[79] Pulmonary function testing can reveal the need for bronchodilators and the presence of obstructive or restrictive lung disease.

The efficacy of preoperative or intraoperative management techniques beyond basic standards of care has not been clearly demonstrated, and well-delivered anesthetic and postoperative care may be the best guarantors of good outcome.[68,69] Because the effect of perioperative red blood cell transfusion versus no transfusion in preventing ACS or other sickle cell complications has not been tested by an adequately controlled study, the efficacy of prophylactic erythrocyte transfusion is controversial. One recent guideline suggests the avoidance of transfusion in low-risk situations, while considering transfusion only for cases assessed as greater risk.[68] If transfusion is undertaken, exchange transfusion aiming to decrease the concentration of hemoglobin S to 30% is no more efficacious than correction of anemia to a hematocrit of 30% in preventing SCD exacerbations but results in more transfusion-related complications.[74] Consequently, if a decision is made to transfuse in the hope of preventing ACS, the target should be a hematocrit of 30% rather than a specific dilution of hemoglobin S.

Sickle cell patients frequently develop postoperative atelectasis. It is unclear if this relates to underlying sickle lung disease, difficulty with analgesia, other causes, or a combination of factors. Pain management can be difficult. Postoperative pain and opioid consumption is often great in SCD patients, and opioid use may lead to respiratory blunting and atelectasis.[84] ACS tends to involve the lower segments of the lung,[73] suggesting an association between atelectasis and ACS. Incentive spirometry can prevent the development of atelectasis and pulmonary infiltrates associated with ACS.[85] Regional analgesia, supplemental nonopioid analgesics, prophylactic incentive spirometry, early mobilization, and good pulmonary toilet may decrease the incidence of atelectasis and ACS.

Treatment of ACS is focused on supporting gas exchange. Supplemental oxygen, noninvasive ventilatory support such as continuous positive airway pressure, or intubation and mechanical ventilation are indicated by the degree of dysfunction. Bronchodilators, incentive spirometry, and chest physiotherapy may be useful in preventing progression of the disease. In the presence of a significant ventilation/perfusion mismatch, correction of anemia can improve arterial oxygenation. Erythrocyte transfusion increases oxygen-carrying capacity, decreases fractional peripheral tissue extraction, and increases returning venous oxygen levels. Because the mean arterial oxygen content in the presence of a shunt is significantly affected by the oxygenation of blood returning from nonventilated parts of the lung, increasing venous oxygen levels can improve arterial oxygen content. Whereas transfusion has not been clearly shown to improve outcome, both exchange and simple transfusion can improve oxygenation.[73]

Summary

Pulmonary complications are a major cause of perioperative morbidity in the pediatric population. Although preexisting pulmonary pathologic processes in children can present significant challenges to anesthetic delivery, a thorough assessment of the problem combined with intelligent anesthetic management allows most children to undergo surgical interventions without long-term adverse sequelae. Consultation with a pediatric pulmonologist is indicated when appropriate for specific problems as outlined in this chapter; a team approach may markedly improve operative and postoperative outcomes.

Annotated References

Accurso FJ: Update in cystic fibrosis 2005. Am J Respir Crit Care Med 2006; 173:944-947
A current review of the pathophysiology of cystic fibrosis

Bishop MJ, Cheney FW: Anesthesia for patients with asthma: low risk but not no risk. Anesthesiology 1996; 85:455-456
A thoughtful editorial on the implications, dangers, and practical implications of asthma

Davis PB: Cystic fibrosis since 1938. Am J Respir Crit Care Med 2006; 173:475-482
A succinct discourse on the evolution of management of cystic fibrosis

Doherty GM, Chisakuta A, Crean P, Shields MD: Anesthesia and the child with asthma. Paediatr Anaesth 2005; 15:446-454
A recent review of the perioperative management of asthma

Firth PG, Head CA: Sickle cell disease and anesthesia. Anesthesiology 2004; 101:766-785
A comprehensive review of anesthetic management of sickle cell disease

National Asthma Education and Prevention Program: Full Report of the Expert Panel: Guidelines for the Diagnosis and Management of Asthma (EPR-3). Bethesda, MD, National Heart, Lung, and Blood Institute, National Institutes of Health, 2007
An extensive review of current evidence on the pathophysiology, diagnosis, and management of asthma

Tait AR, Malviya S: Anesthesia for the child with an upper respiratory tract infection: still a dilemma? Anesth Analg 2005; 100:59-65
A broad review of the data on perioperative upper respiratory tract infections and suggested approaches to management

References

Please see www.expertconsult.com

The Pediatric Airway

Melissa Wheeler, Charles J. Coté, and I. David Todres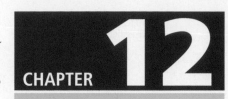

CHAPTER 12

THE DIFFERENCES BETWEEN A child's airway and an adult's dictate differences in anesthetic management techniques. Knowledge of normal developmental anatomy and physiologic function is required to understand and manage both the normal and the pathologic airways of infants and children (Video Clip 12-1, see website). Techniques and principles to assist in this management are reviewed in this chapter.

Developmental Anatomy of the Airway

The classic works by Negus, Eckenhoff, and Fink and Demarest form the foundation of our knowledge about the structure and function of the pediatric and adult airway.[1-3] There are five major anatomic differences between the neonatal and adult airway; these are outlined below.[2-4] In addition, the relatively large head of an infant negates the need to place anything under the head to achieve a proper "sniffing position." The older child will have airway features that represent a transition between these two developmental stages.

Note: Many manufacturers have graciously provided us samples of airway devices so that we could illustrate examples of commonly available equipment. There is insufficient room to illustrate all available devices. Lack of illustration of a device should not be construed as lack of efficacy nor should illustration of a device be interpreted as endorsement. Practitioners are encouraged to use all equipment available and make their own educated decision about what devices provide the most safety and efficacy in their hands.

Tongue

An infant's tongue is relatively large in proportion to the rest of the oral cavity. Thus, it more easily obstructs the airway, especially in a neonate. The tongue is more difficult to manipulate and stabilize with a laryngoscope blade.

Position of the Larynx

An infant's larynx is higher (more cephalad) in the neck, classically described at the level of C3-4, than is an adult's larynx which is at the level of C4-5 (Fig. 12-1). A study that used magnetic resonance imaging (MRI) and computed tomography (CT) to localize airway structures confirmed that the larynx is higher (more cephalad) in children than in adults and noted that the hyoid bone is at the C2-3 level in children from neonate to 2 years of age.[5] Because the larynx is higher (more cephalad) in the neck of an infant, the distances between the tongue, hyoid bone, epiglottis, and roof of the mouth are smaller than in an older child or adult. Thus, the tongue easily obstructs the infant's airway. The proximity of the tongue to the more superior larynx also makes visualization of laryngeal structures more difficult because it produces a more acute angulation between the plane of the tongue and the plane of the glottic opening. Therefore, the infant tongue is also more likely to obstruct the view of the larynx. It is for this reason that a straight laryngoscope blade, which more effectively lifts the tongue from the field of view during laryngoscopy, facilitates visualization of an infant's larynx. This anatomic relationship is further complicated in

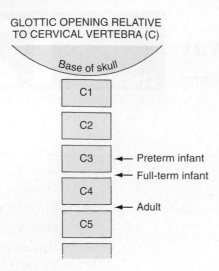

Figure 12-1. In a preterm infant, the larynx is located at the middle of the third cervical vertebra (C3); in a full-term infant, at the C3-4 interspace; and in an adult, at the C4-5 interspace. (Adapted from Negus VE: The Comparative Anatomy and Physiology of the Larynx. Oxford, Butterworth-Heinemann, 1949.)

certain conditions such as the Treacher Collins anomaly and other syndromes associated with mandibular and midfacial hypoplasia that make direct visualization of the glottis difficult and sometimes impossible with standard laryngoscopy (Fig. 12-2). The reason for this difficulty is that with mandibular and

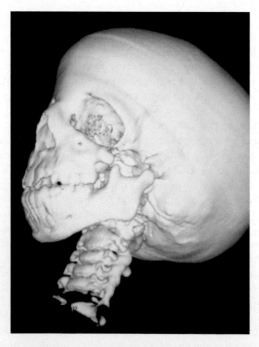

Figure 12-2. This three-dimensional reconstruction of a child with the Treacher-Collins anomaly demonstrates the retrognathic and more posterior position of the mandible, midfacial hypoplasia, and the exaggerated angle and closer proximity between the base of the tongue and the laryngeal inlet (nearly 90 degrees), making direct visualization of the larynx difficult.

midfacial hypoplasia, the base of the tongue is positioned more caudally (known as glossoptosis) and in closer proximity to the laryngeal inlet than normal; the result is an even greater acute angulation between the plane of the tongue and the plane of the laryngeal inlet (often 90 degrees) (Fig. 12-3). In this situation, conventional rigid laryngoscopy results in direct visualization of the esophageal inlet rather than of the laryngeal inlet. In these children, special equipment or special techniques may be required to intubate the trachea.

Epiglottis

An adult's epiglottis is flat and broad and its axis is parallel to that of the trachea (Fig. 12-4), whereas the infant's epiglottis is narrower, omega shaped, and angled away from the axis of the trachea (Fig. 12-5). It is therefore more difficult to lift the infant's epiglottis with the tip of a laryngoscope blade.

Vocal Folds

An infant's vocal folds (cords) have a lower (caudad) attachment anteriorly than posteriorly, whereas in an adult, the axis of the vocal folds is perpendicular to the trachea. This anatomic feature alters the angle at which the tracheal tube approaches the laryngeal inlet and occasionally leads to difficulty in intubation, especially with the nasal approach; the tip of the ETT may be held up at the anterior commissure of the vocal folds.

Subglottis

Classic teaching is that the narrowest part of an infant's larynx is the cricoid cartilage; in an adult, it is the rima glottidis. A study using MRI and CT demonstrated that the immediate subglottic area was the narrowest portion of the airway in young (<2 years) children.[5] Another study of children ages 2 months to 13 years undergoing MRI with propofol sedation and no paralysis demonstrated that the narrowest portions of the pediatric larynx are the glottic opening and the immediate sub–vocal cord level. However, these investigators found no change in the relationships of these dimensions relative to cricoid dimensions throughout childhood.[6] Nonetheless, when a relatively large diameter tube is inserted into the glottic aperture the tube passes through the cords but may become stuck immediately below the cords (e.g., in the subglottic or cricoid ring region; see later).

As discussed earlier, in adults, the classic teaching is that the rima glottidis is the narrowest part of the airway. Thus, an ETT that traverses the glottis passes freely into the trachea because the airway beyond is of larger diameter. However, a study of adult cadaver specimens found that in approximately 70% of cases the narrowest portion of the airway was also in the subglottic region.[7] The range in diameter for adult females was 10 to 16 mm, and for adult males it was 13 to 19 mm. Thus, the likely reason that ETTs pass easily through the glottic opening into the trachea of adults is that, overall, the narrowest portion of the airway is still larger than the most commonly used ETT sizes. This apparent subglottic narrowing in adults is generally not evident unless there is the need to pass a larger-diameter ETT such as a double-lumen tube. In contrast, in a child, it is common for an ETT to pass easily through the vocal folds (glottic opening) but not through the subglottic region (Fig. 12-6; see Video Clip 12-1 [on website]). Thus, one can conceptualize both the adult and pediatric larynx to be somewhat funnel shaped, but this configuration is exaggerated in infants and young children.

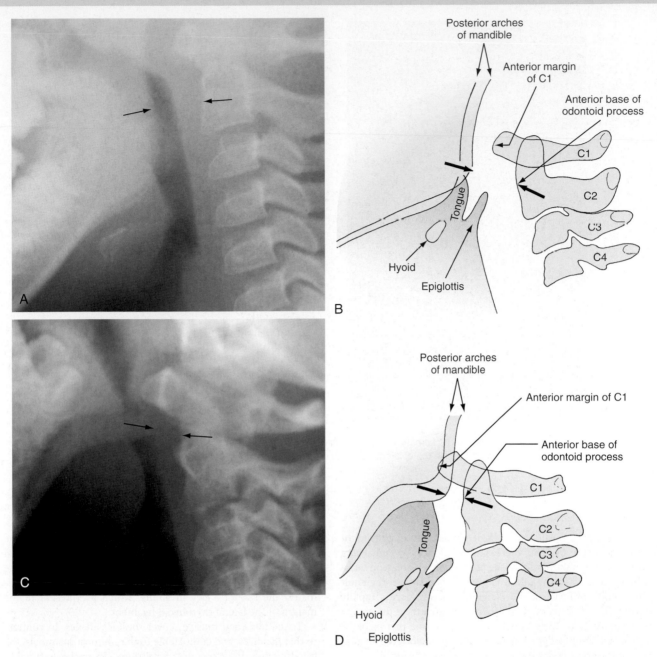

Figure 12-3. The larynx in children with mandibular hypoplasia is located more posteriorly than in children with normal anatomy. **A,** A lateral radiograph of the upper airway including the base of the skull and cervical spine of a normal 7-year-old child; the *arrows* denote the posterior border of the ramus of the mandible and the anterior border of the second cervical vertebra. **B,** A diagrammatic representation of the normal anatomy in **A**. **C,** The same radiographic projection in a 6-year-old child with Treacher Collins syndrome; the *arrows* again denote the posterior border of the ramus of the mandible and the anterior margin of the second cervical vertebra. **D,** A diagrammatic representation of the anatomy in **C**. Note the significantly smaller space between the ramus of the mandible and the second cervical vertebra; the anterior margin of the first cervical vertebra overlaps the posterior margin of the mandible. This extreme posterior location of the tongue and larynx makes direct visualization of the laryngeal inlet nearly impossible in many children with this anomaly because of the acute angulation between the base of the tongue and the laryngeal inlet. (Radiographs courtesy of Donna J. Seibert, MD, John A. Kirkpatrick, Jr., MD, and Robert H. Cleveland, MD.)

The cricoid is the only complete ring of cartilage in the laryngotracheobronchial tree and is therefore nonexpandable. A tight-fitting ETT that compresses the tracheal mucosa at this level may cause edema, reducing the luminal diameter of the upper airway and increasing airway resistance at the time of extubation (post-extubation croup). Because the subglottic region of an infant is smaller than in an adult, the same degree of airway edema is more compromising in the infant. For example, assuming the diameter of the infant cricoid ring or trachea to be approximately 4 mm and the diameter of the adult cricoid ring or trachea to be approximately 8 mm, if 1 mm of edema forms circumferentially (i.e., the diameter of the airway

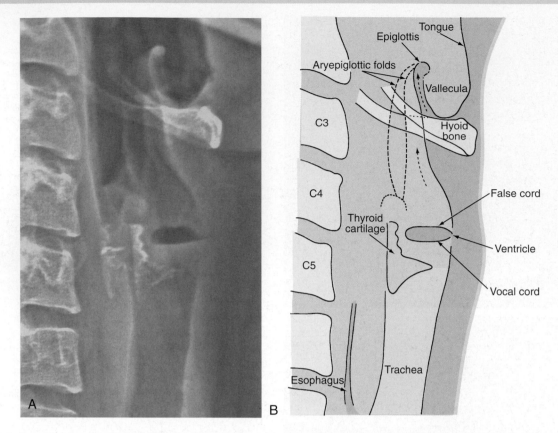

Figure 12-4. Lateral neck xerogram (**A**) and schematic (**B**) of an adult's larynx. Note the relatively thin, broad epiglottis, the axis of which is parallel to the trachea. The hyoid bone "hugs" the epiglottis; there is no subglottic narrowing.

is reduced by 2 mm), the cross-sectional area of the infant airway decreases by 75%, whereas the adult cross-sectional area decreases only 44%. Similarly, the proportional increase in resistance to airflow in the infant is greater than that in the adult (Fig. 12-7).[2] Growth of the subglottic airway occurs rapidly during the first 2 years of life; thereafter, growth of the airway is linear.[8] At 10 to 12 years of age, the cricoid and thyroid cartilages reach adult proportion, thus eliminating both the angulation of the vocal cords and the narrow subglottic area.

The Larynx

Understanding the anatomy and function of the larynx is critical to knowledgeable, safe, and successful management of the airway.

Anatomy

Structure

The larynx is composed of one bone (hyoid) and a series of cartilages (the single thyroid, cricoid, and the paired arytenoid, corniculate, cuneiform cartilages, and triticea cartilages). These cartilages are suspended by ligaments from the base of the skull. The body of the cricoid cartilage articulates posteriorly with the inferior cornu of the thyroid cartilage. The paired triangular

arytenoid cartilages rest on top of, and articulate with, the superoposterior aspect of the cricoid cartilage. The arytenoid cartilages are protected by the thyroid cartilage (Fig. 12-8). The triticea cartilages are rounded nodules of cartilage, approximately the size of a pea in adults, which are present in the margin of the lateral thyrohyoid ligament.

Tissue folds and muscles cover these cartilages. In contrast to that in adults, and comparable to that in most mammals, the cartilaginous glottis accounts for 60% to 75% of the vocal folds' length in children younger than 2 years of age.[8] Contraction of the intrinsic laryngeal muscles alters the position and configuration of these tissue folds, thus influencing laryngeal function during respiration, forced voluntary glottic closure (Valsalva maneuver), reflex laryngospasm, swallowing, and phonation (Fig. 12-9).

The laryngeal tissue folds consist of the following:

- Paired aryepiglottic folds extending from the epiglottis posteriorly to the superior surface of the arytenoids (the paired cuneiform and corniculate cartilages lie within for support and reinforcement)
- Paired vestibular folds (false vocal cords) extending from the thyroid cartilage posteriorly to the superior surface of the arytenoids
- Paired vocal folds (true vocal cords) extending from the posterior surface of the thyroid plate to the anterior projection or vocal process of the arytenoids

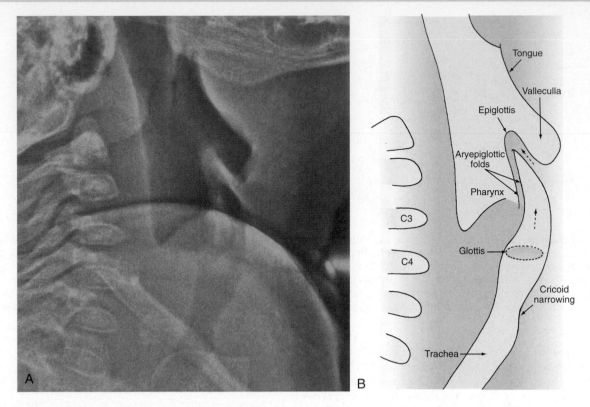

Figure 12-5. Lateral neck xerogram (**A**) and schematic (**B**) of an infant's larynx. Note the angled epiglottis and the narrow cricoid cartilage.

- A single interarytenoid fold (composed of the interarytenoid muscle covered by tissue) bridging the arytenoid cartilages
- A single thyrohyoid fold extending from the hyoid bone to the thyroid cartilage

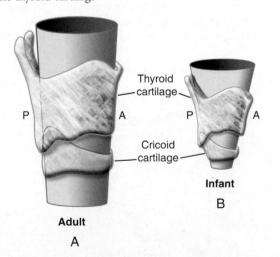

Figure 12-6. Configuration of the larynx of an adult (**A**) and an infant (**B**). Note that both the adult and infant's larynx are somewhat funnel shaped but that this shape is exaggerated in the infant and toddler. The adult laryngeal structures are of such size that most endotracheal tubes pass easily into the trachea. In infants and toddlers, it is common for the endotracheal tube to pass easily through the vocal cords but to become snug at the level of the nondistensible cricoid cartilage. Concern for causing edema at this point resulted in the classic teaching to use uncuffed endotracheal tubes in young children (see text for more details).

Histology

The highly vascular mucosa of the mouth is continuous with that of the larynx and trachea. This mucosa consists of squamous, stratified, and pseudostratified ciliated epithelium. The vocal cords are covered with stratified epithelium. The mucosa and submucosa are rich in lymphatic vessels and seromucous-secreting glands, which lubricate the laryngeal folds. The submucosa consists of loose fibrous stroma; therefore, the mucosa is loosely adherent to the underlying structures in most areas. However, the submucosa is scant on the laryngeal surface of the epiglottis and the vocal cords; therefore, the mucosa is tightly adherent in these areas.[9,10] For this reason, most inflammatory processes of the airway above the level of the vocal cords are limited by the barrier formed by the firm adherence of the mucosa to the vocal cords.[9] For example, the inflammation of epiglottitis is usually limited to the supraglottic structures, and the loosely adherent mucosa explains the ease with which localized swelling occurs (see Figs. 37-3 and 37-4). In a similar manner, an inflammatory process of the subglottic region (laryngotracheobronchitis) results in significant subglottic edema in the loosely adherent mucosa of the airway below the vocal cords, but it does not usually spread above the level of the vocal cords (see Fig. 37-5).[10]

Sensory and Motor Innervation

Two branches of the vagus nerve, the recurrent laryngeal and the superior laryngeal, supply both sensory and motor innervation to the larynx. The superior laryngeal nerve also has two branches: the internal branch provides sensory innervation to the supraglottic region, whereas the external branch supplies motor innervation to the cricothyroid muscle. The recurrent laryngeal nerve provides sensory innervation to the subglottic

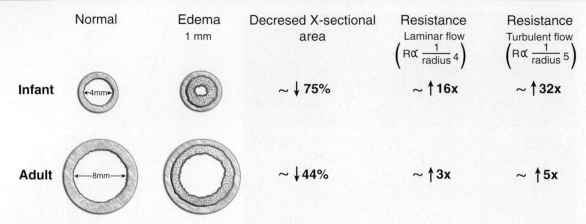

	Normal	Edema 1 mm	Decresed X-sectional area	Resistance Laminar flow $\left(R\alpha \dfrac{1}{radius^4}\right)$	Resistance Turbulent flow $\left(R\alpha \dfrac{1}{radius^5}\right)$
Infant	←4mm→		~ ↓75%	~ ↑16x	~ ↑32x
Adult	←8mm→		~ ↓44%	~ ↑3x	~ ↑5x

Figure 12-7. Relative effects of airway edema in an infant and an adult. The normal airways of an infant and an adult are presented on the left and edematous airways (1 mm circumferential, reducing the diameter by 2 mm) on the right. Note that resistance to airflow is inversely proportional to the radius of the lumen to the fourth power for laminar flow (beyond the fifth bronchial division) and to the radius of the lumen to the fifth power for turbulent flow (from the mouth to the fourth bronchial division). The net result in an infant with a 4-mm diameter airway is a 75% reduction in cross-sectional area and a 16-fold increase in resistance to airflow, compared with a 44% reduction in cross-sectional area and a 3-fold increase in resistance to airflow in an adult with a similar 2-mm reduction in airway diameter.

larynx and motor innervation to all other laryngeal muscles.[10,11] Local anesthetic agents injected to block the superior laryngeal nerve result in anesthesia of the supraglottic region down to the inferior margin of the epiglottis and motor blockade of the cricothyroid muscle, which results in relaxation of the vocal cords. Translaryngeal injection of local anesthetic through the cricothyroid membrane or a specific recurrent laryngeal nerve block is required for infraglottic and tracheal anesthesia.[12-14]

Blood Supply

Laryngeal branches of the superior and inferior thyroid arteries provide the blood supply to the larynx. The recurrent laryngeal nerve and artery lie in close proximity to each other, thus accounting for the occasional vocal cord paresis after attempts to control bleeding during thyroidectomy.[15]

Function

Inspiration

During inspiration, the larynx is pulled downward (caudad) by the negative intrathoracic pressure generated by the descent of the diaphragm and contraction of the intercostal muscles. Longitudinal stretching of the larynx results, thus increasing the distance between the aryepiglottic and vestibular folds as well as the distance between the vestibular and vocal folds. When the intrinsic muscles within the larynx contract, the arytenoids move laterally and posteriorly (rocking backward and rotating laterally), increasing the interarytenoid distance and separating as well as stretching the paired aryepiglottic, vestibular, and vocal folds. Overall, inspiration enlarges the laryngeal opening, both longitudinally (like opening a telescope) and laterally,

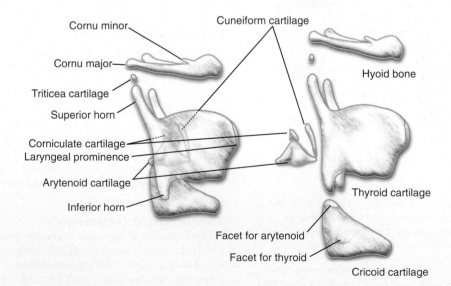

Figure 12-8. Laryngeal cartilages. The natural positions of the laryngeal cartilages are presented on the left, with the individual cartilages separated on the right. (Reprinted by permission from Fink BR, Demarest RJ: Laryngeal Biomechanics. Cambridge, MA, Harvard University Press, © 1978 by the President and Fellows of Harvard College.)

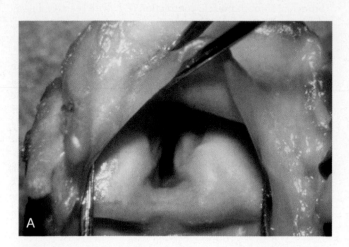

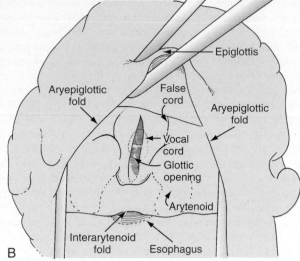

Figure 12-9. Laryngeal anatomy. Larynx of a premature infant (**A**) and schematic (**B**).

allowing the passage of greater quantities of air through the airway.

Expiration

At the end of expiration, the larynx reverts to its resting position, with longitudinal shortening of the distance between the aryepiglottic, vestibular, and vocal folds (closing of the telescope). The arytenoids return simultaneously to their resting position by rotating medially and rocking forward, thus decreasing the interarytenoid distance and reducing the tension on the paired aryepiglottic, vestibular, and vocal folds and causing them to thicken.

Forced Glottic Closure and Laryngospasm

Glottic closure during forced expiration (forced glottic closure or Valsalva maneuver) is voluntary laryngeal closure and is physiologically similar to involuntary laryngeal closure (laryngospasm). Forced glottic closure occurs at several levels. Contraction of the intrinsic laryngeal muscles results in (1) marked reduction in the interarytenoid distance; (2) anterior rocking and medial movement of the arytenoids, causing apposition of the paired vocal, vestibular, and aryepiglottic folds; (3) longitudinal shortening of the larynx, obliterating the space between the aryepiglottic, vestibular, and vocal folds (like complete closing of the telescope). Contraction of an extrinsic laryngeal muscle, the thyrohyoid, pulls the hyoid bone downward (caudad) and the thyroid cartilage upward (cephalad), leading to further closure.[1,3,4,16-19]

Closure of the larynx during laryngospasm is similar to, but not identical with, that described for voluntary forced glottic closure. There are two important differences. First, laryngospasm is accompanied by an inspiratory effort, which longitudinally separates the vocal from the vestibular folds. Second, in contrast to forced glottic closure, neither the thyroarytenoid muscle, an intrinsic muscle of the larynx, nor the thyrohyoid muscle contract; thus, apposition of the aryepiglottic folds and median thyrohyoid folds is minimal. These two differences allow the upper portion of the larynx to be left partially open during mild laryngospasm, resulting in the hallmark high-pitched inspiratory stridor (see Video Clip 12-1 on website).[1,16] Anterior and upward displacement of the mandible ("jaw thrust") longitudinally separates the base of the tongue, the epiglottis, and the aryepiglottic folds from the vocal folds, helping to relieve laryngospasm.[17]

Swallowing

Glottic closure during swallowing is also similar to that which occurs during forced closure of the glottis. Protection of the glottic opening is achieved primarily by apposition of the laryngeal folds and secondarily by upward (cephalad) movement of the larynx. The upward movement of the larynx brings the thyroid cartilage closer to the hyoid bone, resulting in folding of the epiglottis over the glottic opening.[1,16,18,19] With loss of consciousness or deep sedation, the normal protective mechanism of the larynx may be lost or obtunded, thus predisposing to pulmonary aspiration of pharyngeal contents.

Phonation

Phonation is accomplished by alteration of the angle between the thyroid and cricoid cartilages (the cricothyroid angle) and by medial movement of the arytenoids during expiration.[1,11,20] These movements result in fine alterations in vocal fold tension during movement of air, causing vibration of the vocal folds. Lesions or malfunction of the vocal folds (e.g., inflammation, papilloma, or paresis) therefore affect phonation. Phonation is the only laryngeal function that alters the cricothyroid angle.[1] Thus, despite significant airway obstruction during inspiration it may be possible to phonate.

Physiology of the Respiratory System

Obligate Nasal Breathing

Infants are considered to be obligate nasal breathers.[21,22] Obstruction of their anterior or posterior nares (nasal congestion, stenosis, choanal atresia) may cause asphyxia.[23-25] Immaturity of coordination between respiratory efforts and oropharyngeal motor/sensory input accounts in part for obligate nasal breathing.[26] Furthermore, because the larynx is higher (more cephalad) in the neck of an infant and oropharyngeal structures are closer together, during quiet respiration, the tongue rests against the roof of the mouth, resulting in oral airway obstruction.[22] Multiple sites of pharyngeal airway obstruction may also contribute to airway obstruction when attempting to breathe against a partially obstructed upper airway or with relaxation of upper airway muscle tone after sedation or induction of anesthesia.[27-31] As the infant matures, its ability to coordinate respiratory and oral function matures. The larynx enlarges and moves down lower (more caudad) in the neck as the cervical spine lengthens and the infant begins to breathe adequately through the mouth. This maturation occurs by age 3 to 5 months. Studies have shown that the ability to breathe through the mouth when the nares are obstructed is age dependent: 8% of preterm infants 31 to 32 weeks postconceptual age were able to breathe through the mouth in response to nasal occlusion compared with 28% of more mature preterm infants of 35 to 36 weeks postconceptual age.[32] In a second study by these same investigators, approximately 40% of full-term infants could switch from nasal to oral breathing.[33] However, more recent data contradict these earlier data. Slow and fast nasal occlusion was applied to 17 healthy preterm infants (gestational age, 32 ± 1 weeks; postnatal age, 12 ± 2 days). All demonstrated the ability to switch from nasal to oral breathing. These authors attribute the difference in findings to the more extended observation period in their study (>15 sec).[34] The presence of a nasogastric tube may also significantly affect the infant's breathing if the "unobstructed" nasal passage has an existing underlying obstruction.

Tracheal and Bronchial Function

Tracheal and bronchial diameters are a function of elasticity and of distending or compressive forces (Fig. 12-10). An infant's larynx, trachea, and bronchi are highly compliant compared with an adult's and therefore more subject to distention and compression forces.[21,35,36] The intrathoracic trachea is subject to stresses that are different from those in the extrathoracic portion.[35] During expiration, intrathoracic pressure remains slightly negative, thus maintaining patency of the intrathoracic trachea and bronchi (Fig. 12-10B). During inspiration, a greater negative intrathoracic pressure dilates and stretches the *intrathoracic* trachea.[37] The *extrathoracic* trachea at the thoracic inlet is slightly narrowed by dynamic compression that results from the differential between intratracheal pressures and atmospheric pressures. However, the cartilages of the trachea maintain patency of the airway along with the muscles and soft tissues of the neck (Fig. 12-10A). Obstruction of the extrathoracic upper airway that can occur with epiglottitis, laryngotracheobronchitis, or an extrathoracic foreign body alters normal airway dynamics. Inspiration against an obstruction leads to the development of a more negative intrathoracic pressure, thus dilating the intrathoracic airways to a greater degree. Clinically, the net effect is an increased tendency toward dynamic collapse of the extrathoracic trachea below the level of the obstruction. This collapse is maximum at the thoracic inlet, where the greatest pressure gradient exists between negative intratracheal and atmospheric pressures. As a result, inspiratory stridor is prominent (Fig. 12-10C; see also Video Clip 12-1 on website).[35-42] With intrathoracic tracheal obstruction (e.g., a foreign body or vascular ring), stridor may occur during both inspiration and expiration.[43-46] In lower airway obstruction (e.g., asthma or bronchiolitis), significant intrathoracic tracheal and bronchial collapse may occur as a result of the prolonged expiratory phase and greatly increased positive extraluminal pressure

(Fig. 12-10D).[47] In addition, because the airways in children are very compliant, they may be more susceptible to closure during bronchial smooth muscle contraction (e.g., with reactive airway disease). Preterm and term infants may experience airway closure even during quiet respirations.

Avoiding dynamic airway collapse is particularly important. The very compliant trachea and bronchi of an infant or child are prone to collapse, particularly at the extremes of transluminal pressures that may occur when a child is vigorously crying. The susceptibility of a child to these dynamic forces on the airway is inversely related to age, with preterm infants most susceptible and adults least susceptible.[48] For this reason, it is essential that children with airway obstruction remain calm. Skill and understanding are required on the parts of the parents, nursing staff, and physicians. *Sedatives and opioids should be used with caution before insertion of an ETT because they may depress or ablate the life-sustaining voluntary efforts to breathe, resulting in significant morbidity or mortality.*

Work of Breathing

Work of breathing may be defined as the product of pressure and volume. It may be analyzed by plotting transpulmonary pressure against tidal volume. The work of breathing per kilogram body weight is similar in infants and adults. However, the oxygen consumption of a full-term neonate (4 to 6 mL/kg/min) is twice that of an adult (2 to 3 mL/kg/min).[49] This greater oxygen consumption in infants accounts in part for the increased respiratory frequency compared with older children. In preterm infants, the oxygen consumption related to breathing is three times that in adults.[50]

The location of airway resistance differs between infants and adults. The nasal passages account for 25% of the total resistance to airflow in a neonate, compared with 60% in an adult.[22,51] In infants, most resistance to airflow occurs in the bronchial and small airways. This results from the relatively smaller diameter of the airways and the greater compliance of the supporting structures of the trachea and bronchi.[21,52,53] In particular, the chest wall of a neonate is very compliant; the ribs provide less support to maintain negative intrathoracic pressure. This lack of negative intrathoracic pressure combined with the high compliance of the bronchi can lead to functional airway closure with every breath.[54-56] In infants and children, therefore, small-airway resistance accounts for most of the work of breathing, whereas in adults, the nasal passages provide the major proportion of flow resistance.[22,54,55,57-62] In the presence of increased airway resistance or decreased lung compliance, an increased transpulmonary pressure is required to produce a given tidal volume and, thus, the work of breathing is increased. Any change in the airway that increases the work of breathing may lead to respiratory failure. Recall that the resistance component of respiratory work is inversely proportional to the radius of the lumen increased by the power of 4 during laminar flow and to the power of 5 during turbulent flow (a crying child). Because the diameter of the airways in infants is smaller than those in adults, pathologic narrowing of the airways in infants exerts a greater adverse effect on the work of breathing. Increase in the work of breathing may also occur with a long ETT of small diameter, an obstructed ETT, or a narrowed airway. These situations all result in increased oxygen consumption, which in turn increases oxygen demand.[63] The increased oxygen demand is initially met by an increase in respiratory rate, but the increased work of

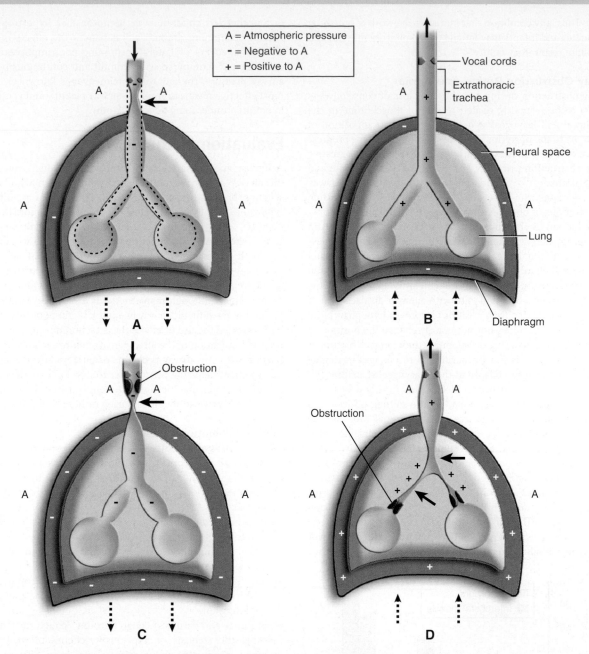

A = Atmospheric pressure
− = Negative to A
+ = Positive to A

Figure 12-10. A, With descent of the diaphragm and contraction of the intercostal muscles, a greater negative intrathoracic pressure relative to intraluminal and atmospheric pressure is developed. The net result is longitudinal stretching of the larynx and trachea, dilatation of the intrathoracic trachea and bronchi, movement of air into the lungs, and some dynamic collapse of the extrathoracic trachea (*arrow*). The dynamic collapse is due to the highly compliant trachea and the negative intraluminal pressure in relation to atmospheric pressure. **B,** The normal sequence of events at end expiration is a slight negative intrapleural pressure stenting the airways open. In infants, the highly compliant chest does not provide the support required; thus, airway closure occurs with each breath. Intraluminal pressures are slightly positive in relation to atmospheric pressure, resulting in air being forced out of the lungs. **C,** Obstructed extrathoracic airway. Note the severe dynamic collapse of the extrathoracic trachea below the level of obstruction. This collapse is greatest at the thoracic inlet, where the largest pressure gradient exists between negative intratracheal pressure and atmospheric pressure (*arrow*).[35] **D,** Obstructed intrathoracic trachea or airways. Note that breathing against an obstructed lower airway (bronchiolitis, asthma) results in greater positive intrathoracic pressures, with dynamic collapse of the intrathoracic airways (prolonged expiration or wheezing [*arrows*]).

breathing may not be sustainable. The end result may be exhaustion, which leads to respiratory failure (carbon dioxide [CO_2] retention and hypoxemia).

The difference in histology of the diaphragm and intercostal muscles of preterm and full-term infants compared with older children also contributes to increased susceptibility of infants to

respiratory fatigue or failure. Type I muscle fibers permit prolonged repetitive movement; for example, long-distance runners through repeated exercise increase the proportion of type I muscle fibers in their legs. The percent of type I muscle fibers in the diaphragm and intercostal muscles change with age (preterm infants < full-term infants < 2-year-old children) (Fig.

12-11). Thus, any condition that increases the work of breathing in neonates and infants may fatigue the respiratory muscles and precipitate respiratory failure.[64-66]

Airway Obstruction During Anesthesia

Airway obstruction during anesthesia or loss of consciousness appears to be primarily related to loss of muscle tone in the pharyngeal and laryngeal structures rather than apposition of the tongue to the posterior pharyngeal wall.[27,28,67,68] The progressive loss of tone with deepening anesthesia results in progressive airway obstruction primarily at the level of the soft palate and the epiglottis.[27,28,31,67,69,70] In children, the pharyngeal airway space decreases in a dose-dependent manner with increasing concentrations of both sevoflurane and propofol anesthesia.[71-73] This reduction in pharyngeal space has been noted primarily in the anteroposterior dimension. As the depth of propofol anesthesia in children increases, upper airway narrowing occurs throughout the entire upper airway but is most pronounced in the hypopharynx at the level of the epiglottis. Extension of the head at the atlanto-occipital joint with anterior displacement of the cervical spine (sniffing position) improves hypopharyngeal airway patency but does not necessarily change the position of the tongue. This observation supports the concept that upper airway obstruction is not primarily due to changes in tongue position but rather to collapse of the pharyngeal structures.[29-31] Pharyngeal airway obstruction also occurs during obstructive sleep apnea in infants and adults.[26,74] The sniffing position has been demonstrated to improve cross-sectional area and to decrease the closing pressure of both the retropalatal and retroglossal space in anesthetized adults with obstructive sleep apnea.[75] The application of continuous positive airway pressure (CPAP) is a common method to overcome such airway obstruction (see Fig. 37-2). During propofol anesthesia in children, CPAP works primarily by increasing the transverse dimension of the airway.[72] This occurs despite the fact that anesthesia obstructs the airway mostly by narrowing the anteroposterior dimension. Chin lift and jaw thrust also improve airway patency in anesthetized children with adenotonsillar hypertrophy.[76-78] Lateral positioning dramatically enhances the effects of these airway maneuvers.[77,78] Lateral positioning alone improves airway dimensions.[79] Compared with chin lift and continuous positive airway pressure, the jaw thrust maneuver is known to be the most effective means to improve airway patency and ventilation in children undergoing adenoidectomy.[76]

Evaluation of the Airway

A history and physical examination with specific reference to the airway should be performed in all children who require sedation or anesthesia. In particular, a history of a congenital syndrome or physical findings of congenital anomaly (e.g., microtia which has been associated with difficult laryngoscopy)[80] should alert the practitioner to the possibility of difficulties with management of the airway. In special situations, radiologic and laboratory studies are required to further evaluate and clarify a disorder revealed by the history and physical examination. Although many methods exist for evaluating and predicting the difficult airway in adults,[81-85] no published studies have assessed the use of any of these techniques in children.[86,87] Routine evaluation of the airway in all children followed by correlation with any airway problems occurring during anesthetic management helps the practitioner to develop experience. This experience then may be used to identify future children who might have airway difficulties during or after anesthesia.

Clinical Evaluation

The *medical history* (both present and past) should investigate the signs and symptoms listed below; a positive history should alert the practitioner to the potential problems that are noted in parentheses (video clips are available on the website for some examples).

- Presence of an upper respiratory tract infection (predisposition to coughing, laryngospasm, bronchospasm, and desaturation during anesthesia or to post-intubation subglottic edema or postoperative desaturation)[88-92]
- Snoring or noisy breathing (adenoidal hypertrophy, upper airway obstruction, obstructive sleep apnea, pulmonary hypertension)
- Presence and nature of cough ("croupy" cough may indicate subglottic stenosis or previous tracheoesophageal fistula repair; productive cough may indicate bronchitis or pneumonia; chronicity affects the differential diagnosis [e.g., the sudden onset of a persistent cough may indicate foreign-body aspiration])
- Past episodes of croup (post-intubation croup, subglottic stenosis)
- Inspiratory stridor, usually high pitched (subglottic narrowing [see Video Clip 12-1], laryngomalacia [see Video Clip 12-1], macroglossia, laryngeal web [Video Clip 12-2], extrathoracic foreign body or extrathoracic tracheal compression)
- Hoarse voice (laryngitis, vocal cord palsy, papillomatosis [see Video Clip 12-1], granuloma [see Video Clip 12-1])
- Asthma and bronchodilator therapy (bronchospasm)
- Repeated pneumonias (incompetent larynx with aspiration, gastroesophageal reflux, cystic fibrosis, bronchiectasis, residual tracheoesophageal fistula, pulmonary sequestration, immune suppression, congenital heart disease)

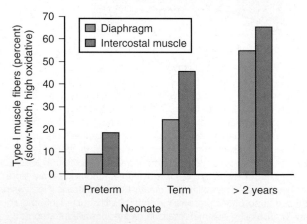

Figure 12-11. Muscle fiber composition of the diaphragm and intercostal muscles related to age. Note that a preterm infant's diaphragm and intercostal muscles have fewer type I fibers compared with term newborns and older children. The data suggest a possible mechanism for early fatigue in preterm and term infants when the work of breathing is increased. (Data from Keens TG, Bryan AC, Levison H, et al: Developmental pattern of muscle fibers in human ventilatory muscles. J Appl Physiol 1978; 44:909-913.)

- History of foreign-body aspiration (increased airway reactivity, airway obstruction, impaired neurologic function)
- History of aspiration (laryngeal edema [Video Clip 12-3], laryngeal cleft [Video Clip 12-4])
- Previous anesthetic problems, particularly related to the airway (difficult intubation, difficulty with mask ventilation, failed or problematic extubation)
- Atopy, allergy (increased airway reactivity)
- History of smoking by primary caregivers (increased airway resistance)[93]
- History of a congenital syndrome (many are associated with difficult airway management)

The *physical examination* should include the following observations:

- Facial expression
- Presence or absence of nasal flaring
- Presence or absence of mouth breathing
- Color of mucous membranes
- Presence or absence of retractions (suprasternal, intercostal, subcostal [see Video Clip 12-1])
- Respiratory rate
- Presence or absence of voice change
- Mouth opening (Fig. 12-12A)

- Size of mouth
- Size of tongue and its relationship to other pharyngeal structures (Mallampati)[84]
- Loose or missing teeth (Fig. 12-12B)
- Size and configuration of palate
- Size and configuration of mandible
- Location of larynx in relation to the mandible (Fig. 12-12C)
- Presence of stridor and if present:
  - Is stridor predominantly inspiratory, suggesting an upper airway (extrathoracic) lesion (epiglottitis, croup, extrathoracic foreign body)?
  - Is stridor both inspiratory and expiratory, suggesting an intrathoracic lesion (aspirated foreign body, vascular ring, or large esophageal foreign body)? (see Video Clip 12-1)
  - Is the expiratory phase prolonged or stridor predominantly expiratory, suggesting lower airway disease?
- Baseline oxygen saturation in room air
- Microtia:
  - Bilateral but not unilateral microtia is associated with difficulty in visualizing the laryngeal inlet (Grade 3 or 4 Cormack and Lehane, see later).[80] Of those with bilateral microtia, 5 of 12 children (42%) had a difficult laryngeal

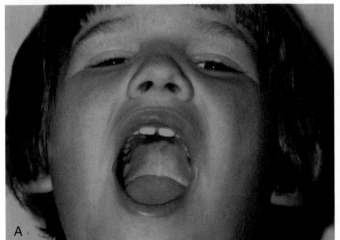

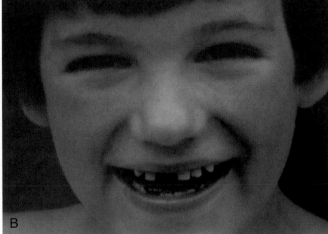

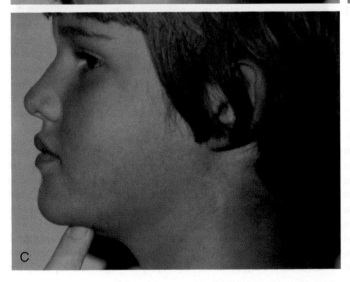

Figure 12-12. A, How far can a child open his or her mouth? Are there any abnormalities of the mouth, tongue, palate, mandible? **B,** Are any teeth loose or missing? **C,** Is the mandible of normal configuration? How much space is there between the genu of the mandible and the thyroid cartilage? This space is an indication of the extent of the superior and posterior displacement of the larynx; there should normally be at least one finger's breadth in a newborn and three finger's breadths in an adolescent.

philosophy consists of advancing the laryngoscope blade under constant vision along the surface of the tongue, placing the tip of the blade directly in the vallecula and then using this location to pivot or rotate the blade to the right to sweep the tongue to the left and adequately lift the tongue to expose the glottic opening. This avoids trauma to the arytenoid cartilages. One can thus lift the base of the tongue, which in turn lifts the epiglottis, exposing the glottic opening. If this technique is unsuccessful, one may then directly lift the epiglottis with the tip of the blade (see Video Clip 12-1 on website). Another approach is to insert the Miller blade into the mouth at the right commissure over the lateral bicuspids/incisors (paraglossal approach). The blade is advanced down the right gutter of the mouth aiming the blade tip toward the midline while sweeping the tongue to the left. Once under the epiglottis, the epiglottis is lifted with the tip of the blade, thereby exposing the glottic aperture. By approaching the mouth over the bicuspids/incisors, dental damage is obviated. This is a particularly effective approach for the infant and child with a difficult airway. Whichever approach is used, care must be taken to avoid using the laryngoscope blade as a fulcrum through which pressure is applied to the teeth or alveolar ridge. If there is a substantive risk that pressure will be applied to the teeth, then a plastic tooth guard may be applied to cover the teeth at risk.

Optimal positioning for laryngoscopy changes with age. The trachea of older children (6 years of age and older) and adults is most easily exposed when a folded blanket or pillow is placed beneath the occiput of the head (5-10 cm elevation), displacing the cervical spine anteriorly.[116] Extension of the head at the atlanto-occipital joint produces the classic "sniffing" position.[99,117,118] These movements align three axes: those of the mouth, oropharynx, and trachea. Once aligned, these three axes permit direct visualization of laryngeal structures. They also result in improved hypopharyngeal patency.[29,31,67,75,117,118] Figure 12-14 demonstrates maneuvers for positioning the head during airway management. In infants and younger children, it is usually unnecessary to elevate the head because the occiput is large in proportion to the trunk, resulting in adequate anterior displacement of the cervical spine; head extension at the atlanto-occipital joint alone aligns the airway axes. When the occiput is displaced excessively, exposure of the glottis may actually be hindered. In neonates, it is helpful for an assistant to hold the shoulders flat on the operating room table with the head slightly extended. Some practitioners have adopted the practice of placing a rolled towel under the shoulders of neonates to facilitate tracheal intubation. This technique is a major disadvantage when the laryngoscopist stands but may be an advantage when he or she is seated, as otolaryngologists usually are.

The validity of the three-axis theory (alignment of the mouth, oropharynx, and trachea) to describe the optimal intubating position in adults has been challenged.[119-122] Some authors challenge the notion that elevating the occiput improves conditions for visualization of the laryngeal inlet based on evidence from both MRI and clinical investigation.[119,121] No comparable studies have been performed in children. An investigation of 456 adults used as their own controls found that neck extension alone was adequate for visualization of the larynx in *most* adults. However, for obese patients or those with limited neck extension, an optimal intubating position was not determined.[119] Others have argued in favor of the superiority of the sniffing position but with varying support of the three-axis theory.[123-129] Even if the

tracheas of only a few patients are intubated more easily when placed in the sniffing position compared with only head extension, the routine application of the sniffing position would appear to remain the best clinical practice.

Laryngoscopy can be performed while the child is awake, anesthetized, and breathing spontaneously, or with a combination of anesthesia and neuromuscular blockade. Most tracheal intubations in children who are awake are performed in neonates, an approach not usually feasible or humane in older awake and uncooperative children. Awake intubation in the neonate is generally well tolerated and, if performed smoothly, is not associated with significant hemodynamic changes.[130] However, data suggest that even preterm and full-term infants are better managed with sedation and paralysis so as to minimize adverse hemodynamic responses.[131-134]

Selection of Laryngoscope Blade

A straight blade is generally more suitable for use in infants and young children than a curved blade because it better elevates the base of the tongue to expose the glottic opening. Curved blades are satisfactory in older children. The blade size chosen depends on the age and body mass of the child and the preference of the anesthesiologist. Table 12-1 presents the ranges commonly used.

Endotracheal Tubes

Since 1967, all materials used in the manufacture of tracheal tubes have been subjected to rabbit muscle implantation testing in accordance with the standards promulgated by the Z79 committee. If the material caused an inflammatory response, it could not be used in the manufacture of tracheal tubes. This resulted in the elimination of organometallic constituents, such as those used in the manufacture of red rubber tracheal tubes.

The selection of a proper size ETT depends on the *individual* child.[135] The only size requirement for a manufacturer is that they standardize the internal diameter (ID) of an ETT. The external diameter (OD) may vary, depending on the material from which the ETT is constructed and its manufacturer. This diversity in external diameter mandates the need to check for proper ETT size and leak around the tube. An appropriately sized uncuffed ETT may be approximated according to the patient's age and weight (Table 12-2).[136] ETTs of half ID size above and below the selected size should be available because of the variability of patient anatomy. The use of the diameter of the terminal phalanx of either the second or fifth digit is unreliable.[137] Children with Down syndrome will often require a smaller than anticipated ETT.[138] After intubation and stabilization of the child, if there is no air leak around the tube below 20

Table 12-1. Laryngoscope Blades Used in Infants and Children

Age	Blade Size		
	Miller	Wis-Hipple	Macintosh
Preterm	0	–	–
Neonate	0	–	–
Neonate-2 years	1	–	–
2-6 years	–	1.5	1 or 2
6-10 years	2	–	2
Older than 10 years	2 or 3	–	3

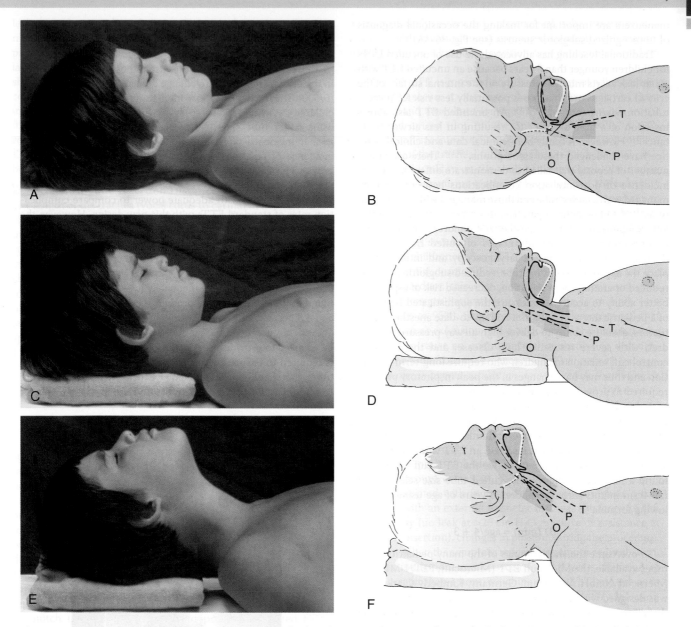

Figure 12-14. Correct positioning for ventilation and tracheal intubation. With a patient flat on the bed or operating table (**A**), the oral (O), pharyngeal (P), and tracheal (T) axes pass through three divergent planes (**B**). A folded sheet or towel placed under the occiput of the head (**C**) aligns the pharyngeal (P) and tracheal (T) axes (**D**). Extension of the atlanto-occipital joint (**E**) results in alignment of the oral (O), pharyngeal (P), and tracheal (T) axes (**F**).

Table 12-2. Endotracheal Tubes Used in Infants and Children*

Age	Size (mm ID)
Preterm	
1000 g	2.5
1000-2500 g	3.0
Neonate-6 months	3.0-3.5
6 months-1 year	3.5-4.0
1-2 years	4.0-5.0
Older than 2 years	(age in years + 16)/4

ID, internal diameter.
*Uncuffed; one half size smaller for cuffed ETT, see text.

to 25 cm H_2O (short-term intubation perhaps as high as 35 cm H_2O) peak inflation pressure (PIP), the ETT should be changed to the next half size smaller. An air leak at this pressure is recommended because it is believed to approximate capillary pressure of the adult tracheal mucosa. If lateral wall pressure exceeds this amount, ischemic damage to the subglottic mucosa may occur.[139] Be aware, however, that if a child is intubated without the aid of muscle relaxants, laryngospasm around the ETT may prevent any gas leak and mimic a tight-fitting ETT.[140] When anesthesia has been deepened, an air leak could become evident. Changes in head position may also increase or decrease the leak.[140] These

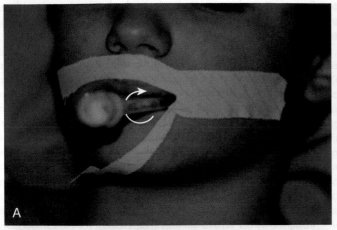

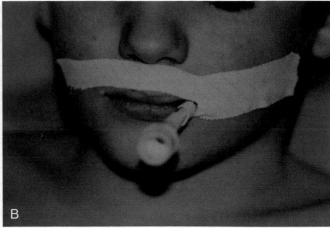

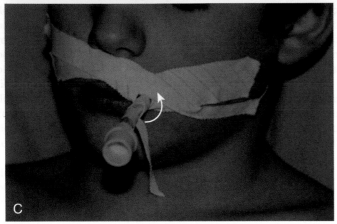

Figure 12-16. Securing the endotracheal tube. After insertion of the oral endotracheal tube and examination for proper position, the area between the nose and upper lip and both cheeks is coated with tincture of benzoin. **A,** After the benzoin is dry, tape that has been split up the middle is applied to the cheek and the endotracheal tube is placed at the division of the split tape. **B,** One half is wrapped circumferentially around the tube, and the other half is applied to the space above the upper lip. **C,** A second piece of tape is applied in similar fashion from the opposite direction. A nasal endotracheal tube may also be secured with this technique.

may have a reduced incidence after prolonged intubation because of the relative immaturity of the cricoid cartilage. At this age, the cartilage structure is hypercellular and the matrix has a large fluid content, making the structures more resilient and less susceptible to ischemic injury.[191]

The pathogenesis of acquired subglottic stenosis results from ischemic injury secondary to lateral wall pressure from the ETT. Ischemia results in edema, necrosis, and ulcerations of the mucosa. Secondary infection results in exposure of the cartilage. Within 48 hours, granulation tissue begins to form within these ulcerations. Ultimately, scar tissue forms, resulting in narrowing of the airway (Fig. 12-17).[192-194] Specimens obtained from partial cricotracheal resection in children were found to have severe and sclerotic scarring with squamous metaplasia of the epithelium, loss of glands and elastic mantle fibers (tunica elastica), and dilation of the remaining glands with formation of cysts. Also, the cricoid cartilage was affected on the internal and external side, with irreversible loss of perichondrium on the inside and resorption by macrophages of cartilage on both sides.[194]

Factors that predispose to subglottic stenosis are intubation with too large an ETT, laryngeal trauma (traumatic intubation, chemical or thermal inhalation, external trauma, surgical trauma, gastric reflux), prolonged intubation (particularly >25 days), repeated intubation, sepsis and infection, chronic illness, and chronic inflammatory disease.[190,195,196]

Laryngeal Mask Airway

The laryngeal mask airway (LMA) has become a standard alternative for airway management during general anesthesia.[197-202]

A variety of types have been introduced into practice since the development of the original, now called the LMA Classic. These include the disposable LMA Unique, the ProSeal LMA (described later), the intubating LMA Fastrach, the Flexible LMA, and the LMA CTrach designed for continuous videoendoscopy of the tracheal intubation procedure (Fig. 12-18). Neither the Fastrach nor the CTrach is available in pediatric sizes. However the Fastrach has been described for use in children who weigh more than 40 kg.[203] The LMA Classic is made of medical-grade silicone and consists of a large-bore tubular structure (barrel) that has a 15-mm adapter at its proximal end and an elliptical mask-like device that fits over the laryngeal inlet at its distal end. All masks are inflated via a valved pilot tube and balloon. The LMA Classic and the ProSeal LMA can be sterilized for reuse up to 40 times. The LMA Classic is available in eight sizes. Guidelines for selecting the appropriate mask for children are based on weight (Table 12-4). A number of other manufacturers have developed similar devices; however, there are minimal comparative data available for children.

The LMA has been used in many types of surgical cases.[204] Some suggest that the LMA can be used for any case in which spontaneous ventilation is appropriate or any case that might reasonably be managed by face mask. Advantages of the LMA over the face mask are that it frees the anesthesiologist's hands for other tasks and that it may be associated with a lesser amount of operating room pollution compared with mask ventilation.[205,206] The use of controlled ventilation with the LMA Classic has also been described.[207,208] However, this practice is more controversial than the use of the LMA Classic in spontaneously

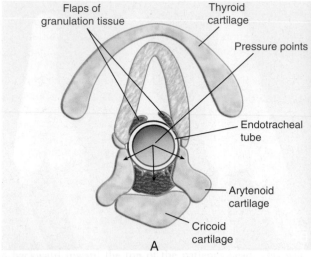

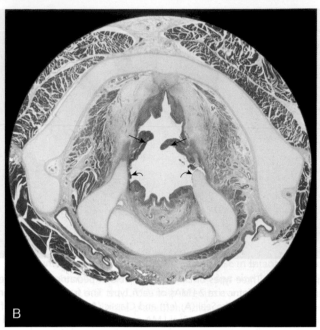

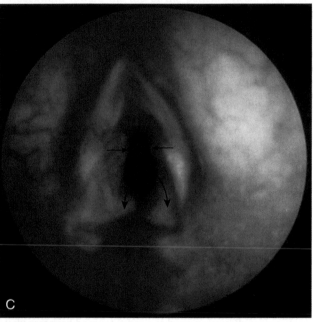

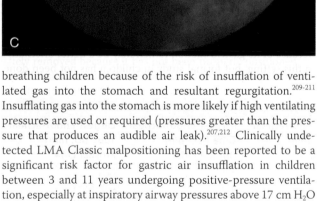

Figure 12-17. The pathogenesis of intubation injuries. **A,** Schemata of a cross section through the glottis. Pressure necrosis causes ulcerations at the vocal processes of the arytenoids with exposed cartilage. Flaps of granulation tissue are present anterior to these ulcerations. **B,** Cross section of the glottis at this same level; *straight arrows* indicate flaps of granulation tissue and *curved arrows* the absence of mucosa and ulcerations with exposed cartilage on the vocal processes of the arytenoids. **C,** Intubation injury to a 2-month-old infant; *straight arrows* indicate granulation tissue and *curved arrows* indicate area of ulcerations (white area). The most severe area of injury is generally at the level of the cricoid cartilage, resulting in subglottic stenosis. (Reproduced with permission from Holinger LD, Lusk RP, Green CG: Pediatric Laryngology and Bronchoesophagology. Philadelphia, Lippincott-Raven, 1997.)

breathing children because of the risk of insufflation of ventilated gas into the stomach and resultant regurgitation.[209-211] Insufflating gas into the stomach is more likely if high ventilating pressures are used or required (pressures greater than the pressure that produces an audible air leak).[207,212] Clinically undetected LMA Classic malpositioning has been reported to be a significant risk factor for gastric air insufflation in children between 3 and 11 years undergoing positive-pressure ventilation, especially at inspiratory airway pressures above 17 cm H_2O peak inspiratory pressure.[213]

More recently, the ProSeal LMA (PLMA) has been introduced. The PLMA has been designed to improve sealing pressures and to provide a conduit for evacuation of stomach contents; thus, it is more appealing for use with positive-pressure ventilation. In sizes greater than or equal to 3, there is a second dorsal cuff to increase the seal pressure of the glottic mask. The dorsal and ventral cuffs communicate, allowing simultaneous inflation by a single pilot balloon. In the smaller sizes there is no second dorsal cuff but the profile of the mask has been altered to improve sealing. The PLMA is reported to be easy to insert, to allow greater airway pressures with posi-

tive-pressure ventilation, and to provide better protection against gastric insufflation.[214] A number of studies support the efficacy of the PLMA for use in children for both spontaneous and controlled ventilation.[215-219] For children, the PLMA is reported to have similar ease of insertion, proper position confirmed by fiberoptic visualization, and similar frequency of mucosal trauma compared with the LMA Classic. However, the advantage is that oropharyngeal leak pressure is greater and gastric insufflation is less common with the PLMA.[216,217,219] For children, the ability to provide pressure support ventilation during PLMA anesthesia also improves gas exchange and reduces work of breathing compared with the application of CPAP.[220] The higher sealing pressure may also protect against aspiration, as described in a case report in which a PLMA successfully channeled regurgitated fluid away from the respiratory tract of a 5-year-old child after inguinal hernia repair.[221]

Flexible diagnostic and therapeutic bronchoscopy, radiation therapy, radiologic procedures, ear/nose/throat surgeries, and ophthalmologic procedures are the most commonly described pediatric indications for the LMA.[202,204,222-225] An advantage of the LMA for securing the airway in ophthalmologic surgery is

and different mechanism for maintaining the airway are discussed next.

Other Supraglottic Airway Devices

The Laryngeal Tube

The Laryngeal Tube (LT) (VBM Medizintechnik, Sulz a. N., Germany) is designed to secure a patent airway during either spontaneous breathing or controlled ventilation. This device is available as either a single lumen for ventilation only or as a double-lumen tube that allows suction of gastric contents through one and ventilation through the other. The system in theory seals the esophagus at the distal end with a small cuff attached at the tip (distal cuff) and a larger balloon cuff at the middle part of the tube (proximal cuff) stabilizes the device and blocks the oropharynx and nasopharynx. The two openings that lie between the cuffs are positioned so that the more distal opening faces the glottis. The cuffs are inflated through a single pilot tube and balloon, through which cuff pressure can be monitored. There are three black lines on the tube near a standard 15-mm connector, which indicate adequate depth of insertion when aligned with the teeth. The nondisposable device is made of silicone (latex free) and is reusable up to 50 times after sterilization in an autoclave. There are four variations of the Laryngeal Tube (LT): standard and disposable; standard laryngeal tube-Suction II and disposable laryngeal tube-Suction II (Fig. 12-19 [see website])[275] It is available in six sizes, suitable for neonates up to large adults (Table 12-5).

The device should be inserted while the child's head and neck are placed either in the sniffing position or in the neutral position. The tip of a well-lubricated LT is placed against the hard palate behind the upper incisors. The device is then slid down the center of the mouth until resistance is felt or the device is almost fully inserted. After connection to the anesthesia circuit, proper placement is ascertained by standard means of assessing ease of ventilation. Some adjustment (usually slight withdrawal) may be required to provide optimal ease of ventilation. Care should be taken not to push the tongue toward the posterior pharynx, to minimize a possible obstruction of the airway. Ease of insertion of the standard LT is reported to be comparable to that of the LMA Classic, although the LT may require more readjustments of its position to obtain a clear airway.[276,277] The incidence of complications with the two devices appears to be similar.[276] The LT may provide a better seal than the Classic LMA.[278] Compared with the PLMA, the LT may be less effective and more difficult to insert.[279-281] Although the LT-suction type may have similar success to the PLMA,[282] little has been published about the use of this device in children.[283-285] An

Table 12-5. Size Selection and Recommended Cuff Volumes for the Laryngeal Tube

Tube Size	Patient's Body Size	Recommended Cuff Volumes (mL)	Connector Color
0 Newborn	<5 kg	10	Clear
1 Infants	5-12 kg	20	White
2 Children	12-25 kg	35	Green
3 Adults: small	<155 cm	60	Yellow
4 Adults: medium	155-180 cm	80	Red
5 Adults: large	>180 cm	90	Purple

Table 12-6. Suggested CobraPLA Size, Weight, Cuff Volume, and Endotracheal Tube Sizes

Size	Patient Weight (kg)	Cuff Volume (mL)	Internal Diameter (mm)	Maximal Size Endotracheal Tube (mm ID)
0.5	>2.5	<8	5.0	3.0
1	>5	<10	6.0	4.5
1.5	>10	<25	6.0	4.5
2	>15	<40	10.5	6.5
3	>35	<65	10.5	6.5
4	>70	<70	12.5	8.0
5	>100	<85	12.5	8.0
6	>130	<85	12.5	8.0

initial report of its use in children ages 2 to 12 years found a successful placement rate of 96% (77/80 children). Complications occurred in 2 children; one had laryngospasm that resolved with deepening of the anesthetic, and the other complained of mild difficulty with swallowing postoperatively.[284] A study comparing the LT with the LMA found it to be less effective for either spontaneous or assisted ventilation and for fiberoptic evaluation of the airway in children younger than 10 years of age.[283] A study of 70 children using sizes 0 to 3 reported failure to place the LT in 12% of children. Failures were caused by inability to ventilate, hypoxemia, gastric insufflation, cough, and laryngospasm or stridor, particularly for children weighing less than 10 kg; thus, the LT was not recommended for children of this size.[285] Although the manufacturer states that a fiberoptic scope may be passed through the device, the openings are of insufficient size to permit passage of an ETT.

The Cobra Perilaryngeal Airway (CobraPLA)

The CobraPLA (Engineered Medical Systems, Inc., Indianapolis, IN) is a disposable supraglottic device marketed for the same indications as the LMA but it creates a seal higher in the hypopharynx using a cylindrical inflatable cuff. The distal end of the device sits over the larynx but the distal end is not inflatable (Fig. 12-20 [see website]).[273,286,287] An initial report comparing the CobraPLA with the LMA found that insertion times, airway adequacy, and number of repositioning attempts were similar. Peak airway sealing pressure was significantly greater with the CobraPLA; the authors concluded that the CobraPLA has better airway sealing capabilities than the Classic LMA.[288] A more recent group of investigators studying the CobraPLA in adults raised concerns about both the design and the safety of this device, particularly during controlled ventilation. After studying 29 patients, investigations were suspended and later stopped after 2 cases of significant pulmonary aspiration occurred in patients while using the CobraPLA.[289] The device is available in eight sizes for infants as small as 2.5 kg (Table 12-6).[286] The distal grill has a long center slit specifically designed to allow passage of a fiberoptic scope and ETT (the size 1/2 Neonate allows easy passage of a 3.5 uncuffed ETT). In a pediatric study the orientation of the larynx as viewed through the CobraPLA using video was obtained in 45 infants and children. An acceptable view of the airway was obtained in all subjects, but the laryngeal view was nearly or completely obstructed by the folding of the epiglottis over the glottic opening in 76.9% of children weighing less than 10 kg. (Note that a similar problem is encountered in approximately 80% of children managed with

Table 12-7. Pediatric Airway Pathology Related to Anatomic Site

Anatomic Site	Etiology	Clinical Condition
Nasopharynx	Congenital	Choanal atresia, stenosis,[23,24] encephalocele[436]
	Traumatic	Foreign body, trauma
	Inflammatory	Adenoidal hypertrophy,[437] nasal congestion[25]
	Neoplastic	Teratoma
Tongue	Congenital	Hemangioma, Down syndrome[438-442]
	Traumatic	Burn, laceration, lymphatic/venous obstruction[112,113,443-448]
	Metabolic	Beckwith-Wiedemann syndrome,[449-453] hypothyroidism, mucopolysaccharidosis,[454-469] glycogen storage disease,[470] gangliosidosis, congenital hypothyroidism
	Neoplastic	Cystic hygroma,[471,472] cystic teratoma
Mandible/maxilla	Congenital hypoplasia	Pierre Robin syndrome,[473-481] Treacher Collins syndrome,[482-486] Goldenhar syndrome,[487,488] Apert syndrome, achondroplasia,[489,490] Turner syndrome,[491,492] Cornelia de Lange syndrome,[493,494] Smith-Lemli-Opitz syndrome,[495-497] Hallermann-Streiff syndrome,[498] Crouzan syndrome[499]
	Traumatic	Fracture,[500] neck burn with contractures
	Inflammatory	Juvenile rheumatoid arthritis[501-505]
	Neoplastic	Tumors, cherubism[506]
Pharynx/larynx	Congenital	Laryngomalacia (infantile larynx),[507] Freeman-Sheldon syndrome (whistling face),[508-512] laryngeal stenosis,[513] laryngocele,[507] laryngeal web,[507] hemangioma
	Traumatic	Dislocated/fractured larynx,[514-519] foreign body,[43,44,520-529] inhalation injury (burn),[443-448] post-intubation edema/granuloma/stenosis,[530-540] swelling of uvula,[112] soft palate trauma, epidermolysis bullosa[541-543]
	Inflammatory	Epiglottitis,[39-41,544-559] acute tonsillitis,[437] peritonsillar abscess,[560,561] retropharyngeal abscess, diphtheritic membrane, laryngeal polyposis[562-567]
	Metabolic	Hypocalcemic laryngospasm[36]
	Neoplastic	Tumors
	Neurologic	Vocal cord paralysis, Arnold-Chiari malformation[568-571]
Trachea	Congenital	Vascular ring,[45,46] tracheal stenosis or complete tracheal rings (see Video Clip 12-10 on website),[572] tracheomalacia[507,513,540,548]
	Inflammatory	Laryngotracheobronchitis (viral),[38,41,42,172,573-575] bacterial tracheitis
	Neoplastic	Mediastinal tumors: neurofibroma,[576] paratracheal nodes (lymphoma)

the Classic LMA as well).[290] The investigators thus suggested extra vigilance to prevent airway obstruction in small children. Also, the grill bars of the CobraPLA were closely opposed to the epiglottis and supraglottic structures in nearly all subjects, and therefore it was suggested that removal of the device in a deeper plane of anesthesia might theoretically minimize laryngeal stimulation. Further study of this device in children, particularly infants, is needed to define its role compared with the LMA.

Conclusions

A variety of supraglottic airway devices are currently available. Some are imitators of the Classic LMA but available at a reduced cost, whereas others are completely new designs. It is wonderful that there is so much new equipment to assist us in the management of children with normal and difficult airways, but there are insufficient data to clearly state that one device or one manufacturer is superior to another.

Airway Management: The Abnormal Airway

Classifying the Abnormal Pediatric Airway

It is important to recognize circumstances that may cause airway obstruction or difficult laryngoscopy. Conditions that predispose to airway problems may be grouped according to anatomic location and may result from congenital, inflammatory, traumatic, metabolic, or neoplastic disorders. Tables 12-7 and 12-8 list the more common pediatric airway problems according to anatomic location. Appendix 12-1 lists the more common pediatric syndromes and associated anesthetic considerations; more complete information may be obtained elsewhere.[291-295]

Table 12-8. Cervical Spine Anomalies*

Etiology	Clinical Condition
Congenital	Down syndrome,[438,577-582] Klippel-Feil malformation,[583] Goldenhar syndrome,[487,488] torticollis
Traumatic	Fracture, subluxation,[514-518,584] neck burn contracture
Inflammatory	Rheumatoid arthritis[501-505]
Metabolic	Mucopolysaccharidosis (Morquio syndrome)[438,454-462]

*Abnormalities of the cervical spine may limit extension and flexion, thereby contributing to the difficulties of airway management; a significant percent of Down syndrome infants have atlantoaxial instability.[581,582]

should be recalled that midazolam takes nearly 5 minutes to achieve peak electroencephalographic effects, therefore necessitating adequate time between incremental doses (see Fig. 48-10).[307,308] Ketamine is generally titrated in doses of 0.25 to 0.5 mg/kg intravenously every 2 minutes. Although there is a large incidence of psychomimetic emergence reactions in adults, these reactions are less common in children, particularly if ketamine is combined with midazolam. Ketamine can cause increased secretions that may increase airway reactivity and interfere with fiberoptic airway management. Administration of an antisialagogue before ketamine and pre-endoscopy suctioning of the airway is strongly recommended to minimize this problem. A number of reports have described dexmedetomidine, administered as the sole sedating agent or combined with low doses of other sedatives/opioids, to be effective for sedation while maintaining spontaneous respirations for awake fiberoptic intubation in adults and children.[309-315] Topical anesthesia can be used in conjunction with sedation or general anesthesia to blunt airway reactivity in those children in whom spontaneous ventilation is preserved. Useful methods to provide topical anesthesia to the airway include: (1) nebulized lidocaine; (2) topical application of local anesthetic sprays, jellies, or ointments; (3) translaryngeal delivery of lidocaine (Video Clip 12-8); (4) "spray as you go" with lidocaine injected onto the surface of the larynx and vocal cords through the channel of a fiberoptic scope usually used for suctioning or administering oxygen; and (5) superior laryngeal nerve block.[305] Caution is required to avoid delivering a toxic dose of local anesthetic. Maximum doses of the local anesthetic are based on the patient's weight and should be calculated in advance (see Table 42-2). Lidocaine seems to have the best safety profile; we limit our maximum dose to 5 mg/kg. We do not recommend the use of Cetacaine spray in children weighing less than 40 kg because it is associated with methemoglobinemia and it is difficult to titrate/limit the dose administered.[86,316] An antisialagogue decreases secretions that can interfere with the effectiveness of topically administered local anesthesia and with flexible fiberoptic techniques.

In addition, the anticholinergic effect of atropine or glycopyrrolate will blunt reflex bradycardia that can occur with airway manipulation.

Many techniques and devices for managing a difficult airway have been recommended. These techniques and devices are reviewed in detail later. Previous experience in normal airways can render these devices valuable adjuncts in difficult airway management.

Finally, if one is unable to intubate the airway, it is important to recognize the limits of one's ability. In this circumstance, do not hesitate to seek assistance from a colleague or request the surgeon to perform a tracheostomy or bronchoscopy. As an alternative, the child can be awakened and referred to a major pediatric center. In an urgent life-threatening situation, LMA placement or percutaneous cricothyroidotomy may be lifesaving (see Unexpected Difficult Intubation, later).[199,223,227,228,317-319]

Documentation

Documentation of the difficult airway is essential to provide useful information for the subsequent time that the child requires sedation/anesthesia. A note in the anesthesia record should clearly address the following issues:

1. Whether or not mask ventilation was attempted and, if so, was there any difficulty
2. Special maneuvers that were required for successful mask ventilation
3. Special maneuvers that were not helpful with mask ventilation
4. Any difficulty with intubation
5. Special techniques that were required for successful intubation
6. Special techniques that were not helpful for intubation
7. Grade of laryngoscopic view of laryngeal structures during rigid laryngoscopy (Fig. 12-22)

In addition to discussion with the family and child, when age appropriate, a letter should be written to the family and child outlining the difficulties and referring them to the Medic

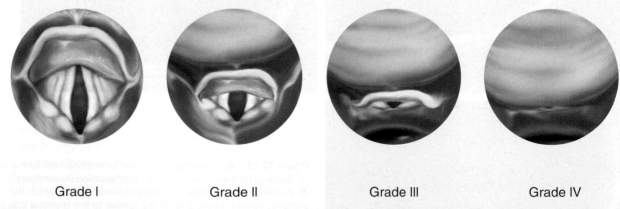

| Grade I | Grade II | Grade III | Grade IV |

Figure 12-22. The laryngoscopic grading system of Cormack and Lehane offers a reasonable means of describing visualization of the larynx. It is useful to grade the degree of visualization during laryngoscopy and how that visualization was achieved (e.g., external cricoid pressure or laryngeal manipulation, the size and configuration of the laryngoscope blade). This provides useful information for the next person attempting laryngoscopy so that he or she has some degree of knowledge regarding what to expect. Grade I is visualization of the complete laryngeal opening; grade II, visualization of just the posterior area; grade III, visualization of just the epiglottis; and grade IV, visualization of just the soft palate. (Reproduced with permission from Cormack RS, Lehane J: Difficult tracheal intubation in obstetrics. Anaesthesia 1984; 39:1105-1111.)

Alert registry.[320] This should be copied and circulated to the medical record and the Medic Alert registry. In the United States, the Medic Alert registry for difficult airway/difficult intubation can be reached at 1-800-432-5378. Similar registries are also being formed internationally.[321] The Medic Alert registration form asks for clinical details about the type of airway difficulty and maneuvers that were successful in management and those that were not. Any practitioner who provides airway management to the registered patient can update this information at any time. Despite the fact that scoring systems used in adults[81-85] have not been thoroughly investigated in children,[86] it is nevertheless useful to describe in detail the view of the larynx one was able to achieve and how it was achieved (e.g., blade type, size, external laryngeal manipulation).

The Unexpected Difficult Intubation

With careful preoperative evaluation and planning, the unexpected difficult pediatric airway should be a rare occurrence. However, the practitioner should always be prepared for this potentially life-threatening event. Because the unexpected difficult airway occurs after beginning an anesthetic (plan A), many of the management decisions required for the anticipated difficult airway have already been made. Of primary importance is maintaining adequate oxygenation while a definitive course of action is pursued (plan B, C, and so on). A reasonable decision tree, based on the American Society of Anesthesiologist's (ASA) difficult airway algorithm is presented in Figure 12-23. An important difference between infants and adults should be noted in this scenario. Because infants have an increased metabolic rate and decreased functional residual capacity, the time between the loss of the airway and resultant hypoxemia with potential secondary neurologic injury is significantly diminished compared with adults.[322] Approximate time to zero oxygen saturation from an inspired oxygen concentration of 90% is 4 minutes in a 10-kg child, whereas the same event in a healthy 70-kg adult takes almost 10 minutes.[323]

Extubation of the Child with the Difficult Airway

Unless a child in whom airway management is difficult requires a tracheostomy for long-term management, he or she will require extubation. Preparation for extubation begins shortly after the airway is secured. Equipment used to secure the airway should be rechecked, quickly returned to functional status, and then left in the operating room until successful safe extubation. Children who had prolonged attempts at intubation or who will have procedures that may lead to airway edema may benefit from a dose of dexamethasone (0.5-1 mg/kg). If significant airway edema is suspected either because of airway management or the type of surgery, consider leaving the child intubated postoperatively until this resolves. The child must be fully awake and have full return of strength and adequate ventilatory effort before extubation is attempted. Consideration should be given to extubation over a ventilating stylet (Airway exchanger, Rapi-Fit, Cook, Inc., Bloomington, IN). The ventilating stylet is a hollow plastic guide with holes on its distal end and an adapter on its proximal end that allows the placement of either a Luer-Lok connector for connection to a jet ventilator or a 15-mm adapter for connection to standard anesthesia ventilating systems (Fig. 12-24 [see website]). It is available in a variety of sizes to allow the exchange of ETTs 3.0 mm ID or larger. This can be used for oxygenation and ventilation and as a guide to reinsert the ETT if the child's ventilatory efforts are inadequate

or if airway obstruction occurs.[324] However, caution is required when using this device for jet ventilation because significant barotrauma has been reported.[325,326] An alternative to jet ventilation is the Enk Oxygen Flow Modulation set (Cook, Inc., Bloomington, IN) that allows flows from a standard low pressure flowmeter to be adjusted by occluding holes in the delivery system with the thumb and forefinger (Fig. 12-25A [see website]). Alternatively, one could cut a side hole in the plastic oxygen delivery tubing to accomplish a similar low pressure oxygen delivery system (see Fig. 12-25B [on website]).

In circumstances in which the child will remain intubated for a prolonged period of time after surgery, it is advisable to have the patient return to the operating room for extubation. Both a surgeon who is prepared to perform rigid bronchoscopy and/or tracheostomy and an anesthesiologist who is familiar with the techniques used for the previously successful airway management should be in attendance.

Special Techniques for Ventilation

Multi-handed Mask Ventilation Techniques

These techniques can provide an effective temporizing measure until the airway is secured or the child is awakened. One person uses both hands to maintain an adequate mask fit, and a second person compresses the ventilation bag (Fig. 12-26). A single person using two hands to optimize the mask fit and the anesthesia ventilator to provide ventilation can replicate this technique.[327] Occasionally, a second person must assist by performing a jaw thrust with one hand while compressing the anesthesia bag with the other. Rarely, a third person may be required to compress the anesthesia bag with two hands (so as to generate a higher peak inflation pressure) while the first person holds the mask with two hands and a second person performs a two-handed jaw thrust.[327]

Laryngeal Mask Airway

The LMA has revolutionized difficult airway management in children. Numerous case reports and extensive clinical experience attest to the value of the LMA for establishing an airway when both ventilation and intubation are extremely difficult or impossible.[298,328-331] The LMA has been described as a tool for use in both the nonemergency (can ventilate/can't intubate) and the emergency pathway (can't ventilate/can't intubate) of the ASA difficult airway algorithm.[296,298] Use has been described in the awake child (LMA insertion in awake infants with Pierre Robin syndrome)[329] and in the anesthetized child with a known or suspected difficult airway. It can be used as the definitive airway in some circumstances, as a conduit for intubation, or as a temporizing airway while other options are pursued (e.g., a surgical airway). Other supraglottic devices have also been reported to be useful in the management of the child with difficult airway, including the CobraPLA[287] and the Laryngeal Tube.[332]

Percutaneous Needle Cricothyrotomy

In 1992, the American Heart Association changed its recommendations for emergency airway management to a percutaneous needle cricothyrotomy over a surgical cricothyrotomy because it was believed that there is less risk of injury to vital structures such as the carotid arteries or jugular veins, particularly in the hands of nonsurgical trained practitioners.[333] In addition, most practitioners can more rapidly perform the

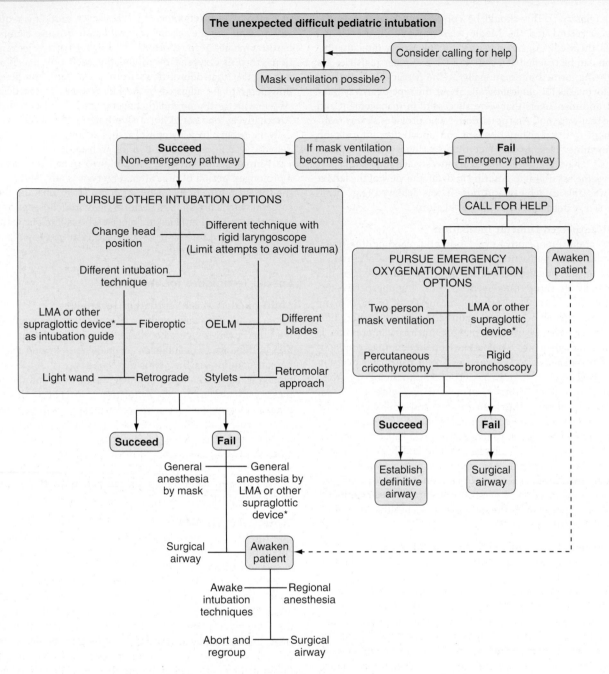

The unexpected difficult pediatric intubation

Consider calling for help

Mask ventilation possible?

Succeed
Non-emergency pathway

If mask ventilation becomes inadequate

Fail
Emergency pathway

CALL FOR HELP

PURSUE OTHER INTUBATION OPTIONS

Change head position

Different technique with rigid laryngoscope (Limit attempts to avoid trauma)

Different intubation technique

LMA or other supraglottic device* as intubation guide — Fiberoptic

OELM

Different blades

Light wand — Retrograde

Stylets

Retromolar approach

Succeed

Fail

General anesthesia by mask

General anesthesia by LMA or other supraglottic device*

Surgical airway

Awaken patient

Awake intubation techniques

Regional anesthesia

Abort and regroup

Surgical airway

PURSUE EMERGENCY OXYGENATION/VENTILATION OPTIONS

Awaken patient

Two person mask ventilation

LMA or other supraglottic device*

Percutaneous cricothyrotomy

Rigid bronchoscopy

Succeed

Fail

Establish definitive airway

Surgical airway

*Consider using PLMA if the child is at risk for aspiration or if high inflation pressures are needed

Figure 12-23. A proposed algorithm for management of the unexpected difficult pediatric airway. LMA, laryngeal mask airway; OELM, optimal external laryngeal manipulation; PLMA, ProSeal LMA. (Modified with permission from Wheeler M: Management strategies for the difficult pediatric airway. Anesth Clin North Am 1998; 16:743-761.)

percutaneous procedure. However, the cricothyroid membrane is of small width in infants and children. Attempts at cricothyrotomy may readily damage cricoid and thyroid cartilages, resulting in subsequent laryngeal stenosis and permanent damage to the speech mechanism. Therefore, this procedure should be reserved for use only under emergency circumstances.[334-338] Because this procedure is rarely utilized, it is recommended that experience be gained with patient simulators or in animal models.[339] A schema of this procedure is presented in

Figure 12-27. A commercial product called the Jet-Ventilation-Catheter (VBM, Robert-Bosch-Str. 7, D-712172 Sulz a. N., Germany) is available in three sizes: 16, 14, and 13 gauge. It consists of a slightly curved puncture needle within a Teflon, kink-resistant cannula nearly identical to an intravenous catheter (Fig. 12-28A). This cannula has two lateral eyes at its distal end and a combined Luer-Lok and 15-mm adapter at its proximal end (Fig. 12-28B). It also has a fixation flange and foam neck tape to secure the airway. *Percutaneous needle cricothy-*

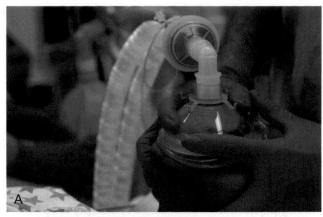

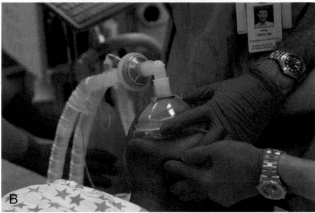

Figure 12-26. A, The two-handed technique for mask ventilation may be useful to improve mask fit and therefore ventilation when the traditional technique is inadequate. One person holds the mask while a second person squeezes the ventilation bag. **B,** Occasionally a third person is required to perform a two-handed jaw thrust (see text). (Reproduced with permission from American Heart Association, American Academy of Pediatrics: Pediatric Advanced Life Support. Elk Grove Village, IL, American Academy of Pediatrics, 1994.)

rotomy provides only a means for oxygen insufflation and does not reliably provide adequate ventilation. In the spontaneously breathing patient, simple delivery of intratracheal oxygen may be sufficient in the short term because hypercarbia is generally well tolerated by healthy children.[335,336,340] A number of children with arterial CO_2 values well above 150 mm Hg have survived neurologically intact when adequate oxygenation was maintained.[340] Thus, simple oxygenation without attempts at ventilation may be all that is required to sustain life (Fig. 12-29). For the child without respiratory effort, there is a need to provide ventilation in addition to oxygenation. An Ambu bag with the pop-off closed can provide limited ventilation through a percutaneous catheter. Extremely high ventilating pressures are required, but mid-tracheal pressures are significantly lower (10 to 16 mm Hg).[336] A percutaneous cricothyrotomy catheter can also be used with a jet ventilation system. Jet ventilation via a catheter passed through a narrow glottic opening has also been described.[341-344] Be aware that if upper airway obstruction is present (e.g., after multiple unsuccessful attempts at rigid laryngoscopy), there will be a limited pathway for egress of air and oxygen and barotrauma may result from insufflation of oxygen or attempts at ventilation. Very serious morbidity and mortality may result from massive subcutaneous emphysema or tension pneumothorax.[345,346] Thus, jet ventilation must be used with extreme caution in infants and children.[347] Another intravenous catheter type emergency airway device is the Emergency Transtracheal Airway Catheter (Cook, Inc., Bloomington, IN) that consists of a 6-Fr reinforced catheter that is advanced over a 15-gauge needle similar to the devices described earlier (Fig. 12-30 [see website]). It should be noted that none of these devices have been examined in controlled trials to confirm their efficacy, in part because these events are so rare. It is for this reason that we recommend training on simulators so that each practitioner can determine what device is best in his or her hands.

A number of percutaneous emergency airway devices are available that use large-diameter but short needles or use a needle, guidewire, and dilator to aid insertion of a percutaneous airway.[339,348-351] The Quicktrach (Rüsch, Inc. Duluth, GA) is a device that consists of a tapered 2- or 4-mm catheter with a fixation flange for securing with cloth tape. A removable plastic stopper is designed to limit the depth of needle insertion. This device requires several steps: puncture, aspiration for air, removal of the stopper, removal of the needle/syringe, and attachment to standard 22-mm connector; a flexible connector is also provided (Fig. 12-31 [see website]).

Other devices that use the Seldinger technique (needle, guidewire, scalpel incision of the skin, and passage of a dilator and tracheostomy tube) are the Arndt and Melker devices (Cook, Inc., Bloomington, IN). These devices provide a 3.0-mm ID airway that is sufficient for ventilation as well as oxygenation (Fig. 12-32 [see website]). However, the time required to insert such devices may be longer than simpler devices and may be inappropriate for immediate rapid establishment of an airway.[351]

Another device, Pertrach (Engineered Medical Systems, Inc., Indianapolis, IN), uses a split needle on a syringe to puncture the cricothyroid membrane (Fig. 12-33 [see website]). A skin incision is made and an introducer with tracheostomy tube (3.0 mm ID) is directed into the trachea while splitting the needle and removing it. The introducer is then removed and the airway is secured with tracheostomy tape. There are no case reports in the literature to determine the ease or difficulty of insertion in children, but the multiple steps required suggest that it may not be a device for emergent establishment of a surgical airway; however, it may be useful in less urgent situations.

Another percutaneous tracheostomy device is the Portex Pedia Trake kit (Fig. 12-34 [see website]). This device uses a scalpel to make a skin incision, followed by introduction of a large needle with a skin dilator, which in theory opens the incision sufficiently to allow passage of an obturator and 3.0, 4.0, or 5.0 mm ID tracheostomy (with or without cuff). This device appears sufficiently complicated so as to not be useful in a "can't intubate/can't ventilate" emergency but might be better suited to an urgent need to establish surgical access to the airway. Other devices with limited pediatric use[352] are kits designed to place a full-sized tracheostomy (e.g., Nu-Trake [International Medical Devices, Inc. Northridge, CA] or Abelson [Gilbert Surgical Instruments, Inc., Bellmawr, NJ]) and may potentially cause tracheal/laryngeal injury in small patients because of the relatively large size of the needle; again, little experience in children is available.[353,354]

Appendix 12-1. Syndromes and Disease Processes with Associated Airway Difficulties

Syndrome	Airway	Cerebral	Cardiac	Renal	Gastrointestinal	Endocrine Metabolic	Musculoskeletal	Anesthetic Considerations
Achondroplasia[490,585-590]	Midfacial hypoplasia, small nasal passages and mouth	Megacephaly ± hydrocephalus due to narrow foramen magnum					Dwarfism, odontoid hypoplasia with atlantoaxial instability	Difficult intubation; Difficult mask airway ± hydrocephalus
Apert syndrome[499]	Maxillary hypoplasia, narrow palate ± cleft palate	Craniosynostosis, flat facies, hypertelorism	± CHD	± Hydronephrosis, ± polycystic kidney	± Esophageal atresia		Syndactyly	Possible difficult intubation; Associated cardiac and renal problems
Arthrogryposis multiplex congenita (multiple congenital contractures)[591]	Associated hypoplastic mandible, cleft palate, Klippel-Feil syndrome, torticollis		± VSD				Thoracolumbar scoliosis	Difficult intubation; Associated cardiac disease; Minimal muscle relaxant required; ± Malignant hyperthermia
Beckwith-Wiedemann syndrome (visceromegaly)[449-453]	Macroglossia: regresses with age; may require partial glossectomy	± Mental handicap due to hypoglycemia	Large heart	Enlarged kidneys	Omphalocele, hepatosplenomegaly	Hypoglycemia up to age 4 months polycythemia	Eventration of diaphragm	Difficult intubation; Asymptomatic hypoglycemia; Omphalocele; Neonatal polycythemia
Cherubism (fibrous dysplasia of jaw)[506]	Bilateral painless mandibular and maxillary swelling may progress to airway obstruction							
Cornelia de Lange syndrome[493,494]	High arch palate, micrognathia, spurs at anterior angle of mandible, large tongue, ± cleft palate, short neck	Mental handicap	± CHD					Difficult intubation; Associated cardiac disease
Craniofacial dysostosis of Crouzon[499]	Maxillary hypoplasia with inverted V-shaped palate, ± large tongue	Ocular proptosis due to shallow orbits, craniosynostosis						Possible difficult intubation; Eye injury

Congenital hypothyroidism	Large tongue	May be mentally handicapped		Hypothermia, hypometabolic	Umbilical hernia	Difficult intubation Hypothermia Decreased drug metabolism
Epidermolysis bullosa[541]	Pressure lesions to mouth and airway Possible microstomia					Need gentle intubation with small tube. Postoperative laryngeal obstruction due to bulla formation
Freeman-Sheldon syndrome (whistling face)[508-512]	Small mouth, high palate	Hypertelorism, ± increased intracranial pressure, ± mental deficiency, ± microcephaly			Craniocarpotarsal dysplasia, Strabismus, kyphoscoliosis, hip/knee contractures	Difficult intubation ± Malignant hyperthermia[511,512]
Goldenhar syndrome (oculoauriculo-vertebral syndrome)[487,488]	Hypoplastic zygomatic arch, mandibular hypoplasia, macrostomia, ± cleft tongue, palate, tracheo-esophageal fistula	Hydrocephalus			Occipitalization of atlas, cervical vertebral defects	Difficult intubation Cervical spine defects
Hallermann-Streiff syndrome (oculo-mandibulo-dyscephaly)[498]	Malar hypoplasia, micrognathia, hypoplasia of rami and anterior displacement of temporomandibular joint, narrow high arch palate					Difficult intubation
Marfan syndrome[592,593]	Narrow facies with narrow palate		Dissecting aortic aneurysm, aortic insufficiency		Scoliosis, kyphosis	Difficult intubation Associated cardiac and pulmonary disease
Mucopolysac-charidoses[456-460,463-466]						
Type IH (Hurler)[461]	Coarse facial features, macroglossia, short neck, tonsillar hypertrophy, narrowing of laryngeal inlet and tracheobronchial tree	± Increased intracranial pressure	Severe coronary artery and valvular heart disease, cardiomyopathy	Hepatosplenomegaly	Joint stiffness, kyphosis, contractures, odontoid hypoplasia and atlantoaxial subluxation	Difficult intubation Postobstructive pulmonary edema

(Continued)

Appendix 12-1. Syndromes and Disease Processes with Associated Airway Difficulties—cont'd

Syndrome	Airway	Cerebral	Cardiac	Renal	Gastrointestinal	Endocrine Metabolic	Musculoskeletal	Anesthetic Considerations
Thalassemia major (Cooley anemia)[595]	Malar hypoplasia causes relative mandibular hypoplasia		Hemosiderosis					May be difficult intubation Anemia Associated cardiac disease
Treacher Collins syndrome[482-486]	Malar, mandibular hypoplasia, ± cleft lip, ± choanal atresia, ± macro- or microstomia		± CHD				± Cervical spine deformity	Difficult intubation Associated cardiac disease
Trisomy 21 (Down syndrome)[438-442,577-582,596-598]	Small mouth, hypoplastic mandible, protruding tongue	Mental handicap	AV communis, VSD, ASD		Duodenal atresia		Hypotonia, cervical spine subluxation	May be difficult intubation Associated cardiac disease Less muscle relaxant required Increased risk of post-intubation stridor
Turner syndrome (Noonan syndrome)[491,492]	Narrow maxilla, small mandible, short neck	Mental handicap	Coarctation of aorta in females, pulmonary artery coarctation in males	Idiopathic hypertension		Hypogonadism		Difficult intubation Associated cardiac disease Hypertension

ASD, atrial septal defect; AV, atrioventricular; CHD, congenital heart disease; VSD, ventricular septal defect.

Anesthesia for Thoracic Surgery

Gregory B. Hammer

CHAPTER 13

General Perioperative Considerations	Techniques for Single-Lung Ventilation in Infants and Children
Ventilation and Perfusion during Thoracic Surgery	Surgical Lesions of the Chest
Thoracoscopy	**Summary**

General Perioperative Considerations

A thorough preoperative evaluation is essential when caring for the child who is scheduled for thoracic surgery. Appropriate imaging and laboratory studies should be performed according to the lesion involved. Guidelines for fasting, choice of premedication, and preparation of the operating room are the same as for other infants and children scheduled for major surgery. After induction of anesthesia, placement of an intravenous catheter, and tracheal intubation, arterial catheterization should be considered for children undergoing thoracotomy as well as those with severe lung disease having thoracoscopic surgery. For thoracoscopic procedures of relatively brief duration in children without significant lung disease, an arterial catheter may not be required. The arterial catheter facilitates monitoring of systemic blood pressure during manipulation of the lungs and mediastinum as well as arterial blood gas tensions during single-lung ventilation (SLV). Placement of a central venous catheter is generally not indicated if peripheral intravenous access is adequate for projected fluid and blood administration.

Inhalational anesthetic agents are commonly administered in 100% O_2 during maintenance of anesthesia. Isoflurane may be preferred owing to less attenuation of hypoxic pulmonary vasoconstriction compared with other inhalational agents, although this has not been studied in children.[1] Nitrous oxide is avoided. Intravenous opioids have a sparing effect on the concentration of inhalational anesthetics required, and, therefore, may limit the impairment of hypoxic pulmonary vasoconstriction. Alternatively, total intravenous anesthesia may be used.

A variety of approaches have been described to prevent and treat pain after videoscopic procedures. Bupivacaine infiltration at incision sites before skin incision has been shown to decrease postoperative pain.[2,3] Bupivacaine infiltration was found to be superior to intravenous fentanyl or tenoxicam in reducing postoperative pain.[4] The combination of general anesthesia with regional anesthesia and postoperative analgesia is particularly desirable for thoracotomy but may also be beneficial for thoracoscopic procedures. This is especially true when thoracostomy tube drainage, a source of significant postoperative pain, is used

after surgery. In addition, regional blockade for postoperative analgesia facilitates deep breathing and coughing, which may limit atelectasis and pneumonia. A variety of regional anesthetic techniques have been described for intraoperative anesthesia and postoperative analgesia, including intercostal and paravertebral blocks, intrapleural infusions, and epidural anesthesia (see Chapters 42, 43, and 44).

Ventilation and Perfusion during Thoracic Surgery

Ventilation is normally distributed preferentially to dependent regions of the lung, so that there is a gradient of increasing ventilation from the least to the most dependent lung segments. Because of gravitational effects, perfusion normally follows a similar distribution, with increased blood flow to dependent lung segments. Therefore, ventilation and perfusion are normally well matched. In infants, however, ventilation is normally distributed to the nondependent areas of the lung and perfusion is more evenly distributed because of their smaller anteroposterior distance that mitigates the effect of gravity. These two effects result in increased ventilation/perfusion ($\dot{V}/\dot{Q}$) mismatch. During thoracic surgery, several factors act to further increase $\dot{V}/\dot{Q}$ mismatch. General anesthesia, neuromuscular blockade, and mechanical ventilation may cause a decrease in functional residual capacity of both lungs. Compression of the dependent lung in the lateral decubitus position may cause atelectasis. Surgical retraction and/or SLV collapse the operative lung. Hypoxic pulmonary vasoconstriction, which acts to divert blood flow away from underventilated lung, thereby minimizing $\dot{V}/\dot{Q}$ mismatch, may be diminished by inhalational anesthetic agents and other vasodilating drugs. These factors apply equally to infants, children, and adults. The overall effect of the lateral decubitus position on $\dot{V}/\dot{Q}$ mismatch, however, is different in infants compared with older children and adults.

In adults with unilateral lung disease, oxygenation is optimal when the patient is placed in the lateral decubitus position with the healthy lung dependent ("down") and the diseased lung nondependent ("up").[5] Presumably, this is related to an increase in blood flow to the dependent, healthy lung and a decrease in blood flow to the nondependent, diseased lung because of the

Table 13-1. Thoracoscopic Procedures in Infants and Children

| Diagnostic inspection |
| Lung biopsy |
| Lobectomy |
| Sequestration resection |
| Cyst excision |
| Lung decortication |
| Foregut duplication resection |
| Thymectomy |
| Patent ductus arteriosus ligation |
| Thoracic duct ligation |
| Esophageal atresia repair |
| Sympathectomy |
| Aortopexy |
| Mediastinal mass excision |
| Anterior spinal fusion |

Table 13-2. Advantages of Thoracoscopic versus Open-Chest Surgery

| Improved surgical visualization |
| Decreased pain |
| Decreased surgical stress |
| Decreased ileus/earlier return to feeds |
| Quicker return to normal activity (parents and child) |
| Shorter hospitalization |
| Fewer long-term complications |
| Cosmetically superior |

hydrostatic pressure (or gravitational) gradient between the two lungs. This phenomenon promotes $\dot{V}/\dot{Q}$ matching in the adult patient undergoing thoracic surgery in the lateral decubitus position.

In infants with unilateral lung disease, however, oxygenation is improved with the healthy lung "up."[6] Several factors account for this discrepancy between adults and infants. Infants have a soft, easily compressible rib cage that cannot fully support the underlying lung. Therefore, functional residual capacity is closer to residual volume, making airway closure likely to occur in the dependent lung even during tidal breathing.[7] When the adult is placed in the lateral decubitus position, the dependent diaphragm has a mechanical advantage because it is "loaded" by the abdominal hydrostatic pressure gradient. This pressure gradient is reduced in infants, thereby reducing the functional advantage of the dependent diaphragm. The infant's small size also reduces the hydrostatic pressure gradient between the nondependent and dependent lungs. Consequently, the favorable increase in perfusion to the dependent, ventilated lung is attenuated in infants.

Finally, the infant's increased oxygen requirement, coupled with a small functional residual capacity, predisposes to hypoxemia. Infants normally consume 6 to 8 mL of O_2/kg/min compared with adult rates of 2 to 3 mL of O_2/kg/min.[8] For these reasons, infants are at an increased risk of significant oxygen desaturation during surgery in the lateral decubitus position.

Thoracoscopy

With the miniaturization of instruments, progress in video technology, and growing experience among pediatric surgeons, video endoscopic surgery of the chest, or thoracoscopy, is being performed for an increasing number of pediatric surgical indications (Table 13-1). Advantages of thoracoscopy include smaller chest incisions, reduced postoperative pain, and more rapid postoperative recovery compared with thoracotomy (Table 13-2, Fig. 13-1).[9,10] Endoscopes that can be passed through a needle are now manufactured, and digital video signals can be electronically modified to yield sharp, detailed, color images with a minimum light intensity. Digital cameras are designed to maintain an image in an upright orientation regardless of how

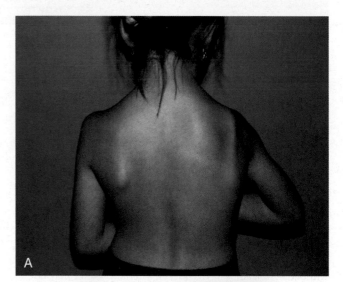

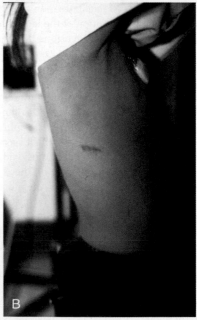

Figure 13-1. A, Significant chest deformity may occur with growth after thoracotomy. **B,** Smaller incisions associated with thoracoscopic surgery result in minimal musculoskeletal changes.

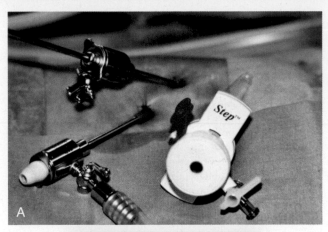

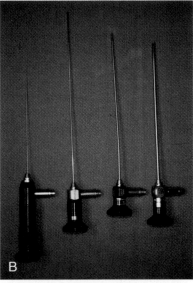

Figure 13-2. A, Thoracoscopic instruments in situ in an infant. **B,** Telescopes for use in infants range in size from 1.2 to 4.0 mm.

bed positioning. Robotic tools can be vocally directed to position telescopes in the surgical field for optimal viewing; these surgical "telemanipulators" facilitate microsurgery in confined spaces even for small infants. Other endoscopic robots are being developed for a wide range of surgical applications.

Thoracoscopy can be performed while both lungs are being ventilated using CO_2 insufflation and placement of a retractor to displace lung tissue in the operative field. However, SLV is extremely desirable during thoracoscopy because lung deflation improves visualization of thoracic contents and may reduce lung injury caused by the use of retractors. There are several different techniques that can be used for SLV in children.

Techniques for Single-Lung Ventilation in Infants and Children

Use of a Single-Lumen Endotracheal Tube
The simplest means of providing SLV is to intentionally intubate the ipsilateral main-stem bronchus with a conventional single-lumen endotracheal tube (ETT).[11] When the left bronchus is to be intubated, the bevel of the ETT is rotated 180 degrees and the child's head is turned to the right.[12] The ETT is advanced into the bronchus until breath sounds on the operative side disappear. A fiberoptic bronchoscope (FOB) may be passed through or alongside the ETT to confirm or guide placement. When a cuffed ETT is used, the distance from the proximal cuff to the tip of the endotracheal tube must be less than the length of the main-stem bronchus so that the upper lobe orifice is not occluded (Fig. 13-3).[13] This technique is simple and requires no special equipment other than a FOB. This may be the preferred

the telescope is rotated. They are also equipped with an optical or digital zoom to magnify the image or give the illusion of moving the telescope closer to the object of interest. The smallest of telescopes use fiberoptics and are less than 2 mm in diameter (Fig. 13-2). Two-millimeter disposable ports, mounted on a Veress needle, are used for introduction of these small instruments. Larger instruments and ports are used in larger children and for more complex cases.

A second area of major advance in video endoscopic surgery is the development of the endoscopic suite in which all necessary wiring is in equipment booms, ceilings, and walls. The manipulation of digital images is controlled by voice or touch-screen command either from the operative field or at a conveniently located station nearby. High-quality digital images are displayed on flat panel monitors that can be positioned within a comfortable viewing range. Remote-controlled cameras can direct any view in the room to any of the monitors or to a remote site. Digital radiographs can be routed from the radiology department to the operating room, and consultants in remote locations can be viewed on monitors in the operating room so that the surgeon can see to whom he or she is speaking. An additional feature of newer endoscopy suites is voice-controlled

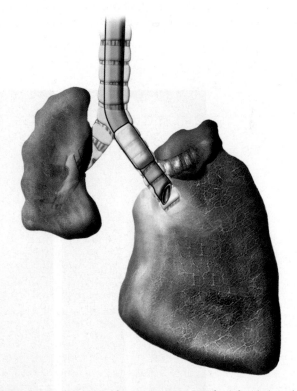

Figure 13-3. Placement of a single-lumen ETT for left-sided single-lung ventilation results in obstruction of the upper lobe orifice if the distance from the proximal cuff to the tip of the ETT is longer than the main-stem bronchus.

technique of SLV in emergency situations such as airway hemorrhage or contralateral tension pneumothorax.

Problems can occur when using a single-lumen ETT for SLV. If a smaller, uncuffed ETT is used, it may be difficult to provide an adequate seal of the intended bronchus. This may prevent the operative lung from adequately collapsing or fail to protect the healthy, ventilated lung from contamination by purulent material or blood from the contralateral lung. One is unable to suction the operative lung using this technique. Hypoxemia may occur due to obstruction of the upper lobe bronchus, especially when the short right main-stem bronchus is intubated.

Variations of this technique have been described, including intubation of both bronchi independently with small ETTs.[14-17] One main-stem bronchus is initially intubated with an ETT, after which another ETT is advanced over a FOB into the opposite bronchus. The disadvantages of these techniques include technical difficulties and trauma to the tracheal and bronchial mucosa. Even after successful bilateral bronchial intubation, the inner diameters of the tubes will be small, limiting gas flow and impeding suctioning of the airways.

Use of Balloon-Tipped Bronchial Blockers

A Fogarty embolectomy catheter or an end-hole, balloon wedge catheter may be used for bronchial blockade to provide SLV (Fig. 13-4).[18-21] Placement of a Fogarty catheter is facilitated by bending the tip of its stylette toward the bronchus on the operative side. A FOB may be used to reposition the catheter and confirm appropriate placement. Various techniques for placing an end-hole catheter outside the ETT have been described. Using one such method, the bronchus on the operative side is initially intubated with an ETT.[18] A guidewire is then advanced into that bronchus through the ETT. The ETT is removed and the blocker is advanced over the guidewire into the bronchus.

An ETT is then reinserted into the trachea alongside the blocker catheter. The catheter balloon is positioned in the proximal main-stem bronchus under fiberoptic visual guidance. Alternatively, if a FOB small enough to pass through the indwelling ETT is not available, fluoroscopy may be used (Fig. 13-5). With an inflated blocker balloon the airway is completely sealed, providing more predictable lung collapse and better operating conditions than with an ETT in the bronchus.

One potential problem with this technique is dislodgement of the blocker balloon into the trachea, blocking ventilation to both lungs and/or preventing collapse of the operative lung. The balloons of most catheters currently used for bronchial blockade have low compliance properties (i.e., low volume, high pressure). They require 1 to 3 mL of air or saline to fully inflate. Overdistention of the balloon can damage or even rupture the airway.[22] A recent study, however, reported that bronchial blocker cuffs produced lower "cuff to tracheal" pressures than double-lumen tubes.[23] When closed-tip bronchial blockers are used, the operative lung cannot be suctioned and continuous positive airway pressure (CPAP) cannot be provided to the operative lung if needed.

When a bronchial blocker is placed outside the ETT, care must be taken to avoid injury caused by compression and resultant ischemia of the tracheal mucosa. The sum of the catheter diameter and the outer diameter of the ETT should not significantly exceed the tracheal diameter. Outer diameters for pediatric-size ETTs are shown in Table 13-3. These numbers provide an estimate of the predicted tracheal diameter, which should approximate the size of the uncuffed ETT predicted to produce a seal in the trachea.

Recently, adapters have been developed that facilitate ventilation during placement of a bronchial blocker through an indwelling ETT.[24,25] Use of a 5-Fr endobronchial blocker that is designed

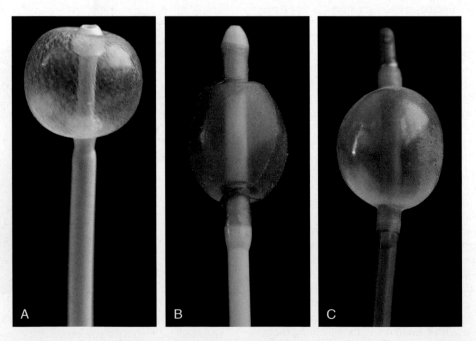

Figure 13-4. A variety of balloon-tipped catheters have been used for single lung ventilation, including an Arrow balloon wedge catheter (**A**), the Cook pediatric bronchial blocker (**B**), and a Fogarty embolectomy catheter (**C**). (Photographs by Michael Chen, MD.)

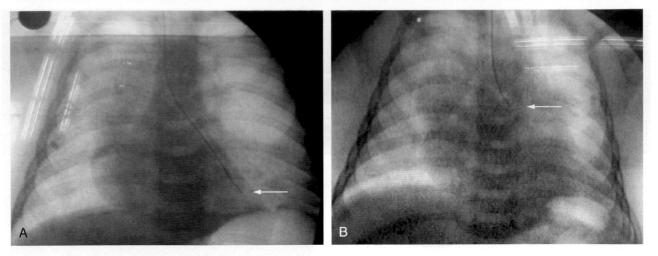

Figure 13-5. A bronchial blocker (*arrow*) is placed in a distal left bronchus (**A**) and withdrawn into the proximal left main-stem bronchus (**B**) under fluoroscopic guidance (*arrow*).

for use in children with a multiport adapter and FOB has been described (Cook, Inc., Bloomington, IN).[26] The balloon is elliptical so that it conforms to the bronchial lumen when inflated. The blocker catheter has a maximum outer diameter of 2.5 mm (including the deflated balloon), a central lumen with a diameter of 0.7 mm, and a distal balloon with a capacity of 3 mL. The balloon has a length of 1.0 cm, corresponding to the length of the right main-stem bronchus in children approximately 2 years of age.[27] The blocker is placed coaxially through a dedicated port in the adapter, which also has a port for passage of a FOB and ports for connection to the anesthesia breathing circuit and ETT (Fig. 13-6). The FOB port has a plastic sealing cap, whereas the blocker port has a Tuohy-Borst connector that locks the catheter in place and maintains an airtight seal. Because oxygen can be administered during passage of the blocker and FOB, the risk of hypoxemia during blocker placement is diminished, and repositioning of the blocker may be performed with fiberoptic guidance during surgery.

When a FOB is used to guide the placement of a bronchial blocker, both the blocker catheter and FOB must pass through the indwelling ETT. The smallest ETT through which the catheter and FOB can be passed must be larger than the sum of the outer diameters of the catheter and the FOB. The 5-Fr Cook bronchial blocker and a FOB with a 2.2-mm diameter, for example, may be inserted through an ETT with an internal diameter as small as 5.0 mm; for children with an indwelling ETT smaller than this, a blocker catheter can be positioned under fluoroscopy (see Fig. 13-5).

Use of a Univent Tube
The Univent tube (Fuji Systems Corporation, Tokyo, Japan) is a conventional ETT with a second lumen containing a small blocker catheter that can be advanced into a bronchus (Fig. 13-7).[28,29] A balloon located at the distal end of this small tube serves as a blocker. Univent tubes require a FOB for successful placement. Univent tubes are now available in sizes with internal diameters as small as 3.5 and 4.5 mm for use in children older than 6 years of age.[30] Because the blocker tube is firmly attached to the main ETT, displacement of the Univent blocker balloon is less likely than when other blocker techniques are used. The blocker tube has a small lumen that allows egress of gas and can be used to insufflate oxygen or suction the operated lung.

One disadvantage of the Univent tube is the large cross-sectional area occupied by the blocker channel, especially in the smaller size tubes. Therefore, Univent tubes have a large outer diameter with respect to their inner (luminal) diameters (Table 13-4). Smaller Univent tubes have a disproportionately high resistance to gas flow.[31] The Univent tube's blocker balloon has low-volume, high-pressure characteristics so mucosal injury can occur during normal inflation.[32,33]

Use of Double-Lumen Tubes
All double-lumen tubes (DLTs) are essentially two tubes of unequal length molded together. The shorter tube ends in the trachea, and the longer tube ends in the bronchus (Fig. 13-8). DLTs for older children and adults have cuffs located on the tracheal and bronchial lumens. The tracheal cuff, when inflated, allows positive-pressure ventilation. The inflated bronchial cuff

Table 13-3. Single-Lumen Endotracheal Tube Diameters

ID (mm)*	OD (mm)	Equivalent French Size
3.0	4.3	13
3.5	4.9	15
4.0	5.5	17
4.5	6.2	19
5.0	6.8	21
5.5	7.5	23
6.0	8.2	25
6.5	8.9	27
7.0	9.6	29
7.5	10.2	31
8.0	10.8	32

*Sheridan Tracheal Tubes, Hudson RCI, Arlington Heights, IL.
ID, internal diameter; OD, outer diameter.
Note: Cuffed tubes have approximately 0.5-mm additional outer diameter.

The high-volume, low-pressure cuffs should not damage the airway, provided the cuffs are not overinflated with air or distended with nitrous oxide. Alternatively, saline may be used to inflate the cuffs.

A disadvantage of DLTs is the need to change the DLT to a single-lumen ETT if mechanical ventilation is required after surgery. This is a particular problem for children in whom tracheal intubation was difficult initially because of anatomic or functional limitations. Even when an airway was not classified as difficult preoperatively, it may become difficult secondary to facial and supraglottic edema, the presence of secretions and/or blood in the airway, and laryngeal trauma from the initial intubation. The use of an ETT exchange catheter may facilitate the exchange of a DLT for a single lumen ETT.[40] These devices are commercially available in a variety of sizes and allow oxygen insufflation and jet ventilation (Cook Critical Care, Inc, Bloomington, IN) (Fig. 12-24A-C).

Several important caveats should be considered before using an ETT exchange catheter. First, it must be small enough to pass through the tracheal lumen of the DLT. This should be tested in vitro before the procedure is performed in vivo. Second, it should never be advanced against resistance, and the clinician must always be cognizant of the depth of insertion; perforations of the tracheobronchial tree have been reported.[41] Third, a jet ventilator should be immediately available in case the new ETT does not follow the ETT exchange catheter into the trachea and the oxygenation via the catheter is needed. The jet ventilator should be preset to a peak inspiratory pressure of 25 psi by an in-line regulator. When passing an ETT over an ETT exchange catheter, a laryngoscope should be used to facilitate passage of the ETT into the trachea. It should be noted that the tip of the ETT may hang up on the laryngeal inlet and may require 90° rotation clockwise or counter-clockwise to successfully pass should this occur.

General Considerations in the Management of Single-Lung Ventilation

Once the ETT, bronchial blocker, or DLT is in place, airway pressures should be confirmed during SLV. If peak airway pressure is 20 cm H_2O during two-lung ventilation with a given tidal volume, inflating pressure should not exceed 40 cm H_2O in SLV when the same tidal volume is delivered during SLV. In general, smaller tidal volumes with increased respiratory rates are used to deliver a somewhat reduced minute ventilation with SLV as with two-lung ventilation. Some degree of permissive hypercapnia is targeted to minimize lung trauma.

After the child has been placed in the lateral decubitus position, proper ETT, bronchial blocker, or DLT position should be reconfirmed because malpositioning may occur when turning the patient. Two-lung ventilation should be maintained for as long as possible before switching to SLV. When SLV is required, an FIO_2 of 1.0 is generally used. Assuming an intact hypoxic pulmonary vasoconstriction response, PaO_2 during SLV should be between 150 and 210 mm Hg.[42] The lungs should be ventilated with a tidal volume of 8 to 10 mL/kg at a ventilatory rate that maintains the $PaCO_2$ between 45 and 60 mm Hg, unless this degree of hypercapnia cannot be tolerated due to other physiologic factors (e.g., concomitant metabolic acidosis). Inadequate tidal volumes may lead to atelectasis in the ventilated lung (reduced functional residual capacity), and increased intrapulmonary shunting, resulting in hypoxemia. Large tidal volumes

may force blood to the nondependent lung (similar to the application of positive end-expiratory pressure), thereby increasing the intrapulmonary shunt.[43,44]

After the institution of SLV, PaO_2 may continue to decrease for up to 45 minutes. Should hypoxemia develop, proper positioning of the indwelling blocker or tube should be reconfirmed by fiberoptic bronchoscopy if possible. Several techniques can be employed to improve oxygenation. The most effective maneuver for improving PaO_2 is the application of continuous positive airway pressure (CPAP) to the nondependent lung.[45] Insufflation of oxygen to achieve a CPAP of 10 cm H_2O, for example, produces alveolar inflation and decreases intrapulmonary shunt fraction. This can usually be accomplished without significant expansion of the lung and interference with surgical conditions. If the PaO_2 continues to decrease despite the application of CPAP to the deflated lung, a malpositioned bronchial blocker or tube should be considered. This may be signaled by a sudden increase in the inflation pressure, a decrease in tidal volume, and/or a change in the capnogram. When a DLT is in place, the surgeon may aid repositioning. The surgeon can palpate the bronchi and manually occlude the main bronchial lumens, thereby guiding the tip of the DLT into the correct position. When the cause of the hypoxemia and/or hypercarbia cannot be readily identified, the balloon or cuff should be deflated and both lungs should be ventilated after informing the surgeon of the problem.

Guidelines for selecting appropriate tubes (or catheters) for SLV in children are shown in Table 13-6. There is significant variability in overall size and airway dimensions in children, particularly in teenagers. The recommendations shown in Table 13-6 are based on average values for airway dimensions. Larger DLTs may be safely used in large adolescents.

Surgical Lesions of the Chest

Neonates and Infants

A variety of congenital intrathoracic lesions for which surgery is required may occur in the neonatal or infancy period. These

Table 13-6. Tube Selection for Single-Lung Ventilation in Children

Age (yr)	ETT (ID)*	BB (Fr)	Univent†	DLT (Fr)
0.5-1	3.5-4.0	2‡		
1-2	4.0-4.5	3‡		
2-4	4.5-5.0	5§		
4-6	5.0-5.5	5§		
6-8	5.5-6.0	5§	3.5	
8-10	6.0 cuffed	5§	3.5	26¶
10-12	6.5 cuffed	5§	4.5	26¶-28¶
12-14	6.5-7.0 cuffed	5§	4.5	32¶
14-16	7.0 cuffed	5, 7§	6.0	35¶
16-18	7.0-8.0 cuffed	7, 9§	7.0	35, 37¶

*Sheridan Tracheal Tubes, Hudson RCI, Arlington Heights, IL.
†Fuji Systems Corporation, Tokyo, Japan.
‡Edwards Lifesciences LLC, Irvine, CA.
§Cook Critical Care, Inc, Bloomington, IN.
¶Teleflex Medical, Research Triangle Park, NC
¶Nellcor, Pleasanton, CA.
BB, bronchial blocker; DLT, double-lumen tube; ETT, endotracheal tube; Fr, French size; ID, internal diameter.

include lesions of the trachea and bronchi, lung parenchyma, and diaphragm.

Tracheal stenosis may be acquired or congenital. Tracheal stenosis occurs most commonly due to prolonged tracheal intubation, often in neonates with infant respiratory distress syndrome associated with prematurity. Ischemic injury of the tracheal mucosa may occur due to a tight-fitting ETT at the level of the cricoid cartilage, which becomes scarred and constricted after a period of time. *Subglottic stenosis* may develop, resulting in stridor after tracheal extubation. Reintubation may be required due to oxygen desaturation and hypercarbia.

Fiberoptic bronchoscopy is used to evaluate the severity of the stenosis and exclude other causes of stridor (e.g., vocal cord paralysis or laryngomalacia). When general anesthesia is required, inhalational anesthesia may be administered via a face mask with the FOB inserted through an adapter in the mask and into the nasopharynx. This is usually performed while the infant breathes spontaneously.[46]

A cricoid split procedure may be performed for infants with acquired subglottic stenosis. After diagnostic bronchoscopy, the infant is either intubated with an ETT or a rigid bronchoscope is left in place during the operation. Anesthesia may be maintained with inhalational agents or an intravenous anesthetic technique, such as with propofol and remifentanil.[47] Typically, an ETT 0.5 mm larger than the original endotracheal tube is placed after the repair.

For infants with severe *congenital tracheal stenosis*, a laryngotracheoplasty may be performed. This procedure involves the placement of a costal, auricular, or laryngeal cartilage graft into the anterior and/or posterior trachea.[48] In some cases, a stent may be positioned within the trachea. These infants may require a tracheal tube and mechanical ventilation for a variable period of time postoperatively. In these cases, sedation, analgesia, and at times neuromuscular blockade are maintained after surgery.

Pulmonary sequestrations result from disordered embryogenesis, producing a nonfunctional mass of lung tissue supplied by anomalous systemic arteries. Patients may present with cough, pneumonia, and failure to thrive; these signs often occur during the neonatal period, and usually before the age of 2 years. Diagnostic studies include computed tomography (CT) of the chest and abdomen and arteriography. Magnetic resonance imaging may provide high-resolution images, including definition of vascular supply. This may obviate the need for angiography. Surgical resection is performed once the diagnosis is confirmed. Pulmonary sequestrations do not generally become hyperinflated during positive-pressure ventilation. Nitrous oxide administration may result in expansion of these masses, however, and should be avoided.

Congenital cystic lesions in the thorax may be classified into three categories.[49] *Bronchogenic cysts* result from abnormal budding or branching of the tracheobronchial tree. They may cause respiratory distress, recurrent pneumonia, and/or atelectasis due to lung compression. *Dermoid cysts* are clinically similar to bronchogenic cysts but differ histologically because they are lined with keratinized, squamous epithelium rather than respiratory (ciliated columnar) epithelium. They usually manifest later in childhood or adulthood. *Cystic adenomatoid malformations* are structurally similar to bronchioles but lack associated alveoli, bronchial glands, and cartilage.[50] Because these lesions communicate with the airways, they may become

overdistended due to gas trapping, leading to respiratory distress in the first few days of life. When they are multiple and air filled, cystic adenomatoid malformations may resemble congenital diaphragmatic hernias radiographically. Treatment is surgical resection of the affected lobe. As with congenital diaphragmatic hernias, prognosis depends on the amount of remaining lung tissue, which may be hypoplastic due to compression in utero.[51]

Congenital lobar emphysema often manifests with respiratory distress shortly after birth.[52] This lesion may be caused by "ball-valve" bronchial obstruction in utero, causing progressive distal overdistention with fetal lung fluid. The resultant emphysematous lobe may compress lung bilaterally, resulting in a variable degree of hypoplasia. Congenital cardiac deformities are present in about 15% of children.[53] Radiographic signs of hyperinflation may be misinterpreted as tension pneumothorax or atelectasis on the contralateral side (Fig. 13-9). Positive-pressure ventilation may exacerbate lung hyperinflation. Nitrous oxide is contraindicated, and isolation of the lungs during anesthesia is desirable.

Congenital diaphragmatic hernia is a life-threatening condition that occurs in approximately 1 in 2,000 live births. Failure of a portion of the fetal diaphragm to develop allows abdominal contents to enter the thorax, interfering with normal lung growth. In 70% to 80% of diaphragmatic defects, a portion of the left posterior diaphragm fails to close, forming a triangular defect known as the *foramen of Bochdalek*. Hernias through the foramen of Bochdalek that occur early in fetal life usually cause respiratory failure immediately after birth owing to pulmonary hypoplasia. Distention of the gut postnatally with bag-and-mask ventilation exacerbates the ventilatory compromise by further compressing the lungs. The diagnosis is often made prenatally, and fetal surgical repair has been described.[54] Neonates present with tachypnea, a scaphoid abdomen, and absent breath sounds over the affected side. Chest radiography typically shows bowel in the left hemithorax with deviation of the heart and mediastinum to the right and compression of the right lung (Fig. 13-10). Right-sided hernias (see Fig. 13-10C) may occur late and manifest with milder signs. In the presence of significant respiratory distress, bag-and-mask ventilation should be avoided and immediate tracheal intubation should be performed.

Because pulmonary hypertension with right-to-left shunting contributes to severe hypoxemia in neonates with congenital diaphragmatic hernia, a variety of pulmonary vasodilators have been used. These include tolazoline, prostacyclin, dipyridamole, and nitric oxide.[55-59] High-frequency oscillatory ventilation has been used in conjunction with pulmonary vasodilator therapy to improve oxygenation before surgery.[60] In cases of severe lung hypoplasia and pulmonary hypertension refractory to these therapies (e.g., $Pao_2 < 50$ mm Hg with Fio_2 of 1.0), extracorporeal membrane oxygenation (ECMO) should be initiated early to avoid progressive lung injury. Improved outcomes have been associated with early use of ECMO followed by delayed surgical repair.[61]

A particularly poor prognosis is predicted if congenital diaphragmatic hernia is associated with cardiac deformities, preoperative alveolar-to-arterial oxygen gradient greater than 500 mm Hg, or severe hypercarbia despite vigorous ventilation.[62,63] Prognosis has also been correlated with pulmonary compliance and radiographic findings.[64,65]

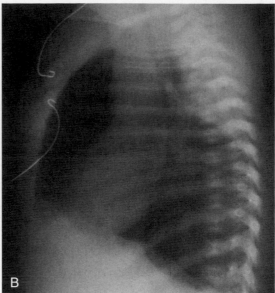

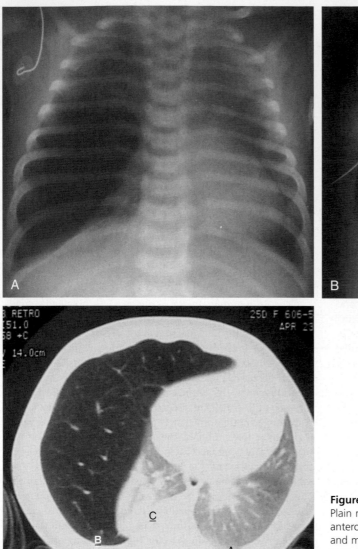

Figure 13-9. Congenital lobar emphysema of the right lower lobe. Plain radiography illustrates hyperlucency of the right lung on the anteroposterior image (**A**) and posterior displacement of the heart and mediastinum on the lateral image (**B**). The CT scan (**C**) demonstrates compression of the left lung (A) and right upper lobe (C) as well as hyperinflation of the right lower lobe (B).

Surgical correction via a subcostal incision with ipsilateral chest tube placement may be performed before, during, or immediately after ECMO.[66,67] In children undergoing surgical repair off ECMO, pulmonary hypertension is the major cause of morbidity and mortality. Hyperventilation to induce a respiratory alkalosis and 100% oxygen may be administered to decrease pulmonary vascular resistance. The anesthetic should be designed to minimize sympathetic discharge, which may exacerbate pulmonary hypertension (e.g., a high-dose opioid technique). The lungs of these infants should be ventilated with small tidal volumes and low inflating pressures to avoid pneumothorax on the contralateral (usually right) side. Both nitric oxide and high-frequency oscillatory ventilation have been used during surgical repair.[68,69] A high index of suspicion of right-sided pneumothorax should be maintained, and a thoracostomy tube should be placed in the event of acute deterioration of respiratory or circulatory function. It is also imperative that normal body temperature, intravascular volume, and acid-base status be maintained. Mechanical ventilation is continued postoperatively in nearly all cases because lung compliance is markedly reduced after surgery.

Failure of the central and lateral portions of the diaphragm to fuse results in a retrosternal defect, the *foramen of Morgagni.* This usually manifests as signs of bowel obstruction rather than respiratory distress. Repair is usually performed via an abdominal incision (see also Chapter 36).

Tracheoesophageal fistula and/or esophageal atresia occurs in approximately 1 in 4000 live births. In 80% to 85% of infants, this lesion includes esophageal atresia with a distal esophageal pouch and a proximal tracheoesophageal fistula.[70,71] The fistula is usually located one to two tracheal rings above the carina. Afflicted neonates present with spillover of pooled oral secretions from the pouch and may develop progressive gastric distention and tracheal aspiration of acidic gastric contents via the fistula. A common association is the VACTERL complex, consisting of vertebral, anorectal, cardiac, tracheoesophageal, renal, and/or limb defects.[72] Esophageal atresia is confirmed when an orogastric tube passed through the mouth cannot be advanced more than about 7 cm (Fig. 13-11). The proximal pouch tube should be secured and continuous suction applied, after which a chest radiograph is diagnostic.

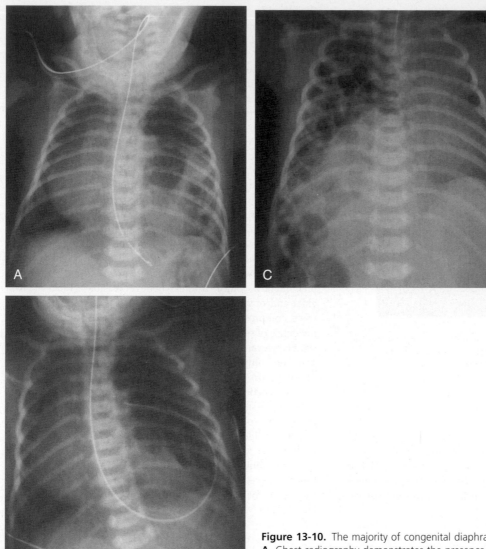

Figure 13-10. The majority of congenital diaphragmatic hernias are left sided. **A,** Chest radiography demonstrates the presence of bowel in the left hemithorax. **B,** A nasogastric tube has been advanced into the stomach. **C,** Congenital diaphragmatic hernias may also occur on the right side.

Mask ventilation and tracheal intubation are avoided before surgery if possible, because they may exacerbate gastric distention and further compromise respiration. Once the trachea is intubated, an attempt is made to occlude the tracheal orifice of the fistula with the tracheal tube. The tip of the tracheal tube is positioned just above the carina by auscultation of diminished breath sounds over the left axilla as the tube is advanced into the right main-stem bronchus, after which the tube is retracted until breath sounds are increased over the left chest (Fig. 13-12A). A small FOB may be passed through the tracheal tube to confirm appropriate placement. Rarely, an emergency gastrostomy is performed due to massive gastric distention. Placement of a balloon-tipped catheter in the fistula via the gastrostomy may be performed under guidance with an FOB to prevent further gastric distention and/or enable effective positive-pressure ventilation in cases of significant lung disease (see Fig. 13-12B).[73] "Antegrade" occlusion of a tracheoesophageal fistula has also been reported with a balloon-tipped catheter advanced through the trachea into the fistula (see Fig. 13-12C).[74] Preoperative evaluation should be performed to diagnose associated anomalies,

particularly cardiac, musculoskeletal, and gastrointestinal defects, which occur in 30% to 50% of infants.[75] A poor prognosis for infants with tracheoesophageal fistula and esophageal atresia has been associated with prematurity and underlying lung disease as well as the coexistence of other congenital anomalies.[76]

Surgical repair usually involves a right thoracotomy and extrapleural dissection of the posterior mediastinum. In most cases, the fistula is ligated and primary esophageal anastomosis is performed ("short gap atresia"). In cases in which the esophageal "gap" is long, the proximal segment is preserved for subsequent staged anastomosis with or without intestinal interposition.[77] The trachea may be intubated with the infant breathing spontaneously or during gentle positive-pressure ventilation with small tidal volumes to avoid gastric distention. If a gastrostomy tube is in place, occlusion of the fistula may be confirmed by cessation of bubbling via underwater tubing connected to the gastrostomy or appearance of CO_2 by gas analysis.[78] Alternatively, the tracheal tube may be positioned in the main-stem bronchus opposite the side of the thoracotomy incision until the fistula is ligated.

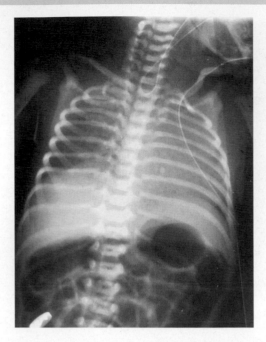

Figure 13-11. Tracheoesophageal fistula with esophageal atresia. Note the feeding tube coiled in the esophageal pouch and presence of a large volume of gas in the abdomen.

Esophageal atresia without connection to the trachea occurs much less commonly. These lesions are generally diagnosed by radiography after inability to pass an orogastric tube, at which time an absence of gas in the abdomen may be noted (see Fig. 36-4). So-called H-type tracheoesophageal fistula without esophageal atresia is relatively rare. Infants with H-type lesions may present later in childhood or adulthood with recurrent pneumonias or gastric distention during positive-pressure ventilation (see Chapter 36).[79]

Childhood

Some of the lesions described earlier may not be diagnosed until childhood. These include pulmonary sequestration, cystic lesions, and lobar emphysema. Other disorders for which thoracic surgery is performed in children, either for definitive treatment or diagnostic purposes, include neoplasms, infectious diseases, and musculoskeletal deformities.

Anterior mediastinal masses include neoplasms of the lung, mediastinum, and pleura. These tumors may be primary or metastatic. Perhaps the most common primary tumors are *lymphoblastic lymphoma*, a form of non-Hodgkin lymphoma, and *Hodgkin disease.* Less commonly, teratomas (germ cell tumors), thymomas, and thyroid, parathyroid, and mesenchymal tumors may manifest as anterior mediastinal masses.[80] Signs and symptoms due to vascular and/or airway compression may include dyspnea, orthopnea, pain, coughing, pleural effusion, and/or superior vena cava syndrome (swelling of the upper arms, face, and neck).[81,82]

Preoperative evaluation should include CT, echocardiography, and flow-volume studies whenever feasible. Tracheal, bronchial, and/or vascular (superior vena cava or pulmonary outflow tract) compression as detected by CT is associated with a high incidence of serious complications during induction of anesthesia.[82] However, CT scans are static pictures that may not identify dynamic compression of an airway or vascular outflow tract. These tumors may occur as extrathoracic or intrathoracic variable obstruction or fixed obstruction. Echocardiography identifies compression of the superior vena cava or pulmonary outflow tract. Flow-volume studies are the most effective investigations to detect evidence of dynamic compression of the airways (see Chapter 11).

Establishing the correct diagnosis often requires a tissue biopsy. More often than not, there is an urgency to secure the tissue for diagnosis because non-Hodgkin lymphoblastic lymphomas, which comprises 30% to 40% of non-Hodgkin lym-

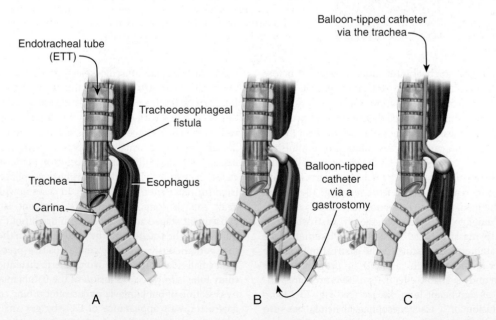

Figure 13-12. Methods for minimizing gastric insufflation in infants with a tracheoesophageal fistula. The tip of the ETT may be placed distal to the fistula in cases in which the fistula is well proximal to the carina (**A**). Alternatively, a balloon-tipped catheter may be placed in the fistula via a gastrostomy (**B**) or the trachea (**C**).

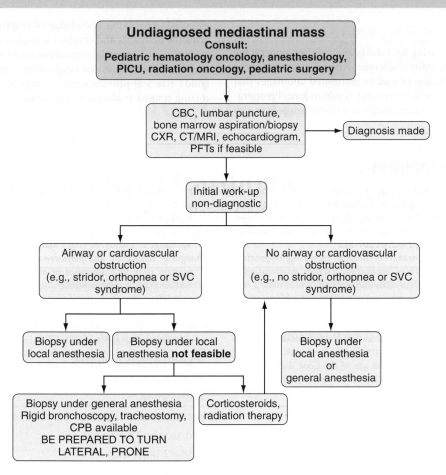

Figure 13-13. Algorithm for management of the child with a mediastinal mass. CBC, complete blood cell count; CXR, chest radiograph; LP, lumbar puncture; PFTs, pulmonary function tests; SVC, superior vena cava.

phoma, has a 12-hour doubling time. A rapid diagnosis and chemotherapy prescription may prevent widespread dissemination of the tumor. Indeed, today the 5-year survival of Hodgkin and non-Hodgkin lymphoblastic lymphoma exceeds 80%. Every effort should be made to secure a tissue diagnosis by lymph node or bone marrow biopsy under local anesthesia, thereby precluding the need for obtaining tissue under general anesthesia and facilitating early treatment. If peripheral tissue diagnosis cannot be obtained and signs of airway and/or circulatory compromise are present, careful consideration should be given to performing a biopsy under local anesthesia, administering a 12- to 24-hour burst of corticosteroids, initiating chemotherapy, and/or treating with limited radiation to decrease the size of the tumor and reduce the risk of life-threatening compression of the airway or major vessels under anesthesia. However, all of these interventions may compromise the ability of pathologists to accurately determine the tissue diagnosis; thus, some oncologists prefer that none of these interventions is used. Corticosteroids effect a reduction in tissue mass of lymphomas by inducing apoptosis in the tumor via a number of mechanisms.[83]

Induction of anesthesia in children with anterior mediastinal masses may be associated with severe airway obstruction and circulatory collapse.[84,85] This may occur even in children without signs or symptoms of respiratory or cardiovascular compromise.[86,87] Recommended anesthetic techniques for children with anterior mediastinal masses include inhalation induction with maintenance of spontaneous respiration.[88] The use of continuous positive airway pressure may help to maintain functional residual capacity that is otherwise reduced under anesthesia.[89] Keeping the head of the bed elevated may decrease the deleterious effects of supine positioning, including cephalad displacement of the diaphragm and secondary reduction of thoracic volume.[90] Keeping the child in a partial or even full right lateral decubitus position may help to maintain airway patency and reduce cardiac and vascular compression. Performing tracheal intubation while deeply anesthetized without the use of muscle relaxants and positive-pressure ventilation may preserve the normal transpulmonary pressure gradient and improve flow through conducting airways.[91-93] The decrease in chest wall tone associated with neuromuscular blockade is thought to increase the risk of severe airways compression.[94] As an alternative to tracheal intubation, use of a laryngeal mask airway has been described.[95] The use of a helium-oxygen mixture has been advocated to allow laminar flow and decrease resistance to gas flow.[95] In the event of tracheal or bronchial collapse under anesthesia, lateral or prone positioning and/or rigid bronchoscopy may be lifesaving. Performing a median sternotomy and cardiopulmonary bypass in this situation has been recommended but may be impractical unless access for partial bypass was established before induction of anesthesia.

Institutions should have an algorithm in place for the evaluation of children with anterior mediastinal masses that includes a multidisciplinary approach (see Fig. 13-13).

Overall, a bicuspid aortic valve (Video Clip 14-1) is the most common cardiac defect, occurring in up to 1% of the population.[9,10] Ventricular septal defects (Video Clip 14-2) represent the next most common congenital lesion,[9,11-15] followed by secundum atrial septal defects (Video Clip 14-3).[9,16] Among the cyanotic conditions, tetralogy of Fallot is the most common, affecting nearly 6% of children with CHD.[17] In the first week of life, however, D-transposition of the great arteries is the most common cause of cardiac cyanosis, because a subset of infants with tetralogy of Fallot will either be acyanotic or mildly desaturated at birth so that their cardiac disease will go undetected until later in life.

Segmental Approach to Diagnosis

A number of classification schemes have been proposed to characterize and categorize the various congenital cardiac malformations.[18-24] The one known as "the segmental approach to the diagnosis of CHD" assumes a sequential, systematic analysis of the three major cardiac segments (atria, ventricles, and great arteries) to characterize the abnormalities in a given patient. The guiding principle of this approach is that specific cardiac chambers and vascular structures have characteristic morphologic properties that determine their identities, rather than their positions within the body.[25] An organized, systematic identification of all cardiac structures or segments and their relationships to each other (connections or alignments between the segments) is carried out to define a given patient's anatomy.[26]

The initial steps to characterize the anomalies and classify a child's cardiovascular disease are to determine the cardiac position within the thorax and the situs of the thoracic and abdominal organs. The position of the heart can be described in terms of its location within the thoracic cavity and the direction of the cardiac apex. For simplicity, the following approach is frequently used. The term *levocardia* indicates that the heart is in the left hemithorax, as is normally the case. *Dextrocardia* specifies that the heart is located in the right hemithorax and *mesocardia* that the heart is displaced rightward but not completely in the right thoracic cavity. It is important to consider that an abnormal location of the heart within the thorax (cardiac malposition) may result from displacement of the heart by adjacent structures or underlying noncardiac malformations (e.g., diaphragmatic hernia, lung hypoplasia, scoliosis). The visceral situs or sidedness of the abdominal organs (liver and stomach) and atrial situs are considered independently. The visceral situs is classified as *solitus* (normal arrangement of viscera; liver on the right, stomach on the left and single spleen on the left), *inversus* (inversion of viscera; liver on the left, stomach on the right), or *ambiguous* (indeterminate visceral position). Abnormal arrangements or sidedness of the abdominal viscera, heart, and lungs suggests a high likelihood of complex cardiovascular pathology. The atrial situs, atrioventricular connections, ventricular looping (referring to the position of the ventricles as a result of the direction of bending of the straight heart tube in early development), ventriculoarterial connections, and relationship between the great vessels are then delineated. Finally, any associated malformations are described, including number and size of septal defects if present, valvar and/or great vessel abnormalities, and so on. Whereas many types of congenital defects fall neatly into this classification scheme, others, such as heterotaxy syndromes (a condition associated with malposition of the heart

and abdominal organs) are often more difficult to precisely define.

Physiologic Classification of Defects

The wide spectrum of cardiovascular pathology in the pediatric age group presents a unique challenge to the clinician who does not specialize in the care of these children. Even for those with a focus or interest in cardiovascular disease, the range of structural defects and the varied associated hemodynamic perturbations can be overwhelming.

Although the segmental approach is extremely helpful in characterizing CHD, there are many instances when a physiologic classification system can facilitate understanding of the basic hemodynamic abnormalities common to a group of lesions, congenital or acquired, and assist in patient management.[27,28] Several pathophysiologic classification schemes have been proposed, including some that categorize structural defects into simple versus complex lesions, consider the presence or absence of cyanosis or whether pulmonary blood flow is increased or decreased, and so on.[29-31] The following classification approach groups pediatric heart disease into six broad categories according to the underlying physiology or common features of the pathologies.

Volume Overload Lesions

Volume overload lesions are typically due to left-to-right shunting at the atrial, ventricular, or great artery levels. In general, if the location of the left-to-right shunt is proximal to the mitral valve (e.g., as is the case in atrial septal defects, partial anomalous pulmonary venous return, or unobstructed total anomalous pulmonary venous return), right heart dilation will occur. Lesions distal to the mitral valve (e.g., ventricular septal defect, patent ductus arteriosus, truncus arteriosus) lead to left-sided heart dilation. Children with atrioventricular septal defects (also known as atrioventricular canal defects) also fit into this category. The magnitude of the shunt and resultant pulmonary to systemic blood flow ratio ($\dot{Q}p:\dot{Q}s$) dictates the presence and severity of the symptoms and similarly guides medical and surgical therapies. Diuretic therapy and afterload reduction are beneficial in controlling pulmonary overcirculation and ensuring adequate systemic cardiac output. Transcatheter approaches or surgical interventions may be required to address the primary pathology associated with ventricular volume overload (see Chapter 20).

Obstruction to Systemic Blood Flow

Lesions characterized by systemic outflow tract obstruction include those with ductal-dependent systemic blood flow. These range from critical aortic stenosis, severe coarctation of the aorta, interruption of the aortic arch, and hypoplastic left heart syndrome. Prostaglandin E_1 infusion maintains ductal patency and ensures adequate systemic blood flow until either surgical or transcatheter intervention is performed in the first few days of life to relieve the systemic outflow tract obstruction. Often, inotropic and/or mechanical ventilatory support is necessary. Many of these infants also have significantly increased pulmonary blood flow with a high $\dot{Q}p:\dot{Q}s$ ratio, requiring diuretic therapy and manipulation of the systemic and pulmonary vascular resistances to control blood flow.

Obstruction to Pulmonary Blood Flow

Lesions with pulmonary outflow tract obstruction include those with ductal-dependent pulmonary blood flow. Pulmonary atresia with intact ventricular septum and critical pulmonary valve stenosis are defects that rely on patency of the ductus arteriosus for pulmonary blood flow. These infants may also require prostaglandin E_1 infusions to manage their cyanosis until the pulmonary outflow tract obstruction is relieved or bypassed.

Parallel Circulation

In the neonate with D-transposition of the great arteries the pulmonary and systemic circulations operate in parallel rather than the normal configuration in series. In this condition, deoxygenated blood from the right ventricle is ejected into the aorta and the left ventricle is in subpulmonary position ejecting oxygenated blood into the lungs. Neonates with this lesion depend on mixing of blood at the atrial, ventricular, or ductal levels. Although an infusion of prostaglandin E_1 can maintain ductal patency, many neonates benefit from a balloon atrial septostomy shortly after birth to create or enlarge an existing restrictive interatrial communication and optimize mixing. This is because mixing at the atrial level is much more effective than either the ventricular or ductal levels.

Single-Ventricle Lesions

This category is the most heterogeneous group, consisting of defects associated with atrioventricular valve atresia (i.e., tricuspid atresia), heterotaxy syndromes, and many others.[32] In some cases, both atria empty into a dominant ventricular chamber (i.e., double-inlet left ventricle); and although a second rudimentary ventricle is typically present, the physiology is that of a single ventricle or univentricular heart. Other cardiac malformations with two distinct ventricles (i.e., unbalanced atrioventricular septal defect) may also be considered in the functional single-ventricle category because of associated defects that may preclude a biventricular repair. A common feature among these lesions is complete mixing of the systemic and pulmonary venous blood at the atrial or ventricular level. Another frequent finding is aortic or pulmonary outflow tract obstruction. These children require careful delineation of their anatomy because each child represents a unique challenge to the practitioner. An important goal in single-ventricle management involves optimization of the balance between the pulmonary and systemic circulations early in life. This relates to the fact that a low pulmonary vascular resistance is an essential prerequisite for later palliative strategies and favorable outcomes. These considerations are also relevant in the anesthetic management of these children during noncardiac surgery.[30,33,34]

Intrinsic Myocardial Disorders

Children with primary cardiomyopathies or other forms of acquired heart disease such as myocarditis are characterized as having heart muscle disease (see later). They frequently have impaired ventricular function, either systolic or diastolic, and benefit from therapies tailored to their particular disease process.

Acquired Heart Disease

Cardiomyopathies

The term *cardiomyopathy* usually refers to diseases of the myocardium associated with cardiac dysfunction.[35,36] These have been classified into primary and secondary forms. The most common types in children are hypertrophic, dilated or congestive, and restrictive cardiomyopathies. Other forms include left ventricular noncompaction[37-39] and arrhythmogenic right ventricular dysplasia.[40] Secondary forms of cardiomyopathies are those associated with neuromuscular disorders such as Duchenne muscular dystrophy, glycogen storage diseases (i.e., Pompe disease), hemochromatosis or iron overload, and mitochondrial disorders. In addition, chemotherapeutic agents such as anthracyclines may result in dilated cardiomyopathies.[41] It is important to understand the basic hemodynamic processes behind the myocardial disease and implications for acute and chronic management.

Hypertrophic cardiomyopathy (HCM) is characterized by ventricular hypertrophy without identifiable hemodynamic etiology resulting in increased myocardial thickness. This is one of the most common forms, accounting for nearly 40% of cardiomyopathies in children.[42-45] The condition represents a heterogenous group of disorders, with the majority of the identified genetic defects exhibiting autosomal dominant inheritance patterns.[46,47] The mutations typically involve genes that encode sarcomeric proteins. This type of cardiac muscle disease is the most common cause of sudden cardiac death (SCD) in athletes, with an overall incidence estimated to be approximately 1% per year, with children and young adults affected most frequently.[48,49] Most children affected by HCM do not have left ventricular outflow tract obstruction (nonobstructive cardiomyopathy). It is unclear if the remaining minority with hypertrophic obstructive cardiomyopathy (HOCM), previously known as idiopathic hypertrophic subaortic stenosis (IHSS), are at an increased risk of SCD as compared with children without obstruction.[44] Hypertrophic cardiomyopathy may also involve the right ventricle.

The diagnosis of HCM begins with a history and physical examination. Most children are identified upon evaluation of a heart murmur, syncope, palpitations, or chest pain. Occasionally, an abnormal electrocardiogram (ECG) leads to referral. An accurate family history is essential. A prominent apical impulse is often present. Auscultation may reveal a systolic ejection outflow murmur that becomes louder with maneuvers that decrease preload or afterload (standing, Valsalva maneuver) or increase contractility. The murmur decreases in intensity with squatting and isometric handgrip. A mitral regurgitant murmur may also be present. An ECG will meet criteria for left ventricular hypertrophy in most children (Fig. 14-1). In some, the ECG findings may be striking (Fig. 14-2). Echocardiography demonstrating a hypertrophied nondilated left ventricle is diagnostic (Video Clip 14-4).[49] In many children, the hypertrophy may be asymmetrical (Video Clip 14-5). Echocardiography is the primary imaging modality for long-term assessment of wall thickness, ventricular dimensions, presence and severity of obstruction, systolic and diastolic function, valve competence, and response to therapy. Other diagnostic approaches such as cardiac catheterization and magnetic resonance imaging (MRI) may add helpful information in some cases.

The care of children with HCM includes maintenance of adequate preload, particularly in those with dynamic obstruction. Diuretics are generally not indicated and will often worsen the hemodynamic state by reducing left ventricular volume and increasing the outflow obstruction. Drugs that augment myocardial contractility (inotropic agents, calcium infusions) are not well tolerated. Patients usually undergo continuous ECG monitoring (Holter recording) and exercise testing for risk stratification.[50] β blockers and calcium-channel blockers are the primary

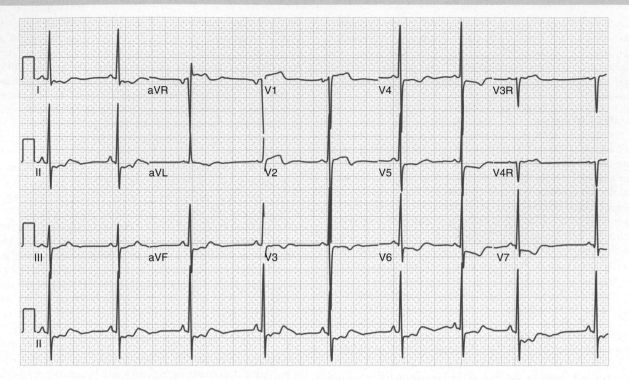

Figure 14-1. ECG in adolescent female with hypertrophic cardiomyopathy demonstrating left ventricular hypertrophy (deep S wave in V_1 and tall R waves over the left precordial leads). There is ST-segment depression and T-wave inversion over the left precordial leads related to repolarization changes associated with left ventricular hypertrophy, also known as a "strain" pattern. Reciprocal ST-segment elevation is noted over the right precordial leads.

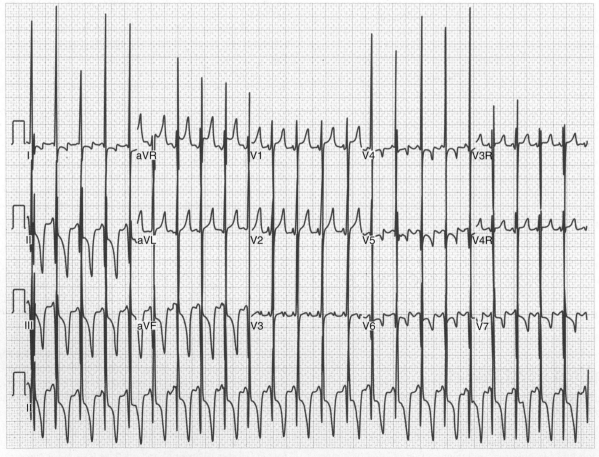

Figure 14-2. Tracing in a patient with Pompe disease, a severe form of hypertrophic cardiomyopathy displaying dramatic right and left ventricular voltages, as well as ST-segment and T-wave abnormalities. The recording is displayed at full standard (10 mm/mV, meaning that the ECG was not reduced in size to fit on the paper) as are all other ECG tracings in this chapter for reference.

agents for outpatient drug therapy.[51] Long-term treatment is individualized and based on the degree of hypertrophy, presence of ventricular ectopy, symptomatology (including syncope and congestive heart failure), family history, and genetic mutation analysis when available. Therapies range widely and include longitudinal observation with medical management of heart failure and arrhythmias, implantation of cardioverter-defibrillators, surgical myotomy/myectomy, transcatheter alcohol septal ablation, and cardiac transplantation. Patients with HCM are usually restricted from participating in competitive sports activities.[50]

Dilated cardiomyopathy (DCM), also known as congestive cardiomyopathy, is characterized by thinning of the left ventricular myocardium, dilation of the ventricular cavity, and impaired systolic function.[52-54] There is a broader range of etiologies than with HCM, ranging from genetic/familial forms with multiple types of inheritance patterns to those caused by infections (adenovirus, coxsackievirus, human immunodeficiency virus[55]), metabolic derangements (thyroid disorders, mitochondrial disorders, carnitine deficiency), toxic exposures (anthracyclines), and degenerative disorders (Becker and Duchenne muscular dystrophy).[56,57] Chronic tachyarrhythmias can also lead to DCM that may or may not improve once the rhythm disturbance is controlled.[58-60]

Most children with DCM present with signs and symptoms of congestive heart failure (tachypnea, tachycardia, gallop rhythm, diminished pulses, hepatomegaly). The chest radiograph typically demonstrates cardiomegaly, pulmonary vascular congestion, and, in some cases, atelectasis (Fig. 14-3). An ECG may identify the likely cause of the cardiac dysfunction in those with cardiomyopathy secondary to rhythm disorders or anomalous origin of the left coronary artery from the pulmonary root. The echocardiogram is essential for diagnosis and characteristically demonstrates a dilated left ventricle and systolic functional impairment (reduced shortening fraction and ejection fraction) (Video Clip 14-6).[61] Therapy in the short term is supportive and aimed at stabilization by controlling congestive heart failure and ventricular dysfunction. Management may include inotropic support (including phosphodiesterase inhibition) and mechanical ventilation. Unlike children with HCM, those with DCM have a volume-loaded, poorly contractile ventricle(s); therefore, gentle diuresis is beneficial. The infusion of large fluid boluses might be poorly tolerated and result in hemodynamic decompensation and cardiovascular collapse. The outcome of children with dilated cardiomyopathy is variable. In most, recovery of left ventricular systolic function occurs; however, others eventually require cardiac transplantation.[62] In a subset of children with severe disease, mechanical circulatory support may be necessary as a bridge to recovery or cardiac transplantation (Fig. 14-4, see Chapter 19).[63-65] Once initial stabilization is achieved, the treatment strategy typically switches to β blockade and afterload reduction with angiotensin-converting enzyme inhibitors.

Restrictive cardiomyopathy (RCM) is the least common of the major subsets of cardiomyopathies (5%) and portends a worse prognosis when it presents during childhood (survival <50% at 2 years from diagnosis).[66-71] The disorder is characterized by diastolic dysfunction related to a marked increase in myocardial stiffness resulting in impaired ventricular filling. Most cases are thought to be idiopathic. The presenting symptoms are generally nonspecific and primarily relate to the respiratory system. Occasionally the diagnosis is made following a

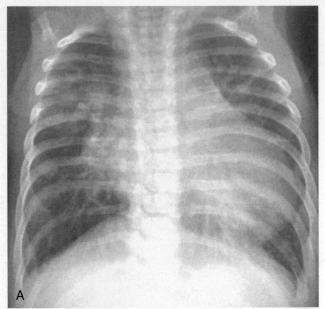

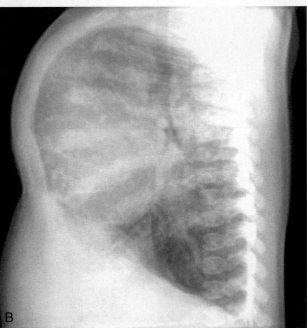

Figure 14-3. Chest radiographs in a young child with dilated cardiomyopathy in the posteroanterior (**A**) and lateral (**B**) projections demonstrating moderate to severe cardiomegaly and pulmonary vascular congestion. The lateral film shows the heart bulging anteriorly against the sternum.

syncopal or near sudden death event. The physical examination may demonstrate hepatomegaly, peripheral edema, and ascites.

The echocardiographic hallmark of RCM is that of severe atrial dilation (due to elevated atrial pressures) associated with normal- to small-sized ventricles (Video Clip 14-7). The marked diastolic dysfunction leads to increased end-diastolic pressures, left atrial hypertension, and secondary pulmonary hypertension. Children with RCM are prone to thromboembolic

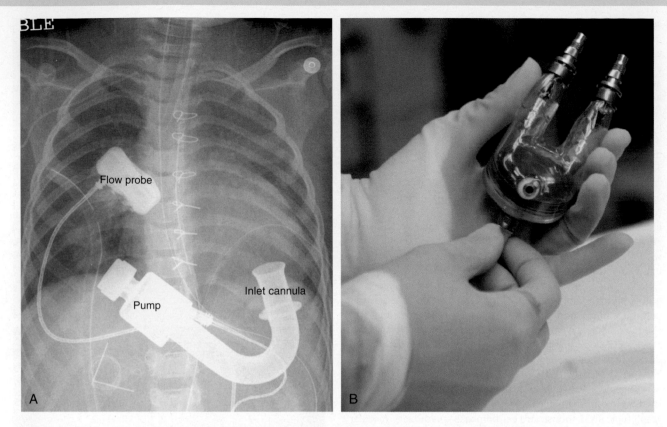

Figure 14-4. Mechanical circulatory assist devices. **A,** Chest radiograph in a child with end-stage dilated cardiomyopathy after placement of a MicroMed/DeBakey Child ventricular assist device for circulatory support while awaiting cardiac transplantation. This miniaturized device includes a titanium pump, inlet cannula (placed in the left ventricle), percutaneous cable, flow probe and outflow graft (placed in the aorta, not radiopaque). **B,** The Berlin Heart ventricular assist device. This device allows for paracorporeal placement and circulatory support in infants and small children. Although not approved by the U.S. Food and Drug Administration, the device has been used under specific guidelines and is available in several European countries.

complications, and anticoagulation therapy is frequently recommended. This is an important consideration during perioperative care as adjustments in the anticoagulation regimen may be necessary. Atrial and ventricular tachyarrhythmias may also occur. Optimal medical treatment is controversial because no specific agents or strategies have been shown to significantly alter outcomes.[71] Similar to children with HCM, diuretics often cause a decrease in the needed preload with detrimental effects on hemodynamics. Inotropic agents are not beneficial because systolic function is typically preserved and the arrhythmogenic properties of inotropic drugs can induce a terminal event. In many centers cardiac transplantation has been effectively utilized.[72,73]

Myocarditis

Myocarditis is defined as inflammation of the myocardium, often associated with necrosis and myocyte degeneration. In the United States it is most often caused by a viral infection. Over the past 20 years the spectrum of viral pathogens causing myocarditis has changed, such that adenovirus, enteroviruses (i.e., coxsackievirus B), and parvovirus have become the most frequent causes of fulminant disease.[74-76] The pathogenesis of

myocyte damage in myocardial inflammatory diseases is quite complex.

The overall incidence of myocarditis is not known because it is frequently underdiagnosed, going unrecognized as a nonspecific viral syndrome. A large 10-year population-based study on cardiomyopathy found an annual incidence of 1.24 per 100,000 children younger than 10 years of age, only a fraction of which represented those with myocarditis.[77] The diagnosis is made utilizing clinical history, physical examination, and imaging modalities. A child with new-onset congestive heart failure or ventricular arrhythmias without evidence of structural heart disease should be considered to have myocarditis until proven otherwise. An ECG will typically demonstrate low-voltage QRS complexes with tachycardia, sometimes ventricular in origin. Chest radiography often shows cardiomegaly with pulmonary vascular congestion (Fig. 14-5). Echocardiography reveals dilated ventricles with impaired systolic function, similar to dilated cardiomyopathy, and is useful in the exclusion of alternative diagnoses, such as pericardial effusion or anomalous origin of a coronary artery, which can present in a similar manner. Myocarditis is generally a clinical diagnosis, because definitive

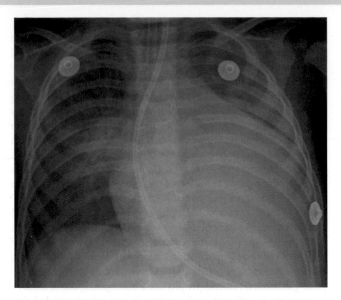

Figure 14-5. Chest radiograph in a child with acute myocarditis. Note the severe cardiomegaly and increased pulmonary vascularity.

confirmation requires the analysis of tissue obtained through myocardial biopsy either in the catheterization laboratory or the operating room (rarely performed).[78]

Many children with myocarditis have subclinical or mild clinical disease, whereas others progress to overt heart failure and/or arrhythmias. Among children with overt heart failure, approximately one third will regain full ventricular function, one third will recover but continue to demonstrate impaired systolic function, and one third will require cardiac transplantation.[79,80] A subset of children, not all of whom initially manifest severe symptoms in the acute period, will progress to develop DCM.

Although no specific therapies have been identified to directly treat the myocardial injury, a variety of strategies have been employed.[81-84] In the past, aggressive inotropic support was used to maintain cardiac output, perfuse vital organs, and prevent metabolic complications. However, increasing inotropy concomitantly increases myocardial oxygen demand and can have detrimental effects. The paradigm has therefore shifted toward diuresis and gentle inotropic support, often with agents such as phosphodiesterase inhibitors (milrinone), to improve myocardial performance without placing a large burden on an already failing heart.[81] Rhythm disturbances should be treated appropriately. Therapy with immune modulation or suppression with intravenous immunoglobulin is the standard of care at many centers.[80,85-87] Mechanical circulatory support may also be required in fulminant disease.[88-93]

Rheumatic Fever and Rheumatic Heart Disease

Acute rheumatic fever and rheumatic heart disease are leading causes of acquired cardiac disease in developing countries, with between 5 and 30 million children and young adults affected worldwide and a mortality rate of 1% to 10%.[94] In the United States, the availability of antibiotics to treat streptococcal pharyngitis has markedly reduced the incidence of this disease but sporadic cases still occur.[95] In children, the peak incidence occurs between 5 and 14 years of age.

Rheumatic fever results from infection by particular strains of group A β-hemolytic *Streptococcus* or *Streptococcus pyogenes*. Both cellular and humoral immune responses to the bacterial antigens cross react with native tissues to result in a multisystemic inflammatory disorder. The incubation period for most strains of group A β-hemolytic *Streptococcus* is typically 3 to 5 days, although some children will present with a more remote history of pharyngitis.

The diagnosis of rheumatic fever is made clinically based on the modified Jones criteria.[96] Major criteria include carditis, polyarthritis, chorea, subcutaneous nodules, and erythema marginatum. Evidence of a prior streptococcal infection along with two major or one major and two minor criteria are required to make the diagnosis in children without prior history of rheumatic fever or echocardiographic evidence of typical valvular involvement. Fever and arthritis are common symptoms. The polyarthritis has a migratory pattern, typically affecting large joints. Cardiac involvement or carditis occurs in nearly 50% of children with their first attack of rheumatic fever. Rheumatic heart disease represents a sequela of the acute process, affecting the mitral and aortic valves most frequently.

Primary prevention of rheumatic fever and rheumatic heart disease begins with prompt recognition and appropriate treatment of the initial streptococcal infection.[97,98] Secondary prevention, with ongoing therapy in individuals with a known history of rheumatic fever, has been shown to be extremely effective at preventing recurrent attacks. Although there is some debate regarding the optimal regimen, intramuscular injections of benzathine penicillin every 3 to 4 weeks appear to be most efficacious.[99]

Finally, in a subset of children with severe cardiac involvement, elective or emergent surgery plays an important role.[100] Valvular disease, rather than global myocarditis, is often the cause of congestive heart failure symptoms; and medical management is, therefore, limited in efficacy. When possible, valve repair rather than replacement is preferred.

Infective Endocarditis

Children with structural or acquired heart disease are at risk for developing infective endocarditis.[101,102] The risk varies from negligible to significant depending on a number of factors but to a great extent is based on the nature of the cardiac condition. The infection results from deposition of bacteria or other pathogens on tissues in areas of abnormal or turbulent blood flow. The diagnosis of endocarditis is made clinically by applying the modified Duke criteria.[103, 104] Major criteria include demonstration of microorganisms and evidence of pathologic lesions. The presentation of the disease may be acute or subacute. New or changing heart murmurs may indicate the development of either regurgitation or obstruction on an affected valve. Among the physical findings in children with endocarditis (part of the minor criteria) are signs of systemic embolization. Splinter hemorrhages (linear streaks under the nail beds), Janeway lesions (painless macules on the hands or feet), Osler nodes (small, painful nodules on the fingers), and Roth spots (retinal hemorrhages with clear centers) may be present. Inflammatory markers, such as erythrocyte sedimentation rate and C-reactive protein levels, are typically elevated, albeit nonspecific. Microscopic hematuria, as a manifestation of renal involvement, is frequently seen.

antiplatelet drugs.[123] Myocardial ischemia and infarction, although infrequent, are important potential complications in children with coronary artery involvement.[120,124] Anesthetic care thus requires careful considerations regarding myocardial oxygen demand and supply; on rare occasion coronary revascularization may be necessary.

Cardiac Tumors

In children, cardiac tumors in general are extremely rare, and thus the natural history and optimal treatment strategies are often determined from limited case series.[125-127] Unlike adults, in whom atrial myxomas represent more than 90% of cardiac tumors, in children they tend to be either rhabdomyomas or fibromas.[128] Less common types include hemangiomas, myxomas (Video Clip 14-9), Purkinje cell tumors, and teratomas. Whereas in adults, most tumors are found in the left atrium, cardiac tumors in children occur in all four cardiac chambers. Malignant primary tumors are extremely rare, and data on their outcomes are even more limited.

Rhabdomyomas are the most common primary cardiac tumors in children. They often involve the ventricular septum and left ventricle and are multiple in the majority of cases.[129] Although they are considered benign, children may present with cardiomegaly, congestive heart failure, arrhythmias, or sudden death. The significance of a rhabdomyoma is determined largely by its size and any obstruction it may cause. Many tumors regress over time or completely resolve; thus, surgery is not indicated unless symptoms are present.[130,131] Many children with cardiac rhabdomyomas have associated tuberous sclerosis.[132,133]

Cardiac fibromas are the second most common type of pediatric primary cardiac tumors.[134] They are typically single and involve the ventricular free wall. In a subset of fibromas, the tumor will invade the conduction system causing atrioventricular nodal disease or arrhythmias.[135] Surgery or cardiac transplantation may be required in some cases.[136,137] The tumors may be very large, so that complete surgical resection may result in severely depressed cardiac function. Partial resections have been found to result in an arrest in growth with good outcomes while sparing cardiac function.[131] The primary concern in the perioperative care of children with cardiac tumors relates to the impact of the mass on hemodynamics (i.e., ventricular filling, patency of outflow tracts) and associated abnormalities of cardiac rhythm.[138]

Heart Failure in Children

Definition and Pathophysiology

Over the last several decades heart failure has been a major field of interest and investigation in adult medicine. Although this entity is less common in children, the interest in heart failure has been the subject of various publications,[139] scientific meetings, and the focus of several textbooks.[140,141] It is important to emphasize that pediatric heart failure results from markedly different causes than those reported in adults.[142] Understanding the cellular basis of heart failure in children, compensatory mechanisms, and therapeutic advances in this area are now at the forefront of pediatric medicine.[139-141,143,144] The discussion that follows highlights a few of the key concepts as they relate to anesthetic practice.

The definition of heart failure has evolved over the years. It is considered not only a pump failure but also a circulatory failure involving neurohumoral aspects of the circulation.[145] A number of conditions may ultimately compromise the ability to generate an adequate cardiac output to meet the systemic circulatory demands. It is important to recognize that heart failure does not necessarily imply impairment of ventricular systolic function but that diastolic heart failure is now an increasingly recognized clinical entity.

Etiology and Clinical Features

Causes of heart failure differ with age. In the perinatal period, cardiac dysfunction is typically related to birth asphyxia or sepsis or may represent an early presentation of CHD. The neonate with heart failure typically presents with clinical signs of a low-cardiac output state. Causes include left-sided outflow obstruction (as in aortic stenosis, aortic coarctation, hypoplastic left heart syndrome), severe valve regurgitation (as seen in Ebstein anomaly), or absent pulmonary valve syndrome.

During the first year of life most cases of heart failure are caused by structural heart disease. Other causes of heart failure are cardiomyopathies secondary to inborn errors of metabolism or acute events such as myocarditis. In infants with heart failure, tachypnea, dyspnea, tachycardia, as well as feeding difficulties and failure to thrive are prominent symptoms.[146] The physical examination is characterized by grunting respirations, rales, intercostal retractions, a gallop rhythm, and hepatosplenomegaly. Frequently, a mitral regurgitant murmur is present.

Beyond the first year of life, heart failure is either a consequence of previous surgical interventions, unpalliated/unrepaired cardiovascular disease, cardiomyopathies, myocarditis, or anthracycline therapy for a malignancy. Occasionally, a child may present with severe ventricular systolic impairment related to ongoing myocardial ischemia as a result of a coronary artery anomaly or rarely due to acquired pathologies such as Kawasaki disease. Older children with heart failure exhibit exercise intolerance, fatigue, and growth failure, whereas adolescents have symptoms similar to adults.

Treatment Strategies

Therapy is tailored to the etiology of the cardiac dysfunction and may include supportive care, mechanical ventilation, inotropic support, afterload reduction, prostaglandin E_1 therapy to maintain pulmonary or systemic blood flow, maneuvers to balance the systemic and pulmonary circulations, catheter-based interventions, or surgery.[147-151] Maintaining organ perfusion is the main goal in acute heart failure therapy. The primary therapeutic agents include catecholamines and inodilators. If the cause of the heart failure is not correctable, treatment consists of the standard drug regimen for chronic heart failure (diuretic therapy, β blockade, angiotensin-converting enzyme inhibition).[152,153] Newer agents that have received increasing attention in the management of pediatric heart failure include nesiritide (a recombinant form of human B-type natriuretic peptide)[154-156] and carvedilol (a third-generation β blocker).[157-159] For all ages, nutrition requires particular attention, because the work of breathing causes high caloric demands in the setting of fluid restriction and often inadequate intake; hypercaloric nutrition through an enteral feeding tube may be required.

Syndromes, Associations, and Systemic Disorders: Cardiovascular Disease and Anesthetic Implications

A wide variety of disorders including those resulting from chromosomal abnormalities, single-gene defects, gene deletion syndromes, as well as known associations (nonrandom occurrence of defects), and teratogenic exposure may manifest as cardiovascular disease. The coexistence of frequently associated multiple organ system comorbidities with cardiovascular disease presents a number of challenges to the anesthesia care provider.

Chromosomal Syndromes

Down Syndrome

Down syndrome is the most frequent chromosomal aberration, occurring with a frequency of 1 in 800 living births. The incidence increases sharply with advanced maternal age. In most children, it is the result of trisomy 21 but it may occur from balanced or unbalanced translocations of chromosome 21 or mosaicism. The phenotypes are indistinguishable. In general, these children are typically smaller than normal for age and craniofacial features include microbrachycephaly, short neck, oblique palpebral fissures, epicanthal folds, Brushfield's spots, small low-set ears, macroglossia, and microdontia with fused teeth. Mandibular hypoplasia and a broad flat nose are typical. A narrow nasopharynx with hypertrophic lymphatic tissue (tonsils, adenoids), in combination with generalized hypotonia, frequently leads to sleep apnea. Other conditions that affect these children include mental retardation, cervical spine disorders with vertebral and ligamentous instability, thyroid disease, leukemia, obesity, subglottic stenosis,[160] and gastrointestinal problems.

Airway issues include the potential for upper airway obstruction due to the presence of a prominent tongue, postextubation stridor,[161] and cervical spine injury.[162-164] Vascular access can be difficult. Subjectively, there is an impression that these children have small vessel sizes, vascular hyperreactivity, and fragile tissue consistency and may suffer from more complications after arterial cannulation.

Cardiovascular defects occur in 40% to 50% of children, so it has been recommended that all children undergo screening for CHD in early infancy.[165,166] The most common lesions include atrioventricular septal defects (Video Clip 14-10), ventricular septal defects, tetralogy of Fallot, and patent ductus arteriosus. Pathology after repair of atrioventricular septal defects is most often related to mitral regurgitation, left ventricular outflow tract obstruction, residual intracardiac shunts, and, rarely, mitral stenosis. Bradycardia under anesthesia occurs commonly.[167] Pulmonary hypertension resulting from either the cardiac pathology or from chronic hypoxemia secondary to upper airway obstruction should be considered in the management of these children.[168] Reduced nitric oxide bioavailability has been reported, leading to endothelial cell dysfunction,[169] possibly explaining the increased pulmonary vascular reactivity in these children with an early and higher incidence of pulmonary obstructive disease, even after corrective cardiac surgery.

Trisomy 18

Also known as Edwards syndrome, trisomy 18 is recognized as the second most common chromosomal trisomy (incidence of 1 in 3500 newborns). Most patients exhibit microcephaly, delayed psychomotor development, and mental retardation.[170] Characteristic craniofacial features include micrognathia or retrognathia, microstomia, malformed ears, and microphthalmia.[171] These abnormalities may affect airway management.[172,173] Skeletal anomalies include clenched fingers and severe growth retardation. Neurologic abnormalities are characterized by developmental delay, hypotonia, and central nervous system malformations. The high mortality rate in children with trisomy 18 is usually related to the presence of cardiac and renal problems, feeding difficulties, sepsis, and apnea caused by neurologic abnormalities.

Cardiovascular disease is present in most children and consists primarily of ventricular septal defects and polyvalvular disease.[174,175] Implications for anesthetic care include the high incidence of congestive heart failure and aspiration pneumonia.[173] These children may require interventions to address associated gastrointestinal or genitourinary anomalies.

Trisomy 13

Trisomy 13, an uncommon autosomal trisomy, is also known as Patau syndrome. The incidence of this chromosomal disorder ranges from 1 in 5,000 to 12,000 live births. Major features of this syndrome include cleft lip and palate, holoprosencephaly, polydactyly, rocker-bottom feet, microphthalmia, microcephaly, and severe mental retardation.[176,177] Nearly all children have associated cardiovascular defects that include patent ductus arteriosus, septal defects, valve abnormalities, and dextrocardia.[175] The overall prognosis for children with this syndrome is extremely poor.

Turner Syndrome

Turner syndrome is a genetic disorder (estimated incidence of 1 in 5,000 liveborn female infants) characterized by partial or complete X chromosome monosomy.[178] There is a high degree of spontaneous abortion among affected fetuses. Features of this syndrome include webbed neck, low-set ears, multiple pigmented nevi and micrognathia, lymphedema, short stature, and ovarian failure.[179] Systemic manifestations include cardiac defects (notably aortic coarctation and bicuspid aortic valve), hypertension, hypercholesterolemia, renal anomalies, liver disease, and inflammatory bowel disease. Obesity is common in older children as well as a high incidence of endocrinologic abnormalities such as hypothyroidism and diabetes.[178,180] Renal anomalies occur in up to one third of children.

Gene Deletion Syndromes

Williams Syndrome

Williams syndrome is a congenital disorder with an incidence of 1 in 20,000 live births. The genetic abnormality responsible for this syndrome in the majority of cases is a chromosomal deletion on the long arm of chromosome 7, altering the elastin gene.[181,182] The absence of this gene is detected by fluorescent in-situ hybridization (FISH). Features of Williams syndrome include characteristic elfin facies, outgoing personality, endocrine abnormalities (including hypercalcemia and hypothyroidism), mental retardation, growth deficiency, and altered neurodevelopment. Associated cardiovascular pathology includes valvar and supravalvular aortic stenosis (Fig. 14-7) and coarctation of the aorta.[183,184] The arteriopathy found in these

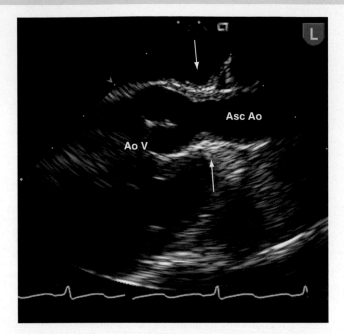

Figure 14-7. Echocardiogram displaying the classic supravalvar aortic narrowing in a patient with Williams syndrome (*arrows*). Ao V, aortic valve; Asc Ao, ascending aorta.

children may also involve the origin of the coronary arteries or other systemic and pulmonary vessels. Diffuse narrowing of the abdominal aorta may occur in association with renal artery stenosis.

Several reports in the literature have described unanticipated events during anesthetic care in these children.[185-187] Two conditions may result in increased anesthetic morbidity and the potential for mortality: coronary artery stenosis leading to myocardial ischemia and severe biventricular outflow tract obstruction. Because the extent of the disease in the affected individual is variable and may have devastating implications, a thorough cardiac evaluation is advisable in all children.[188] On occasion, children may require further evaluation before undergoing anesthetic care.

Children with Williams syndrome may exhibit some degree of muscular weakness; thus, the cautious use and application of muscle relaxants has been suggested.[188] Associated neurodevelopmental delay, attention-deficit disorder, and autistic behavior often requires adequate premedication. A high prevalence of subclinical hypothyroidism has been reported in these children.[189] Renal manifestations include renovascular hypertension, reduced function, and hypercalcemia-induced nephrocalcinosis.

Chromosome 22q11.2 Deletion Syndrome: DiGeorge and Velocardiofacial Syndrome

The 22q11.2 deletion syndrome, with an estimated incidence of approximately 1 in 3,000, encompasses DiGeorge, conotruncal face, and velocardiofacial syndromes. It is also known as CATCH 22 syndrome: an acronym for cardiac defects, abnormal facies, thymic hypoplasia, cleft palate, and hypocalcemia, all of which are commonly present.[190] Cardiac malformations, speech delay, and immunodeficiency are the most common features of the chromosome 22q deletion syndromes. Because no single feature

is overwhelmingly associated with the deletion, it should be considered in any child with a conotruncal anomaly, neonatal hypocalcemia, or any of the less common features when seen in association with dysmorphic facial features.

Cardiac anomalies are often described as conotruncal anomalies; however, outflow tract anomalies are also frequently seen.[191] The remainder of the cardiac defects crosses an enormous spectrum, ranging from hypoplastic left ventricle to vascular rings. Only a minority of children with this chromosomal deletion have a normal cardiovascular system. The immune system is affected in a significant number of children. As a consequence of thymic hypoplasia, children typically have diminished T-cell numbers and function. The immunodeficiency requires the use of irradiated blood products and strict aseptic precautions during vascular access. Neurodevelopmental features include primarily speech delay as well as attention-deficit disorders. Psychiatric disorders are well described in these individuals.[192]

Single-Gene Defects

Noonan Syndrome

Noonan syndrome, an autosomal dominant syndrome, occurs with a frequency of 1 in 1,000 to 2,500 livebirths. It is characterized by distinctive dysmorphic features that include neck webbing, low-set ears, chest deformities, hypertelorism, and short stature.[193] Some male children also have cryptorchidism. The diagnosis of Noonan syndrome depends primarily on clinical features.[194] In neonates, the facial features may be less apparent; however, generalized edema and excess nuchal folds may be present as are seen in Turner syndrome. The facial features are more difficult to detect in later adolescence and adulthood.

The disorder is associated with a high incidence of CHD (~50%), with pulmonary valve dysplasia/stenosis being the most common.[195] Hypertrophic cardiomyopathy may develop during the first few years of life (in 10% to 20% of patients).[196] Clinical problems may also include developmental delay and bleeding diathesis (von Willebrand disease, factors XI and XII deficiency, and thrombocytopenia).[197]

Marfan Syndrome

Marfan syndrome is a multisystem disorder with variable expression resulting from a mutation in the fibrillin gene, a connective tissue protein.[198] It is estimated that about 1 in 10,000 individuals in the United States is affected by this syndrome. Clinical manifestations typically involve the cardiovascular, skeletal, and ocular systems.[199,200] Cardiovascular pathology includes mitral valve prolapse and regurgitation, ascending aortic dilation (Fig. 14-8), and main pulmonary artery dilatation. Dilatation of the sinuses of Valsalva is found in 60% to 80% of adults. The risk of aortic dissection rises considerably with increasing aortic size but may occur at any point in the course of the disease.[201] Cardiac arrhythmias may be related to valvular heart disease, cardiomyopathy, and/or congestive heart failure.

β-blocker therapy and aggressive blood pressure control has been the standard of care in patients with aortic root dilation[202] and should be continued perioperatively. Aortic root replacement in Marfan syndrome has been associated with a greater risk of re-dissection and recurrent aneurysm when compared with other patients who have undergone similar interventions.[203] Therefore, it is wise to maintain hemodynamics near baseline values during anesthetic care even in the postoperative period.

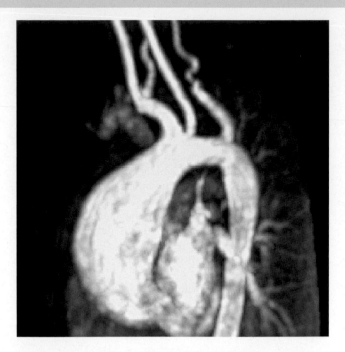

Figure 14-8. Dilated aortic root as displayed by MRI in a patient with Marfan syndrome. There is a marked discrepancy between the diameters of the ascending and descending aorta.

After aortic root surgery some individuals may require chronic anticoagulation therapy. Preoperative hospitalization may be necessary to adjust the anticoagulation regimen in anticipation of surgery. In emergency cases, infusion of coagulation factors and other blood products may be required to offset the anticoagulants. In addition to vascular pathology, children with Marfan syndrome have a predisposition for ventricular dilatation as well as abnormal ventricular function.[204,205]

Several factors can result in pulmonary disease in these children.[206] Chest wall deformities and progressive scoliosis can contribute to restrictive lung disease. In addition, it is thought that the fibrillin defect may affect both lung development and homeostasis impairing pulmonary function. The development of pneumothoraces is relatively common.

Associations

VATER or VACTERL Association

VACTERL association is an acronym given to describe a series of nonrandom anomalies that include vertebral, anal, cardiovascular, tracheoesophageal, renal, and limb defects.[207,208] Up to three fourths of children with VACTERL association have been reported to have CHD. The most common lesions include ventricular septal defects, atrial septal defects, and tetralogy of Fallot. Complex pathology such as truncus arteriosus and transposition of the great arteries occur less frequently.

Vertebral and tracheal anomalies can complicate airway management and regional anesthesia. Approximately 70% of children with VACTERL have vertebral anomalies usually consisting of hypoplastic vertebrae or hemivertebra. These may predispose children to developing scoliosis. Anal atresia or imperforate anus is reported in about 55% of children. These anomalies are usually noted at birth and often require surgery in the first days

of life. Esophageal atresia with tracheoesophageal fistula is found in a large number of affected infants. Low birth weight (<1500 g) and associated cardiac pathology have been identified to be independent predictors of mortality in infants undergoing surgery for esophageal atresia/tracheoesophageal fistula (see Chapter 36). The presence of a ductal-dependent cardiac lesion further increases perioperative morbidity and mortality.[209] Limb defects occur in most children and include absent or displaced thumbs, polydactyly, syndactyly, and forearm abnormalities. These may impact vascular access and monitor placement. Renal defects are noted in approximately 50% of children.

CHARGE Association

CHARGE association is characterized by congenital anomalies that include coloboma, heart defects, choanal atresia, retardation of growth and development, genitourinary problems, and ear abnormalities. The association is estimated to occur in approximately 1 in 10,000 to 12,000 live births. The etiology is unknown, but it has been suggested that deficiency in migration of neural crest cells, deficiency of mesodermal formation, or defective interaction between neural crest cells and mesoderm play a part in these defects of blastogenesis.[210,211] Specific genetic abnormalities have also been identified in some individuals.[212,213]

Cardiac defects occur in as many as 50% to 70% of children and commonly include conotruncal and aortic arch anomalies.[214] Retardation of growth and development is usually due to cardiac disease, nutritional problems, or growth hormone deficiency. The developmental delay often is associated with sensory deficits (vision and hearing loss). Most children have some degree of mental retardation. Anesthetic implications, in addition to the cardiac defects, are focused around the airway.[215] A retrospective review of 50 cases reported upper airway abnormalities in 56% of children apart from choanal atresia and cleft lip and palate.[216]

Other Disorders

Tuberous Sclerosis

Tuberous sclerosis is a genetic disease with an autosomal dominant inheritance pattern and an incidence of approximately 1 in 25,000 to 30,000 births.[217] In a relatively large number of children this can be attributed to spontaneous mutations. This systemic disease primarily presents as cutaneous and neurologic symptoms, but cardiac and renal lesions are frequent findings.

The presence of upper airway nodular tumors, fibromas, or papillomas in affected children may interfere with airway management. Cardiac pathology is frequent and includes cardiac rhabdomyoma in 60% of children and coexisting CHD in 33% of cases.[218-220] Cardiac abnormalities with obstruction to flow, heart failure, arrhythmias, conduction defects, or preexcitation may affect the selection of anesthetic agents. Preoperative evaluation in most cases should include an ECG to exclude arrhythmia, conduction defects, or preexcitation.[218] Blood pressure and renal function should also be assessed. Anticonvulsants should be optimized and continued until the morning of surgery. Generally, baseline medical treatment should be resumed as soon as possible because seizures are the most common postoperative complication.[221] The presence of mental retardation may require the administration of agents such as midazolam or ketamine to facilitate parental separation.

Selected Vascular Anomalies and Their Implications for Anesthetic Care

Aberrant Subclavian Arteries

An aberrant or anomalous subclavian artery usually arises from the descending aorta as a separate vessel distal to the "usual" last subclavian artery in a posterior location. In a left aortic arch the aberrant vessel is the right subclavian artery. In this anomaly the arrangement is as follows: the first branch of the left aortic arch is the right carotid artery, followed by the left carotid and left subclavian arteries. The aberrant right subclavian artery, rather than arising proximally from the innominate artery as the first arch branch, originates distal to the last (left) subclavian artery as the fourth branch and courses behind the esophagus toward the right arm. This variant is one of the most common aortic arch anomalies. It is reported to occur in 0.4% to 2% of the general population and may or may not be associated with CHD.[222] There is a high incidence of this anomaly in children with Down syndrome and an association with ventricular septal defects and tetralogy of Fallot among other lesions. In a right aortic arch, the anomalous left subclavian artery originates distal to the origin of the right subclavian artery (Fig. 14-9). This anomaly may be seen in the context of conotruncal malformations. The diagnosis of an aberrant subclavian artery is made by most currently available imaging modalities.

Implications of this anomaly include the following:

- The presence of an aberrant subclavian artery may influence the location of placement of a systemic-to-pulmonary artery shunt.
- This anomaly should be considered in the selection of a site for arterial line placement if the need for transesophageal monitoring is also anticipated during surgery. The aberrant vessel may be compressed along its retroesophageal course by the imaging probe, resulting in inaccurate readings.[223] It may be wise, regardless of the site of arterial line placement, to monitor the arm supplied by the anomalous vessel by pulse oximetry or other methods during esophageal instrumentation.
- On occasion, an aberrant subclavian artery may be part of a vascular ring.
- Rarely, older children with a left aortic arch and aberrant right subclavian artery and without the findings of a complete vascular ring may complain of mild dysphagia (dysphagia lusorium).

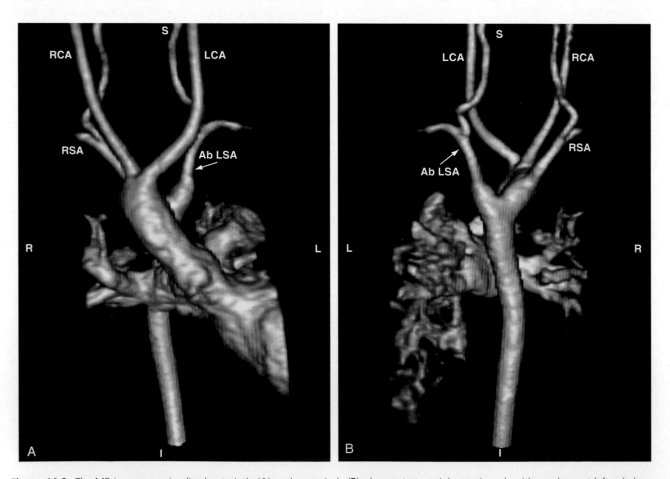

Figure 14-9. The MR images, as visualized anteriorly (**A**) and posteriorly (**B**), demonstrate a right aortic arch with an aberrant left subclavian artery (Ab LSA). The first arch vessel is the left carotid artery (LCA), followed by the right carotid (RCA), and right subclavian artery (RSA). The Ab LSA is the most distal branch originating from the descending aorta and coursing toward the left arm. This vessel may be compressed by a transesophageal echocardiographic probe.

Persistent Left Superior Vena Cava to Coronary Sinus Communication

A persistent left superior vena cava (LSVC) is a form of anomalous systemic venous drainage identified in 4.4% of children with CHD, most frequently those with septal defects.[224] It represents a remnant of the left anterior cardinal vein that typically obliterates during development. If it persists, it remains patent and drains into the right atrium via an enlarged coronary sinus. Bilateral superior vena cavae can be present (Fig. 14-10), or the right superior vena cava might be absent. In the presence of bilateral superior vena cavae the two vascular structures may communicate via an innominate or bridging vein.

Implications of this anomaly include the following:

● In the absence of an innominate vein a catheter placed in the left arm or left internal jugular vein and advanced into the central circulation may rest within the coronary sinus, a potentially undesirable location in a small infant. On chest radiography an unusual course is identified as the catheter courses along the left side of the mediastinum and can be mistaken for intracarotid, intrapleural, or mediastinal locations.

● An LVSC may be of relevance during venous cannulation for cardiopulmonary bypass to ensure adequate venous drainage and optimal operating conditions.

● The presence of an LSVC is important in patients with single-ventricle physiology undergoing palliation involving a cavopulmonary (Glenn) connection(s).

● Association with a dilated coronary sinus. On transesophageal echocardiography it may be confused with other defects, including an ostium primum atrial septal defect (one that lies in the inferior aspect of the atrial septum) and anomalous pulmonary venous return to the coronary sinus.

● On occasion, an LSVC may drain to an unroofed coronary sinus or directly into the left atrium, in which case a right-to-left shunt is present. This may be identified by injection of agitated saline into a left arm or left neck vein while performing an echocardiogram and may be associated with systemic arterial desaturation. This constitutes a risk for paradoxical systemic embolization.

● During cardiac surgery an enlarged coronary sinus may interfere with the administration of retrograde cardioplegia.

● It may confound placement of a pulmonary artery catheter and cardiac output determinations.

Evaluation of the Patient with a Cardiac Murmur

The finding of an incidental murmur during the perioperative period in many cases results in significant distress to the child or family, may trigger additional diagnostic studies including cardiology consultation, and has the potential to delay the scheduled procedure when identified preoperatively. Although cardiac auscultation is a challenging skill that takes many years of practice to master,[225] it is important for the practicing anesthesiologist who cares for children to recognize the main physical findings that may distinguish an innocent cardiac murmur from a pathologic one. In addition, knowledge of several core concepts and red flags can help avoid overlooking potentially important diagnoses.

The majority of normal children, in the range of 90%, will have a murmur at some point in their lives. This is most commonly identified during the neonatal period and early school

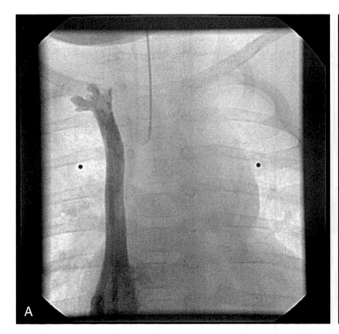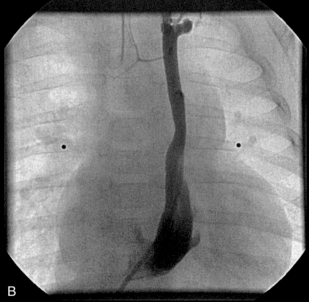

Figure 14-10. Bilateral superior vena cavae. **A,** Angiogram depicting the superior vena cava, normally a right-sided structure, as it drains into the right atrium. **B,** Angiogram in the same child demonstrating drainage of a large left superior vena cava into the coronary sinus. The catheter courses from the inferior vena cava into the right atrium, coronary sinus, and left superior vena cava. Contrast medium into the left superior vena cava demonstrates no innominate (or bridging) vein. A dilated coronary sinus is noted.

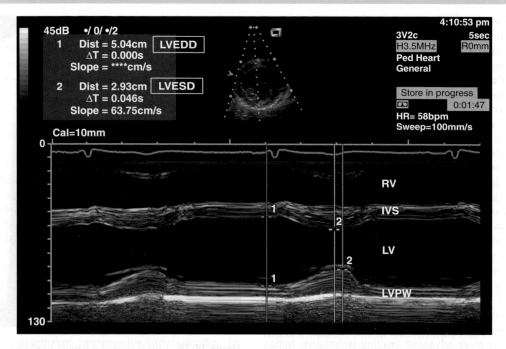

Figure 14-27. M-mode echocardiography allows for determination of left ventricular dimensions and calculation of shortening fraction. RV, right ventricle; IVS, interventricular septum; LV, left ventricle; LVPW, left ventricular posterior wall; LVEDD, left ventricular end-diastolic dimension; LVESD, left ventricular end-systolic dimension.

flow across cardiac valves and great vessels, color flow imaging allows detection of subtle lesions such as small septal defects that can be difficult to identify by standard 2D imaging alone. Traditionally, flow toward the transducer is displayed in red whereas flow away is represented as blue. Turbulent blood flow is associated with increased Doppler velocities and can be readily identified as a mosaic of colors, typically of greenish tint (Video Clip 14-12).

Pulsed- and continuous-wave Doppler represent spectral modalities that complement the color flow data and provide quantitative information. Pulsed-wave interrogation is advantageous in localizing specific sites of stenosis or turbulence but is limited in the magnitude of velocities it can detect. Continuous-wave Doppler, on the other hand, allows for quantification of much higher velocities (see Video Clip 14-12). By using velocities obtained with pulsed- and continuous-wave Doppler, estimates of pressures within various cardiac chambers are possible by applying the simplified Bernoulli equation, which states that the difference in pressure between two locations is approximately four times the square of the velocity of the jet of flow between them:

$$\text{Pressure gradient (in mm Hg)} = 4 \times v^2$$

The applications of 3D echocardiography have been increasingly investigated in the diagnosis of CHD.[280-282] An examination can provide clear and useful volumetric assessments when the images are adequate. A significant advantage of this imaging approach is that it is able to display cardiovascular structures and their interrelationships in detail, in many cases facilitating the understanding of pathologic conditions over 2D imaging. It allows for an enhanced perspective of the margins and geometry of abnormalities, such as septal defects and valvar anomalies. 3D echocardiography may also be particularly useful when

interventions are planned. Technologic advances in a number of areas should allow for improved image quality and shorter acquisition times.

Practical Concepts Regarding the Interpretation of an Echocardiographic Report

Measurements of Cardiac Chambers and Vessel Dimensions
A number of measurements are routinely performed during an echocardiographic examination. These generally include ventricular dimensions such as left ventricular end-diastolic (LVED) and end-systolic (LVES) dimensions, thickness of the interventricular septum and left ventricular posterior wall, as well as measurements of valve sizes and great artery dimensions. To determine whether these are appropriate for the child being examined, the measurements are related to values obtained in normal children matched for body-surface area. In many centers the reports include determinations of Z scores to indicate how many standard deviations the observations are from mean values in a comparative population.

Assessment of Ventricular Function
A number of echocardiographic techniques are able to provide information regarding ventricular performance. Two of the most commonly reported indices of ventricular systolic function involve measurements of the extent of shortening, namely, shortening fraction and ejection fraction.

Shortening fraction (SF) represents the percent of change in left ventricular diameter during the cardiac cycle. This is calculated using the following equation:

$$\text{SF (\%)} = \text{LVED dimension} - \text{LVES dimension/LVED dimension}$$

Values range from 28% to 44%, with a normal mean value of 36%. This index, however, is dependent on ventricular preload and afterload.

Ejection fraction (EF) is the fraction of blood ejected by the ventricle (stroke volume) relative to its end-diastolic volume. In other words, it represents the percentage of blood ejected from the left ventricle with each heart beat. Ejection fraction is derived by volumetric analysis of the left ventricle by means of the following equation:

$$EF\ (\%) = LVEDV - LVESV/LVEDV$$

where LVEDV = left ventricular end-diastolic volume and LVESV = left ventricular end-systolic volume

Normal values vary in the literature but in most studies range between 56% and 78%. A low ejection fraction is generally associated with systolic functional impairment, but cardiac dysfunction may occur in the presence of a normal ejection fraction. Such may be the case of a child with diastolic heart failure.

It is important to also consider that although these functional indices are routinely and easily obtained they have significant limitations. The estimation of ejection fraction is based on geometric assumptions for the elliptical left ventricle. These assumptions thus may not be applicable to a systemic right ventricle or other types of ventricular geometries.[283] There has therefore been an escalating interest in newer echocardiographic approaches and imaging modalities that may provide more sensitive and comprehensive information regarding ventricular performance, even in the absence of clinical disease. Some of the newer techniques being used in the assessment of ventricular function include (1) myocardial performance index (MPI), also known as the Tei index, which combines systolic and diastolic intervals to assess global ventricular function[284-286]; (2) Doppler tissue imaging (DTI) to evaluate intramural myocardial velocities[287]; and (3) strain and strain rate imaging to quantitate the rate of segmental myocardial deformation.[288] Although values in normal children have been established for all of these imaging modalities and alterations in the presence of pathologic conditions have been described,[289,290] additional studies documenting their clinical applications in specific types of cardiovascular pathology are needed.

Estimation of Pressures

When the peak velocity of a tricuspid regurgitant jet is reported, these data can be used to estimate right ventricular systolic pressure and thus pulmonary artery systolic pressure, in the absence of pulmonary stenosis or outflow obstruction (Video Clip 14-13). If, for example, a peak regurgitant velocity of 3 m/sec is recorded across the tricuspid valve, using the simplified Bernoulli equation as discussed earlier, the pressure gradient or difference between the right atrial and right ventricular systolic pressures can be estimated to be $4 \times 3^2 = 36$ mm Hg. If a normal right atrial pressure is assumed (4 to 6 mm Hg), this would predict a right ventricular systolic pressure of approximately 40 mm Hg. Similarly, if the peak or maximal flow velocity across a ventricular septal defect is measured at 4.5 msec, this predicts a pressure gradient of $4 \times 4.5^2 = 81$ mm Hg between the ventricles, implying that the defect is pressure restrictive and the right ventricular and pulmonary artery systolic pressures are relatively low.

Evaluation of Gradients

Estimation of a peak instantaneous gradient is the most clinically useful method for quantifying the severity of obstructions across semilunar valves and outflow tracts. It is derived by application of the simplified Bernoulli equation. These estimates when obtained across the pulmonary valve tend to have a higher correlation with catheterization peak-to-peak gradients than those measured across the aortic valve, where mean gradients (obtained by automated integration of the velocities under a spectral Doppler tracing) are found to have a higher correlation.[291] The mean gradient rather than a peak gradient as determined by Doppler echocardiography is considered a better indicator of the severity of the obstruction across atrioventricular valves and other low-flow venous pathways.

Evaluation of Regurgitant Lesions

Although a number of echocardiographic parameters have been investigated that may facilitate the evaluation of the severity of regurgitant lesions, in most pediatric cardiac centers this remains largely a qualitative assessment. The severity of the pathology is usually characterized as mild, moderate, severe, or combinations thereof when there is overlap among these categories. Serial echocardiographic assessment and comparative data are clinically more meaningful than an isolated report.

Magnetic Resonance Imaging

Cardiovascular MRI/angiography has emerged in recent years as a complementary technology to other traditional imaging modalities (Video Clips 14-14 and 14-15). Benefits have been reported in the assessment of complex pathology,[292,294-298] delineation of systemic and pulmonary vascular anomalies,[297,298] evaluation of global and regional ventricular function,[299] assessment of myocardial viability,[300] and characterization of pulmonary blood supply in children with structural alterations of the pulmonary vascular tree.[301] Particularly interesting applications that may further expand the utility of MRI in cardiovascular medicine include the quantification of left-to-right shunts[302-304] and measurement of blood oxygen saturation.[305] Furthermore, MRI has been found to be of benefit for guiding interventions in pediatric heart disease.[306-308] Most common indications in infants include assessment of complex cardiovascular malformations, delineation of vascular structures (aortic arch, systemic and pulmonary venous drainage), evaluation of possible airway compression, and characterization of cardiac tumors. Despite the significant technical challenges associated with the technique in children, this imaging approach plays an important diagnostic role. In adults with CHD, particularly in those with poor acoustic windows, this is frequently the imaging modality of choice. This may also be the case in children with palliated or repaired CHD.

Although the temporal resolution of MRI is inferior to echocardiography, new sequences and techniques allow for real-time acquisition similar to that of fluoroscopy. Spatial resolution continues to improve as well, particularly with the use of more powerful magnets. An important aspect in the acquisition of MRI data with high spatial resolution is the use of both cardiac and respiratory gating to allow sampling during only specific portions of the cardiac and respiratory cycles. Slow heart rates and low respiratory rates facilitate this process. MRI, in contrast to CT, does not involve radiation exposure, making it preferable for serial examinations that many young children with cardiovascular pathology require. However, MRI examinations are associated with the need for multiple anesthetics and their inherent risks.

Because of the nature of the magnetic fields generated in MRI, the presence of several types of metal, including pacemakers, ICDs, cerebrovascular clips/coils, or recently implanted intracardiac or intravascular coils and devices, are considered contraindications. Some artificial devices such as vascular clips, intravascular stents, and atrial septal defect occluder devices are typically made of titanium, allowing for sequences to be acquired that minimize the artifact produced by the foreign material. Stainless steel, on the other hand, as is found in coils used for occlusion of collateral vessels or a patent ductus arteriosus, generates significant artifacts within the study.

An additional limitation of MRI is the need for patient immobility during long examinations for optimal image quality. In small children this requirement usually necessitates the use of deep sedation/general anesthesia.[309-311] In infants with complex, and often cyanotic, CHD, specialists skilled in the care of children with cardiovascular pathology are often asked to provide care during the procedures. The severity of the cardiovascular disease may add to the challenges presented to the anesthesia care provider in a remote location.[312,313] The lengthy nature of the studies and the significant time requirements to perform postprocessing of the images cause MRI to be much more time intensive for the interpreting physician than other noninvasive imaging modalities.

A significant advantage to this technique is avoidance of harmful radiation inherent to traditional catheterization techniques. As MRI technology improves, with faster scans, increasing availability, and decreasing cost, it will continue to play an increasing role in the diagnosis and longitudinal follow-up of congenital and acquired pediatric heart disease.

Computed Tomography

Cardiac computed tomography (CT), with or without ECG gating, has also become an option among the battery of imaging modalities available to the pediatric cardiologist (Fig. 14-28).[292,296,314,315] The major advantage of CT over MRI is the very rapid scan times, such that, in most children, sedation is minimal or not necessary. With multislice CT detectors, a complete CT of the thorax can be performed in less than 10 seconds; and as new 64-slice detectors become increasingly available, the time required for the study will continue to shorten. A significant drawback of CT is the significant radiation burden, although typically estimated to be similar or slightly higher than a diagnostic cardiac catheterization, and the likely need for iodinated contrast agents with their concomitant risks.

Cardiac CT is not as accurate as MRI for delineation of intracardiac anatomy, but it provides excellent spatial resolution and information on extracardiac vasculature. CT has been reported to be of benefit in the evaluation of aortic arch anomalies and vascular rings, as well as in defining the systemic and pulmonary venous returns. In adult patients, multislice CT provides excellent information on coronary arteries and the presence of atherosclerotic disease; but in infants and children with smaller vessels and more rapid heart rates, these images are more difficult to obtain.

Cardiac Catheterization and Angiography

Cardiac catheterization involves the invasive measurement of intracardiac/vascular pressures and blood oxygen saturation coupled with angiography to assess cardiac anatomy and hemodynamics (Figs. 14-29 and 14-30). Before the era of 2D echocardiography, cardiac catheterization was frequently used for diagnostic purposes. At the present time, with the advances in noninvasive imaging, diagnostic procedures represent a relatively small proportion of these studies. Current indications for cardiac catheterization at most centers include (1) the assessment of physiologic parameters such as pressure and resistance data, (2) anatomic definition when other diagnostic modalities are inadequate, (3) need for electrophysiologic testing/treatment, and (4) when interventions are anticipated.

The majority of catheterizations in the current era involve interventions, ranging from endomyocardial biopsies, to angioplasties and stenting of stenotic vessels, dilation of valves, and conduits, to occlusion techniques for both native defects such as a patent ductus arteriosus, septal defects, or fistulous connections and surgically created defects such as Fontan fenestrations (Fig. 14-31, Video Clip 14-16, see Chapter 20). In some cases,

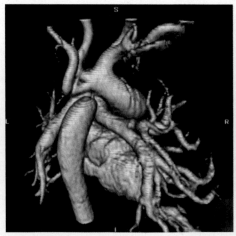 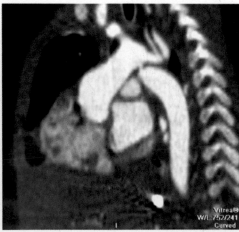

Figure 14-28. These two CT images display the details of the aortic arch anatomy in an infant with severe aortic arch obstruction.

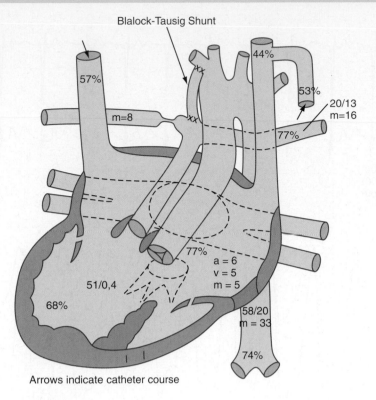

Blalock-Tausig Shunt

57%

44%

53%

20/13
m=16

m=8

77%

77%

a = 6
v = 5
m = 5

51/0,4

68%

58/20
m = 33

74%

Arrows indicate catheter course

Wt 3.3 KG

Diagnosis:
1. Heterotaxy
2. Dextrocardia
3. Complete atrioventricular canal
4. Double outlet right ventricle
5. Pulmonary stenosis, severe
6. L-transposition of the great arteries
7. Interrupted inferior vena cava with azygous continuation
8. Status post innominate to main pulmonary artery shunt
9. Right pulmonary artery isolation

Figure 14-29. Cardiac catheterization. Diagram illustrating the structural abnormalities in a child with complex cardiovascular pathology. Data routinely obtained at cardiac catheterization are depicted, including oxygen saturation determinations, pressure measurements, and hemodynamic calculations. These types of pictorial representations are extremely helpful when caring for children with complex defects.

such as might be the case of critically ill neonates with complex heart disease, catheter-based interventions such as balloon atrial septostomy and other procedures can be lifesaving.

In most children, access to the central circulation is accomplished percutaneously via the femoral approach. Those with occluded femoral veins or with cavopulmonary connections may require venous access through an internal jugular vein. In general, most examinations involve hemodynamic evaluation with recording of pressure data through catheters positioned at various sites of interest. Oxygen saturation data are obtained by reflectance oximetry or blood gas measurement from various cardiac chambers and vessels. It is important to recognize that in contrast to the oxygen saturation calculations derived from a blood gas analysis, reflectance oximetry assessments are actually measured values. This allows for the determination of oxygen content (total amount of hemoglobin in the blood) and, when combined with values of oxygen consumption, for the assess-

ment of blood flows and other calculations (i.e., shunts).[316] Additional data that may be obtained include pressure gradients, cardiac output measurements, and parameters to derive vascular resistances and valve areas.

Fluoroscopy and cineangiography are essential components of most cardiac catheterizations studies. Of the two, cineangiography accounts for the majority of the radiation exposure during the procedure as images are recorded during the injection of contrast material typically at 15 or 30 frames per second.[317] Most angiograms are obtained during biplane imaging by positioning the equipment to obtain optimal views that allow for delineation of the pathology in question (axial angiography) (Video Clip 14-17).[318,319]

Although cardiac catheterization has evolved over the years providing improved safety, it is an invasive procedure involving a number of risks and potential for morbidity and mortality, albeit relatively small. Risks associated with cardiac catheteriza-

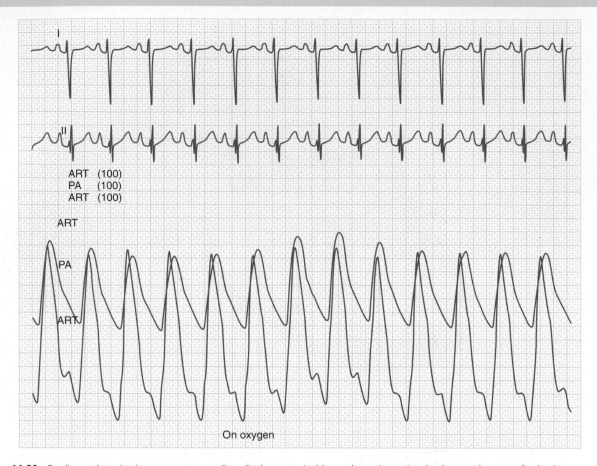

Figure 14-30. Cardiac catheterization pressure recording displays a typical hemodynamic tracing (scales are the same for both pressures). Note that the pulmonary artery systolic pressures are at systemic levels in this child with multiple left-sided obstructions. ART, systemic arterial pressure; PA, pulmonary artery pressure.

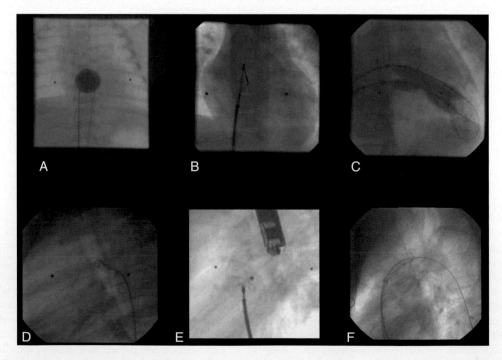

Figure 14-31. Catheter-based procedures. *Upper panel:* (**A**), balloon atrial septostomy; (**B**), blade atrial septostomy; (**C**), mitral balloon valvuloplasty. *Lower panel:* (**D**), placement of ductal occluder device; (**E**), transcatheter closure of secundum atrial septal defect; (**F**), pulmonary artery dilation with stent placement.

tion include excessive blood loss, vascular complications,[320,321] infection, arrhythmias, vascular/cardiac perforation,[322] systemic air embolization, myocardial ischemia, and those associated with the administration of contrast agents. These are more likely to occur in infants and small children.[323] Although transient increases in body temperature may occur after a study, the incidence of endocarditis is extremely rare. Interventional catheterizations, by the nature of the procedures, are associated with a greater rate of complications. However, as transcatheter interventions become safer and more effective, an increasing number of children may obviate the need for surgery, often undergoing procedures on an outpatient basis.[324] New techniques continue to evolve in this field, such as the percutaneous placement of valves,[325] strategies that combine cardiac catheterization and surgical intervention, so-called hybrid procedures,[326-328] and catheter-based interventions during fetal life.[329]

Practical Concepts Regarding the Interpretation of a Cardiac Catheterization Report

Pressure Data

Atrial pressure tracings are characterized by several waves (a, c, and v waves) and descents (x and y). The right atrial pressure is typically "a" wave dominant. The mean right atrial pressure is normally less than 5 mm Hg. In the presence of significant tricuspid valve regurgitation or a junctional rhythm, the "v" wave becomes the dominant wave. The left atrial pressure tracing in contrast to the right atrium, displays "v" wave dominance, which is accentuated during mitral regurgitation. The mean left atrial pressure rarely exceeds 8 mm Hg. The reported values for atrial pressures correspond to the "a" and "v" waves and mean pressures. Ventricular pressures are recorded and reported during systole, at end systole, and at end diastole. For the right ventricle the systolic pressure is normally in the 25- to 30-mm Hg range, with end-diastolic pressure of 5 to 7 mm Hg. The systolic pressure in the left ventricle normally increases with age and should equal the systolic arterial pressure; the end-diastolic pressure is typically less than 10 mm Hg. The pulmonary artery pressure is reported in terms of systolic, diastolic, and mean pressures. The systolic pulmonary artery pressure in a normal child should be equal to the right ventricular systolic pressure, and the mean pulmonary artery pressure should not exceed 20 mm Hg. The pulmonary artery wedge pressure is obtained by advancing a catheter into a distal vessel until this is occluded, reflecting the left atrial pressure. The aortic pressure and contour of the tracing varies depending of the site of interrogation. Typically, there is an increase in the systolic pressure as the catheter navigates toward the peripheral circulation. This phenomenon is known as "pulse wave amplification."

Pressure gradients represent the differences between two distinct sites and can be measured in a number of ways (mean gradient and peak gradient). It is important to consider that a number of factors may affect the determination of pressure gradients. The flow across the lesion is significantly influenced by the severity of the obstruction and the ventricular function.

Shunt Calculations

Shunts are characterized in terms of their direction (left-to-right, right-to-left, bidirectional) and magnitude. Left-to-right shunts can be quantified based on the ratio of the pulmonary ($\dot{Q}p$) to systemic ($\dot{Q}s$) blood flow ratio as follows:

$$\dot{Q}p/\dot{Q}s = \frac{(Sao_2 - MVo_2)}{(PVo_2 - PAo_2)}$$

where Sao_2 = systemic arterial O_2 saturation, MVo_2 = mixed venous O_2 saturation, PVo_2 = pulmonary venous O_2 saturation, and PAo_2 = pulmonary arterial O_2 saturation.

A $\dot{Q}p:\dot{Q}s$ ratio that exceeds 3:1 is considered a significant shunt, although smaller ratios may be associated with significant symptomatology.

Cardiac Output Determinations

The volume of blood ejected by the heart into the systemic circulation, or cardiac output, can be derived in several ways. Thermodilution measurements use saline as an indicator to measure pulmonary blood flow. In the absence of intracardiac shunts this is equivalent to the systemic blood flow or cardiac output (expressed as liters per minute). In the Fick method, oxygen is used as an indicator and cardiac output is obtained by the application of the following formula:

$$\dot{Q}s \text{ (L/min)} = Vo_2 \text{ (L/min)}/Sao_2 \text{ content} - MVo_2 \text{ content}$$

where Vo_2 = oxygen consumption (assumed or measured), Sao_2 = systemic arterial O_2 content, MVo_2 = mixed venous O_2 content, and O_2 content = O_2 saturation $\times$ (1.36 $\times$ 10 $\times$ hemoglobin concentration).

Vascular Resistances

Resistance represents the change in pressure in the systemic or pulmonary circulation with respect to flow. This is expressed as mm Hg/L/min (Wood units) and is usually normalized for body surface area.

The systemic (SVR) and pulmonary vascular resistance (PVR) are derived as follows:

SVR = (aortic mean pressure − right atrial mean pressure)/$\dot{Q}s$

PVR = (pulmonary artery mean pressure − pulmonary capillary wedge pressure or left atrial pressure)/$\dot{Q}p$

Considerations in the Perioperative Care of Children with Cardiovascular Disease

General Issues

The anesthetic care of children with heart disease[330] is challenged by the following factors:
- The remarkable spectrum of disease, from structural defects to acquired pathology
- The wide range of congenital lesions and their underlying physiologic consequences
- The numerous surgical procedures in CHD (Table 14-4) and their hemodynamic implications
- The fact that many parents are unaware of the full extent or details of their child's lesion or abnormalities

At the same time, to optimally care for these patients the following objectives should be met:
- Familiarity with the cardiovascular pathology
- Understanding of the physiologic abnormalities and available therapies

Table 14-4. Surgical Procedures for Congenital Heart Disease

Procedure	Description	Goal/Result
Arterial switch (Jatene) operation	Arterial trunks transected above the level of the semilunar valves, relocated to their appropriate respective ventricles, coronary arteries reimplanted into the neoaortic root	Establishes the normal ventricular-arterial connection (right ventricle to pulmonary artery and left ventricle to aorta)
Atrioventriculoseptal defect (atrioventricular canal) repair	Patch closure of atrial and ventricular communications, reconstruction of atrioventricular valves, closure of cleft in left-sided atrioventricular valve	Eliminates the intracardiac shunt
Blalock-Taussig shunt	Subclavian artery to pulmonary artery communication. Modified implies placement of a graft.	Allows for or increases pulmonary blood flow
Central shunt, Waterston shunt, Pott shunt	Creation of communication between systemic and pulmonary circulations	Allows for or increases pulmonary blood flow
Closure of septal defects	Patch or primary closure of communications at the atrial or ventricular levels	Eliminates the intracardiac shunt
Coarctation repair	Relief of aortic arch obstruction (various approaches)	Establishes patency across the aortic arch
Damus-Kaye-Stansel	End-to-side anastomosis of main pulmonary artery onto the aorta. Necessitates reestablishing pulmonary blood flow via an alternative route (graft from a systemic artery into the pulmonary artery or a right ventricular to pulmonary artery conduit)	Allows for unobstructed systemic outflow in the context of single ventricle associated with obstruction to aortic flow or other settings
Division/ligation of patent ductus arteriosus	Obliteration of the ductus arteriosus	Eliminates shunting at the level of the great arteries
Fontan procedure	Connection that allows for inferior vena cava blood to drain into pulmonary circulation	Separates the pulmonary and systemic circulations in patients with single ventricle physiology. Usually final step in the single-ventricle palliation pathway.
Glenn anastomosis (cavopulmonary connection)	Superior vena cava to pulmonary artery direct anastomosis (bidirectional implies flow from superior vena cava into both pulmonary arteries)	Provides for pulmonary blood flow while unloading the single ventricle. May be first or intermediate step in the single-ventricle palliation pathway.
Konno-Rastan procedure (aortoventriculoplasty)	Enlargement of the left ventricular outflow tract and aortic annulus. The defect created in the ventricular septum to enlarge the outflow tract is repaired with a large patch.	Alleviates subvalvar and valvar aortic obstruction. When the aortic root is replaced by an autologous pulmonary root this is referred to as a Ross-Konno. Alternatively, cryopreserved homograft tissue may be used in the form of an extended root replacement.
Norwood procedure (stage I palliation)	Involves aortic reconstruction, an atrial septectomy, and placement of a systemic-to-pulmonary artery shunt	Addresses systemic outflow tract obstruction by allowing the right ventricle to eject into a reconstructed aorta. The atrial septectomy provides for unobstructed drainage of the pulmonary venous return into the right atrium. The systemic-to-pulmonary artery shunt supplies the pulmonary blood flow.
Pulmonary artery banding	Constrictive band placed around main pulmonary artery	Limits excessive pulmonary blood flow
Rastelli operation	Creation of an intracardiac tunnel that allows for left ventricular output into the aorta while closing a ventricular septal defect and placement of a right ventricular conduit to pulmonary artery	Allows for the left ventricle to eject solely into the aorta at the same time as it abolishes the intracardiac shunting at the ventricular level and provides for unobstructed pulmonary blood flow. The procedure results in separation of the pulmonary and systemic circulations.

Table 14-4 (continued). Surgical Procedures for Congenital Heart Disease

Procedure	Description	Goal/Result
Sano modification of the Norwood procedure	Placement of graft between the right ventricle and main pulmonary artery as an alternative to a modified Blalock-Taussig shunt in the Norwood operation	Provides for pulmonary blood flow
Senning/Mustard procedure (atrial switch)	Intra-atrial baffle procedure	Allows for pulmonary venous blood to be rerouted through the tricuspid valve into the right ventricle (as the systemic chamber that ejects into the aorta). At the same time the systemic venous return is channeled across the mitral valve into the left ventricle, which pumps into the main pulmonary artery.
Tetralogy of Fallot repair	Closure of ventricular septal defect and relief of right ventricular outflow tract obstruction	Eliminates intracardiac shunting at the ventricular level (cyanosis) and addresses the right ventricular outflow tract obstruction (frequently at several levels)
Truncus arteriosus repair	Closure of the ventricular septal defect and establishment of right ventricular to pulmonary artery continuity (usually via a homograft)	Abolishes the intracardiac shunting and restores the normal connection between the ventricles and great arteries
Valvectomy	Valve excision	Relieves valvar obstruction
Valvotomy	Opening of stenotic valve	Relieves valvar obstruction
Valve replacement	Placement of bioprosthetic or mechanical valve	Addresses valvar pathology (obstruction and/or regurgitation)
Valvuloplasty	Valve repair	Relieves valvar regurgitation and/or stenosis

- Recognition of compensatory mechanisms, signs of limited reserve, and potential perioperative risks
- Ability to identify the potential impact of the scheduled intervention/surgical procedure on the patient's underlying condition and anticipate how this will be tolerated

The combination of the daunting challenges and difficult objectives can be intimidating even to the most experienced clinician. Thus, when caring for children with cardiovascular disease, an interdisciplinary approach is desirable and highly recommended, allowing for the formulation and execution of optimal management plans. If available, consultation with the child's cardiologist or primary care physician should include inquiries about the details of the child's disease, overall clinical status, past and current medical treatment, prior surgical interventions, and presence of residual pathology. The interaction between members of the perioperative team should allow the opportunity for an exchange of information, discussion of concerns, and recommendations that may facilitate patient care as well as the development of comprehensive care plans.[331] This is particularly important in the management of children with complex pathologic processes.

A complete medical history and focused examination is essential during the preoperative assessment. In addition to providing the opportunity for evaluation of the child's disease processes, overall clinical status, and functional reserve, this allows for appraisal of issues that may affect anesthetic management (limited vascular access, difficult airway, gastroesophageal reflux, manipulations to manage pulmonary and systemic blood flow and pressures). Available diagnostic studies should be reviewed (e.g., ECG, chest radiograph, echocardiogram, Holter monitor, cardiac catheterization). On occasion, depending on the nature of the procedure, complexity of the disease, and potential impact on perioperative outcome, additional evaluation and/or diagnostic studies may be warranted. In many cases, the anesthesiologist plays a major role in the determination of whether the available information is adequate.

A fundamental goal in the preoperative evaluation is the identification of children who are at increased risk because of cardiac and pulmonary limitations imposed by their cardiovascular disease. After the preoperative visit, the anesthesiologist caring for a child with CHD should have an adequate understanding of the pathophysiology of the cardiac defect and implications of any previous interventions. Abnormal indices that should raise potential concerns include hypoxemia (SpO_2 less than 75%), pulmonary to systemic blood flow ratio ($\dot{Q}p:\dot{Q}s$) exceeding 3:1, outflow tract gradients over 50 mm Hg, pulmonary hypertension (mean pulmonary artery pressure above 30 mm Hg), increased pulmonary vascular resistance index (>2 Woods units · m^2) or polycythemia (hematocrit >60%). In addition, the following clinical states may place children at significant risk for severe cardiopulmonary decompensation during anesthesia and surgery: history of recent congestive heart failure, uncontrolled arrhythmias, severe ventricular dysfunction, unexplained syncope, substantial exercise intolerance, or any condition associated with significant functional cardiac or pulmonary impairment.

Clinical Condition and Status of Prior Repair

Children with CHD may present for anesthetic care before catheter-based or surgical interventions for their cardiovascular disease or after palliation or definitive procedures. It is important to recognize that true "corrective procedures" are those that result in a normal life expectancy and normal cardiovascular reserve.[332] They generally require no further medical or surgical treatment. As such, only a few procedures fulfill these criteria: ligation/division/occlusion of a patent ductus arteriosus and closure of an isolated secundum atrial septal defect. Other interventions or surgical procedures may result in repair or "correction," however not necessarily in normal hemodynamics or life expectancy. In fact, some assume limitation in cardiovascular reserve and the need for close follow-up, further medical management, and potential or additional surgical therapies. In other cases, as in children with palliated CHD, the circulation may still be abnormal. These individuals have been reported to be at a greater risk of adverse perioperative events.[333-335]

The effect or impact to the heart and other systems during previous procedures also requires careful consideration. A number of problems may remain or develop after surgical intervention. These include residual shunts, valvar stenoses or outflow tract obstruction, valvar regurgitation, pulmonary hypertension, arrhythmias, and ventricular dysfunction. Children who require a detailed appraisal of perioperative risks include those with residual significant pathology; suspected or known pulmonary hypertension, single-ventricle physiology (including patients post Norwood procedures, Glenn operations, or Fontan palliations), and after conduit placement or cardiac transplantation (see Chapters 15, 16, and 21).

Summary

Caring for children with heart disease is a major aspect of pediatric anesthesia practice. The spectrum of pathology in the pediatric age group includes a wide range of structural defects as well as varied acquired diseases. The ability to provide optimal care is dependent on an understanding of the basic pathophysiology of the lesions; familiarity with the commonly used diagnostic modalities and their clinical applications; and medical and surgical treatment options available to affected individuals. In this chapter we have presented basic concepts in cardiology that may enhance the overall knowledge of the practicing anesthesiologist in pediatric cardiovascular disease.

Annotated References

Hata T, Todd MM: Cervical spine considerations when anesthetizing patients with Down syndrome. Anesthesiology 2005; 102: 680-685

The review stresses the need for careful preoperative evaluation in children with Down syndrome to identify symptomatic patients with cervical spine anomalies.

Jefferies JL, Denfield SW, Price JF, et al: A prospective evaluation of nesiritide in the treatment of pediatric heart failure. Pediatr Cardiol 2006; 27:402-407

The study evaluated the potential role of recombinant B-type natriuretic peptide (nesiritide) for the treatment of pediatric decompensated heart failure. Nesiritide was associated with improved urine output and functional status, supporting its application in the treatment of pediatric heart failure.

Ikemba CM, Su JT, Stayer SA, et al: Myocardial performance index with sevoflurane-pancuronium versus fentanyl-midazolam-pancuronium in infants with a functional single ventricle. Anesthesiology 2004; 101:1298-1305

The study assessed changes in ventricular function in response to two anesthetic regimens in single-ventricle patients using recently described echocardiographic indices (myocardial performance index and Doppler tissue imaging).

Lang RM, Mor-Avi V, Sugeng L, et al: Three-dimensional echocardiography: the benefits of the additional dimension. J Am Coll Cardiol 2006; 48:2053-2069

The article focuses on the benefits of 3D echocardiography, the realistic and unique comprehensive views of cardiac valves and congenital abnormalities; and the utility in the intraoperative and postoperative settings.

Samyn MM: A review of the complementary information available with cardiac magnetic resonance imaging and multi-slice computed tomography (CT) during the study of congenital heart disease. Int J Cardiovasc Imaging 2004; 20:569-578

The review highlights the applications of cardiac magnetic resonance imaging and computed tomography (CT) in the diagnosis of congenital heart disease.

References

Please see www.expertconsult.com

Anesthesia for Children Undergoing Heart Surgery

Angus McEwan

Preoperative Evaluation

In the United States 40,000 children with congenital heart disease (CHD) are born every year.[1] This represents an incidence of 6 to 8 per 1,000 live births.[2] Children with chromosomal abnormalities such as trisomy 21 (Down syndrome) exhibit a greater incidence of CHD. Having a sibling with CHD increases the risk of CHD, as does the presence of other congenital abnormalities.[3] With improving diagnostic techniques many children with CHD are diagnosed in the prenatal period or early in neonatal life. Associated with this improvement in diagnostic ability is a trend in most centers to undertake definitive repair earlier, with many children being operated on in the neonatal period. Overall, about half of all children undergo cardiac surgery in the first year of life and about 25% undergo surgery in the first month of life.[4,5] The perioperative management of children with complex cardiac defects requires a dedicated team of anesthesiologists, cardiologists, intensivists, surgeons, perfusionists, and nurses. Anesthesiologists caring for these children are challenged by some of the greatest physiologic aberrations encountered in clinical medicine. As a result, anesthesiologists who are responsible for the care of these children require a comprehensive understanding of the physiology and pathophysiology of the heart. The anesthesiologist must be able to adapt to each nuance of pathophysiology that is encountered.

In addition to children with CHD, the pediatric cardiac anesthesiologist may also be responsible for the care of adults with CHD. This group of young adults with "grown up congenital heart disease" is ever expanding as more and more children with CHD survive to adulthood. Although having CHD, they also have some of the comorbidity of older age. The ideal for this group of patients is to be cared for in specialist units, but these are few in number. In the meantime, the care of these patients may well fall to the most qualified physicians and the pediatric cardiac anesthesiologist. In addition, there are children with acquired rheumatic heart disease, those with cardiomyopathy, and those who have undergone heart transplantation who require care from specialists.

Other changes occurring with the specialty is the increasing reliance on echocardiography and magnetic resonance imaging (MRI) in acquiring diagnostic data. At the same time, fewer children are being subjected to diagnostic angiography. However, more interventional cardiac catheterization procedures are being performed. Many conditions that would previously have been treated surgically are now treated in the angiography suite by interventional cardiologists, such as atrial septal defects (ASDs), patent ductus arteriosus (PDA), and ventricular septal defects (VSDs). Other interventions include dilating arteries with balloon catheters with and without stents as well as coiling of aberrant or excessive collateral vessels. The pulmonary artery is commonly ballooned and stented and, increasingly, coarctation of the aorta is treated by ballooning. Stenotic valves are also commonly dilated. These procedures have all led to a "risk transfer," the risk being transferred from the operating room to the angiography suite.[6] Whereas for the individual child there has been a dramatic decrease in morbidity as increasing numbers of conditions are treated in the angiography suite, the risks of complications that occur in the angiography suite have increased as more complex procedures are performed (see Chapter 20).

The Preoperative Visit and Evaluation

The preoperative visit is an important part of the overall anesthetic management of children with CHD.[7] The aims of the preoperative visit include:

- Medical assessment
- Prescribing premedication
- Providing information
- Creating a relationship with the child and family
- Formulating an anesthetic plan

Medical Assessment

It is essential that the anesthesiologist has a clear and detailed understanding of cardiac pathophysiology of each patient and what surgery is to be undertaken. In addition, it is also important to have a clear understanding of any associated congenital abnormalities or medical conditions. The medical assessment includes collation of information from the history, physical examination, and review of imaging and laboratory data. The majority of diagnostic information will be obtained from the medical record. Particular attention should be taken of the echocardiographic, MRI, angiographic, or other imaging data, chest radiograph, and ECGs. Many centers have joint cardiac conferences where decisions about treatment are discussed in a multidisciplinary forum. Reports from these meetings are valuable in the preoperative assessment.

In addition to gathering this specific diagnostic information, a directed history and physical examination should be performed to assess the overall condition of the child. Attention should be directed toward assessing the degree of cardiac failure, cyanosis or risks of pulmonary hypertension, and prior surgical procedures and how this may alter access to the central circulation and the placement of invasive monitors. Also, the general nutritional state of the child should be assessed; poor growth and development are often a sign of severe CHD. Other information should also be sought that may have a bearing on the anesthetic plan. For example, is this repeat surgery and therefore does it require a repeat sternotomy? This has a bearing on line placement because the femoral area should be avoided when possible because femoral bypass may be required. The previous use of aprotinin is important because the risk of anaphylaxis is increased in a second exposure and, particularly, if it has been given in the previous 6 months.[8] The type of surgery to be performed is important. Examples include the fashioning of a Blalock-Taussig shunt; if the shunt is placed on the left, the arterial line should not be placed in the left arm because the trace will be lost or distorted during subclavian cross clamping. If a Glenn shunt is planned, a short internal jugular line will be useful to monitor pulmonary artery pressure after it has been created but should be removed early in the postoperative period so as not to risk the formation of thrombosis in the superior vena cava (SVC).

The presence of any good veins should be sought and marked for the application of local anesthetic cream. This is useful in sick children even if an inhalational induction is planned because it will allow placement of a venous cannula during a very light plane of anesthesia and thus avoid myocardial depression from high concentrations of inhalation anesthetics.

Prescribing Premedication

The use of sedative premedication can be very useful in cardiac anesthesia, but this practice varies widely. There are numerous medications that may be used, and numerous different recommendations exist. Premedication for infants younger than 6 months of age is usually unnecessary. Premedication for older, healthier children who show little anxiety and with whom good preoperative rapport can be established is often also unnecessary. However, there are some older children, particularly if they have undergone previous surgery, who have very real fears about the anesthesia and surgery. In these children, it is very important to address their fears. Sedative premedication may play an important role to ensure anxiolysis at the time of separation from the parents and induction of anesthesia. I prefer to avoid premedication in children with severe congestive heart failure. Cyanotic children such as those with tetralogy of Fallot often benefit from sedative premedication because during induction of anesthesia crying and struggling may worsen cyanosis. However, it is important that these cyanotic children are well supervised after premedication because they have been shown to have a blunted response to hypoxia.[9] In the United States, supplemental premedication is sometimes administered under the direct supervision of the anesthesiologist in the preoperative facility, providing for a calm child and gentle separation from the parents. In the United Kingdom, where induction of anesthesia takes place in a dedicated anesthetic room, parents are present until after the induction, making additional premedication often unnecessary.

The most common medication used for premedication in children is oral midazolam, 0.5 to 1.0 mg/kg.[10] However, the effect of midazolam may be unpredictable and occasionally leads to dysphoria. Numerous other medications have been recommended for this purpose, including ketamine, clonidine, temazepam, and chloral hydrate. The use of these drugs is often dictated by local preferences and is not always evidence based. Table 15-1 outlines the cardiac premedication used at my institution.

Table 15-1. Suggested Oral Premedication for Cardiac Surgery

Age/Weight	Premedication Drug	Dose	Comments
<4 wk	None		EMLA or Ametop only
From 4 wk up to 6 kg	Triclofos	50-75 mg/kg	
6-15 kg	Triclofos	50-75 mg/kg	
>15 kg	Midazolam	0.5-1.0 mg/kg	Maximum 15 mg
	Temazepam	0.5-1.0 mg/kg	Maximum 20 mg

Giving Information

Providing information to the parents and to the child if they are capable of understanding is a key element of the preoperative visit. This information includes the use or not of sedative premedication, the type of induction, fasting times, the type and likely position of invasive lines, the need for a stay in an intensive care unit (ICU) postoperatively, and the likely length of that stay. The use of other monitors such as transesophageal echocardiography (TEE) should be outlined (and any contraindications sought), along with the probability of the need for blood transfusion. Questions about the risk of anesthesia and surgery should be addressed to the satisfaction of the parents (see Chapter 4).

Creating Rapport with the Child and Family

By creating a good relationship with the family, the anesthesiologist can reduce the anxiety of the child and the parents. The family develops a sense of trust, and this can improve their hospital experience.

Formulating an Anesthetic Plan

Having assessed the patient, it will be possible to formulate a detailed anesthetic plan.

Upper Respiratory Tract Infection and Cardiac Surgery

It has been shown that otherwise healthy children undergoing elective non-cardiac surgery in the presence of an upper respiratory tract infection (URTI, Table 15-2) are more likely to suffer respiratory complications. These complications are usually minor, are easily managed, and usually result in minimal morbidity.[11-13] The decision as to whether to proceed with noncardiac surgery in a child with a URTI should be evaluated on an individual basis.

The decision to proceed with cardiac surgery in children is difficult. Children with cardiac failure are prone to multiple URTIs and may have signs that can mimic URTI. In addition, it may be that surgery is relatively urgent and that postponing the surgery exposes the child to an increased risk of sequelae. It has been shown that cardiac surgery in children with a URTI results in a prolonged stay in the ICU and prolonged ventilation times, although overall hospital stay is not prolonged. There is an increased incidence of pulmonary atelectasis and an increase in postoperative bacterial infections. There appears not to be any statistically significant increase in mortality (4.2% URTI vs. 1.6% non-URTI) or long-term sequelae in children with URTI who undergo cardiac surgery. The URTI group was significantly younger and smaller, which may account in part for

the greater but statistically insignificant increased mortality.[14] While this increase in mortality was not statistically significant, it does raise concerns about the risks posed by URTI prior to cardiac surgery. Children scheduled for surgery to perform a Glenn shunt or completion of the Fontan circulation may be at particular risk because any increase in pulmonary vascular resistance (PVR) can adversely affect outcome. It is probably prudent to postpone a procedure in a child with a URTI who is scheduled for elective cardiac surgery. If the surgery is urgent, discussion with the surgical team is required to correctly assess the risks and benefit to the child.

Specific Perioperative Challenges in Pediatric Cardiac Anesthesia

Cyanosis

Children with cyanotic cardiac defects compensate for chronic hypoxia with increased erythropoiesis, increased circulating blood volume, vasodilation, and metabolic adjustments of factors, such as circulating 2,3-diphosphoglycerate (2,3-DPG). These changes allow greater tissue delivery of oxygen. The increase in blood viscosity with polycythemia leads to increased vascular resistance and sludging, which may result in renal, pulmonary, and cerebral thromboses, especially in dehydrated children.[15] Long periods without oral intake both preoperatively and postoperatively should therefore be avoided in children with polycythemia, unless adequate intravenous hydration is provided.

PVR increases more than systemic vascular resistance (SVR) as the hematocrit rises, further decreasing pulmonary blood flow in children who already have a compromised pulmonary circulation. Coagulopathies are common in children with cyanotic CHD and may adversely influence surgical hemostasis.[16,17] When the hematocrit exceeds 65%, excessive viscosity impairs microvascular perfusion and outweighs the advantages of increased oxygen-carrying capacity. Reduction of red blood cell volume has been shown to correct the coagulopathy and also to improve hemodynamics when hematocrit elevations are extreme.[18]

Intracardiac Shunting

In CHD, much of the pathophysiology involves communications between chambers or vessels that are normally separate, resulting in shunting of blood between ventricles, atria, the great arteries, or a combination of these, depending on the nature of the lesion. Management of shunting is a major consideration during anesthesia and requires an understanding of the factors that control shunting.

Dependent and Obligatory Shunts

Rudolph's distinction between dependent and obligatory shunting is very useful for understanding the control of intracardiac shunting.[19] Dependent shunts are those in which size and direction of shunting through abnormal cardiac communications depend on the relationship between PVR and SVR and are thus variable. Dependent shunting occurs between two structures having pressures that are nearly equal or at least having the same order of magnitude. Dependent shunts include PDA, simple atrial or ventricular septal defects (ASD or VSD), aortopulmonary windows, and other systemic-to-pulmonary shunts, such as a Blalock-Taussig shunt.

Table 15-2. Diagnosis of Upper Respiratory Tract Infection

At least two of the following + confirmation by a parent:
  Rhinorrhea
  Sore or scratchy throat
  Sneezing
  Nasal congestion
  Malaise
  Cough
  Fever > 38°C (100.4°F)

Data from Schreiner MS, O'Hara I, Markakis DA, Politis GD: Do children who experience laryngospasm have an increased risk of upper respiratory tract infection? Anesthesiology 1996; 85:475-480.

In contrast, obligatory shunts are those in which shunting is relatively independent of the relationship between PVR and SVR. Resistances tend to be fixed, and blood flow occurs between structures having pressures differing by an order of magnitude. Obligatory shunting occurs between the left ventricle and the right atrium in common atrioventricular (AV) canal defects and between systemic arteries and veins in peripheral arteriovenous fistulas.

Special forms of obligatory shunts occur in complex heart disease when partial or complete obstruction to blood flow occurs along with communications between chambers. In tricuspid or mitral atresia, obligatory shunting occurs between the atria because there is no atrial outlet on the side of the atresia. In aortic or pulmonary atresia, likewise, obligatory shunting occurs between either the atria or the ventricles because there is no ventricular outlet. Although these special types of obligatory shunts are independent of vascular resistances, they can only occur simultaneously with a dependent type of shunt at another level; such an example is a PDA, which provides either pulmonary blood flow in pulmonary atresia or systemic flow in aortic atresia.

When partially obstructive lesions occur simultaneously with communications between chambers, as in pulmonary stenosis with PDA or tetralogy of Fallot, the distinctions between the two types of shunts blur. Similarly, when the pressure differential on two sides of a dependent shunt becomes very great, it takes on the characteristics of an obligatory shunt. However, except in the most complex forms of congenital heart disease, knowledge of the distinctions between various types of shunting described earlier is sufficient when anesthetizing most children with CHD. These distinctions predict how any particular stress or anesthetic manipulations will affect the shunts.

Restrictive Shunts

The foregoing discussion assumes that the intracardiac and great vessel communications are relatively large and nonrestrictive. When communications are small, the size of the defect itself limits shunting and considerations of relative PVR and SVR become correspondingly smaller in determining the amount of shunting. Whenever there is a large pressure differential at the same level of the circulation on either side of a communication, the communication is restrictive; flow is limited across the defect, and other factors determining shunt flow become less important. This is usually the situation in children with mild heart disease that is asymptomatic or minimally symptomatic, such as small ASDs and VSDs or a small PDA.

Dependent Shunting during Anesthesia

In children with dependent shunts, the direction and amount of intracardiac shunting are determined by the circulatory dynamics. Control of circulatory dynamics to minimize the shunt is one major goal of anesthetic management. Because shunting in these children is dependent on the relationship between SVR and PVR, anesthetic management often revolves around control of relative vascular resistances.

In children with dependent right-to-left shunts, decreases in SVR or increases in PVR increase the shunt. In children with dependent left-to-right shunts, increases in SVR and decreases in PVR increase the shunt. In children with bidirectional or balanced shunting, any change in either vascular resistance increases the net shunt away from the side with elevated vascular resistance.

For practical purposes, acute increases in left-to-right shunts during anesthesia are of clinical importance in a number of situations. A substantial "steal" of systemic blood flow by the pulmonary circulation can occur in conditions such as AV canal, truncus arteriosus, and hypoplastic left heart syndrome. Left-to-right shunting is generally well tolerated, except when pulmonary steal leads to systemic hypotension, increasing acidosis or insufficient coronary perfusion. Shunting from right-to-left, because it is accompanied by at least some degree of arterial oxygen desaturation, is more frequently a problem during anesthesia.

Impaired Hemostasis

Hemostasis is impaired after bypass in infants and children. This results from a combination of immature coagulation factor synthesis, hemodilution after bypass, and a complex interaction involving consumption of clotting factors and platelets. At birth, the levels of vitamin K–dependent coagulation factors in healthy full-term neonates are only 40% to 66% of adult values. During the first month of life, these levels increase to 53% to 90% of adult values.[20] However, in children with CHD, especially those with cyanosis or systemic hypoperfusion, coagulation factors often continue to be depressed secondary to impaired hepatic protein synthesis. Although antithrombin III levels are also low, true heparin resistance is rare in infants because of the equal decrease in coagulation factors. At the onset of cardiopulmonary bypass (CPB), the introduction of the prime volume, which is two to three times greater than the child's blood volume, dilutes the factor levels, in particular fibrinogen to 50% and the platelet count to 30%, of pre-bypass levels. This degree of dilution occurs even when the pump circuit is primed with whole blood. Greater dilution may occur when packed red cells are used in the priming volume. Thus, at the conclusion of neonatal bypass, the activity of clotting factors is often extremely low, the fibrinogen level is frequently below 100 mg/dL, and the platelet count may be as low as 50,000 to 80,000/mm^3.[21] In addition to these quantitative changes, platelets undergo functional changes during bypass. Extracorporeal circulation causes a loss of platelet adhesion receptors, activation of platelets, and formation of leukocyte-platelet conjugates. Platelet adhesion receptors are more depressed in children with cyanotic compared with acyanotic cardiac defects. Heparin also impairs platelet function independent of CPB.[22] Cardiac surgery is also associated with significant activation of the fibrinolytic system.[23] Inadequate heparin levels during CPB in children may also contribute to postoperative bleeding because inadequate anticoagulation may allow activation of the hemostatic pathways. This activation causes the consumption of platelets and clotting factors. It has been shown that the standard measurement of anticoagulation, the activated clotting time (ACT), shows a poor correlation with heparin levels in children undergoing CPB.[24] In one study, the use of heparin monitoring and heparin titration was associated with the use of larger doses of heparin but smaller doses of protamine for antagonism. Activation of clotting cascades is also reduced, thus resulting in less bleeding in the postoperative period.[25] As a result of this multifactorial coagulopathy, blood loss is a greater problem in children than in adults and is a particular problem in neonates and small infants (see Chapter 17).[26]

Strategies to Reduce Bleeding after Bypass

In an effort to normalize factors and platelets to effective levels, some centers utilize fresh whole blood in the cardiopulmonary circuit prime. In adult patients and an in-vitro aggregation study, transfusion of fresh whole blood provided equal or greater hemostatic and functional benefit versus transfusion of platelet concentrates. In children, transfusion of fresh whole blood less than 48 hours from harvest is associated with less blood loss compared with transfusion of reconstituted whole blood (packed erythrocytes, fresh frozen plasma, and platelets).[27] However, fresh whole blood is often difficult to obtain. Furthermore, the units must be refrigerated for 24 to 48 hours while donor screening is performed and this storage causes significant platelet injury. Insistence on fresh whole blood places tremendous pressures on the transfusion service and donor center to coordinate the matching of donor types with recipient needs.

Alternatively, individual component therapy may be utilized. Platelets should be used first in treating coagulopathy after bypass in children and when given in a dose of 10 mL/kg will usually correct the clotting defect. Furthermore, platelets may be administered if bleeding persists and the platelet count is less than 100,000/mm³.[28] If platelets are required, one might also anticipate that cryoprecipitate will also be required. This follows because if platelets are substantially reduced, the other important factors such as fibrinogen (II) and factor VIII will also be reduced. In addition to high levels of fibrinogen, cryoprecipitate contains high levels of factor VIII and von Willebrand factor as well as factor XIII. Fibrinogen and von Willebrand factor are required for platelet adhesion and aggregation to occur. Platelet adhesion and aggregation are the fundamental first steps in primary hemostasis (see Chapter 10). The subsequent step of platelet degranulation "switches on" the entire coagulation cascade and cannot take place without adhesion and aggregation.[29] Use of fresh frozen plasma in the infant may result in excessive dilution of red cell mass and platelets, and there is no evidence that it is effective in treating this type of coagulopathy.[30]

Transfusion guidelines have been described in adults and have been shown to reduce postoperative bleeding and transfusion requirements.[31,32] However, similar guidelines have not been forthcoming in children and practice appears to be more empirical. This is a less than ideal situation, and more work is urgently needed to produce well-validated guidelines. The thromboelastogram (TEG) and the platelet count may be used to identify which children are likely to bleed after cardiac surgery.

Antifibrinolytics

The antifibinolytics used in pediatric cardiac surgery include ε-aminocaproic acid (EACA), tranexamic acid (TA), and aprotinin. EACA and TA are both lycine analogues that have been shown to reduce bleeding after cardiac surgery in adults and children.[33,34] They do not appear to have any anti-inflammatory activity, and the doses for use in pediatric cardiac surgery have not been clearly established. Aprotinin is a serine protease inhibitor that is well studied in adults. Many studies had shown it to significantly reduce bleeding, reduce the time taken to extubation, shorten ICU stay and reduce overall mortality.[35] However, subsequent studies have contradicted these earlier findings.[35a] The same volume of evidence has not yet been produced in children, although there are a number of studies that do suggest it is effective in reducing bleeding and that it also reduces length of time on the ventilator and reduces ICU stay.[36-39] It may be that the doses used in pediatric studies do not take into account the large pump prime to blood volume difference

that occurs when children are placed on the bypass circuit. Mossinger and associates[40] have shown that if a pump prime dose is used that is based on the size of the pump prime, rather than on the size of the child, plasma aprotinin levels are similar to those seen in adults. When this dosing regimen is used, postoperative bleeding is reduced, lung function is improved, and time to extubation is reduced. Aprotinin is expensive and there is a risk of anaphylaxis particularly if the child has been previously exposed to aprotinin. There is also a concern that it may be associated with thrombosis. Recently, a large study in adults undergoing revascularization surgery reported that there was a significantly increased risk of renal failure or stroke.[41] In addition, these same investigators reported an increase in 5-year mortality in adults after the use of aprotinin in revascularization surgery.[42] Also, in a large prospective randomized multicenter study involving more than 2,000 adults comparing antifibrinolytics, aprotinin was shown to increase 30 day mortality by one third compared with TA or EACA.[42a] There is no evidence to date that suggests that this is true in children, however, following these studies it is very likely that aprotinin will no longer be available for use in cardiac surgery. (see Chapter 18).

Topical Agents

The use of topical agents to promote clot formation and reduce bleeding in children after cardiac surgery is becoming increasingly widespread. They have been shown to significantly reduce bleeding in children.[43]

Ultrafiltration

Ultrafiltration is a process that removes ultrafiltrate from a child during and after CPB. It provides many benefits, including increasing the hematocrit, concentrating the clotting factors and platelets, increasing blood pressure and reducing PVR, and removing inflammatory mediators in the ultrafiltrate. It has been shown to significantly reduce bleeding after cardiac surgery in children.[44,45]

Desmopressin

Desmopressin acts by increasing plasma levels of factor VIII and von Willebrand factor. It has been shown to be effective in reducing bleeding after CPB in adult cardiac surgery.[46] Unfortunately, similar studies in children failed to demonstrate that desmopressin is as effective in reducing either bleeding or transfusion requirements.[47]

Anesthetic Management of Surgery Requiring Cardiopulmonary Bypass

Monitoring

Noninvasive monitoring during pediatric cardiac surgery includes pulse oximetry, five-lead electrocardiography, an automated blood pressure cuff, a precordial or esophageal stethoscope, continuous airway manometry, inspired and expired capnography, anesthetic gas and oxygen analysis, multiple-site temperature measurement, and volumetric urine collection. The pulse oximeter is especially important when managing children with congenital cardiac disease, and at least two probes should be placed on different limbs in the event that one should fail during the procedure. In children with cyanotic congenital heart disease, conventional pulse oximetry overestimates arterial oxygen saturation as saturation decreases.[48] This error tends to be worse with severe hypoxemia.[49] When monitoring children with shunting across the ductus arteriosus, a probe should be placed on a right hand digit to measure preductal oxygenation and a second probe should be placed on a toe or foot to measure postductal oxygenation (children with a right-sided aortic arch may require the probe to be placed on a left-hand digit). Children undergoing repair of coarctation of the aorta should be monitored with a pulse oximeter on the right upper limb, because it may be the only reliable monitor during the repair; and both pre- and post-coarctation blood pressure cuffs should be placed. These two cuffs may be cycled, and the differential noted, before and after surgical correction.

Monitoring end-tidal carbon dioxide tension (PET_{CO_2}) is of value in most children. However, in children with cyanotic-shunting cardiac lesions, PET_{CO_2} measurement may be less reliable because of ventilation-perfusion mismatching.[50] Arterial blood gases are the most accurate measure of the adequacy of ventilation and oxygenation. To provide for rapid decision-making, it is very helpful to have the blood gas analysis machine located in or immediately near the cardiac operating room.[51]

Monitoring of ionized calcium levels in arterial blood is essential during cardiac surgery or other surgical procedures in which significant quantities of citrated blood are infused rapidly or when entire blood volumes are replaced. Neonates are particularly prone to disturbance of their ionized calcium level when citrated blood is infused, and those with limited cardiac reserve tolerate ionized hypocalcemia poorly because of greater sensitivity to the myocardial effects of citrate infusion.[52] The total serum calcium value by itself is misleading in this regard.

Temperature monitoring during CPB is a critical guide to adequate brain cooling and to appropriate rewarming before separation from bypass. Because it is not practical to measure brain temperature directly, surrogate measuring sites are utilized. The tympanic membrane, esophagus, and rectum should all be monitored. Of these sites, the esophagus most closely matches the true brain temperature whereas the tympanic and rectal sites overestimate the brain temperature.[53,54] The rectal temperature is a useful guide during the rewarming phase.

After induction of anesthesia, an arterial catheter should be placed in those children who will undergo CPB. The radial artery may generally be percutaneously cannulated with relative ease even in infants. Prior arterial cannulation, prior placement of a Blalock-Taussig shunt, or coarctation of the aorta may interfere with accurate radial artery pressure measurements. Children with trisomy 21 may have radial anomalies that make cannulation of the radial artery challenging. *In small infants, the femoral arteries are frequently used for arterial access; in addition, the axillary arteries are commonly used. The use of the brachial artery is generally avoided because it is an end artery.* Catheters placed in the dorsalis pedis or posterior tibial artery often provide inaccurate hemodynamic data, especially after separation from bypass, and it may even become difficult to sample blood for laboratory testing. In the rare circumstance that peripheral arterial cannulation cannot be accomplished, the surgeon may place a catheter in the internal mammary artery after sternotomy and a sterile monitoring line may be passed over the drapes.

Central venous lines can be very useful in children with cardiac disease. For cardiac surgical procedures, there are two commonly used methods of obtaining central access; the deci-

sion of which to use may be determined in part by institutional bias. In the first method, the cardiac surgeons usually expose the heart quickly and have it available for inspection and estimation of filling pressures. Central lines can be readily established from the field and handed off to the anesthesia team. These transthoracic central lines are useful but still carry a small amount of risk.[27] In the second method, percutaneous insertion of central venous lines may again reflect institutional bias, but the method is particularly indicated for long, complex procedures, especially when access to the infant is limited or the heart is not exposed. Percutaneous cannulation of the central circulation through either the internal jugular approach or the subclavian approach has been demonstrated to be safe.[28] However, it is important to appreciate that insertion of central venous lines through the internal jugular or subclavian route may fail or may be associated with pneumothorax, hemorrhage, and hematoma formation after puncture of major arteries.[28-30] Cannulation of the external jugular vein may avoid some of these serious complications when the catheter can be successfully threaded into the central circulation.[31] Increasingly, ultrasound-guided techniques are being employed to establish central venous access. The use of ultrasound-guided central venous cannulation in adults is associated with fewer complications and a greater success rate. The evidence for this in children has not been forthcoming, but it is likely that the use of ultrasound in the placement of central venous catheters will be even more important in children (see Chapter 49). In the United Kingdom, the use of ultrasound for the placement of these lines is spreading.

In children with unrestrictive ventricular or atrial septal defects, including hearts with a single ventricle or single atrium, central venous pressure is equivalent to left ventricular filling pressure. Cannulation of vessels that drain into the SVC should be approached with caution in children with univentricular anatomy who may undergo the Fontan procedure because thrombosis of the SVC can be a devastating complication in these children. In such circumstances, the femoral veins may be the preferred site for venous pressure monitoring.

Pulmonary arterial catheters in children with intracardiac defects usually provide little more information than a simple central line, are difficult to insert without fluoroscopy, and may not provide meaningful measurements of cardiac output and as a result are rarely used in pediatric cardiac patients.

Transesophageal Echocardiography (TEE)

The use of perioperative echocardiography during pediatric cardiac surgery has become the standard of care in the United States.[55,56] In adult practice, anesthesiologists generally perform the TEE; however, in pediatric cardiac surgery the TEE is more commonly performed by the pediatric cardiologist. This may to some extent reflect the increased complexity of congenital lesions and the difficulty in accurately assessing these lesions and their repairs. TEE has been shown to be cost effective when used routinely during pediatric cardiac surgery.[57] The use of TEE can have a significant impact on surgical and medical management. In one large study, a second bypass run was undertaken in 7.3% of cases based on the findings of the TEE. In addition, there was a surgical alteration in management of 12.7% and medical alteration in 18.5%. Furthermore, it has been shown that pediatric cardiac anesthesiologists can perform the vast majority of pre- and post-bypass TEE provided they have received adequate training.[58] The introduction of small probes with multiplane capability has greatly increased the use of TEE even in infants and neonates.[59,60] In 1999, a survey of centers in the United States indicated that 93% used intraoperative echocardiography and all but one used TEE.[61] The American Society of Echocardiography and the Society of Cardiovascular anesthesiologists have published guidelines for performing a comprehensive intraoperative TEE in adults[62] and children.[63]

Although the use of TEE in children is generally safe, complications do occur and may be more common in small infants.[64] Complications include damage to the mouth, oropharynx, esophagus, and stomach. Other complications include hemodynamic disturbance as a result of compression of the left atrium or other structures. Interference with the airway also occurs in a small number of cases. This includes inadvertent extubation, right main-stem intubation, and compression of the endotracheal tube. However, the overall incidence is small, around 2%.[65] Information gathered from the TEE examination takes place both before and after bypass and may be divided broadly into two categories. These include hemodynamic assessment and monitoring and structural diagnostic information. Hemodynamic information includes information about ventricular function and filling.[66] Diagnostic information relates to confirmation or otherwise of preoperative findings and post-bypass assessment of the adequacy of the surgical repair.

Induction of Anesthesia

In the United Kingdom, induction of anesthesia takes place in an anesthetic room, which is immediately adjacent to the operating room, and the parents are almost always present for induction. Very commonly anesthesia will be induced while the child is sitting with or being held by a parent. It is possible to involve some parents to the extent that they can actually hold the mask for the child as he or she is anesthetized. Once the child is asleep, he or she is transferred to the anesthetic trolley where the trachea is intubated and venous and arterial access is secured. This practice is different from most centers in North America where induction of anesthesia takes place in the operating room.

Induction of anesthesia can be achieved using either an intravenous or inhalational technique. The type of induction should be tailored to both the child and the cardiac defect. If intravenous access has already been established, an intravenous induction is preferred. If intravenous access has not been achieved, a decision is made about the optimal induction technique. In severely ill children, it is advisable to obtain intravenous access before induction of anesthesia. The use of local anesthetic cream such as EMLA or Ametop is very helpful in reducing the pain of injection. The use of local anesthetic cream is also very helpful if an inhalational induction is to be used because it will allow the insertion of an intravenous cannula during a much lighter plane of anesthesia. This requires that the appropriate veins are selected during the preoperative visit and that clear instructions are given to nursing staff about where the cream is to be applied.

The most common inhalational induction agent is sevoflurane. It has replaced halothane as the induction agent of choice. However, despite sevoflurane's apparent better safety profile compared with halothane, it is still easy to overdose the child with CHD and produce bradycardia, hypotension, and apnea. It is therefore important that it is carefully titrated and that the concentrations are rapidly reduced when an adequate level of anesthesia is achieved. In children who are cyanosed with a right-to-left shunt and a reduction in pulmonary blood flow, inhalational inductions will be much slower than in children without cyanosis. Indeed, as the solubility of the inhalational agent decreases, right-to-left shunting may be sufficiently large so as to preclude either a rapid induction or achievement of a deep level of anesthesia (see Chapter 6). The addition of nitrous oxide can aid an inhalational induction in two ways. First, because it is odorless it can be started before the introduction of the sevoflurane, allowing the child to be somewhat sedated before the stronger smelling agent is started. Second, it allows for a smoother and more rapid induction compared with sevoflurane alone. Concentrations of up to 70% nitrous oxide can be used to smooth induction of anesthesia even in cyanosed children, but the nitrous oxide should be replaced with air and oxygen or 100% oxygen as soon as intravenous access is obtained and a muscle relaxant has been given. It is not always necessary to use a mask for an inhalational induction because cupped hands are often more acceptable to the child, particularly one who is frightened of "the mask." It is important to tell the child about each event before it happens and to show them on yourself, a parent, or toy animal. You should also offer the child the opportunity to hold the mask or if accompanied by a parent offer the child the choice of the parent holding the mask. Good premedication will often aid this process (see Chapter 4).

In sick children in whom it may be preferable to use an intravenous induction, various options are available. For example, in neonates with coarctation of the aorta or with hypoplastic left heart syndrome who are not ventilated before coming to the operating room, one approach is to administer fentanyl in a dose of 2 to 3 µg/kg followed by pancuronium and then a very low dose (sedative dose) of sevoflurane or isoflurane. Fentanyl obtunds the hypertensive response to intubation, and the pancuronium maintains cardiac output by maintaining the heart rate. The very low dose volatile agent provides the sedation/anesthesia. In older children, etomidate is a very good induction agent, providing stable hemodynamics, although it does cause pain on injection. Ketamine is also widely used for intravenous induction in neonates as well as in older children. Ketamine maintains or increases blood pressure, heart rate, and cardiac output. Although the exact mechanism of these effects of ketamine is not known, it may be that ketamine stimulates the release of endogenous stores of catecholamines, although it is a negative inotrope in the denervated heart.[67] It may be that this negative inotropic effect makes ketamine a poor choice in children in whom catecholamine stimulation may already be maximal, such as in severe cardiomyopathy. It may also be a poor choice if tachycardia is undesirable, such as in the case of aortic stenosis. Ketamine can be used intramuscularly or orally, which makes it useful when intravenous access is difficult.

Monitoring should ideally be applied before induction begins, but applying monitoring can upset the child and this can be detrimental (e.g., the child with tetralogy of Fallot who begins to cry and precipitates a "tet spell"). It is probably preferable to start the induction as soon as possible after applying the monitors.

Sevoflurane or isoflurane may provide another advantage by offering a degree of ischemic preconditioning both to the heart and also to other organs, particularly the brain and kidney. In a double-blind study of adult patients undergoing coronary bypass grafting, exposure to 4% sevoflurane for 10 minutes before cross clamping reduced the degree of myocardial dysfunction and renal damage postoperatively.[68] It is thought that the same effect is seen in children.[69]

Maintenance of Anesthesia

Maintenance of anesthesia in children with CHD depends on the preoperative status and the response to induction of anesthesia. Whether inhalation agents, additional opioids, or other intravenous agents are used for maintenance depends on the tolerance of the individual child and postoperative plans for ventilatory management. If a primary opioid-based anesthetic is chosen, additional opioid should be administered on initiation of CPB to offset dilution from the pump prime and maintain adequate opioid plasma levels. Awareness during adult cardiac surgery has been reported when amnestic agents are not utilized. Although small children may be unable to describe such events, the potential for awareness during pediatric cardiac surgery should not be underestimated. To prevent awareness, isoflurane may be administered via the membrane oxygenator with an anesthetic vaporizer or intravenous midazolam 0.2 mg/kg may be administered. Alternatively propofol may be given by infusion during the bypass period to reduce the possibility of awareness.

Institution and Separation from Bypass

Before initiation of CPB, the surgeon will request that heparin is given. After administration of heparin (preferably flushed through a central venous catheter), the ACT should be checked *before the initiation of bypass.* The ACT measurement should be at least three times the baseline; if aprotinin is used, the ACT should be even longer. When bypass is started, any additional anesthetic drugs should be administered and positive-pressure ventilation is stopped. Both hypertension and hypotension may complicate bypass. Blood pressure may be controlled within the normal range using α-adrenergic blockers or agonists. Phenylephrine is commonly used to increase blood pressure, and phentolamine is often used to lower blood pressure. The child is usually cooled at this stage, using the nasopharyngeal temperature as a guide. Cardioplegia is given by the perfusionist after cross clamping the aorta to stop the heart and provide cardioprotection during the period of ischemia. This is usually repeated every 20 to 30 minutes, although it will not be required if the surgery is performed while the heart is beating. Myocardial damage is related to both the duration of the aortic cross clamping and the effectiveness of the myocardial protection.

At an appropriate time during the surgery, the cross clamp is removed and perfusion to the heart is restored. The heart will usually start to beat in normal sinus rhythm, although this is not always the case. Various degrees of heart block are common after heart surgery and it is most frequently associated with the administration of cardioplegia. As the heart is reperfused for a longer time, and the effects of cardioplegia are reduced, normal sinus rhythm is usually restored. However, heart block may result from damage to the conducting system during surgery.

After the release of the cross clamp, any inotropes or vasodilators that are required are usually started. Rewarming may have begun before release of the cross clamp, but more usually the child is rewarmed only after release of the clamp.

When the child has adequately rewarmed, as reflected by a normal core and minimal core-peripheral temperature difference, good heart function has returned, the child's lungs are adequately ventilated, and any inotropes required have been started, the child is ready to be separated from bypass. If a TEE probe is in place, the heart should be scanned for the presence of any air. If air is present, further de-airing should occur before attempting to come off bypass. In the initial stages after separat-ing from bypass, additional volume can be administered by the perfusionist via the aortic cannula, usually under the direction of the surgeon or anesthesiologist. Many centers at this point would institute modified ultrafiltration. This involves taking arterial blood from the aortic cannula and passing this blood through the ultra-filter. This blood, which is oxygenated and warm is then reinfused into the right atrium. When this process is complete, a thorough TEE examination can be undertaken. When the team is satisfied with the TEE result, the surgeon will ask for protamine to be administered. *Before this is done, both the perfusionist and the surgical team should be informed that protamine is about to be administered. The surgeons should remove any pump suckers from the field and the perfusionist should stop all pump suction. This is to ensure that no protamine enters the bypass circuit in case it is necessary to go back on bypass for any reason.* The ACT can now be checked along with blood gas analysis. The ACT should return to pre-bypass levels. Any blood products required are usually given after the administration of protamine, and these are usually given while the surgeons are achieving hemostasis. As soon as the chest is closed the child can then be transferred to the cardiac ICU.

Control of Systemic and Pulmonary Vascular Resistance during Anesthesia

In some children with hypoplastic left heart syndrome (HLHS) who present for a Norwood procedure, excessive blood flow to the lungs resulting from a relatively low PVR and a relatively high SVR "'steals'" blood from the systemic circulation, leading to hypotension, myocardial ischemia, and progressive acidosis. However, when the reverse happens and PVR is relatively high compared with SVR, the child develops progressive desaturation. Similar pathophysiology exists with other duct-dependent circulations and to some extent with other shunting lesions. It can prove difficult to manipulate SVR and PVR predictably. The reasons for this are that (1) control of PVR is poorly understood, (2) vasoactive drugs usually are distributed on both sides of the circulation, and (3) pharmacologic attempts to modify shunting have produced unpredictable results.[70] Despite these problems, a number of techniques have proved useful in manipulating relative PVR and SVR. Potent inhalation anesthetics appear to reduce SVR more than PVR. PVR is decreased in children by increasing inspired oxygen to 100% and by hyperventilation to a pH of 7.6 or greater. Positive end-expiratory pressure, acidosis, hypothermia, and the use of 30% or less inspired oxygen can increase PVR. Vasoconstrictors such as phenylephrine increase SVR more than PVR and therefore are acutely effective in reducing right-to-left shunting and increasing left-to-right shunting in the operating room.

During cardiac surgical procedures, a direct method of selectively increasing PVR or SVR is to have the surgeon place partially obstructing tourniquets around pulmonary arteries or the aorta to increase resistance so that flow to the opposite side of the circulation increases. SVR can be increased similarly during abdominal surgery with aortic clamps if greater systemic pressures are needed to perfuse the lungs through a systemic-to-pulmonary-artery shunt. Although these are only temporary measures, they may be useful to reestablish a better relative balance of resistances and a more normal physiology in a deteriorating clinical situation.

Anesthetic Drugs Used in Pediatric Cardiac Anesthesia

Inhalation Agents

Sevoflurane

Sevoflurane is now the induction agent of choice in pediatric anesthesia.[71,72] It is associated with little myocardial depression or dysrhythmias.[73-75] It has specific advantages over halothane when used in children with CHD, particularly in children younger than 1 year of age and in cyanosed children.[76] In contrast to halothane, sevoflurane causes no reduction in heart rate at 1.0 and 1.5 MAC in healthy children compared with awake values.[77] However, at larger concentrations it can cause slowing of the heart rate and respiratory depression. Both of these features are important in children with CHD because a slow heart rate will reduce cardiac output and hypoventilation will lead to hypercarbia and hypoxia and can lead to rises in PVR. In the absence of nitrous oxide, sevoflurane causes less depression of myocardial contractility than halothane during induction of anesthesia in children. Sevoflurane does cause a mild decrease in SVR, but, in common with halothane and isoflurane, it does not perturb the shunt between the right and left sides of the heart through an ASD or VSD when it is given in standard anesthetic concentrations in 100% oxygen.[78] Sevoflurane has also been reported to cause conduction abnormalities in susceptible patients.[79] It should also be used with great caution in children with severe ventricular outflow tract obstruction (see Chapter 6).[80]

Isoflurane

At equipotent concentrations, isoflurane causes similar hemodynamic depression in neonates and infants when compared with halothane. Isoflurane is generally not used for induction of anesthesia because of the high frequency of laryngospasm (greater than 20%).[81] Inadequate ventilation because of laryngospasm or other causes quickly leads to large increases in PVR secondary to hypoxemia and hypercarbia. This increase in PVR and the resulting pulmonary hypertension is poorly tolerated in small children with heart disease, especially in the presence of right-to-left shunting (see Chapter 6).

Halothane

In the United States and the United Kingdom, the use of halothane has all but ceased but is still widely used in other parts of the world. It is included here for completeness. Uptake of halothane in infants younger 3 months of age is more rapid than it is in adults. Thus, anesthetic concentration probably increases more rapidly in the myocardium of an infant as well.[82] Although the effects of halothane on the human neonatal myocardium are unknown, it has been shown that young rats have a reduced cardiovascular tolerance for halothane but require greater amounts for anesthesia.[83] Studies have shown a significant incidence of hypotension with bradycardia in infants with normal cardiovascular systems during induction with halothane.[84] During induction of anesthesia in normal infants, halothane decreases the cardiac index to 73% of awake values at 1.0 minimal alveolar concentration (MAC) and to 59% at 1.5 MAC.[85] The MAC for halothane in infants 1 to 6 months of age is the greatest of any age group.[86] This increased anesthetic requirement in infants, combined with the immaturity of their cardiovascular system, explains in part, the relative cardiovascular intolerance for halothane in infants. Atropine has been used intramuscularly before induction to partially compensate for the myocardial depression of halothane by reducing bradycardia and hypotension. Although halothane may produce some degree of hypotension, an increase in arterial saturation in children with cyanotic congenital heart disease may occur.[87]

A careful induction with sevoflurane is usually well tolerated in children with mild to moderate heart disease. However, large concentrations of potent inhalation agents may be an unwise choice for induction in young infants with severe cardiac disease. In children of any age with marginal cardiovascular reserve and in those with severe desaturation of systemic arterial blood due to right-to-left shunting, inhalational anesthetic-induced myocardial depression and systemic hypotension are poorly tolerated. A more appropriate use of these anesthetic agents in children with severe heart disease is the addition of low concentrations of the inhalation agent to control hypertensive responses after an intravenous induction (see Chapter 6).

Nitrous Oxide

Nitrous oxide should be avoided for maintenance of anesthesia in children with CHD because of the risk of enlarging intravascular air emboli and the potential to increase PVR. Nitrous oxide may expand microbubbles and macrobubbles, thus increasing obstruction to blood flow in arteries and capillaries. In all children with right-to-left shunts, there is a potential for these bubbles to be shunted directly into the systemic circulation. Thus, care must be taken to ensure that no air bubbles are accidentally injected into the veins. Adverse outcomes after coronary air embolism are exacerbated in the presence of nitrous oxide.[88] Additionally, the hemodynamic effects of venous air embolism are increased by nitrous oxide, even without paradoxical embolization.[89] In children with preexisting right-to-left shunts, paradoxical air embolism is clearly a potential problem; but even those with large left-to-right shunts can transiently reverse their shunts. This is especially true during coughing or a Valsalva maneuver, when the normal transatrial pressure gradient is reversed. Several studies have demonstrated right-to-left shunting of microbubbles of air after injection of saline into the right atrium during these maneuvers.[90-92] Because coughing and Valsalva maneuvers may occur during anesthetic induction, even the most rigorous attention to avoiding air bubbles in intravenous lines may not prevent some small amounts of air from reaching the systemic circulation. Microbubbles have also been observed after CPB.[93]

Nitrous oxide is reported to increase PVR in adults.[94,95] However, in a 50% inspired concentration it does not appear to affect PVR or pulmonary artery pressure in infants.[96] Nitrous oxide does mildly decrease cardiac output at this concentration.[97] It has been suggested that the use of nitrous oxide should be avoided in children with limited pulmonary blood flow, pulmonary hypertension, or depressed myocardial function. In the well-compensated child who does not require 100% inspired oxygen, nitrous oxide (generally at concentrations of 50%) may be used during induction of anesthesia but then discontinued before tracheal intubation. If reduced inspired oxygen is indicated to maintain an appropriate balance between PVR and SVR after tracheal intubation, air may be added to the inspired gas mixture (see Chapter 6).

Intravenous Induction Agents

Ketamine

The cyclohexamine derivative ketamine is a dissociative anesthetic agent. It is a good analgesic agent and increases blood pressure, heart rate, and cardiac output. Although the exact mechanism of the stimulation of blood pressure and heart rate has not been established, it is believed to stimulate the release of endogenous stores of catecholamines. Ketamine exerts a negative inotropic effect on the denervated heart.[98] I believe that this combination makes a poor choice in children in whom catecholamine stimulation may already be maximal, such as in severe cardiomyopathy. It is also a poor choice in circumstances in which tachycardia is undesirable, such as in a child with aortic stenosis. Ketamine is thought to have minimal effect on PVR in children with congenital heart disease as long as the airway and ventilation are well preserved,[99,100] although it has been reported to occasionally increase PVR in children undergoing cardiac catheterization. Ketamine is quite a versatile anesthetic that may be administered both intramuscularly or orally when intravenous access is difficult or an inhalational induction is contraindicated. The usual intravenous dose of 2 mg/kg produces a very predictable response, although an intramuscular dose of 8 to 10 mg/kg (combined with intramuscular midazolam, 0.1 mg/kg) is less predictable. The use of ketamine varies greatly from one institution to another, with some units using it extensively whereas others use it rarely (see Chapter 6).

Etomidate

Etomidate is a very safe drug with an $LD_{50}:ED_{50}$ of 26.[101] This figure implies that the lethal dose is 26 times the effective dose. It is a short-acting anesthetic with little effect on systemic blood pressure, heart rate, and cardiac output after a single dose in healthy children.[102] Etomidate has a favorable hemodynamic profile even when used in shocked children and appears to have a low risk of clinically important myoclonus or status epilepticus.[103,104] The major concern about etomidate is the increased mortality reported when it is administered as a continuous infusion. This very grave side effect has been attributed to adrenal suppression.[105-107] The inhibition of steroid synthesis occurs not only after a prolonged infusion but also after single dose of etomidate and has created a controversy about its use as an anesthetic agent in some jurisdictions (see Chapter 6).[108]

Propofol

Propofol is a rapidly acting intravenous hypnotic agent that may be administered as a single dose or continuous infusion. It has no analgesic properties. Propofol has mild antiemetic properties.[109] Its short duration of action is the result of rapid redistribution and metabolism, which also allows the drug to be given by continuous infusion without accumulation. After an induction dose of propofol in children, SVR, blood pressure, and cardiac output decrease. The effect on heart rate is variable. The ED_{50} for propofol in infants and small children is greater than it is in adults.[110-112] If propofol is given very slowly, then smaller doses are required, although the induction time increases. The slower infusion also results in more stable hemodynamics.[113] Pain on injection and involuntary movement after intravenous propofol have been concerns that have been overcome (see Chapter 6). Although propofol can be used safely in children with CHD, it is generally avoided as an induction agent in children with severe CHD disease because of its effects on SVR and

blood pressure. It should be avoided in those with a fixed cardiac output such as severe aortic or mitral stenosis because it may cause severe hypotension. It can be used by infusion during CPB to reduce awareness and may be particularly useful if an early extubation is planned (see Chapter 6).

Opioids

Fentanyl

As in adults with severe cardiac disease, intravenous fentanyl combined with pancuronium and either 100% oxygen, or air and oxygen, provides an excellent induction technique in very sick children with CHD. The inclusion of intravenous midazolam or another amnestic agent is strongly urged to avoid awareness. In neonates and infants, the use of high-dose opioid anesthesia provides excellent hemodynamic stability, with suppression of the hormonal and metabolic stress response.[114,115] When fentanyl or other opioids are combined with nitrous oxide, the negative inotropic effects of nitrous oxide may be evident, particularly in sicker children.[116] The high-dose fentanyl technique is effective in preterm neonates undergoing ligation of a PDA.[117] In high-risk full-term neonates and in older infants with severe CHD, the high-dose fentanyl technique in doses of up to 75 µg/kg, combined with pancuronium, maintains stable hemodynamics during induction, tracheal intubation, and surgical incision.[118] Oxygen saturation levels are also well maintained and often improve during induction, even in cyanotic children.[119] Cardiac index, SVR, and PVR in infants given 25 µg/kg of fentanyl do not change significantly.[120] Specifically, combining pancuronium with fentanyl is desirable as the vagolytic effects of pancuronium offset the potential vagotonic effects of fentanyl. The hemodynamic stability reported in infants with the combination of high-dose fentanyl and pancuronium may not be replicated when other muscle relaxants are used (see Chapter 6).[121]

Sufentanil

Sufentanil (5-20 µg/kg), an alternative to fentanyl, is 5 to 10 times more potent than fentanyl but has a large margin of safety.[122] It is highly lipophilic and is rapidly distributed to all tissues. It is infrequently used in CHD in infants and children.

Remifentanil

Remifentanil is an ultra-short-acting opioid that is rapidly metabolized in the plasma and tissue by nonspecific esterases to an inactive metabolite. It has a very brief elimination half-life with a context-sensitive half-life of only 9 minutes, independent of the duration of infusion. In pediatric cardiac surgery it is an attractive alternative to fentanyl that provides intense analgesia during the most stimulating parts of surgery but facilitates rapid awakening and weaning from mechanical ventilation without residual opioid effect. Furthermore, its pharmacodynamics are unaffected by CPB.[123] It provides stable hemodynamic conditions in children, although there is a tendency toward bradycardia and systemic hypotension.[124-126] It has no negative inotropic effect even in the failing heart.[127] One significant concern about remifentanil is the development of acute tolerance with increasing analgesic requirements after discontinuing remifentanil.[128-130] Some studies have suggested that this is not clinically important.[131] Remifentanil is also used for prolonged sedation of children in the ICU. Many units have moved toward early extubation and discharge from the ICU after cardiac surgery, also called "fast tracking," and remifentanil is a useful drug in this setting (see Chapter 6). Consideration must be given to transitioning to a longer-acting opioid before discontinuation of remifentanil.

Muscle Relaxants

Pancuronium has been studied in depth in children with CHD. When administered over a 60- to 90-second interval, pancuronium maintains heart rate and blood pressure.[132] An intubating bolus dose of pancuronium may produce tachycardia and an increase in cardiac output. This bolus dose effect is sometimes desirable to support cardiac output in infants in congestive heart failure because their stroke volume is fixed. Pancuronium may be the muscle relaxant of choice when high-dose opioid techniques are used to offset the vagotonic effects of opioids such as fentanyl. Other muscle relaxants are also widely used in infants and children, particularly if they are to be extubated either in the operating room or early in the ICU.

Regional Anesthesia

The use of regional anesthesia to provide pain relief during and after cardiac surgery in adults reduces the stress response to surgery and may also reduce morbidity and mortality. In adults undergoing cardiac surgery, the benefits of regional anesthesia include earlier extubation, fewer respiratory complications, a reduction in renal failure, and fewer strokes, as well as less myocardial damage after CPB.[133-135] In animals, thoracic epidural anesthesia using local anesthetics reduces myocardial damage after coronary occlusion.[136] The same benefits may be achieved by using intrathecal (spinal) analgesia. High spinal anesthesia using bupivacaine reduces the stress response to CPB and β-adrenergic dysfunction and improves cardiac performance after cardiac surgery in adults.[137] Good research into regional anesthesia and analgesia in pediatric cardiac surgery is limited. Caudal morphine has been used to provide postoperative analgesia. Caudal morphine produced good analgesia for about 6 hours and reduced the analgesic requirement for up to 24 hours.[138] There are some retrospective studies in children[139,140]; one was a case review in 50 children and the other was a retrospective study of 200 children. In the latter study, all children were targeted for early tracheal extubation and a variety of regional anesthetic techniques were used. Time to extubation, control of pain, incidence of respiratory depression, other complications, and length of hospital stay were determined. There were no deaths. Eighty-nine percent of the children were tracheally extubated in the operating room, 4.1% of whom required reintubation within 24 hours. Adverse effects of regional anesthesia included emesis (39%), pruritus (10%), urinary retention (7%), postoperative transient paresthesia (3%), and respiratory depression (1.8%). The incidence of peridural hematoma was zero. The rate of adverse effects was less when the thoracic catheter epidural approach was used as compared with various caudal, lumbar epidural, and spinal approaches. Hospital duration of stay was not affected by the presence of regional anesthetic complications. Although this study appears to indicate that regional analgesia is safe, the numbers in the study are too small to conclude that regional analgesia is safe for cardiac surgery.

The use of regional anesthesia in cardiac surgery for children remains controversial.[141,142] The main concern is the risk of bleeding and the potential for disastrous neurologic complications. The risks may be greater in children than in adults because of the presence of collateral vessels, increased venous pressure, coagulopathy related to cyanosis, and the use of aspirin. There remain many unanswered questions, such as the true incidence of epidural hematoma in children, the time delay required between placement of the epidural catheter and full anticoagulation, and the correct management if a bloody tap occurs. Ho and associates have estimated the risk of epidural hematoma during cardiac surgery in adults to be 1:1000 and 1:2400 for spinal and epidural block, respectively.[143] Whether the risks are similar or greater in children cannot be determined because, to date, the numbers of children involved in studies are too small. A large randomized prospective study to evaluate a true risk-benefit without bias is needed; until this information is available, various commentators have advised great caution with the use of regional analgesia for cardiac surgery and some have suggested that it may not be possible now to perform the study required because of ethical considerations.[144]

"Fast Tracking"

"Fast tracking" refers to abbreviating the perioperative period of children undergoing cardiac surgery. It should include every phase of the child's journey from referral and preoperative evaluation to less invasive surgery, early weaning from respiratory support and extubation, and early discharge from the ICU and hospital.

Early extubation of pediatric patients after cardiac surgery has been shown to offer advantages in terms of cost as well as reduced morbidity associated with longer ICU stays.[145-149] The success of this approach depends on the close teamwork of a multidisciplinary team, with every member of the team working toward the same goal. Successful fast tracking usually requires the development of care pathways to ensure that the quality of patient care is not compromised.[150] Early extubation and discharge from the ICU requires preplanning and the adoption of a technique that facilitates this goal. The use of very large doses of fentanyl is not appropriate; various alternative techniques have been used, including smaller doses of fentanyl in combination with inhalational agents[151,152] or the use of remifentanil either in combination with inhalational agents or with propofol. Others have advocated regional anesthesia as a means of speeding extubation, but this remains controversial. It is also important to choose a muscle relaxant with a shorter duration of action than pancuronium to ensure that it is easy to reverse the neuromuscular block at the end of surgery. Other important considerations to ensure that early extubation is a success include adequate pain relief in the form of intravenous paracetamol (where available), patient-controlled or nurse-controlled analgesia, and antiemetics because nausea appears to be more of a problem in children who are extubated early.

Some clinicians advocate extubating the trachea in the operating room, whereas others advocate waiting until the child is in the ICU. Delaying extubation until the child is in the ICU may save time in the operating room and may reduce the risks of cardiovascular instability, bleeding, and hypothermia.[153] Despite these concerns, many units frequently extubate children in the operating room after cardiac surgery with good results.

Cardiopulmonary Bypass

This is covered in Chapter 17 and will not be discussed further here.

Stress Response to Cardiac Surgery

Cardiac surgery and CPB are altered physiologic conditions associated with exaggerated stress responses characterized by the release of numerous metabolic and hormonal substances, including catecholamines, cortisol, growth hormone, prostaglandins, complement, glucose, insulin, and β-endorphins.[154,155] The cause of the elaboration of these substances is multifactorial: contact of blood with foreign surfaces, low perfusion pressure, anemia, hypothermia, myocardial ischemia, low levels of anesthesia, and nonpulsatile flow. Other factors that contribute to the increase in stress hormones are delayed renal and hepatic clearance and exclusion of the pulmonary circulation during extracorporeal circulation.[156]

Neonates of all viable gestational ages, as well as older infants and children, have nociceptive systems that are sufficiently developed and integrated with brainstem cardiovascular control centers to trigger both humoral and circulatory responses to pain and stress.[157] Substantial humoral, metabolic, and cardiovascular responses to painful and stressful stimulation during surgery have been documented in neonates of all gestational ages and older infants.[158,159] Hormonal stress responses in neonates subjected to cardiac and noncardiac operations are threefold to fivefold greater than those in adults after similar surgeries. Circulatory responses to stressful stimuli in children include systemic and pulmonary hypertension.

Humoral stress responses are particularly extreme during and after cardiac surgery. These responses are characterized by increases in circulating catecholamines, glucagon, cortisol, β-endorphins, growth hormone, and insulin. In these studies, circulating concentrations of catecholamines increased by as much as 400% over baseline preoperative concentrations. This is evidence of a massive activation of sympathetic outflow in response to surgical stimulation. Some of these responses may continue for several days postoperatively.[160]

It has been suggested that such extreme stress responses and neuroendocrine activation may be associated with greater mortality and morbidity during the postoperative period. In adults, intraoperative adrenergic activation of 50% above baseline is associated with significant postoperative alterations in β-adrenergic receptor function, including increased β-receptor density and decreased receptor affinity. Mortality among adults with severe congestive failure is associated with increased levels of hormones regulating cardiovascular function, including aldosterone, epinephrine, and norepinephrine.[161] In neonates undergoing cardiac surgery, increased concentrations of stress hormones are associated with increased hospital mortality.

The metabolic response to stress in children includes increased oxygen consumption, glycogenolysis, gluconeogenesis, and lipolysis. These metabolic responses cause substantial intraoperative and postoperative catabolism. The metabolic stress responses after comparable operative stresses in neonates exceed those in adult patients and result in substantial alterations in metabolic balance and levels of various metabolic substrates. These metabolic responses are usually related to changes in plasma cortisol, catecholamines, and other counter-regulatory hormones such as glucagon and growth hormone. The most prominent clinical effects that result from activation of these processes are perioperative hypoglycemia and hyperglycemia, lactic acidemia, and negative nitrogen balance extending well into the postoperative period. Neonates and infants tolerate such metabolic derangements poorly. Their impaired tolerance is the result of a relative lack of endogenous reserves of carbohydrates, proteins, and fats, the large metabolic cost of rapid growth, a high obligate requirement for glucose by the relatively large brain, the immature hormonal control of intermediary metabolism, and the limited functional capabilities of immature enzyme systems in the metabolic organs. Thus, severe stress responses superimposed on the "normal" neonatal and infant physiology may be poorly tolerated. However, it remains unclear whether these metabolic alterations might provide some beneficial effects toward mobilizing the bodily resources to provide a metabolic milieu for healing tissues or whether they are purely maladaptive, resulting in detrimental effects on postoperative outcome.

Another factor is the potential effect of stress-induced hyperglycemia on the neurologic outcome. Neonates and young infants are capable of substantial rates of glucose production, mainly from glycogenolysis and gluconeogenesis during stress. This can result in substantial hyperglycemia during major surgery in neonates. Such hyperglycemic responses may be associated with poorer neurologic outcome, particularly after a period of cerebral ischemia.[162] The use of high doses of fentanyl (>50 µg/kg) has been shown to reduce the hormonal stress response and resultant hyperglycemia and may lessen the risk of neurologic injury.[163]

In sufficient doses, opioids can blunt the stress responses in neonates, infants, and adults.[164-166] This blunting results in a more normal, homeostatic humoral and metabolic milieu in the circulation by reducing neuroendocrine activation and levels of regulating hormones. In infants, the use of high-dose opioids for major surgical procedures and postoperative sedation substantially attenuates the neuroendocrine response to surgically induced pain and stress. Catecholamine release that results from intraoperative stress responses may predispose the vulnerable myocardium to dysrhythmias. In neonates with HLHS, sudden ventricular fibrillation occurred in 50% of neonates during surgical manipulation until high doses of fentanyl were introduced as the primary anesthetic agent.[167] With the use of high-dose opioids, intraoperative ventricular fibrillation has virtually disappeared as a problem in this group of neonates.[168] In several studies, opioids have been shown to increase the ventricular fibrillation threshold in isolated cardiac Purkinje fibers and to alter action potential duration similar to that with class III antiarrhythmic agents.[169,170] Thus, even electrophysiologic events in the neonatal heart, in addition to humoral and hemodynamic responses, may be altered by using high-dose fentanyl anesthesia to attenuate the effects of pain and stress in neonates.

Reducing the Stress Response to Surgery and Bypass

Corticosteroids

Corticosteroids are used in many centers in an attempt to reduce the inflammatory response to surgery and bypass.[171] However, there is a huge variability in the formulation of the corticosteroids used, the doses, the timing of administration, and the indications for their use. The literature lacks adequate evidence for the use of corticosteroids, although there are a number of small studies in humans and animals that suggest they confer a benefit.[172,173] Many authors have called for a large multicenter study to determine the benefit of corticosteroids before bypass and for the optimal dose and timing.[174]

Aprotinin

Aprotinin, which was originally used to reduce bleeding after CPB, is now also appreciated to was shown to confer significant anti-inflammatory effect.[175-179] In adults, it was shown to reduce mortality and length of ICU stay.[180] In children, it improves pulmonary function in the postoperative period and also reduces the time to extubation and ICU stay.

Allopurinol

Allopurinol is thought to provide protection against oxygen free radicals during reperfusion by inhibiting xanthine oxidase. It reduces oxygen free radical production and may reduce neurologic and cardiac damage after deep hypothermic cardiac arrest.[181] This strategy does not appear to have developed widespread use.

Ischemic Preconditioning

It is now accepted that the heart is capable of short-term rapid adaptation to brief ischemia such that during a subsequent, more severe ischemic insult, myocardial necrosis is delayed. The infarct-delaying properties of ischemic preconditioning have been observed in all species studied. Five minutes of ischemia is sufficient to initiate preconditioning, and the protective period lasts for 1 to 2 hours. Laboratory experiments have demonstrated that the stimulation of adenosine receptors initiates preconditioning and the intracellular signal transduction mechanisms involve protein kinase C and adenosine triphosphate (ATP)–dependent potassium channels, although there may be some differences between species. An analysis of studies on myocardial infarction in humans has demonstrated that some adults who report having had angina in the days before infarction have a better outcome after their infarction in part due to the ischemic preconditioning. More direct evidence has come from an investigation of adults undergoing percutaneous transluminal angioplasty in whom the ST-segment changes induced by balloon inflation were more marked during the first inflation than the second. In adults undergoing coronary artery bypass grafting, the decline in ATP content during the first 10 minutes of ischemia was reduced in those subjected to a brief preconditioning protocol.[182-186] It is now thought that it may be possible to protect organs other than the heart by ischemic preconditioning.

It may even be possible to protect organs "remotely" by producing a period of ischemia in one area such as a limb, which then confers protection to "remote" organs.[187] Cheung and coworkers have demonstrated that the use of a blood pressure cuff to produce short periods of limb ischemia can produce beneficial effects on the heart, lungs, and generalized inflammatory response.[188]

Glucose-Insulin and Potassium

The use of glucose-insulin and potassium has been advocated for more than 40 years in adult cardiac surgery. It is thought to protect the myocardium from the effects of ischemia caused by aortic cross clamping.[189-192] Its effects have not been studied in children undergoing cardiac surgery.

Anesthetic Considerations for Specific Cardiac Defects

Specific discussion of anesthetic considerations for repair of every form of congenital heart disease is beyond the scope of this chapter. However, a brief discussion of the problems that may be encountered during repair of the more common congenital heart lesions is presented. It is useful however to group lesions together because the management principles can be applied more generally within groups (Table 15-3).

"Simple" Left-to-Right Shunts

These shunts result in increased pulmonary blood flow. If the shunt is large, blood flow to the lungs can be threefold to fourfold greater than normal, resulting in volume loading of the right side of the heart. This, in turn, leads to right atrial enlargement and right ventricular hypertrophy perhaps associated with tricuspid and pulmonary regurgitation. This combination results in cardiac failure (Table 15-4).

Medical management of these children includes the use of diuretics sometimes in combination with digoxin. If pulmonary blood flow is large and left untreated, pulmonary vascular disease begins to develop, resulting in pulmonary hypertension.

Table 15-3. Classification of Congenital Heart Disease

"Simple" Left-to-Right Shunt: Increased Pulmonary Blood Flow
Atrial septal defect (ASD)
Ventricular septal defect (VSD)
Patent ductus arteriosus (PDA)
Endocardial cushion defect (e.g., atrioventricular septal defect [AVSD])
Aortopulmonary window (AP window)
"Simple" Right-to-Left Shunt: Decreased Pulmonary Blood Flow with Cyanosis
Tetralogy of Fallot (TOF)
Pulmonary atresia
Tricuspid atresia
Ebstein anomaly
Complex Shunts: Mixing of Pulmonary and Systemic Blood Flow with Cyanosis
Transposition of great arteries (TGA)
Truncus arteriosus
Total anomalous pulmonary venous drainage (TAPVD)
Double-outlet right ventricle (DORV)
Hypoplastic left heart syndrome (HLHS)
Obstructive Lesions
Aortic stenosis
Mitral stenosis
Pulmonary stenosis
Coarctation of aorta
Interrupted aortic arch

Table 15-4. Clinical Features of Cardiac Failure in Children

Failure to thrive
Difficult feeding
Breathlessness
Recurrent chest infection
Tachycardia
Cardiac murmur
Hepatomegaly
Cardiomegaly
Pulmonary plethora
Wheezing

In the early stages the changes are reversible, but in time, the changes may become irreversible.[193-198] Eisenmenger's syndrome refers to severe pulmonary hypertension that leads to suprasystemic pulmonary artery pressures that cause the shunt to reverse, leading to cyanosis. The previous left-to-right shunt becomes a right-to-left shunt. At this point the child's condition becomes inoperable. Increasingly, definitive surgery is being performed at a younger age to reduce the risk of developing pulmonary vascular disease. If early definitive surgery is not possible, a pulmonary artery band is applied to reduce pulmonary blood flow. This is performed through a sternotomy incision but without the need for CPB. This provides the infant the opportunity to grow, postponing the need for definitive surgery without increasing the risk of developing pulmonary hypertension. In the presence of significantly increased pulmonary blood flow, pulmonary vascular disease is often severe and irreversible by 1 year of age. Definitive surgery should be performed between 3 and 6 months of age to avoid this complication.

Atrial Septal Defect

Atrial septal defect is a common heart defect in children, occurring in 1:1500 live births and accounting for approximately 10% of all CHD.[199] Several different types of ASDs exist.

- Patent foramen ovale (PFO). A PFO is a normal fetal communication between the two atria that usually closes soon after birth. In up to 30% of people the PFO remains patent; PFO is usually left untreated in children.
- Primum ASD (Fig. 15-1A); this is located in the inferior part of the atrial septum close to the AV valve and may be associated with a cleft mitral valve. This is a variant of AV septal defect (AVSD).
- Secundum ASD (Fig. 15-1B); this is found in the region of the fossa ovalis and results from a deficiency in the septum secundum.
- Sinus venosus ASD (Fig. 15-1C); this occurs high in the atrial septum often close to the opening of the SVC. It may be associated with partial anomalous pulmonary venous drainage.
- Coronary sinus ASD (unroofed coronary sinus); a defect in the atrial wall allows blood to flow from the left atrium to right atrium through the coronary sinus.
- Common atrium: there is complete absence of the atrial septum. The AV valves may be abnormal or unaffected.

Many ASDs can now be closed using a percutaneous, transcatheter device. PFO and secundum ASDs are most commonly closed using this technique.

Anesthetic Considerations

- These children can frequently be extubated on the operating table or early in the ICU and smaller doses of opioid can be used. Alternatively, short-acting drugs such as (remifentanil) by infusion possibly in combination with propofol are useful if early extubation is planned.
- The problems of postoperative pulmonary hypertension are seldom encountered.

Ventricular Septal Defect

This is the most common congenital defect in children, occurring in 1.5 to 3.5 per 1,000 live births and accounting for 20% of CHD in children (Fig. 15-2A).[200] Four types are described: subarterial (5%), perimembranous (80%), inlet (5%), and muscular (10%). If the flow through the VSD is small, it is referred to as "restrictive," whereas if the flow is large, it is called "unrestrictive." It is now possible to close a small percent of VSDs using a percutaneous, transcatheter device.

Anesthetic Considerations

- Inotropic support may be required postoperatively.
- Postoperative pulmonary hypertension may be a problem if the left-to-right shunt has been significant preoperatively or if the surgery is undertaken late.

Atrioventricular Septal Defect

These lesions are also known as AV canal defects or endocardial cushion defects and result from a defect in the AV septum. They occur in about 0.2 per 1,000 live births and account for about 3% of CHD. They are commonly associated with trisomy 21. They may come associated with other cardiac lesions such as tetralogy of Fallot and DiGeorge syndrome (Table 15-5).

Two common types of AVSD exist:

- Partial AVSD. This usually consists of a primum ASD with a cleft in the anterior mitral valve leaflet (Fig. 15-1A).
- Complete AVSD. This consists of a large septal defect with both atrial and ventricular components and a common AV valve (Fig. 15-2B).

Further description of AVSD refers to "balanced" or "unbalanced," depending on whether the AV valve is stenotic or atretic or if some of the valve chordae are straddling (i.e., crossing to the other side of) the ventricular septum. The hemodynamic effects associated with AVSD include shunting at the atrial or ventricular level and AV valve regurgitation.

Anesthetic Considerations

- If the child has trisomy 21, the anesthetic implications of this need to be managed.
- Inotropes are frequently required.
- Postoperative pulmonary hypertension may occur.
- TEE is particularly helpful in assessing the repair of the left AV valve.
- Heart block may occur postoperatively.

Aortopulmonary Window

This rare CHD defect in which there is a communication between the main pulmonary artery and the ascending aorta accounts for 0.1% of CHD (Fig. 15-3). The defect is classified depending on its size and exact position into four types.[201] A left-to-right shunt is usually present. These children present in heart failure and are at risk of developing pulmonary vascular

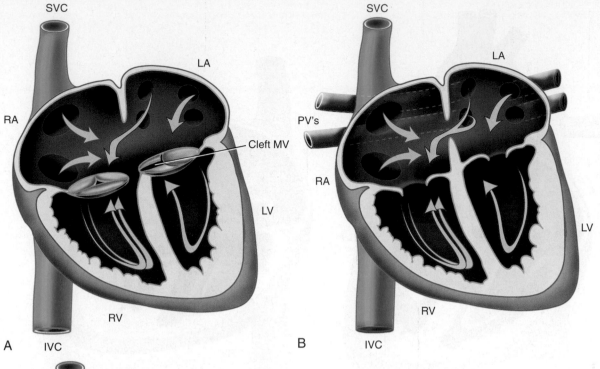

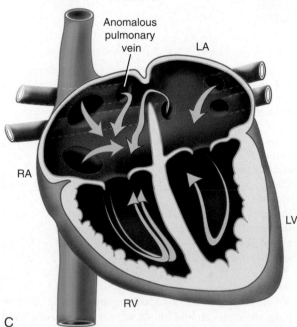

Figure 15-1. A, Diagram of primum ASD with great vessels removed showing left-to-right shunt through defect and cleft of the mitral valve, also called a partial AVSD. **B,** Diagram of secundum ASD with great vessels removed showing left-to-right shunt through the defect. **C,** Diagram of sinus venosus ASD showing left-to-right shunt through defect close to superior vena cava and also an anomalous pulmonary vein draining to right atrium. SVC, superior vena cava; IVC, inferior vena cava; RA, right atrium; RV, right ventricle; LA, left atrium; LV, left ventricle; MV, mitral valve; PV's, pulmonary veins. (Adapted with permission from May LE: Pediatric Heart Surgery: A Ready Reference for Professionals; Milwaukee, WI, Maxishare, 2005.)

disease if not treated early. It is frequently associated with other anomalies both cardiac and noncardiac:

- VACTERL
- CHARGE
- CATCH-22 association
- DiGeorge syndrome

Anesthetic Considerations

- Postoperative pulmonary hypertension may be problematic.
- Inotropes may be required.

Patent Ductus Arteriosus

The ductus arteriosus, a remnant from the fetal circulation, extends from the descending aorta to the main pulmonary artery and usually closes soon after birth. However, it remains patent in approximately 1 in 2,500 live births and accounts for about 10% of all CHD (Fig. 15-4). In the fetus, blood from the right ventricle is directed into the pulmonary artery but because of the high PVR it flows into the descending aorta. After birth, however, the PVR decreases and blood flows from the aorta to the lungs. PDA is common in preterm infants, and its presence may explain an ongoing requirement for mechanical ventilation.

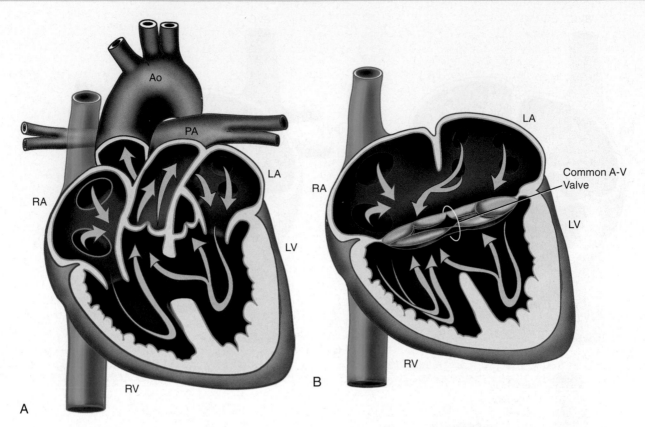

Figure 15-2. A, Diagram of ventricular septal defect showing left-to-right shunt. **B,** Diagram of complete atrioventricular septal defect (AVSD) with great vessels removed showing left-to-right shunt through both atrial and ventricular components of the defect and also a single common atrioventricular valve. RA, right atrium; RV, right ventricle; LA, left atrium; LV, left ventricle; PA, pulmonary artery; Ao, aorta. (Adapted with permission from May LE: Pediatric Heart Surgery: A Ready Reference for Professionals; Milwaukee, WI, Maxishare, 2005.)

In these small infants, a left thoracotomy is required to ligate or divide the PDA. It may also occur in older children; but, at this age, percutaneous closure by an interventional cardiologist is the preferred approach. The anesthetic implications are similar to those of other lesions described with left-to-right shunts preoperatively.

In many centers PDA closure in preterm infants who weigh less than 1000 g and who are already mechanically ventilated is undertaken in the neonatal intensive care unit (NICU). This avoids the need to transfer these very small infants to the operating theater and the associated problems, particularly hypothermia.

Preoperative requirements include:
- Crossmatched blood
- Antibiotics (risk of endocarditis)

Table 15-5. Clinical Features and Concerns of DiGeorge Syndrome

Absent or small thymus
T-cell abnormality with associated immunodeficiency
Hypoparathyroidism with associated hypocalcemia
Dysmorphic features, particularly small mouth
Increased surgical morbidity and mortality
Irradiated blood products needed to prevent graft-versus-host disease

- Vitamin K

Particular perioperative risks include:
- Difficult ventilation or desaturation because of lung retraction
- Tearing of PDA with massive hemorrhage
- Inadvertent ligation of aorta or pulmonary artery
- Endocarditis
- Paradoxical air embolism

Monitoring

This should include all the standard monitors, but in addition two pulse oximeters should be placed, one on the right hand and one on a lower limb. If the pulse is lost from the lower limb during a test clamping of the duct, this might indicate that the aorta has been clamped inadvertently.

Invasive blood pressure monitoring is helpful if already established or if it can be placed reasonably quickly but is not absolutely necessary.

Monitors used in nonoperating room sites may not be compatible with the electrocautery equipment, thus resulting in loss of monitoring whenever the cautery is utilized. Additionally, the NICU may not have end-tidal carbon dioxide monitors, thus necessitating that such a device be brought from the operating room to the NICU. Other essential anesthetic equipment such as blood warmers, drug infusion pumps, and operating room intravenous and blood transfusions systems may also need to be brought to the NICU.

Anesthetic Considerations

- A dedicated intravenous line for fluids and drugs with a long (100-150 cm) low-caliber extension to allow access from a distance (space around the cots in NICU is limited)
- High-dose opioids
- Muscle relaxation
- The tracheal tube should have only a small air leak. A large leak will make ventilation difficult during lung retraction (recheck security and correct position of the tip of the tube before starting surgery).
- Intercostal nerve block by surgeon at completion of surgery
- Glucose-containing fluids maintained at basal rates

"Simple" Right-to-Left Shunts

Tetralogy of Fallot

Tetralogy of Fallot is the most common cyanotic CHD defect and accounts for 6% to 11% of CHD. The four features of the tetralogy (Fig. 15-5) are:

- VSD
- Overriding aorta
- Right ventricular outflow tract obstruction (RVOTO)
- Right ventricular hypertrophy

The RVOTO ranges from mild to severe, and the level of the obstruction also varies. Commonly, a dynamic subpulmonary

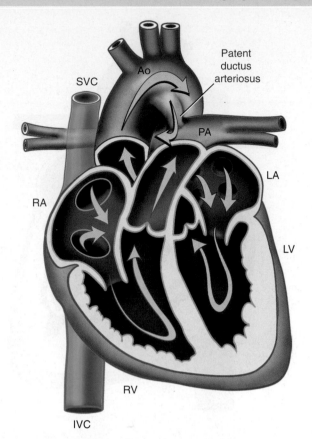

Figure 15-4. Patent ductus arteriosus showing left-to-right shunt. RA, right atrium; RV, right ventricle; LA, left atrium; LV, left ventricle; PA, pulmonary artery; Ao, aorta. (Adapted with permission from May LE: Pediatric Heart Surgery: A Ready Reference for Professionals; Milwaukee, WI, Maxishare, 2005.)

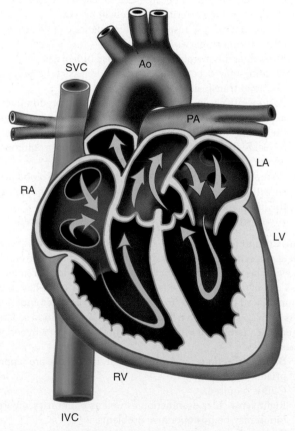

Figure 15-3. Diagram of aortopulmonary window showing left-to-right shunt through the defect. SVC, superior vena cava; IVC, inferior vena cava; RA, right atrium; LA, left atrium; PA, pulmonary artery; Ao, aorta. (Adapted with permission from May LE: Pediatric Heart Surgery: A Ready Reference for Professionals; Milwaukee, WI, Maxishare, 2005.)

infundibular obstruction is present. Dynamic narrowing of the infundibulum is frequently the cause of hypercyanotic "spells," also known as "tet spells," in which there is an increase in the shunting of blood from right to left. However, the RVOTO may also be at the level of the pulmonary valve or main or branch pulmonary arteries. Indeed, pulmonary atresia may exist as a variant of TOF. Children with pulmonary atresia who have well-developed pulmonary arteries derive their pulmonary blood supply from a PDA. By contrast, those with hypoplastic pulmonary arteries derive their pulmonary blood supply from major aortopulmonary collateral arteries.

The right-to-left shunt and cyanosis observed in children with TOF results from a combination of the RVOTO and VSD. The degree of hypoxemia depends on the relationship between the RVOTO and the SVR that determines the degree of right-to-left shunting. TOF may be associated with a large number of other cardiac and extracardiac anomalies. Extracardiac anomalies include DiGeorge syndrome and trisomy 21.

Hypercyanotic "Spells"

These episodes of cyanosis occur in 20% to 70% of untreated children. They may be initiated by crying or feeding, and they may occur during anesthesia. The cause of these spells is unclear, but metabolic acidosis, increased Pco_2, circulating catecholamines, and surgical stimulation are implicated.

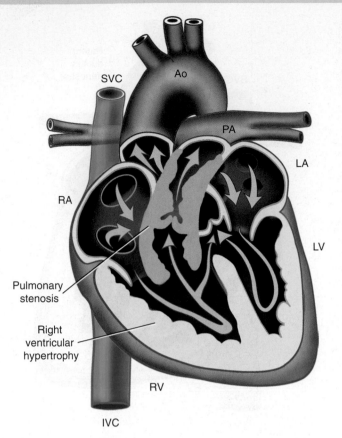

Figure 15-5. Tetralogy of Fallot. This diagram shows the features of the tetralogy: VSD, overriding aorta, right ventricular hypertrophy and pulmonary stenosis. Shown here is both pulmonary and subpulmonary obstruction. The result is right-to-left shunting resulting in cyanosis. AVC, superior vena cava; RA, right atrium; RV, right ventricle; LA, left atrium; LV, left ventricle; PA, pulmonary artery; Ao, aorta. (Adapted with permission from May LE: Pediatric Heart Surgery: A Ready Reference for Professionals; Milwaukee, WI, Maxishare, 2005.)

Management includes:
- 100% oxygen
- Hyperventilation
- Intravenous fluid bolus
- Sedation (e.g., fentanyl)
- Sodium bicarbonate
- Vasoconstriction
  - Norepinephrine, 0.5 µg/kg bolus then 0.1 to 0.5 µg/kg/min
  - Phenylephrine, 5 µg/kg bolus then 1 to 5 µg/kg/min (larger bolus doses may be required in small preterm infants)
- β blockers to relax infundibular spasm and reduce heart rate
  - Propranolol, 0.1 to 0.3 mg/kg bolus

Surgical Management

The optimum surgical management of children with TOF remains controversial. The choice is between initial palliation with a systemic-to-pulmonary shunt followed by a complete repair when the infant is older versus complete repair during the neonatal or early infant period. Currently, the trend is toward early complete repair.[202,203] Complete repair involves closure of the VSD and relief of the RVOTO. The relief of the RVOTO most commonly involves a transannular patch that involves a right ventriculotomy. Right ventricular dysfunction is a particular problem after repair, and a degree of pulmonary regurgitation is almost always present. Junctional ectopic tachycardia is a particular risk after complete correction.

Anesthetic Considerations

Systemic-to-Pulmonary Shunt. Most frequently this will be a modified Blalock-Taussig shunt; this is a shunt from the subclavian artery to a branch pulmonary artery.
- Child usually a neonate or small infant
- Sedative premedication useful to prevent crying during induction, which may provoke hypercyanotic spell
- Risk of hypercyanotic spell during induction and surgery
- Inhalational or intravenous induction appropriate
- Surgery usually through a thoracotomy (left or right) but may be through sternotomy
- CPB not required
- Arterial and central venous access required
- Endotracheal tube should be "snug" with no air leak because lung retraction during surgery makes ventilation very difficult.
- Arterial line should not be in the arm on the side that the shunt will be placed because the subclavian artery will be clamped and the arterial pressure will be lost.
- Hemodynamic and respiratory disturbance can be problematical during surgery.
- The surgeon may request a small dose of heparin.
- Bleeding may occur after clamps are released; be prepared for blood transfusion.
- Postoperatively pulmonary blood supply is predominantly dependent on the size of the shunt. If the shunt is too small the infant will remain with a low saturation; if the shunt is too large the infant may develop heart failure or pulmonary edema.
- Pulmonary blood flow also depends on systemic blood pressure; the greater the blood pressure, the more blood flows to the lungs and the higher is the saturation.
- A period of postoperative ventilation may be required.

For Complete Repair. If the child is scheduled for early complete correction with no systemic pulmonary shunt, the child is likely to be a neonate or small infant. These children remain at risk for hypercyanotic spells. If, however, the child has had a shunt placed previously, he or she is likely to be older and much less likely to suffer from a hypercyanotic episode. Good sedative premedication is more important in those at risk of a hypercyanotic episode.
- Both intravenous and inhalational induction are appropriate.
- CPB is required.
- Right ventricular dysfunction as well as pulmonary regurgitation may be postoperative problems.
- Too much inotrope may worsen RVOTO postoperatively by dynamic narrowing of RVOT.
- Milrinone may be particularly useful because it promotes diastolic relaxation of the stiff right ventricle.
- Pyrexia and excessive β-adrenergic stimulation may help precipitate junctional ectopic tachycardia postoperatively.

- Surgeons will frequently measure right ventricular pressure to assess quality of the repair.
- Perioperative echocardiography is useful in assessing repair and right ventricular function.

Complex Shunts. In complex shunts there is mixing of pulmonary and systemic blood flow with cyanosis.

Transposition of the Great Arteries

Transposition of the great arteries is common and accounts for about 6% of all CHD. It frequently occurs as an isolated lesion and is rarely associated with extracardiac anomalies. The operation most commonly performed in these infants is the arterial switch operation (ASO), the short- and long-term results of which have improved to such an extent that children with a good repair can expect a normal life.

TGA refers to the situation in which the aorta arises from the morphologic right ventricle and the pulmonary artery arises from the morphologic left ventricle (Fig. 15-6). This is known as ventriculoarterial (VA) discordance, and the atria are related to the ventricles in the normal way (i.e., AV concordance). This results in two circulations that run in parallel rather than in series, which is the normal anatomic arrangement. Without some mixing of the two circulations, the systemic circulation

would remain completely deoxygenated. However, some mixing does occur through the PDA or through a VSD that is present in approximately 25% of cases. If there is no VSD and mixing is inadequate, ductal patency is maintained after birth with the use of intravenous prostaglandin infusion, and a balloon atrial septostomy is performed urgently in the neonatal period.

In TGA with intact ventricular septum, it is important to perform the ASO early in the neonatal period, preferably in the first 2 to 3 weeks of life because the left ventricle is exposed only to the pressure of the pulmonary circulation. The longer this situation is allowed to continue, the less the left ventricle is able to adapt to the work required to pump blood at systemic pressure after the ASO. If, however, there is an unrestrictive VSD, both the left and right ventricles are exposed to systemic blood pressure and the left ventricle is better conditioned to perform the work of the systemic ventricle after the ASO.

If not treated, the majority of infants with TGA die in the first year of life from hypoxia and heart failure. Pulmonary vascular disease develops early in these infants and contributes to this high mortality.[204,205] The mechanism for the early development of pulmonary vascular disease is complex and not simply related to high pulmonary blood flow; however, the presence of a VSD further accelerates this process. This means that these infants are at risk of developing pulmonary hypertensive crises in the postoperative period.[206]

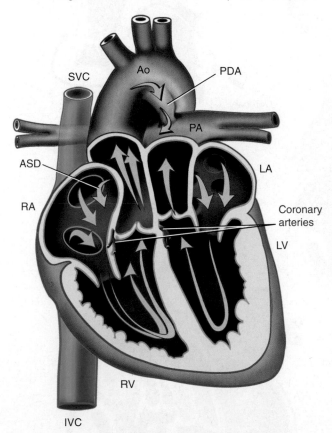

Figure 15-6. Diagram of transposition of the great vessels (TGA). Shown here is TGA with intact ventricular septum. The aorta arises from the right ventricle, and the pulmonary artery arises from the left ventricle. The coronary arteries are shown arising from the aorta. These children are cyanosed. SVC, superior vena cava; IVC, inferior vena cava; Ao, aorta; RA, right atrium; RV, right ventricle; LA, left atrium; LV, left ventricle; PA, pulmonary artery. (Adapted with permission from May LE: Pediatric Heart Surgery: A Ready Reference for Professionals; Milwaukee, WI, Maxishare, 2005.)

Surgical Options

Arterial Switch Operation. This is the operation of choice if the intracardiac anatomy is appropriate. The ASO involves transecting the two main arterial trunks distal to their respective valves and "switching" them to produce VA concordance (Fig. 15-7). It also involves disconnecting the coronary arteries from the "old" aorta and reconnecting them to the neo-aorta. This restores anatomic and physiologic normality. The coronary anatomy varies widely in TGA but must be well assessed preoperatively because moving the coronary arteries to the neo-aorta is the most difficult and most crucial part of a successful outcome after the ASO. In a proportion of cases, the coronary arteries run in the wall of the aorta (intramural), and this poses particular difficulties for the surgeon. Clearly, ventricular function after surgery depends largely on unrestricted flow in the coronary arteries.

Mustard and Senning Procedures. The Mustard or Senning procedures are atrial switch procedures. These involve the use of intra-atrial baffles to redirect deoxygenated blood from the venae cavae to the left atrium, left ventricle, and pulmonary artery and oxygenated pulmonary venous blood to the right atrium, right ventricle, and aorta. They create AV discordance, restore physiologic but not anatomic normality, and leave the physiologic right ventricle as the systemic ventricle. These procedures were performed as definitive procedures before the arterial switch became successful but are rarely used today as definitive repairs. They are still, however, used as palliation in those children with TGA, VSD, and pulmonary vascular disease.[207] In these cases the VSD is left open.

Rastelli Procedure. The Rastelli procedure is used in children with TGA, VSD, and left ventricular outflow tract obstruction (LVOTO). The basis of the procedure is to close the VSD in such a way as to direct blood from the left ventricle to the aorta. The

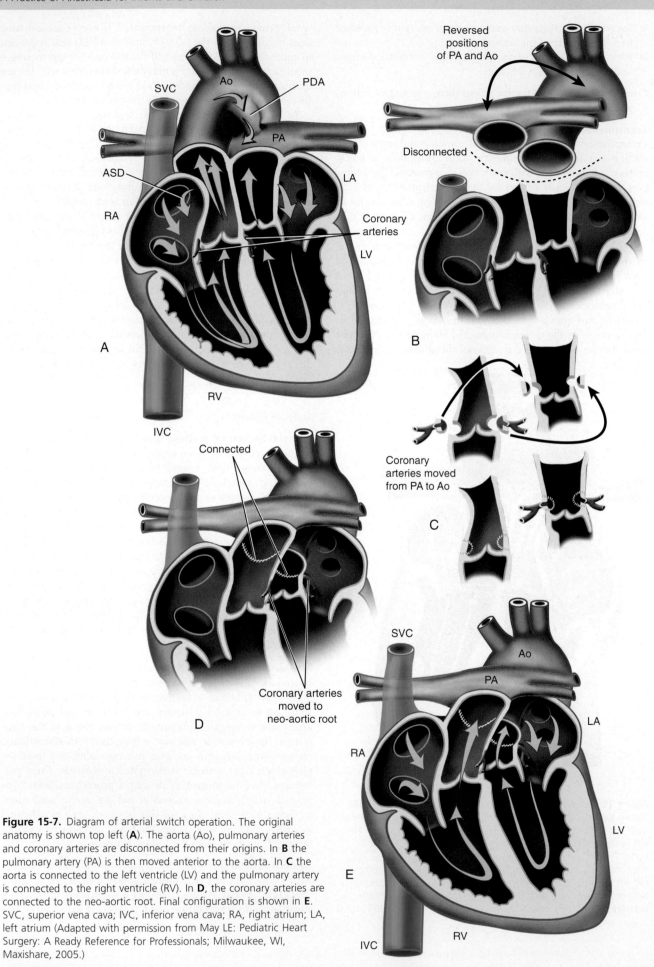

Figure 15-7. Diagram of arterial switch operation. The original anatomy is shown top left (**A**). The aorta (Ao), pulmonary arteries and coronary arteries are disconnected from their origins. In **B** the pulmonary artery (PA) is then moved anterior to the aorta. In **C** the aorta is connected to the left ventricle (LV) and the pulmonary artery is connected to the right ventricle (RV). In **D**, the coronary arteries are connected to the neo-aortic root. Final configuration is shown in **E**. SVC, superior vena cava; IVC, inferior vena cava; RA, right atrium; LA, left atrium (Adapted with permission from May LE: Pediatric Heart Surgery: A Ready Reference for Professionals; Milwaukee, WI, Maxishare, 2005.)

pulmonary artery is ligated just distal to the pulmonary valve, and a valved conduit is inserted from the right ventricle to the pulmonary artery. The result of this is continuity between the left ventricle and aorta and between the right ventricle and the pulmonary artery. In addition the LVOTO (subpulmonary area) is bypassed. In the past, the Rastelli procedure was performed at 2 to 3 years of age with a Blalock-Taussig shunt performed for palliation in the neonatal period. However, there is now a trend toward neonatal Rastelli repair without the need for a shunt.

Anesthetic Considerations for the Arterial Switch Procedure
- Neonate in the first few weeks of life
- Inhalational or intravenous induction
- Invasive arterial and central venous lines required. If VSD closure is required, bicaval cannulation may be required for CPB and internal jugular central venous pressure may interfere with this and a femoral central venous pressure line may be preferable. If no VSD is present, a single venous cannula in the atrium will be used for CPB and the internal jugular vein can be used.
- Myocardial ischemia in the period after the cross clamp is removed may be related to coronary air emboli or poor coronary anastomoses. A generous perfusion pressure after removal of cross clamp will encourage flushing air from coronary arteries. If ischemia is thought to be due to an anatomic problem with the coronary arteries, they should be reanastomosed immediately.
- TEE is useful in assessing adequate de-airing, myocardial function, and adequacy of coronary anastomoses.
- Post CPB myocardial dysfunction may be due to one or more of the following:
  - An inherently poor left ventricle
  - Poor myocardial protection
  - Poor coronary transference
  - Coronary air
- Pulmonary hypertension is possible and one needs a high index of suspicion
- Inotropes are almost always required. Dopamine or epinephrine can be used, and milrinone is a particularly useful agent in these cases because of its inodilation.
- Left atrial dilation should be avoided if possible. This is because after the repair the pulmonary artery is anterior to the aorta and close to the origin of the coronaries. Left atrial dilation causes pulmonary hypertension and dilation of the pulmonary artery, which may distort or compress the coronary arteries. Every effort should be made to keep the left atrial pressure low, and this includes giving fluid boluses very carefully. A left atrial monitoring line is often left in place.
- Post-bypass coagulopathy
- Aprotinin frequently used

Truncus Arteriosus

Truncus arteriosus is a rare congenital heart defect that occurs in about 0.7 per 1000 live births and accounts for about 1% of all CHD. The basic lesion is that of a common arterial outlet for the aorta and pulmonary artery associated with a single valve and a VSD (Fig. 15-8). There are three types described, depending on how the pulmonary arteries arise from the aorta and on the size of the aorta. Blood mixes at the arterial level with a resultant high pulmonary blood flow. This leads to heart failure and the early development of pulmonary hypertension. As

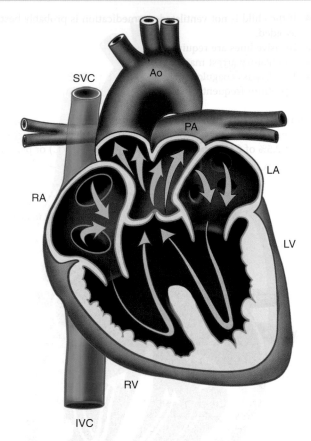

Figure 15-8. Diagram of truncus arteriosus showing common truncal valve and mixing of red and blue blood. SVC, superior vena cava; IVC, inferior vena cava; Ao, aorta; RA, right atrium; RV, right ventricle; LA, left atrium; LV, left ventricle; PA, pulmonary artery. (Adapted with permission from May LE: Pediatric Heart Surgery: A Ready Reference for Professionals; Milwaukee, WI, Maxishare, 2005.)

a result, surgery must be performed early in life to prevent pulmonary hypertension from becoming irreversible. Truncus arteriosus is associated with DiGeorge syndrome. Irradiated blood products should be used and calcium levels carefully monitored.

Surgical repair involves separating the systemic from the pulmonary circulation and closure of the VSD. This involves disconnecting the pulmonary artery/arteries from the aorta and repairing the truncal valve. The pulmonary arteries are then connected to the right ventricle usually with a valved conduit. Circulatory arrest may be required. Early postoperative mortality is high and varies from between 5% and 25%. Factors that particularly influence mortality are truncal valve stenosis, coronary abnormalities, and low birth weight.

Anesthetic Considerations
- Small neonate in the first month of life
- High-risk procedure
- Presence of heart failure
- Risk of postoperative pulmonary hypertensive crisis
- Patients may already be intubated and ventilated and may already be on inotropes

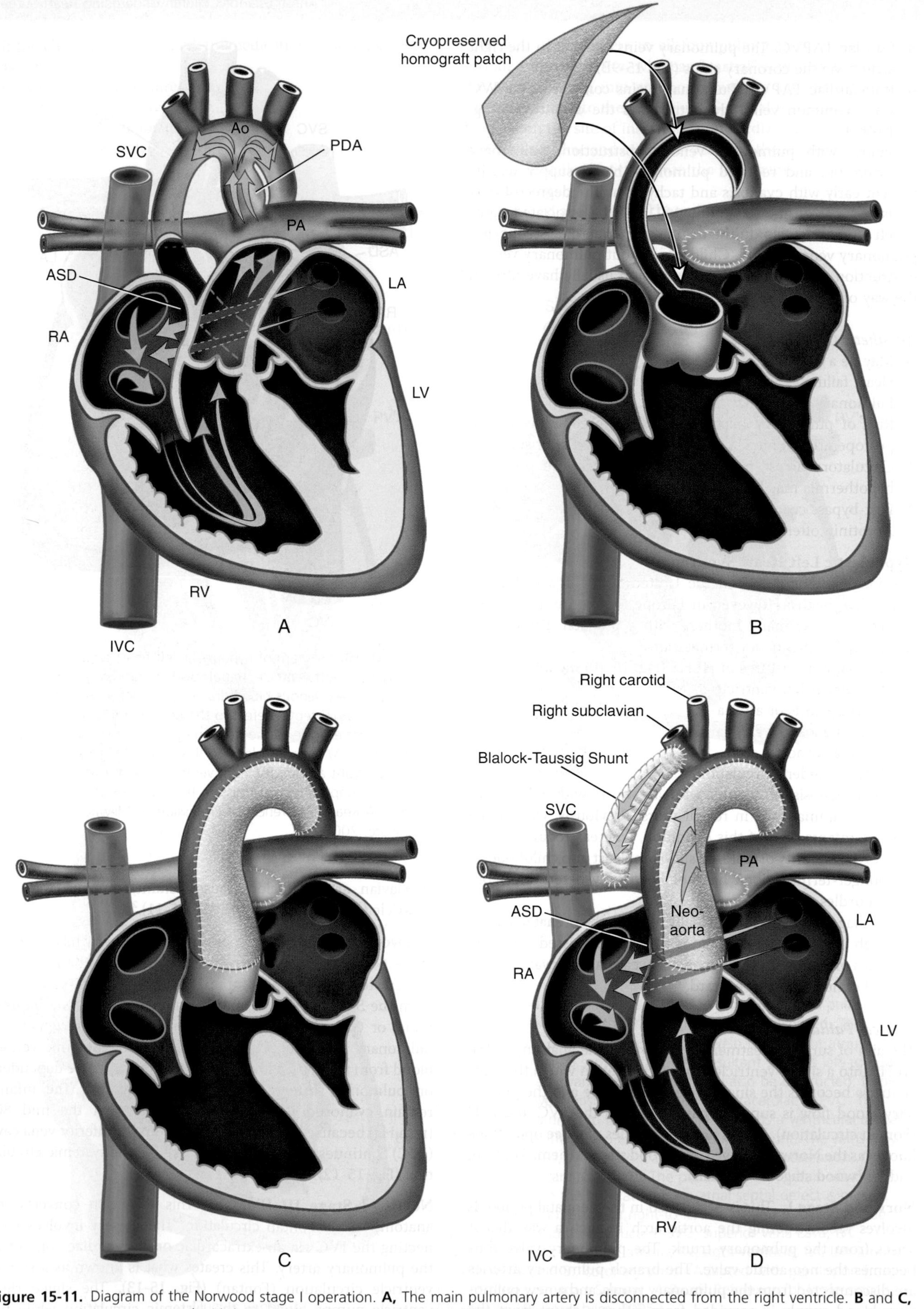

Figure 15-11. Diagram of the Norwood stage I operation. **A,** The main pulmonary artery is disconnected from the right ventricle. **B** and **C,** The aortic arch is reconstructed with homograft and connected to the right ventricle, which becomes a single ventricle. **D,** Pulmonary blood is then supplied by a Blalock-Taussig shunt from the subclavian artery to the pulmonary artery. The children remain cyanosed. PDA, patent ductus arteriosus; SVC, superior vena cava; IVC, inferior vena cava; Ao, aorta; RA, right atrium; RV, right ventricle; LA, left atrium; LV, left ventricle; PA, pulmonary artery. (Adapted with permission from May LE: Pediatric Heart Surgery: A Ready Reference for Professionals; Milwaukee, WI, Maxishare, 2005.)

valve[...]
How[...]

Coarctatio[...]
Coarctatio[...]
and accou[...]
lesion is of[...]
The follow[...]
however, o[...]
such as VS[...]
malities. Th[...]
ductal, dep[...]
The most c[...]
preductal t[...]
collateral c[...]
glandin to[...]
ductal coa[...]
collateral v[...]
is importar[...]
erals and i[...]
aortic cros[...]
two groups[...]
preductal [...]
ventricular[...]
older than[...]
better left[...]
poor left [...]
Femoral pu[...]
acidosis. D[...]
sures in the[...]
sis) may in[...]

Anesthetic [...]
For neona[...]
- These i[...]
  They sh[...]
  gist sho[...]
  well.
- Some i[...]
  may be[...]
  not be.[...]
- Intraver[...]
  glandin[...]
  inductic[...]
  tanyl (u[...]
  this wit[...]
  be omit[...]
- Inotrop[...]
  be avail[...]
- Ideally,[...]
  allow b[...]
  clampir[...]
  during [...]
  the coa[...]
  cross c[...]
  because[...]
- A centr[...]
- Surgery[...]
  withou[...]
  tilation[...]
  trachea[...]

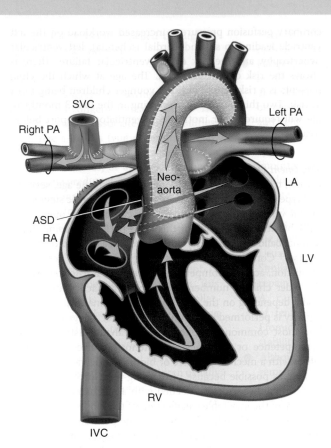

Figure 15-12. Diagram of Norwood stage 2 (hemi-Fontan) operation. The Blalock-Taussig shunt is disconnected, and a Glenn shunt is created by connecting the superior vena cava to the pulmonary artery. SVC, superior vena cava; IVC, inferior vena cava; RA, right atrium; RV, right ventricle; LA, left atrium; LV, left ventricle; PA, pulmonary artery. (Adapted with permission from May LE: Pediatric Heart Surgery: A Ready Reference for Professionals; Milwaukee, WI, Maxishare, 2005.)

pulmonary blood supply is provided by passive flow by systemic venous blood from the SVC and IVC. It is essential that PVR remains low because any increase in PVR will dramatically reduce pulmonary blood flow. It is common for a small hole (fenestration) to be created between the extracardiac conduit and the right atrium so that if the PVR rises, blood will be directed to the right atrium and allow cardiac output to be maintained. In this situation, the child becomes cyanosed but cardiac output is maintained, a much safer situation than a low cardiac output state. Postoperatively, increased systemic venous pressure may cause pleural effusions, enlarged liver, or protein-losing enteropathy. Later, if PVR remains consistently low, the fenestration can be closed with a transvenous device.

The long-term problem in these children is that the morphologic right ventricle that becomes the systemic ventricle fails over time. The only recourse in these children is for heart transplantation.[210,211]

Anesthetic Considerations
For stage I Norwood:
- It is essential that the anesthesiologist understands the anatomy and physiology of HLHS.

- It is important to maintain the balance between systemic and pulmonary circulation by balancing PVR and SVR. If the PVR decreases, blood flow will be directed away from the systemic circulation and the lungs will be flooded. This results in hypotension and hypoperfusion with increasing acidosis. If PVR increases cyanosis will increase. Before anesthesia, these infants are best managed spontaneously breathing in room air with a prostaglandin E_1 infusion to maintain ductal patency. However, if mechanical ventilation is required, it is important to maintain normal/high $Paco_2$ and very low Fio_2, usually with air.
- Air should be available for transfer to the operating room, or a self-inflating bag should be used.
- High-dose opioid technique is preferred.
- Venous access is gained via the femoral or umbilical veins. The internal jugular is avoided because narrowing of the SVC would jeopardize the Glenn shunt.
- Profound hypothermia may be required.
- Postoperative myocardial dysfunction is common, and inotropes will be required.
- Balancing systemic and pulmonary blood flow is an issue after bypass as well. Some centers use the long-acting α-adrenergic blocker phenoxybenzamine after bypass to reduce

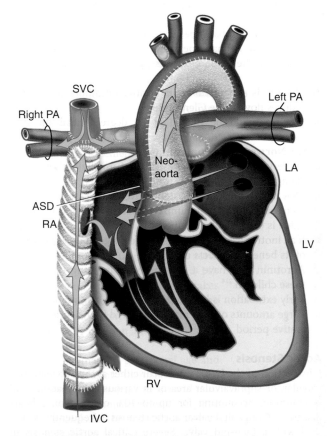

Figure 15-13. Diagram of Norwood stage 3 (Fontan) operation. The Fontan circulation is created by connecting the inferior vena cava to the pulmonary artery with a conduit. A fenestration is shown between the conduit and the right atrium. SVC, superior vena cava; IVC, inferior vena cava; RV, right ventricle; LA, left atrium; LV, left ventricle; PA, pulmonary artery. (Adapted with permission from May LE: Pediatric Heart Surgery: A Ready Reference for Professionals; Milwaukee, WI, Maxishare, 2005.)

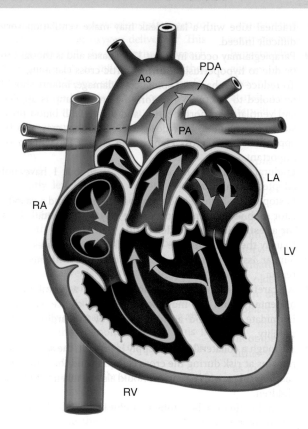

Figure 15-14. Diagram of interrupted aortic arch. The patent ductus arteriosus (PDA) supplies the body below the interruption. RA, right atrium; RV, right ventricle; LA, left atrium; LV, left ventricle; PA, pulmonary artery. (Adapted with permission from May LE: Pediatric Heart Surgery: A Ready Reference for Professionals; Milwaukee, WI, Maxishare, 2005.)

late. Mortality is increased with small size or acidosis preoperatively and if there are associated cardiac lesions.[227]

Anesthetic Considerations
- Small sick neonate
- DiGeorge syndrome (particularly hypocalcemia and need for irradiated blood products)
- High-dose opioid technique usual
- Ideally, blood pressure should be monitored above and below the interruption, but this is often difficult in practice.
- Deep hypothermic circulatory arrest may be used.
- Aprotinin is useful.
- Post-bypass coagulopathy
- Anticipate poor renal function postoperatively.

- There is a risk of postoperative pulmonary hypertensive crises.

These infants are likely to require reoperation to deal with recurrent LVOTO, which may occur at any level. Restenosis of the repaired aortic arch can be dilated with transluminal balloon dilatation.

Transport and Handover to Pediatric Intensive Care Unit

Once surgery is completed cardiac surgical patients need a period of intensive care. The first phase of this care is the transport of the children from the operating room to the PICU. This is a potentially hazardous time and requires good organization, teamwork, and appropriate equipment. Guidelines exist for the safe transport of these children.[228] The transport of these children to the PICU can be defined as the preparatory phase, the transport phase, and the stabilization phase.[229] The preparatory phase is when the estimated time of arrival in the PICU is communicated with the PICU. During this time, the bed space is prepared, ventilator and monitors are configured in an appropriate way, and any additional interventions that may be required are made ready. In my institution, a form is sent to the PICU that indicates the child's age and weight, the ventilator settings that will be required, the number of transducers that will be required, and the infusions that are running. After arrival in the PICU two basic tasks need to be undertaken: transfer of technology and transfer of information. It is better to allow the technology transfer to occur before the information handover. This includes ensuring that all the monitors are connected and working appropriately, that the ventilator is connected and delivering adequate ventilation, that all infusions are working, and that drains and urinary catheter are all in place with baseline readings noted. When this has been accomplished, the handover of information can start. This should be done with a single handover with all the appropriate personnel present and should include information given by the anesthesiologist and surgeon. In my institution a checklist is followed to ensure that no important information is omitted. It is important to avoid a large number of handovers being given between individuals rather than a single comprehensive handover with all the relevant personnel present.

Acknowledgment

The author wishes to thank Paul R. Hickey, Richard L. Marnach, Dolly D. Hansen, Robert W. Reid, and Frederick A. Burrows for their prior contributions to this chapter.

Annotated References

Arnold DM, Fergusson DA, Chan AK, et al: Avoiding transfusions in children undergoing cardiac surgery: a meta-analysis of randomized trials of aprotinin. Anesth Analg 2006; 102:731-737

In a meta-analysis of the use of aprotinin in children, these researchers found that the majority of published studies were of poor quality. They also noted that there were very wide differences in the doses used in children. Although they could not find any convincing evidence for the use of aprotinin in children, they commented that there was an urgent

need for further high-quality studies to determine the role of aprotinin in children undergoing cardiac surgery.

Andropoulos DB, Stayer SA, Diaz LK, Ramamoorthy C: Neurological monitoring for congenital heart surgery. Anesth Analg 2004; 99:1365-1375

This is a wide-ranging review of cerebral monitoring during cardiac surgery in children. The section on the use of cerebral oximetry is particularly relevant to clinical practice.

Bettex DA, Pretre R, Jenni R, Schmid ER: Cost-effectiveness of routine intraoperative transesophageal echocardiography in pediatric cardiac surgery: a 10-year experience. Anesth Analg 2005; 100:1271-1275

Bettex and coworkers showed in a retrospective study of 580 pediatric patients undergoing cardiac surgery that the use of routine intraoperative TEE was cost effective. They identified 33 children who required a second bypass run on the basis of the intraoperative TEE. The authors estimate that the savings per child were in the region of $690 to $2130.

Hoffman TM, Wernovsky G, Atz AM, et al: Prophylactic intravenous use of milrinone after cardiac operation in pediatrics (PRIMA-CORP) study. Prophylactic Intravenous Use of Milrinone After Cardiac Operation in Pediatrics. Am Heart J 2002; 143:15-21

In this large multicenter prospective randomized double-blind study it was shown that the use of milrinone in high doses (75 μg/kg bolus over 60 minutes followed by 0.75 μg/kg/min infusion) in infants undergoing complex congenital cardiac operations reduced the incidence of low cardiac output syndrome in the postoperative period.

Kern FH, Morana NJ, Sears JJ, Hickey PR. Coagulation defects in neonates during cardiopulmonary bypass. Ann Thorac Surg 1992; 54:541-546

Kern and colleagues showed that hemodilution is an important if not the most important factor in the development of post-bypass coagulopathy in neonates. They showed that platelets and coagulation factors were dramatically reduced as soon as the neonate was placed on CPB and were not significantly reduced further during CPB.

Malviya S, Voepel-Lewis T, Siewert M, et al: Risk factors for adverse postoperative outcomes in children presenting for cardiac surgery with upper respiratory tract infections. Anesthesiology 2003; 98:628-632

These investigators have shown that children with an upper respiratory tract infection at the time of cardiac surgery are at risk for more complications in the postoperative period and have a longer stay in the ICU. These children need very careful assessment before surgery, and the risk-benefit for the child must be considered.

Mangano DT, Tudor IC, Dietzel C: The risk associated with aprotinin in cardiac surgery. N Engl J Med 2006; 354:353-365.

Mangano and associates reported a large observational study in adult patients undergoing revascularization surgery. They reported an increase in renal failure, myocardial infarction, heart failure, stroke, and encephalopathy. This study has been criticized for not being a randomized study. These effects have not been shown in children, but it has created an unease about the use of aprotinin in children. It is important that well-designed, independent, large studies are carried out in children to establish the role of aprotinin.

Naik SK, Knight A, Elliott M: A prospective randomized study of a modified technique of ultrafiltration during pediatric open-heart surgery. Circulation 1991; 84(5 Suppl):III422-III431

Naik and colleagues were the first to report the use of modified ultrafiltration (MUF) after CPB in children. They showed a number of beneficial effects, including reduced total body water, higher hematocrit, higher blood pressure, less postoperative bleeding, and less requirement for inotropes. MUF is now used in many centers worldwide and has a number of benefits.

References

Please see www.expertconsult.com

Cardiac Physiology and Pharmacology

CHAPTER 16

Avinash C. Shukla, James M. Steven, and
Francis X. McGowan, Jr.

Cardiovascular Physiology

At birth, the normal neonatal cardiovascular system rapidly undergoes major alterations in the pattern of circulation. Although these changes are most dramatic in the first hours of life, the maturation process of the heart and circulation continues over the ensuing few years. In addition to the differences in pharmacokinetics discussed elsewhere in this text, neonates and infants manifest different cardiovascular pharmacodynamic responses to anesthetic drugs. An understanding of neonatal cardiovascular maturation will enable anesthesiologists caring for neonates and infants to anticipate their responses to perioperative management strategies.

Structural malformations of the cardiovascular system remain among the most common birth defects. In addition to the profound changes occurring during transitional circulation at birth, these infants are subjected to a variety of additional abnormal cardiovascular loading conditions imposed by the structural abnormality. Because congenital heart disease (CHD) often accompanies other organ system malformations, these children may present for a variety of noncardiac procedures. In addition, early cardiac interventions have created a new population of infants and young children who have undergone major reconstructive cardiac surgery. Despite interventions designed to minimize the physiologic burdens imposed by CHD, many of these "repairs" leave significant hemodynamic residua and sequelae (see Chapter 21). Anticipating these results and their functional consequences should constitute a substantial component of anesthetic planning and management.

Acquired cardiovascular disease is significantly less common in children than in adults. Generally these cases represent manifestations of systemic diseases that attack the integrity of cardiac structures, conduction system, or myocardium. Many cases represent progressive ailments that are significantly less amenable to surgical intervention than CHD. Nevertheless, such children with acquired cardiovascular disease also present for a variety of cardiac and noncardiac procedures.

In this chapter we provide a foundation for the physiologic and pharmacologic implications germane to the anesthesiologist caring for children. The added consequences of CHD and acquired heart disease are included.

Fetal Circulation

Unlike the normal postnatal circulatory pattern, which functions as a "series" circuit of pumps (i.e., the ventricles) and resistance beds (i.e., the pulmonary and systemic circulations), the fetal circulation behaves more like a "parallel" circuit. Both the right and left ventricles provide systemic blood flow. An anatomic illustration reveals that admixture of blood occurs at a variety of fetal connections (Fig. 16-1).[1,2] Relatively oxygenated blood returns from the placenta via the umbilical vein and crosses the ductus venosus to enter the inferior vena cava. A differential streaming effect causes much of this more saturated blood to cross the foramen ovale into the left atrium, thereby providing the most oxygenated blood for the cerebral circulation (Fig. 16-2A). Only 10% of the right ventricular output courses through the pulmonary circulation in utero (Fig. 16-2B). The remaining right ventricular output crosses the ductus arteriosus to provide the preponderance of systemic flow beyond the aortic arch.

Fetal Circulation

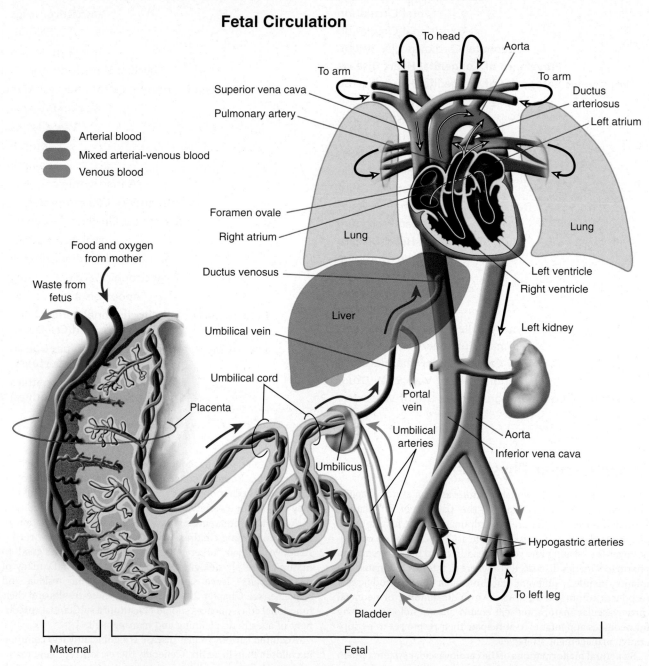

Figure 16-1. Course of the fetal circulation in late gestation. Note the selective blood flow patterns across the foramen ovale and the ductus arteriosus. (From Greeley WJ, Steven JM, Nicolson SC, et al: Anesthesia for pediatric cardiac surgery. In Miller RD [ed]: Anesthesia, 5th ed. Philadelphia, Churchill Livingstone, 2000, vol 2, pp 1805-1847.)

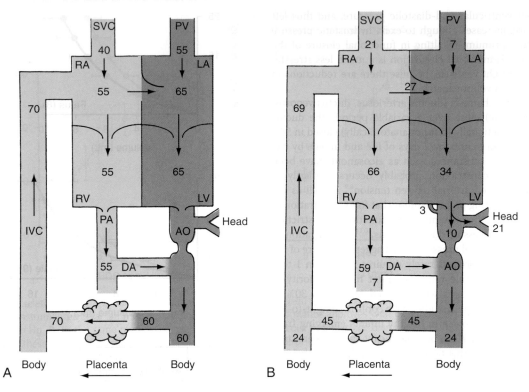

Figure 16-2. Fetal circulation in the late gestation lamb. **A,** The numbers indicate the percent of oxygen saturation. The oxygen saturation is the greatest in the inferior vena cava (IVC), representing flow that is primarily from the placenta. The saturation of the blood in the heart is slightly greater on the left side than on the right side. **B,** The course of the circulation. The numbers represent the percentage of combined ventricular output. Some of the return from the IVC is diverted by the crista dividens in the right atrium (RA) through the foramen ovale into the left atrium (LA), where it meets the pulmonary venous return (PV) and passes into the left ventricle (LV) and is pumped into the ascending aorta. Most of the ascending aortic flow goes to the coronary, subclavian, and carotid arteries, with only 10% of combined ventricular output passing through the aortic arch (indicated by the narrowed point in the aorta) into the descending aorta (AO). The remainder of the IVC flow mixes with return from the superior vena cava (SVC) and coronary veins (3%) and passes into the right atrium (RA) and right ventricle (RV) and is pumped into the pulmonary artery (PA). Because of the increased pulmonary resistance, only 7% of the blood passes through the lungs (PV), with the rest passing through the ductus arteriosus (DA) and then to the descending aorta to the placenta and lower half of the body. (Modified from Rudolph AM: Congenital Diseases of the Heart. Chicago, Year Book Publishers, 1974, pp 1-48; from Freed MD: Fetal and transitional circulation. In Fyler DC [ed]: Nadas' Pediatric Cardiology. Philadelphia, Mosby–Year Book, 1992, pp 57-61.)

A parallel circulatory pattern enables disparities in volume output between right and left ventricles while admixture of relatively oxygenated and deoxygenated blood occurs. Right ventricular volume output is nearly twice the left ventricular volume output, because the left ventricle receives only the diminutive pulmonary venous return in addition to that which traverses the foramen ovale from the right atrium.[1,3] Conversely, the right atrium receives all the systemic venous return in addition to the placental return via the umbilical vein. As a lacunar organ, the placenta does not fully oxygenate the blood passing through. Thus, the greatest oxygen saturation observed in the fetal circulation reaches 70% to 80%. The adaptive alterations in hemoglobin binding and other factors, such as increased 2,3-diphosphoglycerate (2,3-DPG), promote adequate tissue oxygen delivery.[4]

Transitional Circulation

At birth, a variety of humoral, biochemical, and physiologic changes occur abruptly. First, the placental circulation is eliminated shortly after the lungs expand. Second, expansion of the lungs to a normal functional residual capacity results in optimal geometric relationship of the pulmonary microvasculature. Third, air entering the lungs causes a marked reduction in alveo-

lar P_{CO_2} and increase in alveolar P_{O_2}. Each of these three factors acts in concert to markedly reduce pulmonary vascular resistance.[2,5,6] The net effect is a substantial increase in pulmonary blood flow, thereby augmenting pulmonary venous return to the left heart. In conjunction with the elimination of the low-resistance umbilical circulation, the left ventricle is suddenly subjected to increased volume load and afterload (Table 16-1).

Table 16-1. Hemodynamic Changes at Birth

Right Ventricle	Left Ventricle
Decreased afterload:	Increased afterload:
Decreased pulmonary vascular resistance	Placenta eliminated
Ductal closure	Ductal closure
Decreased volume load:	Increased volume load:
Eliminated umbilical vein return	Increased pulmonary venous return
Output diminished 25%	Output increased nearly 50%
	Transient left-to-right shunt at ductus

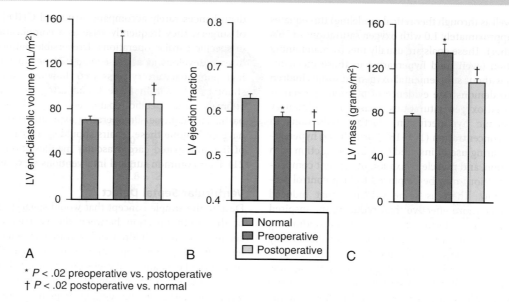

* *P* < .02 preoperative vs. postoperative
† *P* < .02 postoperative vs. normal

Figure 16-8. Postoperative changes following closure of ventricular septal defect (VSD). Echocardiographic evaluation of 23 children an average of 2 years after closure of a simple VSD. **A,** Left ventricular end-diastolic volume (LVEDV). **B,** Left ventricular ejection fraction (LVEF). **C,** Left ventricular mass. Each graph depicts baseline values and postoperative values in the subjects as compared with normal control subjects. Although these results demonstrate a return toward normal, they remain significantly abnormal even 2 years postoperatively. (Data from Jarmakani JM, Graham TPJ, Canent RVJ: Left ventricular contractile state in children with successfully corrected ventricular septal defect. Circulation 1972; 45:I102-I110; and Jarmakani JM, Graham TP Jr, Canent RV Jr, et al: The effect of corrective surgery on left heart volume and mass in children with ventricular septal defect. Am J Cardiol 1971; 27:254-258.)

include arrhythmia, baffle obstruction, and right (systemic) ventricular dysfunction.[54] Followed for 15 years, virtually none of these children remain consistently in sinus rhythm (Fig. 16-9A).[55] Sick sinus syndrome, atrial tachyarrhythmias, and sudden death constitute the most common arrhythmias in these children.[56] Long-term outcome studies have also identified right ventricular failure in 10% to 15% of children after intra-atrial repair of D-TGA (Fig. 16-9B).[57-59]

In the past 15 years, the arterial switch operation has supplanted intra-atrial repairs for D-TGA. Although the frequency of serious sequelae appears significantly reduced, the follow-up period has not been comparable to that of the Mustard or Senning operations.[60,61] Early experience with the arterial switch operation demonstrated postoperative supravalvar obstruction of the aorta or, more commonly, the pulmonary artery.[62] Reports of abnormal coronary flow patterns or coronary flow response to vasodilators have begun to emerge.[63-65] Questions have arisen regarding the long-term function of the neoaortic valve, which was a pulmonary valve during embryologic development.[61,65] For reasons that remain incompletely understood, children with D-TGA demonstrate significantly increased risk of pulmonary vascular disease.[66] Occasionally, this serious sequela occurs despite early corrective repair (see Chapter 21).[67]

Fontan Operation

As the only physiologic repair option for children with a single ventricle, the Fontan operation accomplishes several desirable objectives.[68] Systemic venous return is diverted directly into the pulmonary arteries and oxygenated blood returns to the heart for circulation to the body. As such, the Fontan operation establishes a series circulatory pattern and nearly normal systemic oxygen saturation and limits the pressure and volume load imposed on the single ventricle to that which would be expected of a normal systemic ventricle. These children exhibit marked sensitivity to any condition that might impede pulmonary blood flow. Their ability to increase cardiac output is limited to their capacity to augment pulmonary blood flow passively, requiring moderately increased systemic venous pressure. Exercise testing confirms significant reduction in maximal capacity (Fig. 16-10B).[69,70] Outcome studies conducted on children who underwent the Fontan operation in the 1970s and 1980s revealed progressive deterioration in functional status (Fig. 16-10A) and ongoing mortality, suggesting that this procedure must be considered palliative.[71] Many modifications to the procedure have evolved during the past 25 years to improve outcome.[72-74]

Apart from their progressive deterioration in cardiac function, limited reserve, and exquisite sensitivity to factors that might impede pulmonary blood flow, children who have survived a Fontan operation may demonstrate a variety of sequelae in the context of anesthesia and noncardiac surgery. Preservation of preload represents a central objective in preserving pulmonary blood flow and hence cardiac output. Similarly, ventilatory strategies that minimize pulmonary vascular resistance and management that preserves ventricular function act together to promote pulmonary flow. Atrial arrhythmias and sick sinus syndrome commonly complicate the outcome of children after the Fontan operation.[56,75] Serosal effusions of the pericardial, pleural, and peritoneal spaces may detract from optimal early and intermediate-term outcome. Taken together, these late manifestations of Fontan physiology contribute to make these children among the most fragile candidates for subsequent noncardiac surgery (see Chapter 21).

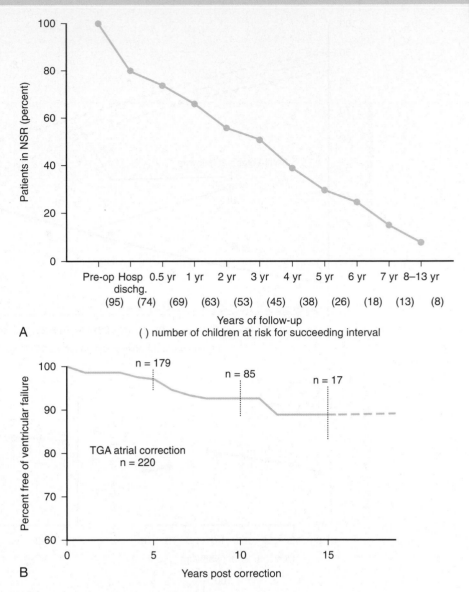

Figure 16-9. Long-term follow-up of children with transposition of the great arteries (TGA) after "physiologic" atrial repairs. **A,** Graph depicts Holter monitoring of 95 children 3 months to 13 years after the Mustard operation. The prevalence of subjects who consistently remain in normal sinus rhythm (NSR) is less than 10% when followed more than 8 years. **B,** Kaplan-Meier graph depicting the percent of children from systemic (right) ventricular failure between 1 month and 20 years after a Senning operation. NSR, normal sinus rhythm; TGA, transposition of great arteries. (**A** from Hayes CJ, Gersony WM: Arrhythmias after the Mustard operation for transposition of the great arteries: A long term study. J Am Coll Cardiol 1986; 7:133-137; **B** from Turina MI, Siebenmann R, von Segesser L, et al: Late functional deterioration after atrial correction for transposition of the great arteries. Circulation 1989; 80[Suppl I]: I162-I167. Reprinted with permission from the American College of Cardiology.)

Acquired Heart Disease

In children, acquired heart disease occurs significantly less commonly than CHD. These findings tend to represent manifestations of systemic disorders. They may accompany inherited diseases (e.g., Down syndrome and Marfan syndrome), inflammatory processes (e.g., Kawasaki disease), or infection (e.g., endocarditis). The disease process may afflict the myocardium, valves, or vasculature. As such, the anesthetic management centers on minimizing pathophysiologic hemodynamic loading conditions and preserving myocardial function and vital organ perfusion. A discussion of the more common systemic diseases follows.

Down Syndrome

At least 40% of neonates with trisomy 21 (Down syndrome) present with CHD. The characteristic distribution of malformations reveals that nearly 50% are endocardial cushion defects, with VSD, tetralogy of Fallot, and patent ductus arteriosus accounting

for the majority of the rest.[76,77] Pulmonary vascular disease may develop more rapidly in infants with Down syndrome and CHD, although the mechanism remains controversial.[78-80]

Marfan Disease

Marfan disease is an autosomal dominant connective tissue disorder that produces progressive dilation of the cardiac valve annulus structure, ultimately resulting in regurgitation.[81] Mitral valve dysfunction occurs early, ultimately affecting as many as 68% of children with Marfan disease.[82,83] Functional aortic valve involvement rarely occurs before the second decade of life.[84] In addition, medial disruption in the aorta predisposes these children to aneurysm formation. Aortic disease can also include the coronary arteries.

Kawasaki Disease

Kawasaki disease is an acute febrile inflammatory disease that leaves residual aneurysms in a variety of vessels, including coronary arteries. Kawasaki disease has become the leading cause of

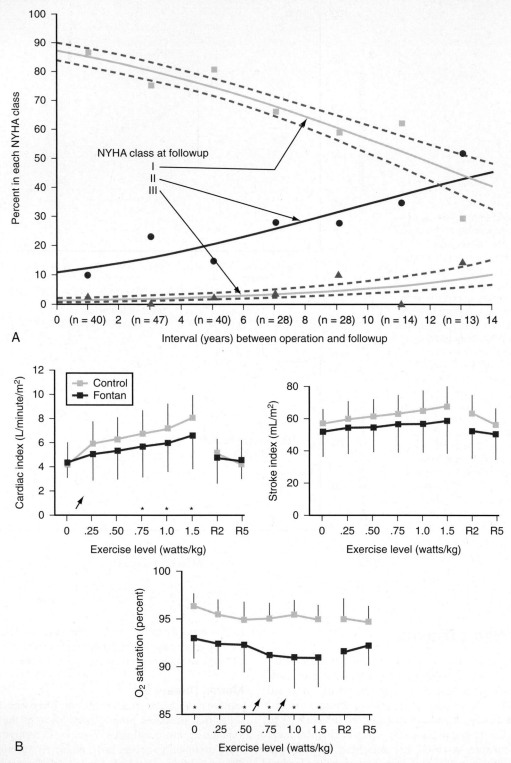

Figure 16-10. A, Symptomatic outcomes of 334 survivors of Fontan operations followed for 1 month to 20 years. Graph illustrates the change in New York Heart Association (NYHA) classifications I (*blue squares*), II (*purple circles*) and III (*brown triangles*) over time. Although most children exhibit good functional status (NYHA class I) immediately after surgery, mild functional limitations evolve over time. Broken lines indicate 70% confidence intervals. **B,** Exercise studies (cardiac index, stroke index, and oxygen saturation vs. exercise level) of 42 children after Fontan operation (*purple squares*) compared with normal control subjects (*blue squares*). Although the protocol was designed to achieve modest targets, significant differences emerged in the capacity of Fontan children to increase cardiac output with exercise and systemic arterial oxygen saturation remained below normal throughout. The primary reason for the inability to increase cardiac output appears to be an inability to increase pulmonary blood flow and consequently systemic ventricular filling. Potential reasons for decreased arterial saturation include intrapulmonary shunting due to arteriovenous malformations and ventilation/perfusion imbalance. (R2, two minutes after exercise; R5, five minutes after exercise. *Arrows* refer to the significance (p < 0.05) of contrasts between consecutive exercise levels). (**A** from Fontan F, Kirklin JW, Fernandez G, et al: Outcome after a "perfect" Fontan operation. Circulation 1990; 81:1520-1536; **B** from Gewillig MH, Lundstrom UR, Bull C, et al: Exercise responses in children with congenital heart disease after Fontan repair: Patterns and determinants of performance. J Am Coll Cardiol 1990; 15:1424-1432. Reprinted with permission from the American College of Cardiology.)

acquired heart disease in children in the United States.[85] As many as 40% of children demonstrate cardiac involvement in the acute febrile stage of the illness, including myocarditis, pericardial effusion, or arrhythmia.[85-87] Coronary aneurysms develop in 20%, causing myocardial infarction and death in as many as 3% to 4%.[85] Although many coronary aneurysms regress over time, some produce ischemia, infarction, and, occasionally, rupture.[87-89]

Endocarditis

Although rheumatic heart disease is rare in the United States, it represents a predominant cause of acquired valve disease worldwide, with 85% of cases affecting the mitral valve.[90,91] Bacterial endocarditis still occurs in association with bacteremia from a variety of sources.[92] Complex cardiac surgical procedures in young infants have dramatically changed the incidence and spectrum of children afflicted with bacterial endocarditis.[93] Approximately 40% of endocarditis episodes develop in postoperative cardiac surgery children, with over 80% having some preexisting CHD or acquired cardiac disease.[94] Residual valve dysfunction requires individual assessment (see Tables 14-1 and 14-2).

Inflammatory Collagen Vascular Diseases

A variety of systemic inflammatory diseases have an impact on the pericardium, myocardium, or conduction system. As many as 50% of children with systemic lupus erythematosus exhibit cardiac manifestations.[95] These include pericardial inflammation or effusion, myocarditis, valve dysfunction, and conduction system abnormalities. An inflammatory myocarditis and cardiomyopathy can also be a prominent feature of human immunodeficiency virus infection and its treatment in children.

Primary Pulmonary Hypertension

Pulmonary vascular disease that develops independent of CHD represents a particularly virulent process that progresses rapidly to death. In young children, no strong gender association emerges, although it is predominantly a disease of females from adolescence onward (4 : 1 ratio). Vasodilator therapy rarely provides more than brief palliation. Although lung transplantation offers some benefit, the 2-year survival rate is only 60%.[96-99]

Cardiovascular Pharmacology

Rational Use of Vasoactive Drugs

Selection of appropriate inotropic and vasopressor therapies depends on several factors, including the clinical situation, underlying cardiac abnormalities, and perfusion requirements of other organs. The major goal is to improve oxygen delivery to the tissues. As such, the primary focus is on improving myocardial pump function, systemic blood flow, and tissue oxygenation. Oxygen-carrying capacity (i.e., hemoglobin) should also be considered carefully in this regard. When deciding on specific agents or regimens, other factors include optimizing heart rate, contractility, and afterload. In certain congenital heart lesions, appropriate balance of systemic and pulmonary blood flow is also important (see later).

Drugs that are catecholamines or have catecholamine-like effects remain the most commonly used inotropic and vasoconstrictor drugs. It is likely that improvements in cardiac output in neonates in response to drugs such as dopamine or dobuta-

mine are due to increases in both heart rate and contractility. Some evidence exists in infants and in young children after cardiac surgery that the increases in cardiac output produced by dopamine and dobutamine may be more related to a positive chronotropic effect than to an increase in the intrinsic contractile state.[100-102] With few exceptions, drugs that primarily increase afterload, such as α-adrenergic agonists, have limited use in children. This occurs mainly because large increases in afterload without corresponding improvements in contractile state are poorly tolerated by infants and children, particularly in the context of significant underlying contractile dysfunction.

Practical Considerations for the Use of Vasoactive Agents

Commonly used drugs, their doses, and a summary of their effects on selected cardiac functions are given in Table 16-4. Much of this information has been empirically derived from studies in adults. There is limited information about the effects of commonly used vasoactive drugs in children at different ages and limited information about the effects of these drugs in various pathophysiologic states. Factors that are likely to provide unique responses to inotropic and vasoconstrictor drugs in neonates and infants include altered pharmacokinetics; differences in receptor types, number, and function; and variability in drug delivery. Substantial variations in measured plasma concentrations, as well as the volume of distribution, have been noted in children receiving inotropic agents, such that as much as a 10-fold range in plasma concentrations has been noted for a given infusion rate.[103,104]

Substantial variability can be observed in the serum concentration of a particular inotrope that is required to produce a given effect. Some of these pharmacodynamic differences are related to receptor maturation and function. It appears that, for example, β-adrenergic receptors are at high density in the term and young infant but their coupling to adenyl cyclase may be incomplete.[24,105] In addition to developmental changes, controlled in part by thyroid hormone, β-receptor and adenyl cyclase activity is diminished in response to sustained administration of exogenous β agonists as well as increased endogenous catecholamines. The latter is a complication of moderate to severe heart failure and other forms of severe stress such as sepsis.[106-108]

The effects of prolonged β-adrenergic stimulation in neonatal myocardium are not quite as clear. Catecholamines may upregulate adrenergic receptor number or function, or both, in infants, perhaps in part owing to mimicking of the normal developmental program of increasing sympathetic nervous system activity as term approaches.[109] With further maturation in early postnatal life, β-adrenergic receptor density declines. The impact of different pathophysiologic states on these processes is unclear overall. For example, congestive heart failure, cardiopulmonary bypass, and ischemic reperfusion all lead to decreased β-receptor and adenyl cyclase expression and activity.[110-113] Increased β-receptor density and greater receptor-stimulated adenyl cyclase activity have been shown in the myocardium of infants with tetralogy of Fallot.[114]

One must pay particular attention to technical issues when administering vasoactive infusions to infants. Infusion preparations for infants are usually rendered in a very concentrated form to limit the amount of volume infused and use "nonstandard" dilutions. Hence, the potential for dose or concentration

Table 16-4. Inotropics and Vasopressors

Agent	Dose (IV)	Comments
Dopamine	2-20 µg/kg/min infusion	Primary effects at β_1, β_2, and dopamine receptors, somewhat related to dose; lower doses (2-5 µg/kg/min) can increase contractility and also have direct dopaminergic receptor effect to increase splanchnic and renal perfusion; increasing doses increase contractility via β effects and also increase likelihood of α-mediated vasoconstriction; effects depend on endogenous catecholamine stores.
Dobutamine	2-20 µg/kg/min infusion	Relatively selective β_1 stimulation; also potential β_2 stimulation, tachycardia, and vasodilation, especially at higher doses (>10 µg/kg/min); may be less potent than dopamine, especially in immature myocardium; no significant α-adrenergic effects; tachydysrhythmias perhaps more likely than with dopamine; effects independent of endogenous catecholamine stores.
Epinephrine	0.02-2.0 µg/kg/min infusion	Primary β effects to increase contractility and vasodilation at lower (0.02-0.10 µg/kg/min) doses; increasing doses (>0.1 µg/kg/min) accompanied by increased contractility and also increased α-mediated vasoconstriction; may be best choice to augment contractility and perfusion, especially in situations of severely compromised ventricular function, shock, or anaphylaxis.
Isoproterenol	0.05-2.0 µg/kg/min infusion	Pure, nonselective β-agonist; significant inotropic, chronotropic (β_1 and β_2) and vasodilatory (β_2) effects; may be an effective pulmonary vasodilator in some children; tachycardia and increased myocardial oxygen consumption may be dose limiting; tachydysrhythmias may also occur; bronchodilator.
Phenylephrine	1-10 µg/kg bolus, 0.1-0.5 µg/kg/min infusion	Pure α-mediated vasoconstriction; no increase in contractility.
Amrinone	0.75-1 mg/kg repeated twice, maximum 3 mg/kg. Neonates and infants may require loading doses of 2-4 mg/kg and infusions of 10 µg/kg/min.	Increases cyclic adenosine monophosphate by phosphodiesterase inhibition; positive inotropy, positive lusitropy, and smooth muscle vasorelaxation; hypotension; reversible thrombocytopenia.
Milrinone	50-75 µg/kg loading dose, 0.5-1.0 µg/kg/min infusion	Similar to amrinone (antiplatelet effects may be less).
Calcium chloride	10-20 mg/kg/dose (slowly)	Positive inotropic and direct vasoconstricting effects; inotropy significant only if ionized calcium is low and/or ventricular function is depressed by other agents; can slow sinus node; increases electrophysiologic abnormalities from hypokalemia and digoxin.
Calcium gluconate	30-60 mg/kg/dose (slowly)	
Digoxin	Total digitalizing dose (TDD): Premature: 20 µg/kg Neonate: 30 µg/kg (1 month) Infant: 40 µg/kg (<2 years) Child: 30 µg/kg (2-5 years) Over 5 years: 20 µg/kg Maintenance: 2.5-5 µg/kg q12h	TDD given in divided doses: $\frac{1}{2}$ TDD followed by $\frac{1}{4}$ TDD q8-12h × 2 increases cardiac contractility; slows sinus node and decreases atrioventricular node conduction; long half-life (24-48 hr) that is prolonged by renal dysfunction; numerous drug interactions; toxicity includes supraventricular tachycardia, atrioventricular block, ventricular dysrhythmias; symptoms include drowsiness, nausea, vomiting; and toxicity exacerbated by hypokalemia.

error is substantial. One study at a tertiary care children's hospital demonstrated that the actual concentration of prepared solutions varied significantly.[115] The high concentration relative to child size means that small errors (either in calculation or infusion pump flow rate) can significantly affect the actual amount of drug delivered. The corresponding slow infusion rate can also lead to a delay in drug delivery (see Chapter 53). Ensuring that the pump drive mechanism is actually delivering drug at the distal end of the infusion tubing, connecting the infusion tubing as close to the child as possible, and using a carrier infusion delivered at constant rate are among ways to decrease variability and increase efficacy of drug infusions. Carrier infusion rate is also probably important: rates in excess of 5 mL/hr (which may be at odds with attempts to limit total

volume administered) are probably necessary to effect rapid (<~10 minutes) changes in the concentration of drug delivered to the infant when using most standard infusion tubing and setups.

Balancing Parallel Circulations

Several groups of children require careful attention to the balance between systemic and pulmonary blood flow ($\dot{Q}p:\dot{Q}s$). Examples include children with hypoplastic left heart syndrome (who have ductal-dependent systemic blood flow), those with critical aortic coarctation (who have ductal-dependent systemic blood flow), those with large ventricular septal or atrioventricular (AV) canal defects (who have potential for left-to-right shunting and systemic hypoperfusion), and children with palliative and surgical systemic-to-pulmonary artery shunts (e.g., Blalock-Taussig shunt).

As noted earlier, maintaining ductal patency with prostaglandin E_1 (see later discussion) is necessary in the treatment of many of the lesions with obstruction to pulmonary or aortic blood flow. At times, atrial septostomy is also required to ensure adequate intracardiac mixing in children with a single-ventricle physiology. Children with ductal-dependent systemic blood flow require careful balancing of systemic vascular resistance and pulmonary vascular resistance to maintain adequate systemic perfusion and appropriate but not excessive oxygenation. In these children, hyperventilation, alkalosis, and hyperoxia can decrease pulmonary vascular resistance, increase pulmonary blood flow, and lead to systemic hypoperfusion, oliguria, and metabolic acidosis. From a practical standpoint, systemic oxygen saturations of 75% to 80% and normal to mildly increased $PaCO_2$ are reasonable goals. Occasionally, reducing the inspiring oxygen concentration below 0.21 by adding nitrogen to inspired air or adding inspired CO_2, requiring mechanical ventilation and heavy sedation or muscle relaxation to avoid compensatory hyperventilation, is necessary to control pulmonary blood flow in these children. Usually, however, appropriate ventilation at low FIO_2 and normal to mild hypercarbia is sufficient to maintain an appropriate balance of systemic and pulmonary blood flow. Occasionally, low-dose inotropic support is also required to optimize systemic perfusion.

Similar considerations apply in children with the potential for large left-to-right cardiac shunting. Here again, one wants to control those factors that decrease pulmonary vascular resistance to also control the magnitude of the left-to-right shunt and avoid excessive pulmonary blood flow, decreased systemic perfusion, and potential worsening of pulmonary vascular congestion.

Children with decreased pulmonary blood flow resulting in cyanosis depend on the balance of pulmonary vascular resistance to systemic vascular resistance, as well as overall cardiac output, to achieve adequate oxygenation. Pulmonary blood flow will typically be through either natural (e.g., patent ductus arteriosus) or surgically created systemic-to-pulmonary arterial communications. Increased pulmonary vascular resistance or decreased systemic vascular resistance compromises pulmonary blood flow in children with shunt-dependent pulmonary flow. In children dependent on surgical systemic-to-pulmonary artery shunts for pulmonary blood flow, pulmonary blood flow is positively affected by increasing cardiac output and systemic vascular resistance and by decreasing pulmonary vascular resistance. Shunt size and patency are, of course, important factors as well.

Cardiac output has a direct influence on systemic arterial oxygen saturation in single-ventricle and other types of mixing lesions because of its effect on venous oxygen saturation. For example, reduced cardiac output leads to reduced venous oxygen saturation. This results in reduced systemic arterial oxygen saturation, owing to the mixing of less saturated venous blood in children with right-to-left shunts or complete mixing lesions. Conversely, improvements in arterial oxygen saturation can be achieved in these children by optimizing cardiac output as well as oxygen content (e.g., increasing hemoglobin in children who are relatively anemic).

Other forms of congenital cardiac lesions can be approached with a similar level of understanding of their underlying patho-physiology. Outflow obstruction (e.g., aortic stenosis) is characterized by increased pressure work, development of chamber hypertrophy, and reduced ability to increase cardiac output in response to increased demand. Therapeutic goals for these children include ensuring adequate preload and maintaining heart rate at a sufficiently slow rate so as to allow adequate time for chamber filling and ejection. Right ventricular outflow obstruction may benefit from reducing afterload on the right ventricle (i.e., reducing pulmonary vascular resistance). In general, systemic vascular resistance should be maintained in a setting of either right or left ventricular outflow obstruction. In the case of fixed aortic outflow, this approach is necessary to ensure adequate coronary perfusion. Right ventricular outflow obstruction leads to right ventricular hypertrophy. Adequate systemic blood pressure is necessary to ensure coronary perfusion to the hypertrophic right ventricle. It is noteworthy that a substantial percentage of total coronary flow to the right ventricle occurs during systole.

Children with significant ventricular dysfunction, for example due to dilated cardiomyopathy (see later), are functioning at the extremes of the Laplace and Frank-Starling relationships. The practical implications are that myocardial wall tension is maximal; subendocardial perfusion is easily compromised; and even relatively minor alterations in heart rate, contractility, preload, and afterload can lead to rapid and, at times, irreversible myocardial decompensation. Disturbances of cardiac rhythm and conduction are also poorly tolerated in such children. Preload augmentation may not reliably increase cardiac output and may, in fact, lead to further ventricular dilation and AV valve regurgitation. Either bradycardia or significant tachycardia may also be poorly tolerated. Inotropic support, along with careful afterload reduction, may improve cardiac performance in such children with severely compromised pump function.

The effects of mechanical ventilation should also be considered.[116,117] Pulmonary vascular resistance is increased at either very large or very small lung volumes. In the former situation, large lung volumes are associated with increased intrathoracic pressures that are transmitted to the pulmonary vasculature. Alveolar overdistention, increased intrathoracic pressures, and large lung volumes compress alveolar capillaries, increasing pulmonary vascular resistance and right ventricular afterload.[118] At the other extreme, hypoventilation and significantly reduced lung volume can increase pulmonary vascular resistance by leading to hypoxia, hypercarbia, and atelectasis. Significantly impaired right ventricular function can compromise left ventricular function by the mechanism of ventricular interdependence. Appropriate positive-pressure ventilation may improve the performance of the systemic ventricle by mechanisms that include decreased afterload, decreased work of breathing, and improvements due to better oxygenation or ventilation. These benefits may more than offset any reduction in performance due to the effects of positive pressure on venous return or other parameters.

Vasoactive Drugs

Dopamine

Dopamine continues to be the most frequently used inotropic agent in neonates, infants, and children. It has activity at α, β, and dopaminergic receptors. Dopamine augments cardiac contractility through two mechanisms. First, it directly stimulates

States. Its properties are generally similar to those of the other members of its class.[150,167] Improvements in indirect indices of cardiac function such as mixed venous oxygen saturation, ventricular filling pressures, and systemic arterial blood pressure were afforded by enoximone in infants after cardiac surgery. A reduced length of hospital stay was also observed in these infants.[168] Enoximone was also useful to support cardiac function and potentially reduce pulmonary vascular resistance in children after cardiac transplantation.[169]

Digoxin

Digoxin remains the most frequently administered oral inotropic agent. Its use in children with congestive heart failure due to large left-to-right shunts has been questioned on the basis that it preserves apparent myocardial contractility in the presence of progressive ventricular dilatation.[170,171] Its efficacy in improving right ventricular dysfunction due to pulmonary hypertension has also been debated.

Digoxin has both direct and indirect effects. Its direct effects are mediated via inhibition of the membrane sodium-potassium ATPase. This mechanism leads to inhibition of outward sodium ion flux. The resulting increased intracellular sodium concentration stimulates the membrane sodium-calcium exchanger, producing increased intracellular calcium and positive inotropic effect. The indirect effects of digoxin are mediated by stimulation of the parasympathetic nervous system. The parasympathetic effects of digoxin result in slowing of atrial and AV node conduction. This drug can also be given to slow the ventricular response in atrial flutter and atrial fibrillation and to treat supraventricular tachycardia (SVT) (see later).

Because digoxin has a slow distribution phase after oral administration and a long elimination half-life (up to 1 to 2 days in neonates and young infants), a loading dose is usually administered (Table 16-5). Renal dysfunction can significantly prolong the elimination half-life. Therapeutic digoxin levels are between 0.5 and 2.0 ng/mL. Intravenous and oral dosing

Table 16-5. Antihypertensives and Vasodilators*

Drug	Dose (IV)	Comments
Propranolol	0.05-0.2 mg/kg slowly	Nonselective β blockade; bradycardia, hypotension, worsening of myocardial pump function; atrioventricular block; hypoglycemia; bronchospasm; depression; fatigue
Labetalol	0.1-0.4 mg/kg/dose; 0.25-1.0 mg/kg/hr infusion	Nonselective β blockade; selective α blockade; ratio of α to β blockade is 1:7 for intravenous form; doses (0.1 mg/kg) can be repeated every 5-10 minutes until desired effect achieved; side effects are similar to those of propranolol.
Esmolol	100-500 μg/kg loading dose (over 5 minutes); 50-250 μg/kg/min infusion	Relatively selective β blockade; short elimination half-life (7-10 minutes); hypotension, especially during bolus administration; if less than desired response after 5 minutes, can repeat or double bolus dose, followed by doubling infusion rate; non–organ-based metabolism by plasma and red blood cell esterases; infusion concentrations >10 mg/mL may predispose to venous sclerosis; dilute infusion at high rates increases risk of volume overload.
Sodium nitroprusside	Start at 0.5-1.0 μg/kg/min infusion; Maximum 6-10 μg/kg/min	Potent direct smooth muscle relaxation; dilates both arteriolar resistance and venous capacitance vessels; hypotension potentiated by hypovolemia, inhalation anesthetics, other antihypertensives; variable pulmonary vasodilation; potential cyanide toxicity; reflex tachycardia; check cyanide and thiocyanate levels if >4 μg/kg/min infused and/or used >2-3 days.
Nitroglycerin	0.5-10 μg/kg/min infusion	Direct smooth muscle relaxation; predominantly dilates venous capacitance vessels, modest effects on arterial resistance at larger doses; weak antihypertensive effects; variable pulmonary vasodilation; used to facilitate cooling and rewarming during cardiopulmonary bypass.
Phentolamine	0.05-0.1 mg/kg dose; 0.5-5 μg/kg/min infusion	Selective α blocker, produces mainly arteriolar vasodilation; some direct vasodilation with mild venodilation.
Enalaprilat	5-10 μg/kg/dose q8-24h	Long duration of effect; angioedema, renal failure, hyperkalemia; potential problematic hypotension with anesthetic agents (see text)
Hydralazine	0.1-0.2 mg/kg bolus q6h	Maximum 20 mg/dose; direct-acting smooth muscle (predominantly arteriolar) vasodilation; long effective half-life; tachyphylaxis; reflex tachycardia; lupus-like syndrome; drug fever; thrombocytopenia
Prostaglandin E₁	0.05-0.1 μg/kg/min infusion	Direct smooth muscle relaxation, relatively specific for ductus arteriosus; variable pulmonary and systemic vasodilation; apnea in neonates

*All drugs should be started in the lower dose range and titrated to effect.

regimens are the same, although the onset of electrophysiologic effects from intravenous dosing may be much more rapid (5 to 20 minutes).

Drug interactions with digoxin are extremely numerous. It should be assumed that just about any drug administered along with digoxin would affect the absorption and clearance of digoxin, usually necessitating a reduction in digoxin dose. The likelihood of digoxin toxicity increases with serum levels above 3 ng/mL.[172] Symptoms of toxicity include drowsiness, nausea, and vomiting. Various conduction abnormalities and SVT are the most frequent cardiac rhythm manifestations of digoxin toxicity in infants and young children. Older children and adults are more likely to experience AV block, ventricular dysrhythmias, junctional tachycardia, and premature ventricular contractions. Hypokalemia, specifically intracellular potassium depletion as would occur for example with long-standing diuretic use, exacerbates the proarrhythmic effects of digoxin.

Calcium

The role, mechanisms of action, and potential for deleterious consequences of intravenous calcium administration continue to be controversial.[173] It is the ionized calcium concentration that is important for myocardial function. Calcium is a positive inotrope, particularly when administered in the presence of ionized hypocalcemia. It may also improve ventricular contractility when left ventricular function is depressed by halothane, β-adrenergic blockade, or disease (e.g., sepsis).[174,175] In the presence of a normal myocardium and normal ionized calcium concentrations, the effects of intravenous calcium administration on contractility are much more modest.[176] Another area of controversy has to do with the effects of intravenous calcium administration on peripheral vascular resistance, with both increases and decreases in systemic vascular resistance having been found in response to intravenous calcium.[177] Calcium most likely increases pulmonary vascular resistance.

There is evidence in adults that the primary effect of calcium administered after cardiac surgery is to increase systemic vascular resistance and mean arterial pressure with little to no effect on intrinsic myocardial contractility.[173,178] In fact, the increase in afterload, if not accompanied by a corresponding increase in contractility, may only serve to decrease stroke volume and cardiac output. Calcium may cause or exacerbate reperfusion injury and cellular damage by mechanisms that include activation of calcium-dependent proteases and phospholipases and organellar damage due to cellular calcium overload.[179,180] These concerns are particularly relevant in children immediately after cardiac surgery. Intravenous calcium may also attenuate the β-adrenergic effects of concurrently administered epinephrine.[173]

The role of intravenous calcium administration in neonates and young infants, both alone and after cardiac surgery, is more complicated. Preterm and term neonates have erratic calcium handling and are prone to ionized hypocalcemia.[181,182] The neonatal myocardium is more sensitive to ionized hypocalcemia than is the adult myocardium, owing to reduced intracellular calcium stores, immaturity of sarcoplasmic reticulum calcium handling mechanisms, and greater dependency on transmembrane calcium flux for excitation-contraction coupling.[183] Furthermore, the need to administer substantial volumes of citrated and albumin-containing blood products (both of which bind calcium) and other fluids in the post–cardiopulmonary bypass

setting increases the likelihood of ionized hypocalcemia.[184] The most prudent approach includes awareness of the greater dependency of the immature myocardium on extracellular calcium, monitoring ionized calcium concentrations, and careful administration to maintain normal or, at most, mildly increased ionized calcium concentrations. This approach is particularly needed in neonates and those with diminished left ventricular function. Administration of large bolus doses of calcium immediately on reperfusion of the heart after a period of ischemia is probably ill advised because of the potential to exacerbate reperfusion injury and even cause myocardial contracture.

Extravasation of calcium can cause local venous irritation and significant tissue necrosis. It has been suggested that calcium gluconate has the potential to cause less harm in this regard than does calcium chloride. Either the gluconate or chloride form should be administered via a centrally positioned catheter whenever possible. Both calcium chloride and calcium gluconate raise ionized calcium concentrations to an equal extent when administered on the basis of equal amounts of elemental calcium.[185] Calcium may cause significant slowing of AV conduction and should be administered cautiously in children with sinus bradycardia or junctional rhythm. Care must also be exercised when administering calcium to children receiving digoxin, particularly in the presence of concurrent hypokalemia, because intravenous calcium will exacerbate the potential for digoxin-induced dysrhythmias in this setting.

Triiodothyronine

Triiodothyronine hormone (T_3) is essential for the maturation of sarcolemmal calcium channels, myosin, actin, and troponin. In addition, hypothyroid rats demonstrate reduced numbers of β receptors, as well as a reduction in stimulatory secondary messenger protein density with an increase in inhibitory secondary messenger protein density. T_3 is mostly produced by monodeiodination of thyroxine. This process is inhibited by surgery, hypothermia, catecholamines, propranolol, and amiodarone. Thus, postoperative T_3 levels are reduced.

T_3 replacement acts via two pathways, intranuclear and extranuclear. Intranuclear effects include an increase in mitochondrial density and respiration, an increase in contractile protein synthesis, and an upregulation in β adrenoceptors. Extranuclear effects include an improvement in glucose transport, increased stimulation of L-type calcium channels with subsequent calcium mobility, and increased efficiency in calcium reuptake with subsequent improvement in diastolic relaxation.

A randomized, double-blind, placebo-controlled study of T_3 administration in children undergoing both simple and complex cardiac surgery demonstrated that the group that received T_3 had better myocardial function and a decreased stay in the intensive care unit.[186] T_3 improves contractility without any associated increase in oxygen consumption. In addition, this group demonstrated no delay in recovery of thyroid function secondary to exogenous administration. The dose of T_3 used was 2 µg/kg on day 1 followed by 1 µg/kg from day 2 to day 12.

Calcium-Sensitizing Agents

Calcium-sensitizing agents represent a relatively new class of drugs with inotropic properties. They continue to undergo preclinical evaluation. Perhaps one of the best studied and closest to more widespread use is levosimendan. Although its mechanism of action is not entirely clear, it appears to act by maintaining the conformation of the calcium-binding site of troponin C in its active conformation, which shifts the calcium binding-concentration relationship toward increased binding (i.e., more binding at lower intracardiac calcium concentrations). Contraction is thereby enhanced for a given cytosolic calcium concentration. One advantage, therefore, over other types of inotropes is that greater myocardial contractility is produced with minimal increase in oxygen demand. The concept of increasing sensitivity to calcium rather than increasing cellular calcium concentrations is also attractive because of the deleterious effects of increased cytosolic calcium concentrations on oxygen consumption, mitochondrial function, and activation of various calcium-dependent proteases and phospholipases (e.g., during ischemia-reperfusion).

Levosimendan also stimulates membrane and mitochondrial potassium-sensitive adenosine triphosphate (K_{ATP}) channels. The former dilates both coronary and peripheral vasculature. Opening mitochondrial K_{ATP} channels is likely to be an important mechanism of pharmacologic (and anesthetic) preconditioning and potential cytoprotection. Interestingly, and for reasons that are not entirely clear, levosimendan either has no effect on lusitropy (diastolic relaxation) or in fact is positively lusitropic. At much greater concentrations, it does inhibit phosphodiesterase III, but this effect does not appear to be relevant at clinical concentrations. Unlike some other agents (e.g., dopamine, amrinone, milrinone), its efficacy as a positive inotrope appears to be maintained in the abnormal myocardium. Both its mechanism of action and experience thus far indicate limited, if any, potential to stimulate arrhythmias.[187]

Clinical effects include improved cardiac output, reduced ventricular filling pressures, and decreased pulmonary vascular resistance during the acute treatment of adult patients with either stable or decompensated heart failure.[188-190] Case reports and small case series also suggest improved cardiac performance in the postcardiotomy, postbypasss setting, including beneficial responses in adult patients who appeared to be poorly responsive to other inotropes. Current studies suggest a 6- to 12-μg/kg loading dose followed by an infusion of 0.05 to 0.2 μg/kg/min. The drug's elimination half-life is approximately 1 hour. There is at least one metabolite that has prolonged (~80 hr) effects, which may, in part, account for observations of sustained benefit after discontinuation of the drug. There are limited data available regarding its use in children or immature animal preparations. One recent study in a relatively small, heterogeneous group of inotrope-dependent children with acute or end-stage heart failure demonstrated significant reductions in the use of inotropes in both groups and improved ejection fraction in those with acute heart failure.[191] These early data and its mechanisms(s) of action suggest the need for further study in children and a likely indication for use in infants and children with decreased myocardial performance from a variety of causes, including after cardiac surgery, myocarditis, and sepsis.

Brain Natriuretic Factor and Nesiritide

Brain natriuretic peptide (BNP) is a member of the natriuretic peptide family, which includes atrial natriuretic peptide (ANP, BNP, and C-type NP). These peptides together play a large role in maintaining hemodynamic and neurohumoral equilibrium. BNP is secreted from cardiac ventricles in response to increased stimulation of cardiac stretch receptors and increased wall tension and acts mostly via natriuretic peptide receptors (NPR)

present in large vessels and kidneys. Once stimulated, NPR receptors promote diuresis, natriuresis, and vasodilation and inhibit the renin-angiotensin-aldosterone system. BNP is used as a marker for heart failure in adults and also as a method for monitoring progress to anti–congestive heart failure therapies. The utility of these indices in children is less obvious. Indeed, two recent studies attempting to determine the predictive value of BNP in acute heart failure in children came to opposing conclusions.[192,193]

Nesiritide is a recombinant form of BNP. It acts via the same receptors with the same end results. Studies suggest that patients with decompensated heart failure may benefit from nesiritide by improving cardiac output, reducing pulmonary capillary occlusion pressure, and dilating the arterial and venous vessels with a minimal increase in heart rate or myocardial oxygen consumption. Although nesiritide reduces mean arterial pressure in children after cardiac surgery, more extensive studies are required before determining its usefulness and safety in children.[194-196]

β-Blocking Agents

There are several indications for the use of β blockers in children, including control of hypertension (both acutely in a perioperative period and chronically), treatment of cyanotic spells and right ventricular outflow obstruction in tetralogy of Fallot, reduction of left ventricular outflow obstruction in hypertrophic cardiomyopathy, control of heart rate in thyrotoxicosis and pheochromocytoma, and control of SVT (see later).[197] Important distinctions include β-receptor subtype selectivity, variability in half-life and metabolism, and intrinsic sympathomimetic activity. "Selective" β blockers lose their selectivity at increased plasma concentrations.

Propranolol

Propranolol is one of the most frequently used β blockers in children. Typical oral doses start at 0.25 to 0.5 mg/kg every 6 hours, titrated every 3 to 5 days; usual dose 2 to 4 mg/kg/day. A sustained-release form is available for older children who are able to swallow pills. Intravenous propranolol is administered at doses of 0.01 to 0.1 mg/kg over several minutes; this may be increased if necessary. Bradycardia and hypotension can be serious sequelae, particularly in infants or after intravenous administration. In addition to bradycardia, propranolol may cause conduction block at the AV node and worsen pump function in congestive heart failure. Other important side effects include fatigue, depression, and lethargy. Interactions with the β_2 receptor may exacerbate bronchospasm and predispose children to hypoglycemia. Propranolol is primarily metabolized in the liver. Significant population variability in its kinetics has been noted. Metabolism is also affected by factors that alter hepatic blood flow and hepatic metabolic enzyme activity. Its major metabolite, 4-hydroxypropranolol, is also bioactive.

Atenolol

The use of atenolol has been increasing in children. It is more selective for the β_1-adrenergic receptor subtype than propranolol. The elimination half-life is 8 to 12 hours. There is little hepatic biotransformation, and there are no active metabolites. The typical starting dose is 0.8 to 1.5 mg/kg/day in one or two doses daily, with an upper limit in the range of 3 mg/kg/day. No intravenous form is available. Atenolol does not cross the blood-brain barrier, and thus some of the limiting side effects common to propranolol are absent. At large doses, β_1 selectivity is probably lost, leading to the potential to exacerbate bronchospasm and hypoglycemia.

Esmolol

Esmolol is a relatively selective β_1-adrenergic blocker with several unique features. Its onset is rapid, it can easily be titrated to a desired end point, and its effects are rapidly terminated via metabolism by red cell and plasma esterases.[198,199] The drug has been particularly useful for the acute control of perioperative hypertension, as well as for treatment of supraventricular tachyarrhythmias (see later). Loading doses between 100 and 500 µg/kg given over 1 to 5 minutes are followed by maintenance infusions of 50 to 100 µg/kg/min. If the desired response is not achieved, the infusion rate is then typically doubled every 5 minutes until a desired response is achieved.

Specifics on pediatric dosing are limited at present. A maximum loading dose of 500 µg/kg and infusion rates of 250 to 300 µg/kg/min are currently suggested. A major potential side effect of esmolol is hypotension, particularly during bolus therapy. As noted earlier, esmolol rapidly distributes and has a very short elimination half-life of 7 to 10 minutes that is unaffected by organ blood flow or disease. Thus, hypotension is usually short-lived, but therapy with vasopressors may occasionally be required until it resolves.[200]

Labetalol

Labetalol has nonselective β-adrenergic blocking properties and is also a selective α-adrenergic receptor blocker. The ratio of α to β blockade efficiency is 1:3 and 1:7 after oral and intravenous administration, respectively. The primary use of labetalol in children is to control hypertension. The drug has been given intravenously to treat hypertensive crisis, to control hypertension after aortic coarctation repair, and as an adjunct to induce controlled hypotension during surgery.[201,202] Typical doses are 0.1 to 0.4 mg/kg given every 5 to 10 minutes until the desired effect is achieved; 0.25 to 1 mg/kg/hour infusion. The elimination half-life of labetalol is 3 to 5 hours.

Vasodilators

Vasodilators are used in children to control blood pressure during and after surgery, to treat systemic and pulmonary hypertension, and to decrease afterload on either the systemic or pulmonary ventricle, thereby improving pump function. Vasodilators are also given during cardiopulmonary bypass to reduce systemic vascular resistance to improve regional perfusion and facilitate rapid and even core cooling and rewarming.

Several different types of vasodilators are currently employed in children for these purposes. The most common are direct-acting nitrosovasodilators such as sodium nitroprusside and nitroglycerin. These drugs directly relax vascular smooth muscle to cause vasodilation. Hydralazine is another direct-acting smooth muscle vasodilator that is occasionally given to children to reduce blood pressure. α-Adrenergic blockers, such as phentolamine and phenoxybenzamine, are also used occasionally to acutely reduce blood pressure and systemic vascular resistance in the perioperative period. The latter blockers are more frequently employed during cardiopulmonary bypass. Angiotensin-converting enzyme (ACE) inhibitors may also be useful to help control blood pressure. Prostaglandin E_1 (PGE_1) is a direct-acting vasodilator with the unique property of being able to dilate the ductus arteriosus and maintain its patency. Prostacy-clin and inhaled nitric oxide are further additions that possess relatively selective pulmonary vasodilating capabilities.

Sodium Nitroprusside

Sodium nitroprusside is used to reduce afterload and blood pressure before, during, and after a wide variety of procedures.[203] For example, it is used intraoperatively and postoperatively to control systemic hypertension during and after repair of aortic coarctation and after correction of other forms of left ventricular outflow tract obstruction. The reduction in afterload may improve performance of a dysfunctional ventricle, particularly in combination with a positive inotropic agent.[204,205] The ability of nitroprusside to successfully treat pulmonary hypertension is variable.[206-208]

Sodium nitroprusside is an extremely potent vasodilator that acts directly on smooth muscle to cause dilation. Its effects reduce cardiac preload as well as afterload. Onset of effect is rapid (within minutes), and offset is similarly rapid. The effect ends within 1 to 2 minutes of terminating the infusion. Because of its potency, it should always be administered with an infusion pump in conjunction with direct continuous arterial pressure monitoring. The starting dosage is 0.5 to 1 µg/kg/min. This can be increased to achieve the desired effect. The hypotensive effects of nitroprusside are potentiated by hypovolemia, inhalation anesthetics, and drugs that inhibit increases in sympathetic tone and renin release, for example, propranolol and ACE inhibitors, respectively. These effects result from reflex increases in sympathetic tone and plasma renin activity that follow nitroprusside-induced vasodilation.

Adverse effects of sodium nitroprusside include cyanide and thiocyanate toxicities, rebound hypertension, inhibition of platelet function, and increased intrapulmonary shunting. Rebound hypertension is most likely due to activation of the aforementioned reflex mechanisms. It can usually be avoided by slowly tapering the infusion rather than abruptly discontinuing it. Toxicity may occur when more than 1 mg/kg of sodium nitroprusside is administered in less than 3 hours or when more than 0.5 mg/kg/hr is administered over 24 hours. A blood cyanide concentration of approximately 400 µg/dL has been associated with death in a child. Cyanide and thiocyanate toxicities are rare but may be more likely in neonates and young infants, as well as in those with impaired hepatic or renal function (see also Chapter 10).[209,210]

Cyanide production results from the metabolism of sodium nitroprusside. Free cyanide is then conjugated with thiosulfate by rhodanase in the liver to produce thiocyanate. A major mechanism of cyanide toxicity is via binding to cytochrome oxidase in the mitochondrial electron transport chain, thereby preventing mitochondrial respiration and ATP production. Signs of toxicity include tachyphylaxis, as well as an increase in mixed venous oxygen saturation and metabolic acidosis. In children who have received prolonged (>24 hours) or high-dose infusions of nitroprusside, as well as those with organ dysfunction, it may be advisable to measure blood cyanide concentrations. Serum thiocyanate concentrations may also be measured. Thiocyanate concentrations may increase when renal function is abnormal. Central nervous system dysfunction may occur when thiocyanate concentrations reach 5 to 10 mg/dL. Treatment of cyanide toxicity consists of intravenous infusion of sodium nitrite, 5 to 10 mg/kg over 5 minutes, and sodium thiosulfate, 150 to 450 mg/kg over 15 minutes. In children with abnormal renal function in whom stimulating the production of thiocyanate from thiosulfate may be contraindicated, administration of hydroxocobalamin has been recommended.

Nitroglycerin

Nitroglycerin is primarily a venodilator that acts on venous capacitance vessels. It has a substantially smaller effect on arteriolar smooth muscle, and its ability to attenuate an increased pulmonary vascular resistance is variable. Compared with nitroprusside, it is relatively ineffective as an antihypertensive agent. It has a short half-life and no significant toxic metabolites. Similar to nitroprusside, it may increase intrapulmonary shunting and cause platelet dysfunction. Nitroglycerin is typically administered in doses from 0.5 to 3.0 μg/kg/min. Effects occur within 2 minutes of starting nitroglycerin and resolve within 5 minutes of discontinuing it. Mild decreases in blood pressure may be observed at doses exceeding 2 to 3 μg/kg/min.

Nitroglycerin has found some favor during cardiopulmonary bypass to facilitate rapid and effective cooling and rewarming, as well as to improve tissue blood flow. Nitroprusside and nitroglycerin may differ substantially with regard to their effects on the microcirculation. Because it primarily reduces arteriolar tone and primarily dilates precapillaries, microvascular blood flow and tissue perfusion may be more diminished by nitroprusside, particularly in the presence of reduced arterial blood pressure, as seen during many phases of cardiopulmonary bypass.[211] In contrast, because nitroglycerin dilates both pre- and postcapillaries with equal efficacy, capillary perfusion is more likely to remain stable or even be enhanced in the presence of nitroglycerin compared with nitroprusside.[212,213]

Phentolamine and Phenoxybenzamine

Both of these drugs are α-adrenergic blocking agents with little selectively for α-receptor subtype. Their primary effect is to decrease resistance on the arterial side of the circulation, although both possess weak venodilating capabilities. Phentolamine is usually administered by infusion at 0.5 to 5 μg/kg/min, whereas phenoxybenzamine is administered orally in a dose of 0.1 to 0.3 mg/kg every 6 hours. The elimination half-life of phenoxybenzamine is much greater than phentolamine. The potent arteriolar dilating effects of phenoxybenzamine and its prolonged elimination half-life have been found to be advantageous by some for use as vasodilators during cardiopulmonary bypass.

Angiotensin-Converting Enzyme Inhibitors

ACE inhibitors are being administered with increasing frequency to children. They may be used in the perioperative setting to help control arterial blood pressure in the context of aortic coarctation repair or relief of left ventricular outflow obstruction. They are also given on a more long-term basis to reduce afterload on the systemic ventricle and to improve ventricular performance in children with congestive heart failure and single-ventricle physiology. Captopril, enalapril, and lisinopril are the ACE inhibitors most often used in children at this time, although there is little pediatric specific information. Side effects common to all ACE inhibitors include angioedema, acute renal failure, and hyperkalemia. A severe angioedema reaction has occasionally been fatal. Monitoring renal function and the serum potassium concentration are indicated.

The contribution of ACE inhibitors to anesthetic-induced hypotension remains controversial. Reports on both sides of this argument can be found. Angiotensin receptor blocking agents such as losartan can produce significant and refractory hypotension with standard anesthetic induction techniques.[214,215] Because of the potential risk of significant and refractory hypotension, which is usually unresponsive to volume expansion and requires substantial pressor treatment, it is our practice to discontinue the long-acting ACE inhibitors 1 day before surgery.

Captopril

Captopril has a relatively brief elimination half-life (<2 hours), is metabolized in the liver, and is then excreted by the kidney.[216] Oral dosing in neonates is 0.05 to 0.1 mg/kg every 8 to 24 hours, titrated up to 0.5 mg/kg every 6 to 24 hours. Infants initially receive 0.2 to 0.3 mg/kg every 6 to 8 hours. This can be titrated toward a maximum dose of 6 mg/kg/day in four divided doses. Older children may receive 0.025 to 0.25 mg/kg every 6 hours. The brief duration of effect, necessitating more frequent dosing, has led to increased use of the longer-acting ACE inhibitors (enalapril and lisinopril) in children.

Enalapril

Enalapril is metabolized in the liver to its active form, enalaprilat. Enalapril is the only ACE inhibitor currently available in the United States that has an intravenous formulation. Its safety and efficacy in infants and young children have not been established. Intravenous dosing in adults has been described at 0.6 to 1.5 mg/dose every 6 hours. Both enalapril and lisinopril are eliminated by the kidney. The duration of their hypotensive actions averages 24 hours but can last up to 30 hours.

Hydralazine

Hydralazine was frequently used in the past to control blood pressure in children. In contrast to adults, its ability to control pulmonary hypertension in children was disappointing.[217] Hydralazine directly relaxes smooth muscle without known effects on receptors. It reduces cardiac afterload but may cause significant reflex tachycardia. With long-term use, it may also cause fluid retention, requiring concurrent administration of a diuretic. Long-term oral hydralazine is given occasionally to treat systemic hypertension in children. Oral dosing is in the range of 0.2 to 0.75 mg/kg every 6 hours. The maximum dose is 7.5 mg/kg/day. Its use to control systemic blood pressure and afterload in children for the long term has largely been replaced by ACE inhibitors. It may also be administered intravenously to control blood pressure and reduce afterload. Intravenous doses are administered as a bolus of 0.1 to 0.2 mg/kg not to exceed 25 mg. The effects of intravenous hydralazine on pulmonary vascular resistance are also variable.[217,218] Tachyphylaxis to the antihypertensive effects of intravenous hydralazine may occur. Important side effects include a drug-related fever, rash, pancytopenia, and lupus-like syndrome. The elimination half-life of the drug is approximately 4 hours, but the effective biologic half-life may be substantially greater owing to significant binding of the drug to vascular smooth muscle.

Prostaglandin E₁

The major use of PGE$_1$ is to establish or maintain patency of the ductus arteriosus in infancy. It is best able to reopen a closing ductus in neonates up to 1 to 2 weeks of age but may occasionally be effective even in older infants.[10,219]

The use of PGE$_1$ to establish or maintain ductal patency is beneficial when the lower body is supplied by right-to-left ductal flow, as in cases of interrupted aortic arch, critical aortic stenosis, and hypoplastic left heart syndrome. Conversely, a patent ductus arteriosus can supply pulmonary blood flow from the aorta in lesions such as pulmonary atresia, tricuspid atresia, and severe tetralogy of Fallot. Side effects of PGE_1 include systemic hypotension, apnea, increased risk of infection, and central nervous system irritability.[220] PGE_1 infusions are usually begun at 0.05 µg/kg/min and may be increased to 0.1 µg/kg/min or more. The risk of apnea is related in part to infusion rate. Intubation and ventilation are often required with infusion rates greater than 0.05 µg/kg/min. PGE_1 has been utilized to treat primary or acquired pulmonary hypertension with varying degrees of success.[221-223]

Inhaled Nitric Oxide

An important development in the treatment of pulmonary hypertension is inhaled nitric oxide gas, which can be delivered directly to the pulmonary circulation. Nitric oxide is made endogenously and is an endothelium-derived relaxing factor that acts on guanylate cyclase in vascular smooth muscle to produce smooth muscle relaxation.[224] Endogenous nitric oxide in the vascular system is produced by endothelial cell nitric oxide synthase. Nitric oxide synthases convert the amino acid L-arginine into nitric oxide and the byproduct L-citrulline. Nitric oxide then diffuses into the subjacent vascular smooth muscle. It produces relaxation by acting on smooth muscle guanylate cyclase to produce cyclic guanosine monophosphate, which acts on a series of protein kinases and reduces intracellular calcium levels to inhibit muscle contraction (see Fig. 36-1). Nitric oxide diffusing in the other direction from the endothelial cell into the blood vessel lumen can decrease the adhesiveness of white blood cells and platelets. Nitric oxide in the blood is rapidly bound by oxyhemoglobin, which is then oxidized to methemoglobin. From this reaction, nitric oxide is inactivated and nitrite and nitrate are released in the blood. Red blood cell methemoglobin is subsequently reduced back to hemoglobin. The rapid binding and inactivation of nitric oxide in the blood means that inhaled nitric oxide has a minimal effect on the systemic circulation and functions as a very specific pulmonary vasodilator.

Significant reductions in pulmonary vascular resistance from inhaled nitric oxide have been demonstrated in adults with mitral stenosis, in neonates with persistent pulmonary hypertension of the neonate, in lung transplant recipients, and in children after surgical repair of a variety of CHDs.[225-229] The efficacy of inhaled nitric oxide is in large part related to the ability to deliver it into the alveolus, which is in close proximity to the pulmonary vascular smooth muscle. Effects on the systemic circulation are minimal because of rapid inactivation by reaction with oxyhemoglobin in the blood.

Inhaled nitric oxide has found several uses in children with CHD. In the cardiac catheterization laboratory, it is used to assess reactivity of the pulmonary vasculature to vasodilation in children with pulmonary hypertension. It can, therefore, help distinguish between children with fixed pulmonary vascular obstructive disease and those with a reversible component to pulmonary hypertension, thereby facilitating operative planning and management.

In the postoperative period after the repair of CHD, nitric oxide can be used to reduce pulmonary vascular resistance and thereby improve cardiopulmonary performance. Experience

thus far suggests that children with two ventricles who have increased left atrial pressure or its pathophysiologic equivalents (e.g., mitral stenosis, severe congestive heart failure, cardiomyopathy, large left-to-right shunts, total anomalous pulmonary venous drainage) are those who will most likely respond to nitric oxide in the postoperative period with a significant decrease in pulmonary vascular resistance. Children with single ventricle physiology are less likely to improve pulmonary blood flow and oxygenation after nitric oxide. Interestingly, some children who do not respond to nitric oxide immediately after cardiopulmonary bypass in the operating room respond to nitric oxide with significant reductions in pulmonary vascular resistance several hours later. Nitric oxide is administered in concentrations of 1 to 80 ppm in oxygen with a specially adapted ventilator. Inspired gas is monitored for greater oxides of nitrogen, which are toxic. Blood methemoglobin concentrations should also be assessed when a child has been receiving long-term inhaled nitric oxide therapy.

Prostacyclin

Continuous intravenous infusion of epoprostenol has been used effectively for many years in children with pulmonary artery hypertension of any cause. It improves hemodynamics by reducing pulmonary artery pressure, increasing cardiac output, and increasing oxygen transport, as well as improving symptoms such as exercise capacity and dyspnea.[230] It has been used with excellent results in the treatment of primary pulmonary hypertension and irreversible acquired pulmonary hypertension in CHD; in children awaiting heart, lung, or heart-lung transplantation; in children with primary pulmonary hypertension; in neonates with persistent pulmonary hypertension; and in pulmonary hypertensive crises.[96,97,231-235] The fact that children who were initially nonresponders may respond after prolonged use of nitric oxide suggests that its mechanism of action involves a degree of remodeling, although no absolute mechanism has been elucidated as yet. Unfortunately, epoprostenol is chemically unstable at room temperature and has an elimination half-life of only 1 to 2 minutes. It is thus administered using a specific delivery system that necessitates central venous access. Complications related to its use include local infection, line sepsis, catheter dislodgement, and pump malfunction. Several of these problems may lead to severe acute pulmonary hypertensive crises. Thus, alternate mechanisms of delivery have been sought.

Oral Prostacyclin Analogues

Beraprost sodium is an oral prostacyclin analogue that is currently licensed for use in Japan. It is more stable chemically than epoprostenol and has a more prolonged elimination half-life. It nonetheless requires dosing three to four times per day, reaching its peak blood concentration at 30 minutes. Two double-blind studies conducted to date showed no significant long-term benefit, but there may still be a role for this drug in combination therapy because improvements have been observed in the exercise capacity in children with idiopathic pulmonary artery hypertension.[236,237]

The inhaled prostacyclin analogue iloprost is another prostaglandin I_2 analogue that can be delivered both intravenously and also by ultrasonic nebulizer. Unfortunately, it still has a very brief elimination half-life of 15 to 20 minutes, which thus requires nebulized treatments six to nine times each day. In adult studies, iloprost has been shown to be beneficial in patients with

nant factor VIIa also activates platelets, adding to the potential benefit of this agent in significant hemorrhage. Thus, this therapy is intuitively attractive for the treatment of surgical bleeding.

There are several case reports of rFVIIa therapy in infants and children undergoing cardiac surgery.[49,50] One report described a series of 9 children (median age 9 years) who had simple cardiac repairs with moderate bleeding in the first 3 hours postoperatively (5.8 mL/kg/hr chest tube output), which decreased to 2 mL/kg/hr in the 3 hours after administration of a single dose of rFVIIa.[50] Because of its high cost, and the paucity of data in children undergoing cardiac surgery, rfVIIa should be reserved for life-threatening hemorrhage unresponsive to other measures. A dose of 90 µg/kg, repeated up to two additional times, can be used.

Sickle Cell Disease

Sickle cell disease (SCD) presents one of the most common hemoglobinopathies among patients of African-American or West Indian origin. This leads to the substitution of valine for glutamic acid in position 6 of the β-hemoglobin chain. SCD is represented by a homozygous genotype (HbSS) with fractional concentrations of HbS in the range from 70% to 90%. Sickle cell trait (SCT), on the other hand, is a heterozygous manifestation (HbAS) and may be as common as 10% in the previously mentioned population. The diagnosis is made by hemoglobin electrophoretic studies (see Chapter 9).

Children with SCD are at a particular risk for perioperative complications.[51,52] Sickling can be triggered by hypoxia, dehydration, acidosis,[53] hypothermia, stress, and infections. Hypoxia induces opening of a Ca^{2+}-activated K^+ channel that causes intracellular dehydration.[54] Chain formation occurs and leads to increased blood viscosity with vaso-occlusion. Opening of the Gardos channel is an important mechanism of sickle cell dehydration, which is temperature dependent, with greater potassium efflux at lower temperatures.[55] Shrinkage of sickle erythrocytes may also result from activation of a K^+/Cl^- cotransport pathway under acidotic conditions.[56] Activation of this pathway can be blocked by increasing the abnormally low level of intracellular magnesium in sickle erythrocytes. The use of magnesium and hydroxy urea in the perioperative period therefore seems to be beneficial.[57]

CPB, particularly for more complex surgical procedures, may involve periods of low flow or even circulatory arrest, as well as hypothermia with consequent local vasoconstriction, hypoxemia, and acidosis. There is some evidence that CPB can be safely undertaken in SCD.[58] Flow conditions are an important determinant of sickle erythrocyte adherence to endothelium. Under low-flow conditions sickle cell adhesion to endothelium increases with contact time in the absence of endothelium activation or adhesive proteins, whereas under venular flow conditions sickle cell adhesion occurs only after endothelial activation. During CPB, both low-flow conditions and endothelial activation may occur. Multiple triggers of sickling are likely to occur during CPB, and close attention should be paid to the conduct of all aspects of bypass.

In the past, routine exchange transfusion has been recommended to prevent these complications.[59] More recent experience provides evidence that not all children require an exchange transfusion.[60] The growing evidence of the harmful effects of blood transfusion adds to the need to carefully reconsider routine exchange transfusion.[61] For uncomplicated bypass

surgery without periods of cardiac arrest, the omission of exchange transfusion has led to good outcomes.

Guidelines have been proposed for the perioperative management of children with sickle cell disorders.[60] The key points are the avoidance of hypothermia if possible with tepid or warm CPB; blood transfusion only for a drop in hematocrit below 20%; maintenance of intravascular volume and body temperature while on CPB; the avoidance of vasopressors, postoperative multimodal pain therapy; and early incentive spirometry to prevent pulmonary complications.[62] In our practice, we utilize cerebral near-infrared spectroscopy (NIRS) to help determine an acceptable hematocrit for the individual child.

For children undergoing hypothermia, successful management with[63] and without[64] partial or complete exchange transfusion on bypass has been reported. Exchange transfusion can occur preoperatively or on initiation of CPB.[65] For exchange transfusion, the extracorporeal circuit is primed with blood and the usual components. Upon CPB start, the child's blood volume is drained into storage bags and processed. The platelet-rich plasma is reinfused at the end of CPB, and the concentrated sickle cells are discarded. Platelet and plasma sequestration in conjunction with exchange transfusion reduces the need for postoperative transfusion and protects the platelets from the negative effects of CPB.[66]

There seems to be no consensus as to a suitable target HbS. Reducing the absolute level of HbS may be of greater benefit than achieving a particular ratio of HbA to HbS because those remaining may still precipitate.[67] In SCD, exchange transfusion has been shown to favorably affect cerebral tissue oxygenation.[68] Exchange transfusion will decrease both the proportion and absolute amount of HbS; it may also have favorable effects on hypoxic pulmonary vasoconstriction.[68] In this context, these children may benefit from continuous hemofiltration to reduce inflammatory mediators and improve pulmonary recovery.[69] Inhaled nitric oxide also has been suggested as an adjunct for the prevention of sickle cell crisis. It may improve the binding of oxygen, thereby reducing the formation of sickle cells; reduce pulmonary hypertension; and improve pulmonary function without adverse effects on normal hemoglobin.[70]

A Perspective on Blood Preservation: Cardiopulmonary Bypass in Jehovah's Witness Patients

Jehovah's Witnesses differ from other religious groups in their conscious objection to decline the therapeutic infusion of blood and blood components. They refuse the transfusion of any primary blood components (PRBCs, platelets, and plasma) as well as predisposed autologous blood. Individual choices that can be made are the acceptance of fractions of blood such as albumin and globulins, dialysis, cell savage, and acute normovolemic hemodilution.

Acute isovolemic reduction of hemoglobin down to 5 g/dL is tolerated in healthy individuals under anesthesia and does not appear to reduce tissue oxygenation significantly.[71] Reduction of oxygen delivery to 7 to 8 mL/kg/min under resting conditions does not lead to an oxygen debt and is compensated by increased extraction, an increase in cardiac index, and a subsequent decrease in systemic vascular resistance.[72,73] In a retrospective study of the tolerance of low hemoglobin levels in Jehovah's Witness patients it was reported that all patients who died had hemoglobin concentrations of less than 5 g/dL.[74] A safe limit of hemodilution in children has not been established. One report showed that hemodilution up to 50% in acyanotic children appears to be safe.[75] In cyanotic children, however, the limit was estimated to be around 40%. If this level of hemodilution is exceeded, hemodynamic instability and inadequate oxygen transfer can occur. Evidence suggests that hematocrit levels of 21.5% on CPB compared with 27.8% leads to significantly improved neurodevelopmental outcome.[76]

The most important and simplest way to avoid transfusion in the setting of cardiac surgery is to limit blood loss. Unnecessary and reduced amounts of blood sampling help to preserve blood.[77] Pharmacologic agents such as aprotinin and tranexamic acid reduce the risk of perioperative blood loss.[78] Hormonal stimulation of erythropoiesis with recombinant erythropoietin is another strategy acceptable to Jehovah's Witnesses. The administration of erythropoietin in the cardiac surgery setting has been shown to reduce the risk of exposure to allergenic blood.[79] However, the associated rise in hematocrit with erythropoietin use may be potentially thrombogenic and could lead to an increase in the incidence of perioperative venous thromboembolism. The cost of using erythropoietin can be large, and cost analysis suggested that its use in cardiac surgery was not cost effective.[80]

Intraoperative recovery of blood with a cell salvage device is also acceptable to many Jehovah's Witnesses. This involves the removal by suction of blood from the operative field followed by washing, filtering, and return of red blood cells to the patient. A randomized controlled trial of intraoperative cell salvage in cardiothoracic surgery has demonstrated a reduction in red blood cell transfusion and an increase in postoperative hemoglobin.[81]

Acute normovolemic hemodilution (ANH) involves the preoperative removal of a volume of blood from the patient with the simultaneous administration of crystalloid or colloid to maintain circulating volume.[82] The collected blood is then reinfused during the operation. Some Jehovah's Witnesses find this process acceptable, especially if the blood line is not detached from the patient. ANH has other advantages, including lower costs, because the blood does not need compatibility testing; reduced possibility of administrative error; and a saving in patient time (see Chapter 10). The development of artificial red cell substitutes could potentially abrogate the need for compatibility testing as well as vastly reduce infection risks with none of the immunomodulatory side effects of allogenic blood.[83] Some of these products would also be acceptable to Jehovah's Witness families. Substitutes include perfluorocarbons, hemoglobin solutions, intramolecular crosslinked hemoglobin, and liposome encapsulated hemoglobin. None of these has reached clinical practice. Lastly, autologous retrograde priming has been used in Jehovah's Witness patients and can further reduce the hemodilutional effects of the prime.[82,84]

In the great majority of adult patients, open-heart surgery can be performed without administration of blood or blood components. In children and small infants weighing less than 5 kg, bloodless open-heart surgery is more complicated. Preoperative iron supplementation (6 mg/kg/day) and erythropoietin (200-400 U/kg/wk) have been used successfully to augment preoperative hemoglobin levels.[85]

Modern bypass circuits allow the reduction of priming volumes to less than 200-300 mL. Main components that are amenable to volume reduction on a regular circuit are the size and length of the lines, small oxygenators and arterial filters, and priming the hemofilter for modified ultrafiltration with blood from the venous line after CPB. Line volumes, for example, may vary between 1.73 mL per 10 cm of a 3/16-inch tubing versus 0.75 mL per 10 cm of a 1/8-inch tubing. The limiting factor, however, is the necessary flow. For a 3/16-inch arterial line, a maximum flow of 1.8 L/minute was established as the point at which the Reynolds number reaches a value of 1000, indicating a change to turbulent flow. Modified ultrafiltration at the end of CPB through a fluid warmer line to prevent heat loss or continuous ultrafiltration has been used. The venous line and the reservoir are emptied before discontinuation of bypass, the field is suctioned, and all blood is retransfused through the arterial line. Decannulation is achieved and protamine is given as usual. Crystalloid cardioplegia should be evacuated from the field by an external sucker to prevent dilution of the pump volume.

Postoperative care involves minimal blood sampling and only on special indications. Noninvasive monitoring allows uncomplicated weaning from the ventilator.[86] The first report of successful outcomes in Jehovah's Witness children with congenital cardiac defects was in 1985;[87] 110 children older than 6 months of age successfully underwent operation, with a perioperative mortality rate of 5.3%. Only one death was attributed to blood loss. A weight less than 5 kg is considered by some as a contraindication for open-heart surgery and palliative procedures were advocated in the past.[88] For some lesions, however, no palliation is possible. The development of miniaturized circuits, preoperative optimization, use of high-dose aprotinin, vacuum-assisted drainage to allow smaller tubing and cannula sizes, as well as the use of modified ultrafiltration, enabled the safe expansion of surgery into the neonatal population. Individualized heparin level based anticoagulation management further results in a reduction of coagulation problems, blood loss, and transfusion requirements.[89] The addition of desmopressin, 0.3 µg/kg, also not proven, is believed by some to improve platelet activity and stimulate the release of von Willebrand factor after protamine infusion.

All of the aforementioned considerations are important in approaching the Jehovah's Witness patient; however, at Texas Children's Hospital, Jehovah's Witness children are not treated differently with regard to blood transfusion practice than any other child. Cerebral NIRS is utilized to help determine the safe hemoglobin level for the individual child at all phases of surgery. Consent for blood transfusion in this situation is a complicated issue, because the legal status of children is different from that of an adult. Each institution must develop a legal informed consent process for blood transfusion for Jehovah's Witness children, in consultation with local legal authorities, social work and ethic groups, and representatives of the Jehovah's Witness faith. Currently we have a release of liability form for the parent to sign stating that he or she requests that blood products not be used but that acknowledges they may be needed to treat his or her child. The parent further agrees to release and hold harmless the physicians and hospital for any liability associated with blood transfusion. This form was developed in conjunction with the local Jehovah's Witness church representatives, and in our practice this has been accepted by more than 95% of parents and has obviated the need for more extreme measures such as temporary child protective services custody during the perioperative period, which was our former practice.

Myocardial Protection

Myocardial protection during cardiac surgery has evolved over the years. Melrose and colleagues introduced the concept of chemical cardioplegia in 1955.[90] Before the popular use of chemical cardioplegia, topical cardiac hypothermia was used. In the late 1970s and early 1980s, the concept of cold hyperkalemic blood cardioplegia was introduced.[91] Potassium concentrations in cardioplegic solutions ranging from 12 to 30 mEq/L are typically used to achieve cardiac standstill within 1 to 2 minutes under hypothermic conditions, with higher concentrations (or longer induction times) required for normothermic conditions. Myocardial edema after bypass and global ischemia can be reduced by a number of strategies that involve modifying the conditions of delivery and composition of cardioplegia solutions as they affect the movement of intracellular and interstitial fluid. In contrast to studies in adults, most studies conducted in newborns have shown little difference between blood and crystalloid cardioplegia.[92,93] Hypothermia also decreases myocardial oxygen consumption. The benefits of this approach appear to be optimal at myocardial temperatures between 24° C and 28° C. Avoidance or reduction of myocardial edema occurs by limiting the pressure of cardioplegia infusions and by providing moderately hyperosmolar cardioplegia solutions that contain blood. Buffering the acidosis that results from ischemia is achieved by including tromethamine (THAM), histidine-imidazole, or both in the cardioplegia solution. Close management of myocardial calcium balance to avoid extremes of intracellular hypercalcemia or hypocalcemia, especially during reperfusion, is very important.[94,95] The addition of magnesium may solve this dilemma by preventing damage from higher cardioplegic calcium concentrations by its action as a calcium antagonist.[95,96] This prevents mitochondrial calcium overload as a consequence of reperfusion injury. Magnesium also prevents the influx of sodium into the postischemic myocardium, which is exchanged for calcium during reperfusion.

Every cardiac program has their own philosophy regarding cardioplegia and myocardial protection. At Texas Children's Hospital we use plain crystalloid cardioplegia. The prime blood gas and electrolytes should mimic physiologically to the child's arterial blood gas as closely as possible. If whole blood or packed cells are added to the prime, the target hemodilution range should be 28% to 30%; the prime should be recirculated continuously and warmed between 35.0° and 36.5° C before initiation of bypass. In neonates and infants, albumin is added to the cardioplegic solution to maintain an appropriate colloid osmotic pressure. This may decrease edema formation of the arrested heart. In children undergoing circulatory arrest, long cross clamp times, and large pump suction return cases, 20 mg/kg methylprednisolone is used up to a maximum of 500 mg, to reduce the production of inflammatory mediators that result in myocardial dysfunction. Table 17-3 summarizes the Texas Children's Hospital protocols for cardioplegia and myocardial protection.

Phases of Cardiopulmonary Bypass

Surgical cases requiring CPB are divided into several basic phases.

Pre-Bypass Period

This phase begins with surgical incision and lasts through initial dissection and preparation for cannulation. During this period transesophageal echocardiography (TEE) is performed to confirm the diagnosis and establish a basis for post-bypass comparison.

Cannulation and Initiation of Bypass

After sternotomy and mediastinal dissection, the aorta is cannulated, along with either the right atrium, if single venous drainage is planned, or the superior and inferior venae cavae for bicaval venous drainage. A large dose of heparin (300-400 units/kg) is administered intravenously, and the adequacy of anticoagulation is measured using the ACT *before initiating CPB*. The target ACT level is usually 480 seconds, but in the presence of aprotinin, a target of 600 seconds is desirable because of this

Table 17-3. Cardioplegia Solution

Cardioplegia Base Solution (385 mL)

Contains		Contents	
Sodium chloride BP	3.54 g/L	Sodium	23 mmol
Anhydrous glucose BP	6.65 g/L	Potassium	15 mmol
Potassium chloride	2.92 g/L	Calcium	0.35 mmol
Mannitol	6.54 g/L	Chloride	39 mmol
Calcium chloride	135 mg/L	Glucose	2.52 g
Mannitol	2.48 g		
Approximate pH 4.5			
275 mOsm/L			

Cardioplegia Buffer Solution

Contains		Contents	
Sodium carbonate	9.37 g/L	Sodium carbonate	0.28 g
Sodium bicarbonate	27.0 g/L	Sodium bicarbonate	0.81 g

Table 17-3. Cardioplegia Solution—cont'd

Uses of Cardioplegia Solution During Cardiopulmonary Bypass

Children weighing <10 kg
  385 mL Cardioplegia base solution
  26 mL Cardioplegia buffer solution
  100 mL 25% Albumin
  Note: This is usually delivered at a pressure of 30 mm Hg for newborns and 30-40 mm Hg for older infants.

Children weighing >10 kg
  385 mL Cardioplegia base solution
  100 mL 0.9% Sodium chloride
  10 mL 25% Mannitol
  5 mL 8.4% Sodium bicarbonate

Note: This is usually delivered at a pressure of 30-60 mm Hg. A good guide is to note the end-diastolic pressure of each child before bypass. This will be a guide to the normal filling pressure of the coronary arteries. When aortic incompetence is present, the CPS flow may need to be increased.

Administration of Cardioplegia Solution

For all patients:

Temperature	8°C-12°C
Initial dose	110 mL/m^2/min for 4 min
Subsequent doses	110 mL/m^2/min for 2 min

Note: Following the initial dose, cardioplegia is to be delivered every 20 minutes during the cross clamp period unless otherwise indicated by the surgeon. The perfusionist will remind the surgeon of the need for cardioplegia and keep track of the time. Because of the nature of the surgical procedure, it may be necessary to deliver cardioplegia directly into the coronary ostia via a hand-held delivery system. In this case the surgeon will direct the perfusionist. Close attention should be paid to the delivery line pressures.

Examples of Primes

Neonate: Whole Blood, if available, otherwise reconstituted

Whole blood	225 mL
Plasmalyte A	50 mL
0.45% NaCl	125 mL
Heparin	2500 units
NaH$_2$CO$_3$	5 mEq
CaCl$_2$	250 mg

Pediatric: Packed Red Blood Cells

PRBCs	250 mL
Plasmalyte A	300 mL
0.45% NaCl	75 mL
25% Albumin	100 mL
Heparin	3500 units
NaH$_2$CO$_3$	20 mEq
CaCl$_2$	300 mg

Adult: Crystalloid Prime

Plasmalyte A	700 mL
0.45% NaCl	600 mL
25% Albumin	100-200 mL (volume varies depending on the size of the patient)
5% Dextrose	40 mL
Heparin	5000 units
NaH$_2$CO$_3$	40 mEq
CaCl$_2$	300 mg
KCl	2.4 mEq

agent's effect on the test measurement. High levels of ACT are maintained on CPB with the addition of heparin to the prime and as needed because larger doses of heparin lead to a reduced degree of consumptive coagulopathy, which translates into reduced blood product therapy requirements.[89] Other methods of measuring anticoagulation include the Hepcon system (a plasma heparin concentration assay), which may allow for more accurate titration of heparin and protamine dosages.[97] The thromboelastogram may also be utilized as a baseline measure of the coagulation system and then may be repeated on bypass with heparinase added to more objectively assess each child's anticipated need for coagulation products.[98] An improved preservation of the hemostatic system with subsequent reduction of blood loss and a reduction in transfusion requirements has been demonstrated after maintenance of high heparin levels during CPB.[99] The additional maintenance of high ATIII concentrations may further contribute to a reduction of hemostatic activation.[100]

In most centers, bicaval cannulation is used for all but the smallest children (<2 kg) to prevent venous return from interfering with the surgical field. A gradual transition to full CPB is then performed to minimize myocardial stress, using a prime that has essentially the same composition as the child's blood with regard to temperature, pH, calcium, potassium, and hematocrit. CPB flows of 150 mL/kg/min are used for infants weighing less than 10 kg, and 2.4 L/min/m^2 is used for children weighing more than 10 kg. Flow rates may be reduced during periods of hypothermia (see later), although many centers now prefer to maintain greater flows throughout the bypass period. Misplaced cannulas can lead to significant morbidity. Obstruction of the inferior vena cava (IVC) by a misplaced IVC cannula can lead to increased venous pressure, which causes ascites and decreased perfusion pressure in mesenteric, hepatic, and renal vascular beds. Misplacement of the cannula in the superior vena cava (SVC) can result in increased venous pressure in the cerebral venous system. Subsequent cerebral edema results from inadequate venous drainage and a consequent reduction in cerebral blood flow, potentially resulting in ischemia. Arterial cannula misplacement can also occur. If the cannula inadvertently slips beyond the takeoff of the right innominate artery, preferential perfusion to the left side of the brain can be observed. This can be detected on the NIRS monitor, which may be an important monitor, particularly in pediatric cardiac surgery.[101]

The presence of any anomalous systemic-to-pulmonary shunts can lead to shunting of blood away from the systemic circulation, through the pulmonary circuit, and then through the venous cannula to the CPB machine. Thus, the systemic perfusion is shunted away from the body in a futile circuit back to the CPB machine. Anatomic lesions where such shunting can occur include an unrecognized patent ductus arteriosus and large aortopulmonary collaterals as found in pulmonary atresia. Bypass flow needs to be adjusted to compensate for these shunts.

Cooling Phase

Systemic cooling is utilized for nearly every case. Hypothermia is classified as mild (30°C-36°C), moderate (22°C-30°C), or deep (17°C-22°C). In general, lower temperatures are used for more complex operations that carry a greater potential for requiring periods of low-flow bypass or circulatory arrest. Cooling is primarily achieved extracorporeally through the heat exchanger in the bypass circuit, although some surgeons also request that ice be applied to the head.

Aortic Cross Clamping and Intracardiac Repair Phase

The aorta is cross clamped, with the heart then rendered asystolic after infusion of a high-potassium cardioplegia solution into the aortic root.

Deep Hypothermic Circulatory Arrest or Selective Cerebral Perfusion Phase

If circulatory arrest is to be used, it is initiated after a slow cooling period of at least 20 minutes, and an attempt is made to limit the total duration of deep hypothermic circulatory arrest (DHCA) to less than 40 minutes. Special bypass techniques (see later) have been developed to avoid the necessity of using DHCA and may also be performed during this time.

Removal of Aortic Cross Clamp and Rewarming Phase

After completion of the intracardiac repair and de-airing of the heart, the aortic cross clamp is removed, allowing reperfusion of the myocardium. Optimally, normal sinus rhythm and myocardial contractility are restored during this time, while the child is slowly rewarmed. During rewarming, surgery is completed, inotropic and vasoactive agents are started, and ventilation begins. Hemofiltration and blood transfusion are used to achieve the desired hematocrit. Left atrial and/or pulmonary artery monitoring lines, if indicated, are placed at this time, as are temporary atrial and ventricular pacing wires. If the child is incompletely rewarmed before separation from CPB, a significant afterdrop with precipitous post-bypass reduction in core body temperature can occur. This would lead to vasoconstriction, shivering, increased oxygen consumption, and acidosis. However, postischemic hyperthermia can lead to delayed neuronal cell death.[102] Mild degrees of hypothermia and certainly the avoidance of hyperthermia are essential in the perioperative period.[103] In children, rectal temperature mostly reflects peripheral temperature. One study showed that the temperature of the foot was more sensitive than the temperature of the hand.[104] Another study revealed that for anatomic or physiologic reasons, temperature gradients in the toes develop more readily than those in the fingers.[105] Several endpoints have been proposed, such as nasopharyngeal temperatures greater than 35.0°C, bladder temperature greater than 36.2°C, or skin temperatures greater than 30°C[106,107]; we use an endpoint of 35.5°C rectal temperature.[108]

Separation from Bypass

The child's core body temperature, hematocrit, and metabolic parameters should be optimized before attempting separation from CPB. Careful observation for left-sided air, confirmation with the TEE, and concurrent ECG changes continue throughout the weaning process, with the child in Trendelenburg position and the aortic root vented. CPB flow is then gradually reduced to zero, while volume is added to the child from the venous reservoir until optimal filling pressures are achieved.

Post-Bypass Period

This phase lasts until chest closure and transfer to the ICU have been accomplished. During this time, modified ultrafiltration

(MUF) may be performed for 10 to 15 minutes after cessation of CPB. Cardiac function and the quality of the surgical repair are assessed via TEE, and, if found to be satisfactory, protamine is then administered to neutralize residual heparin. The usual dose of protamine is 1.0 to 1.3 mg/100 units of heparin given at the onset of bypass. Limiting protamine to this dose prevents overdosing of protamine with its associated effects on platelet function (reduction of the interaction of glycoprotein Ib receptor interaction with von Willebrand factor).[109] If the ACT is still elevated or prime blood is given back to the child, an additional 25% of the initial dose of protamine is added and the ACT is rechecked. However, particularly in infants, the administration of protamine and the persistent treatment of a suspected incomplete heparin reversal should not distract and delay the treatment of other commonly associated post-bypass coagulopathies such as thrombocytopenia, platelet dysfunction, and other coagulation factor deficiencies.

Protamine reactions are much less frequent in children younger than 16 years of age and are reported as 1.76% to 2.88%.[110] Independent risk factors are a female gender, a larger protamine dose, and smaller heparin doses. Type I reactions or effects during administration are rare and adding calcium does not change the hemodynamic consequences of injection.[111] Fortunately, severe anaphylactic reactions (type II) or catastrophic pulmonary vasoconstriction (type III) are rare but have been observed by us and others.[112] Administering the protamine over no less than 5 minutes reduces the severity and precipitous nature of any protamine reaction.

Unstable neonates and small infants may have their sternums temporarily left open, with surgical closure planned 24 to 72 hours later when cardiac function has improved and myocardial edema diminished.

Because CPB can have a multitude of adverse physiologic effects, attempts are made to minimize both the duration of CPB and ischemic (aortic cross clamp) time; thus, as much of the surgery as possible is performed outside of these phases. In general, physiologic responses to bypass are more extreme with decreasing age and size of the child. The neonate experiences a greater degree of hemodilution on bypass and colder temperatures on bypass and frequently requires longer aortic cross clamp times, all of which can result in a greater inflammatory response. Table 17-4 summarizes clinical management issues during the major phases of CPB.

Particular Aspects of Management on Cardiopulmonary Bypass

pH-Stat Versus α-Stat Management

Some degree of hypothermia is utilized for nearly every cardiac operation to slow the metabolism and oxygen consumption of all organs, particularly the brain and heart.[113] During cooling, the carbon dioxide contained in blood becomes more soluble and its partial pressure decreases. The $Paco_2$ sensed by the body decreases as body temperature decreases, with the result that at a core temperature of 17°C to 18°C, if pH and $Paco_2$ have not been corrected for temperature, the body is experiencing a pH of about 7.6 and $Paco_2$ of 15 to 18 mm Hg (Fig. 17-2).[114] This very low $Paco_2$ causes cerebral vasoconstriction, particularly during the cooling phase of bypass, which in turn leads to less

Table 17-4. Checklist for Bypass Management

Before CPB

1. Check temperature; maintain normothermia during induction and preparation.
2. Supplement premedication.
3. Ensure noninvasive monitoring: blood pressure, ECG, pulse oximetry, stethoscope.
4. Perform inhalational induction after preoxygenation; intravenous induction, if cannula is in place.
5. Peripheral intravenous placement(s)
6. Relaxation and ventilation
7. Intubation and mechanical ventilation according to shunt lesion (CO_2, O_2 control)
8. Monitoring:
   a. Arterial line and central venous line
   b. ECG electrodes
   c. Bladder catheter
   d. Temperature probes
   e. TEE probe (in infants >3 kg)
9. Positioning
10. Deepening of anesthetic level
11. Antifibrinolytics and corticosteroids, as indicated
12. Heparin, 300-400 U/kg, before arterial cannulation
13. Check activated clotting time >400 sec.
14. Supplement anesthetics on initiation of bypass.

During CPB

1. Stop ventilation and drips when full flow is reached.
2. Inspect head perfusion.
3. Evaluate quality of perfusion (perfusion pressure, central venous pressure, diuresis, arterial blood gases, temperature gradient).
4. Prepare for separation
   a. Drips (inotropic drugs, calcium)
   b. Pacemaker
   c. Blood products
5. Set and control temperature and rewarming (heating blanket, room temperature).
6. Zero transducers
7. Check arterial blood gases in preparation for discontinuation of CPB; correct abnormalities.
8. Suction and ventilate.

After CPB

1. Separate when
   a. Temperature >35.5°C
   b. Stable rhythm or pacing
   c. Heart contracting well
2. Fine-tune blood pressure; consider direct blood pressure measurement for hypotension at the aortic cannula; volume ± drips.
3. Consider modified ultrafiltration.
4. Check arterial blood gases.
5. Evaluate with transesophageal echocardiography for residual defects.
6. Give protamine, 1-1.2 mg/100 IU heparin.
7. Check activated clotting time and arterial blood gases.
8. Chest closure and recheck arterial blood gases.
9. Transport to the intensive care unit.

of α receptors rather than to the half-life of the drug.[141] Phenoxybenzamine improves the CPB flows and decreased metabolic acidosis as well as the cellular response to stress after CPB. Phenoxybenzamine, used as part of a treatment strategy after stage 1 palliation for hypoplastic left heart syndrome, has been associated with improved outcome.[142,143] Phenoxybenzamine was more effective than sodium nitroprusside in improving peripheral circulation, as shown by temperature gradients intraoperatively.[144] In addition, phenoxybenzamine improved tissue perfusion and increased CPB flow, as evident by a decreased base deficit in comparison with sodium nitroprusside. Phenoxybenzamine increases the flow on CPB to achieve the same mean arterial pressure. Greater CPB flows are associated with an improved oxygen delivery, which can improve patient outcome.[145] Excessive α blockade can be antagonized by vasopressin.[146]

Phentolamine is a nonselective competitive α_1 and α_2 catecholamine receptor blocker. It has a half-life of 19 minutes and is eliminated mainly by the kidneys. Through postsynaptic α_1 and α_2 receptor inhibition it has a vasodilating and hypotensive effect that can improve cardiovascular parameters and metabolic acidosis during CPB management.[147] In children receiving phentolamine, increasing lactate levels at the end of the CPB period show a steady state toward the end of the surgery, whereas it continues to rise in patients who did not receive phentolamine.[147] These findings suggest that the use of phentolamine limits lactic acid production during the hypothermic period and aids the disposal of lactic acid from tissues. Seelye and associates called the physiologic state after hypothermia the "oxygen debt repayment" period in infants.[148] Although it has a beneficial effect on CPB management, the potential harmful effects of phentolamine, especially on the brain, have still not been fully elucidated. One study provided evidence that phentolamine increases S100B protein and a parameter indicative of altered cerebrovascular resistance, the pulsatility index in the middle cerebral artery, in infants given phentolamine during open-heart surgery.[149]

Nitroprusside has been used as an easily titratable agent with α-blocking capacity. One study examined the effect of perioperative sodium nitroprusside application in 25 neonates undergoing an arterial switch operation for transposition of the great arteries.[150] In comparison to the pre-bypass values, a similar increase in the concentration of S100B protein was found 2 hours after the termination of CPB in the sodium nitroprusside–treated and nontreated neonates, which decreased over the subsequent 48 postoperative hours. However, significantly reduced post-bypass serum levels of S100B protein were found in the sodium nitroprusside–treated group after 24 and 48 hours of treatment.

Nitroglycerin has been used with the same success. The only proven benefit over other agents is its nitric oxide donation capacity.[151] In Japan, high-dose chlorpromazine has been used as part of a low-resistance strategy during CPB for the Norwood procedure.[152]

We routinely use phentolamine, 0.1 to 0.2 mg/kg, to provide normal CPB flow and mean arterial pressure in the range of the diastolic pressure. In exceptional circumstances like the arterial switch operation or Norwood procedures, we use phenoxybenzamine 0.25 mg/kg. If hypotension develops on bypass, we increase the flow up to 150% of predicted and examine the acid-base status in conjunction with cerebral oxygenation and mixed venous saturations. Often, severe hemodilution with oxygen

debt is the cause and should be treated as such. After exclusion, we treat the hypotension carefully with vasoconstrictors, knowing that normal systemic pressures will not restore splanchnic hypoperfusion[153] and that vasoconstrictors will often lead to a greater base excess. One study demonstrated that vasoconstrictor treatment results in more sodium bicarbonate to treat the acidosis and is associated with a later time to extubation and return of bowel function.[154]

Conventional Ultrafiltration and Modified Ultrafiltration

Ultrafiltration involves placing a hemofilter (similar to those used for continuous arteriovenous or venovenous hemofiltration in the ICU) in the CPB circuit and has become the standard of care for nearly all congenital heart surgery programs.[155] Conventional ultrafiltration (CUF) is performed during CPB, with the filter placed between the arterial and venous sides of the CPB circuit. The hemofilter has thousands of fibers with pores, which allow water, electrolytes, and small molecules to be filtered out of the blood. Suction is applied to the hemofilter on CPB, and an ultrafiltrate of plasma is produced. Advantages of ultrafiltration include the ability to increase the hematocrit, fibrinogen, plasma proteins, and platelet count,[156,157] without necessitating further blood transfusion, the ability to remove excess free water and sodium (which contribute to excess intravascular volume, tissue edema, pulmonary and myocardial edema), as well as the ability to correct acid-base and electrolyte imbalances and to remove small molecules, such as interleukins and tumor necrosis factor-α (TNF-α) in particular,[158] which are involved in the post-bypass inflammatory process.[159,160] This improves systolic and diastolic function of the myocardium and reduces endothelial dysfunction in the systemic and pulmonary vasculature.[160,161] Pulmonary function is better preserved, probably owing to a slight reduction in interleukin-6 (IL-6) and thromboxane-B_2 (TXB$_2$),[162] even though this is not a consistent finding in the literature.[163,164] Endothelin-1 (ET-1), another mediator of pulmonary damage and hypertension, was not reduced by any filtration method.[164] Clinically, however, any ultrafiltration method seems to benefit children, especially those undergoing complex repairs, neonates, and children with preexisting pulmonary hypertension.[163]

Modified ultrafiltration (MUF) is performed for 10 to 15 minutes immediately after the conclusion of CPB. It can be performed in an arteriovenous manner with a hemofilter placed between the aortic cannula and the IVC cannula or in a venovenous fashion using bicaval cannulation or an internal jugular venous catheter.[165] It was developed in 1991[166] as an alternative method to reduce the side effects of CPB. CUF during bypass is often limited by the minimal venous reservoir levels and requires the addition of crystalloid or colloid to be able to continuously remove cytokines during ultrafiltration. During MUF, blood passes out of the aorta, through the hemofilter, and is returned through the IVC cannula. The theoretical advantage of MUF over conventional ultrafiltration is that only the child's blood volume is filtered, yielding a more efficient system for achieving the goals just outlined. The disadvantages are that the child remains heparinized, body temperature may decrease during the process (unless the circuit is modified to include the heat exchanger).[167] It requires extra time, an aortic cannula is needed that can obstruct the aorta in small infants, and acute intravascular volume shifts may occur at a time when the child is prone to hemodynamic instability. Opposite to the expected effects of fluid removal, MUF actually increases arterial pressures despite decreasing filling pressures and improving myocardial performance.[168]

There is increasing evidence that the use of ultrafiltration reduces bypass-related postoperative morbidity. Outcome studies have demonstrated that ultrafiltration improves myocardial and pulmonary function, lessens tissue edema, allows faster weaning from mechanical ventilation, and decreases the need for inotropic support.[169] The reduction of inflammatory transmitters is only temporary because the levels of cytokines are similar after 24 hours.[170]

Although each method has its proponents, and some centers perform both techniques in the same children, controlled comparative studies revealed no difference in outcome between MUF and CUF.[169,171] We routinely use a balanced ultrafiltration technique for all cases on CPB because it removes fluids and cytokines, as well as reduces lactate, which can aggravate reperfusion injury.[172]

Pre-Bypass Anesthetic Management

The objectives of the anesthetic management of children before bypass include maintenance of normal sinus rhythm and ventricular function and avoidance of extreme increases in heart rate, ventricular contractility, and pulmonary vascular resistance (PVR). The duration of the pre-bypass period varies greatly, particularly in children who have had previous surgeries, and maintaining hemodynamic stability for prolonged periods of time can often be challenging. Adequate anesthetic depth should be ensured to avoid increases in sympathetic stimulation and hypercyanotic spells, and temperature homeostasis should be maintained to avoid cardiac arrhythmias, especially when the duration of the pre-CPB surgical dissection is protracted. For children undergoing repeat sternotomy, blood products with an appropriate-capacity blood warmer should be readily at hand in case of emergent need.

Neonates and children who have been receiving total parenteral nutrition preoperatively receive an infusion of 5% or 10% dextrose before CPB, with frequent monitoring of glucose levels to avoid hypoglycemia or hyperglycemia. Older children receive Plasmalyte, a balanced electrolyte solution, at a reduced maintenance rate, allowing the administration of 5% albumin, if necessary, for volume augmentation.

The placement of purse-string sutures before cannulation, as well as the actual cannulation of the great vessels before CPB, can often precipitate arrhythmias, hypotension, and arterial desaturation, especially in small infants and children. It is not unusual for volume replacement to be necessary during placement of the cannula; and if the aortic cannula is already in place, it is our practice to coordinate the administration of volume between the anesthesiologist and perfusionist while the surgeon completes cannulation. Calcium chloride, 10 mg/kg, is also frequently useful to support hemodynamics at this time.

Anesthesia on Cardiopulmonary Bypass

Changes in Pharmacokinetics

The initiation of CPB introduces additional volume to the intravascular space (hemodilution). This greatly affects drug distribution, plasma concentrations, and elimination. The major factors responsible for this are hemodilution and altered plasma protein binding,[173] hypotension, hypothermia,[174] pulsatility,[175] isolation of the lungs from the circulation, and uptake of anesthetic drugs by the bypass circuit.[176,177] Drugs in the blood exist in the free (unbound and therefore the active form) or plasma bound (inactive form bound to protein, e.g., albumin) forms and therefore are subject to marked changes with alterations in plasma protein levels. CPB alters all these factors, which makes description of pharmacokinetic parameters during CPB problematic. The greatest changes occur within 5 minutes of initiation of CPB. The addition of the prime volume immediately reduces the protein concentration, and the ratio of bound-to-free drug in the circulation changes. A reduction in red blood cell concentration occurs, and this reduces the free drug concentrations. This will reduce the amount of drug available for interaction with the receptors. Most studies show a reduction in total drug concentration in plasma with little change in free drug concentration over time, whereas on CPB other than the transient (<5 minutes) reduction at initiation of CPB[178] it would appear that the greatest risk for unwanted "lightening of anesthesia" is within this time frame and additional doses of fentanyl, muscle relaxant, and midazolam are generally administered just before or with the onset of CPB. The explanation for why free drug levels are sustained during CPB is that the volume of distribution (Vd) for most anesthetic agents is large relative to the volume of the CPB prime and serves as a huge reservoir for drug after intravenous administration. A decrease in the plasma concentrations of medications as a result of hemodilution shifts drugs down their concentration gradient from tissue to plasma. Hypothermia contributes to the changes in plasma concentrations primarily by depressing enzyme function and slowing the metabolism of medications. Drug metabolism is diminished during hypothermia; enzyme activity is halved for every 10°C reduction in temperature. This may increase the free drug available for binding. When normothermia is reestablished, reperfusion of tissues might lead to washout of drug sequestered during the hypothermic CPB period. This may explain the secondary increases in plasma concentrations of opioids reported during the rewarming phase. pH-stat management also affects the degree of ionization and protein binding of certain medications, leading to increased free fractions (active) of these medications. During CPB, the lungs are out of circuit and medications that are taken up by the lungs (e.g., opioids) are sequestered during CPB. These medications are released when systemic reperfusion is established and concentrations are transiently increased. The volume of distribution of many drugs is expanded due to the priming volume of the bypass circuit, especially with neonates and small infants, where the priming volume is often greater than the child's blood volume. Finally, medications may be taken up by various components of the CPB circuit itself.

Changes in Pharmacodynamics

The pharmacodynamic effects of anesthetic agents are affected primarily via the central nervous system, which undergoes major changes during CPB. For example, hypothermia during CPB reduces anesthetic requirements. Hypothermia causes a host of other effects, including decreases in receptor affinity (e.g., decreased opioid receptor affinity[179] and nicotinic acetylcholine receptor sensitivity),[180] increases in both the pharmacokinetic and pharmacodynamic effects of neuromuscular receptor blocking agents, thus enhancing their effects at the neuromus-

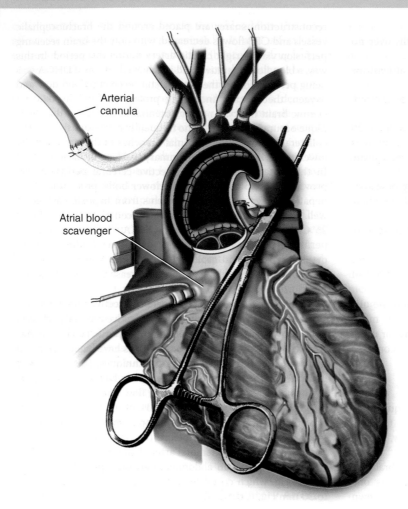

Arterial
cannula

Atrial blood
scavenger

Figure 17-5. Selective cerebral perfusion for the Norwood stage I palliation for hypoplastic left heart syndrome. Arterial inflow for bypass is provided by a small polytetrafluoroethylene graft sewn to the right innominate artery. Instead of deep hypothermic circulatory arrest, flow is provided to the brain at low rates, while the brachiocephalic vessels and descending thoracic aorta are snared, providing a bloodless operating field. (From Pigula FA, Nemoto EM, Griffith BP, Siewers RD: Regional low-flow perfusion provides cerebral circulatory support during neonatal aortic arch reconstruction. J Thorac Cardiovasc Surg 2000; 119:331-339.)

closed. Additionally, myocardial edema has been implicated as a causative factor in the frequent decline in myocardial function that occurs 6 to 12 hours after conclusion of CPB. Inflammatory mediators also affect the responsiveness of the myocardium to catecholamines by interfering with their binding to the cell surface receptors,[216] rendering exogenously administered drugs such as dopamine and epinephrine, as well as the child's endogenous catecholamines, less effective at increasing cardiac output in the perioperative period.

Mechanisms for prevention and treatment of myocardial dysfunction include the use of ultrafiltration and anti-inflammatory drugs such as corticosteroids and aprotinin.[217,218] The prophylactic use of noncatecholamine inotropic agents such as milrinone has also been shown to prevent low cardiac output syndrome in infants, even if cardiac function is adequate in the immediate postoperative period.[219]

Systemic and Pulmonary Vasculature Effects

The inflammatory response to CPB often produces mediators that directly increase pulmonary and systemic vascular resistance. These include interleukins, leukotrienes, and endothelin.[220] Indeed, when pulmonary artery pressure is measured directly, it is often significantly increased immediately after bypass, even if surgical results are optimal. This increase can be extremely detrimental in children with large left-to-right shunts,

those undergoing cardiac transplantation secondary to dilated cardiomyopathy, and those undergoing bidirectional cavopulmonary anastomosis, where right ventricular output depends on maintaining low PVR. Prevention and treatment of increases in PVR include maintaining an adequate depth of anesthesia, ventilating with 100% oxygen, and judicious use of hyperventilation. Milrinone will increase right-sided heart output via its actions as both an inotropic agent and a pulmonary vasodilator. When PVR is significantly elevated, inhaled nitric oxide is often used to assist in the early postoperative period.[221] Although effective, its cost is not inconsequential, and because PVR almost always decreases with time, nitric oxide is generally reserved for selected cases of pulmonary hypertension. Other simpler, less expensive treatments are being investigated for the treatment of significant pulmonary hypertension after bypass, including oral or intravenous sildenafil[222,223] and inhaled nebulized prostacyclin.[224]

Pulmonary Effects

The lungs are not ventilated during CPB and are usually totally collapsed by intention, with the ventilator circuit disconnected, especially in small infants. This leads to significant atelectasis. The lungs are also at least partially ischemic during the bypass period, resulting in decreased production and alveolar levels of surfactant after CPB.[225] In addition, reperfusion injury (pulmonary edema or hemorrhage after a sudden increase in pulmonary flow) can also occur after creation of a systemic-to-pulmonary artery shunt or pulmonary artery unifocalization. Inflammatory mediators liberated by the bypass run also predispose to increases in smooth muscle tone and resistance and can result in bronchospasm.[226]

In addition to complement, endotoxins and certain cytokines can also activate neutrophils and attract them toward sites of inflammation.[227] In animal studies, endotoxin-induced lung injury can lead to rapid (within 45 minutes) accumulation of neutrophils within lung capillaries. Activation of neutrophils, with upregulation of adhesion molecules, neutrophil adhesion to the endothelium of lung vessels, and endothelial damage through proteases, appears to be the main step of the underlying pathophysiologic mechanism (Fig. 17-6). Macrophages play an important role in the evolution of the inflammatory acute lung injury through the secretion of cytokines, cytotoxic metabolites, and chemoattractants for leukocytes. At the clinical level, acute respiratory distress syndrome (ARDS) is often only one part of multiorgan failure and lung injury should be seen as part of a more general state of systemic inflammation. The reported prevalence of ARDS after CPB in adults is 0.5% to 1.7%; the incidence in children is unknown. Interesting enough was the failure of general hypothermia at 28°C to prevent the loss of ATP and the accumulation of lactate in lungs.[228] Different methods that aim to protect the lungs during CPB, such as continuous lung perfusion, pneumoplegia, and nitric oxide ventilation at lung reperfusion prevent more severe hemodynamic deterioration and preserve reactivity of the pulmonary vasculature but fail to prevent pulmonary dysfunction.

The severity of pulmonary dysfunction after CPB can be measured via changes in the alveolar-arterial oxygenation gradient, intrapulmonary shunt, degree of pulmonary edema, pulmonary compliance, and PVR. Treatment of pulmonary atelectasis includes measures that decrease inflammatory mediators, careful reinflation of the lungs when weaning from bypass (by administering several vital capacity breaths), gentle but thorough suctioning of the endotracheal tube, and prophylactic use of inhaled bronchodilators before separation from CPB. Using these measures, pulmonary function has been shown to improve immediately in most children with large left-to-right shunts, with the duration of CPB seemingly having little effect on pulmonary outcomes.[229] Thus, CPB itself has little effect on pulmonary function in most children. There is still an occasional child, however, who experiences classic "pump lung" ARDS, caused by the factors noted earlier. Treatment is supportive as for anyone with ARDS.

Neurologic Monitoring and Effects of Cardiopulmonary Bypass on the Brain

Cerebral monitoring can help to detect those children who are at risk for neurologic sequelae after bypass, promptly recognize and treat changes in cerebral blood flow/oxygenation, evaluate the effect of therapeutic interventions on cerebral physiology, optimize brain protection during the vulnerable periods of CPB, and potentially improve short- and long-term neurologic outcomes.[230]

Near-infrared spectroscopy is a monitor that measures brain tissue oxygenation. This device noninvasively measures the concentration of oxyhemoglobin and deoxyhemoglobin and determines the cerebral tissue oxygen saturation. The cerebral

oximeter probe, a light-emitting diode, is placed on the skin of the forehead and uses near-infrared light similar to a pulse oximeter that measures the hemoglobin oxygen saturation. Commercially available devices use two different wavelengths (730 and 810 nm) that pass through brain tissue 2 to 5 cm beneath the probe in the frontal cortex. The light absorbed by extracranial tissues is subtracted from the total signal (detected by the distal electrode), leaving only the intracranial contribution. The monitor displays a numerical value for the regional cerebral oxygen saturation (rSo_2), the ratio of oxyhemoglobin to total hemoglobin in the light path. rSo_2 is a measure of local microcirculatory oxygen supply-demand balance and is reported on a scale from 15% to 95%. It has been assumed from anatomic models that 75% of the cerebral blood volume in the light path is venous and 25% is arterial. One study verified this in children with congenital heart disease by directly measuring the jugular venous bulb and arterial oxygen saturations and comparing these with the cerebral oxygen saturation measured with NIRS.[231] The actual ratio in children varied widely, but on average the venous to arterial ratio was 85 : 15. All devices measure both the arterial and venous blood oxygen saturations. Accordingly, this device does not provide a measure of the jugular venous bulb oxygen saturation ($Sj\bar{v}o_2$). A corollary of this is that maneuvers that increase arterial oxygen saturation (e.g., increasing Fio_2) increase cerebral oxygenation as measured by these devices, although the $Sj\bar{v}o_2$ may remain unchanged. In a study of 40 infants and children with congenital heart disease who were undergoing cardiac surgery or catheterization, NIRS correlated poorly with $Sj\bar{v}o_2$ measurements, except in infants younger than 1 year of age.[232] In contrast, in a study of 30 children undergoing cardiac catheterization, NIRS correlated very well with $Sj\bar{v}o_2$ ($r = .93$).[233] These data suggest that NIRS is a useful indicator of trends in cerebral oxygenation in individual infants and children.

Neurologic Monitoring for Low-Flow Hypothermic Bypass

Transcranial Doppler (TCD) ultrasonography has been used to determine the threshold of detectable cerebral perfusion during low-flow CPB. *TCD velocities reveal trends or changes in cerebral blood flow and not absolute values.* One report studied 28 neonates undergoing the arterial switch operation using α-stat blood gas management.[136] Their study suggested that NIRS and TCD may be useful to determine the minimum acceptable bypass flow level for an individual neonate during low-flow hypothermic bypass. Blood flow becomes insufficient at bypass flow rates less than 30 mL/kg/min.[136,234] Inadequate blood flow to the brain during this technique could be undetected without such monitoring, and low-flow bypass may confer no advantage to the brain over DHCA in some patients. Long-term outcome studies of this monitoring strategy are not available.

Neurologic Monitoring for Deep Hypothermic Circulatory Arrest

Despite clinical and experimental evidence that periods of DHCA that exceed approximately 40 minutes are associated with an increased risk of adverse long-term neurologic and developmental outcomes, this technique is still widely used in congenital heart surgery. Recent recommendations for improving outcome after DHCA, based on both animal and clinical studies, include using pH-stat blood gas management, low temperatures of 15°C to 18°C, long cooling periods of no less than

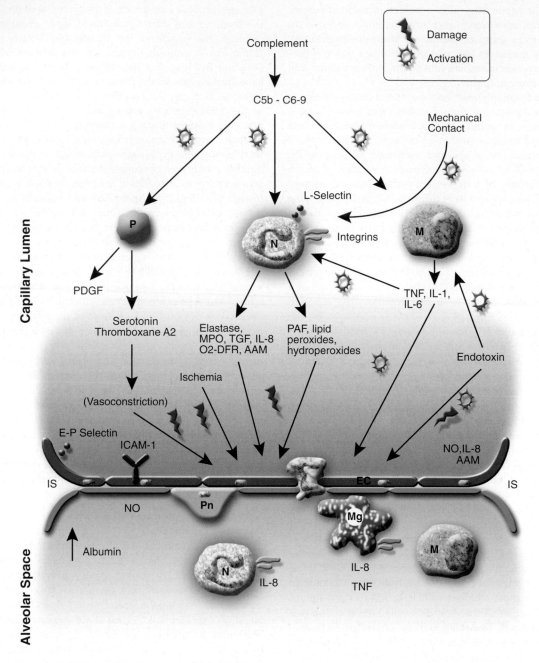

Figure 17-6. Leukocytes, endothelial cells (EC), and humoral inflammatory mediators have been shown to play an important role in the cardiopulmonary bypass–induced lung injury. Complement activation and complement-independent mechanical injury activates leukocytes, which, in their turn, secrete several inflammatory mediators, such as proteases and cytokines. Complement, cytokines, and ischemia-reperfusion also activate endothelial cells. Endotoxin, probably released from intestinal bacteria, exerts similar effects on leukocytes and endothelium. This process leads to disruption of endothelial and epithelial integrity and allows albumin, plasma, and activated leukocytes to enter the interstitial and alveolar space, causing tissue edema and reducing pulmonary compliance and blood oxygenation. AAM, arachidonic acid metabolites; ICAM-1, intercellular adhesion molecule-1; IL, interleukin; IS, interstitial space; LPS, lipopolysaccharide; M, monocyte; Mg, macrophage; MPO, myeloperoxidase; N, neutrophil; NO, nitric oxide; O_2-DFR, oxygen-derived free radicals; P, platelet; PAF, platelet-activating factor; PDGF, platelet-derived growth factor; Pn, pneumocyte; TGF, tumor growth factor; TNF, tumor necrosis factor. (From Asimakopoulos G, Smith PL, Ratnatunga CP, Taylor KM: Lung injury and acute respiratory distress syndrome after cardiopulmonary bypass. Ann Thorac Surg 1999; 1107-1115.)

20 minutes, and higher hematocrit (e.g., approximately 30% vs. the traditional 20% or less). During DHCA, rSo$_2$ predictably decreases to a nadir 60% to 70% (relative change) below baseline values obtained before bypass. The nadir is reached at 10 to 20 minutes, after which there is no further decrease.[235] At this point

it appears that there is no additional oxygen uptake by the brain. Several studies suggest the potential for near-infrared cerebral oximetry to determine the safe conduct and duration of DHCA in the individual child. Kurth and colleagues studied 26 infants and children undergoing surgery with bypass and DHCA. They found that three children with low rSo$_2$ had acute postoperative neurologic changes—seizures in 1, and prolonged coma in 2.[235] In these 3 children, the increase in rSo$_2$ was much less after the onset of CPB (average 3% relative increase vs. 33% increase in children without neurologic deficit) and the duration of cooling before DHCA shorter than in the 23 children without neurologic changes. In a neonatal pig model the time of the nadir of rSo$_2$ values during DHCA correlated with neurologic outcome: a longer period without apparent oxygen uptake by the brain correlated with a greater incidence of adverse neurologic outcome. The maximum safe duration without additional brain oxygen uptake at 17°C was 30 minutes.[133] Interestingly, this time period appears to correlate with clinical and experimental studies, suggesting that 40 minutes is the safe duration for circulatory arrest (see Fig. 17-3). When circulatory arrest is initiated at greater temperatures (e.g., 25°C) there is a faster decrease in rSo$_2$, and the nadir is achieved sooner.[236] Reperfusion results in an increase in rSo$_2$ to levels observed at full bypass flow before DHCA. Based on these data, our current practice is to reperfuse after the NIRS nadir has been reached for a period of 20 to 25 minutes.

Neurologic Monitoring for Regional Low-Flow Cerebral Perfusion

Regional low-flow cerebral perfusion (RLFP) (also known as selective cerebral perfusion or antegrade cerebral perfusion) uses a polytetrafluoroethylene (PTFE) graft or a small aortic cannula as arterial inflow to the right innominate artery for neonatal aortic surgery such as the Norwood stage operation or aortic arch advancement. The other brachiocephalic vessels and descending thoracic aorta are snared, resulting in a bloodless operating field. The brain is perfused through the right innominate and right vertebral arteries only. This approach significantly reduces or eliminates the use of DHCA for these operations and preserves brain perfusion, potentially improving neurologic outcome. Initial descriptions of this technique used the pressure in the radial artery or a predetermined bypass rate of 25 to 30 mL/kg/min as an estimate for the bypass flow during RLFP without neurologic monitoring. When flow rate was estimated on the basis of NIRS monitoring in individual children, it was determined that 20 to 25 mL/kg/min was required.[206] However, NIRS was applied only to the right side of the skull (i.e., brain), the same side as the sole arterial inflow. Using a pH-stat blood gas strategy for RLFP, we noted that the majority of our children had an rSo$_2$ of 95% (the maximum reading on the rSo$_2$ scale) when we used the left radial artery pressure of 20 to 25 mm Hg as the target for bypass flow. These patients were theoretically at risk for excessive cerebral perfusion. Therefore, we performed a study using both NIRS and TCD of the right cerebral hemisphere, to determine if TCD could be used as a guide to RLFP flow rate.[211] Bypass flow rate was adjusted to achieve a cerebral blood flow volume within 10% of baseline (e.g., TCD was used to determine necessary flow). The estimated flow rate, 63 mL/kg/min (range, 24 to 94 mL/kg/min), proved to be significantly greater than that estimated in the earlier studies. This flow rate did not correlate with the pressure in the right or left radial artery. The rSo$_2$ was well maintained in all children, leading us to conclude that TCD was a useful monitor to ensure adequate but not excessive cerebral blood flow during RLFP. Because RLFP perfuses the brain through a single arterial inflow vessel, questions have arisen about the adequacy of cerebral blood flow

and oxygenation to the left cerebral hemisphere. Although the circle of Willis is expected to be intact without stenoses in neonates, 10% of healthy full-term neonates exhibit deviations from normal flow patterns. Two studies concluded that although cerebral blood flow and oxygenation were adequate to both cerebral hemispheres in neonates during RLFP, bilateral monitoring, at least of NIRS, may be warranted.[211,237]

Systemic Inflammatory Response Syndrome (SIRS)

In cardiac surgery, SIRS is thought to result from four main sources of injury: (1) contact of the blood components with the artificial surface of the bypass circuit, (2) ischemia-reperfusion injury, (3) endotoxemia, and (4) operative trauma. Inflammatory cytokines, together with endothelial activation and endothelial-leukocyte interactions, appear to play an important role in the induction of this systemic inflammatory response.

Exposure of blood to the artificial materials in the bypass circuit—plastics, polypropylene oxygenator fibers, and metal suction devices—initiates a cascade of inflammatory responses, including activation of the complement system, the kallikrein system, and the coagulation system.[215] As a result, interleukins, tumor necrosis factor, endotoxin, heat shock protein, and many other inflammatory mediators are released into the circulation. Leukocyte activation also results in secretion of inflammatory mediators, such as proteases and cytokines such as TNF-α and IL-1, which are secreted early in the evolution of the inflammatory process. This chemokine-mediated increased leukocyte activation constitutes an important link in the chain of the propagation of the inflammatory response (see Fig. 17-6).

This inflammatory response is counterbalanced by a complex system of inhibitors such as IL-10 and soluble cytokine receptors.[238] Also, the inflammatory response of the neonate may be more exaggerated than that of the infant or older child,[239] justifying a more aggressive approach to its modulation in the neonate (see later).

A number of novel treatments have been studied, including monoclonal antibodies for inflammatory products such as complement, endotoxin, and tumor necrosis factor. Although theoretically attractive, no clinical difference has been noted with any of these treatments.

Effective treatments used every day in the operating room and ICU include:

- Use of corticosteroids[240]
- Ultrafiltration[217] (see earlier)
- Aprotinin[218] (see earlier)
- Leukocyte depletion[241]: leukocyte-depleted blood prime and in-line arterial filter; initiate bypass using normoxic management (Fio$_2$ of 21%) in cyanotic infants.

Corticosteroids interrupt the inflammatory response at several levels by entering cell nuclei and changing the rate of transcription of inflammatory molecules. Increasing evidence suggests that glucocorticoids act by regulating transcription or translation of anti-inflammatory cytokines, such as IL-10, and altering expression of other proteins, such as endothelin-1 and inhibitor κB.[242,243]

Because these processes take time to develop, the effects of corticosteroids are not immediate, taking up to several hours.[244] Thus, the common practice of adding corticosteroids to the CPB prime will not fully prevent the inflammatory response[245]; to be effective, corticosteroids may need to be administered 4 or more hours before the onset of CPB.

Coagulation Effects

Blood coagulation is frequently abnormal after CPB for several reasons. The inflammatory cascade activates the coagulation system, resulting in factor consumption and fibrinolysis, which, in turn, breaks down existing blood clots, leading to increased bleeding.[15] Treatment is adequate heparinization, reversal with protamine, and the use of aprotinin to inhibit fibrinolysis and improve platelet function.[29] In addition, the smaller the child, the greater the dilution of clotting factors by the bypass prime, and the greater the risk for low concentrations of clotting proteins and fibrinogen postoperatively. Platelets are also degranulated and consumed by the CPB circuit, leading both to low platelet counts and nonfunctioning platelets.[15] The smaller the infant, the greater the duration of bypass, and the more complicated the surgery, the greater the incidence of coagulopathy after bypass. Efforts to minimize the post-bypass coagulopathy in infants includes priming the CPB circuit with fresh whole blood for small infants if available or packed cells plus fresh frozen plasma (FFP) if fresh whole blood cannot be obtained.[18,246] Treatment involves administration of platelets to small infants as the first line of therapy, followed by cryoprecipitate to replace fibrinogen and FFP to replace clotting factors. If these factors are not effective after correcting coagulation parameters such as platelet count, prothrombin/PTT, fibrinogen, and thromboelastogram, then surgical bleeding may be the cause and surgical reexploration may be warranted.[247] Factor VIIa has also been used as a last resort in children who have significant post-bypass bleeding.[49]

Hepatic, Renal, and Gastrointestinal Effects

The liver, kidneys, and gastrointestinal tract, like the brain and heart, may be rendered ischemic by prolonged CPB, DHCA, or low cardiac output syndrome. Renal function is compromised on CPB. This is manifested by the appearance of proteinuria and impaired tubular cellular function immediately after CPB. Renal dysfunction from ischemia is also common. Low urine output may occur secondary to secretion of antidiuretic hormone, a response to surgical stress. However, the latter appears to be transitory and usually resolves spontaneously.[248] The incidence of acute renal dysfunction after congenital heart surgery with bypass is 17%, ranging from 0.7% for ASD closure to 59% for arterial switch operations.[249] Deep hypothermic cardiac arrest subjects the kidney to additional ischemia reperfusion injury.[250] Acute renal failure after CPB is uncommon in children, with fewer than 3% requiring dialysis perioperatively.[249,251] Infants who undergo cardiac surgery routinely receive diuretics or a peritoneal dialysis catheter, the latter prophylactically in some instances.[252,253] Although some have attributed the improved survival with early peritoneal dialysis to the prevention of fluid overload, others have attributed it to a more rapid clearance of CPB-induced proinflammatory cytokines.[254] Further study is required to clarify the mechanism of action of early peritoneal dialysis. In our center, neonates and children with a complex heart defect usually receive peritoneal dialysis immediately postoperatively to prevent fluid overload.

Recovery of hepatic and gastrointestinal function follows hemodynamic recovery but may require several days. Therapy is mainly supportive with increasing oxygen delivery, initiating parenteral nutrition, and awaiting return of function before restarting enteral feedings. Splanchnic and renal perfusion can be monitored noninvasively using somatic oximetry. Somatic oxygenation may predict renal dysfunction and predict organ failure. Interventions based on the somatic NIRS may improve outcome.[255]

Immune System Effects

Leukocytes are activated by the CPB circuit, although their numbers may be depleted by leukocyte filters, which are sometimes used to attenuate the inflammatory response. Despite the theoretical potential that this may increase the risk of infection or neutrophil function, this has not been observed in published studies or clinical practice.[256]

Endocrine System Effects

The magnitude of the inflammatory and endocrine responses after cardiac surgery depends in part on the duration of the surgical procedure and CPB.[257] In children undergoing brief operating times, postoperative blood concentrations of cortisol, adrenocorticotropic hormone, and β-endorphins are significantly greater than those in children undergoing prolonged operation times. In contrast, the serum concentrations of the proinflammatory cytokines IL-6, IL-1β, and TNF-α are similar in the two groups. Adrenocorticotropic hormone and cortisol concentrations correlated positively with the blood concentrations of IL-1β, IL-6, and TNF-α in the group of children with prolonged operation times.

The plasma concentrations of both epinephrine and cortisol increase after cardiac surgery.[258] In children, pre- and post-bypass cortisol and norepinephrine increase significantly during isoflurane anesthesia when 2 μg/kg of fentanyl is used rather than 25, 50, 100, or 150 μg/kg.[259] No significant increase in the blood concentrations of these hormones occurred with any of the fentanyl doses of 25 μg/kg or greater. In addition to cardiovascular stability, continued use of high doses of opiates during bypass minimizes the stress responses and stabilizes hemodynamics during and after bypass.[260] Also, growth hormone, glucose and insulin, lactate, glutamate, aspartate, and free fatty acid concentrations increase after cardiac surgery, whereas total triiodothyronine concentrations decrease.[261]

Transport to the Intensive Care Unit

Extreme vigilance is required during transfer of the child from the cardiac operating room to the ICU. Monitoring of ECG, arterial, venous and atrial pressures, and end-tidal CO_2 and pulse oximetry must be maintained continuously; the battery charge of the monitor and the infusion pumps should be checked beforehand to prevent monitor failure and interruption of the infusions of vasoactive medications. Resuscitation drugs, airway equipment, and blood products should accompany the child to the ICU. Before leaving the operating room, a report should be given to the ICU staff. Children who are transported with tracheal tubes in situ are usually ventilated manually during transport via a Jackson-Rees circuit, with either 100% oxygen or, for those who require an FIO_2 less than 1.0, an oxygen-air blender. For children who require nitric oxide, a respiratory therapist should assist with transport to ensure that no interruptions in therapy occur and that a smooth transfer occurs in the ICU as well. On arrival in the ICU, vital signs are confirmed, all monitoring devices are transferred sequentially to the ICU monitors and rechecked to ensure they are in working order, and a detailed report is given to the ICU staff.

Summary

Cardiopulmonary bypass is a necessary technique for intracardiac and major extracardiac surgery on the great vessels. CPB induces a multitude of physiologic and inflammatory derangements, but, through extensive experience and research, these ill effects can be largely mitigated by a number of evidence-based strategies. Therefore, outcomes after CPB have improved dramatically, and CPB is no longer a barrier to accomplishing complex congenital heart surgery, even in neonates.

Annotated References

Andropoulos DB, Stayer SA, McKenzie ED, Fraser CD Jr: Regional low-flow perfusion provides comparable blood flow and oxygenation to both cerebral hemispheres during neonatal aortic arch reconstruction. J Thorac Cardiovasc Surg 2003; 126:1712-1717

Regional low-flow cerebral perfusion (RLFP), a technique designed to avoid deep hypothermic circulatory arrest, was studied in 20 neonates undergoing the Norwood stage I palliation or aortic arch reconstruction. When RLFP flow is guided by transcranial Doppler ultrasound flow velocity, and near-infrared cerebral oximetry, both right and left cerebral hemispheres have comparable flow velocity and oxygenation values; therefore, this technique can support the whole brain when adequate bypass flows are used.

Carrel TP, Schwanda M, Vogt PR, Turina MI: Aprotinin in pediatric cardiac operations: a benefit in complex malformations and with high-dose regimen only. Ann Thorac Surg 1998; 66:153-158

One of the few controlled studies of aprotinin in pediatric cardiac surgery. Reduction in blood loss, transfusion requirement, and fibrinolysis was seen with a high-dose aprotinin regimen for the arterial switch operation only; it was not effective for tetralogy of Fallot or ventricular septal defect.

du Plessis AJ, Jonas RA, Wypij D, et al: Perioperative effects of alpha-stat versus pH-stat strategies for deep hypothermic cardiopulmonary bypass in infants. J Thorac Cardiovasc Surg 1997; 114:991-1000

In this study 182 neonates and infants were randomized to pH-stat or α-stat CPB strategy. Important trends or statistically significant improved outcomes were seen with pH-stat management for deaths, EEG seizures, return of EEG activity, acidosis, hypotension, inotropic support, and length of mechanical ventilation. These improvements were most significant for arterial switch operation patients.

Jonas RA, Wypij D, Roth SJ, et al: The influence of hemodilution on outcome after hypothermic cardiopulmonary bypass: results of a randomized trial in infants. J Thorac Cardiovasc Surg 2003; 126:1765-1774

One hundred thirteen infants randomized to a target hematocrit of 20% (actual 21.5%) versus 30% (actual 28%) on CPB had lower neurodevelopmental outcome scores at age 1 year: 82 on the Psychomotor Development Index of the Bayley Scales of Infant Development with lower hematocrit versus 90. The lower hematocrit children also had a greater incidence of scores more than 2 SD below the mean (29% vs. 9%).

Miller BE, Mochizuki T, Levy JH, et al: Predicting and treating coagulopathies after cardiopulmonary bypass in children. Anesth Analg 1997; 85:1196-1202

This is the classic article describing the reason for post-CPB bleeding in infants and children. Platelet defects are the most important cause and the first blood product to administer; hypofibrinogenemia is the second most important, and fibrinogen is the next most important blood product, with fresh frozen plasma ineffective or possibly worsening bleeding.

Wypij D, Newburger JW, Rappaport LA, et al: The effect of duration of deep hypothermic circulatory arrest in infant heart surgery on late neurodevelopment: the Boston Circulatory Arrest Trial. J Thorac Cardiovasc Surg 2003; 126:1397-1403

Neurodevelopmental outcomes were assessed with a battery of 6 tests in 155 eight-year olds who had a neonatal arterial switch operation, utilizing α-stat bypass management, hematocrit of 20% on bypass, and varying duration of DHCA at 18° C. Neurodevelopmental outcomes were not adversely affected for the group as a whole until the DHCA time exceeded 41 minutes (95% lower confidence limit 32 minutes).

References

Please see www.expertconsult.com

Medications for Hemostasis

Adam Skinner and Andrew Wolf CHAPTER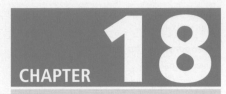

IN RECENT YEARS, CONSIDERABLE attention has been paid to minimizing perioperative blood loss, early identification of coagulation abnormalities, and developing techniques that reduce or even abolish the need for allogenic blood and blood components. This has been driven by several factors: the outcome benefits of limiting blood loss and restoring lost blood back to the circulation, the pathophysiologic effects associated with exogenous stored blood products, and the risk of bacterial, viral, or prion transmission from blood and its components. Children are particularly vulnerable in that immunocompetence has not been fully established and early exposure may have lifelong impact. These issues are particularly heightened in pediatric cardiac surgery owing to the constraints associated with cardiopulmonary bypass (CPB) surgery, its effects on platelet sequestration, and the balance between coagulation and fibrinolysis. Techniques used in cardiac surgery such as hypothermia and insertion of prosthetic material necessitate heightened awareness and clinical manipulation of hemostasis. Bleeding after CPB surgery in children has been shown to be an important cause of morbidity,[1,2] and the hazards associated with surgical re-exploration and the complications of avoidable exposure to allogenic blood products are well recognized.

Minimizing blood loss with meticulous surgical technique is central to blood preservation, but increasingly it is understood that many other factors can have major importance not only in preventing blood loss but also in promptly reestablishing effective coagulation when it has failed (Table 18-1).

In this chapter we review the general principles of hemostasis and how it relates to general pediatrics, particularly for procedures associated with major blood loss, while emphasizing the principles and practice of hemostasis as they relate to pediatric cardiac surgery.

Physiology of Coagulation

The Traditional Model of Coagulation

Before considering the hematopoietic disturbance during major surgery and CPB, it is important to review the models of coagulation to interpret the coagulation investigations available and to be able to appropriately manage the coagulopathic child (see Chapters 9 and 10).

Hemostasis depends on the successful balance between the coagulation, complement, and fibrinolytic pathways, with complex interactions between plasma proteins, platelets, blood flow, viscosity, and the endothelium. The first event to control bleeding is vessel contraction and the formation of a hemostatic plug at the site of vessel damage; von Willebrand factor (vWf) binds to the subendothelium, exposing multiple binding sites for platelets to adhere, activate, and aggregate. The coagulation cascade describes the complex biochemical processes leading to the formation and deposition of a strong cross-linked fibrin mesh throughout the platelet plug.[3] The traditional coagulation cascade, shown in Figure 18-1, describes the biochemical interactions of the coagulation enzymes and cofactors that lead to a "burst" of thrombin generation.[4] This thrombin has multiple functions, including the cleavage of fibrinogen to form fibrin. The enzymes involved in the coagulation cascade belong to a family of proteases known as serine proteases and are represented in the diagram as Roman numerals. These serine proteases have a common mechanism of enzymatic action that requires serine, aspartic acid, and histidine within the active site.[3]

The components of the extrinsic and common pathways are reflected in the laboratory as the prothrombin time (PT), whereas the components of the intrinsic and common pathways are reflected as the activated partial thromboplastin time

Table 18-1. Causes of Excessive Bleeding after Pediatric Cardiac Surgery

Preoperative Causes

Liver immaturity

Congenital coagulopathy

Poor nutrition

Cyanotic congenital heart disease

Drugs: prostaglandin E_1, aspirin, clopidogrel

Intraoperative Causes

Surgical Insult

Inadequate surgical hemostasis before bypass

Inflammatory cascade, fibrinolysis, etc.

Cardiopulmonary Bypass

Inflammatory cascade
  Ongoing fibrinolysis
  Increased vascular permeability
  Capillary damage

Hemodilution
  Platelet reduction
  Clotting factor reduction
  Fibrinogen reduction

Complement activation

Platelet abnormality

Fibrinogen reduction

Disseminated intravascular coagulation

Post Cardiopulmonary Bypass

Inadequate surgical hemostasis

Acidosis

Hypothermia

Hypocalcemia

Excessive blood transfusion and clotting factor dilution

Inadequate reversal of heparin with protamine

Excess protamine

Inadequate reversal of heparin in transfused pump blood

(aPTT).[5] This traditional model of coagulation supports tests of coagulation in the laboratory; however, this cascade has flaws as a model of the hemostatic process in vivo. For example, it fails to describe why hemophiliacs (with factor VIII or IX deficiency) bleed when they have an intact factor VIIa/tissue factor that is a key enzyme in the extrinsic pathway. It also does not explain why those with a factor VII deficiency have a serious bleeding tendency when all these children have an intact "intrinsic" system.[5]

The Modified Cell-Based Model of Coagulation

To achieve effective hemostasis, a platelet plug needs to form at the site of vessel injury. In addition, the procoagulant factors need to remain localized to the injured site to avoid widespread clotting activation. This is achieved through changes at the cell surface. A modified cell-based model has therefore been developed to more fully explain the process of coagulation.[5]

The cell-based model describes the localization of the procoagulant reactions at the site of specific cell surfaces, with the intrinsic and extrinsic pathways occurring simultaneously on different cells. Different cells possess different procoagulant and anticoagulant properties; these are incompletely understood in some cases, but platelets and tissue factor (TF)–bearing cells are central to the process. Keeping these cells separated is partly responsible for avoiding inappropriate coagulation while the endothelium is intact.[5] The described phases of coagulation are overlapping and involve initiation, amplification, and propagation.[6]

Initiation

Coagulation is initiated by a membrane-bound lipoprotein called tissue factor. This is usually expressed on subendothelial TF-bearing cells such as stromal fibroblasts; in the absence of vessel injury it is therefore separated from the vessel lumen. After injury, a complex is formed between TF and factor VIIa (TF/VIIa), which activates factors IX and X. Factor Xa in association with cofactor Va forms "prothrombinase" complexes on the surface of the TF-bearing cell, which activates a small amount of thrombin (factor II)[7] (Fig. 18-2). The purpose of this small generation of thrombin and Xa is to activate platelets and factors V and VIII. This process is augmented by recombinant factor VIIa.

Tissue factor plasminogen inhibitor (TFPI) and antithrombin III (ATIII) provide a localizing function on factor Xa by inhibiting any Xa that becomes dissociated from the TF-bearing cell. Factor IXa is not localized to the cell in the same way.

Subclinical levels of IX and X activation occur in the absence of tissue injury without causing clot formation. The process only leads to amplification when damage to the vasculature allows intravascular platelets and FVIII/vWF to adhere to the extravascular TF-bearing cells.[5]

Amplification

Small quantities of thrombin are generated on the TF-bearing cells. This sets up the subsequent propagation phase during which thrombin is generated in large quantities (Fig. 18-3). This thrombin has many major functions:

- Activation of platelets—exposing receptors and binding sites for clotting factors
- Activation of cofactors V and VIII on the activated platelet surface, thereby releasing vWF to mediate additional adhesion and aggregation at the injury site
- Activation of factor XI to XIa[8]
- Activation of factor XIII (fibrin stabilizing factor) and promotion of fibrin crosslinking
- Cleaving fibrinopeptides A and B from fibrinogen (forming fibrin)

Propagation

Propagation occurs on the surface of activated platelets that are recruited to the site in large numbers. Activated factor IX (from both initiation phase and provided by factor XI on the platelet) binds to VIIIa. The resultant IXa/VIIIa complex activates factor X on the platelet surface. This Xa associates with Va and forms the prothrombinase complex. This causes a "burst" of thrombin generation to cause clot via fibrinogen (Fig. 18-4).[5]

This explains why hemophiliacs bleed despite having a normal FVIIa/TF complex; the Xa formed on the TF-bearing cell during the initiation phase is broken down by ATIII and TFPI if it dissociates from the TF-bearing cell. It is therefore unable to activate the "burst" of thrombin generation that normally occurs in

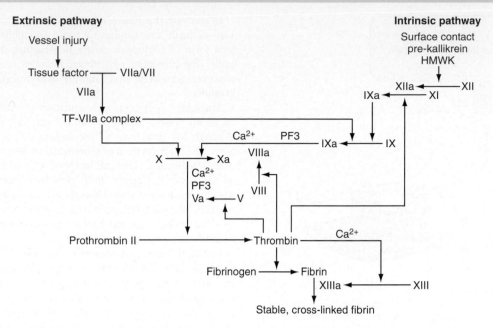

Figure 18-1. The traditional view of the coagulation cascade. The extrinsic pathway is described as a factor VIIa/tissue factor–dependent pathway, and the intrinsic pathway has been described as a factor VIII–dependent pathway. The common pathway is started by the activation of factor X to Xa and leads to the formation of stable cross-linked fibrin. (HMWK = high molecular weight kininogen; PF3 = platelet factor 3.)

this propagation phase. The Xa needs to be generated on the platelet itself via the IXa/VIIIa complex.[5]

Of note, an alternative pathway is initiated by contact factors (XII, XI, pre-kallikrein, and high molecular weight kininogen [HMWK]). It is of no physiologic importance in terms of coagulation activation; however, it provides important acceleration loops through feedback activation of factors VIII, IX, and XI.[9]

Clot Inhibition

The clot is confined to the site of injury by direct and indirect thrombin inhibitory systems. The direct system comprises antithrombin (AT), α_2-macroglobulin and heparin cofactor II

(HCII). AT and HCII are accelerated in the presence of heparin.

Various indirect systems inhibit thrombin, such as the protein C/protein S/thrombomodulin (TM) and the TFPI systems. Thrombin binds to TM at an intact endothelial cell and can therefore no longer cleave fibrinogen to form fibrin. The TM/thrombin complex is also neither able to activate platelets nor activate factors V and VIII. Instead, this complex activates

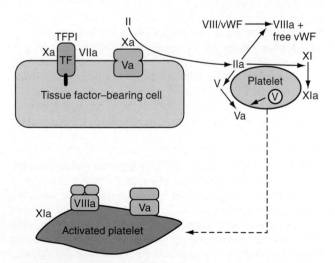

Figure 18-3. Amplification. Small amounts of thrombin set the stage for large-scale generation of thrombin in the propagation phase. Small amounts of thrombin activate platelets as well as other important coagulation enzymes and cofactors. (From Hoffman M: Remodeling the blood coagulation cascade. J Thromb Thrombolysis 2003; 16:17-20.)

Figure 18-2. Initiation. The TF/VIIa complex on the tissue factor–bearing cell activates factors IX and X. The factor Xa/Va is known as the "prothrombinase" complex that forms small amounts of thrombin. (From Hoffman M: Remodeling the blood coagulation cascade. J Thromb Thrombolysis 2003; 16:17-20.)

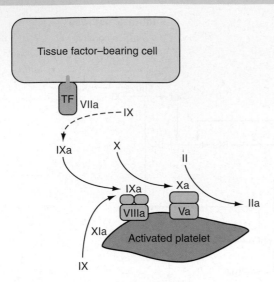

Figure 18-4. Propagation. Factor Xa is formed locally by the VIIIa/IXa complex on the surface of the activated platelet. The resulting Xa/Va prothrombinase complex causes a burst of thrombin generation. (From Hoffman M: Remodeling the blood coagulation cascade. J Thromb Thrombolysis 2003; 16:17-20.)

protein C, which binds to the cofactor protein S and inactivates factors Va (on the surface of endothelial cells and platelets) and VIIIa.[5,9] TFPI bound to endothelial surfaces can form complexes with FXa that inhibit FVIIa. Thrombin generation is therefore inhibited.[9]

Developmental Coagulation

The hemostatic system in the neonate rapidly matures toward that of the adult.[10] One must consider how the coagulation systems mature in the child to interpret coagulation tests and use appropriate modalities to manipulate hemostasis in vivo.

All fetal coagulation factors are produced independently of the mother; fibrinogen starts to be formed as early as 5.5 weeks of gestational age, and blood can clot at 11 weeks. The introduction of microassays in the 1980s allowed for the determination of reference ranges for the coagulation factors beginning at 19 weeks of gestational age.[9,11,12] In general, there are four fundamental differences between the coagulation systems in the infant and the adult[10]:

- Concentrations of components of the hemostatic system
- The turnover rate of various components of the coagulation cascade
- The rate of synthesis
- Differences in the overall ability to generate and regulate the key enzymes thrombin and plasmin

Despite the upregulation of coagulation factors at birth, the vitamin K–dependent factors II, VII, IX, and X in the neonate are only 50% of adult values; this leads to a slightly prolonged PT or international normalized ratio (INR).[9] The contact factors HMWK, prekallikrein, and factors XI and XII are also approximately 50% of adult values.[9,10] The reduced contact factors account for a disproportionally prolonged aPTT. The reduced concentration of factors at birth is probably explained by reduced synthesis of factors by the liver. However, the levels increase rapidly, reaching approximately 80% of adult values by 6 months of age.[9,13]

In contrast, the plasma levels of fibrinogen and factors V and VIII at birth are similar to those in adults, although the fetal form of fibrinogen differs in structure from that of the adult. The physiologic significance of this is not clear.[9] vWF concentrations in the first 2 months of life are greater than those in adults.[14]

The inhibitor systems of coagulation also differ from adults. At birth, plasma protein C and S are 35% of adult values, although the fetal form of the protein differs from the adult form. The concentration of protein C does not reach adult levels until adolescence. Neonatal levels of AT and HCII are 50% of adult values; they reach adult levels by 6 months of age. The α_2-macroglobulin value, however, is increased at birth and remains increased throughout childhood; it is postulated that this may be one of the mechanisms that protects young children from thromboembolic complications.[15]

Finally, thrombin generation in vitro is reduced in children to approximately 75% of adult values,[15] but there is difficulty in interpreting the apparent discrepancy between the sufficient hemostasis seen in vivo and these laboratory thrombin generation assays. It still remains to be clarified whether neonates and children are more susceptible to bleeding[9]; however, the risk of thromboembolic complications appears to increase with age.[15]

With the reduced plasma concentrations of many procoagulant and anticoagulant proteins in infants there still appears to be an effective hemostatic balance; healthy fetuses, neonates, and children do not suffer hemorrhage in the presence of minor challenges. This is consistent with the thromboelastogram studies of healthy children younger than 2 years of age; no defects in coagulation were noted using this test compared with adults, indicating an intact hemostatic system.[2] Another thromboelastogram study reported that infants younger than 1 year of age with complex congenital heart disease have an intact and balanced coagulation-fibrinolytic system but at a "lower level" than healthy children. This has been interpreted as a reduction in hemostatic potential with less reserve.[16]

Alterations in Hemostasis During Pediatric Cardiac Surgery

Routine Anticoagulation

Heparin

Heparin remains the most effective anticoagulant to facilitate CPB.[17] It is an acidic molecule consisting of sequential saccharide units with multiple sulfate groups. These groups give it a negative charge. The saccharide sequence gives heparin its affinity for ATIII. The binding of heparin to lysine sites on ATIII causes a conformational change at the arginine reactive ATIII center. This results in an increase in ATIII potency by increasing the inhibition of thrombin and factors IXa, Xa, XIa, and XIIa by a factor of 1000.[18,19]

For reasons of speed and convenience, heparin therapy is most frequently guided by the activated clotting time (ACT). The ACT is an inexpensive rapid on-site test in which a small sample of blood is mixed with a coagulation activator such as celite, kaolin, or diatomaceous earth. It is used to guide heparin therapy. When this clot is stable the ACT is recorded, with a normal value being between 80 and 140 seconds. A number greater than 400 seconds is required for CPB, although heparin-coated CPB circuits may allow lower values than this.[19]

There are limitations to the use of the ACT; first, the ACT is altered by hypothermia, hemodilution, platelet activation, activation of the hemostatic system, and aprotinin therapy.[20,21] Accordingly, it does not accurately reflect the heparin levels. One study found that as soon as children go on CPB the heparin levels decreased by 50% as a result of hemodilution, even though the ACT doubled.[22] Second, in the bleeding child, the ACT is unable to differentiate between bleeding due to excess heparin or to other acquired hemostatic defects.[22] Alternatively, antifactor Xa or antithrombin assay would give a better guide to heparin levels but this would be much slower to perform; practical application of these tests is limited at present.

Heparinization does not completely abolish the production of thrombin. Low-grade ongoing thrombin production leads to ongoing activation of the coagulation cascade, platelets, fibrinolysis, and the endothelium. One study[22] found that using common pediatric heparin regimens (300 units/kg before CPB, then 100 units/kg to keep ACT >450 sec) 50% of children on CPB had low levels of heparin (<2 units/mL); the levels were significantly less than those in adults.[23] The greater degree of hemodilution is largely responsible for this. It is suggested that reduced levels of heparinization (<2 units/mL) on CPB is a major factor responsible for activation of coagulation and fibrinolysis.[22] The ideal method to achieve adequate thrombin inhibition is unknown.[24]

Despite heparin continuing to provide the "cornerstone" in anticoagulant therapy in cardiac surgery, these studies highlight some of the limitations of its actions; namely, the continued thrombin generation and activity during CPB reflects the inability of the heparin-ATIII complex to inactivate fibrin-bound thrombin. It also does not inhibit thrombin-induced platelet activation. Therefore, a thrombus is still an active reservoir of thrombin that activates platelets and amplifies coagulation.[25] In the future, direct thrombin inhibitors such as hirudin and bivalirudin may be free of these limitations. At present, however, there are scant reports of the use of hirudins in children, making dosing and monitoring difficult.[26]

Side effects from the use of heparin are uncommon; hypotension can occur due to a reduction in ionized calcium or, rarely, anaphylaxis. A benign transient decrease in the platelet count can occur, although heparin-induced thrombocytopenia is a thrombotic condition that must be considered.

Overall, effective heparinization during CPB decreases excessive bleeding and transfusions[24] whereas excess heparin is rarely a cause of postoperative bleeding using the above regimen.[22] Although heparin is easily and inexpensively reversed by protamine, "inadequate heparin reversal" can still contribute to post-bypass coagulopathy.

Reversal of Anticoagulation with Protamine

Protamine is a positively charged polypeptide derived from salmon sperm. It neutralizes heparin by forming an ionic bond with heparin. The resultant complex is removed by the reticuloendothelial system. The most appropriate dosing regimen has yet to be determined.[27] The fixed dose of protamine traditionally used in adult and pediatric practice fails to take into account the range of concentrations of heparin that occurs in infants and children on CPB.[24,28]

Excessive protamine has been associated with catastrophic pulmonary hypertension and hemorrhagic pulmonary edema in children. It is also known that protamine can be associated with coagulation abnormalities; an increasing ACT occurs at a protamine-heparin ratio of 2.6:1, and platelet aggregation occurs with a minimal excess in protamine.[29] Although some studies on titrating protamine regimens in adults demonstrated encouraging results in terms of reduced bleeding,[30] others failed to demonstrate differences in transfusion requirements.[31]

The clearance of protamine is more rapid than heparin, and "heparin rebound" is described as tissue-bound heparin redistributed to the vascular endothelium and muscle.[24] The clinical significance of this is unclear; it has not been associated with a deterioration in surgical stasis.

The diagnosis of heparin rebound is also challenging; the ACT is not a specific measure of excessive heparin, although the advent of the parallel heparinase ACT has addressed this issue but it is not universally available. The ACT is also poor at detecting heparin at low concentrations (<0.5 unit/mL).[32] The aPTT and PT are similarly nonspecific in that they may be increased after CPB in the absence of heparin.[33] The thromboelastogram does not reliably detect heparin rebound if the heparin concentration is small.[34] The titration method of protamine appears to be a sensible approach but difficult to administer. In view of this and the absence of clear clinical benefit, most anesthesiologists continue to give protamine empirically at a protamine-heparin ratio of between 1 to 1.3:1.

Overall, laboratory tests are neither 100% sensitive nor specific and are also too slow to guide the anesthesiologist. Near-patient testing (ACT and thromboelastogram) could act as a useful and practical guide, but their limitations need to be appreciated.

Failure of Hemostasis Associated with Cardiac Surgery

Complex abnormalities occur in the coagulation system in cardiac surgery owing to the profound surgical insult, hypothermia, acid-base disturbance, blood transfusion, anticoagulants, CPB (contact activation, platelet dysfunction and hemodilution), and, in some cases, deep hypothermic cardiorespiratory arrest. The paradox after CPB is that some hematologic events tip the balance toward a bleeding tendency, whereas others tip the balance toward a prothrombotic state.[35] There is also a complex interaction between the inflammatory cascade and endothelium with the components of the coagulation system[25]; the complex relationship between the proinflammatory and anti-inflammatory components of the inflammatory response and the clinical sequelae after CPB remain to be fully understood.

Antecedent drugs such as aspirin or other antiplatelet drugs such as clopidogrel can also exacerbate bleeding. The clinician must balance the risk of perioperative bleeding against the risk of drug discontinuation when deciding if and when to withhold the drug before surgery. Prostaglandin E_1 can inhibit platelet aggregation acting in synergy with endothelial cell–derived factors (nitric oxide and prostacyclin) at clinically relevant concentrations.[36] It is obviously not possible to stop the prostaglandin E_1 infusions in most cases because the children are dependent on its use to maintain ductal patency.[16]

In the child with cyanotic congenital heart disease, hemostasis is further impaired due to polycythemia, low platelet count and altered function,[16] reduced factors V, VII, and VIII, and increased fibrinolysis. The degree of derangement is related to the degree of cyanosis.[37,38]

Despite improvements in design and materials of the CPB circuit, abnormal activation of the coagulation and fibrinolytic systems persist. The normal balance of coagulation and fibrinolysis is particularly delicate in children and more susceptible to exogenous perturbations.[38] Shortly after CPB is started in children, all hemostatic proteins decrease by an average of 56% due to dilution. Because of the relative volume of the circuit in relation to the size of the child, it is not surprising that the magnitude of the effect of hemodilution is greater than data from adults.[22] A study in adult cardiac patients suggested that these reductions in coagulation factor concentrations after cardiac surgery contribute to bleeding and are clinically significant.[39]

In adults, the platelet count is also reduced on CPB by approximately 50%.[40] This is also attributed primarily to dilution, although other factors include organ sequestration, mechanical disruption, and adhesion to the circuit.[41] The platelet count is known to decrease during CPB in children, but the nidus is often not low enough to account for the prolonged bleeding time observed.[22] Such an observation also leads to the suggestion that significant platelet dysfunction occurs.[42]

Plasma proteins are denatured at blood-air interfaces such as cardiotomy suction or the oxygenator. This further reduces the availability of coagulation factors. Low-grade consumption of coagulation factors continually occurs on CPB.[19] This is one explanation for a worsened postoperative coagulopathy after a prolonged bypass.

The major mechanism for activation of the coagulation cascade during CPB is believed to be the "extrinsic" TF pathway, which is activated as a result of surgical trauma and inflammation (see Fig. 18-1).[19,43,44] Inflammatory mediators such as tumor necrosis factor (TNF) and interleukin (IL)-1 induce expression of TF on endothelial cells and monocytes. The intrinsic coagulation system is also activated when factor XII is adsorbed onto the surface of the CPB circuit, causing activation of complement, neutrophils, and the fibrinolytic system via kallikrein.[19]

Diffuse microvascular coagulation and thrombin production during CPB leads to activation of fibrinolysis. Total plasminogen activator causes conversion of plasminogen to plasmin. The plasmin cleaves fibrinogen, fibrin, and fibrin-fibrin dimers, leading to the production of fibrin split products and D-dimers. These increase vascular permeability, inhibit thrombin, and destroy some clotting factors.

A number of factors contribute to the development of bleeding in children undergoing cardiac surgical procedures (see Table 18-1). Induced hypothermia is frequently employed for systemic organ protection in pediatric cardiac surgery. Hypothermia causes dysfunction of both platelets and coagulation factors. It also delays functional recovery of platelets.[45] The platelet count is also decreased due to sequestration in splanchnic tissues. Other effects on coagulation include increased ATIII and anti–factor Xa activity, slowed clotting factor activation, and increased endothelial TF release. From adult data, perioperative blood loss and the need for transfusions decreases during normothermia.[19]

The blood loss in the first 24 hours after cardiac surgery can vary between 15 and 110 mL/kg, although the risk of excessive blood loss is greater among those weighing less than 8 kg, younger than 1 year of age, and children undergoing complex surgery.[46] The common preoperative and intraoperative risk factors for excessive bleeding are summarized in Table 18-2. Blood loss and transfusion requirements in pediatric cardiac

Table 18-2. Common Predictive Factors for Bleeding

Preoperative	Intraoperative
Age <1 or weight <8 kg	Individual surgeon
High hematocrit	Complex surgery
Congestive heart failure	Low platelet count during CPB
Repeat sternotomy	Prolonged CPB
Congenital and preoperative acquired coagulopathy	Duration of hypothermia on CPB
Cyanotic congenital heart disease	Deep hypothermic cardiac arrest

CPB, cardiopulmonary bypass.
From Williams GD, Bratton SL, Ramamoorthy C: Factors associated with blood loss and blood product transfusions: a multivariate analysis in children after open-heart surgery. Anesth Analg 1999; 89:57-64.

surgery vary inversely with age: neonates bleed more and receive more products per kilogram than any other age group.[47] There are some correlations between coagulation tests before and during CPB and postoperative blood component transfusion requirements, although the sensitivity and specificity of the tests are not sufficient to justify routine coagulation tests while on CPB. Of all the tests, a platelet count of ≤108,000/mm³ while on CPB yielded the greatest sensitivity (83%) and specificity (58%) for predicting excessive blood loss.[48]

Perioperative Blood Conservation Strategies

Blood conservation strategies begin with the meticulous attention to surgical hemostasis before CPB when the intrinsic coagulation mechanism is intact, the child's temperature is normal, and the inflammatory cascade has not been activated. After surgery, it is then important to distinguish blood loss treatable by physical means (surgical bleeding) from blood loss treatable by medical intervention (nonsurgical bleeding) and to promptly reestablish the physiologic conditions necessary for hemostasis. Additionally, there are strategies described in adult and pediatric anesthesia to reduce the need for transfusion of allogenic blood and blood products: optimizing blood transfusion practices, increasing red blood cell mass, and decreasing red cell loss (see Chapter 10). A discussion of artificial oxygen carriers is beyond the scope of this chapter.

Optimizing Blood Transfusion Practices

By optimizing national and local blood transfusion practices, it is possible to modify the use of blood products. Many factors need to be considered and documented before products are administered; an isolated hemoglobin concentration is insufficient to trigger an automatic transfusion. We must consider the child's pathology, cardiovascular variables, measures of tissue perfusion, and the potential for postoperative bleeding.[49] The physiologic and hematologic differences between adults and children imply that transfusion guidelines in adults should not be directly extrapolated to children, and the differences should be appreciated.[50] Autologous pre-donation is effective in adults because it reduces exposure to homologous blood products. There are practical difficulties in children that limit its use: the blood-letting process is technically difficult, regular blood collection bags contain too much anticoagulant, and the process may be stressful to children.[38]

Increasing Red Blood Cell Mass

For anemic children, two techniques, iron therapy and erythropoietin, have been effective in increasing the red cell mass. Oral iron (6 mg/kg/day) may take months to correct an iron-deficiency anemia, which may be impractical. Oral iron should be combined with vitamin C to increase the efficiency of gastrointestinal absorption. Modern intravenous preparations of iron carry a reduced risk of anaphylactoid reactions compared with older preparations. They have a peak response at 10 days.[51] There are no official guidelines for the preoperative use of erythropoietin (EPO) in children, although a number of regimens have been published.[49] To achieve a target hemoglobin concentration, EPO should be given intravenously or subcutaneously once or twice weekly for 3 weeks preoperatively after 3 weeks of oral iron therapy. EPO is available in two formulations, liquid or lyophilized. The liquid recombinant EPO is prepared with trace concentrations of albumin to prevent adsorption of the hormone to the glass. The lyophilized formulation is freeze-dried 100% EPO that is albumen free, and it is this formulation that is always suitable for Jehovah's Witnesses (available from Boehringer-Mannheim, Germany). Cost and practicalities may limit its use in many centers. Although a low preoperative hematocrit is a risk factor for requiring blood transfusion, it is not known to be an independent risk factor for a postoperative coagulopathy. The use of EPO increases the mean volume of autologous blood cells that could be collected preoperatively, but the cost is substantial (U.S. $340 per child excluding manpower and indirect costs).[52]

Decreasing Red Cell Loss

There are many nonsurgical approaches to decreasing red cell loss. In noncardiac surgery, techniques are commonly used to reduce intravascular hydrostatic pressure, such as patient positioning, avoidance of fluid overloading, and controlled hypotension. Neuraxial blockade in gynecologic, urologic, and orthopedic surgery also reduces blood loss.[53]

The efficacy of preoperative hemodilution is yet to be established in adults. In children, further problems limit its use. The young child and infant cannot sufficiently increase its stroke volume to compensate for a reduction in oxygen-carrying capacity during hemodilution. Furthermore, the high percentage of fetal hemoglobin in the younger than 4-month-old infant limits peripheral oxygen delivery and may not allow tolerance of a low hematocrit. In the infant older than 4 months of age, the reduction in hematocrit that occurs physiologically may render the technique inapplicable.[38]

Cell salvage and autotransfusion have had limited use in children weighing less than 20 kg. The minimum volume of collected blood required before washing and retransfusion has been approximately 300 mL until recently. In small children, transfusion may therefore be required before washed salvaged blood can be used. Moreover, the recovery yield of small volumes of shed blood is poor because most is absorbed on swabs. Recently, extremely small capacity (55 mL) bowls have been developed. If, however, the bowl is not completely filled, the unit of blood produced could be of variable hematocrit and quality.[38] Another device known as a continuous autotransfusion device allows effective processing of low volumes (<100 mL) with predictable quality and hematocrit.[38] This device is not yet widely available.

After CPB, the red cells in the extracorporeal circuit must be concentrated to avoid fluid overload when retransfused. Modified ultrafiltration (MUF) alone increases the hemoglobin concentration to more than 20 g/dL, although the solution for retransfusion may contain a high concentration of free hemoglobin and heparin.[54] Modern perfusion methods and materials may improve the quality of this blood. A higher-quality solution can be produced from the circuit by using an autotransfusion device to wash the residual volume in the circuit. The resultant blood for retransfusion has an increased hemoglobin concentration (20 g/dL) with much of the heparin and free hemoglobin removed.[38]

Medications Used for Hemostasis

The pathophysiology of coagulopathies in children after cardiac surgery is complex, and the etiology is multifactorial (see Table 18-1). It is not surprising therefore that no single blood component or drug treatment can reverse the abnormal clotting profile seen after CPB. As described earlier, it is important when possible to distinguish between surgical and nonsurgical causes of bleeding. This sometimes can be difficult, particularly in the presence of hypotension and a low cardiac output state, when surgical bleeding may not be easily identified. The anesthesiologist should attempt to restore normal physiologic variables such as body temperature, serum [Ca^{2+}], and acid-base balance. The difficulties of confirming that the heparin-associated anticoagulation has been adequately reversed is discussed earlier, but attention to these details allows excessive bleeding to be assessed more analytically. MUF after CPB has been used to remove excess body water and inflammatory mediators and attenuate the dilutional coagulopathy of CPB.[55,56] It has been shown to reduce blood and coagulation factor transfusion requirements as well as facilitate earlier extubation and earlier removal of the chest tube.[57] Further management consists of provision of blood and blood products that can restore elements of hemostasis and pharmacologic intervention. Laboratory or operating room testing of blood can provide information to aid directed therapy.

Blood Products

In the postoperative period, platelets and other blood products such as fresh frozen plasma (FFP) and cryoprecipitate are the mainstay of treatment for excessive bleeding.[58] Frequently these are administered on a largely empirical basis; laboratory tests describe only parts of the coagulation process[16] and are practically too slow to direct the anesthesiologist in real time as to the requirement for blood components. The thromboelastogram (TEG) is a dynamic whole-blood test that is frequently used as a near-patient test to assess clot elasticity properties and hence more precisely delineate the bleeding and homeostasis profile. In particular, thrombin formation disorders (r phase), fibrinogenesis disorders (K phase), and platelet function (MA phase) can be inferred from the TEG and hence guide blood component administration (Fig. 18-5).[58] The TEG should be performed on whole blood within 6 minutes of taking the sample.[59] Despite this, it still takes considerable time to give useful information in the time frame required in pediatric surgery, but various tech-

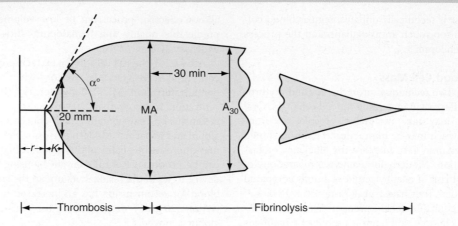

Figure 18-5. Thromboelastogram image describing the viscoelastic properties of the clot. The A_{30} in the diagram refers to the percent reduction in maximum amplitude (MA) at 30 minutes. (From: Rajwal S, Richards M, O'Meara M: The use of recalcified citrated whole blood—a pragmatic approach for thromboelastography in children. Pediatr Anesthes 2004; 14:656-660.)

niques have been used to accelerate this process, including the use of celite or TF-activated heparin–modified TEGs. It has been suggested that these can be taken before coming off CPB to give useful information when needed in the early post-bypass phase.[60]

To determine which blood product should be administered in a clinical situation, an algorithm has been developed for use in adults. This technique has been proven to be effective in reducing the proportion of adults who require platelet and FFP transfusion compared with a non–TEG-directed control group (Fig. 18-6). All adults in the study received prophylactic ε-aminocaproic acid (EACA).[61] Although the TEG has been found to provide useful information in children, it is unclear whether its use leads to a reduction in blood component administration. Although briefly discussed here, blood products are discussed in detail in Chapters 9 and 10.

Whole Blood/Packed Red Blood Cells

Red cells are most commonly administered as citrated packed red cells. There are some benefits to transfusing whole blood in children, although its availability largely limits its widespread use.[62] It is preferable to use fresh blood that is less than 1 week old in neonates because the reduction in 2,3-diphosphoglycerate in older blood could reduce oxygen delivery.[38] Hyperkalemia is a significant risk in neonates who receive older blood, particularly if it is cold and administered rapidly through a central venous access.[63] It has recently been shown in adult cardiac surgery that transfusion of older blood (mean age 20 days) associated with higher mortality, prolonged intubation, and increased incidence of renal failure and sepsis compared to newer blood (with mean age 11 days).[64]

Fresh Frozen Plasma

Fresh frozen plasma is the fluid portion of whole blood that is separated and frozen within 8 hours of collection. The stability of the clotting factors is related to the temperature and duration of storage. Most clotting factors remain stable for 3 months if stored at −24°C or below.[65] FFP has all of the clotting factors at their normal concentrations when administered within 6 hours of thawing. After that interval, the levels of the labile factors, V and VIII, begin to diminish. FFP contains no platelets. It should be ABO compatible with the recipient's red cells, although it can be taken from an AB donor if the recipient's blood type is unknown.[62] The most frequent reason for perioperative administration of FFP is the dilution of clotting factors secondary to massive blood transfusion, although it is also frequently given without clear

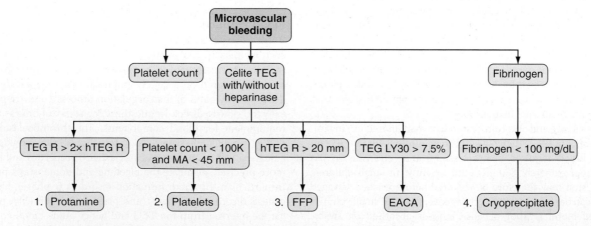

Figure 18-6. Algorithm to direct blood component therapy in adults. hTEG, heparinase-activated TEG; R, reaction time; LY30, lysis index at 30 minutes (percent reduction of maximum amplitude [MA] at 30 minutes); FFP, fresh frozen plasma; EACA, ε-aminocaproic acid. A pediatric TEG algorithm is yet to be developed. (From Shore-Lesserson L, Manspeizer HE, DePerio M, et al: Thromboelastography-guided transfusion algorithm reduces transfusions in complex cardiac surgery. Anesth Analg 1999; 88:312-319.)

hematologic indications. At the same time, one must always recognize that an infected unit of FFP may contain a greater viral load than packed red blood cells (PRBCs) and thus run a greater risk of transmitting human immunodeficiency virus.[66]

When administering large volumes of FFP, it is important to recognize that there is more citrate in FFP than there is in whole blood or citrated PRBCs. If the metabolic capacity of the liver to metabolize the sodium citrate is exceeded, citrate toxicity can occur, leading to hypocalcemia, hypomagnesemia, and a metabolic alkalosis (because the metabolic derivative of citrate is bicarbonate). This has many implications of particular importance to the neonate. First, hypocalcemia can contribute to a coagulopathy itself. Second, the neonate is particularly poor at metabolizing citrate. As a result of the reduced sarcoplasmic reticulum in the heart, the neonate depends on ionized calcium for contraction and relaxation of the myocardium. Consequently, neonates are prone to myocardial dysfunction during citrate-induced ionized hypocalcemic states, particularly when calcium-channel blocking inhalational agents are used. These problems may be minimized by limiting the speed of infusion of FFP to 1 mL/kg/min and by administering prophylactic doses of calcium during the transfusion (see Chapter 10). Consideration should also be given to the dose of inhalational agent because the negative effect of inhaled agents on myocardial contractility is dose dependent.[50,67]

Frequently, FFP is given empirically for bleeding in major surgery. In some cases, the PT has also been used to guide therapy. Despite common use of this test, a study in adults examined the effect of FFP transfusion on those with mild abnormalities in PT (13.1 to 17 seconds). They found that the PT was reduced halfway to normal values in only 15% of patients, and was completely normalized in only 0.8%. It is difficult to interpret how this translates to clinical bleeding tendency. Of note, this study also reported six suspected transfusion reactions of 191 transfusions.[68]

Platelets

Platelets are essential in controlling surgical bleeding. In the surgical environment, the most common causes of low platelets or abnormal function include dilution after massive blood loss and transfusion, platelet function inhibitors such as clopidogrel and aspirin, and disseminated intravascular coagulation (DIC). The effect of CPB on platelet function and number is discussed earlier. Uncommonly, heparin-induced thrombocytopenia occurs and should be considered whenever significant thrombocytopenia is observed.

There is no clear-cut threshold for the transfusion of platelets. The decision to transfuse platelets must follow consideration of a balance of risk (including alloimmunization, infection, allergy, and transfusion-related acute lung injury) against the benefit of reducing morbidity associated with blood loss.[69] In practice, the threshold for transfusion of platelets depends on the etiology and clinical observation of abnormal bleeding. An ongoing consumption of platelets such as DIC may require a platelet transfusion at a greater platelet level than a child with dilutional thrombocytopenia due to massive transfusion.[62]

Clinically, performing a formal bleeding time in the operating room is usually impractical, and there is no currently available platelet function test post CPB.[69] Consequently, the clinician can use only clinical observations, laboratory platelet counts, and thromboelastography as a guide.[62]

A common dosing regimen for platelet transfusion is 0.1 to 0.3 unit/kg. This often produces an increment of 20,000 to 70,000/mm^3. With ongoing blood losses and dilution, a larger dose may be required. Apheresis-obtained platelets contain the equivalent of 6 to 8 standard units.[70] Because the platelets are from a single donor, this process may reduce the probability for disease transmission and increase the initial increment of platelet count. Repeated transfusion leads to antibody production and reduced half-life of subsequent platelet transfusions. It must be remembered that platelets should be agitated to prevent clumping and not refrigerated once released from the blood bank. It is also important to be proactive in arranging for platelets to be available before the start of surgery if heavy bleeding is anticipated. Remember, not all blood banks have platelets readily available. Platelets should be administered through a large-pore (>150 µm) filter to avoid adsorption of the platelets onto the finer mesh filters.[71] Platelets are suspended in plasma, thereby reducing the need for FFP. Four to 5 units of platelets contain clotting factors equivalent to 1 unit of FFP.

In children with low platelet counts before surgery, it is important to give the platelets close to the start of surgery to ensure the greatest levels at the time of peak demand.[62]

Cryoprecipitate

When FFP is thawed at cold temperatures (1°-6°C), an insoluble portion of the plasma precipitates. The supernatant is then removed, leaving the cryoprecipitate (approximately 15 mL) to be refrozen to −18°C. Each bag of cryoprecipitate provides approximately 100 units of factor VIII:C, 200 mg of fibrinogen, as well as vWf and factor XIII. It is used for the following:

- Hypofibrinogenemia (particularly in the context of massive hemorrhage and transfusion)
- Massive hemorrhage and transfusion
- DIC
- von Willebrand disease (unresponsive to desmopressin)
- Factor XIII deficiency
- Hemophilia when concentrates of factor VIII are unavailable (rare)

Cryoprecipitate is usually given in clinical practice when excessive postoperative bleeding has responded poorly to routine procedures (FFP, platelets, temperature and electrolyte correction). At this time, formal coagulation studies may be underway but empirical correction of presumed factor deficiencies may need to precede evidence from the laboratory.

Antifibrinolytics

A number of drugs aimed at reducing bleeding and transfusion requirements have been investigated. Most commonly, antifibrinolytics are used as prophylactic measures and recombinant factor VIIa has been used as "rescue" therapy in emergency situations. Other treatment modalities are briefly discussed below. Commonly, the classes of antifibrinolytics are

1. Synthetic lysine analogues such as ε-aminocaproic acid (EACA) and tranexamic acid (TXA)
2. Protease inhibitors (aprotinin and nafamostat).

There is good evidence that antifibrinolytics improve hematologic function and reduce bleeding in the adult population[72-76]; they have been shown to reduce rates of surgical re-exploration and transfusion of homologous blood products.[77] The evidence is less clear in infants and children. In view of the relative ease at which the fibrinolytic/coagulation system can be imbalanced by CPB in children, theory would suggest that antifibrinolytics such as aprotinin would exhibit even more benefit in pediatric surgery. Despite this, data are conflicting but the commonly used agents are discussed here.

Synthetic Lysine Analogues: Tranexamic Acid and ε-Aminocaproic Acid

Tranexamic acid (*trans*-4-aminomethyl-cyclohexane carboxylic acid [TXA]) and ε-aminocaproic acid (6-aminohexanoic acid [EACA]) have been shown to reduce blood loss effectively; this appears to be clear in cyanotic children. Importantly, the doses need to be sufficient to compensate for:

● The hemodilution of the extracorporeal circuit[78]
● The increased volume of distribution and clearance in children[79]

EACA is Food and Drug Administration (FDA) approved for enhancing hemostasis when fibrinolysis contributes to bleeding.[80] TXA has more specific FDA approval for the short-term treatment or prophylaxis of dental bleeding in hemophiliacs,[81] although many anesthesiologists use it for many cardiac and noncardiac major blood loss cases. Tranexamic acid and EACA are synthetic antifibrinolytic amino acid derivatives. They form reversible complexes with plasminogen and plasmin by binding to lysine-binding sites.[82,83] They prevent the proteolytic action of plasmin on fibrin; hence, there is an inhibition of fibrinolysis at the surgical wound (Fig. 18-7). They also prevent plasmin

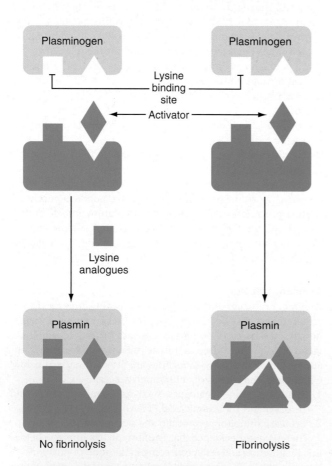

Figure 18-7. Diagrammatic representation of the mode of action of the synthetic lysine analogues tranexamic acid and ε-aminocaproic acid. (From Mahdy AM, Webster NR: Perioperative systemic hemostatic agents. Br J Anaesth 2004; 93:842-858.)

degradation of glycoprotein Ib receptors.[3] It has been suggested that the two drugs are qualitatively similar,[84] although EACA inhibits plasmin to a lesser extent. In cardiac surgery, tranexamic acid has a 6 to 10 times greater potency for inhibiting fibrinolysis than EACA.[78] Importantly, lysine analogues should not be used in DIC because they may increase intravascular thrombosis. The reason is that these drugs inhibit both circulating free plasmin and fibrin-bound plasmin and therefore interfere with the dissolution of clots in small blood vessels, thus worsening the intravascular thrombosis. This contrasts to aprotinin, which spares fibrin-bound plasmin.[3] Although some suggest that TXA has no appreciable effect on platelet numbers and platelet function,[85] others argue that both TXA and EACA prevent plasmin degradation of platelet glycoprotein Ib receptors.[86,87] EACA may also exert an effect of neutralizing plasmin by causing release of α_2-antiplasmin.[88]

Lysine Analogues in Noncardiac Surgery

The extent of intraoperative transfusion requirement during scoliosis surgery is difficult to predict from preoperative investigations; however, factors such as surgical hemostasis, extent and duration of surgery, intraoperative mean arterial pressure, and patient positioning may dramatically affect the amount of bleeding. Children with secondary scoliosis also have a tendency to bleed more than the idiopathic group (see Chapter 30).[82] The cause of nonsurgical bleeding is thus multifactorial, including dilution of clotting factors with infusion of large crystalloid volumes and accelerated fibrinolysis.[84] One can therefore postulate the potential benefit of an antifibrinolytic. The dilutional factor as a contributor of coagulopathy is believed to be particularly important in the secondary scoliosis group.[89]

In one pediatric scoliosis study, the authors used a relatively high dose of TXA (100 mg/kg on induction followed by 10 mg/kg/hr infusion during the case). There was an overall reduction in blood loss of 41% compared with the control group.[82] Among the children who did not have idiopathic scoliosis, the reduction was 48%. Despite this, equal numbers of children in the TXA and control groups received red cell transfusions. There was also an insignificant reduction in the amount of transfused blood, although the study may have been underpowered to answer this question. Among the secondary scoliosis patients there was a 42% reduction of transfusion requirement in the TXA-treated group.[82] In this study, postoperative blood loss was not published, although the use of TXA was an independent predictor of reduced blood loss. A significant reduction in blood loss was not observed in another scoliosis study using only a 10-mg/kg bolus followed by 1 mg/kg/hr, but a significant reduction in packed cell transfusion (by 28%) was observed in the TXA group. That study concluded 24 hours after surgery.[90]

EACA has been used in children undergoing liver transplantation with variable results. Specifically, low dose EACA infusions are widely used to treat severe bleeding in liver transplantation, even though no trials have established such a role for it in children.

Lysine Analogues in Cardiac Surgery

In adults, lysine analogues given prophylactically reduced bleeding after CPB by 30% to 40%.[3,77,91] However, a recent review closely examining the evidence concluded that TXA has not consistently shown evidence of reducing erythrocyte transfusions. There are no substantial data to support the use of EACA in cardiac surgery.[92] In children, it is equally difficult to interpret the studies due to the different dosing regimens used.

Regarding TXA in pediatric cardiac patients, a dose of 100 mg/kg bolus followed by 10 mg/kg/hr has been studied[78] in children undergoing repeat sternotomy. An additional dose of 100 mg/kg was also given at the start of CPB. This regimen reduced the total blood loss by 24% over the first postoperative 24 hours. There was also a 38% reduction in transfusion requirement. A smaller dose (50 mg/kg) regimen demonstrated only a modest reduction in blood loss among a subgroup of preoperative cyanotic patients.[93] This apparent reduced effect of the lower dose regimen is consistent with the studies in pediatric scoliosis patients and also the dose-response relationship of TXA observed in adult cardiac surgery.[94]

EACA is commonly used in children undergoing cardiac surgery,[79] as well as for children on extracorporeal membrane oxygenation (ECMO). Empirical dosing regimens appear to be safe, but the efficacy of EACA appears to be variable. The first controlled trial of EACA in pediatric cardiac patients in 1974 used a 75-mg/kg loading dose and a 15-mg/kg/hr infusion. The results showed greatest benefit in children with cyanotic heart disease with a blood loss reduction of 42%.[95] A more recent study used a 150-mg/kg bolus followed by a 30 mg/kg/hr infusion in high-risk cardiac surgery. This led to a reduction in surgical blood loss with better TEG platelet function (in terms of maximum amplitude [MA]), although there was no reduction in transfusion requirement or postoperative blood loss as measured by chest tube drainage.[96] It is reasonable to conclude that the different dose regimens contributed significantly to the variability in the results. However, using pharmacokinetic principles and the few published clinical trials, it is possible to suggest reasonable dosing regimens in children (see later).

Pharmacokinetics of Lysine Analogues and Dosing Regimens

Tranexamic acid has a volume of distribution of 9 to 12 L in adults.[97] Most of the drug is excreted unchanged by the kidney, so the dose should be reduced in renal failure. The terminal elimination half-life is about 2 hours. As expected, however, the pharmacokinetics of TXA are significantly affected by CPB. In the adult, a 30-minute bolus dose of 12.5 mg/kg followed by 6.5 mg/kg/hr with 1 mg/kg added to the prime maintains the concentration of TXA greater than 334 μmol.[98] However, because the "therapeutic" concentration of TXA is not completely clear, particularly in children, it is difficult to interpret these figures in terms of therapeutic effect. In a recent study that compared dosing regimens in children undergoing CPB, dosing regimens that involved multiple doses to compensate for the changes in volume of distribution caused by CPB (10 mg/kg before, during, and after CPB) were more effective than a larger single bolus (50 mg/kg) at the start of surgery in terms of sternal closure time, blood loss, and blood product requirement.[99]

About 35% of EACA undergoes hepatic metabolism to adipic acid. Most of the drug, however, is excreted unchanged by the kidneys. The terminal elimination half-life is 1 to 2 hours.[100] A pharmacokinetic study in children demonstrated a greater weight-adjusted volume of distribution compared with adults before, during, and after CPB.

Redistribution rates in children were greater than in adults and unaffected by CPB. Based on this, a greater dosing regimen was suggested: 75 mg/kg over 10 minutes, 75 mg/kg in the CPB, and 75 mg/kg/hr as an infusion. This would maintain levels of EACA above the presumed "therapeutic" concentration of 260 μg/mL.[79] As with TXA, the therapeutic concentration required is not clear, but these triple-dosing regimens appear to be clinically effective in children. One study used three doses of 100 mg/kg EACA before, during, and after CPB, which clearly demonstrated a significant reduction in postoperative blood loss, reduced blood and platelet transfusion requirements, and reduced re-exploration rate compared with control subjects.[101]

Adverse Effects of Synthetic Lysine Analogues

As with any antifibrinolytic agent, one of the most worrisome complications is thrombosis, but, unlike aprotinin, the lysine analogues (TXA or EACA) have failed to show an increased risk of renal, cardiac, or cerebral events in adult cardiac surgery patients.[102] Two meta-analyses in adults concluded that prophylactic lysine analogues in cardiac surgery reduced postoperative bleeding by 30% to 40% without increasing the incidence of thromboembolic complications.[77,91] However, thromboses have been reported in nonsurgical hypercoagulable states.[83] Despite occasional anecdotes, there is no clear-cut evidence that the incidence of thrombosis is increased with either of the lysine analogues. Both TXA and EACA appear to have a very low incidence of serious side effects such as anaphylaxis.

ε-Aminocaproic Acid Adverse Effects

The most common acute side effect of EACA is hypotension usually associated with rapid intravenous administration. Rash, nausea, vomiting, weakness, retrograde ejaculation, myopathy, and rhabdomyolysis have been less frequently reported associated with longer-term use.[97] EACA is teratogenic, so it is contraindicated in pregnancy.[103]

Tranexamic Acid Adverse Effects

Rapid intravenous administration of TXA can cause hypotension. Oral administration only can be associated with gastrointestinal side effects. In an adult study, the effects of continuing TXA administration for 12 hours postoperatively were compared with intraoperative administration only. No advantage was reported in terms of blood loss or transfusion reduction, although there was an association with some renal dysfunction in the prolonged infusion group.[104]

Although the authors cannot currently recommend the use of TXA or EACA as "routine" in all procedures involving moderate blood loss, it could potentially be useful to reduce blood transfusions in high-risk children who require surgery such as for secondary scoliosis and repeat sternotomy in cardiac cases. The paucity of prospective studies precludes support for a wider application at present.

Serine Protease Inhibitors: Aprotinin and Nafamostat

Aprotinin is the most widely studied of all the antifibrinolytics. It provides the most consistent efficacy in reducing bleeding and transfusion requirements in cardiac and hepatic patients.[92]

It is a naturally occurring 58-residue polybasic polypeptide; its antifibrinolytic activity occurs due to its ability to form reversible enzyme-inhibitor complexes and inhibit circulating plasmin, trypsin, chymotrypsin, kallikrein, thrombin, and activated protein C.[86,105,106] The mechanism of actions has recently been reviewed.[107] It is indicated for the prevention and treatment of the bleeding diatheses associated with profibrinolytic states. Its effect on platelets is controversial; it has been proposed that it mitigates platelet dysfunction on CPB by preserving glycoprotein Ib and glycoprotein IIb/IIIa function at the platelet surface.[108] Other studies have challenged this, suggesting that aprotinin does not alter platelet function.[3,109,110] Aprotinin may also indirectly inhibit platelet activation on CPB by inhibiting plasmin and other mediators.[111]

At high doses specifically, aprotinin has many anti-inflammatory properties[3]:

- It inhibits kallikrein and complement[112]
- It inhibits the release of TNF-α, IL-6, and IL-8.[113]
- It inhibits endogenous nitric oxide synthase induction[114]
- It decreases CPB-induced leukocyte activation[112]
- It inhibits monocytes and granulocyte adhesion molecule upregulation[115]

Aprotinin is available as a clear colorless solution in a concentration of 10,000 KIU (kallikrein inhibitor units) per milliliter: 1 KIU is defined as the amount of aprotinin that decreases the activity of two biological kallikrein units by 50%,[97] with 1 mg equivalent to 7,143 KIU. Although the manufacturers recommend central venous administration, aprotinin is frequently administered into peripheral veins in children due to the practical requirement of using the limited number of central line lumen for administration of medications such as inotropes. Peripheral administration of aprotinin has not been reported to cause adverse events in children.

The clinical indications for its use are highly variable, and its routine use is controversial. In children, it is reserved for procedures with high risk of major blood loss during and after open-heart surgery with extracorporeal circulation and for those in whom optimal blood conservation during open-heart surgery is an absolute priority. It is also indicated for life-threatening hemorrhage due to hyperplasminemia, such as after thrombolytic therapy, in acute promyelocytic leukemia, and during mobilization of some malignant tumors.[116] It has also been used off-label in high blood loss procedures such as scoliosis surgery[117,118] and liver transplantation.

CPB is associated with a diffuse inflammatory response causing subtle or overt end organ damage and a predisposition to bleeding.[119] Several serine protease enzymes are key mediators in the initiation and amplification of this inflammatory response,[120] so it would be reasonable to suppose that a serine protease inhibitor such as aprotinin would benefit the adult and pediatric cardiac population. Moreover, in children undergoing open cardiac procedures, the disruption of normal hemostatic mechanisms is even more potent than it is in adults. One would therefore expect that blocking coagulation and fibrinolysis with aprotinin would be particularly effective in children. The studies, however, have yielded conflicting results.[38] Some studies have suggested the routine use of prophylactic aprotinin to be of no benefit in simple pediatric cardiac surgery,[121] whereas high dose aprotinin has been shown to be effective in complex cardiac operations in children weighing less than 15 kg.[122] Other studies showed that high-dose (30,000 KIU/kg pre-CPB, then 50,000 KIU on CPB) aprotinin reduced the number of transfused units after CPB in children weighing less than 10 kg,[123] although another failed to demonstrate any benefit in primary operations and a nonsignificant trend in benefit in those children older than 1 year old having repeat procedures.[124]

A more recent retrospective nonrandomized controlled study examined the effect of high-dose aprotinin in children having repeat sternotomy or those younger than 6 months of age.[125] The large doses were based on dose per surface area; 240 mg/m^2 (maximum 280 mg) was given after central and arterial line placement as well as an additional 240 mg/m^2 into the pump prime and 56 mg/m^2/hr as an infusion. Aprotinin significantly reduced operative closure time and trended toward requiring fewer red blood cell unit exposures. There was no difference in terms of platelet or FFP exposures when compared with controls, although the aprotinin group required significantly fewer ventilator days in the postoperative period. It was postulated that the anti-inflammatory properties of aprotinin were responsible for this observation. Notably, there were no thrombotic or anaphylactic complications in the children who received aprotinin.

A meta-analysis examined the effect of aprotinin on the proportion of children transfused, the volume of blood transfused, and the amount of chest tube drainage, citing 12 trials that included 626 children. Aprotinin reduced the proportion of children who received red cell/whole blood transfusions by 33%. Surprisingly, the effect of aprotinin on the proportion of children who received red cells remained significant in the subgroup of those undergoing primary sternotomy. It also remained significant in the children who weighed more than 10 kg and in one study in those who weighed less than 10 kg. Remarkably, aprotinin did not significantly affect the volume of blood transfused or the amount of postoperative chest tube drainage.[105] Because most bypass circuits were primed with blood, it may be that the number of overall donor exposures was not reduced.

As with the studies on lysine analogues, this apparent lack of clarity regarding the efficacy of aprotinin in children may reflect differing doses used in the studies, differing regimens of bypass circuit boluses, and differing empirical regimens of blood product administration. The dose-dependent effect apparently observed in the lysine analogues appears to also occur with aprotinin on closure time, transfusion requirements, intensive care, and hospital days in children having repeat sternotomy procedures.[126]

Pharmacokinetics of Aprotinin

Aprotinin rapidly redistributes into the extracellular space after intravenous administration. It is metabolized in the proximal renal tubules and eliminated in a biphasic pattern: a rapid phase half-life of 40 minutes and a slower phase half-life of 7 hours.[3,100]

A pharmacokinetic study of aprotinin in children undergoing CPB examined aprotinin concentrations after administration of weight-based dosing (25,000 KIU/kg bolus pre-CPB, 35,000 KIU/kg in CPB prime, and 12,500 KIU/kg/hr infusion). It demonstrated significant variability in aprotinin concentration among children of different age and weight (Fig. 18-8).[127] Although there was considerable variation in plasma concentration of aprotinin there was a correlation with weight at 5 minutes after administration and 5 minutes after cardiopulmonary bypass (Figs. 18-9 and 18-10).

This study can provide one possible explanation as to why there are such inconsistent results from aprotinin trials in children. Using a dose-per-weight regimen, the smaller children may fail to achieve therapeutic levels of aprotinin in terms of plasmin inhibition and the possible anti-inflammatory effects (a low concentration of aprotinin, e.g., <200 KIU/mL, would be insufficient to inhibit contact activation on the CPB circuit). To

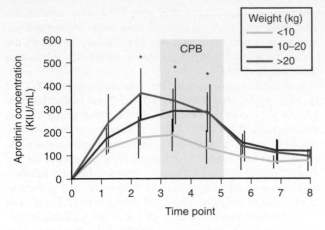

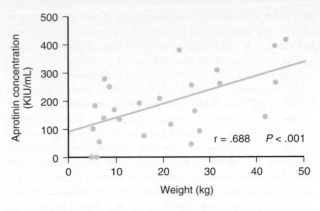

Figure 18-10. Correlation of aprotinin concentration with weight 5 minutes after start of CPB. (From Oliver WC, Fass DN, Nuttall GA, et al: Variability of plasma aprotinin concentrations in pediatric patients undergoing cardiac surgery. J Thorac Cardiovasc Surg 2004; 127:1670-1677.)

Figure 18-8. Graph of aprotinin concentration against time for different weights, demonstrating variability of concentration when a dose per weight is given in children. *Time points:* 1 = baseline, 2 = 5 minutes after aprotinin, 3 = 5 minutes after CPB, 4 = 30 minutes of CPB, 5 = 60 minutes of CPB, 6 = discontinuation of CPB, 7 = 1 hour after discontinuation of bypass, 8 = 4 hours after CPB. (From Oliver WC, Fass DN, Nuttall GA, et al: Variability of plasma aprotinin concentrations in pediatric patients undergoing cardiac surgery. J Thorac Cardiovasc Surg 2004; 127:1670-1677.)

achieve "target" concentrations of aprotinin, aprotinin should be given as a dose per body surface area, as opposed to dose per kilogram. This would result in a 2.5 times greater dose in neonates than would otherwise be given.[38] A recent qualitative literature review suggested that an initial loading dose of at least 30,000 KIU/kg is required, followed by an infusion. The pump prime dose should be based on the volume of the pump rather than the weight of the patient.[128]

Adverse Effects of Aprotinin

Despite the possible reduction in bleeding and exposure to donor blood components there is concern over potential serious side effects of aprotinin. Although aprotinin continues to be used in cardiac and scoliosis surgery, its use in adults has declined after publication of a multicenter observational study in which it was compared with EACA, TXA, and placebo in

4374 adults. This study reported that aprotinin was associated with a 181% increased risk of stroke or encephalopathy, a 55% increased risk of myocardial infarction, and a doubling of the risk of renal failure.[102,*] EACA and TXA have not been associated with these thrombotic risks. In children, only much smaller studies have been performed although the largest review does not suggest an increased risk of thrombosis.[129] For specific surgery such as Fontan and other procedures, thrombosis is a significant cause of early and late morbidity and mortality, although the role of aprotinin in thrombotic complications in children is unclear.[130]

Unlike lysine analogues, animal studies have shown that aprotinin has a high affinity for the kidneys. After free glomerular passage, aprotinin binds selectively to the brush border of the proximal tubule. By means of pinocytosis, it then enters and accumulates in the cytoplasm and inhibits kallikrein, rennin, and prostaglandin synthesis.[102] High kallikrein activity occurs normally during conditions of renal ischemia and hypothermia; with aprotinin the deep cortical and medullary perfusion and its autoregulation is impaired. This is worsened by a dose-dependent renal afferent vasoconstriction. These factors explain the focal tubular necrosis that can occur.[102] Furthermore, animal studies suggest that aprotinin causes macrovascular and microvascular thrombosis by interfering with the synthesis and release of endothelial nitric oxide.[131,132] Eight pediatric studies investigating apportioning have reported renal outcomes; four have failed to show a difference in postoperative creatinine. With the power of these studies being small, no conclusion can be reached with regard to the renal safety of aprotinin in children.[128]

As with many polypeptides, anaphylactic reactions can occur with aprotinin. Reactions can range from mild (no intervention required) to severe (long-lasting hypotension despite vasopressors). The reported incidence of adverse reactions in children varies, but the largest reported experience with aprotinin found 1 reaction from 2202 primary exposures (0.05%) and 6 reactions from 453 reexposures (1.3%). There were no severe reactions

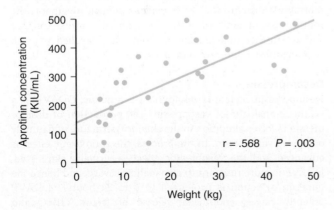

Figure 18-9. Correlation of aprotinin concentration with weight of child 5 minutes after administration. (From Oliver WC, Fass DN, Nuttall GA, et al: Variability of plasma aprotinin concentrations in pediatric patients undergoing cardiac surgery. J Thorac Cardiovasc Surg 2004; 127:1670-1677.)

*Some conclusions of this paper have been questioned for reasons such as failure to control for the treatment center or how comorbidity and transfusions affected outcomes.

after 1998 attributed to factors such as elimination of use in recently exposed patients.[133] Many studies report the incidence and severity of reaction to be less than that of adults. This may be due to the immature neonatal immune system.[128]

In order to predict those who are at high risk of anaphylaxis from reexposure to aprotinin, both skin testing and anti-aprotinin IgG have been measured. Unfortunately, neither measurement is effective, as both tests have a poor predictive value.[129,134] Various measures have been taken to reduce the incidence of anaphylaxis from aprotinin: preadministration of histamine (H1 and H2) antagonists, test dose preceding the bolus load, and avoidance of reexposure within 6 months of the previous dose. The use of a test dose is controversial, as anaphylaxis can occur to a test dose[135,136]; furthermore, a negative test dose does not exclude the possibility of subsequent anaphylaxis. Nonetheless, many clinicians advocate its use. Some suggest waiting at least 20 minutes between test dose and bolus does.[137] There are insufficient data with regard to the preventative effect of H1/H2 antagonists or steroids.[136] The only current solid recommendations with regard to preventing anaphylaxis are:

- Test dose and initial loading dose are not given until it is possible to rapidly initiate CPB (package insert).
- Avoiding the use of aprotinin within 12 months of previous exposure (FDA recommendation)[138]

When considering the use of aprotinin, it is important to balance the possible benefits of blood loss reduction, anti-inflammatory effects, reduced donor unit exposure, and reoperation rate against the known serious side effect profile. Measures can be taken as described earlier to reduce this risk, although serious morbidity and mortality can occur despite these risk-reducing strategies. The overall safety of aprotinin has been scrutinized by the FDA, with safety reviews in 2006 and again in 2007. It remained approved until a recent trial in adults suggested aprotinin was associated with a possible increase in mortality. At the time of this writing, aprotinin has been withdrawn from the US market pending review.

Nafamostat is a synthetic protease inhibitor. It inhibits thrombin, factors Xa and XIIa, kallikrein, plasmin, and complement factors C1r and C1s. It preserves platelet function on CPB and acts as an antifibrinolytic, anti-inflammatory, and anticoagulant agent. Although it has proven to be beneficial in liver transplantation and CPB, the sample sizes in the studies of nafamostat were very small. Furthermore, there is no experience with this medication in Europe or the United States.[3] In view of its lack of widespread availability, it is not discussed further in this chapter.

Which Antifibrinolytic in Pediatric Cardiac Surgery?

The wide variation in study design and dosage of all three drugs makes comparison very difficult. Before using a prophylactic antifibrinolytic, it is important to balance the risks and benefits of each drug in the context of the individual patient and the type of surgery. A meta-analysis of adult cardiac patients concluded that both EACA and low-dose aprotinin significantly reduced blood loss by 35%, and high-dose aprotinin reduced blood loss by 53% compared with placebo. The proportion of patients who were transfused after EACA and high-dose aprotinin was similar, although the re-exploration rate was significantly reduced only in the high-dose aprotinin group.[71] In an adult study that compared the inflammatory markers after aprotinin and EACA, the increase in the proinflammatory and anti-

inflammatory interleukins IL-6 and IL-10 were significantly attenuated only after aprotinin.[139] One study highlighted the increase in complication rate after aprotinin compared with the lysine analogues.[102] It is not possible to confidently extrapolate these data to children.

In pediatric cardiac surgery, low-dose aprotinin (10,000 KIU/kg followed by 10,000 KIU/kg/hr) has been compared with EACA, 100 mg/kg on induction, in the pump prime and on weaning CPB. There was a significant reduction in postoperative blood loss and in transfusion requirements in both groups compared with control but no significant difference between the two drugs.[140] These data are difficult to interpret because substantively larger doses of aprotinin are frequently used in current practice. More recently, TXA, 100 mg/kg before, during, and after CPB was compared with aprotinin, 30,000 KIU after induction, 30,000 KIU in the pump, and 30,000 KIU after weaning off bypass. There was a significant reduction in the time to sternal closure, transfusion requirements, and blood loss compared with control but no significant difference between the two drugs. Interestingly, when the two drugs were combined at the same doses they showed no additional benefit.[141]

When EACA (100 mg/kg on induction, in the pump, and post CPB) and TXA (10 mg/kg on induction, in the pump, and post CPB) were compared with placebo, fewer blood products were required and there was a smaller incidence of re-exploration with both drugs compared with placebo but no difference between the two drugs.[142]

If no significant difference has been noted between the antifibrinolytics in terms of blood loss, transfusion, time to sternal closure, or re-exploration rate using standard dosing regimens, the choice of antifibrinolytic will depend on the side effect profiles and cost. It is not clear how the larger doses of aprotinin commonly used today compare with the lysine analogues. Despite the reduced incidence of side effects such as anaphylaxis and thrombotic complications after lysine analogues when compared with aprotinin, many choose to use high-dose aprotinin regimens in high-risk complex pediatric cardiac surgery because it remains the most extensively studied drug. The effects of aprotinin in reducing the inflammatory response and possibly preserving platelet function are often cited as further reasons for its use. The "hard" benefits of aprotinin or lysine analogues in children in terms of surgical re-exploration, hospital stay, and mortality are far from clear. It remains difficult to support the routine use of antifibrinolytics in pediatric cardiac surgery without further independent randomized controlled trials to examine these important outcomes.

Desmopressin

Desmopressin acetate (1-desamino-8-D-arginine; DDAVP) is a synthetic analogue of vasopressin. The production of desmopressin involves alteration in the chemical structure of naturally occurring vasopressin. In the process, the antidiuretic effect is enhanced and the vasopressor effect is virtually eliminated. DDAVP is more resistant to enzymatic cleavage, and hence the duration of action is prolonged to 6 to 24 hours.[97] DDAVP potently causes endothelial release of factor VIII:C and VIII:vWf. It has been used in mild hemophilia, von Willebrand disease, coagulopathy of uremia, and liver failure and in adults undergoing cardiac and spinal fusion surgery.

During the early phase of coagulation, platelets bind via the glycoprotein receptor Ib to vWf on the damaged endothelium.

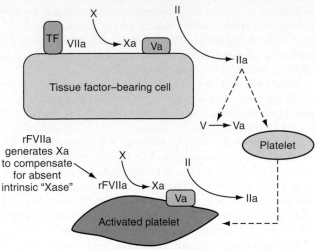

rFVIIa GENERATES Xa ON THE PLATELET
SURFACE IN HEMOPHILIACS

Figure 18-11. Schematic representation of the cell-based coagulation model and the proposed mechanism of how rFVIIa can potentially improve coagulation in hemophiliacs. At supraphysiologic concentrations, rVIIa can bind to the phospholipid membranes of activated platelets where it activates factor X independent of the tissue factor pathway, causing a large rise in thrombin at the platelet surface. It can therefore compensate for a lack of factor VIII or IX and possibly explain its effectiveness in platelet function disorders. (From Welsby IJ, Monroe DM, Lawson JH, Hoffmann M: Recombinant activated factor VIIa and the anaesthetist. Anaesthesia 2005; 60:1203-1212.)

Intravenous desmopressin releases vWf, thus enhancing the binding of platelets to damaged endothelium. The maximum effect of desmopressin is observed at a dose of 0.3 μg/kg. It must be given *after* cessation of the extracorporeal circuit to prevent unwanted platelet activation.[38]

Several meta-analyses of its use in adults have been published, the most recent showing that desmopressin was associated with a small reduction in blood loss but no benefit in terms of repeat sternotomy, proportion of patients requiring transfusion, or mortality.[77] It was also associated with a 2.4-fold increase in risk of myocardial infarction.

In children, 0.3 μg/kg failed to demonstrate any benefit for both non–high-risk[143] and high-risk cardiac surgery.[144] Younger children are not as capable of releasing vWf from endothelial storage sites as older children, and the maximal release of vWf caused by the operative stimulus cannot be enhanced by desmopressin.[145] Potential adverse sequelae from desmopressin use includes fluid retention, hyponatremia, tachyphylaxis, tachycardia, and mild hypotension.[146] Desmopressin is therefore not currently recommended in pediatric surgery,[38] although one could postulate that it could be reserved for those with ongoing bleeding with evidence of platelet function abnormalities such as prolonged bleeding time or decreased MA values on a TEG.[147]

Factor VIIa

Recombinant activated factor VII (rVIIa) is known to be a safe and effective treatment for and prevention of hemorrhage in hemophiliacs with circulating inhibitors to replacement factors. It is also used in patients with Glanzmann thrombasthenia refractory to platelet transfusion.[148] Regulatory approval has been granted in Europe and the United States for these conditions.

Based on our understanding of the cell-based coagulation process discussed earlier, it is possible to demonstrate how activated rVIIa can potentially restore, in part, thrombin generation and effect hemostasis in many anesthetic and intensive care settings. Overall, the mechanism of action of rVIIa has been attributed to a combination of its ability to increase or restore thrombin production in TF-rich areas and to augment the generation of factor Xa on the platelet and monocyte surfaces (Fig. 18-11).[148] The therapeutic effects of factor rVIIa begin at doses up to 10 times greater than physiologic concentrations of the endogenous factor. It is therefore not simply a "replacement" therapy of a deficient factor.[149]

Using the above model, the theory behind the mechanism of action of rVIIa to reduce bleeding in many surgical situations is delineated. Figure 18-12 demonstrates the theoretical mechanisms by which rVIIa can improve hemostasis.

It is proposed there will be further indications for factor VIIa as rescue therapy in the future (Fig. 18-13),[150] judging by the number of case reports of the many "off-label" uses in adult and pediatric practice that are becoming popular where conventional therapy has failed (Table 18-3).[151-163]

rVIIa does not produce a hypercoagulable state in vitro,[164] and in clinical practice only 18 spontaneous thrombotic complications have been reported after over 400,000 doses.[148] Although this is probably an underestimate of the true incidence, the Hemophilia Research Society of North America has described a less than 1% incidence of adverse reactions related to treatment.[165] This is likely related to the rVIIa dependence

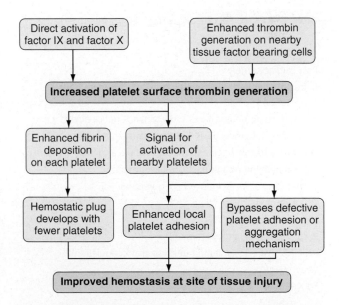

Figure 18-12. Theoretical mechanisms by which recombinant activated factor VII could increase thrombin generation and fibrin deposition that may lead to improved hemostasis. (From Welsby IJ, Monroe DM, Lawson JH, Hoffmann M: Recombinant activated factor VIIa and the anaesthetist. Anaesthesia 2005; 60:1203-1212.)

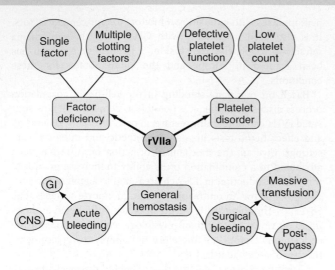

Figure 18-13. Proposed possible future indications for recombinant factor VIIa. (From Barcelona SL, Thompson AA, Coté CJ: Intraoperative pediatric blood transfusion therapy: a review of common issues: II. Transfusion therapy, special considerations and reduction of allogenic blood transfusions. Pediatr Anesth 2005; 15:814-830.)

on surface-located TF, rendering thrombin and clot generation injury-site specific. This does not explain however how rVIIa increases platelet activation when it is added to hemophilic blood in the absence of tissue factor[166] and can shorten the aPTT (TF-independent) as well as the TF-dependent PT.[167] The explanation of this apparent anomaly may lie in the finding that rVIIa can activate factor Xa on the surface of platelets[149] and monocytes[168]; these processes are not dependent on the presence of tissue factor. Hence, it is proposed that rVIIa augments the activation of factor X in both a TF-dependent and TF-independent manner.[148]

Table 18-3. Case Reports of Successful Off-Label Use of Recombinant Factor VIIa

Traumatic liver injury[145]

Post cardiac surgery[146-148]

Refractory hemorrhage during extracorporeal membrane oxygenation[149]

Intraventricular hemorrhage and vitamin K deficiency[147]

Necrotizing enterocolitis and abdominal hemorrhage[147,150,151]

Pulmonary hemorrhage and methylmalonic acidemia[147]

Pulmonary hemorrhage post cardiac surgery[152]

Herpes simplex virus–induced coagulopathy[151]

Acute or chronic liver failure[153,154]

Liver transplantation[155]

Postoperative hepatoblastoma[146]

AML-M2 with disseminated intravascular coagulation[146]

Head injury[156]

Polytrauma[157]

Note: Most cases were for refractory hemorrhage; however, in some cases it was used for the correction of coagulopathy or non-overt disseminated intravascular coagulation. Note that the rVIIa is used in addition to conventional therapy, but it has been given early to prevent fluid overload with continued use of blood products.

It is to be expected that case report descriptions are subject to positive reporting bias; well controlled studies are lacking,[142] particularly in the pediatric populations. For many emergency indications for VIIa, a randomized controlled trial may be very difficult to perform. With these caveats in mind, a case series showed a reduced blood loss and reduced requirement for blood products. Of interest, rVIIa has helped distinguish surgical bleeding from that of a thrombocytopathy.

With numerous on- and off-label potential indications for rVIIa, the dose regimen is yet to be firmly established. Another difficulty is that there is no satisfactory laboratory test to monitor the effectiveness of rVIIa.[148,169] Factor VII coagulant activity does not always predict efficacy.[170] Although it is known that the PT, aPTT, and TEG improve after rVIIa is given in liver surgery,[171] it cannot reliably be used to determine a dosing regimen. If the main effect of rVIIa is at the site of injury, clinical observation still remains the best indication of efficacy.[148] The dose used often closely relates to the dose indicated in hemophilia patients (90 units/kg); however, in practice this often relates to the size of the child because the high cost of rVIIa deters some clinicians from opening a second vial in the absence of clear dosing guidelines.[171]

The pharmacokinetics of rFVIIa differs between adults and children. The terminal elimination half-life in children is smaller (1.3 vs. 2.7 hr), and the clearance is greater (67 vs. 37 mL/kg/hr) than in adults.[172] It appears that rVIIa does not accumulate in neonates, nor does it result in excessive thrombotic complications at high doses. After prophylactic rVIIa 100 μg/kg was given every 4 hours for 72 hours to 10 preterm infants between 23 and 28 weeks of gestational age, there were two umbilical artery catheter thromboses and no embolic events. There were no other treatment-related side effects. Clinicians are yet to be guided on both dose and indications for use by well-conducted clinical trials.[173]

Currently, the decision on when and where to use rFVIIa for children with uncontrolled bleeding continues to be one that must be made by the individual clinicians, assisted by their hospital pharmacotherapeutics and transfusion committees.[174]

There has been very little published work on the use of prophylactic rFVIIa in the pediatric surgical setting. A recent double-blind placebo-controlled study in children younger than 1 year old with congenital heart disease examined the prophylactic use of low dose (40 μg/kg) rFVIIa (in addition to conventional therapy). No benefit was demonstrated in terms of time to chest closure, volume, or type of blood product transfused, although the mean postoperative prothrombin time was significantly less in the rFVIIa group (14.5 seconds) compared with control (20.4 seconds).[175]

Summary

It is easier to understand the mechanisms of hemostatic agents when one considers the cellular-based model of coagulation. Currently, the medications are used to prevent bleeding in children who are at high risk. Decisions to use or not use a hemostatic agent requires that we balance the benefits and the risks (e.g., anaphylaxis, thrombotic complications) of each agent in the context of the individual child. The evidence of this risk-benefit ratio is far from clear, and at the time of writing there has been no adequately powered placebo-controlled prospective studies to investigate the safety of lysine analogues or factor VIIa in cardiac, hepatic, or orthopedic surgery in adult or pediatric populations. A recent trial* in adult cardiac patients comparing aprotinin with the lysine analogues has been stopped due to an apparent increase in mortality in the aprotinin treated group. This follows shortly after the publication of a meta-analysis concluding aprotinin does not increase the risk of thrombosis or death.[176] The situation in children remains even less clear.

*Blood conservation using antifibrinolytics: a randomized trial in a cardiac surgery population—the BART study; publication of the details of this study is awaited.

Meticulous surgical hemostatic technique is essential to prevent bleeding. This occasionally requires the combination of an antifibrinolytic with topical hemostatic agents such as thrombin or fibrin sealants.[177] General correction of factors such as inadequate heparin reversal, temperature, calcium, and acid-base disturbance or replacement of blood components necessary for hemostasis are essential considerations before entertaining the use of medications such as rVIIa. In terms of specific drugs for hemostasis, antifibrinolytics can be useful in routine practice; however, the clinical indications and criteria for their use are variable and controversial.[178] Recombinant factor VIIa is expensive, and it currently remains as an "off license" rescue therapy for life-threatening hemorrhage when other approaches have failed.

Annotated References

Eaton MP: Antifibrinolytic therapy in surgery for congenital heart disease. Anesth Analg 2008; 106:1087-1100

A clear review on the use of antifibrinolytics in children for cardiac surgery. The author illustrates the difficulties in drawing quantitative conclusions from the varied trial designs.

Hoffman M: Remodeling the blood coagulation cascade. J Thromb Thrombolysis 2003; 16:17-20

Hoffman explains the difficulties associated with the "old model" of coagulation cascade. The paper contains an excellent step-by-step discussion of the cellular based model of coagulation.

Kovesi T, Royston D: Pharmacological approaches to reducing allogeneic blood exposure. Vox Sang 2003; 84:2-10

The authors review and critically analyze the evidence concerning the use of aprotinin, EACA, tranexamic acid, DDAVP, and rFVIIa.

Mangano DT, Tudor IC, Dietzel C: The risk associated with aprotinin in cardiac surgery. N Engl J Med 2006; 354:353-365

A frequently cited large observational study on the use of aprotinin, this adult study suggested an increased incidence of thrombotic complications and renal failure. The authors seriously questioned the safety profile of aprotinin in adult cardiac patients. The methodology and

interpretation has been questioned by some; we would therefore also like to direct the reader to the correspondence that followed:

Ferraris VA, Bridges CR, Anderson RP: Aprotinin in cardiac surgery. N Engl J Med 2006; 354:1953-1957 (Correspondence)

Brown JR, Birkmeyer NJO, O'Connor GT: Aprotinin in cardiac surgery. N Engl Jf Med 2006; 354:1953-1957 (Correspondence)

Levy JH, Ramsay JG, Guyton RA: Aprotinin in cardiac surgery. N Engl J Med 2006; 354:1953-1957 (Correspondence)

Mangano DT: Aprotinin in cardiac surgery. N Engl J Med 2006; 354:1953-1957 (Correspondence)

Webber TP, Grosse Hartlange MA, Van Aken H, Brooke M: Anaesthetic strategies to reduce perioperative blood loss in paediatric surgery. Eur J Anaesthesiol 2003; 20:175-181

This is an overview of current strategies for reducing blood loss in children. The authors discuss pros and cons of various techniques, including practical limitations of cell salvage.

Welsby IJ, Monroe DM, Lawson JH, Hoffmann M: Recombinant activated factor VIIa and the anaesthetist. Anaesthesia 2005; 60:1203-1212

This is a very good overview of the mechanisms and use of rFVIIa.

References

Please see www.expertconsult.com

Cardiac Assist Devices

Laura K. Diaz and Anthony Chang

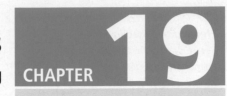

THE NUMBER OF CHILDREN surviving with congenital heart disease is increasing yearly as pharmacologic and surgical therapies for their care continue to improve. As a result, an expanding cohort of children exist who have survived initial palliative surgical procedures but have eventually progressed to end-stage heart failure.[1] These infants and children, together with those diagnosed with cardiomyopathies or myocarditis, often require mechanical circulatory support (MCS) for bridging to myocardial recovery or cardiac transplantation, making the use of mechanical circulatory assistance an increasingly important component of care in pediatric intensive care units (ICUs). Data from the Randomized Evaluation of Mechanical Assistance for the Treatment of Congestive Heart Failure Trial (REMATCH) demonstrated prolonged survival and increased quality of life in adult patients with end-stage heart failure who received MCS.[2] Unfortunately, the number and type of mechanical support devices available for children remain limited, particularly for children weighing less than 20 kg in the United States.[3] Recent initiatives by the National Heart, Lung, and Blood Institute to support the development of MCS devices for infants and children offer promising alternatives for the future care of these children.[4]

CHAPTER 19

Initiation of Mechanical Circulatory Support

Indications and Contraindications

Failure of the myocardium despite maximal medical therapy to provide sufficient cardiac output for adequate support of end organ perfusion results in the need for mechanical support of the circulation (Table 19-1). Depending on the child's clinical condition and the indication for initiation of support, it may then be utilized either as a bridge to myocardial recovery or cardiac transplantation. Although MCS devices have been approved for use as destination therapy in adults, this option is not currently available for pediatric patients.[2]

Mechanical support in children is most often required due to intrinsic failure of the myocardium. Preoperative cardiopulmonary stabilization may occasionally be required in children with profound hypoxemia and/or cardiovascular collapse due to hypercyanotic spells, pulmonary hypertensive crises, obstructed total anomalous pulmonary venous connection, or malignant dysrhythmias.[5,6] Extracorporeal membrane oxygenation (ECMO) has also been successfully utilized in the cardiac catheterization laboratory, both preemptively before high-risk interventional procedures[7] and as a rescue technique for those with catheter-induced complications or persistent low cardiac output or hypoxemia.[8]

Postcardiotomy myocardial dysfunction can manifest as either early failure (inability to wean from cardiopulmonary bypass) or late failure (sustained postoperative low cardiac output syndrome) with poor end-organ function, continuing elevation of serum lactate levels greater than 0.75 mmol/L/hr, and low mixed venous oxygen saturations and escalating inotropic support.[9] It is essential to rule out the presence of residual surgical lesions, coronary insufficiency secondary to surgical manipulation, or mechanical problems such as cardiac tamponade before initiating MCS to increase the likelihood of patient survival.[10] Ungerleider and colleagues described the use of routine MCS in all children after a stage I Norwood procedure to optimize postoperative cardiac output.[11] Other cardiac pathophysiologic processes such as acute myocarditis or cardiomyopathy, coronary ischemia, end-stage heart failure due to chronic cardiomyopathies or congenital heart defects, and graft rejection after cardiac transplantation may also warrant the use of MCS. Noncardiac indications for MCS include severe hypothermia, sepsis/shock, children with a critical airway (tracheal stenosis), drug toxicity, and near-drowning.[12]

Contraindications to implementation of MCS should be considered on a case-by-case basis. Advanced multisystem organ failure, severe neurologic damage or intracranial hemorrhage, severe coagulopathy, and extreme prematurity are

Table 19-1. Indications for Mechanical Circulatory Support

Preoperative Stabilization

Severe cyanosis/hypercyanotic spells

Pulmonary hypertensive crises

Myocardial dysfunction

Malignant dysrhythmias

Sepsis

Postcardiotomy Patients

Failure to wean from cardiopulmonary bypass

Late postcardiotomy failure (prolonged low cardiac output syndrome)

Stage I palliation for hypoplastic left heart syndrome

After ALCAPA repair

Malignant dysrhythmias

Bridge to Myocardial Recovery

Acute myocarditis

Cardiomyopathy

Acute cardiac transplant rejection

Bridge to Transplantation

Direct bridge to transplantation

Bridge-to-bridge (short- to long-term support)

Noncardiac Indications

Near-drowning

Severe hypothermia

Drug toxicity

Critical airway (tracheal stenosis)

Sepsis/shock

ALCAPA, anomalous origin of the left coronary artery from the pulmonary artery.

blood cell count (CBC), platelet count, prothrombin time (PT), partial thromboplastin time (PTT), activated clotting time (ACT), plasma hemoglobin, antithrombin III, fibrinogen, and thromboelastogram (TEG). A minimum of two units of packed red blood cells should be available, preferably cytomegalovirus-negative, leukocyte-reduced, and irradiated, because all children should be considered potential cardiac transplant candidates. In infants, ultrasonography of the head is useful before considering institution of MCS. Anesthesiologists are frequently involved during the cannulation procedure, and all arterial and central venous lines, as well as the endotracheal tube, should be well secured and the ventilator easily accessible.

The emergent use of ECMO for pediatric cardiac patients experiencing cardiac arrest with failure of conventional resuscitation methods has become increasingly common in pediatric ICUs (see Chapter 40).[15-17] Acceptable neurologic outcomes have been described in pediatric patients after cardiopulmonary resuscitation (CPR) of up to 3 hours in duration before institution of ECMO,[18] and a retrospective study found no difference between survivors and nonsurvivors when the length of CPR before ECMO cannulation was evaluated.[19] A dry circuit can be kept ready for rapid deployment, with crystalloid prime used during initiation of support and addition of blood products (packed red blood cells and fresh frozen plasma) as soon as they become available. During continuing resuscitative efforts before beginning mechanical support, multiple doses of vasoconstrictors should be avoided if possible, acidosis should be corrected, and ice may be placed around the head to provide cerebral protection. Ultimately, the restoration of cardiac output, even with a low hematocrit, is the most important factor for successful resuscitation and long-term survival of these children.[20,21]

Mechanical Circulatory Support Devices

In pediatric practice, the size of the child and the type of support required (cardiopulmonary vs. cardiac) are the most important considerations when choosing an MCS device (Table 19-2). Factors of secondary importance are the indication for, and expected duration of, support, as well as the desired endpoint: bridge to surgery, recovery, or transplantation. Certain devices, such as the intra-aortic balloon pump (IABP), ECMO, and centrifugal pump are best utilized for less than 2 to 4 weeks, and in certain circumstances they may serve as a "bridge to bridge" for institution of a long-term mechanical support device.[22]

A ventricular assist device (VAD) may be defined most simply as a mechanical pump attached between the heart and either the aorta or pulmonary artery to circulate blood when one or both ventricles are no longer capable of adequately maintaining circulation. In short, a VAD is a pump supporting a failing ventricle and may be used for right, left, or biventricular support. Isolated ventricular dysfunction with adequate oxygenation, as seen in acute myocarditis, acute rejection after cardiac transplantation, or dilated cardiomyopathy, is the ideal cardiac pathology for VAD support. ECMO, on the other hand, provides full cardiopulmonary support and may be superior to VAD support for children with pulmonary hypertension, complex congenital heart lesions involving intracardiac shunts, or respiratory failure and/or severe hypoxemia (Fig. 19-1).

generally judged to be contraindications. Additionally, the presence of certain chromosomal abnormalities, multiple congenital anomalies, or existing infections may influence decision-making.[13] A determination should also be made before instituting support regarding the expected outcome: is the child likely to recover; and if not, will he or she be a suitable candidate for cardiac transplantation.

Timing and Preparation for the Initiation of Support

As experience with the use of pediatric circulatory support continues to grow, it has become clear that early institution of support is preferable to better preserve end-organ function and maximize the opportunity for recovery or bridge to transplantation. Although firm criteria for the institution of support have not yet been developed, a review of the outcomes of 17 children who required mechanical circulatory assistance at Texas Children's Hospital between 1995 and 2002 revealed no correlation between the duration of support and the mortality rate, suggesting that earlier institution of MCS does not negatively impact patient survival.[14]

During routine preparation for MCS, baseline laboratory hematologic studies should be obtained, including a complete

Table 19-2. Mechanical Circulatory Support Devices: Advantages and Disadvantages

Device	Advantages	Disadvantages
ECMO	No patient size limitations Cardiopulmonary support Central or peripheral cannulation Relatively inexpensive Extensive pediatric experience	Short-term support Increased bleeding and thromboembolic complications More complex circuit Nonpulsatile flow No patient mobility Need for trained personnel
Centrifugal VAD	No patient size limitations Right, left, or biventricular support Simpler setup than ECMO Less anticoagulation than ECMO Better ventricular unloading than ECMO	Short-term support No respiratory support Nonpulsatile flow No patient mobility Direct cannulation of the heart required
Thoratec	Pulsatile flow Right, left, or biventricular support Extubation/ambulation possible	BSA >1.2 m^2 Sternotomy required for implantation
Berlin Heart EXCOR and MEDOS/HIA-VAD	No patient size limitations Pulsatile flow Right, left, or biventricular support Extubation/ambulation possible Long-term support possible	Not currently available in the United States Sternotomy required for implantation
MicroMed DeBakey Child VAD	Noiseless pump No compliance chamber No artificial valves Fewer moving parts Small blood-to-device interface Long-term support possible	BSA >0.7 m^2 Only left ventricular support

BSA, body surface area; ECMO, extracorporeal membrane oxygenation; VAD, ventricular assist device.
From Diaz LK, Andropoulos DB: New developments in pediatric cardiac anesthesia. Anesthesiol Clin North Am 2005; 23:655-676.

Short-Term Support

Intra-aortic Balloon Pump

Intra-aortic balloon pumps are support devices with a balloon ranging from 2.5 to 20 mL in size mounted on a 4.5- to 7-Fr catheter that may be inserted either via the femoral artery or, in infants, via the ascending aorta. The balloon inflates during diastole, forcing blood toward the heart and increasing blood flow to the coronary arteries, and deflates before systole, decreasing ventricular afterload. Cardiac output is augmented by 10% to 20%, whereas left atrial pressure, left ventricular end-diastolic pressure, and pulmonary artery pressure are all decreased.

Anatomic contraindications to use of the IABP include patent ductus arteriosus, aortic insufficiency, aortic aneurysm, and recent aortic surgery. Technical limitations in children consist of size constraints, the increased distensibility and compliance of the aorta in children, and the difficulty of synchronizing pump function with an infant or child's rapid heart rate,[23] although utilization of M-mode echocardiography–timed IABP in infants and children to assist with cardiac synchronization has been described.[24] A recent review of 24 children ranging in age from 7 days to 17 years who received IABP support revealed a survival to hospital discharge rate of 62.5%, but the potential for serious or fatal complications such as mesenteric ischemia, limb ischemia, or arterial injury exists.[25] Although IABP support can be useful in children, support should be initiated early while ventricular function is still capable of sustaining adequate cardiac output.[26] The most important limitation to the use of IABP is the need for intrinsic left ventricular function because the balloon pump will only augment, and not replace, ventricular output and can only support the left ventricle.

Extracorporeal Membrane Oxygenation

Initially reported for use in treatment of cardiac failure in children by Bartlett in the late 1970s,[27] ECMO is the preferred strategy for mechanical support in neonates with biventricular failure or cardiopulmonary failure. It may also be utilized for mechanical support during interhospital transport of patients and rapid resuscitation/rescue of patients during cardiac arrest.[28] ECMO remains the MCS modality with the most pediatric usage, with over 5,000 neonates and children having received ECMO for cardiac indications according to the 2004 Extracorporeal Life Support Registry Report.[29] Although ideal for rapid rescue support, ECMO support can be maintained only for 1 to 3 weeks before increasing complications and poor outcomes limit its usefulness.[30]

A typical ECMO circuit is composed of either a roller pump with a servoregulatory mechanism for controlling circuit flow or a centrifugal pump; a hollow fiber or membrane oxygenator; a heat exchanger; and venoarterial cannulas attached to the patient. Jacobs and coworkers described the use of a modified ECMO circuit composed of a heparin-coated circuit, a BioMedicus centrifugal pump (BioMedicus, Eden Prairie, MN), a hollow fiber membrane oxygenator, a flow probe, and a hema-

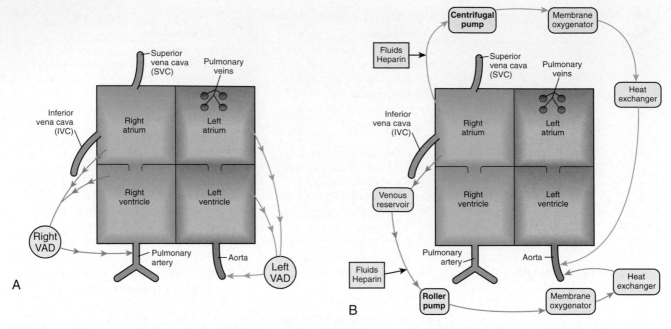

Figure 19-1. A, Right and left ventricular assist circuits. For biventricular assist both RVAD and LVAD circuits are utilized. **B,** Venoarterial ECMO circuits utilizing either a venous reservoir and roller pump, or a centrifugal pump without a reservoir.

tocrit/oxygen saturation monitor allowing the circuit to be set up and primed in 5 minutes for rapid resuscitation.[16] Most hospitals that support such a service have trained personnel readily available that can assist with implementing and maintaining ECMO therapy. Versatility is one of the advantages of ECMO; venoarterial cannulation in postcardiotomy patients may be transthoracic via the right atrial appendage and aorta, or it may be achieved with a transcervical approach via the right internal jugular vein and common carotid artery or via the femoral artery and vein in larger patients. Heparin-bonded circuitry is often used to minimize surface-induced complement activation, platelet dysfunction, and anticoagulation requirements.[31]

In addition to versatility in cannulation, other advantages of ECMO include the lack of patient size limitations, the ability to institute support either in the pediatric ICU or the operating room, the ability to ultrafiltrate or hemodialyze children during mechanical support, and the ability to provide biventricular cardiopulmonary support. Rapid deployment ECMO for pediatric cardiac patients has yielded very acceptable survival rates.[16] A review of 27 children who underwent venoarterial ECMO for cardiac indications, both nonsurgical and postcardiotomy, revealed an overall survival rate of 59%; of note, 56% were undergoing CPR at the time ECMO support was instituted and, of these, 73% survived.[32] Hemodynamic benefits of ECMO support include decreased right ventricular preload and pulmonary artery pressures. Due to the re-entry of blood into the aorta an increase in afterload often occurs and may require pharmacologic afterload reduction therapy such as milrinone, nitroprusside, hydralazine, or phenoxybenzamine.

Several management options exist for children with single ventricle physiology and shunt-dependent pulmonary circulation who receive ECMO support. Jaggers and colleagues reviewed the outcomes of 10 children who underwent single-

ventricle palliation and subsequently required ECMO support. Significantly greater survival rates were observed in children in whom the aortopulmonary shunt was left open during ECMO.[33] Adequate alveolar ventilation must be provided, however; and greater ECMO flow rates are generally necessary to maintain adequate pulmonary and systemic circulations. In children with low pulmonary vascular resistance, pulmonary blood flow may prove to be excessive and limitation of shunt flow may become necessary. Children with single-ventricle physiology have demonstrated favorable survival rates after ECMO support when compared with other cardiac patients who required circulatory support.[32] ECMO has been particularly successful in children with single-ventricles who develop acute shunt thrombosis or transient depression of ventricular function.[34]

Disadvantages of ECMO include the complex circuitry, the need for more systemic anticoagulation than that required by VADs, the necessity for both a blood prime and frequent transfusions, and decreased pulmonary blood flow. Compared with other support modalities, ECMO circuitry is complex and requires full-time supervision by trained personnel. Left atrial decompression may occasionally be inadequate, requiring either the placement of a left atrial vent or an atrial septostomy. Inadequate unloading of the left atrium can lead to mitral regurgitation and pulmonary edema or hemorrhage and can also minimize the chances of myocardial recovery when the left ventricle is not sufficiently unloaded. Moderate levels of ventilatory support must be maintained to ensure that well-oxygenated blood is provided to the coronary arteries, and the child must remain intubated and sedated throughout the period of ECMO support.[35] Survivors of ECMO support also have greater rates of neurologic impairment than those supported with VADs, with poorer outcomes noted in younger children with more complex disease.[36]

Centrifugal Pumps

Currently utilized centrifugal pumps include the BioMedicus, CentriMag (Levitronix, Zurich, Switzerland), RotaFlow (Jostra, Hirrlingen, Germany), and the Capiox (Terumo, Ann Arbor, MI). The term *centrifugal pump* is not always synonymous with VAD, because centrifugal pumps may also be used with an oxygenator to construct an ECMO circuit. Without an oxygenator, they may be used for right, left, or biventricular support (except in infants, when size limitations can preclude the presence of two pumps[37]) and offer the advantage of excellent ventricular unloading and decreased wall stress, optimizing the chances of myocardial remodeling and recovery. Unloading the left ventricle can also decrease left ventricular cavity size and improve septal configuration, resulting in improved tricuspid valve function and right ventricular inflow.[38] If used as a VAD without an oxygenator and heat exchanger, reduced systemic anticoagulation is required compared with ECMO usage.

Centrifugal pumps offer the advantage of decreased trauma to red blood cells and a less pronounced systemic inflammatory response compared with roller pumps.[39] A centrifugal VAD spins, creating a vortex, with negative pressure at the inlet drawing blood into the cone and positive pressure at the outlet allowing ejection at the base (Fig. 19-2). Cardiac output from a centrifugal pump depends on preload, afterload, and the rotational speed of the pump. Because increases or decreases in preload and afterload can affect pump flow without changes in the rotational speed, a flow probe is necessary. Excessive negative inlet pressures (hypovolemia) must be avoided because air can be entrained into the circuit. The lowest pump speed possible to maintain desired flow is used to maximize pump efficiency and minimize hemolysis. Compared to ECMO, centrifugal pumps are less expensive and have faster setup times, reduced priming volumes, and less anticoagulation requirements. Disadvantages of centrifugal pumps include the potential for thrombus formation in the circuit, nonpulsatile flow, and limited duration of usage (usually <3 weeks). Additionally, children must remain sedated and immobilized while receiving centrifugal pump support.

In an attempt to simplify postoperative management and improve neurologic outcomes, Shen and colleagues have advocated the use of routine VAD support after stage I Norwood palliation without the use of an oxygenator, allowing the aortopulmonary shunt to act as the sole source of pulmonary blood flow and allowing maintenance of lower levels of anticoagulation. Twenty-three children received VAD support for an average of 3 days after initial palliative surgery, with no attempt made to balance systemic and pulmonary circulations. Lactate levels were used to guide VAD flows, with support weaned as lactate levels normalized. Eighty-seven percent of children survived to hospital discharge, and neurodevelopmental testing performed before a bidirectional Glenn procedure was normal in all survivors.[40]

Excellent outcomes with centrifugal VAD support have been reported in children who required postcardiotomy ventricular MCS of limited duration, such as those with anomalous origin of the left coronary artery from the pulmonary artery, and in those with ventricular failure due to cardiomyopathy.[41] In addition, fewer postsupport neurologic complications were noted in children who received VAD support compared with those who received ECMO for similar indications.[1]

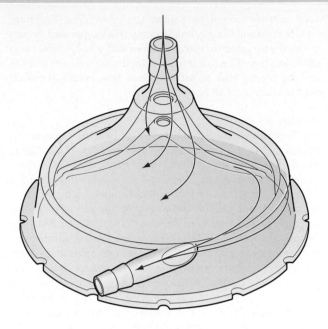

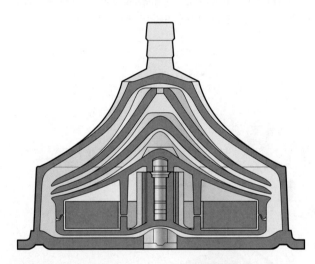

Figure 19-2. Centrifugal pump. (From Karl TR, Kirshbom PM, Horton SB: Mechanical circulatory support in infants and children. In Nichols DG, Ungerleider RM, Spevak PJ, et al [eds]: Critical Heart Disease in Infants and Children, 2nd ed. St. Louis, Mosby/Elsevier, 2006.)

Intermediate- to Long-Term Support

Pulsatile Pumps

Pulsatile pumps are VADs that make chronic support of the circulation possible while also allowing tracheal extubation, the use of enteral nutrition, and ambulation for the child. They are paracorporeal and either pneumatically or electromechanically driven. Like centrifugal pumps, pulsatile VADs enjoy several advantages over ECMO: they are simpler in design, less expensive, and require lower levels of anticoagulation. Pulsatile VADs may be used for left, right, or biventricular support of the circulation. Unlike the previously discussed devices, pulsatile pumps are suitable for intermediate- to long-term mechanical circulatory support, but their use in infants and children has been severely limited by patient size constraints. Currently, no U.S. Food and Drug Administration (FDA)-approved devices are widely accepted for use in children with a body surface area (BSA) less than 0.7 m². Internationally, the Berlin Heart EXCOR and the Medos HIA pulsatile systems have been successfully used in children of all ages.[42,43]

Thoratec

The Thoratec ventricular assist system (Thoratec Corporation, Berkeley, CA) is a pneumatically driven pump with a 65-mL blood sac, Björk-Shiley tilting disc valves, and exteriorized inflow and outflow cannulas (Fig. 19-3). Inflow may be from either the left atrium or left ventricular apex, with outflow to the aorta. Pump output, depending on the cannula size and length, may vary from 5 to 7 L/min.[44] The Thoratec VAD may be operated in three modes: synchronized to the child's underlying heart rate, asynchronous with a set rate programmed into the device, or fill-to-empty, in which the device fills to a set volume before ejection. Although use of the Thoratec has been described in children as small as 17 kg,[45] the risk of thromboembolic events is greater in smaller children, because lower blood flow in the relatively oversized device can lead to stasis and thrombus formation.[46] Children with congenital heart disease and/or left atrial cannulation are at greater risk for neu-

rologic complications during Thoratec support.[47] The use of a fixed-rate mode with an increased stroke rate of 80 to 90 strokes per minute and partial stroke volumes is currently recommended because it is associated with fewer cerebrovascular events in these children. Initial anticoagulation for the Thoratec VAD initially consists of a heparin infusion, whereas long-term protocols generally utilize warfarin (Coumadin) and aspirin, with maintenance of an international normalized ratio (INR) of 2.5 to 3.5.[48]

Reinhartz and colleagues summarized worldwide experience with the Thoratec paracorporeal VAD in 209 children younger than 18 years of age, ranging from 17 to 118 kg and with a BSA of 0.7 to 2.3 m². Overall survival to discharge was 68%, but subgroups with cardiomyopathies and myocarditis had greater survival rates than those children with congenital heart disease. Device configuration and the type of support used (LVAD vs. BiVAD) were not correlated with negative patient outcomes.[49]

Berlin Heart EXCOR

First used in adults in 1987,[50] the Berlin Heart EXCOR (Berlin Heart AG, Berlin, Germany) is a pulsatile, paracorporeal pump currently manufactured in three pediatric sizes (10, 25, and 30 mL) and three adult sizes (50, 60, and 80 mL) (Fig. 19-4A).

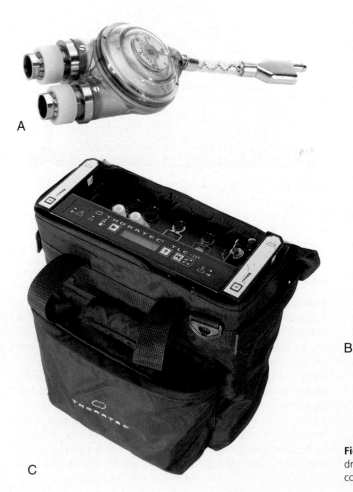

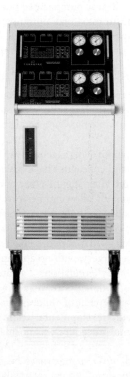

Figure 19-3. (A) Thoratec ventricular assist device. **(B)** Thoratec dual drive console. **(C)** Thoratec portable VAD driver. (Images provided courtesy of Thoratec Corporation.)

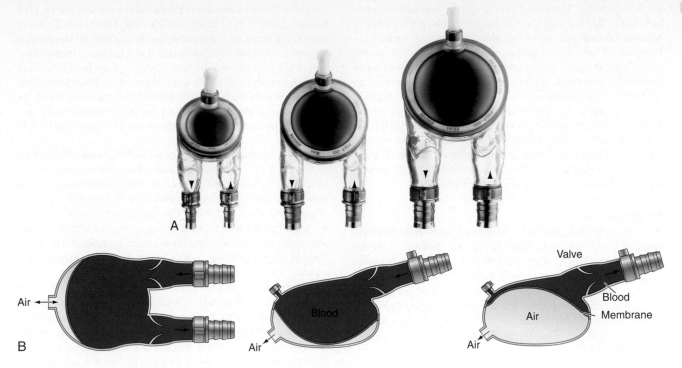

Figure 19-4. A, Berlin Heart EXCOR ventricular assist device in pediatric and adult sizes. **B,** A flexible diaphragm in three layers divides the pump chamber into an air chamber and a blood chamber. (From Hetzer R, Potapov E, Stiller B, et al: Improvement in survival after mechanical circulatory support with pneumatic pulsatile ventricular assist devices in pediatric patients. Ann Thorac Surg 2006; 82:917-925.)

The pediatric version was first used in 1992[51] and has since been successfully employed in 11 European countries in neonates and infants with a BSA as low as 0.2 m^2.[42] The device has not received FDA approval in the United States, but use by emergency exemption in the United States and Canada has grown dramatically since 2000.

The Berlin Heart EXCOR consists of a pneumatically driven translucent polyurethane pump, trileaflet polyurethane inlet and outlet valves, and silicone inflow and outflow cannulas. All blood-contacting surfaces, including the polyurethane valves, are heparin-coated (Carmeda AB, Upplands Vasby, Sweden). A flexible diaphragm in three layers divides the pump chamber into an air chamber and a blood chamber (see Fig. 19-4B), with the two diaphragm layers facing the air chamber serving as driving membranes and the third seamless blood membrane passively moved by the driving membranes.[52] The Berlin Heart EXCOR has been successfully used to provide univentricular (left or right) or biventricular support even in infants and may be operated in a synchronous, asynchronous, or fill-to-empty mode. A rechargeable battery is available that can provide up to 5 hours of independent power supply for adult-sized pumps, but power requirements are greater for pediatric pump operation owing to the greater flow resistance with small-diameter cannulas and greater pump rates.[53]

Although initial outcomes were not as favorable in infants and children with congenital heart disease,[54] more recently survival rates of 70% have been reported for children younger than 1 year of age, even those requiring prolonged support. Improvements in survival were attributed to the development of optimized miniaturized apical cannulas, the addition of heparin-coated tubing allowing lower anticoagulation levels, the use of dipyridamole and aspirin after the first week of support, and continued experience with surgical and intensive care management with utilization of TEGs and platelet function tests to modify anticoagulation.[42] Hetzer and colleagues in Berlin described a cohort of 70 infants and children younger than 18 years of age with circulatory failure resistant to pharmacologic management who received mechanical support with the Berlin Heart EXCOR for periods of time ranging from several days to 14 months, with 78% survival-to-discharge in infants younger than 1 year of age.[55] It is important to note, however, that children with existing intracardiac shunts were not candidates for Berlin Heart EXCOR support and instead were treated with ECMO.

In addition to pulsatile flow, major benefits of Berlin Heart EXCOR support include the ability to tracheally extubate children, allow enteral nutrition, and optimize patient mobility during chronic support. In addition to these advantages, transfusion of blood products during MCS is less in children supported with the Berlin Heart EXCOR when compared with those supported with ECMO. In a study comparing 30 children receiving Berlin Heart EXCOR support to 34 children on ECMO support, transfusion requirements for platelets, red blood cells, and fresh frozen plasma were significantly less in Berlin Heart

EXCOR patients. The overall mortality rate was also noted to be lower in Berlin Heart EXCOR patients.[56] Since the advent of heparin-bonded coating to all blood-contacting surfaces in 1994, ACTs have been maintained in the 140- to 160-second range, with the clear pump tubing allowing early detection of developing thrombus. TEGs and activated PTT are used to monitor anticoagulation status, along with platelet aggregation tests to monitor the use of aspirin and dipyridamole. Antithrombin III levels are closely monitored and substituted if the levels fall below 70%.[52] Pump exchange may be necessary if thrombus formation occurs in the valves, but the authors reported no complications from this procedure in 15 years of adult and pediatric experience with the EXCOR.[57]

MEDOS System

The MEDOS/HIA (MEDOS Medizintechnik AG, Stolberg, Germany) VAD was first utilized in 1997 for children.[58] Like the Berlin Heart EXCOR, the MEDOS/HIA provides a pulsatile, paracorporeal pump in several different sizes for children. It differs from EXCOR in that the left ventricular pumps offer 10% greater stroke volumes than the corresponding right ventricular pumps.[59] Survival has been reported to be 57% in children from younger than 1 year to 16 years awaiting cardiac transplantation.[60]

Axial Flow Devices

The most recent advance in pediatric mechanical circulatory support systems took place in March 2004 with the first use of the MicroMed DeBakey VAD *Child* (MicroMed Technology Inc, Houston, TX), an axial flow device currently available for use in the United States for children 5 to 16 years of age via FDA Human Device Exemption (HDE). The MicroMed DeBakey VAD *Child* is the first intracorporeal device with FDA approval for provision of left ventricular MCS as a bridge to transplantation in the pediatric population. Children must have New York Heart Association (NYHA) class IV end-stage heart failure that is refractory to medical management, be currently listed for cardiac transplantation, and have a BSA between 0.7 m² and 1.5 m² to be considered candidates for DeBakey VAD *Child* support.[61]

Initially developed by Dr. Michael DeBakey and collaborators at the National Aeronautics and Space Administration, the MicroMed DeBakey VAD *Child* is an implantable titanium axial flow pump that weighs approximately 4 ounces and is capable of pumping over 10 L/min. Changing electromagnetic fields drive the pump's only moving part, an impeller with six blades with eight magnets hermetically sealed in each blade (Fig. 19-5). The MicroMed DeBakey VAD *Child* is placed via median sternotomy utilizing cardiopulmonary bypass. A titanium inlet cannula is sutured into the apex of the left ventricle via a circular core ventriculotomy, and a 12-mm gel-weave outflow graft is then anastomosed to the ascending aorta.[61] A percutaneous cable containing the pump power and flow probe cables passes through the skin to the Clinical Data Acquisition system. A separate case, the VADPAK, contains a pump controller and two 12-volt batteries in a portable carrying case that can allow 5 to 8 hours of patient mobility.[62]

Like a centrifugal pump, the MicroMed DeBakey VAD *Child* pump function is dependent on preload and afterload. Decreases in preload can cause emptying and collapse of the ventricle,

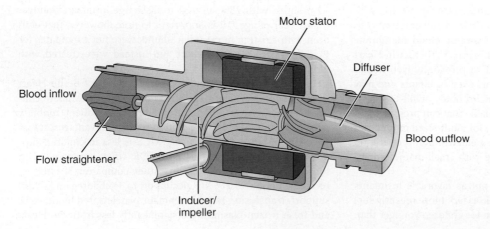

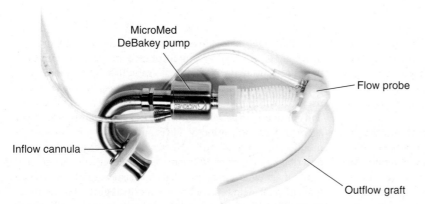

Figure 19-5. MicroMed DeBakey *Child* ventricular assist device. (Images provided courtesy of MicroMed Cardiovascular, Inc.)

whereas elevations in afterload initially result in reductions in forward flow and ultimately can lead to regurgitant flow. In initial clinical experience with the MicroMed DeBakey VAD *Child*, anticoagulation management has proved to be more challenging than in adult patients and modifications to adult protocols have been necessary. A heparin infusion is used immediately after device placement, transitioning later to warfarin and aspirin therapy, with a target INR of 2.5 to 3.5.[63] In one child, recurrent pump thrombosis also required the use of oral clopidogrel and monitoring of platelet function tests until cardiac transplantation was accomplished.[61]

Axial pumps offer several advantages over pulsatile pumps, including their small blood-to-device interface, the lack of a compliance chamber or artificial valves, and fewer moving parts. They are quieter than pulsatile pumps, which is a decided advantage for the child. Axial pumps can also allow some pulsatile flow to occur as the ventricle recovers, and cardiac output can increase in response to increased patient activity. The major disadvantages for children are the continuing size limitations for placement and the fact that the device provides only left ventricular support.

Outcomes

The only available forms of mechanical circulatory support for infants and small children in the United States continue to be ECMO and centrifugal VAD. Whereas adults generally have isolated left ventricular failure, children more often require true cardiopulmonary support due to hypoxemia, pulmonary hypertension, or concurrent right ventricular failure. For children who require short-term cardiopulmonary support, ECMO is the modality of choice. Although bilateral ventricular support via the use of both right- and left-sided centrifugal pumps can be achieved, it should be noted that this technique requires four cannulation sites as opposed to two for ECMO, making it less optimal for very small infants. Centrifugal VAD is, therefore, best used for the treatment of isolated univentricular failure.

When feasible, the use of centrifugal VAD offers several major advantages over ECMO. First, the lack of an oxygenator simplifies the circuit, lessening anticoagulation requirements as well as trauma to blood elements. Second, ECMO-supported patients have been shown to suffer higher rates of neurologic impairment than patients supported with VADs, particularly in younger children with more complex heart disease.[36] Additionally, evidence suggests that the superior ventricular decompression and physiologic rest provided by VAD support may promote myocardial recovery in children with acute myocarditis or dilated cardiomyopathy by allowing normalization of ventricular geometry and reverse remodeling.[64-66]

Regardless of the type of MCS chosen, the indication for and timing of initiation of support appear to be major factors in outcome. Overall survival with all devices has been greater in children who required support secondary to acute myocarditis or dilated cardiomyopathy as compared with children who received support due to congenital heart defects or postcardiotomy failure.[67] In comparing survival in children supported with either ECMO or VAD, similar rates of weaning from support and survival to discharge were reported. Irrespective of the type of support used, failure of return of adequate ventricular function within 48 to 72 hours of institution of support was a negative prognostic indicator.[1] If significant improvement in myocardial function has not been observed within this time frame, the child should be evaluated for potential cardiac transplantation.[8,68]

Children awaiting cardiac transplantation who are experiencing progressive multiorgan dysfunction have been shown to benefit from the use of pulsatile VADs with potential recovery of pulmonary, renal, and hepatic function.[69] A recent multi-institutional study reviewed the outcomes of 99 children bridged to cardiac transplantation with MCS, comparing them to 2,276 children listed for transplantation during the same era who did not require MCS. Several significant findings emerged, most importantly the lack of difference in survival rates between VAD-supported and the non–VAD-supported children and the lack of difference in survival rates between children who required biventricular support versus left ventricular support. The data also showed an increasing trend in the number of children undergoing transplantation who received VAD support and an increase in the use of long-term MCS devices in the most recent era. Patients with long-term devices were significantly more likely to survive to transplantation than those with short-term devices. Ten of the children were "double bridged" from ECMO to VAD support before transplantation, with 9 of these children then undergoing successful transplantation. Not surprisingly, the subgroups of smaller, younger patients and those with congenital heart disease had less successful outcomes.[70]

Perioperative Management and Complications of Mechanical Circulatory Support

Hemodynamics

During ECMO support, central venous pressure should remain low if adequate venous drainage is being achieved. Left atrial pressure should be closely monitored and can be estimated via echocardiographic evaluation of atrial septal position. An increase in left atrial pressure may indicate incomplete unloading of the left atrium and ventricle, potentially requiring a blade and/or balloon atrial septostomy[71] or surgical placement of a left atrial vent. Anatomic issues such as the presence of aortopulmonary collateral vessels, aortic insufficiency, or a patent ductus arteriosus can also result in a persistently increased left atrial pressure.

Increased arterial pressures and systemic vascular resistance during ECMO can be due to large pump flows, but other causes such as unrecognized seizure activity, inadequate pain or sedation management, and hypothermia should also be considered. High systemic vascular resistance during ECMO support can be pharmacologically managed with nitroprusside, nitroglycerin, or milrinone infusions. In general, mean arterial pressures should be maintained at a level appropriate to the child's size and body weight.

Unlike ECMO support, support of the left ventricle with a VAD requires maintenance of effective right ventricular output to provide adequate left ventricular preload. Right ventricular failure, pulmonary hypertension, and arrhythmias can all limit left ventricular filling and must, therefore, be aggressively treated.[72] Other potential causes of inadequate left ventricular filling include cannula malposition or low intravascular volume. Evaluation of central venous pressure can be used to evaluate volume status, and serial echocardiograms are useful for ongoing assessment of right ventricular function and estimation of right

child's condition at the time of surgery, the presence of preoperative multiorgan failure, and the need for cardiopulmonary bypass with cross-clamping of the aorta have all been shown to increase perioperative risk.[87]

A comprehensive preoperative evaluation of the child is essential. Knowledge of the underlying etiology necessitating MCS and the length of the child's illness are crucial, along with evaluation of other potential multiorgan dysfunction, including neurologic, hematologic, renal, hepatic, and pulmonary issues. Review of current drug therapy, particularly the duration and degree of current inotropic support, anticoagulation protocols, sedation regimens, cardiac function, intravascular volume status, and the presence and degree of preoperative hemorrhage, is essential. Physical examination should encompass the airway and both current vascular access as well as the availability of sites for potential vascular access.

Preoperative laboratory evaluation should include CBC with platelet count, electrolytes, blood urea nitrogen and creatinine levels, PT/PTT, and liver function tests. Levels of B-type natriuretic peptide (BNP) produced in the myocardium serve as a marker of ventricular overloading and have been shown in adult and pediatric patients with congenital heart disease to correlate with the degree of ventricular dysfunction.[88] Serial BNP levels in pediatric patients supported with ECMO have also been used to predict clinical outcomes, with greater BNP levels noted after termination of ECMO support in nonsurvivors than in children who ultimately survived.[89]

Useful preoperative coagulation data includes recent TEG results, fibrinogen levels, and platelet function tests if available. The most recent echocardiography data should be reviewed along with a recent chest radiograph. Blood products, including packed red blood cells, platelets, cryoprecipitate, and fresh frozen plasma, should be available at the bedside or in the operating room, with provision for continuing supply of products as needed. The use of antifibrinolytic agents and appropriate antibiotic prophylaxis should be discussed with the surgeon.

Standard American Society of Anesthesiologists monitoring should be employed before the induction of anesthesia. If not already in place, the use of arterial and central venous lines is warranted for virtually all cases involving MCS. In children who have been in the ICU for a prolonged time, or those undergoing current resuscitation, the placement of additional vascular access lines can be quite challenging and may occasionally require surgical assistance. For children already on a mechanical support device, it is important to be aware that VAD ejection is usually asynchronous with the child's underlying heart rate, yielding a discrepancy between the observed electrocardiographic and the arterial line waveform. Multiple peripheral intravenous lines are useful for the administration of volume and blood products.

During induction of anesthesia, preoperative inotropic and vasoactive therapy should be maintained and care should be taken to avoid changes in preload, afterload or heart rate. Etomidate is generally the optimal induction drug for children with severely compromised ventricular function because it does not result in myocardial depression at clinically relevant concentrations.[90] Judicious doses of opioids and benzodiazepines may be added, while the choice of a neuromuscular blocking agent is often dictated by the consideration of preexisting hepatic or renal compromise. Adequate depth of anesthesia should be ensured before endotracheal intubation to avoid abrupt increases in pulmonary vascular resistance, particularly in children with marginal right ventricular function. In children undergoing device placement, induction drugs should be given incrementally because circulation and onset time will be abnormally slow owing to depressed ventricular function. Children may frequently exhibit decreased responsiveness to β-adrenergic agonists due to depletion of myocardial catecholamines.[91] Hypotension on induction of anesthesia and decreased responsiveness to catecholamines may also be observed in children who have been chronically receiving angiotensin-converting enzyme inhibitors for afterload reduction preoperatively.[92-94] For children already on VAD support, appropriate pump function will continue independently of the induction drugs used as long as adequate preload is maintained.

Opioids, benzodiazepines, and neuromuscular blocking agents are generally used for anesthetic maintenance before ECMO cannulation or initiation of cardiopulmonary bypass for VAD implementation, with the express goal of maintaining adequate cardiac output and resultant systemic perfusion to end organs. Trends in serum lactate levels, mixed venous hemoglobin-oxygen saturations, and the presence or absence of metabolic acidosis are useful indices for evaluating the adequacy of cardiac output.

Unless contraindicated by patient size or the presence of gastrointestinal bleeding, a transesophageal echocardiographic (TEE) probe should be placed after the induction of anesthesia for use throughout the procedure. Initial TEE examination is important for determining the presence of any intracardiac shunts that would require closing before initiation of MCS. The competence of the aortic valve should also be evaluated, because more than trivial insufficiency can result in recirculation of blood through an LVAD. The mitral valve should also be examined for significant stenosis that could limit left ventricular inflow. After device placement, TEE helps in ensuring that adequate cardiac de-airing has occurred as well as in ongoing evaluation of ventricular function. TEE is also useful after device placement for monitoring the orientation of intracardiac cannulas and decompression of the left atrium and ventricle after pump activation.

For children undergoing placement of an LVAD, as the venous line from the CPB circuit is occluded the pump speed will be gradually increased. If LVAD flow (and rate when fill-to-empty mode is utilized) is less than desired, the major areas of concern are hypovolemia or poor right ventricular function. The right ventricle should be monitored closely for signs of dysfunction or failure. In children with preexisting right ventricular dysfunction, pulmonary vasodilatory agents such as milrinone, prostaglandin E_1, or nitric oxide[95] should be aggressively utilized to optimize right-sided heart function. Children with low pressures and signs of vasodilatory shock may require infusions of vasopressin, epinephrine, or norepinephrine for circulatory support. In addition, adequate volume loading and VAD output should be ensured.

Tracheal extubation is not an option for those undergoing ECMO or centrifugal VAD support, but children receiving pulsatile VADs or axial pumps may be considered candidates for extubation. Timing of extubation will depend on the child's preoperative condition, degree of preexisting pulmonary dysfunction, length of the surgical procedure, extent of postoperative bleeding, and maintenance of appropriate hemodynamic parameters.

Future Directions

Although options for prolonged mechanical circulatory support in infants and children remain limited in the United States, great progress in the care of these children has been made with the development of pulsatile pumps such as the Berlin Heart EXCOR in Europe. In response to the demonstrated need for appropriate devices to provide MCS to all pediatric patients, the National Heart, Lung, and Blood Institute introduced a Pediatric Circulatory Support Initiative in 2002 to foster development of devices suitable for children between 2 and 25 kg. Technical goals for proposed systems included the following: (1) ability to be deployed and functioning in less than 1 hour; (2) minimal priming volume; (3) variable cannulation strategies; (4) minimization of exposure to blood products, and (5) capability of providing support for up to 6 months.[4]

Five proposals were awarded in early 2004, allowing for development of an implantable mixed-flow VAD for children up to 2 years of age, a mixed-flow VAD capable of intravascular or extravascular implantation, a compact pediatric cardiopulmonary assist system, an apically implanted axial-flow device, and a pulsatile-flow VAD. Continued development and testing of these devices over the next 5 years should yield exciting possibilities for the future care of all pediatric cardiac patients. The National Institutes of Health–sponsored Interagency Registry for Mechanically Assisted Circulatory Support (INTERMACS), started in 2005, will also aid in delineating and facilitating the role of mechanical circulatory support in all children, with pediatric data collection that began in 2006.[96]

Annotated References

Baldwin JT, Borovetz HS, Duncan BW, et al: The National Heart, Lung, and Blood Institute Pediatric Circulatory Support Program. Circulation 2006; 113:147-155

An overview of the NHLBI Pediatric Circulatory Support Program and the five devices currently under development.

Deiwick M, Hoffmeier A, Tjan TD, et al: Heart failure in children—mechanical assistance. Thorac Cardiovasc Surg 2005; 53(Suppl 2): S135-S140

A review article summarizing the use of ECMO versus VAD support in children as well as the use of pulsatile VAD support in children.

Dickerson HA, Chang AC: Perioperative management of ventricular assist devices in children and adolescents. Semin Thorac Cardiovasc Surg Pediatr Card Surg Ann 2006; 9:128-139

An excellent review article discussing the various types of MCS available for children as well as perioperative issues in caring for patients requiring VAD support.

Duncan BW: Pediatric mechanical circulatory support. ASAIO J 2005; 51:ix-xiv

A description of current ECMO usage along with brief discussions of centrifugal pumps, pulsatile pumps, and the future of pediatric circulatory support.

Hetzer R, Potapov EV, Stiller B, et al: Improvement in survival after mechanical circulatory support with pneumatic pulsatile ventricular assist device in pediatric patients. Ann Thorac Surg 2006; 82:917-924

A review of children supported with the Berlin Heart EXCOR, documenting improved survival in patients younger than 1 year due to earlier device implantation, cannula modifications and improved coagulation monitoring.

Hines MH: ECMO and congenital heart disease. Semin Perinatol 2005; 29:34-39

A summary of the indications for ECMO in congenital heart disease, as well as techniques, equipment, management, and potential complications.

Karl TR, Horton SB, Brizard C: Postoperative support with the centrifugal pump ventricular assist device (VAD). Semin Thorac Cardiovasc Surg Pediatr Card Surg Ann 2006; 9:83-91

An excellent review of the use of centrifugal VAD support, along with indications and clinical management.

Kirklin JK, Holman WL: Mechanical circulatory support therapy as a bridge to transplant or recovery (new advances). Curr Opin Cardiol 2006; 21:120-126

A review article summarizing currently available and emerging support devices for children and adults.

Merkle F, Boettcher W, Stiller B, Hetzer R: Pulsatile mechanical cardiac assistance in pediatric patients with the Berlin Heart ventricular assist device. J Extra Corpor Technol 2003; 35:115-120

A detailed description of the Berlin Heart EXCOR and initial outcomes.

Thourani VH, Kirshbom PM, Kanter KR, et al: Venoarterial extracorporeal membrane oxygenation (VA-ECMO) in pediatric cardiac support. Ann Thorac Surg 2006; 82:138-145.

An article describing the use of ECMO for resuscitation in pediatric cardiac patients and outcomes in both univentricular and biventricular patient subsets.

References

Please see www.expertconsult.com

Interventional Cardiology

Andrew J. Davidson, Adam Skinner, and Geoffrey K. Lane

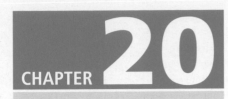

CHAPTER 20

THE USE OF CATHETERIZATION in the care of children with congenital heart disease (CHD) was first described by Dexter and colleagues in 1947[1] and has evolved from a physiologic assessment tool, to a technique to define anatomic relationships, and now to a therapeutic modality. The first interventional procedure, balloon atrial septostomy, was described by Rashkind and Miller in 1966,[2] and, since then, interventional cardiology has been an evolving discipline. As echocardiography and MRI diagnostic capabilities have increased there has been a decline in the need for purely diagnostic cardiac catheterization.[3,4] However, technologic advances and more sophisticated equipment have increased the scope for interventional procedures. The patient population has also changed as more children with CHD are surviving longer. As the surgical management of CHD has evolved, it has also introduced a new spectrum of surgical complications. Some surgical operations have been replaced altogether by interventional procedures. At the same time, some interventional procedures have facilitated more complex heart surgery.[5] This shift in practice and population has had important implications for the anesthetic management of these children.[6] Procedures are more diverse, and patients can vary from moribund neonates to healthy adolescents. There are no simple anesthesia recipes for all children and all heart conditions; for each case, the anesthetic must fit the child and the procedure.

In this chapter we first outline the main procedures performed in interventional cardiology, then describe the potential issues and complications with which an anesthesiologist must be aware, and, finally, address the principles and details of anesthetic techniques.

Procedures Performed

Diagnostic Catheterization

Diagnostic catheterization allows the accurate documentation of pressure and oxygen content from all regions of the circulation. The interpretation of these hemodynamic data allows quantification of the degree of intracardiac shunting and calculation of the vascular bed resistances. This information is necessary to assess the suitability of a child to undergo either palliative or reparative surgery for congenital heart lesions. Expected values for hemodynamic variables are listed in Table 20-1. There are no absolute values for these parameters, and they vary depending on the age of the child.

The use of angiocardiography to define anatomy is waning given the widespread use of noninvasive imaging modalities such as echocardiography, computed tomography, and magnetic resonance imaging.

Interventional Catheterization

At many centers interventional catheterization now accounts for more than 60% of cases of cardiac catheterizations.

Atrial Septostomy

This procedure improves the mixing of oxygenated and deoxygenated blood at the atrial level in newborns with

Table 20-1. Normal Values in Diagnostic Cardiac Catheterization

Structure	Value
Right atrium	3-5 mm Hg (mean)
Right ventricle	20-25/3-5 mm Hg (systolic/end-diastolic)
Pulmonary artery	12-15 mm Hg (mean)
Pulmonary artery	7-10 mm Hg (mean)
Left ventricle	65-110/3-5 mm Hg (systolic/end-diastolic)
Aorta	65-110/35-65 mm Hg (systolic/diastolic)

D-transposition of the great vessels. Children with this disorder are born with ventriculoarterial discordance whereby the right ventricle pumps deoxygenated blood to the aorta and the left ventricle pumps oxygenated blood to the main pulmonary artery. Enlargement of the foramen ovale by atrial septostomy improves the mixing of oxygenated and deoxygenated blood, resulting in increased systemic oxygen saturation. This procedure can be performed in the catheterization laboratory with fluoroscopic guidance, or it can be easily and safely undertaken at the bedside in the intensive care unit utilizing echocardiographic guidance.[7] Either a femoral venous or umbilical venous approach can be used. The drawback with the umbilical venous route is the often encountered difficulty in traversing the ductus venosus to secure access to the inferior vena cava. The major risks with this procedure are vessel injury, paradoxical embolism, arrhythmia, and cardiac perforation.

Atrial Septal Defect Closure

With the development of specifically designed closure devices, this endovascular therapy for closure of the atrial septal defect (ASD) is now one of the most commonly performed procedures. The technique is intended for closing secundum ASDs, that is, defects located in the region of the fossa ovalis. Defects falling outside this area, such as sinus venosus and primum ASDs, are not suitable for percutaneous closure. To warrant closure, children need to demonstrate clear evidence of volume loading of the right-sided heart structures along with a defect that is unlikely to close spontaneously in the short to medium term. The choice of closure device depends on both the size and the margins of the defect. In general, there are two design types for closure devices with either a centering or a noncentering design (Fig. 20-1). The choice of one design type over another is based more on clinician preference than scientific performance, although currently the Amplatzer Atrial Septal Occluder (AGA Medical Corporation, Golden Valley, MN) has the capability to close a wider range of defect sizes.[8-10] Daily aspirin in a dose of 3 to 5 mg/kg is recommended for a minimum period of 6 months after implantation of either type of device. The main complications associated with ASD closure include vessel injury, cardiac arrhythmia, cardiac perforation, and device embolization.[11] Atrial septal closure devices have also been used to close surgically created fenestrations between the atrium and venous conduits after a Fontan operation. This is only undertaken when the fenestration is no longer required.

Ventricular Septal Defect Closure

Ventricular septal defect (VSD) closure presents a technically greater challenge than ASD closure and is associated with a greater risk. The VSDs most suitable for device closure are those in the midmuscular septum or those closer to the apex.[12] With further refinement of the implantation technique and equipment, this approach has been undertaken with perimembranous defects.[13,14]

During device closure of VSDs a snare is placed in the right side of the heart to capture a guidewire that has been passed across the VSD from the left ventricle. The guidewire is then brought outside the body to form an arteriovenous rail. The delivery sheath for the VSD device is then advanced over the wire to approach the VSD from the right side of the heart. For anterior and high muscular defects, the wire is best snared and brought out via the femoral vein, whereas for defects in the mid

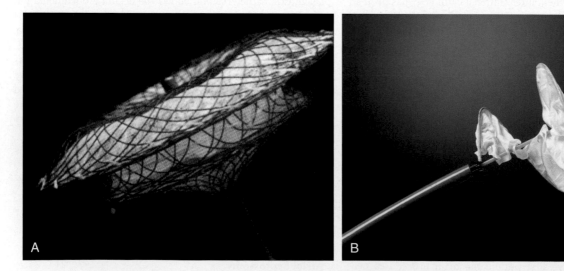

Figure 20-1. Devices for closure of atrial septal defect. **A,** The Amplatzer Atrial Septal Occluder (courtesy of AGA Medical Corporation, Golden Valley, MN). **B,** The HELEX[1.5] Septal Occluder (courtesy of W.L. Gore & Associates, Flagstaff, AZ).

to low muscular septum the wire is best snared and exteriorized from a jugular venous approach (Fig. 20-2). Complications include dysrhythmias, blood loss, valve dysfunction, and device embolization.[15,16]

Patent Ductus Arteriosus Closure

Closure of patent ductus arteriosus (PDA) was the second specific intervention developed for children with congenital heart disease and continues to be a common procedure performed using techniques that are similar to the original methods pioneered by Rashkind and associates.[17] The customary approach

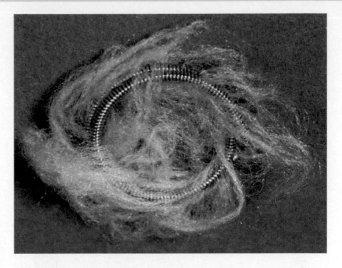

Figure 20-3. Coil used for patent ductus arteriosus closure.

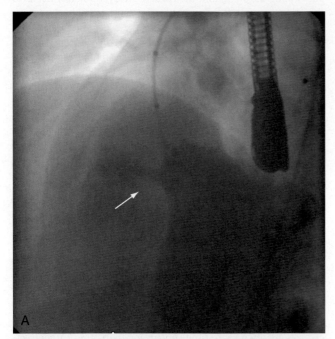

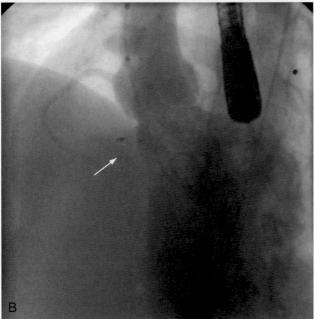

Figure 20-2. A, Angiography of ventricular septal defect (VSD) device before deployment. *Arrow* shows contrast agent passing through VSD. **B,** Appearance of same region (*arrow*) after deployment of the device.

is to perform an aortogram to define the size and geometry of the PDA. Based on this information a choice is made between using either a stainless steel coil(s) or an occluder device to close the communication.[18] Most interventional cardiologists implant a stainless steel coil to close a PDA with a minimal size (no greater than 3 mm). The approach can be performed either retrograde or antegrade.[19] To lessen the chance of coil embolization during implantation, several techniques have been described to offer controlled release of the coils.[20-22] For the larger PDA, most interventional cardiologists would implant an occluder device because this lessens the risk of a significant residual shunt. The major risks associated with this procedure are vessel injury and device/coil embolization. Coils are also used to close major aortopulmonary collateral vessels (Figs. 20-3 and 20-4) (Video clips 20-1 and 20-2).

Balloon Dilation and Stent Implantation

Balloon angioplasty techniques are used to dilate stenotic aortic, mitral, tricuspid, and pulmonary valves or stenotic segments of the aorta or of the pulmonary arteries. In neonates, membranous atresia of the pulmonary valve may be crossed with either the stiff end of a guidewire[23] or, more recently, interventional cardiologists have used radiofrequency catheters.[24] After both techniques, the valve is dilated with a balloon that is approximately 120% the size of the annulus. Balloon angioplasty of stenotic pulmonary valves in children beyond infancy is often a "curative" procedure, whereas balloon valvuloplasty of critical pulmonary stenosis in the neonate often requires reintervention in later infancy. The potential hemodynamic behavior of the child depends on the nature of the lesion; a neonate with duct-dependent critical stenosis and little antegrade flow will tolerate balloon dilation well because there is little disruption of the cardiac output, whereas neonates and infants with less critical stenosis can suffer significant reductions in cardiac output when the balloon is inflated, especially if the ductus arteriosus is not patent. Older children tend to tolerate balloon valvuloplasty surprisingly well,[25] with life-threatening hypotension being uncommon.[26]

In contrast to pulmonary balloon valvuloplasty, aortic balloon valvuloplasty is usually only a palliative procedure, with most children eventually requiring surgery. Balloon dilation of aortic stenosis in the neonate is a high-risk procedure. These infants

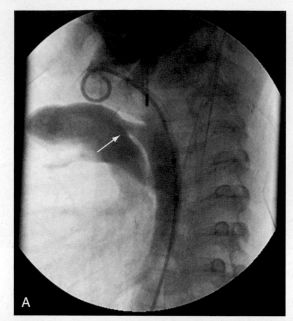

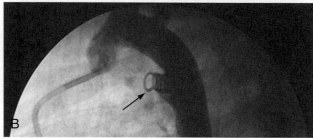

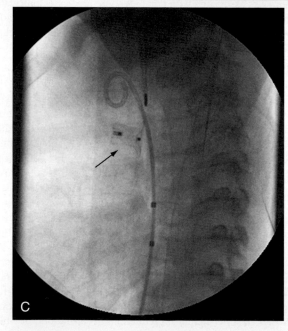

Figure 20-4. A, Lateral angiography demonstrating patent ductus arteriosus (PDA). *Arrow* shows PDA between aorta and pulmonary artery. The angiography catheter is in the proximal aorta. **B,** Lateral angiography after closure of PDA with coil. *Arrow* shows coil in PDA. **C,** Lateral fluoroscopy after closure of PDA with device. *Arrow* shows device in PDA.

often present in a low cardiac output state requiring ventilation, inotropic support, and PGE_1 infusion to maintain ductal patency. Catheterization can be complicated by arrhythmias (including asystole), the development of significant aortic regurgitation, which may require surgical intervention, and sudden death due to acute coronary ischemia.[25] The complication rate in older children is less, with transient hypotension, bradycardia, and left bundle branch block seen commonly.

Stents are sometimes implanted across focal areas of persistent stenosis in both the systemic and pulmonary circulations. The technique of stent implantation requires great precision in positioning the stent, and the cardiac interventionalist needs to take into account the inevitable shortening that occurs with stent implantation when selecting a device for a particular lesion. The major complication encountered with stent implantation, in addition to those of balloon angioplasty, is stent malposition and potential dislodgement. Rarely, late aneurysm formation has been reported after stenting the aorta for coarctation.

Electrophysiologic Catheterization

Endocardial catheters that record an electrocardiogram first became available in the early 1960s. Endovascular techniques were developed as an alternate to surgery to treat certain forms of tachycardia. These therapies initially utilized direct current energy and subsequently have made use of radiofrequency energy and, more recently, localized freezing techniques. Tachycardia may be treated by this technique in children with both structurally normal hearts and those who have dysrhythmias after surgery for CHD.[25] Ablative procedures now account for close to 20% of all cardiac catheterization procedures. The technique requires specialized equipment and specially trained staff as well as the use of multiple catheters to measure the electrical signals within the heart at any given point in time. These procedures are often more time consuming than other catheterization procedures. The success of the therapy varies depending on the mechanism of the tachycardia, the location of the aberrant pathway, and the technique for interrupting the aberrant pathway. Ablation of ectopic foci in general has a good success rate and low complication rate.[27,28] The main risks with this procedure are heart block, cardiac perforation, vessel injury, and stroke.

Choice of Vessel Access

The most common access approach for cardiac catheterization is the femoral route. Femoral venous catheterization avoids the risk of pneumothorax, and it is easier to access than the internal jugular vein (IJV) in the nonanesthetized child. In children who are likely to have a cavopulmonary shunt as a surgical palliation, avoiding routine cannulation of the IJV will decrease the risk of compromising the superior vena cava (SVC). However, there are occasions when IJV access is required, such as during VSD closures, investigating patients after cavopulmonary connections, and when the cardiac interventionalist is unable to obtain access via the femoral veins. In neonates, the umbilical vein may be used, although cardiac interventionalists must recognize the potential difficulty in crossing the ductus venosus. The patency of the ductus venosus can be assessed by ultrasound before the procedure to avoid unnecessary manipulation of the umbilical vein. An alternate option is for transhepatic puncture. This route has been used both for temporary access during catheterization and for more long-term vascular access.[29]

Complications of the Procedures

Interventional cardiology can be associated with significant morbidity and mortality. Complications attributable to the procedure, or the physiology of the child, occur far more frequently than purely anesthesia-related problems. An important prerequisite for providing quality anesthetic care is having a complete understanding of the diagnosis and management of the anticipated complications. Complications such as tamponade, dysrhythmia, embolism, and rupture may be sudden and without warning. The anesthesiologist must be vigilant and maintain communication and rapport with the cardiologist throughout the procedure. The availability of surgical, cardiologic, and anesthesiologic backup is certainly preferable, and standard procedures for emergencies should be in place. Some authors have advocated that the ability to place children on unanticipated cardiopulmonary bypass (CPB) or extracorporeal membrane oxygenation (ECMO) should be available.[16] Although this therapy is available in major referral hospitals, it may not be an option in some centers. It is for this reason that institutions need to develop policies regarding the nature of the procedures that can be undertaken locally (based on experience and infrastructure) and the children who require referral to centers that are better equipped to address more complex procedures.

Overall Mortality

Despite the increased complexity of interventional procedures, the mortality is steadily decreasing. A report from the early 1960s found an overall mortality of 0.44%,[30] but more recent data show an overall mortality of 0.08%,[31] 0.14%,[30,31] and 0.39%.[26] All reviews note a relatively high mortality among infants and neonates in particular.[26,30,32] Explanations for this include a reduced physiologic reserve, presence of uncorrected or partially palliated congenital heart defects, increased risk of obstruction to great vessels and cardiac chambers, and greater susceptibility to catheter-induced damage in infancy.[26] The preponderance of mortality in neonates is, however, diminishing; one institution reported a decrease in mortality in neonates from 6.7% to 0.9% during a span of 20 years. The explanations cited for this decrease were noninvasive imaging that reduced the number of neonates who required cardiac catheterization, improved management of the critically ill child, correction of metabolic abnormalities, use of prostaglandin E_1, and improved catheters and support equipment such as temperature control.[30]

Overall Morbidity

Complications are frequently categorized into major, minor, and "incidental."[26,32] Major complications are potentially life-threatening events that require intervention, that is, any event requiring surgical intervention or a significant permanent lesion resulting from the procedure (e.g., cerebral infarct). Minor complications are events that are transient and resolve with specific treatment (e.g., transient arterial thrombosis). An incident is an event that has no effect on the patient's condition and requires minimal or no treatment (e.g., transient hypotension responding to volume infusion). The incidence of major complications is between 1.4%[32] and 2.6%,[33] and for minor complications it is between 6.8%[32] and 7.5%.[33] The overall complication rate has remained stable for the past 20 years.[33]

In general terms, three groups are at high risk for complications: young age, low weight, and those undergoing interventional as opposed to diagnostic procedures (with balloon interventions carrying the highest risk).[30,32,33] The incidence of vascular access complications after interventional procedures is reported to be three times greater than the rate for diagnostic procedures[32]; this may be related in part to the use of larger-diameter catheters during interventional procedures compared with purely diagnostic procedures. It is worth noting that closure of PDA and balloon atrial septostomy carry a low overall risk.[26,30]

Vascular Complications

Vascular complications are the most common and broadest category of complications.[30] They may be acute, leading to unexpected hemodynamic instability, or delayed, leading to longer-term morbidity. Factors that contribute to unexpected hemodynamic instability are multifactorial and include the child's condition, blood loss, dysfunction of a valve, arrhythmias, tamponade, vessel rupture, balloon dilation, catheter-induced interruptions in blood flow or coronary perfusion, and malposition of devices.

Arterial Thrombosis/Occlusion

Femoral artery occlusion due to thrombosis is one of the most common complications after femoral cannulation.[34] The true incidence of arterial compromise is unknown,[30] although Kocis and coworkers reported that after femoral arterial cannulation 32% of infants had compromised blood flow to the leg as measured by Doppler studies.[35] Clinically, the incidence of arterial compromise is 2.4% to 3.7%.[30,32] Infants undergoing dilational interventional procedures are at particularly high risk.[36] The incidence of these complications can be reduced by minimizing the size of the sheath, systemic heparinization, and avoidance of arterial entry by using alternative techniques to enter the left side of the heart.[30] Despite the widespread use of intravenous heparin for prophylaxis against arterial occlusion there is no agreement on the appropriate dosage. Commonly, 50 to 100 IU/kg is used, but schedules vary.[25] Larger doses than these have not been shown to reduce the incidence of arterial compromise.[34]

In the majority of cases in which there is a reduced or absent pulse due to catheterization, it is either self-resolving or managed with anticoagulation or thrombolysis therapy.[30,32,36] Although the requirement for surgical intervention is rare, the most common indications for surgical intervention are arterial tear or avulsion, arterial thrombosis (including iliac arteries), or arterial pseudoaneurysm.[36] Occasionally, despite medical therapy and a well-perfused lower limb, a pulse may be persistently reduced. There is little information to help us predict how and when a reduced pulse may cause delay in limb growth,[30] although cases are reported.[36]

Venous Thrombosis/Occlusion

Although venous thrombosis is a well-known complication of central venous access, the incidence after cardiac catheterization is unclear. Isolated cases of femoral or iliofemoral venous occlusions with limb edema have been published as part of large series,[30,32] with the incidence of symptomatic venous occlusion from these studies being less than 0.3%. All of these children responded to heparin therapy without the need for further intervention.[32] Like arterial thrombosis, the use of smaller catheters and heparin prophylaxis during catheterization procedures may reduce the incidence of venous thrombosis, although the incidence of long-term venous occlusion or insufficiency after cardiac catheterization is unclear.

Vessel Rupture/Perforation/Dissection

Vessel rupture can either occur at the site of vessel entry or at the site of intervention. It is a rare but potentially catastrophic event. One death was reported in a series of 4,454 catheters due to intra-abdominal hemorrhage after rupture of a femoral vein in a neonate.[26] Arterial or venous perforation was responsible for four major complications and six minor complications in a series of 4,952 procedures, whereas significant groin hematoma was noted in 25 cases.[30] Femoral artery injuries may require surgical consultation and exploration.

There are also reports of vessel perforation at the site of intervention, particularly with balloon interventions. Ruptures have been reported most often after balloon dilation of branch pulmonary arteries[4,25] but also along the ascending aorta and arch after balloon dilation of the aortic valve. Depending on the site of tear, rupture may cause hemopericardium and/or hemothorax.[36] Intrapulmonary hemorrhage is usually self-limiting. If rupture or hemorrhage occurs, then avoid hypertension, intubate the trachea (if the airway is not already secured), and antagonize any circulating heparin. Pulmonary artery disruption after balloon dilation may manifest as hemoptysis. Increased blood flow after balloon dilation of pulmonary vessels may lead to unilateral pulmonary edema, which may present as hemoptysis. On occasion, arterial dissection may occur,[36] as well as aneurysm and pseudoaneurysm formation.

Cardiac Tamponade and Perforation

Cardiac tamponade is an uncommon complication of cardiac catheterization. However, when it occurs, it can be responsible for significant morbidity and mortality. The incidence of cardiac tamponade in three large series was 0.1%,[30] 0.04%,[26] and 0%.[32] In one series of 4,952 patients, tamponade was responsible for two deaths: one neonate after a balloon atrial septostomy and one 4-year old after a recent Fontan procedure for branch pulmonary artery stent insertion.

Although tamponade is uncommon, perforation is not uncommon. The atrial appendage and right ventricular outflow tract are the sites most commonly perforated,[36] although the left ventricle has been punctured.[37] Perforation of the heart is described during many procedures, including balloon and blade atrial septostomy, balloon dilation of the mitral valve,[4] and attempted radiofrequency perforation of membranous pulmonary atresia.[5]

Signs that are suggestive that perforation has occurred include wires appearing in unexpected places, atypical contrast appearance, lack of a return to baseline blood pressure after catheter-induced tachycardia, and hemodynamic instability. Echocardiography should always be immediately available to confirm any suspicion of perforation or tamponade. If it occurs, a cannula can be placed in the pericardium to remove blood that can then be given back to the child via the femoral venous catheter. If the tamponade is not controlled with catheter drainage, then the cardiac surgeons should be notified and an operating room prepared.

Damage or Dysfunction of a Valve

Damage to a valve is not particularly common, although it is more likely to occur with a balloon valvuloplasty procedure than with other procedures.[36] The primary complication is the creation of excessive regurgitation. The hemodynamic consequences of such a defect are more significant on the systemic side of the circulation than on the pulmonary side.[5,36] The mechanism of injury is most commonly leaflet avulsion during dilation, although the leaflet can be inadvertently perforated by the guidewire with the likelihood of significant further damage to the leaflet with advancement of the angioplasty catheter and its subsequent inflation. Emergency repair is occasionally required.[36] Injuries to the atrioventricular valves have rarely been reported. The placement of wires and large sheaths across atrioventricular valves and septal defects can cause severe hemodynamic disturbance. This is particularly true during implantation of VSD occluder devices.[15,25] ASD and PDA occlusions are less likely to produce significant hemodynamic disturbance.[25] On rare occasion the implanted ASD and VSD devices can adversely affect the functioning of one or another of the atrioventricular valves.

Blood Loss

Blood loss may be sudden with rupture of vessels or more often slow and insidious due to multiple blood samples and loss associated with catheter exchanges. Anemia may be difficult to detect in a dark room and a covered patient. Significant loss is more likely to occur during procedures for closure device insertion. Laussen and colleagues reported that with 86 VSD closure devices, blood transfusion was required in 54% of cases.[15]

Dysrhythmias and the Catheterization Laboratory

Transient dysrhythmias are common during cardiac catheterization.[26] Dysrhythmias are usually mechanically induced and, on most occasions, repositioning the wire or catheter resolves the dysrhythmia. Other causes of rhythm abnormality include coronary air embolism, electrolyte imbalance, and hypercarbia. Although they are usually minor complications, dysrhythmias are one of the most common causes of major complications, with a frequency being reported of between 2.6%[30] to 3.6%.[32] Infants have the highest incidence of rhythm disturbance. A defibrillator, a pacing device, and antiarrhythmic agents must be present in the cardiac catheter suite. Doses of any unfamiliar antiarrhythmic drugs should always be double checked or determined before the procedure.

Types of Dysrhythmias

Dysrhythmias may be atrial or ventricular in origin or involve degrees of heart block. Atrial arrhythmias such as supraventricular tachycardia or atrial flutter frequently resolve spontaneously, but persistent atrial dysrhythmias can be treated pharmacologically or with overdrive pacing. They rarely progress to major events.[30,32] Cassidy and coworkers reported atrioventricular block in 0.4% of cases, of which a fourth required pacing (although all patients were in sinus rhythm by discharge from hospital).[32] First- or second-degree atrioventricular block is well tolerated at all ages. When complete heart block occurs, it generally resolves shortly after the procedure and rarely persists.[30] Device closure for VSD has a high incidence (10.5%) of severe junctional bradycardia or complete heart block; nearly half of these children require pacing or isoproterenol.[15] Transient left bundle-branch block has been reported after dilation of the aortic valve.[25]

Overall, the incidence of ventricular tachycardia/fibrillation is approximately 0.2%.[30,32] However, Laussen and colleagues reported that 30% of children having VSD device placement had serious dysrhythmias and hypotension (requiring catheter withdrawal), of which 8.5% were ventricular arrhythmias requiring lidocaine or cardioversion.[15] Even relatively low risk procedures carry a risk of dysrhythmias. Balloon atrial septostomy is frequently accompanied by rhythm disturbances. Typically these are transient, but rarely they can be permanent or even fatal.[4]

Cardioversion

Tachyarrhythmias (atrial, supraventricular, and ventricular), bradycardias, atrioventricular block, and bundle-branch blocks have all been described after cardioversion. Factors that influence the incidence of tachyarrhythmias include the underlying rhythm disturbance and cardiac disease, metabolic derangement, drugs (e.g., digoxin), and the strength of shock. Histologic injury to the myocardium is rare when the starting power for cardioversion is set for 0.5 J/kg.[25] Systemic and pulmonary emboli are extremely rare in children compared with adults, in whom the incidence is 1% to 2%. Cardioverting children with pacemakers is becoming more common, and this can be done safely providing the electrode pads are placed a distance from the generator and the pacemaker circuits and programming mode are checked afterward.

Cyanosis

The etiology of cyanosis when it occurs in the catheterization laboratory may be either respiratory or circulatory in origin. A transesophageal echocardiographic (TEE) probe can cause hemoglobin desaturation by compressing the bronchi or vessels, pressing on the trachea, or precipitating bronchospasm. These events are common in children weighing less than 10 kg.[25] Pneumothorax is rare but documented.[32] Hypercarbia, acidosis, excessive positive-pressure ventilation, contrast media, and hypoxia can all increase pulmonary vascular resistance, which may lead to increased shunting and cyanosis. Hypercyanotic "spells" are frequently noted,[30] particularly in infants with unoperated tetralogy of Fallot. In one study, 12% of children with Fallot tetralogy exhibited a hypercyanotic episode within 12 hours of catheterization despite adequate hydration, sedation, and the use of nonionic contrast media.[32]

Embolization

Air, thrombus, misplaced devices, and fragments of catheters can all result in embolization.

Device and Balloon

In an older report of 1,457 interventional cases, 18 devices embolized, of which 3 required surgical removal, 8 were removed in the catheterization laboratory, and 7 were of no hemodynamic consequence and were left in situ. Devices that embolized included coils, duct umbrellas, an atrial defect occluder, and endovascular stents.[30] Improvements in device design are reducing the risk for embolization; for example, for ASD devices the risk has fallen from 11.1% to less than 1.1%.[4,38]

Balloon rupture was common in the past, although rarely produced intimal damage or embolic phenomena.[36] Today, balloon fragmentation is uncommon as a result of technologic improvements in material and design. To minimize this risk, an inflation device with attached manometer is recommended to ensure that the pressure does not exceed the burst pressure of the balloon.

Thrombus or Dislodged Material

Thrombus may be dislodged from devices or catheters, and balloon dilation may dislodge calcium, intimal lining from conduits, and thrombus from surgical systemic-pulmonary shunts.[4]

Air

Gas emboli may occur via sheaths and catheters, burst balloons, or anesthetic infusion lines. Air embolus (as well as blood loss) is a known risk during interventional procedures where there are many wire and catheter exchanges.[25] Balloons are dilated with a weak contrast mixture; and in view of the occasional occurrence of balloon rupture, it is important to make sure all gas bubbles are eliminated from the contrast mix syringe and catheter before dilation is undertaken. Balloons used for flotation tip catheters should be filled with CO_2 rather than air to minimize the potential embolic effect should the balloon burst. All intravenous lines, injections, and infusions must be strictly free of air bubbles because these sources can cause embolic occlusion of arterial vessels causing cerebral or myocardial ischemia in children with right-to-left mixing. Nitrous oxide should be avoided because it may expand any air embolism.

Contrast Toxicity

Adverse reactions to intravascular contrast are relatively uncommon, but it is essential that the anesthesiologist detect and manage a contrast-mediated reaction early to minimize morbidity or mortality. Reactions are often classified into idiosyncratic (unpredictable reactions independent of dose or concentration, e.g., anaphylaxis) or chemotoxic (related to dose and physiologic characteristics, e.g., osmolality). The pathophysiology of most reactions, however, is complex.[39]

There is reasonable evidence that severe anaphylactoid reactions to contrast media are not IgE mediated, but this does not explain the increased risk among atopic and asthmatic individuals. Many mechanisms have been proposed, including direct mast cell activation and degranulation, complement activation, inhibition of various enzyme systems, and binding to plasma proteins with conformational change.

Acute Reactions

Acute reactions to contrast agents can vary from mild to severe. Flushing, nausea, pruritus, vomiting, headache, and urticaria occur in 1% to 3% of patients receiving nonionic contrast.[40] These reactions are usually mild and self-limiting, requiring no specific treatment. Intermediate effects can manifest as moderate hypotension and bronchospasm as well as more severe degrees of the mild reactions. Severe reactions can include convulsions, laryngeal edema, dysrhythmias, and cardiac arrest. The likelihood of reaction varies with the type of contrast material, with low osmolar (non-ionic) solutions having considerably lower risk. The incidence of severe reactions with high osmolar (ionic) contrast is 0.2% to 0.06%, whereas reaction to low osmolar contrast is five times less common.[39] Reactions are more common when contrast medium is given through an arterial access compared with a venous access. Acute reactions should be managed as per anaphylaxis protocols (intravenous fluid, epinephrine, corticosteroids, and histamine-1 and histamine-2 antagonist therapy). Prophylaxis with corticosteroids and antihistamines should be considered only if there is a well-documented previous history of acute reaction to a nonionic contrast material. If there is a history of reaction to nonionic contrast material, then other modalities of imaging such as magnetic resonance imaging should be strongly considered. Occasionally, staining of the myocardium by contrast material has been observed, although this does not appear to confer any significant consequences.[32]

Delayed Reactions

Delayed reactions to both ionic and nonionic media are well described, with an incidence in one study of 8%.[41] Manifestations of such reactions include flu-like illness, parotitis, nausea and vomiting, abdominal pain, headache, and rashes. The pathophysiology is unknown.

Renal Adverse Reactions and Prevention

The term *contrast media nephrotoxicity* (CMN) refers to an increase in serum creatinine concentration by more than 25% or 0.5 mg/dL within 3 days of receiving intravenous contrast media in the absence of another cause.[39,41] The underlying mechanism is not clear. It is generally accepted that the contrast media reduces renal perfusion and is toxic to the tubular cells, but the specific pathology remains elusive.

CMN occurs almost exclusively in children with preexisting renal damage. Children with CHD undergoing coronary angiography with low osmolar contrast media may develop some slight glomerular effects and reversible tubular dysfunction, but no long-term effects have been demonstrated. Despite this, any child with reduced renal perfusion such as dehydration or cardiac failure should be regarded as at risk for CMN. It has also been suggested that neonates, infants, and children receiving more than 5 mL/kg of a contrast agent are at increased risk for CMN.[42]

Many interventions have been given prophylactically to prevent CMN, including normal saline/half-normal saline hydration, administration of N-acetylcysteine (NAC), mannitol, theophylline, calcium-channel blockers, diuretics, dopamine, dopamine-1 receptor antagonists, endothelin receptor antagonists, atrial natriuretic peptide, angiotensin-converting enzyme inhibitors, and prostaglandin E_1.[43,44] Although preliminary studies with NAC have been promising, no interventions have been more effective than normal saline hydration. To minimize the risk of CMN, the lowest possible dose of contrast agent should be used.[43,44] Furthermore, when possible, potentially nephrotoxic drugs should be stopped at least 24 hours before the procedure.[45]

Gadolinium-based contrast materials are considered non-nephrotoxic in the normal MRI dose of up to 0.3 mmol/kg.[45] However, there is some evidence that the increased doses required for cardiac angiography may still confer adverse renal effects.[46]

Neurologic Events

Both central and peripheral neurologic damage can occur as a complication of the catheterization procedure. In one prospective study, 0.38% children suffered a neurologic complication.

The incidence of neurologic complications is significantly greater after interventional procedures compared with diagnostic procedures.[47]

Central Nervous System

An ischemic cerebrovascular event may occur as a result of embolization, damage to the carotid artery, or acute low cardiac output states causing hypoxic-ischemic encephalopathy.[32,47] Thrombotic emboli may originate from any site in which there is endovascular or endocardial damage from the inner surface of the catheter or an implanted device. Factors that increase the risk during interventional procedures include large catheter size, more numerous vascular punctures, and longer procedures.[47] However, embolic strokes can follow an unremarkable catheterization procedure as well. The most common complication of an embolic stroke appears to be convulsion and hemiplegia. Patients with this type of stroke often have a full recovery.[47] Seizures have also been reported from lidocaine toxicity.[48] The outcome is more guarded after hypoxic-ischemic encephalopathy that occurs due to a period of low cardiac output.[47]

Peripheral Nervous System

As with any prolonged procedure under general anesthesia, it is crucial to consider pressure areas and traction forces on nerves such as the brachial plexus. Low cardiac output states associated with cardiac catheterization can augment the risk. Frequently, the arms are extended above the head to improve the lateral views of the heart. Brachial plexus injury is common in these circumstances[25,49] and is an important cause of nerve injury malpractice lawsuits.[50] At-risk positions should be accepted only if the cardiologist clearly indicates it is required. If it is necessary to abduct the arms and flex the elbows, it is important to make sure that the elbows are elevated at least 15 cm above the level of the table and there is no excessive stretch on the neck to exacerbate traction on the brachial plexus.[49,51] Passive movement may help reduce injury but increases the risk of dislodging monitoring equipment or the airway. If such positions are required it should be noted in the anesthesia record that this was the request/requirement of the cardiologist.

Radiation

There is a risk of radiation to both the child and staff. Radiation overexposure can lead to scarring and skin injury as well as cellular injury, mutation, cell death, leukemia, bone cancer, thyroid cancer, and birth defects.[52] The general principle with regard to radiation exposure is "ALARA" or "ALARP," which means *as low as reasonably achievable/practical*; this principle needs to be taken in the context of obtaining adequate diagnostic images.

Patient Radiation Exposure

This is a particularly important consideration in children owing to their higher radiosensitivity compared with adults. Moreover, a greater proportion of their body is irradiated during procedures. Complex interventional procedures require long fluoroscopy times with multiple angiographic/fluoroscopic acquisitions.[53] Children undergoing electrophysiologic studies are particularly at risk of long fluoroscopy times.

When estimating the lifetime risk of cancer from radiation exposure, the patient's age and weight need to be considered as well as the duration and effective dose of radiation exposure. The risk for adult coronary angiography is 6% per Sievert, and the average dose is about 10 mSv, which gives an increased risk of 0.06%.[54] In contrast, infants require lower exposure due to their low weight but have an increased sensitivity. An infant has a lifetime cancer risk of 11% to 15% per Sievert. Therefore, if an infant is exposed to approximately 20 mSv (e.g., 1 hour of fluoroscopy and seven digital acquisition runs), the lifetime cancer risk is 0.03%.[54]

Staff Radiation Exposure

Most exposure comes from "scatter" from the beam entry point on the patient. Lesser amounts come from the x-ray tube and intensifier. The need for staff protection is well established and is accomplished with the wearing of lead "aprons" as well as using thyroid shields, goggles, and suspended mobile glass lead screens for the head and neck. Operators should all have monitoring devices to monitor exposure, and only essential personnel should be present in the unprotected area.

Hypothermia and Hyperthermia

The procedure is often prolonged, increasing the need for close temperature monitoring. Children may become hypothermic, which could exacerbate blood loss or dysrhythmias, or they may become hyperthermic, which may exacerbate any neurologic injury.

Endocarditis

Antibiotic prophylaxis against endocarditis for routine diagnostic cardiac catheterization varies among centers. All children scheduled for insertion of implantable devices should receive prophylactic antibiotics during the procedure, and most centers continue to recommend endocarditis prophylaxis for a minimum of 6 months after implantation of a device. Although most centers do not routinely administer antibiotics for angioplasty procedures, there is usually a residual flow disturbance after the procedure that warrants ongoing endocarditis prophylaxis.

Future Directions in Procedures

The main limitation in the use of catheterization techniques in younger/smaller children has been the delay in the development of equipment of appropriate size. To overcome this difficulty, clinicians have developed hybrid procedures to permit current catheter-based techniques to be utilized in infants and small children. Examples of this collaborative approach between surgeon and interventional cardiologist include per ventricular closure of muscular ventricular septal defects[55] and hybrid stage 1 palliation for hypoplastic left heart syndrome (off-pump placement of a PDA stent and creation of an unrestricted ASD).[56] The next great challenge that we face is to develop equipment and techniques that can be used in conjunction with magnetic resonance imaging.[57] This would provide clear benefits to minimize radiation exposure to both children and staff. However, there are significant technical obstacles that need to be overcome before it will fully replace catheterization laboratories utilizing ionizing radiation.

Anesthesia

Who and How

The aims of anesthesia care for pediatric interventional cardiology are:

- Ensure the child is not distressed
- Provide optimal conditions for accurate diagnostic measures *and/or* successful completion of any intervention
- Manage the complications and significant derangements that may occur in the child's cardiovascular physiology during the procedure

These aims may require general anesthesia or on occasion may be met with deep sedation. The care of these children may be provided by a nurse anesthetist, general pediatric anesthesiologist, or specialized cardiac pediatric anesthesiologist depending on the complexity of the child's condition and qualifications of the practitioner. Because deep sedation can easily merge into general anesthesia, current guidelines sensibly suggest that deep sedation should be supervised by someone skilled at providing anesthesia as well as sedation.[58] This person should be skilled at resuscitation of children with CHD and must not be the proceduralist. The choice of sedation versus general anesthesia and seniority of anesthesiologist should match the procedure and the child. Increasingly, there are fewer diagnostic procedures and more interventional procedures. This change is reflected in a shift from sedation toward general anesthesia and the increasing role of specialized cardiac pediatric anesthesiologists.[59] Anesthesia providers for these children must have a high level of experience in pediatric anesthesia and a thorough understanding of pediatric cardiology and CHD. They must clearly understand the physiology, the procedure, and potential complications.

Preprocedural Assessment and Management

Children scheduled for elective interventional cardiology are often admitted to the hospital on the day of the procedure. Ideally, all these children should have an anesthesia assessment at the same time as their preprocedural cardiologic workup. An efficient and complete anesthesia assessment requires good coordination and communication between cardiology and anesthesia units. The anesthesia preoperative assessment should include a thorough understanding of the known anatomy and cardiac function and clear details of the planned procedure or intervention.

Up to 25% of children with CHD have syndromes or other anomalies that may affect their anesthesia care and require a thorough assessment of all relevant systems. These children may have had previous cardiac surgery or several other interventions. Obtaining intravenous access may be very difficult in some of these children. Children with CHD are likely to have had several previous anesthetics, and the family may be very well informed about their child's condition, hospital process, and anesthesia. Preoperative assessment should include discussion about sedative premedication, parental presence, and mode of induction (see Chapters 1 and 4).

Interventional cardiology procedures may involve considerable physiologic trespass, and some children may also have limited cardiac reserve. Therefore, these children should be in optimal health whenever possible. Intercurrent illness or infection may bias cardiorespiratory diagnostic values, increase risk of endocarditis, and increase risk of anesthesia complications such as laryngospasm. The urgency of the procedure, the cardiovascular status of the child, and the extent of the procedure should be considered carefully before proceeding for a child with an intercurrent illness.

Anatomy and Function

When assessing the anatomy and function there are four primary questions that may affect anesthesia management:

- Where does the blood go?
- What is the ventricular function?
- How reactive is the pulmonary circulation?
- Is there a stenosis, either fixed or dynamic?

The answer to these questions will help the anesthesiologist answer these potentially critical clinical management questions:

- How well is hyperoxia or hypoxia tolerated?
- What will be the effect of increased sympathetic stimulation or vasodilation and/or reduction in myocardial contractility?
- What are the likely causes of cardiovascular collapse and how should they be managed?

The primary questions can be answered from the record, details of previous surgery, and, most importantly, a recent echocardiography. Very poor function may be easily discovered in the history and physical examination, but moderate levels of dysfunction may not be offered or easily detected clinically.

Blood should be taken for a hematocrit evaluation and cross-matched for possible rapid transfusion. Premedication may consist of paracetamol for postprocedural analgesia and, if needed, sedation with oral midazolam (0.5 mg/kg) or ketamine (up to 5 mg/kg). Larger doses of sedative premedications may be used to provide more reliable or greater sedation if heavy sedation is mandatory, but large doses may cause delayed recovery or significant sedation after the procedure. Care should be taken that these children do not become excessively dehydrated. Fasting times should be adequate but not excessive, and in select children, a preprocedural intravenous line should be started. Topical anesthesia creams can be used if an intravenous induction is planned. Finally, to plan the optimal anesthetic, the anesthesiologist must have a clear understanding of exactly what the cardiologists are hoping to achieve and what conditions the cardiologist needs.

The Environment

Cardiac catheterization laboratories are often remotely located from the main operating room complex, limiting availability of immediate assistance and increasing transport times to and from central recovery areas. Ideally, cardiac catheterization laboratories should be located adjacent to cardiac theaters to facilitate rapid management of complications. For some cases ECMO and cardiopulmonary bypass circuits should be nearby and immediately available. Blood gas analysis should be rapidly available, and blood should be immediately available for urgent transfusion for interventional procedures such as balloon dilation and device insertion.

The cardiac catheterization laboratory is a hostile environment for anesthesiologists. Access to the child may be limited by the anteroposterior and lateral x-ray cameras, sterile drapes, and radiation protection devices. The x-ray cameras are bulky and may be unexpectedly moved for oblique views, different fields, or greater magnification. The lighting is often subdued to enhance viewing of the radiographs (Fig. 20-5).

Great care must be taken to secure all monitoring and the tracheal tube or laryngeal mask, before draping begins or the x-ray cameras are positioned. Access to the child during the procedure is limited and hazardous. Blind manipulation under

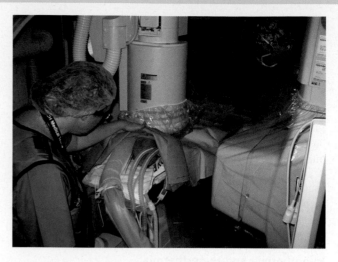

Figure 20-5. Typical setup of a catheterization laboratory showing limited access to a child.

the drapes can result in dislodging monitors or the tracheal tube. Moving cameras are a hazard to the anesthesiologist and may also dislodge anesthesia monitoring, the tracheal tube, and airway circuit.

The Cardiac Patient

The management of anesthesia for children with CHD is discussed in detail in other chapters (see Chapters 14 to 16). Important considerations include the potential for myocardial dysfunction and poor ventricular function reserve. This may be a particular problem in children with hypertrophied right ventricles operating at near-systemic pressures or with volume-loaded dilated ventricles.

Another important consideration is pulmonary hypertension and the reactivity of the pulmonary circulation. The pulmonary resistance is particularly important in a number of situations:

- Children may have increased reactivity such as in neonates or children with primary pulmonary hypertension.
- Children may have chronically increased pulmonary artery pressures and minimal right ventricular reserve.
- Children may have balanced circulations such as after a Norwood procedure in which increases or decreases in pulmonary vascular resistance may lead to spiraling hypoxia or systemic ischemia and acidosis.
- Children may have low pressure pulmonary circulations such as cavopulmonary shunts or after Fontan surgery.

Choice of Anesthesia

The choice of anesthesia should be determined by the three factors linked to the aims stated earlier. The ideal anesthesia cocktail should:

- Ensure the child is not distressed
- Provide optimal conditions for accurate diagnostic measures or successful completion of any intervention
- Minimize any risk inherent in children with abnormal cardiovascular physiology

A wide variety of anesthesia agents and techniques have been used in pediatric interventional cardiology. The choice will, to some extent, be determined by the procedure and the pathology.

Sedation

The difference between deep sedation and general anesthesia is imprecise and controversial, especially in small children in whom consciousness and memory are harder to measure (see Chapter 48). When considering the suitability of sedation or general anesthesia, the important issues to consider are:

- Does immobility need to be guaranteed?
- What will be the level of stimulation?
- Do oxygen and carbon dioxide levels need to be controlled?
- What will be the cardiovascular effects of the anesthesia agents?
- How likely is significant physiologic trespass?
- What will be the duration of the procedure?

Sedation is associated with a degree of movement that may make some procedures difficult or potentially dangerous, such as in device placement or balloon dilation. Stimulating procedures such as balloon dilation may make smooth sedation difficult. Sedation is poorly tolerated if the arms need to be placed above the head for long periods or if the procedure is prolonged. As for any other procedure, sedation for interventional cardiology is unwise if the child has obstructive sleep apnea or airway abnormalities. If significant cardiovascular complications are likely due to either the procedure or the status of the child, then control of the airway with general anesthesia may be safer. For all children, if sedation is used there must be provision for rapid and expert transition to general anesthesia.

Sedation techniques have evolved over the past 2 decades, resulting in much more effective and titratable strategies today. Since the 1950s the classic "lytic cocktail" consisting of intramuscular meperidine, promethazine, and chlorpromazine has been the standard for sedation.[60] However, this cocktail has a high incidence of both failure and oversedation as well as an incidence of sterile abscess.[61] Oral ketamine and midazolam have been shown to provide more reliable sedation but still result in episodes requiring respiratory support.[62] In theory, intravenous ketamine is an excellent choice for sedation because it provides a stable or increased heart rate and blood pressure and has little, if any, effect on the pulmonary vascular resistance. However, prolonged recovery and dysphoric reactions may be problematic.[63] Intravenous ketamine has been successfully used alone or in combination with midazolam[64] or propofol.[65] Propofol is also widely used for sedation but, compared with ketamine, propofol causes a greater reduction in both systemic blood pressure and systemic vascular resistance, with no effect on pulmonary vascular resistance. This may increase a right-to-left shunt or in diagnostic procedures may attenuate the gradient across a stenosis, making the decision to dilate the stenosis more difficult.[63,66,67] Compared with propofol sedation, a combination of ketamine with propofol produces similar sedation with less cardiovascular depression.[68] Recently, dexmedetomidine has been proffered for sedation for children undergoing cardiac catheterization, although it may not provide sufficient sedation by itself.[69] When combined with ketamine, dexmedetomidine was inferior to propofol and ketamine.[70]

In sedated children, the use of topical local anesthesia cream to facilitate venous access may be of benefit.[71] Spinal anesthesia has been described as an alternative to sedation or general anesthesia in high-risk infants younger than 6 months of age when the procedure is expected to take less than 90 minutes.[72]

Sedation is often used to avoid the potential effects of general anesthesia on diagnostic measures. However, as the diagnosis shifts to intervention, this argument assumes less relevance. Also, deep sedation may be associated with significant respiratory changes[62,73] and hypoxia[67] in some children. These changes could have as much an effect on the circulation as general anesthesia agents, limiting the theoretical advantage of sedation. Both general anesthesia and sedation may alter hemodynamics and intracardiac shunts.[62,67]

General Anesthesia

If general anesthesia is required for diagnostic procedures, the aim should be to maintain normal inspired oxygen, normal arterial carbon dioxide, and minimal direct hemodynamic effects. Positive-pressure ventilation will more easily maintain carbon dioxide levels than spontaneous ventilation, but positive-pressure ventilation will also decrease preload to pulmonary and systemic atria, increase afterload on the right ventricle, and decrease afterload on the left ventricle. Provided the child can maintain adequate oxygenation and normal carbon dioxide tension during sedation/general anesthesia, spontaneous ventilation is often preferred.

There is no general anesthetic agent that is definitely superior. Using physiologic and theoretical arguments, there is evidence for and against volatile or intravenous anesthesia but there are no outcome studies to provide strong evidence for either technique. Certainly, great care should be taken to avoid myocardial depression or vasodilation due to excessive doses of volatile of intravenous anesthetics. For this reason, some argue against inhalational induction, although it can also be argued that the use of total intravenous anesthesia is unwise given the wide variability in children. Nitrous oxide should be avoided if there is an element of reversible pulmonary hypertension and to avoid expansion of gas bubbles.

Etomidate may have a role in children with significant compromise because it has little hemodynamic effect on systemic or pulmonary pressures or resistances.[74] Remifentanil may offer advantage in cardiac procedures owing to the short context-sensitive half-time that allows rapid awakening at the completion of the procedure, although it is an opioid and lacks the sedation qualities of other medications. Concerns remain over the theoretical risks of bradycardia, hypotension, and chest wall rigidity with this opioid.[75,76] In some cases postprocedural sedation may offer an advantage in reducing patient movement and thereby reducing the risk for dislodgement of the clot at the catheterization site.

Opioids are not usually needed for interventional cardiology and may contribute to postanesthesia nausea and vomiting. Adequate infiltration with local anesthesia around the femoral vessels can significantly limit the degree of stimulus and in competent hands should not impair ease of vessel access. However, earlier reports of local anesthetic toxicity in children undergoing cardiac catheterization has led to a moratorium on the use of local anesthetics in the cardiac catheterization laboratory in some centers.

Radiofrequency ablation procedures may be of protracted duration and require an immobile child. They may also precipitate arrhythmias, requiring defibrillation. For these reasons general anesthesia is preferred. General anesthetic agents have effects on conduction that may affect the generation of pre-excitation and automatic tachycardia. Good clinical data are scant; however, it appears that for pre-excitation, isoflurane and sevoflurane have little effect at less than 1 MAC, whereas propofol and opioids have no demonstrable effects at any dose. In contrast, automatic tachycardia may be suppressed by high doses of opioids and propofol. In a prospective randomized trial no difference was found between isoflurane- and propofol-based anesthesia in duration of anesthesia or effectiveness of ablation.[77]

Principles of Technique

Attention to detail is the essential component of providing safe anesthesia for children with reduced ventricular reserve and critical pulmonary circulations. The most frequent error precipitating adverse events is providing inadequate anesthesia. Hemodynamic consequences of light anesthesia, or hypoxia due to laryngospasm, are poorly tolerated in children with pulmonary hypertension. Hypoxia or hypercapnia may lead to increasing pulmonary vascular resistance, which may, in turn, increase the shunt and further worsen the hypoxia. Increased pulmonary hypertension may also lead to significant decreases in pulmonary compliance, further increasing hypoxia and precipitating a downward spiral.[78] Another cause for an adverse outcome is the use of unfamiliar anesthetic technique. For example, it is foolhardy to first try the use of remifentanil in a child with primary pulmonary hypertension. Although there are theoretical grounds to support the use of one drug or another, the most important feature of anesthesia in children with CHD is to carefully use techniques that are reliable and familiar. This reinforces the need for these children to be anesthetized only by those with sound knowledge and experience with the physiology and procedures. Careful anesthesia entails attention to preprocedural anxiolysis, fluid management, full monitoring, expert assistance, and taking extra time to deliver anesthesia drugs slowly or in incremental doses to avoid overpressure or excessive blood levels.

The procedures often involve long periods of very little painful stimulation with occasional painful moments such as sheath change or balloon dilation. These moments can be anticipated provided good communication is maintained between the cardiologist and the anesthesiologist. During dilation of the aortic arch or aortic valve, it is prudent to have an arterial line (preferably right radial) to allow continuous blood pressure monitoring. The reader should be aware that dilation of vessels, whether they are arterial or venous, is quite painful and may cause coughing or significant patient discomfort if the child is only sedated.

TEE is increasingly used as part of diagnostic procedures or during device placement. TEE can be painful, requiring a deeper plane of anesthesia (i.e., the addition of opioids or neuromuscular blockade or both). TEE requires an endotracheal tube to provide a patent airway; care must be taken to hold the tube during manipulations of the TEE probe because TEE manipulations and the gel required can easily dislodge endotracheal tubes.

Coughing and straining on extubation may increase the risk of bleeding. For this reason deep extubation may be preferred. The advantages of deep extubation must be balanced with the risks of hypoxia and hypercapnia with loss of airway control or laryngospasm that may ensue if the endotracheal tube is removed before the child is fully awake. Postoperative delirium and restlessness can increase the risk of bleeding. Children should have sufficient analgesia to prevent postoperative distress. This is usually provided with paracetamol and local anesthetic infiltration.

To provide rapid resuscitation, reliable intravenous access is essential in these children. Using leg veins may not be ideal if the femoral veins are occluded with thrombosis or catheters. Similarly, pulse oximetry and noninvasive blood pressure cuffs should not be placed on the legs.

The Future

Anesthesia for interventional cardiac catheterizations will become more challenging as new interventions are found for sicker children and as more cardiology procedures are performed in combination with open surgery or magnetic resonance imaging. More children are likely to need anesthesia as opposed to sedation, and the specialist pediatric cardiac anesthesiologists will be spending an increasing proportion of their time in interventional cardiology suites.

Annotated References

Arnold PD, Holtby HM: Anesthesia for the cardiac catheterization laboratory. In Andropoulos DB, Stayer SA, Russell IA (eds): Anesthesia for Congenital Heart Disease. Malden, MA, Blackwell Futura, 2005, pp 407-426

A very good and readable source for a more detailed description of the subject.

Bennett D, Marcus R, Stokes M: Incidents and complications during pediatric cardiac catheterization. Paediatr Anaesth 2005; 15:1083-1088

Cassidy SC, Schmidt KG, Van Hare GF, et al: Complications of pediatric cardiac catheterization: a 3-year study. J Am Coll Cardiol 1992; 19:1285-1293

Vitiello R, McCrindle BW, Nykanen D, et al: Complications associated with pediatric cardiac catheterization. J Am Coll Cardiol 1998; 32:1433-1440

All important papers describing the complications in pediatric cardiac catheterization.

Friesen RH, Alswang M: Changes in carbon dioxide tension and oxygen saturation during deep sedation for paediatric cardiac catheterization. Paediatr Anaesth 1996; 6:15-20

An important paper outlining a significant issue with sedation techniques.

Javorski JJ, Hansen DD, Laussen PC, et al: Paediatric cardiac catheterization: innovations. Can J Anaesth 1995; 42:310-329

An excellent but slightly dated review of the subject.

Reddy K, Jaggar S, Gillbe C: The anaesthetist and the cardiac catheterisation laboratory. Anaesthesia 2006; 61:1175-1186

A good and recent review of anesthesia for adult and pediatric cardiac catheterization.

References

Please see www.expertconsult.com

Anesthesia for Noncardiac Surgery in Children with Congenital Heart Disease

CHAPTER 21

Wanda C. Miller-Hance

OVER THE PAST SEVERAL decades significant advances in diagnostic and interventional cardiology, surgical techniques, cardiopulmonary bypass, anesthetic management, and critical care have dramatically altered the natural history of congenital heart disease (CHD). The net result of these refinements has been a decrease in morbidity and mortality in affected children and improved quality of life. As life expectancy continues to increase and survival rates further improve, an escalating number of pal-liated and "repaired" children with CHD will need to undergo noncardiac surgery or other procedures unrelated to their heart disease. Because children with CHD are operated on at earlier and earlier ages, this group represents the majority of children with CHD that an anesthesiologist would most likely encounter during elective or emergent noncardiac surgery. In some cases, children may require noncardiac surgery before undergoing procedures to repair their cardiovascular pathology. In others, the condition may not require or be amenable to surgical intervention. The care of children with CHD is becoming more frequent in all diagnostic and surgical settings.

A wide spectrum of extracardiac anomalies has been described in children with CHD.[1-5] Furthermore, a high incidence of chromosomal syndromes and genetic disorders are associated with CHD. The reported prevalence of associated malformations is between 10% and 33%.[6-8] The organ systems most often affected include musculoskeletal, central nervous, renal-urinary, gastrointestinal, and respiratory. Although many extracardiac malformations are relatively minor and have limited or no clinical implications, a substantial proportion of children with CHD have significant noncardiac comorbid conditions.[9] These pathologic and disease processes may necessitate surgical intervention. In addition, other routine ailments and conditions that require surgical intervention may afflict these children. The challenges of caring for children with CHD are magnified by the diversity of structural malformations, each with specific physiologic perturbations, hemodynamic consequences, and severity. This is further complicated by the variety of therapeutic strategies, both medical and surgical, that are characteristic of this pediatric population. The net effect is an individualized and tailored anesthetic prescription for most children with CHD.[10,11]

Clinical outcome in CHD depends on the nature of the anatomic abnormalities and the possibility of successful palliation or "correction."[12] Children who have had palliative surgery continue to have abnormal cardiovascular anatomy and physiology. The primary goal of the surgical intervention is to favorably influence the natural history of the defect and decrease the likelihood of the severe consequences of the disease. The abnormal circulation in these children is associated with an increased risk of adverse events during emergent or elective noncardiac surgery.[13-16] The expectations of reparative, corrective, or definitive procedures are to improve hemodynamics and cardiac function and minimize long-term ill effects of an abnormal circulation, thus improving overall clinical outcome. Although the pathologic process may have been surgically treated, the cardiovascular system should not be considered normal. *In fact, true surgical "correction" may be the exception rather than the rule in CHD.* In other words, repair of a congenital cardiac pathologic process should not be equated to a "cure" for most children. Despite these considerations, in those with good hemodynamic results, the risks associated with noncardiac surgery may not vary significantly from children without CHD. They are generally considered to be doing well clinically, have a good functional status, require few or no medications, have no exercise restriction, and undergo routine surveillance. These children require no to minimal adjustments in perioperative care from that which is routinely administered. In others, however, residual abnormalities exist. In some who are less fortunate, a pathologic process may remain or develop after cardiac surgery related to the primary disease or therapy. This may lead to severe cardiovascular and/or pulmonary impairment. These residua and sequelae may necessitate further medical and/or surgical interventions and may increase perioperative morbidity during noncardiac surgery.[17] The management of these children is influenced by a number of factors but, to a significant extent, by a residual pathologic process and associated hemodynamic perturbations.[18,19]

Many publications have examined the anesthetic implications for children and adults with CHD undergoing noncardiac surgery.[10,18-32] However, only a limited number of studies have provided data regarding perioperative outcomes.[33-37] In contrast to the extensive adult literature regarding perioperative cardiac assessment and risk stratification during noncardiac surgery leading to the development of guidelines aimed at improving clinical outcomes, the lack of rigorous scientific data on this subject in the pediatric age group has made an equivalent effort challenging, in part because of the rapid development of alternative therapies and major corrective interventions earlier in life.[38]

In this chapter, general principles of anesthetic practice are reviewed with a focus on preoperative assessment, intraoperative management, and postoperative care for children with CHD having noncardiac surgery. Because anesthetic management is significantly influenced by a number of factors, including the particular structural abnormalities, pathophysiologic consequences of the defect(s), functional status, potential residua, sequelae, and long-term outcome, this discussion addresses fundamental concepts in this regard. In addition, specific perioperative considerations in children with CHD and issues applicable to high-risk patient groups are reviewed.

Preoperative Assessment

A detailed preoperative evaluation is indispensable for identifying and anticipating factors that may place a child with CHD at increased anesthetic risk (Table 21-1).[39,40] An important goal of this assessment is to gather information regarding the nature of the cardiovascular disease and prior therapeutic interventions. A determination of functional status is based on clinical data. The history and physical examination, in addition to the laboratory data and ancillary tests (i.e., an up-to-date echocardiogram), provide complementary information regarding anatomic or hemodynamic status, allowing for risk assessment. Based on this clinical assessment and consideration of the major pathophysiologic consequences, a systematic, detailed, organized plan should be formulated for anesthetic and perioperative management. In some cases, the preoperative evaluation may establish

Table 21-1. Potential Risk Factors in Children with Congenital Heart Disease for Noncardiac Surgery

Young age (infancy)
Single-ventricle physiology or complex defects
Congestive heart failure
Hypoxemia
Long-standing cyanosis
Ventricular dysfunction
Anticoagulation therapy
Syncope
Arrhythmias
Pulmonary hypertension/pulmonary vascular disease
Unrepaired pathology
Significant sequelae or residua
Older age at the time of cardiac intervention
"Older" type of cardiac surgical procedure
Major noncardiac surgery

the need to delay or defer elective noncardiac surgery or other interventions.

History and Physical Examination

As in all children undergoing anesthesia, the history and physical examination are essential components of a thorough preoperative evaluation. In addition to the specifics regarding the present illness and planned procedure, the history should focus on the status of the cardiovascular system. Relevant information includes the type of cardiovascular disease and comorbid conditions, medications, allergies, prior hospitalizations, surgeries, anesthetic experiences, and complications. Symptomatology including tachypnea, dyspnea, tachycardia, dysrhythmias, and fatigue should be sought. Feeding difficulties and diaphoresis may represent significant symptoms in infants, whereas decreased activity level or exercise intolerance may be of concern in older children. Palpitations, chest pain, and syncope should be characterized. The history should include an assessment of growth and development (i.e., evaluation of the child's growth chart), because these may be affected in children with CHD. Failure to thrive suggests ongoing cardiorespiratory compromise. Those with decompensated disease, complex pathologies, associated genetic defects, or other syndromes may be particularly vulnerable. Recent illnesses such as intercurrent respiratory infections or pulmonary disease may increase the potential for perioperative complications and require careful appraisal of the risk-benefit ratio in elective cases.[41,42]

The physical examination should include the child's weight and height. Vital signs, including heart rate, respiratory rate, hemoglobin-oxygen saturation, and blood pressure, should be documented. If the child is known or suspected to have, or has been treated for any form of aortic arch obstruction or has had any systemic-to-pulmonary shunt, upper and lower extremity as well as right and left upper extremity blood pressure recordings and palpation of the quality of pulses should be documented. These examinations may also provide information regarding patency of arterial beds and may be useful regarding site selection for blood pressure monitoring. Emphasis should be given to the airway and cardiovascular system, with particular attention to any changes from previous examinations. General appearance should include the child's level of activity, breathing pattern, level of distress if any, and presence of cyanosis. Respiratory evaluation should note the quality of the breath sounds and indicate the presence or absence of labored breathing, intercostal retractions, wheezing, rales, or rhonchi. Abnormalities may suggest congestive symptoms or a pneumonic process. Cardiac auscultation should include assessment of heart sounds, pathologic murmurs, and gallop rhythms. The presence of a thrill, representing a palpable murmur, should be noted. The abdomen should be examined for the presence of hepatosplenomegaly. Assessment of the extremities should include examination of pulses, overall perfusion, capillary refill, cyanosis, clubbing, and edema. Noncardiac anomalies or pathology that may affect anesthetic care (e.g., a specific syndrome complex, a potentially difficult airway, gastroesophageal reflux) should be noted.

An important objective of the preoperative evaluation is to identify children with functional cardiopulmonary limitations imposed by their cardiovascular pathology. Symptoms and signs consistent with congestive heart failure, cyanosis, hypercyanotic episodes, and compromised functional status, as suggested by significant exercise intolerance or syncopal episodes, should raise concerns for the potential of perioperative problems. The pediatric cardiologist should provide information regarding the nature and severity of the cardiovascular pathology, an impression of the child's overall clinical status, and an assessment of prior complications. In addition, the cardiologist should assist in the identification of children at high risk and optimize their preoperative clinical condition. The perioperative care teams should be alerted to any particular concerns that may affect the care of the child. The anesthesiologist should have a detailed understanding of the child's cardiac defect, pathophysiologic consequences, nature of the medical and surgical therapies applied, functional status, and implications for perioperative management. Although the surgical team may not have an in-depth understanding of the child's cardiovascular disease, by sharing the details of the surgical plan and potential issues that are anticipated or may arise with the anesthesiologist, problems may be anticipated and proactively addressed.

Ancillary Studies and Laboratory Data

A recording of the systemic arterial saturation by pulse oximetry (SpO_2) should be obtained as a baseline value when the child is calm and breathing room air. Acceptable values depend on many factors that include the particular cardiac abnormalities, whether the child has a two- versus a one-ventricle circulation, the preoperative versus postoperative status with respect to the cardiac pathology, and the stage in the palliative pathway for those undergoing such strategy. In general, children who have undergone definitive procedures should be expected to have normal to near-normal SpO_2 ($\geq 95\%$). After palliative interventions, SpO_2 values typically range between 75% and 85%.

The extent of laboratory testing largely depends on the type, anticipated duration, and complexity of the surgery. The preoperative tests most commonly obtained include hematocrit, hemoglobin, electrolytes, and coagulation tests. In cyanotic children, a complete blood cell blood count provides the determination of polycythemia, microcytic anemia, and thrombocytopenia. Prothrombin time, partial thromboplastin times, and international normalized ratio (INR) provide an indication of clotting ability. It is important to consider in children with increased red blood cell mass and relatively small plasma volumes that the collection of coagulation specimens requires sampling tubes that adjust the amount or concentration of citrate to prevent artifactual prolongation of coagulation studies. In those receiving diuretic therapy, digoxin, or angiotensin-converting enzyme inhibitors, the determination of serum electrolytes may be useful. Blood typing and crossmatching should be performed based on the anticipated blood loss.

A recent electrocardiogram (ECG) should be reviewed for any changes from prior studies (particularly regarding criteria consistent with chamber dilation and/or ventricular hypertrophy), the presence of rhythm abnormalities, and findings suggestive of myocardial ischemia. If an arrhythmia is noted, further evaluation regarding potential etiology is warranted because this may reflect an underlying hemodynamic abnormality that may affect the perioperative course. A continuous ECG recording (Holter monitor) and further evaluation may be indicated in the child with a history of rhythm disturbance, palpitations, or syncope or an ECG suggestive of significant ectopy or arrhythmia. An exercise tolerance test or treadmill study may be warranted if there is concern about myocardial ischemia, as may be the case in the child with aortic stenosis, coronary artery anomalies, or exercise-induced arrhythmias.

Review of a recent chest radiograph, including a lateral view, provides information regarding cardiac size, chamber enlargement, and pulmonary vascularity. Prior studies such as echocardiograms (particularly a recent echocardiogram), cardiac catheterizations, electrophysiologic procedures, and magnetic resonance imaging should be reviewed. In some cases, it may be necessary to obtain further diagnostic information before proceeding with the planned elective procedure if there are symptoms that merit additional investigations or issues of concern. These evaluations should be coordinated with the child's cardiologist. It is also important to consider whether the child may benefit from cardiac catheterization for diagnostic purposes or from interventions to address significant structural, functional, or hemodynamic abnormalities before the anticipated procedure. In addition to providing potentially helpful information, the clinical status of the child can be substantially improved in many cases by such interventions. This may be of significant benefit when the anticipated procedure is considered to be a major intervention.

One of the goals of the preoperative evaluation is to obtain the most diagnostic information with the fewest tests and the least risk, discomfort, and expense to the child. The anesthesiologist is particularly suited to determine which tests are appropriate for optimal perioperative planning and if additional data are needed.

Informed Consent

The physicians involved in the care of the child should meet with the patient and family to explain and answer questions regarding the surgical procedure and anesthetic plan, as well as to discuss the benefits and risks involved. Although surgery in children with CHD, particularly in those with uncorrected defects, may carry an increased risk, it may not be possible to define the specific contribution of each of the involved factors to the overall risk. The preoperative consultation provides the opportunity to alleviate patient and parental anxiety.

Fasting Guidelines

Although the optimal period of fasting in children undergoing surgery has been the subject of some debate, most centers follow established guidelines to reduce the risk of aspiration.[43-46] In general, the same fasting guidelines are applicable to children with CHD with a few additional considerations. In some children the intravenous administration of maintenance fluids to ensure adequate hydration may be required if the fasting period is prolonged. This is particularly important in small infants, those with obstructive lesions, cyanotic disease, or single-ventricle physiology. Maintenance of adequate hydration and ventricular preload may limit potential detrimental hemodynamic changes associated with anesthesia and surgery.

Medications

Children with CHD may be receiving medications such as digoxin, diuretics, vasodilators, anticoagulants, antiarrhythmics, or immunosuppressants (post–cardiac transplantation). Although there may be an occasional exception, such as diuretic or anticoagulation therapy, there is usually no need to discontinue chronic medications before surgery. In fact, it is often important to continue these drugs until the time of surgery and

in most centers children are allowed to take scheduled oral medications with small amounts of water preoperatively.

Intraoperative Management

Anesthesia and surgery impose additional stresses on the cardiovascular system and provoke compensatory mechanisms to maintain homeostasis. Therefore, it is important to assess the child's physiology and cardiovascular reserve to anticipate his or her ability to increase cardiac output to meet metabolic demands. This information, along with the nature and complexity of the surgery, will help decide the extent of monitoring required. It is also relevant to use this information to choose anesthetic agents and techniques that will have the least impact on the child's cardiovascular system. It is imperative to be prepared to intervene promptly if decompensation occurs. Good communication between the surgeon, cardiologist, anesthesiologist, and nursing teams during the entire perioperative period is of utmost importance in children with complex disease.

General Considerations

Anesthesia Care Provider

The anesthetic care should be provided by an experienced individual who is familiar with children with CHD, the planned operative procedure, and the surgeon's usual approach. The most important factor that an anesthesiologist can offer this group of children is a comprehensive understanding of the anatomic abnormalities, pathophysiology of the cardiac malformation, and how this may be affected by the anesthetic and surgical procedure. A familiarity with the most likely residua and sequelae is essential.[17] Adequate communication among all physicians involved is critical because this enhances the likelihood of best possible outcomes.

Premedication

The use of premedication to provide sedation and anxiolysis is routine before most surgical procedures in children because most experience some degree of fear or anxiety. This facilitates parental separation, entry into the operating room, placement of monitors, and induction of anesthesia. The cardiorespiratory effects of premedication in children may be influenced by underlying systemic disease.[47-51]

Commonly used premedications include oral or intravenous benzodiazepines, opioids, and small amounts of hypnotic agents. Alternatives include the intramuscular, intranasal, and rectal routes. Children with hemodynamic decompensation may require little or no premedication. Caution should also be exercised in those with a history of cardiovascular pathology associated with significant increases in pulmonary artery pressure/pulmonary arteriolar resistance because hypoventilation and hypoxemia may further increase pulmonary vascular tone. Conversely, children who are subject to hypercyanotic episodes or those with catecholamine-induced arrhythmias may benefit from heavy premedication. In selected children (e.g., infants, those with cyanotic heart disease), oxygen saturation monitoring after premedication and the administration of supplemental oxygen as necessary have been recommended.[49]

Intravenous Access

Secure intravenous access is mandatory for administration of fluids and medications during anesthetic care. In most children with CHD, intravenous access is established after an inhalational induction. However, in those considered at high risk, such as children with severe outflow tract obstruction, moderate to severe cardiac dysfunction, pulmonary hypertension, or potential for hemodynamic compromise, consideration should be given for placement of intravenous access before induction of anesthesia or very early in the process. The size of the intravenous catheter should be determined by the anticipated fluid requirements. If poor peripheral access is present, central venous access might be necessary, particularly given the potential for large intravascular volume shifts, while also allowing central venous pressure monitoring. Placement of a central venous catheter may be assisted by audio Doppler or two-dimensional ultrasound guidance (see Chapter 49). In the small infant with single-ventricle physiology, central venous cannulation with catheter placement in the superior vena cava may be undesirable in view of concerns of potential venous obstruction that may impact pulmonary blood flow or subsequent surgical palliation. In these children a small catheter or alternate approach (femoral venous access) should be considered. In children with an existent or potential right-to-left shunt, all air must be removed from intravenous infusion tubing. In general, air filters may be difficult to use in the operating room because they may restrict the volume of intravenous fluids or blood administered in emergency situations, but they may be useful in the preoperative and postoperative periods.

Emergency Drugs

In view of the potential for hemodynamic instability in some children with CHD that may occur under any circumstance and at any time, drugs for emergency situations should be prepared or immediately available to the anesthesiologist providing care.

Monitoring

A basic principle of intraoperative monitoring is to use techniques or devices that provide useful information to help with clinical decision-making and to avoid monitors that are distracting or redundant. Basic monitoring involves observation of the child, including skin color, capillary refill, respiration, pulse palpation, events on the surgical field, and color of shed blood. Standard noninvasive monitors used during most surgical interventions include oscillometric blood pressure assessment, electrocardiography, pulse oximetry, capnography, and temperature monitoring. In addition, a precordial stethoscope can be extremely helpful to monitor for changes in heart tones that may suggest early hemodynamic compromise. In the child with CHD, relatively sophisticated and invasive monitoring may be needed. The level of monitoring required is influenced by the child's cardiovascular pathology, clinical condition and functional status, and the complexity and duration of the surgery or procedure being performed.

Arterial Blood Pressure Assessment

Basic blood pressure monitoring begins with pulse palpation. An automated blood pressure cuff is used in most children. The selection of monitoring site may be influenced by vascular anomalies (e.g., aortic arch pathology, aberrant origin and course of aortic arch vessels) or prior surgical interventions (e.g., Blalock-Taussig shunt, arterial cutdown). Direct systemic blood pressure monitoring via an indwelling arterial catheter may be necessary in some cases for beat-to-beat assessment and for blood gas analysis. In children, this is usually accomplished after induction of anesthesia. Arterial cannulation can be achieved percutaneously in most circumstances with a low risk of complications (see Chapter 49). Use of the radial arteries is preferable, particularly in the neonate, to minimize catheter-related vascular problems. The decision regarding the need for invasive monitoring is largely based on the child's clinical condition and nature of the surgical procedure.

Electrocardiography

An ECG is used to monitor heart rate, cardiac rhythm, and ST-segment analysis. Usually one or multiple leads are displayed. Most systems use two leads: standard lead II for arrhythmia monitoring plus inferior ischemia detection, and precordial lead V_5 for lateral ischemia detection. Arrhythmias may occur as a result of hypoxia, electrolyte imbalances, acid-base abnormalities, intravascular/intracardiac catheters, and surgical manipulations near or around the thorax. Ischemia may be evident on direct examination of the ECG or ST-segment analysis.[52] Although in the adult population this is associated with worsened outcome, the implication in children is unknown.[53,54] Because ectopic foci may develop follow cardiac surgery, observation of arrhythmias intraoperatively may be the first clinical manifestation; such observations should be documented and discussed with the child's cardiologist postoperatively.

Pulse Oximetry

Monitoring of arterial oxygen saturation is particularly useful in infants, cyanotic children, and those with complex anatomy or significant hemodynamic compromise. In addition to providing continuous assessment of hemoglobin-oxygen saturation and heart rate, the pulse oximetry waveform may also indicate the adequacy of peripheral perfusion and cardiac output.[55,56] Other parameters that may be reflected by the SpO_2 include intracardiac or great artery level shunting and pulmonary blood flow. Placement of an oximeter probe is well tolerated, even in uncooperative children, and it is typically one of the earliest monitors applied during anesthetic induction.

Capnography

Capnography is essential to confirm proper placement of the endotracheal tube and aids in assessing adequacy of ventilation, and in the recognition of certain pathologic conditions such as bronchospasm, airway obstruction, and malignant hyperthermia. In spontaneously breathing sedated children receiving supplemental oxygen via nasal cannula, capnography may also be feasible for end-tidal or exhaled carbon dioxide ($PETCO_2$) concentration monitoring. A prospective observational study in children undergoing cardiac catheterization with sedation administered by nonanesthesiologists found that monitored end-tidal CO_2 values provided a reasonable estimate of arterial blood CO_2 values.[57] Although the absolute value for $PETCO_2$ may not be as reliable as in the presence of an endotracheal tube, the capnograph waveform confirms the presence or absence of respirations and air exchange. End-tidal CO_2 monitoring also provides a gross index of pulmonary blood flow. It should be recognized that in children with cyanotic heart disease, $PETCO_2$ values may underestimate arterial carbon dioxide tension ($PaCO_2$) measurements owing to altered pulmonary blood flow and ventilation-perfusion mismatch.[58,59]

Temperature Monitoring

Temperature should be routinely monitored during most procedures. Although temperature swings are usually not profound, some children may become significantly hypothermic, particularly the small neonate, owing to the large body surface area/body weight ratio and decreased subcutaneous tissue. This may influence oxygen delivery (increased oxygen consumption) and emergence from anesthesia, cause detrimental changes in hemodynamics, and affect hemostasis.

Urinary Output Measurements
The production of urine is a useful index of the adequacy of renal perfusion and cardiac output. Urine output is usually monitored during cases involving major fluid shifts or blood loss, or if the surgical procedure will be prolonged. No specific value for urine output is necessarily predictive of good renal function in the postoperative period.

Transesophageal Echocardiography
Various reports have documented the utility of transesophageal echocardiography as a monitoring device in high-risk adults undergoing noncardiac procedures.[60-71] Although sporadic reports have demonstrated the utility of transesophageal echocardiography in children undergoing noncardiac surgery, the overall contribution or application of this modality in the pediatric age group in this particular setting has not been well defined and requires further evaluation.[72]

Selection of Techniques and Agents
A number of anesthetic regimens have been used in children with CHD undergoing noncardiac interventions and studies that require deep sedation or immobility, such as cardiac catheterization, electrophysiologic evaluation, and magnetic resonance or other diagnostic imaging. Although a formula or recipe cannot be provided, the anesthetic techniques and agents used for a particular situation should be selected in consideration of the procedure to be performed, the child's disease process and functional status, and the impact of the hemodynamic effects of the anesthetic and procedure on the pathophysiologic process. Factors such as age, physical characteristics, and preferences of the anesthesiologist must be taken into consideration. The primary goals of anesthetic management with respect to the cardiovascular system are to optimize systemic oxygen delivery, maintain ventricular function within expected parameters for the individual patient, and ensure the adequacy of cardiac output. An essential concept while caring for these children is their potential decreased cardiovascular reserve and reduced tolerance for perioperative stress and alterations of the balance between pulmonary and systemic blood flow during anesthesia and surgery. A carefully titrated anesthetic, regardless of the specific agents, is advisable.

Anesthetic Technique
General anesthesia has the advantages of wide acceptance, ease of application, and relative certainty of effect. It is the appropriate choice for most children undergoing noncardiac surgery. Disadvantages include a greater potential for wide fluctuations in the hemodynamics and a prolonged recovery period. The intravenous route allows for rapid induction of anesthesia. If intravenous access is not present, an inhalation induction may be performed. Inhalational or volatile anesthetics dilate vascular beds and lower sympathetic responsiveness. These are all desirable goals in most children, even those with heart disease, because adequate myocardial function and a reactive sympathetic nervous system are usual. However, some children may

have decreased myocardial performance and require a high resting sympathetic tone to maintain systemic perfusion. Potent inhalation agents in this setting may lead to further impairment of ventricular function, decreased sympathetic tone, and, potentially, cardiovascular decompensation. These children, as well as others with a relatively fixed cardiac output, may require a technique that combines several drugs (balanced technique) to achieve anesthesia while minimizing the risk of hemodynamic compromise. A potent opioid/amnestic agent/muscle relaxant technique usually causes little myocardial depression and tends to leave sympathetic responsiveness intact while providing analgesia, amnesia, and a motionless child.

Regional anesthesia has been demonstrated to be safe and effective in children with CHD (see Chapter 42).[73-76] Advantages of regional anesthesia, such as epidural and spinal techniques, include an effect largely limited to the surgical site, decreased number of systemic medications, potentially shorter overall recovery period, and, generally, a more pleasant experience for the child. Use of these techniques, however, is limited in small children and may not always be effective. Regional anesthesia retains the potential for hemodynamic compromise, particularly in hypovolemic children or those with a fixed cardiac output, and is generally contraindicated in those with coagulation defects. The administration of agents into the caudal space such as local anesthetics, opioids, or other adjuvants (e.g., clonidine) may attenuate the sympathetic outflow associated with surgical manipulation and noxious stimuli and facilitate postoperative pain management.

The choice of technique also affects termination of the anesthetic and emergence. Anesthetics performed with fewer agents are inherently simpler and are usually easier and more predictable to terminate. The availability of ultra-short-acting opioids, such as remifentanil, has facilitated the use of a high-dose opioid-relaxant technique and avoided the need for postoperative ventilation solely related to residual respiratory depressant effects of high-dose opioids. It is important to recognize that ventricular function, as well as the presence of intracardiac shunts, can significantly affect both uptake and distribution of volatile anesthetics and the kinetics of intravenous medications (see Chapter 6).

Inhalational Agents
The use of volatile anesthetics has been at the forefront of pediatric anesthesia practice for many years.[77] A number of inhalational agents are available with varying induction, recovery, and safety characteristics.[78] Halothane was considered for many decades the primary agent for inhalation induction in children in combination with oxygen and nitrous oxide. However, with the introduction of sevoflurane in the mid 1990s, it has replaced halothane for induction of anesthesia in many centers. The safety and efficacy of halothane and sevoflurane in infants and children with CHD during cardiac surgery demonstrated twice as many episodes of hypotension, as well as moderate bradycardia and emergent drug use in those who received halothane compared with sevoflurane.[79] Based on these data and other studies that have demonstrated potential benefits of sevoflurane regarding hemodynamic stability and minimal impact on myocardial performance, sevoflurane has been advocated as the preferred anesthetic for children, particularly those with heart disease.[80-85] Nonetheless, in some jurisdictions and under some conditions, halothane remains the primary anesthetic for chil-

dren. Experience has suggested that it can be used in children with heart disease provided careful attention is paid to a slow, titrated induction and that spontaneous respirations are maintained (see Chapter 6).

Intravenous Agents

Propofol is one of the most frequently used medication for intravenous sedation and general anesthesia. The administration of this medication has been reported in children with CHD undergoing cardiac catheterization, electrophysiologic testing, and magnetic resonance imaging.[86-88] Propofol has also been used during procedures such as cardioversion, pericardiocentesis, chest tube placement, and transesophageal echocardiography.[89]

The hemodynamic effects of propofol in children have been investigated in those with normal hearts as well in those with cardiovascular disease. An echocardiographic study in infants with presumably normal hearts undergoing elective surgery demonstrated that propofol did not alter heart rate, shortening fraction, rate-corrected velocity of circumferential fiber shortening, or cardiac index after intravenous induction.[90] However, propofol decreased arterial blood pressure to a greater extent than thiopental, an effect attributed to a reduction in afterload. A comparison of propofol and ketamine during cardiac catheterization found that propofol caused a transient decrease in mean arterial pressure and mild arterial oxygen desaturation in some children.[91] The investigators concluded that propofol was a practical alternative for elective cardiac catheterization in children, being preferable to ketamine in view of the significantly more rapid recovery. Another investigation in 30 children with CHD undergoing cardiac catheterization demonstrated significant decreases in mean arterial blood pressure and systemic vascular resistance during propofol administration.[86] No changes in heart rate, mean pulmonary artery pressure, or pulmonary vascular resistance were observed. In children with intracardiac shunts, the net result of propofol was a significant increase in the right-to-left shunt, a decrease in the left-to-right shunt, and decreased pulmonary-to-systemic blood flow ratio, resulting in a statistically significant decrease in the PaO_2 and arterial oxygen saturation (SaO_2), as well as reversal of the shunt direction from left-to-right to right-to-left in two patients. They also demonstrated that propofol can lead to further desaturation in children with cyanotic heart disease.

The effects of propofol have also been examined in children undergoing electrophysiologic testing and radiofrequency catheter ablation for tachyarrhythmias. It has no significant effect on sinoatrial or atrioventricular node function or accessory pathway conduction in Wolff-Parkinson-White syndrome.[92,93] However, a study documented that ectopic atrial tachycardia may be suppressed during propofol administration in children.[94]

Collectively, these data suggest that the judicious use of propofol may be a reasonable option in children with adequate cardiovascular reserve who can tolerate mild decreases in myocardial contractility and heart rate and mild to moderate decreases in systemic vascular resistance. The effects of propofol on the direction and magnitude of intracardiac shunts may be an important consideration in children with cyanotic heart disease and may influence the hemodynamic assessment of those undergoing evaluation of pulmonary-to-systemic blood flow ratios.

Thiopental, a rapidly acting barbiturate, has been used for many years for induction of anesthesia. Several investigations have documented the cardiovascular responses of this agent in the pediatric age group. In children with normal hearts, cardiac index remains unchanged, although shortening fraction decreases and alterations in load-independent parameters of contractility are reported.[90] The myocardial depressant properties of barbiturates are well documented, as well as its effects on venodilation and blood pooling in the periphery. These data suggest that some children who receive thiopental may be at risk for hemodynamic instability. Some recommend that thiopental should be used with caution, particularly in those with limited reserve and/or high sympathetic tone.

Etomidate, a carboxylated imidazole derivative, has anesthetic and amnestic properties but no analgesic effects. This agent demonstrates favorable qualities over other intravenous drugs due to its lack of effect on hemodynamics.[95,96] This, combined with laboratory and clinical data that support minimal effects on myocardial contractility, makes this drug a particularly desirable agent in critically ill children and in those with limited cardiovascular reserve.[97] Despite these benefits, several undesirable side effects are associated with the use of this agent. These include pain on intravenous administration, myoclonic movements that may mimic seizure activity, and inhibition of adrenal steroid synthesis perioperatively.[98,99] Although used primarily as an induction agent, etomidate has been administered for sedation of children during cardiac catheterization and in other settings.[100-102]

Ketamine is a "dissociative" anesthetic agent administered via the intravenous, intramuscular, and oral routes. In view of its sympathomimetic effects, resulting in an increased heart rate, blood pressure, and cardiac output, ketamine has been widely used in children with heart disease, particularly the younger age groups. Because of its effects on systemic vascular resistance, ketamine may be considered a suitable choice in children with right-to-left shunts because pulmonary blood flow would be enhanced. This is in contrast to inhalational agents, which by causing systemic vasodilation may decrease pulmonary blood flow in the presence of an intracardiac communication and potentially worsen the degree of cyanosis. In clinical use, however, oxygen saturation typically increases with both agents. Additional favorable properties of ketamine include the intense analgesia it produces at subanesthetic doses and the fact that the drug is relatively devoid of respiratory depressant effects.

Several investigations have addressed the concern of potential detrimental changes in pulmonary vascular tone resulting from ketamine administration. Two of these studies demonstrated no significant effect in pulmonary arterial pressures or pulmonary vascular resistance at doses used clinically.[103,104] Regarding its effect on myocardial performance, in-vitro studies have shown a direct myocardial depressant effect both in animal species and the failing adult human heart. This is thought to be the result of inhibition of L-type voltage-dependent calcium channels in the sarcolemmal membrane and may be a consideration in critically ill infants with severely impaired cardiac reserve. Additional undesirable effects of ketamine include emergence reactions, excessive salivation, vomiting, and increased intracranial pressure.

Opioids and *benzodiazepines* are widely used medications in pediatric anesthesia practice. Opioids attenuate the neuroendocrine stress response associated with anesthesia and surgery.[105,106]

After repair of congenital heart defects, these medications have been shown to blunt the stress response in the pulmonary circulation elicited by airway manipulations.[107] Commonly used opioids include the naturally occurring morphine and codeine; semisynthetics such as hydromorphone and meperidine; and synthetic agents such as fentanyl, alfentanil, sufentanil, and remifentanil. Morphine administration may be associated with histamine release and hypotension. The synthetic opioids are devoid of these effects and provide excellent hemodynamic stability with minimal changes in heart rate and blood pressure in children with CHD.[108] In general, the primary consideration of opioid administration relates to their central respiratory depressant effects because their primary cardiovascular manifestations are minimal. Benzodiazepines provide sedation and amnesia during the perioperative period. Midazolam has a short duration of action and faster clearance compared with diazepam and lorazepam. Midazolam administration may allow for a reduction in the inspired concentration of volatile anesthetic agents, which is a desirable feature in children with labile hemodynamics or in those considered at high risk for the myocardial depressant properties of inhalational anesthetics. Studies regarding the effects of benzodiazepines in children with CHD are limited.[109]

Muscle relaxants facilitate endotracheal intubation and prevent reflex movement during surgery if the anesthetics alone are insufficient. All inhalational anesthetics potentiate the effects of nondepolarizing muscle relaxants. These medications have varying onset and duration of action and hemodynamic effects. The cardiovascular and autonomic effects of muscle relaxants have been characterized mainly in adults with acquired cardiovascular disease.[110-113] In general, the choice of relaxant is based on the need for surgical relaxation, to facilitate endotracheal intubation, their hemodynamic side effects, and the anticipated duration of surgery.

Induction of Anesthesia

Induction of anesthesia in children with CHD can be accomplished using one of several techniques. The most common approaches consist of the inhaled and intravenous routes. The intramuscular route (i.e., ketamine administration) may be preferable in some cases, particularly in the uncooperative, developmentally delayed, or combative child who will not accept an oral premedication or intravenous catheter placement. Other less common induction techniques include subcutaneous, intranasal, and rectal administration of agents. These various approaches may also be used in combination (see Chapter 4).

An intravenous induction of anesthesia is preferable in some children (those at risk for acute hemodynamic decompensation) because of a potentially greater safety margin. In addition to the ability to titrate medications and rapidly correct hemodynamic alterations, other benefits include the speed of effect, although this may be slowed in children with large left-to-right shunts due to recirculation of the drug in the lungs. Left-to-right shunting results in a less concentrated amount of anesthetic agent reaching the brain and delayed onset of action. Right-to-left shunts speed intravenous induction because a significant portion of the medication directly enters the systemic circulation and, thus, more rapidly reaches the brain.

If intravenous access is not present, an inhalational induction is performed in most cases. A carefully titrated inhalational induction and early placement of an intravenous catheter is generally safe even in children with moderate hemodynamic disturbances, particularly after premedication has been given. This produces loss of consciousness, with acceptable conditions for establishing intravenous access. Inhalation induction may be delayed in cyanotic children and in those with right-to-left shunts because the decreased pulmonary flow limits the rate of increase of the concentration of inhalational anesthetics in the arterial blood. The rapidity of an inhalation induction is increased by low cardiac output because the anesthetic partial pressure in the alveoli increases as less anesthetic is removed by the slow-moving blood in the pulmonary vasculature (see Chapter 6). Left-to-right intracardiac shunts have limited effects on the speed of induction of inhaled anesthetics.

Maintenance of Anesthesia

After induction, anesthesia can be maintained using either an inhalation or intravenous technique. A combination of inhalational and intravenous anesthetics (opioid and muscle relaxant) is frequently used. The same inhalational agent administered for induction may be continued or a different anesthetic or technique may be selected for maintenance. In children with CHD, anesthesia may result in hemodynamic instability regardless of the technique, agents, or experience of the anesthesiologist. Some children may not tolerate even minor alterations in hemodynamics associated with anesthesia or surgical manipulations. Factors that may lead to cardiovascular collapse in the marginally compensated child include hypovolemia, relative anesthetic overdose, increased vagal tone, positive-pressure ventilation, myocardial ischemia, arrhythmia, anaphylaxis, alteration in $Paco_2$ (altering the balance between systemic and pulmonary blood flow), hypoxemia, and airway obstruction. The anesthesiologist should be prepared to manage these rare but occasionally unavoidable occurrences.

Emergence from Anesthesia

Most children undergoing noncardiac surgical interventions are expected to awaken immediately at the completion of the procedure or shortly thereafter. This usually involves reducing and then discontinuing intravenous or inhalational anesthetics, antagonizing neuromuscular blockade, and removing the endotracheal tube, if present. Ensuring the return of protective reflexes and monitoring the adequacy of the airway and respiration are especially important considerations.

Postoperative Care

The postoperative management of the child with CHD involves many of the same physiologic principles applicable to intraoperative care. The extent of the postoperative care, optimal place for recovery, and need for monitoring and hospitalization depends, in large part, on the type and extent of the surgery and the child's clinical condition. Immediately after surgery most children are awakening from anesthesia and recovering from muscle relaxants, which may impose various stresses and hemodynamic changes. Adequate oxygenation and ventilation along with airway protection must be ensured and may need to be provided if the child cannot manage these functions on his or her own. It is of paramount importance to avoid significant hypoventilation during this time because this may negatively affect pulmonary vascular tone and overall hemodynamics in vulnerable children with CHD. Analgesia and, at times, sedation are important postoperatively. This may be a challenging issue in the child who requires noncardiac surgery soon after a prolonged hospitalization in view of the high likelihood for tolerance to sedative/analgesic drugs.

Observation and physical examination provide a great deal of information regarding respiratory status, cardiac function, and systemic perfusion during the postoperative period. Adequacy of oxygenation and ventilation can also be assessed with noninvasive monitoring and blood gas analysis. Monitoring urine output may be helpful.

It is important to monitor hemoglobin or hematocrit values as a measure of oxygen-carrying capability in cases in which significant blood loss may have occurred. Serum electrolytes are screened if fluid shifts may have taken place during the surgical and postoperative periods. Particular attention should be given to the avoidance of hypokalemia in children receiving digoxin. Serum glucose levels should be followed in neonates and small infants and/or dextrose-containing fluids administered as appropriate. Determination of ionized calcium levels may be indicated in those with a history of DiGeorge sequence, because hypocalcemia is a feature of this syndrome. The required fluid replacement is dictated by the child's heart defect, type of surgery performed, and insensible volume losses (see Chapters 8 and 10).

Perioperative Problems and Special Considerations

The potential perioperative problems that may be encountered while caring for children with CHD who require noncardiac interventions are numerous. These relate to multiple factors, including the particular cardiac defect(s) and its pathophysiologic ramifications, the child's functional status, and the nature/complexity of the surgical intervention. In addition, a variety of patient subsets, circumstances, and unique scenarios require particular considerations. Because it is not feasible to detail in a comprehensive manner all possible problems and special considerations, this section highlights a few of these issues to serve as a framework.

Hypotension

Hypotension that occurs during noncardiac surgery may be related to hypovolemia secondary to prolonged fasting, volume loss, arrhythmia, anesthetic agents, myocardial dysfunction, or mechanical influences associated with the operative procedure. A suggested practical diagnostic and therapeutic approach is to consider factors that may affect ventricular preload, contractility, afterload, and the assessment of cardiac rhythm. Although the management of hypotension should be guided primarily by the causative factor, acutely increasing blood pressure by the administration of volume and an appropriate vasopressor, if indicated, often restores adequate perfusion while definitive therapy is instituted. Ensuring adequate intravascular volume with a fluid challenge often helps in restoring perfusion and blood pressure, especially in hypovolemic patients. A pure α-adrenergic agent such as phenylephrine increases systolic blood pressure without further increases in heart rate. Some children are unable to tolerate any degree of myocardial depression or reduction in sympathetic outflow and require continuous inotropic support or vasopressor infusions throughout and after the operative procedure.

Cyanosis

The presence of cyanosis is a common finding among defects characterized by limited pulmonary blood flow or intracardiac mixing. As surgical management strategies evolve to target the youngest of infants, the effects of cyanosis may be limited in these children. However, in those children who require delayed surgery, palliation, or staged correction of their defects, the effects of cyanosis may be of long duration. Chronic hypoxemia affects all major organ systems. Compensatory mechanisms that attempt to provide adequate systemic oxygen delivery in the presence of chronic hypoxemia include polycythemia, increases in blood volume, alterations in oxygen uptake/delivery, and neovascularization. Despite the favorable effects of the adaptive responses, these alterations may also be detrimental. Polycythemia, the most significant compensatory response, is associated with increases in blood viscosity and red cell sludging. The common occurrence of iron-deficiency anemia in cyanotic children further enhances hyperviscosity and the unfavorable consequences of this condition. In addition, a number of hemostatic abnormalities have been documented as a result of hypoxemia and erythrocytosis that may affect the coagulation system and increase perioperative risks.[114,115] This is compounded by increased tissue vascularity, with a large number of blood vessels per unit of tissue. Additional factors that may account for a bleeding diathesis in cyanotic children include thrombocytopenia, altered platelet function, and clotting factor abnormalities.[116-119]

The increased blood viscosity in children with cyanosis is associated with stasis and a risk for thrombotic events.[120] If the hematocrit exceeds 65% preoperatively, some clinicians would advocate phlebotomy to lower the hematocrit to 60% to 65%.[121] This reduces sludging of red blood cells and enhances tissue oxygen delivery. If blood is removed by preoperative phlebotomy, it may be kept for autologous transfusion during the perioperative period.

It is important to maintain adequate preoperative hydration in children with cyanotic CHD, many of whom should be encouraged to drink clear liquids liberally while following recommended fasting guidelines. If this is not possible, consideration should be given to the administration of maintenance fluids by the intravenous route. Care should also be taken to avoid prolonged venous stasis. Adequate hydration and systemic vascular tone should be ensured throughout the surgery.

Cyanotic children are at risk for paradoxical embolic events, mandating meticulous attention to intravenous lines during fluid or drug administration. In fact, it would be reasonable to advocate this approach as a routine for all patients with CHD, regardless of the nature of the structural abnormalities. The addition of air filters to intravenous tubing should not replace vigilance in avoiding the introduction of air into these lines.

Tetralogy Spells

Tetralogy spells, or hypercyanotic episodes, result from decreased pulmonary blood flow in children with significant dynamic right ventricular outflow tract obstruction. In general, these are relatively rare during noncardiac surgery, probably because general anesthesia attenuates the triggers. Occasionally, however, cyanosis may occur without warning in response to obscure stimuli. Whatever the cause, worsening cyanosis generally implies increases in dynamic obstruction and exacerbation of the right-to-left shunting. Factors that decrease systemic blood pressure and systemic vascular resistance such as hypovolemia and extreme vasodilation should be avoided. Therapy includes increasing blood volume, inspired oxygen concentrations, and systemic vascular resistance, often with phenylephrine. Lowering inspiratory ventilatory pressures may also lead to clinical improvement. Additional therapies include increasing the level of sedation or anesthetic depth and β-adrenergic blockade. The pulmonary vascular resistance does not play a major role in the physiology of hypercyanotic episodes in tetralogy of Fallot, although acute increases may account for cyanosis in children with other cardiac anomalies.

Congestive Heart Failure
In infants, congestive heart failure is most often due to ventricular volume overload resulting from intracardiac communications at the ventricular level or left-to-right shunts between the great arteries (e.g., patent ductus arteriosus, aortopulmonary window). In some cases this may be related to severe valvular regurgitation or obstructive lesions. Older children and adults with CHD may have heart failure symptoms as a result of poor myocardial contractility, in which case cardiac output may be compromised and not able to meet the systemic demands. In children with significant pulmonary vascular congestion, positive-pressure mechanical ventilation may be necessary before and after surgery. In cases of elective surgery, it may be of significant benefit to optimize medical therapy and/or address the particular defect(s) before the planned procedure.

Ventricular Dysfunction
Ventricular dysfunction, either right-sided, left-sided, combined, regional, or global, may be present in children with CHD. This may be of a temporary nature in those who have undergone surgery or permanent in some cases. The pathology is classified as systolic in origin if contractile function is primarily impaired or as diastolic if abnormal relaxation or ventricular compliance is present. In some children impairment in both systolic and diastolic function is found. The etiology of ventricular dysfunction is frequently multifactorial and may result from factors such as age at operation and chronicity of the cardiac workload (either pressure or volume); may be secondary to the primary disease, myocardial hypertrophy, ischemia, or cyanosis; or occur as a direct effect of surgery (ventriculotomy, cardiopulmonary bypass, ischemic time or circulatory arrest).

Ventricular Pressure Overload
Pressure overload typically results from residual or recurrent muscular, valvar or distal outflow obstruction, or elevated pulmonary artery pressure and/or vascular resistance. In children with abnormal distal pulmonary arterial beds, for example, the hypoplastic vessels may not be amenable to surgical repair, although associated defects may have been satisfactorily addressed. This results in increased proximal pulmonary artery and right ventricular pressures and compensatory myocardial hypertrophy. Right ventricular pressure may exceed systemic values and compromise left ventricular function because septal shift may impair left ventricular filling or result in obstruction to systemic outflow. Abnormal pressure loads to the right ventricle may also result from progressive conduit stenosis after procedures that involve outflow tract reconstructions. Because of the anticipated need in children for successive conduit replacements, these surgical interventions are delayed as much

as feasibly possible. This implies long-standing pressure loads on the myocardium with associated wall hypertrophy and potentially some element of ischemia until criteria for surgical intervention have been fulfilled.

Whether the altered loading conditions affect the right or left ventricle primarily, the result is an increased demand due to the increased wall tension. This implies an increased susceptibility of the ventricular myocardium to the supply-and-demand relationship, a reduced tolerance for factors that may alter this fine balance, and an increased risk of ischemia.

Ventricular Volume Overload
Ventricular volume overload, as manifested by increased left atrial pressure, left ventricular end-diastolic, and stroke volumes, is a common feature in many children with unoperated CHD. Long-standing volume overload results in atrial enlargement, ventricular dilation, and cardiomegaly. In the postoperative child, residual valvar regurgitation may be associated with altered loading conditions that, if significant, may result in congestive symptoms and ventricular dysfunction. The palliated single-ventricle patient may be particularly vulnerable to conditions associated with ventricular volume overload (e.g., shunts).

Myocardial Ischemia
A number of factors have been implicated in the etiology of myocardial ischemia in children with CHD. These include chronic hypoxemia, increased systolic and diastolic wall stress, and decreased coronary perfusion secondary to low diastolic pressures in the presence of large systemic-to-pulmonary shunts. Conditions that may be associated with myocardial ischemia include lesions such as anomalous origin of the left coronary artery from the pulmonary artery and increased blood viscosity associated with cyanosis. The deprivation of myocardial perfusion may result in ventricular dysfunction and subsequent development of myocardial fibrosis in these children.

Altered Respiratory Mechanics
Chronically increased pulmonary blood flow and pulmonary artery pressures may result in progressive pulmonary vascular changes, increases in pulmonary vascular resistance, and alterations in lung mechanics. The primary effects on respiratory mechanics relate to increased airway resistance and decreased lung compliance. These alterations may have detrimental respiratory consequences in children with inadequate palliation or residual shunts. In some children, left atrial dilation may lead to respiratory compromise (air trapping, atelectasis) due to bronchial compression.

Pulmonary Hypertension and Increased Pulmonary Vascular Resistance
Pulmonary hypertension is a relatively common feature of unoperated CHD that may persist or develop after surgery. In the unoperated child, the increased pulmonary artery pressures are likely related to increased pulmonary blood flow. One of the benefits of early correction is a reduction in pulmonary artery pressures and a reduced incidence of pulmonary vascular reactivity after cardiac surgery. A less frequent entity is that of increased pulmonary vascular resistance. It is important to consider whether this is of a reactive or fixed nature. In some cases both components may be present. This information is derived

Table 21-2. Factors Known to Increase Pulmonary Vascular Tone

Hypoxemia
Hypercarbia
Acidemia
Hypothermia
Atelectasis
Transmitted positive airway pressure
Stress response/stimulation/light anesthesia

from formal invasive evaluations and vasodilator testing, aimed at addressing this question.

Although pulmonary hypertension is a feature of many cardiac anomalies, only a minority of children these days are susceptible to acute pulmonary hypertensive crisis due to a reactive pulmonary vascular bed. In a child with an intracardiac communication that allows for shunting, acute increases in pulmonary artery pressure may be suggested by acute arterial desaturation, bradycardia, and/or systemic hypotension. In the absence of an intracardiac shunt, elevations of pulmonary artery pressures or resistance result in increased right ventricular afterload, unfavorable leftward shifting of the interventricular septum leading to compromised left ventricular filling, and decreased cardiac output.

A number of factors influence pulmonary vascular tone, resulting in increased right ventricular afterload, tricuspid regurgitation, right ventricular dilation, and left ventricular dysfunction (Table 21-2). Therapy is directed toward decreasing pulmonary artery pressures with sedation, hyperventilation, hyperoxygenation, and treatment of acidosis. Acute pulmonary hypertensive crises might require the use of selective pulmonary vasodilators such as inhaled nitric oxide or other agents, as well as inotropic therapy to support right ventricular function. Manipulation of pulmonary hemodynamics is challenged by the difficulty of directly measuring pulmonary artery pressures in children. Management of these critical situations requires a thorough understanding of the pathophysiologic process and a great deal of clinical judgment. Because of the potential significant morbidity and even mortality in children with a history of severe pulmonary hypertension, an in-depth consideration of the risk-benefit ratio of the planned procedure and its impact on the overall quality of life is essential.

Infective Endocarditis

The American Heart Association recently published revised guidelines for the prevention of infective endocarditis (see Chapter 14).[122] The new guidelines recommend that routine antibiotic prophylaxis is no longer needed for many children with CHD although it was suggested in the past. In addition, the administration of antibiotics solely to prevent endocarditis is no longer recommended for children undergoing genitourinary or gastrointestinal tract procedures.

The new guidelines target individuals at increased risk for a poor outcome if they develop endocarditis. Based on the review of scientific evidence preventive antibiotics for dental procedures are now recommended for children with:

- Prosthetic cardiac valve
- History of infective endocarditis

- Congenital heart disease
  - Unrepaired cyanotic CHD (including palliative shunts and conduits)
  - Completely repaired congenital heart defect with prosthetic material or device, whether placed by surgery or by catheter intervention, only for the first 6 months after the procedure
  - Repaired CHD with residual defects at the site or adjacent to the site of a prosthetic patch or prosthetic device (which inhibit endothelialization)
- Cardiac transplantation recipients who develop cardiac valvulopathy

Systemic Air Embolization

The presence of shunts in children with CHD allows for potential right-to-left shunting and paradoxical systemic air embolization. This risk is further enhanced by the presence of increased right-sided pressures or pulmonary vascular resistance in association with many cardiovascular malformations. Because this may lead to catastrophic consequences, it is imperative to ascertain the presence of, or likelihood for, intracardiac/vascular shunting or assume that this may potentially be the case in most children and consider appropriate precautions.

Anticoagulation

Anticoagulants, antiplatelet drugs, and thrombolytic agents are increasingly being utilized in the pediatric age group, particularly in those with CHD.[123-127] Decisions regarding management of children receiving these drugs during noncardiac surgery are primarily influenced by the nature of the procedure, urgency of the intervention, specific drug therapy, and expected effects/laboratory data. The major concern relates to the potential for bleeding. Recommendations regarding optimal management of anticoagulation in patients on warfarin (Coumadin) therapy during the perioperative period vary widely.[128-130] The various strategies are quite heterogeneous, and the lack of consensus is related to the paucity of randomized trials addressing this issue. The problem is further complicated in children owing to the lack of guidelines specific to pediatric practice.[131] In general, if the indications for anticoagulation are for native valve disease or atrial arrhythmias, the risk of a major thromboembolic event is considered relatively low and warfarin may be discontinued 1 to 2 weeks before the day of surgery. In those with mechanical prosthetic valves, the risk of thromboembolic events is considered greater. Many recommend discontinuation of oral anticoagulation a few days before surgery,[128] allowing the prothrombin time to return to at least 20% of normal. Administration of parenteral vitamin K or clotting factors including fresh frozen plasma may be required to restore the prothrombin time within an acceptable range, especially in those with liver disease and in emergency cases. Some experts advise preoperative hospitalization, particularly in high-risk individuals such as those with mitral or combined valve prostheses, in order to discontinue warfarin therapy and to initiate a heparin infusion, which is continued up until a few hours before surgery. Others suggest that low-molecular-weight heparin might be a better option over unfractionated heparin because the perioperative conversion from warfarin therapy can be accomplished without the need for hospitalization.[129] Anticoagulation is usually reinitiated after 24 hours in children with valvular prostheses, and this may be achieved with either a continuous heparin infusion or intermittent subcutaneous injections. The advantage of heparin is the ability to rapidly reverse the drug effect with protamine sulfate if bleeding complications occur. Oral anticoagulants are reinitiated 2 to 3 days after surgery if there are no bleeding concerns and the child is able to swallow oral medications. Although it has been suggested that there is no need to discontinue anticoagulation therapy for minor procedures, such as dental or ophthalmologic surgery in adults, guidelines for children are less clear.

The risk of bleeding from the surgical intervention versus the potential for thromboembolism from a lowered anticoagulant dose determines to what extent and for what duration the anticoagulant therapy should be reduced. In some cases, the cardiologist and surgeon may decide to temporarily switch to aspirin therapy before and after the surgery. There is disagreement regarding whether antiplatelet therapy is preferable to anticoagulation in children with prosthetic aortic valves or after certain surgical interventions.[132-135]

Conduction Disturbances and Arrhythmias

Acute rhythm disturbances may occur with the use of any anesthetic agent or technique and may be related to a variety of factors. A preoperative history or pathology associated with arrhythmias requires consideration of the risk-benefit ratio while administering agents with vagolytic or sympathomimetic properties. Bradycardia may occur during induction of anesthesia, laryngoscopy, and endotracheal intubation, particularly in infants and those with Down syndrome.[136] In most cases, the bradycardia is self-limited and requires no therapy. Drugs such as atropine, epinephrine, and isoproterenol, if needed, are generally effective in the treatment of bradycardia unless the bradycardia is caused by hypoxia or associated with advanced heart block. Atrioventricular block that fails to respond to chronotropic drugs may require transthoracic or transvenous pacing (see Chapter 14).

Several types of congenital pathologies are associated with a high likelihood of rhythm abnormalities and/or arrhythmias. These have the potential for acute hemodynamic deterioration and increase perioperative risk. If feasible, this should be evaluated fully before the surgery. Conduction system abnormalities and rhythm disturbances may occur following cardiac surgery in children. This may be a direct result of the procedure or may subsequently develop due to the inadequacy of the palliation or repair. Because the incidence of cardiac arrhythmias is more prevalent among specific surgical subgroups, anticipation for this occurrence and planning for management is advocated. Sinus node dysfunction, for example, may occur after extensive atrial baffling procedures, such as Mustard or Senning operations, or after the Fontan procedure. In some children, but particularly in those with single-ventricle physiology or significant functional impairment, loss of sinus rhythm may negatively affect the adequacy of cardiac output. Preparation should include the availability of appropriate medications and immediate access to devices suitable for management of conduction abnormalities/arrhythmias.

Pacemakers and Implantable Cardioverter-Defibrillators

An in-depth discussion of perioperative considerations in children with implanted devices can be found in Chapter 14. Briefly, it should be emphasized that perioperative consultation with a cardiologist/electrophysiologist is essential when caring for those with implanted pacemakers or defibrillators. Device interrogation and programming is required in most cases before the planned procedure. The purpose would be to avoid potential problems with pacemaker malfunction related to electromagnetic interference (electrocautery). Chronotropic agents and backup pacing modalities (transvenous, epicardial, transcutaneous) should be readily available and carefully considered in the event of pacemaker malfunction associated with an inadequate underlying heart rate. Capture thresholds can be affected by pharmacologic agents (i.e., increased by amiodarone), and this should be considered in children who are receiving antiarrhythmic drug therapy. A magnet should be accessible to allow for asynchronous pacing if required. Perioperative ECG monitoring is essential, as well as modalities that confirm pulse generation during pacing (esophageal stethoscope for assessment of heart sounds, pulse oximetry, invasive arterial blood pressure monitoring). Implanted devices should be interrogated and reprogrammed after a surgical procedure.

Nerve Palsies

Surgery for CHD is associated with risks of injury to the recurrent laryngeal and phrenic nerves. These injuries may be transient or permanent. Recurrent laryngeal nerve injuries may result in abnormal phonation or airway difficulties and lead to aspiration, particularly in small infants. Diaphragmatic palsies resulting from phrenic nerve injuries are associated with abnormal lung mechanics and limited pulmonary reserve, both of which may account for perioperative complications during noncardiac surgery.

Eisenmenger Syndrome

Eisenmenger syndrome is characterized by irreversible pulmonary vascular disease and cyanosis related to reversal in the direction of an intracardiac or arterial level shunt.[137,138] This is unlikely to occur in the current surgical era, but it may occasionally occur in an older child, adolescent, or adult with CHD. Morbidity in these individuals relates to problems associated with chronic cyanosis and erythrocytosis. They may suffer from thromboembolic events, cerebrovascular complications, and hyperviscosity syndrome. Other problems include hemoptysis, gout, cholelithiasis, hypertrophic osteoarthropathy, and decreased renal function. Variables associated with poor outcome include syncope, elevated right ventricular end-diastolic pressure, and significant hypoxemia (systemic arterial oxygen saturation <85%). Life expectancy is significantly shortened, with a reported survival rate of 80% at 10 years, 77% at 15 years, and 42% at 25 years.[139] Most patients succumb suddenly, probably from ventricular tachyarrhythmias. Surgical modalities that have been advocated in selected patients include combined heart and lung transplantation,[140] as well as lung transplantation alone.[141]

Despite the overall poor prognosis, a number of reports have documented successes with a variety of anesthetic techniques and agents.[142-146] A published review of anesthesia and surgery in patients with Eisenmenger syndrome identified an overall mortality rate of 14%. Regional anesthesia was associated with a perioperative mortality rate of 5%, whereas those receiving general anesthesia had a mortality of 18%. The investigators concluded, however, that mortality in this patient group was most likely a result of the surgical procedure and disease rather than the anesthesia.[145] Nevertheless it is vital that the family and patient, if of appropriate age, understand these risks before undertaking any procedure requiring anesthesia or deep sedation.

Post–Cardiac Transplant Recipients

Cardiac transplantation is considered a viable option in certain children and adolescents with end-stage cardiac pathology as a result of either congenital or acquired disease.[147] A major consideration in the care of these children relates to the issue of the lack of external nerve supply of the transplanted heart. The physiology of the denervated heart implies that the usual autonomic regulatory mechanisms are not operational, increasing the vulnerability of transplanted children to hemodynamic alterations.[148] In addition, compensatory responses may be delayed, further increasing the potential for compromise.

In the transplanted heart, the resting heart rate is faster than normal owing to the loss of parasympathetic inhibition. Critical determinants of cardiac output in these individuals include the systemic venous return and maintenance of an adequate heart rate. During the early post-transplant period, heart rate is supported by exogenous chronotropes or pacing. Subsequently, heart rate is driven by circulating endogenous catecholamines. Regardless of the time interval from transplantation, while caring for these children medications with chronotropic properties should be available as well as drugs with direct action on the myocardium and vasculature. Emergent cardiac pacing modalities should be readily accessible.

Chronic immunosuppression in children who have undergone transplantation presents a number of issues during noncardiac surgery. First is the concern regarding the administration of multiple medications, particularly immunosuppressant agents, throughout the perioperative period, in addition to the potential need for "stress" dose corticosteroids, a controversial subject. Second is the fact that immunosuppressive therapy is associated with side effects that may affect various organ systems. Cyclosporine administration, for example, increases systemic arterial blood pressure, potentially influencing hemodynamics. The drug is also responsible for renal dysfunction. Anesthetic management must consider potential alterations in hepatic and renal function. Third, there is the need for strict practice of an aseptic technique in the presence of a compromised immune system.

An additional anesthetic consideration is the potential for graft vasculopathy (small vessel coronary artery disease). Because older children/adolescents with ongoing myocardial ischemia may not experience anginal symptoms, it is reasonable to assume that most of these children are at risk for ischemic events, particularly those who are several years after transplantation.

Perioperative Stress Response

The typical physiologic response to painful stimuli in normal children consists of an increase in heart rate and blood pressure and a transient decrease in Pao_2. These normal patterns, however, may be detrimental to children with unoperated CHD or those who may have undergone interventions. Tachycardia may shorten diastolic filling time and diminish cardiac output. Hypertension may compromise increases in ventricular afterload. The reduced ability of the postoperative child with CHD to increase cardiac output in response to stimulation and their limited maximal exercise capacity have been well documented for a number of cardiac malformations.

Outcomes of Noncardiac Surgery

There is a paucity of data regarding the risks of noncardiac surgery and anesthesia in children with CHD. However, the available information raises some concerns. A review of 110 children with CHD who underwent 135 anesthetic procedures over a period of a year reported adverse events in 47% and more than a single adverse event in a significant number of children.[33] The subject of perioperative rhythm abnormalities was examined prospectively in 70 children with CHD and a history of ventricular arrhythmias. Continuous monitoring documented a 35% and 87% incidence of intraoperative and postoperative ventricular arrhythmias, respectively.[149] Other studies have demonstrated cyanosis, treatment for congestive heart failure, poor health, and young age as risk factors.[34] A retrospective database review in a large number of children also documented that these risks involved both major and minor interventions.[36]

Specific Congenital Heart Defects

The anesthetic management of children with CHD undergoing noncardiac surgery is significantly influenced by the specific nature of the cardiovascular malformation(s), associated pathophysiology of the lesion(s), extent of palliative/definitive procedure, and presence of complications associated with the primary pathology or treatment. This section addresses relevant anatomic features and hemodynamic consequences of selected cardiac defects because this is essential in the formulation of appropriate management strategies. In addition, potential residua, sequelae (Table 21-3), and long-term outcome of these lesions are discussed, focusing on their implications for perioperative care.

Atrial Septal Defects

Anatomy and Pathophysiology

Defects in the interatrial septum or atrial septal defects (ASDs) (see Fig. 15-1B) are among the most common congenital cardiac anomalies in childhood. Based on their location, several types of defects are identified as follows:

1. *Ostium secundum or fossa ovalis defect* (most common type). This results from a deficiency in the region of the fossa ovalis (region of the septum primum or area near or at the mid aspect of the interatrial septum). An association with mitral valve prolapse and/or mitral regurgitation is well recognized.[150-152]

2. *Ostium primum defect,* regarded as a form of atrioventricular septal (canal or endocardial cushion) defect (see Fig. 15-1A).[153] This is characterized by a deficiency in the inferior portion of the interatrial septum and is frequently associated with a commissure or "cleft" in the anterior leaflet of the mitral valve, potentially resulting in varying degrees of regurgitation.

3. *Sinus venosus defect,* usually located in the superior aspect of the interatrial septum, just below the region where the superior vena cava joins the right atrium (superior vena cava type of sinus venosus defect) (see Fig. 15-1C).[154] A less common equivalent defect may occur posteriorly at the inferior vena cava to right atrial junction (inferior vena cava type of defect). These defects are frequently associated with anomalous pulmonary venous drainage.[155]

Table 21-3. Potential Long-Term Issues after Interventions for Selected Congenital Heart Defects

Atrial Septal Defects

- Residual intracardiac shunt
- Persistent right ventricular dilation and abnormal motion of interventricular septum
- Atrial arrhythmias/ventricular dysfunction if late repair
- Pulmonary venous obstruction (sinus venosus defect associated with anomalous pulmonary venous return)
- Mitral valve problems/left ventricular outflow tract obstruction (ostium primum defect with cleft mitral valve)
- Development of pulmonary vascular disease (rare)

Atrioventricular Septal Defects

- Mitral valve problems (regurgitation/stenosis)
- Left ventricular outflow tract obstruction
- Residual intracardiac shunts
- Atrioventricular block/conduction abnormalities
- If prior palliation with pulmonary artery banding, this may have resulted in inadequate protection of pulmonary vasculature or distortion of pulmonary artery anatomy
- Pulmonary hypertension may persist

Coarctation of the Aorta

- Systemic hypertension
- Residual/recurrent obstruction
- Death in untreated pathology related to heart failure, aortic rupture/dissection, infective endarteritis/endocarditis, premature coronary artery disease, or cerebral hemorrhage
- Endocarditis risk with concomitant aortic valve disease

Coronary Artery Anomalies

- May go unsuspected for a period of time
- Myocardial ischemia
- Ventricular dysfunction
- May present as syncope or lead to sudden death

D-Transposition of the Great Arteries

- Residual pathology (intracardiac shunts, outflow tract obstruction)
- After atrial baffle procedure: baffle leak, obstruction of systemic or pulmonary venous pathways, progressive right ventricular dilation/failure, tricuspid regurgitation, sinus node dysfunction, atrial arrhythmias
- After arterial switch operation: aortic root dilation, aortic regurgitation, supravalvar stenosis (pulmonary or aortic), coronary insufficiency

Ebstein Anomaly

- Progressive tricuspid regurgitation and right-sided volume overload
- Right ventricular dysfunction
- Atrial tachyarrhythmias
- Potential for paradoxical right-to-left shunting in the presence of an interatrial communication
- Valve repair/replacement may be necessary

Interrupted Aortic Arch

- Residual intracardiac defects
- Subaortic obstruction
- Residual/recurrent aortic arch obstruction

Left Ventricular Outflow Tract Obstruction

- Residual/recurrent obstruction
- Aortic regurgitation/aortic root dilation
- Risk of endocarditis
- Ventricular dysfunction
- Potential subendocardial ischemia if ongoing ventricular pressure overload
- Coronary ostial stenosis, diffuse arteriopathy (supravalvar aortic stenosis)
- Need for reoperation in those with bioprosthetic or mechanical valves/conduits
- After Ross procedure: autograft/right ventricular homograft failure, progressive aortic root dilation, aortic regurgitation

L-Transposition of the Great Arteries (Congenitally Corrected Transposition of the Great Arteries

- Residual defects (shunts, outflow tract obstruction)
- Systemic (right) ventricular dilation, dysfunction, failure
- Left-sided (tricuspid) valve regurgitation
- Atrioventricular block/arrhythmias

Patent Ductus Arteriosus

- Residual/recurrent shunting
- Increased pulmonary vascular resistance (rare in current surgical era)

Right Ventricular Outflow Tract Obstruction

- Residual/recurrent obstruction resulting in ventricular pressure overload
- Pulmonary regurgitation may require intervention
- After right ventricular to pulmonary artery conduit: need for reoperation related to conduit failure

Single Ventricle

- After aortopulmonary shunt: shunt stenosis with associated hypoxemia, ventricular volume overload, systemic ventricular dilation, distortion of pulmonary artery anatomy, pulmonary hypertension
- After bidirectional Glenn connection/hemi-Fontan procedure: progressive cyanosis due to venous collaterals or other vascular communications allowing for venous pathways to bypass the pulmonary circuit or due to the development of pulmonary arteriovenous malformations (more likely with classic Glenn anastomosis)
- After Fontan procedure: increased venous pressures, right atrial hypertension (with atriopulmonary connection), sinus node dysfunction, atrial rhythm disturbances, atrioventricular valve regurgitation, hepatic dysfunction, thrombotic complications, coagulation defects, protein losing enteropathy, progressive systemic ventricular dilation/dysfunction

Table 21-3 (continued). Potential Long-Term Issues after Interventions for Selected Congenital Heart Defects

Tetralogy of Fallot	*Truncus Arteriosus*
• Residual/recurrent pathology (intracardiac shunts, right ventricular outflow tract obstruction, distal pulmonary artery bed abnormalities)	• Residual intracardiac shunting
	• Revision of right ventricular to pulmonary artery reconstruction (for stenosis/regurgitation)
• Progressive pulmonary regurgitation with need for re-intervention (right-sided heart dilation and/or dysfunction)	• Truncal (aortic) valve stenosis/regurgitation
• Arrhythmias in association with poor hemodynamics	*Ventricular Septal Defect*
• Syncope/sudden death (presumably arrhythmogenic in nature)	• Potential residual defect(s)
• Restrictive right ventricular physiology	• Risk of endocarditis (diminishes with time after repair)
	• Aortic regurgitation
	• In rare cases of increased pulmonary vascular resistance, this may not improve postoperatively.

4. *Coronary sinus defects* (relatively rare) consist of a communication between the left atrium and mouth of the coronary sinus. These are commonly associated with an unroofed coronary sinus and persistent left superior vena cava that drains directly into the left atrium, accounting for a right-to-left shunt.[156]

5. *Other entities* that allow for interatrial shunting include a patent foramen ovale (PFO) at one end of the spectrum and a confluent or common atrium at the other. A PFO has been identified in as many of 25% of individuals. The presence of this communication may have implications for perioperative care.[157,158] A common atrium is characterized by complete or near-total absence of the interatrial septum and may be a finding in complex CHD.

An atrial communication allows for mixing of the pulmonary and systemic venous returns. A shunt in the left-to-right direction allows for pulmonary venous blood to enter the right atrium. The magnitude of interatrial shunting relates to the size of the defect, relative ventricular compliances, and pulmonary artery pressures. A clinically significant defect results in right-sided volume overload. A pulmonary-to-systemic blood flow ratio ($\dot{Q}p{:}\dot{Q}s$) that exceeds $2{:}1$ and the potential detrimental effects of chronic right ventricular volume overload are considerations for intervention.

Potential Residua, Sequelae, and Long-Term Outcome
Surgical closure of ASDs in childhood provides excellent results and almost normal long-term survival.[159-162] Surgical mortality is essentially negligible for isolated secundum defects. Minimally invasive techniques using a limited median sternotomy may result in faster postoperative recovery and improved cosmetic results. Normal ventricular function should be anticipated after repair of these defects. Rarely, children may demonstrate persistent right ventricular dilation and abnormal ventricular septal motion postoperatively. However, this may not be associated with a functional deficit.[163] Late repair of defects may lead to the development of atrial arrhythmias and ventricular dysfunction as a result of chronic volume overload. The abnormally increased pulmonary blood flow, if defect closure is delayed, may be a risk factor for the development of pulmonary vascular disease later in life, although this rarely occurs. The transcatheter route may be considered as an alternative to the surgical approach for closure of secundum ASDs in selected children, with excellent success rates reported par-

ticularly for relatively small communications (see Chapter 20).[164-168] Complications are relatively rare and may occur in association with the intervention or at a later time.[169]

Morbidity after surgical closure of ostium primum defects relates primarily to mitral valve dysfunction (mitral regurgitation) and, rarely, to left ventricular outflow tract obstruction.[170-174] In the majority of children, outcomes are favorable after repair at an early age.

After closure of sinus venosus defects, potential problems include the presence of residual shunts, pulmonary venous obstruction, or loss of sinus node function.[175-177] The repair of coronary sinus defects consists of patch closure of the atrial communication at the mouth of the coronary sinus.[178] In this approach a small right-to-left shunt remains as deoxygenated blood from the coronary sinus continues to drain directly into the left atrium. If a connection between the left superior vena cava and left atrium is present, a variety of surgical approaches are available to allow for redirection of the abnormal systemic venous return. In most children with atrial communications, significant postoperative sequelae are unlikely to occur and outcomes are generally good. Thus, in the majority of cases no major repercussion from the repaired defect should be expected for anesthetic care.

Ventricular Septal Defects

Anatomy and Pathophysiology
Ventricular septal defects (VSDs) are the most common of all congenital cardiac anomalies, excluding a bicuspid aortic valve (see Fig. 15-2A).[179] These can be found in isolation or within the context of other structural malformations. Large defects require early attention for symptomatology related to congestive heart failure or pulmonary hypertension. VSDs have a greater rate of spontaneous closure in childhood.[180,181]

Various classification schemes have been proposed for these defects based on their anatomic location, size, restrictive or nonrestrictive nature, and hemodynamic significance.[182,183] The scheme noted here categorizes defects into four major morphologic types based on their anatomic location. In some cases, however, the boundaries of a defect may extend beyond the margin of a particular region of the ventricular septum into another.

1. *Perimembranous defects* (most common type) are located in the membranous region, under the septal leaflet of the

tation, residual shunts, and the presence of abnormal communications between the systemic and pulmonary vascular beds (aortopulmonary collaterals). Ventricular pressure loads, on the other hand, may result from residual or recurrent right ventricular outflow tract or obstruction to the pulmonary artery bed. This is associated with right ventricular hypertension, myocardial hypertrophy, and reduced ventricular compliance.

Conditions that may require re-intervention include pulmonary regurgitation of significant severity, residual or recurrent pulmonary outflow tract obstruction, and residual hemodynamically significant intracardiac shunts. Catheter-based procedures may be effective in the management of obstruction of the pulmonary vasculature and have been applied to rehabilitate the vascular tree in cases of significant underdevelopment. Children who have undergone right ventricular to pulmonary artery reconstruction by means of placement of an extracardiac conduit eventually develop conduit failure (stenosis and/or regurgitation) requiring reoperation.[244] Aortic root dilation can lead to increasing degrees of regurgitation and the need for surgical intervention.

In the past, most children underwent definitive repair at an older age, consisting of an extensive right ventriculotomy to facilitate resection of the infundibular obstruction and closure of the VSD. A significant number were also subjected to procedures that included placement of a large patch that encompassed the subpulmonic region, valve annulus, and supravalvar region (transannular patch). Although effective in relieving the obstruction, this invariably resulted in pulmonary regurgitation, which, although reasonably well-tolerated, is known to progress over time. On late follow-up, pulmonary regurgitation has been a significant cause of morbidity and, if not addressed, may result in progressive right ventricular dysfunction due to significant volume overload, ventricular arrhythmias with its associated disability, and even death. In recognition of the long-term morbidity linked to severe pulmonary regurgitation, the surgical strategy for this defect has undergone appraisal and modification over the years.[245] The current approach involves avoidance of an extensive ventriculotomy, if feasible, limiting the infundibular incision and avoiding or limiting the size of the transannular patch. Although these refinements have led to overall improvements in postoperative outcomes, the preoperative evaluation of children after repair of TOF for noncardiac surgery should include inquiries regarding exercise tolerance, as an indicator of functional status, in addition to an appraisal of right ventricular function, residual pathology, potential rhythm abnormalities, and conduction disturbances. Magnetic resonance imaging has become an extremely helpful imaging modality to evaluate right ventricular systolic function, quantitate the severity of pulmonary regurgitation, and evaluate the distal pulmonary vascular bed. Electrophysiologic testing and programmed ventricular stimulation may be indicated to refine antiarrhythmic drug therapy, for ablation of arrhythmia foci, and/or implantation of a cardioverter-defibrillator system.

Postoperatively, a subset of children with tetralogy develop a pattern that is characterized by right ventricular diastolic noncompliance, known as "restrictive right ventricular physiology." This is associated with a reduced likelihood of progressive pulmonary regurgitation and right ventricular dilation. In these children, the right ventricle operates at a greater end-diastolic pressure and they demonstrate superior exercise performance in addition to a reduced likelihood of developing ventricular rhythm abnormalities.[246]

Perioperative goals in the child with TOF, pulmonary regurgitation, and right ventricular dysfunction after definitive intervention include optimizing right ventricular filling, maintaining/supporting right ventricular function (i.e., avoiding agents with detrimental effects on systolic function, instituting inotropic therapy), and minimizing factors that may further increase right ventricular work (i.e., increased pulmonary vascular resistance, increased peak inspiratory pressures). It is important to take into account that any detrimental factor that may affect the right ventricle may also negatively affect the left ventricle due to ventricular interdependence, and, by decreasing left ventricular filling and function, may compromise cardiac output. In children with restrictive right ventricular physiology the myocardial supply-to-demand relationship is of particular importance because the stiff, poorly compliant right ventricular myocardium may not tolerate alterations in this balance and may be vulnerable to decreases in subendocardial oxygen delivery.

D-Transposition of the Great Arteries

Anatomy and Pathophysiology
In D-transposition of the great arteries (D-TGA) the aorta arises from the anatomic right ventricle and the pulmonary artery arises from the left ventricle (see Fig. 15-6). This anomaly accounts for the most common cause of cyanotic heart disease during the neonatal period. Associated defects include a VSD, left ventricular outflow tract obstruction, and coronary artery anomalies.

In D-TGA the systemic and pulmonary circulations operate in parallel rather than in series as is normally the case, resulting in cyanosis. Mixing at the atrial, ventricular, or ductal level is essential for survival. Initial management in most infants includes prostaglandin E_1 therapy to maintain ductal patency and enhance intercirculatory mixing. If restrictive, the interatrial communication may require enlargement by balloon atrial septostomy.

Because comorbidities requiring noncardiac surgical care are unlikely to occur in the majority of neonates with D-TGA, most of the anesthetic concerns before surgical correction apply to diagnostic procedures or interventions in the cardiac catheterization laboratory. Considerations for anesthetic management primarily relate to cyanosis and heart failure (more likely to occur in infants with coexistent large VSDs). An inadequate communication for intercirculatory mixing may account for profound hypoxemia, potentially progressing to metabolic acidosis due to compromised tissue oxygenation. Less commonly, a high pulmonary vascular resistance may account for severe cyanosis despite prostaglandin E_1 therapy and an adequate anatomic communication.

Potential Residua, Sequelae, and Long-Term Outcome
The standard surgical approach for this defect several decades ago consisted of an atrial baffle (atrial switch) or redirection procedure (such as the Mustard or Senning operations). This accomplished physiologic correction by allowing systemic venous blood to drain into the left ventricle and pulmonary artery, while pulmonary venous blood was rerouted through the tricuspid valve into the right ventricle and aorta. The right ventricle remained as the chamber ejecting against systemic afterload. These procedures provided relief of cyanosis and reasonably good survival.[247] However, in the long term they led to complica-

tions such as sinus node dysfunction and the development of atrial rhythm disturbances. In these individuals, the likelihood of sinus rhythm significantly decreased over time, whereas the incidence of junctional rhythm, intra-atrial reentry tachycardia/ atrial flutter, and other complex atrial arrhythmias dramatically increased with age.[248] The abnormal afterload resulted in progressive right ventricular dilation, tricuspid (systemic atrioventricular valve) annular dilation, associated regurgitation, and eventual right ventricular dysfunction/failure.[249-251] This, in addition to the rhythm abnormalities and conduction defects, was thought to account for sudden death in a number of individuals later in life. Other problems included progressive obstruction of venous pathways and intracardiac shunting through atrial baffle leaks. It is not surprising that reduced exercise tolerance, as well as abnormal right and left ventricular responses to exercise, have been documented in these patients.[252]

The complications associated with atrial redirection procedures prompted the evolution of a new surgical strategy for this lesion. At present, the arterial switch operation (Jatene procedure) is the standard surgical approach in neonates with D-TGA. The repair establishes a normal, concordant relationship between the ventricles and their respective great arteries, achieving anatomic correction. The procedure involves transection of the arterial trunks above the level of the semilunar valves, anastomotic connections to their appropriate outflows, translocation of the coronary arteries to the neoaortic root, and, if present, closure of intracardiac communications (see Fig. 15-7A-D). Normal physiology is restored, allowing for the left ventricle to become the systemic pump. This operation is performed during the neonatal period with relatively low mortality and almost absent late mortality.[253] Long-term outcomes are generally very favorable.[254-256] Early in the surgical experience supravalvar pulmonary obstruction related to the anastomotic site was a common occurrence; however, modifications in surgical techniques have significantly reduced the need for catheter-based interventions or reoperation for this complication. A less common problem is obstruction across the aortic suture line. Mild neoaortic root dilation and trivial to mild aortic regurgitation are frequently identified by echocardiography during follow-up, but, in general, are not considered to have major hemodynamic implications. Ventricular function is normal in the majority of cases.[257]

Most children undergoing noncardiac surgery after the arterial switch operation have been managed as those without structural or functional abnormalities, without reported ill events. However, there is some concern for coronary complications in these children that may not be readily evident clinically or by routine surveillance methods. Investigations have demonstrated postoperative regional left ventricular wall motion abnormalities, evidence of myocardial perfusion defects, and pathologic changes in the coronary vasculature, suggesting that some children may be at risk for coronary insufficiency.[258-262]

Congenitally Corrected Transposition of the Great Arteries

Anatomy and Pathophysiology

This defect, also known as L-transposition of the great arteries (L-TGA), is characterized by malposition of the great vessels and ventricular inversion (atrioventricular and ventriculoarterial discordance). In children with this anomaly, the right atrium empties into an anatomic left ventricle that then contracts into the pulmonary trunk. The left atrium opens into an anatomic right ventricle that, in turns, ejects into the aorta. The aorta is typically oriented in a leftward and anterior position with respect to the pulmonary artery.

Cyanosis is absent because the circulations are considered to be physiologically corrected. The anatomic right ventricle functions as the systemic pump. Associated defects are frequently present and include pulmonary outflow tract obstruction, a ventricular communication, and tricuspid (left-sided) abnormalities. In some individuals this lesion may remain undetected until the onset of arrhythmias or syncope, owing to complete atrioventricular block or the effects of concomitant pathology.[263]

Potential Residua, Sequelae, and Long-Term Outcome

Without associated defects, children with corrected transposition may do well for many years. The development of complete atrioventricular block is common with increasing age.[264] Selected children, particularly those at a young age or with coexistent defects that maintain left ventricular pressure at systemic levels, may be suitable candidates for a surgical intervention that restores the left ventricle as the systemic chamber.[265] This complex repair, known as the double-switch operation or a variation thereof, combines redirection of the systemic and pulmonary venous flows in an atrial baffle procedure with the arterial switch operation. This strategy, however, may not affect mortality compared with conservative management.[266]

Issues that require long-term surveillance in children with congenitally corrected transposition include right ventricular performance and tricuspid valve competency, in view of the chronic pressure and, possibly, volume overload. Late right ventricular systolic impairment and progressive tricuspid regurgitation culminating in heart failure may occur.[267] The overall long-term survival of individuals with this condition is substantially reduced compared with age-matched controls.[268,269]

Truncus Arteriosus

Anatomy and Pathophysiology

This malformation is characterized by a single arterial trunk that gives rise to the aorta, pulmonary root, and coronary arteries (see Fig. 15-8). A ventricular communication is almost always present underneath the single arterial root or truncal valve. Various anatomic types are identified according to the origin of the pulmonary arteries from the arterial trunk.[270,271] Associated pathology includes a right aortic arch, aortic arch interruption, abnormalities of the truncal valve (abnormal number of cusps, stenosis, regurgitation), and coronary artery anomalies. Approximately one third of children with truncus arteriosus have DiGeorge syndrome (see Chapter 14).

The clinical features of the neonate with this defect are largely dependent on the status of the pulmonary vasculature. If the resistance is relatively high, the infant is well compensated. However, the normal decline in pulmonary vascular resistance leads to symptomatology related to pulmonary overcirculation and congestive heart failure symptoms. This accounts for the fact that most infants require surgical intervention early in life. Truncus arteriosus represents one of the structural malformations associated with a significant risk for adverse events before correction, because balancing of the pulmonary and vascular resistances may be quite challenging.[272] The physiology that characterizes a low pulmonary vascular resistance and a significant "runoff" setting is that of a high arterial oxygen saturation, low diastolic arterial pressures potentially leading to myocardial ischemia, systemic hypotension, impaired cardiac output, and hypoperfusion of distal beds.

Potential Residua, Sequelae, and Long-Term Outcome

The typical surgical procedure for this lesion consists of detaching the main pulmonary artery segment from the truncal root, repairing the ensuing vessel wall defect, patch closure of the VSD allowing for left ventricular output through the arterial root, and placement of an extracardiac right ventricular to pulmonary artery conduit. Alternate approaches to establishing right ventricular to pulmonary continuity have been used without the use of conduits.[273] Neonates undergoing truncus arteriosus repair have excellent survival rates.[274-276] Actuarial survival rates of 90% at 5 years, 85% at 10 years, and 83% at 15 years were observed in a series of 165 patients observed since 1975.[277] Late complications include conduit failure, residual or recurrent pulmonary artery obstruction, and truncal valve problems. Truncal valve dysfunction may require repair or replacement.

Ebstein Anomaly

Anatomy and Pathophysiology

The classic findings in Ebstein anomaly of the tricuspid valve include a large "sail-like" anterior leaflet and apically displaced septal and posterior leaflets.[278,279] This results in tricuspid regurgitation and an atrialized portion of the right ventricle. An interatrial communication is frequently present, in some cases allowing for right-to-left shunting and clinical cyanosis. The spectrum of the disease is remarkably variable.[280] Some children have minimal or no symptoms, whereas others may have severe tricuspid regurgitation resulting in intractable congestive heart failure. A neonatal presentation implies a major clinical problem and generally portends a poor prognosis. Symptoms in older children include cyanosis, palpitations, dyspnea, and exercise intolerance. Initial symptoms may be related to supraventricular tachycardia.

Potential Residua, Sequelae, and Long-Term Outcome

A number of children with Ebstein anomaly require only medical care. Interventions such as tricuspid valve surgery, closure of interatrial communications, and procedures to ablate arrhythmias may occasionally be indicated. In contrast to the adult age group, children are unlikely to require valve replacement.[281] A cavopulmonary or Glenn connection (so-called one and a half ventricle repair) has been proposed as an approach to decreasing right-sided volume overload associated with severe tricuspid valve regurgitation and right ventricular dysfunction.[282,283]

Interrupted Aortic Arch

Anatomy and Pathophysiology

Interrupted aortic arch is an uncommon malformation characterized by discontinuity between the ascending and descending thoracic aorta (see Fig. 15-14). Ductal patency is essential for perfusion of systemic beds distal to the area of interruption. This anomaly is described in terms of the site of interruption as type A if it occurs distal to the left subclavian artery; type B if it is between the left carotid and left subclavian arteries and; type C if it is between the carotid arteries. Type B interruption is the most common variant, followed in frequency by types A and C.

Interrupted aortic arch is usually associated with a VSD. This is, in many cases, a posteriorly malaligned defect resulting in subaortic obstruction. Associated defects include a right aortic arch, aberrant origin of a subclavian artery, and truncus arteriosus. A high incidence of DiGeorge syndrome is found in affected children.

The neonatal presentation relates to aortic arch obstruction (congestive heart failure, poor perfusion, cardiovascular collapse/shock) as the ductus arteriosus closes, and occasionally to differential cyanosis. Immediate therapy includes stabilization of the infant and initiation of prostaglandin E_1 therapy. In the selection of sites for blood pressure monitoring and pulse oximetry, it is important to consider the site of the interruption, as well as the presence of coexistent anomalies that may influence this choice. An adequate response to prostaglandin E_1 therapy generally implies no significant gradient between the areas proximal and distal to the obstruction and an oxygen saturation differential (higher values in beds supplied proximal to the interruption, lower distally).

Potential Residua, Sequelae, and Long-Term Outcome

In the majority of infants, a surgical intervention is necessary during the first few days of life. The current approach favors a one-stage repair.[284,285] The goal is to establish aortic arch continuity and to address coexistent defects. Survival after complete neonatal repair in uncomplicated cases is excellent at most high-volume cardiac centers.[286] Complications after repair mainly involve the left ventricular outflow tract and aortic arch. Aortic outflow tract obstruction is primarily related to subaortic narrowing and/or a hypoplastic aortic valve annulus. This may require reoperation and potentially left ventricular outflow tract enlargement (Konno). In some cases this may culminate in an aortic root and/or valve replacement or a Ross-Konno procedure.

Congenital Anomalies of the Coronary Arteries

Anatomy and Pathophysiology

Congenital anomalies of the coronary arteries include those in which there is an abnormal origin of one of the main branches, aberrant course, or pathologic communications that involve the coronary circulation.[287,288] The most common anomalies detected during childhood include anomalous origin of the left main coronary artery from the pulmonary artery (ALCAPA), coronary to pulmonary artery fistulas, and coronary cameral fistulas (connection between a coronary artery and cardiac chamber). Although anomalous origins of the coronary arteries from the incorrect (controlateral) sinus of Valsalva are rare in asymptomatic children and adolescents, a prevalence of 0.17% has been described in a study that prospectively evaluated a large pediatric population.[289] In some instances, a major coronary artery courses between the great arteries. This may be associated with compromised coronary blood and myocardial ischemia during exercise, as the arterial roots dilate to accommodate the increased stroke volume.

The clinical presentation varies according to the nature of the anomaly. Infants and young children with ALCAPA may exhibit severe ventricular dysfunction and mitral valve regurgitation considered to be largely ischemic. Children with fistulous coronary artery connections may present with a heart murmur or evidence of ventricular volume overload. If the volume load is significant, congestive heart failure symptoms may be present.

Other coronary artery anomalies may manifest as myocardial ischemia, causing exertional syncope or chest pain, and in some cases arrhythmias leading to a near-death event.

Potential Residua, Sequelae, and Long-Term Outcome

After surgical intervention for ALCAPA most children demonstrate significant recovery of myocardial function. Others continue to exhibit alterations in myocardial performance, may develop dilated cardiomyopathy, and, if severe, may require eventual cardiac transplantation. A small proportion of children reach adulthood without symptoms or any intervention. Coronary artery fistulas resulting in congestive symptoms may be referred for catheter-based or surgical interventions to abolish left-to-right shunting. Anginal complaints, myocardial infarction, and sudden death are potential risks when an aberrant coronary artery courses between the arterial trunks. The risk is greater when the left coronary artery originates from the right sinus of Valsalva and courses between the aorta and the right ventricular outflow tract. Sudden death is most likely to occur during or immediately after relatively strenuous exercise. The anesthetic implications of coronary artery anomalies primarily relate to the underlying ventricular dysfunction, potential for myocardial ischemia, and effects of ventricular volume overload.

Single Ventricle

Anatomy and Pathophysiology

A number of congenital cardiac defects compose the single-ventricle (univentricular heart) spectrum. Defects include those with ventricular hypoplasia (HLHS), an atretic atrioventricular valve (tricuspid atresia), and selected lesions with an abnormal atrioventricular connection (double-inlet left ventricle). Other malformations with two distinct ventricles may also be considered in the functional single-ventricle category due to associated defects that preclude a biventricular circulation (i.e., unbalanced AVSD).

Single-ventricle physiology is characterized by complete mixing of the systemic and pulmonary venous circulations at the atrial and/or ventricular levels. Aortic or pulmonary outflow tract obstruction is a common feature in these pathologies. An important management strategy before final palliation involves optimizing the balance between the pulmonary and systemic circulations.

A number of surgical procedures may be utilized in the palliation pathway in children with a functional single-ventricle physiology.

Aortopulmonary Shunt

Infants with limited or ductal-dependent pulmonary blood flow require the creation of a connection between the systemic and pulmonary circulations. This most commonly takes the form of an aortopulmonary shunt, by placement of a Gore-Tex graft between the right subclavian and right pulmonary arteries (modified right Blalock-Taussig shunt). In some cases, the connection is created between another arch vessel and either the right or left pulmonary arteries. The goal of this procedure is to augment or allow for pulmonary blood flow. Potential problems at either side of the spectrum include shunt malfunction associated with reductions in pulmonary blood flow and congestive heart failure related to excessive pulmonary blood flow and ventricular volume overload. A number of factors determine blood flow across an aortopulmonary shunt, with systemic arterial pressure playing a major role.

Pulmonary Artery Band

Placement of a pulmonary artery band results in limitation of pulmonary blood flow in children with minimal to no restriction. This allows for the pulmonary vascular bed to be protected from high flow and high pressure, an essential requirement for subsequent strategies in the management of the child with a functional single ventricle.

In addition to being inadequate (too loose or too tight), distortion of the proximal branch pulmonary arteries may result from pulmonary artery band placement. The primary considerations in these children relate to the presence of an intracardiac communication, associated shunting, ventricular volume load, the consequences of ventricular hypertrophy developed as a response to the mechanical limitation of pulmonary blood flow, and issues associated with coexistent defects. In a few children, pulmonary artery banding may lead to ventricular dysfunction and the development of, or an increase in the severity of, atrioventricular valve regurgitation.

Norwood Procedure

In infants with HLHS, its variants, and other lesions with similar hemodynamic consequences, systemic blood flow is largely dependent on patency of the ductus arteriosus. Cerebral and coronary blood flow is provided in retrograde fashion across a typically hypoplastic transverse aortic arch. A key strategy in the management of these infants before cardiac surgery is to optimize systemic perfusion and the balance between the pulmonary and systemic circulations. Alteration of this balance may manifest with signs of inadequate systemic output (as evidenced by hypotension, lactic acidosis, decreased urine output) within the context of a high systemic arterial oxygen saturation, reflecting relative excessive pulmonary blood flow. In this setting, maneuvers that increase pulmonary vascular resistance are indicated to improve hemodynamics. Measures employed include limiting inspired oxygen concentrations, the administration of subambient gas mixtures (accomplished by increasing inspired nitrogen concentrations), and increasing the partial pressure of carbon dioxide (P_{CO_2}) either by hypoventilation or increasing the inspired carbon dioxide. A comparison of hypoxia versus hypercarbia in infants with HLHS under conditions of anesthesia and paralysis demonstrated that although $\dot{Q}p:\dot{Q}s$ falls in both conditions, inspired CO_2 was more effective than hypoxic gas mixtures at increasing parameters associated with improved systemic output, such as systemic arterial blood pressure and oxygen delivery.[290] In most cases, the administration of inspired CO_2 is favored over hypoventilation as a means of increasing pulmonary vascular resistance and overall clinical condition. This is accomplished by the addition of CO_2 into the inspiratory limb of the anesthesia circuit using either a CO_2 cylinder or by adjusting the corresponding flowmeter in the anesthesia machine if one is available.

The Norwood procedure is considered the first step of the three stages in the palliation pathway for these infants with univentricular cardiac malformations.[291] The surgical intervention, also referred to as stage I single-ventricle palliation or reconstruction, is typically performed within the first few days of life. This consists of (1) aortic reconstruction or creation of a neoaorta, establishing continuity between the native main pulmonary artery and aortic arch to provide for unobstructed systemic outflow from the right ventricle, (2) the creation of an unrestricted atrial communication by means of an atrial septectomy, and (3) establishing a source of pulmonary blood flow (see Fig. 15-11).[292] For many years, pulmonary blood flow was established by fashioning a modified Blalock-Taussig shunt. However, in recent years, a right ventricular to pulmonary artery conduit (Sano modification) has been developed as an alternate approach to the Blalock-Taussig shunt to provide pulmonary blood flow and as a means to improve immediate postoperative hemodynamic stability. An ongoing multicenter randomized controlled study is underway to establish if one strategy is superior.[293,294] As an alternative to this procedure a hybrid stage I strategy has been applied to selected high risk neonates. During this approach both branched pulmonary arteries are banded via a median sternotomy and a stent is delivered across the ductus arteriosus via a puncture in the main pulmonary artery puncture under fluoroscopic guidance.[295,296]

Outcomes after the Norwood procedure vary among institutions; good results imply operative survival in 85% to 90% of infants.[297] Immediate postoperative problems include systemic hypoxemia, decreased myocardial performance, and excessive pulmonary blood flow. Monitoring of mixed venous oxygen saturation has been found to be helpful in balancing the pulmonary and systemic circulations in this setting. Occasionally, aortic arch obstruction occurs and, less commonly, the atrial septum becomes restrictive. Interstage mortality accounts for attrition among Norwood survivors.[298] Among infants who have undergone placement of a right ventricular to pulmonary artery conduit, stenosis of the conduit associated with progressive cyanosis may account for significant interstage morbidity and often requires intervention or early second-stage palliation.

The anticipated arterial oxygen saturation after stage I surgery should be within the 75% to 85% range. Regarding perioperative care, blood pressure monitoring should consider the potential presence of a Blalock-Taussig shunt that may compromise ipsilateral subclavian artery flow. An important aspect is the fact that in these infants the right ventricle ejects into both the pulmonary and systemic circulations. Although this is a more stable arrangement as compared with the pre-Norwood procedure, it remains a relatively fragile parallel circulation. These infants display little tolerance to even the most common childhood conditions, and ailments such as dehydration, febrile illnesses, or other stresses may have catastrophic consequences.

Glenn Anastomosis/Hemi-Fontan Procedure

A cavopulmonary connection or Glenn procedure (stage II palliation) consists of the creation of a direct anastomosis between the superior vena cava and one of the pulmonary artery branches (see Fig. 15-12). This is considered an intermediary step in the sequential diversion of the systemic venous blood into the pulmonary vasculature in children with single-ventricle physiology. The original or "classic" operation consisted of an end-to-end anastomosis of the transected superior vena cava onto a disconnected right pulmonary artery.[299] Unfortunately, this was complicated by increasing desaturation attributed in many cases to the development of pulmonary arteriovenous fistulae. The current approach is to attach the superior vena cava to the right pulmonary artery in end-to-side fashion with preservation of pulmonary artery continuity (bidirectional cavopulmonary anastomosis [BCPA]). Depending on the specific anatomic

abnormalities, a left or bilateral BCPAs may be indicated. This intervention assumes a low pulmonary vascular resistance; thus, the procedure is performed beyond the neonatal period, typically between 3 and 8 months of age.

As an alternative approach to this second-stage palliation, a hemi-Fontan procedure may be performed. This entails (1) anastomosis of the superior vena cava to the pulmonary artery confluence and (2) placement of a patch between the cavopulmonary anastomosis and common atrium. The patch allows for systemic venous return from the superior vena cava only to be diverted into the pulmonary circulation and not to enter the heart directly. Ligation of the systemic to pulmonary artery connection (shunt or conduit) is performed as part of stage II palliation, whether a BCPA or hemi-Fontan procedure is undertaken.

The second-stage intervention requires a low pulmonary vascular resistance because of the passive nature of the pulmonary blood flow. Thus, the procedure is typically performed between 3 and 8 months of age after the normal neonatal fall in pulmonary vascular resistance. This operation provides adequate palliation to a significant number of infants at an early age while conferring favorable hemodynamic benefits.[300] Diverting a portion of the systemic venous return directly into the pulmonary bed reduces the output requirements of the single ventricle while resulting in a decrease in the ventricular volume load and myocardial work.

Anesthetic care of these children should consider the passive nature of the pulmonary blood flow and the importance of maintaining adequate intravascular volume (minimal fasting) to enhance pulmonary blood flow, in addition to limiting significant increases in pulmonary vascular tone. Pulmonary blood flow, and thus systemic arterial oxygenation, is significantly influenced by the interplay between pulmonary artery pressure (equal to the pressure in the superior vena cava), pulmonary venous pressure, and pulmonary vascular resistance. The expected systemic arterial oxygen saturation typically ranges between 75% and 85%. Although factors that increase pulmonary vascular resistance may negatively influence pulmonary blood flow, the observation has been made that early after BCPA, moderate hypercapnia with respiratory acidosis improves arterial oxygenation and reduces oxygen consumption, enhancing overall oxygen transport in these children.[301] Hyperventilation has been demonstrated to potentially decrease cerebral oxygenation and should be avoided.[302] Postoperative issues of concern include the presence of hypoxemia related to the development of collateral vessels that bypass the pulmonary circulation, atrioventricular valve regurgitation, and impaired ventricular function.

Fontan Procedure

The Fontan procedure is the final step (stage III reconstruction) in the eventual separation of the pulmonary and systemic circulations in children with a functional single ventricle. This surgical intervention, frequently performed between 3 and 5 years of age, allows for passive blood flow from the inferior vena cava into the pulmonary vascular bed, while bypassing the heart and achieves a circulation in series (see Fig. 15-13). A fenestration, or communication, between the systemic venous pathway and physiologic common atrium may be created in some cases, serving as a "pop off" that allows for right-to-left shunting, thereby providing for cardiac output not to be solely dependent on pulmonary blood flow. Although the Fontan procedure has evolved into numerous modifications over the years, a common feature is the separation of the pulmonary and systemic circulations and the relief of hypoxemia.[303] Pulmonary blood flow occurs without an intervening ventricular chamber being critically dependent on the transpulmonary pressure gradient (or driving pressure across the pulmonary bed) and influenced by pulmonary vascular resistance. This, in turn, determines cardiac output, again emphasizing the importance of adequate hydration and maintenance of central venous pressure.

A number of anatomic and hemodynamic variables impact Fontan physiology. Critical factors include unobstructed systemic venous return, status of the pulmonary vasculature (anatomy, pulmonary artery pressure and resistance), low intrathoracic pressures, systemic atrioventricular valve competency, systemic ventricular function, unobstructed systemic outflow, and atrial contribution to ventricular filling (sinus rhythm/atrioventricular synchrony).[304] Long-term problems in these children relate to sinus node dysfunction, loss of atrioventricular synchrony, atrial arrhythmias, atrioventricular valve regurgitation, ventricular dysfunction, venous pathways obstruction/thrombotic complications, and symptomatology related to a chronic low cardiac output state.[305] Long-standing increases in systemic venous pressures in children after the Fontan procedure have been linked to morbidity that includes hepatic dysfunction, coagulation defects, protein-losing enteropathy, and rhythm disturbances. The quality of life after the Fontan operation may be compromised by a late decline in functional status, reoperations, arrhythmias, and thromboembolic events.[306-311] Exercise tolerance is affected in most children and represents limited cardiopulmonary reserve, as manifested by an inability to increase cardiac output to meet metabolic demands associated with increased work. In some cases surgical revision to a more hemodynamically favorable Fontan modification is indicated.[312,313]

Several considerations are of critical relevance to the perioperative care of children with Fontan circulation. Factors that influence cardiac output such as ventricular preload, atrioventricular synchrony, contractile function, afterload, and stress response are of utmost importance in this population because even mild alterations in of any of these parameters may adversely impact hemodynamics. Ensuring the adequacy of hydration, preserving sinus rhythm, and limiting the stress response represent key goals. Maintenance of adequate ventricular function may require the administration of inotropic agents, such as dopamine or milrinone perioperatively. Because systemic venous pressures are typically elevated, the potential for bleeding and its effects on ventricular filling should be considered. The likelihood of blood loss and ensuing hemodynamic instability is exacerbated by the presence of coagulation defects in these children.[314] In addition, the potential for end-organ dysfunction related to chronically decreased organ perfusion, particularly the renal and hepatic systems, should be considered and may require interventions to minimize perioperative morbidity. The immediate availability of drugs/devices appropriate for cardiac rhythm/arrhythmia management is recommended.

Regarding the airway and ventilatory management, various principles apply after the Fontan operation. Although spontaneous ventilation favors phasic pulmonary flow patterns in these children, controlled ventilation is preferable (using the minimum mean intrathoracic pressures necessary) in most cases. This minimizes the potential detrimental effects of factors such as hypoventilation, atelectasis, hypoxemia, hypercarbia, and respiratory acidosis on pulmonary vascular resistance during spontaneous ventilation, potentially limiting passive drainage of systemic venous blood into the pulmonary circulation. The aim should be to maintain pH and Pco_2 within the normal range and arterial oxygen saturation close to baseline. The latter may depend on the presence or absence of a fenestration and the degree of right-to-left shunting. The institution of positive-pressure ventilation, however, may negatively impact pulmonary blood flow and cardiac output. Mechanical ventilation with large lung volumes may impair pulmonary blood flow as increases in mean intrathoracic pressures transmitted to the pulmonary vascular bed increase pulmonary artery pressures, as well as decrease systemic venous return. The judicious use of mechanical ventilatory support is therefore warranted. Suggested parameters include smaller than usual tidal volumes and low positive-end expiratory pressures, allowing delivery of the lowest mean airway pressure possible and normal to relatively low inspiratory times (normal to slightly prolonged inspiratory to expiratory ratios). Although adequate minute ventilation may require increases in the respiratory rate, the potential detrimental effects of very fast rates should also be considered. The goals are to maintain adequate lung volumes, functional residual capacity, and optimal gas exchange.

Summary

Noncardiac surgery in children with CHD can usually be accomplished in a safe and effective manner. A thorough understanding of the child's cardiovascular anatomy and physiology is essential to guide appropriate preoperative, intraoperative, and postoperative management and to achieve the best possible outcomes. Many children with CHD have undergone complete repair in infancy, with resultant normal or near-normal hemodynamics at the time of noncardiac surgery. A carefully administered anesthetic will be tolerated in most of these children. Special attention must be paid to preoperative assessment to identify children at increased risk, particularly those whose defects have not been repaired or who have undergone palliative interventions. Children with a history of congestive heart failure, cyanosis, pulmonary hypertension, young age, or significant residual or sequelae should be considered at potentially higher risk of perioperative morbidity.

An important objective of caring for children with a history of CHD is to diminish cardiac-related morbidity and minimize the likelihood of an adverse outcome. An interdisciplinary approach is highly desirable to accomplish this goal. The application of perioperative strategies that might limit the risks of anesthesia and surgery should be a combined effort of all health care providers involved. Anticipation of these risks can decrease the likelihood of complications and facilitate prompt and appropriate treatment if and when difficulties are encountered. Good communication among the perioperative team members is of utmost importance.

Acknowledgment

We wish to thank Dr. Maureen A. Strafford for her prior contributions to this chapter.

Annotated References

Bacha EA, Daves S, Hardin J, et al: Single-ventricle palliation for high-risk neonates: the emergence of an alternative hybrid stage I strategy. J Thorac Cardiovasc Surg 2006; 131:163-171

The study proposed that a less-invasive hybrid approach would be beneficial for stage I palliation of high-risk neonates with hypoplastic left heart syndrome or related anomalies. Hospital survival was 78.5% (11 of 14) among neonates undergoing this approach, suggesting that this may be a valid option in this patient population.

Baum VC, Barton DM, Gutgesell HP: Influence of congenital heart disease on mortality after noncardiac surgery in hospitalized children. Pediatrics 2000; 105:332-335

The investigation evaluated the incremental risk of congenital heart disease on mortality after noncardiac surgery in children. Short-term and 30-day mortality was increased in these patients (30-day mortality odds ratio 3.5; 95% confidence limit, 3.2-3.9). Mortality was also increased in children with congenital heart disease in the two youngest age groups, for the 100 most common operations, and for 10 relatively minor operations. Children with more severe forms of heart disease had higher mortality than did children carrying less serious cardiac diagnoses.

Carmosino MJ, Friesen RH, Doran A, Ivy DD: Perioperative complications in children with pulmonary hypertension undergoing noncardiac surgery or cardiac catheterization. Anesth Analg 2007; 104:521-527

A retrospective review of medical records was conducted of children with pulmonary hypertension who underwent anesthesia or sedation for noncardiac surgical procedures or cardiac catheterizations from 1999 to 2004. Two hundred fifty-six procedures were performed in 156 patients. The study concluded that children with suprasystemic pulmonary artery pressures have a significant risk of major perioperative complications, including cardiac arrest and pulmonary hypertensive crisis.

Coté CJ, Wax DF, Jennings MA, et al: End-tidal carbon dioxide monitoring in children with congenital heart disease during sedation for cardiac catheterization by non-anesthesiologists. Pediatr Anesth 2007; 17:661-666

This prospective observational study compared end-tidal carbon dioxide values with blood gas carbon dioxide measurements in children sedated by non-anesthesiologists during cardiac catheterization. It was found that end-tidal carbon dioxide monitoring provides a reasonable reflection of blood CO_2 values if the expired gas-sampling catheter is taped in place after ensuring a good waveform.

Torres AJ, DiLiberti J, Pearl RH, et al: Noncardiac surgery in children with hypoplastic left heart syndrome. J Pediatr Surg 2002; 37:1399-1403

The authors examined outcomes of children with hypoplastic left heart syndrome undergoing noncardiac surgical procedures. They reported that even minor surgical interventions were associated with considerable mortality (overall mortality for all procedures of 19%), indicating that these children should be considered a high-risk group.

Williams GD, Jones TK, Hanson KA, Morray JP: The hemodynamic effects of propofol in children with congenital heart disease. Anesth Analg 1999; 89:1411-1416

The hemodynamic effects of propofol were examined during elective cardiac catheterization in 30 children with congenital heart disease. The main hemodynamic effect of propofol in this patient population was a decrease in systemic vascular resistance. In children with intracardiac shunts this resulted in a decrease in the ratio of pulmonary-to-systemic blood flow, and in those with cyanotic heart disease it can lead to arterial desaturation.

References

Please see www.expertconsult.com

The Brain and Glands

Essentials of Neurology and Neuromuscular Disease

Peter Crean and Elaine Hicks

Introduction

Disorders of the nervous system are common in childhood and variable in their manifestations. They may lead to interventions that initially require anesthesia for diagnostic procedures and subsequently for surgery for complications of the diseases themselves. In addition, children with these disorders are subject to the same acute illnesses as other children, such as acute appendicitis. Many neurologic disorders exert profound effects on other body systems that function under complex autonomic control. For example, dysfunction of bulbar musculature may predispose to the risk of aspiration in the perioperative period because protective reflexes may be incomplete. In addition, medications being taken for chronic conditions may interact with anesthetic agents. There are specific ways in which anesthetic agents may interact with an underlying disorder, and this problem is becoming better understood with advances in molecular genetics. It is therefore essential that the anesthesiologist has an understanding of the underlying neurologic/neuromuscular condition and its impact on anesthetic management to optimize perioperative outcomes.

General Considerations

The term *neurologic disorder* encompasses a wide variety of conditions that may have extremely mild or very serious effects (Table 22-1).[1-5] These disorders are especially likely to be associated with a degree of physical, cognitive, or a combined disability. It is important to realize that many children with severe physical disabilities have normal intelligence and are competent to make decisions about treatment options. Those who are mildly cognitively impaired may well wish to be consulted about treatment choices; adolescents in particular must be involved in decision-making.[6] This is especially important in managing individuals with chronic disorders who are accustomed to thinking about health issues and who often have strong and well-defined opinions about how they wish to be treated.[7]

When planning an anesthetic for such individuals, one must become knowledgeable about them and their conditions. Assumptions should not be made about their level of comprehension or about how they and their parents view the choices available.[8] In addition, whereas in former times it may have been acceptable practice for children with chronic neurologic disorders to be excluded from the full range of therapeutic options, it is now essential that these are considered.[9]

Parents of children with chronic disorders of all types are usually accustomed to dealing with health care situations and will often have thought carefully about the implications of various treatments. Generally, they know their child best and are usually most qualified to make decisions by proxy; however, this is not universally the case. Widespread use of the Internet in particular has assisted many parents in becoming extremely knowledgeable about their child's condition and about potential interventions.[10] Their aims are usually entirely appropriate, and this may assist doctors in their task of collaboration with patients and parents in determining the best management of a child's condition. On occasion, however, the information obtained has been from an unreliable source and may be inaccurate, inap-

Table 22-1. Neurologic Disorders

Condition	Prevalence	Reference
Cerebral palsy: all types	2.2/1,000 live births	1
Epilepsy	5-10/1,000 all ages	2
Central nervous system tumors	1-5/1,000 all ages	3
Neuromuscular disorders (all ages)	1/2,900 total population	4
Congenital myopathy	1/28,600	
Duchenne muscular dystrophy	1/12,000 (males)	
Myotonic dystrophy	1/12,000	
Limb girdle dystrophy	1/90,000	
Spinal muscular atrophy	1/74,000	
Mitochondrial disorders	11.5/100,000 (all ages)	5

propriate for this particular child, or simply incorrect.[11] The ramifications of misinformation can precipitate difficult situations for professionals, especially when there is a perceived disparity between what parents desire and what the child desires or what the clinician considers to be in the child's best interest. It is usually the surgical team who will be most involved in the process of obtaining informed consent, but the anesthesiologist must participate in the dialogue because the anesthetic may be that part of the treatment that carries the greatest risk.

Children with a neurologic disorder usually have a regular physician overseeing their care, either a pediatrician or a pediatric neurologist, and it is important that this doctor participate in the decision-making process. Ideally, the surgeon should establish contact with the child's regular pediatric specialist and the anesthesiologist as soon as surgery is contemplated, informing them of the proposed operation and seeking their opinions to optimize management before, during, and after the procedure. In this way, the child may glean the greatest benefit from the expertise available for his or her care and the parents will have the advantage of being able to review and discuss the plan with a familiar and trusted clinician who has a thorough knowledge of their child. It may be appropriate for additional input to be accessed to assist with clear communication. There may be other professionals closely involved with the child and family such as a social worker. In complex cases or when major surgery is proposed for a severely disabled child, the best practice may include a multidisciplinary meeting of the surgeon, anesthesiologist, pediatrician, and the parents. This can be invaluable in ensuring that accurate and consistent information is efficiently shared, along with an opportunity for questions and answers. At the time of surgery, parents should be involved. If appropriate, the parents may accompany the child to the operating room and may be reunited with the child as soon as he or she recovers consciousness (see also Chapter 4).

Although elective surgery has a time scale that should permit careful decision-making, emergencies do not. Those clinicians who are responsible for providing emergency care to children must have the knowledge and skills required to manage children with neurologic disorders. A preoperative assessment may be required on an urgent basis; a parent-held record of diagnoses and treatment is extremely helpful when available. It is of paramount importance that concurrent medications and previous reactions are documented and that any history of complications such as respiratory insufficiency, electrolyte disturbance, or cardiac, renal, or hepatic dysfunction is elicited before induction of anesthesia. A specific management plan for seizure medications is particularly important for children who are likely to develop ileus postoperatively and thereby require a change from oral to intravenous medications.

Static Neurologic Disorders

Cerebral Palsy

Cerebral palsy (CP) may be defined as a disorder of movement and posture due to a static encephalopathy. CP is caused by a cerebral insult in the immature brain that occurred prenatally, perinatally, or during infancy.[12] It may be classified according to a combination of its severity, its distribution, and the nature of the motor deficit. The nature of the neurologic features and the extent and type of distribution depend on the site and size of the lesion. Early research into the etiology of CP mostly involved detailed neuropathologic studies and was therefore mainly confined to those cases with fatal outcomes. With the advent of modern imaging techniques, especially high-resolution ultrasound and magnetic resonance imaging (MRI), understanding of the pathogenesis of CP has advanced dramatically.[13,14]

The clinical features of CP are classified most commonly according to the type of motor deficit, its distribution, and the severity of the deficit (Table 22-2). Involvement of a single limb is referred to as monoparesis, involvement of both limbs on one side of the body is referred to as hemiparesis, involvement of both lower limbs as diparesis, of three limbs as triparesis, and of all four limbs as tetraparesis (quadriparesis). The motor deficit may manifest as hypotonia, spasticity, or extrapyramidal features such as choreoathetoid/dystonic movements or ataxia. A descriptive classification includes neurologic deficit and distribution (e.g., spastic diparesis, dystonic hemiparesis). Hypotonia is a frequent feature in infancy even when the ultimate pattern is spasticity as the neurologic features evolve over the first few months of life. With aging, patterns of spasticity or extrapyramidal movements evolve often over several years. Low tone often persists in the axial (neck and trunk) musculature with increasing and variable tone in the limbs.

Hypotonic CP usually affects the whole body and is generally associated with significant learning disability. These children are very dependent and have a high incidence of complications such as joint contractures, scoliosis, epilepsy, feeding dysfunction, and recurrent respiratory infections. They are usually relatively immobile, nonambulant, and nonverbal. Although their predominant feature may be low muscle tone, this is most marked in the axial musculature so that head control is poor and the trunk is floppy. Low muscle tone may change with age, evolving

Table 22-2. Cerebral Palsy

Type/Etiology	Motor Deficit	Distribution	Complications
HYPOTONIC Syndromic Dysgenesis Insult: hypoxia-ischemia	Low axial tone Variable limb tone Deep tendon reflexes usually increased	Diffuse	Learning disability Contractures Epilepsy Feeding dysfunction Hearing/vision impairment Respiratory infections
SPASTIC Insult: hypoxia-ischemia, vascular	Increased tone: pyramidal type Increased deep tendon reflexes	Monoparesis Diparesis Hemiparesis Triparesis Tetraparesis	

CHOREOATHETOID
Insult: hypoxia-ischemia;
   neonatal hyperbilirubinemia;
   metabolic
	Involuntary movement: often a
	   mixture of chorea athetosis
	   dystonia
		May be diffuse (tetraparesis) or
		   confined to one or more limbs
		Often coexists with spasticity
			Hearing impairment
			Contractures
			Intellect often maintained

ATAXIC
Cerebral dysgenesis
	Ataxia usually generalized
	   truncal and limb
	May coexist with spasticity
		May be diffuse but often
		   associated with diparesis
			Few, may be mild

into high muscle tone. When this occurs, the tone in the limbs may increase or vary in severity with a degree of asymmetry commonly found.[15] Primitive reflexes may persist with pronounced startle and grasp reflexes, as well as brisk deep tendon reflexes. The etiology of hypotonic CP includes a large number of conditions such as genetic syndromes, metabolic disorders, and cerebral insults that occurred at any time in the prenatal, perinatal, or postnatal infant period.

The spectrum of hypertonic CP may vary from very mild or even asymptomatic to very severe. While tone may be low in infancy, the ultimate pattern of upper motor neuron signs with typical patterns of muscle weakness and spasticity may become present by the second year of life. The presentation may be manifested by delay in achieving motor milestones, abnormal patterns of tone and posture, or related symptomatology, such as falling or toe-walking. In those children who develop hemiparetic features, the first sign may be asymmetry of motor function.

Extrapyramidal type CP may manifest primarily as a disorder of involuntary movements of choreoathetoid type: writhing limb and trunk patterns or of dystonia with involuntary posturing of affected parts of the body. These features commonly coexist to some extent with pyramidal deficits of either hypotonic or spastic predominance. Thus the expression "mixed CP" may be applied.

In those children with a predominantly ataxic clinical presentation, a cerebral malformation often in the cerebellum may be identified on imaging and, on occasion, other features of a syndromic disorder (see Table 22-2).

In those whose bulbar function does not allow continued oral feeding, a gastrostomy tube may be required. Careful assessment by an expert speech and language therapist, often with a full multidisciplinary feeding team, is the norm. Difficulties with swallowing feeds of varying thickness and fluids in addition to any tendency to aspirate can be assessed using feeding videofluoroscopy. Gastroesophageal reflux is very common in children with neurologic disorders and may be resistant to medication and/or thickened feeds. Many of these children suffer from recurrent aspiration and reduced pulmonary reserve as a result. Fundoplication may be indicated if conservative measures fail. Immobility, underhydration, and poor diet predispose to bowel stasis and constipation, which may become severe with impaction occurring on occasion. Thus, the child with CP may have a mild neurologic deficit or a severe multisystem disorder. The perioperative management of such children needs to take into account the many complicating factors that make surgery and anesthesia care a challenge.[16]

Orthopedic surgical procedures are frequently performed in children with CP to release contractures due to shortened muscle or joint deformities. Postoperative immobility may be aggravated by plaster casts on the affected limb or limbs and may predispose to respiratory complications. Botulinum toxin is commonly used to reduce muscle spasm in afflicted children. Although this treatment may not require sedation in some children, the need for repeated treatments and the use of a nerve stimulator to confirm correct placement of the needle may necessitate the use of sedation.[17] Scoliosis, which frequently develops in children with CP, often requires surgery to prevent further deterioration in lung function and to stabilize the spine to facilitate ambulation and sitting.

Ear, nose, and throat surgery may be required for the common illnesses of childhood such as recurrent tonsillitis, adenoidal hypertrophy, or secretory otitis media. In those children with significantly poor oropharyngeal function, drooling may be a major problem. If treatment with hyoscine patches is ineffective, salivary gland surgery may be considered. In the most severely disabled children, obstructive sleep apnea may complicate their already compromised respiratory function, necessitating a tracheostomy.[18]

Children who are unable to communicate verbally pose a particular challenge. They require staff with appropriate skills and training in the preoperative preparation process who can review specifically the most useful methods of pain assessment with both the child and parents. Perioperative problems encountered include temperature instability, muscular spasms, seizures, and respiratory difficulty.[16] Severely compromised children may be optimally managed postoperatively with admission to the pediatric intensive care unit to provide maximum support and aggressive respiratory care and, if stable, transfer to a setting of less intense monitoring thereafter.

Malformations of the Nervous System

Malformations are very common in pediatric neurologic practice and a frequent cause of early mortality. The central nervous system (CNS) is developing very rapidly from the appearance of the neural plate in the 2-week embryo until several years after birth. The etiology of CNS malformations is largely uncertain, with timing more than the nature of the insult being of importance in the type of malformation. Causative agents include maternal drugs such as sodium valproate, which is associated with neural tube defects; infections such as cytomegalovirus, which can cause various cerebral lesions depending on the time in gestation of the infection; toxins such as alcohol; or genetic disorders. Historically, because diagnostic investigation was very limited, postmortem examination was required to demonstrate the neuropathologic changes causing the clinical disorder whereas now MRI can provide adequate images to enable a diagnosis in many instances (e.g., cortical dysplasia).[19]

Cranial and Spinal Dysraphism (Neural Tube Defects)

Cranial Dysraphism

Anencephaly is a lethal disorder that results from a failure of formation of the neural tube that leads to disorganization of neural elements and absence of skull formation.[19] Some deep cerebral structures may remain intact, and the brainstem may develop normally. With the latter, normal respiration and cardiovascular functions may develop, enabling the infant to survive for hours or days. Other structures in the head and brain, including the eyes, face, and pituitary gland, may develop abnormally. Interestingly, the incidence of anencephaly in the population appears to be decreasing. This has been attributed to an increasing awareness of the need for and use of prenatal folic acid supplementation, improved prenatal diagnosis, and to more readily available services to terminate pregnancy.

Encephalocele is a herniation of neural tissue and meninges through deficient skin and bony structure either anteriorly or posteriorly. The site of the lesion varies with geographic location, with anterior encephaloceles being more frequent in Asia and posterior encephaloceles occurring more often in the West. They are frequently associated with other cerebral malformations, such as agenesis of the corpus callosum. Cranial meningocele occurs less frequently and may have coverings of abnormal skin or unusual hair growth.

Anterior encephaloceles may be sited in various locations and may be associated with anomalies of underlying brain or orbital structures or pituitary gland. Nasofrontal encephaloceles may manifest late in life with nasal obstruction or a cerebrospinal fluid leak. These defects are at risk of being damaged during surgery for nasal obstruction if their origin is not recognized before the surgery, or they may serve as a nidus of meningeal infection, especially if they are traumatized.

Posterior encephaloceles may contain cerebral or cerebellar tissue that herniates through a bony defect in the posterior cranium. These defects carry a poor prognosis for long-term survival. Most infants die, and in survivors severe neurodevelopmental disability is very common. Hydrocephalus is present in the majority of these cases.[20] On occasion, encephaloceles may represent part of a recognized syndrome, associated with other malformations of the head and neck, such as cleft palate, microphthalmia, and other midline defects.

Spinal Dysraphism

Spinal dysraphism refers to a group of conditions in which there is abnormal or incomplete formation of the midline structures over the back.[19] Skin, bony, and neural elements may be involved singly or in combination. Congenital malformations of the spinal cord may exist in isolation or in association with brain anomalies. These defects may present at birth, as in the case of the more severe and open lesions (spina bifida) or later in childhood if the skin overlying the spinal defect is intact, as in spina bifida occulta. Those who develop a Chiari malformation (see later) may present with cervical cord or bulbar deficits, placing them at risk for respiratory embarrassment. Children with spinal cord lesions are at increased risk of sensory deficits, making meticulous skin care and positioning essential to prevent pressure sores and damage to neuropathic joints.

Spina bifida occulta occurs in the absence of herniation of neural tissue or coverings so that the overlying skin appears to be intact and normal. In many cases, however, there is an associated superficial defect such as a hairy patch or a dermal sinus (sacral dimple) that may communicate with the meninges or attach to the spinal cord or a lipoma that causes a fatty swelling overlying the bony defect. The spinal cord may be tethered by internal connection to such structures, making it vulnerable to trauma at surgery and during growth, especially at puberty. The spinal cord itself may be abnormally formed with bony spurs, known as diastematomyelia, which potentially damage the cord during growth as the neural tissue grows at a slower rate than the surrounding bone. Such infants may not be candidates for a caudal block since the spinal cord may end at an unusually low position.

Management of spinal dysraphism requires prompt and early diagnosis with MRI, which is the method of choice for demonstrating the site, extent, and nature of the pathologic process. In infants and young children with no neurologic deficit, these lesions may be managed conservatively, with regular monitoring of clinical signs, including neurologic (i.e., development of a wide-based and/or unsteady gate), urologic (i.e., incontinence), and orthopedic findings (asymmetric leg growth) to complement serial MRI examination. The long-term objective is to avoid the development of a neurologic deficit, because once one is established it may be irreversible. The resultant urologic and orthopedic difficulties could result in permanent disability and morbidity. In those with neurologic deficits, neurosurgery may be required to arrest or reverse the evolving deficit.

Spina bifida cystica is the most common type of spinal dysraphism in which an obvious lesion is present on the back. These defects may be diagnosed antenatally or at birth. The abnormally developed spinal cord may be covered either by a layer of meninges (meningocele) or uncovered (myelomeningocele). In myeloschisis the lesion is flat and in myelomeningocele it is bulging, but otherwise these are the same lesion. Associated features of spina bifida cystica include hydrocephalus, which may cause oculomotor palsy, vocal cord palsy with inspiratory stridor, macrocephaly, dysphagia, and neck weakness. Paraparesis is frequently present, with the degree of weakness depending on the level and extent of the lesion, including neurogenic bladder and bowel with renal insufficiency, trophic limb changes, and pressure sores. Joint contractures and scoliosis are also common in many of these children, as are learning disabilities and visual or hearing impairment.

Optimal management of children with spina bifida cystica actually consists of prevention of the spina bifida and early treatment if it occurs. Preventive measures, which are available in many countries worldwide, have resulted in a dramatic decrease in the prevalence of this defect.[21] The cause of spinal dysraphism is considered to be multifactorial, with genetic and environmental factors being the most important. Preconceptual vitamin supplementation has markedly reduced the prevalence of neural tube defects in children. Antenatal screening followed by termination of pregnancy in those cases that test positive has further reduced the prevalence.[22] It is possible that in the future routine scanning for fetal malformations may replace the need for tracking maternal α-fetoprotein levels. When such a defect occurs at birth, it is optimally managed in a specialist center by a multidisciplinary team (pediatrician, neurologist, neurosurgeon, orthopedic surgeon, and others) that can anticipate, prevent, and treat complications as well as assist in the child's long-term care. Good teamwork also requires that the parents are involved in the planning and decision-making for the child's care; and as the child matures (if age and developmentally appropriate) the child should also be included in all decisions related to his or her treatment and any interventions.

Chiari Malformations

Chiari malformations of the nervous system may coexist with other anomalies and manifest in the neonatal period or later in the early decades of life (Table 22-3).

Syringomyelia

This defect results from cavitation within the spinal cord lined by glial cells. Its diagnosis has been greatly simplified by the use of MRI, in which images of the spinal cord and the tubular fluid space within are readily obtained.[19] The pathogenesis of syringomyelia remains unclear, although it is known to complicate a number of pathologic conditions such as rare familial cases, congenital malformations (see earlier), trauma, and meningeal infection. It has also been reported as an apparently coincidental finding in completely normal individuals with no symptoms or signs and no etiologic cause. The classic presenting signs of such defects relate to those of a central cord lesion with dissociated sensory loss usually in the upper limbs causing loss or impairment of pain and temperature sensation, which may cause

trophic changes in the fingers and Charcot joints and may progress to paralysis and hyporeflexia later in life. The lower limbs may exhibit pyramidal signs; and, on occasion, the lesion may extend upward (syringobulbia) and produce lower brainstem signs, such as stridor and laryngospasm (vocal cord palsy). Spinal deformity causes scoliosis at an early stage. Treatment is controversial, especially if the lesion is asymptomatic, and may rest mainly with treatment of associated disorders because progression may be slow or absent.

Hydrocephalus

Hydrocephalus is a condition that results from either overproduction or impaired drainage of cerebrospinal fluid (CSF) from the brain.[20] In practice, overproduction is an uncommon cause for hydrocephalus but is most often due to tumors of the choroid plexus. In contrast, obstruction to CSF drainage is the far more common cause of hydrocephalus. It can occur anywhere in the circulatory path of CSF within the brain. Hydrocephalus can also be categorized according to the site of obstruction: internal hydrocephalus occurs when CSF cannot flow out of the ventricular system, whereas external hydrocephalus occurs when the CSF cannot be resorbed at the arachnoid villi. Consideration of the underlying cause is necessary to plan for the appropriate intervention to resolve the hydrocephalus. To ascertain the cause, detailed imaging and possibly genetic testing may be required. Irrespective of the level of obstruction to CSF flow, the pressure within the cranium gradually increases as CSF accumulates, unless the cranial sutures have not fused. In the latter instance, the sutures will widen as the pressure within the dura increases, resulting in persistently open fontanelles and failure to fuse the cranial bones. However, if the sutures have fused, obstruction to CSF flow will increase intracranial pressure (ICP), causing headache and vomiting; and if this progresses unabated, it may lead to a reduced level of consciousness, oculomotor palsies, sluggish pupillary light reactions, bradycardia, and eventually respiratory arrest. Diagnosis of hydrocephalus is confirmed by imaging techniques, with computed tomography (CT) being the most rapid and readily available technique in the acute situation, although MRI provides higher quality images of cerebral morphology. Treatment to relieve obstructive hydrocephalus usually requires shunting of CSF to either an external drain (external ventricular drain [EVD]) on a temporary basis or an internal shunt within the brain (third ventriculostomy): brain to peritoneum or brain to right atrium for a more permanent solution. Acute hydrocephalus is a medical emergency and

Table 22-3. Chiari Malformations

Type	Main Features	Associated Abnormalities	Neurologic Features
Chiari I	Downward displacement of cerebellar tonsils; elongation of IV ventricle and lower brainstem	Platybasia, basilar impression, syringomyelia, hydrocephalus	Later onset > age 12 years, cervical cord signs: tetraparesis, sensory deficits of upper limbs
Chiari II	Downward displacement of cerebellar vermis/tonsils alongside cervical cord, kinking of cord at C2-3 level	Myelomeningocele in most, brainstem anomalies, aqueduct stenosis	Present as neonate, macrocephaly, increased intracranial pressure, cranial nerve palsies, cord signs
Chiari III	Downward displacement of cerebellum into posterior encephalocele, elongation of IV ventricle	Posterior defects: cervical spina bifida ± cranium bifidum	Present as neonate with signs of hydrocephalus ± brainstem and cervical cord signs
Chiari IV	Cerebellar hypoplasia	Generally none	± Ataxia

is fatal if not promptly treated. ICPs may become very high if the accumulation of CSF has been gradual, and the risk of decompensation is significant despite a less acute or dramatic presentation. Lower-grade obstruction may present less acutely as headache, vomiting, somnolence, lower limb spasticity, ataxia, visual failure, strabismus, or seizures.

Disorders of Ventral Induction

Holoprosencephaly is an undivided forebrain of varying severity.[19] There are three types:

- Lobar: there is almost complete separation of the hemispheres (i.e., almost complete absence of the corpus callosum).
- Semilobar: the two hemispheres are divided posteriorly, with interhemispheric connections present anteriorly; the corpus callosum is absent anteriorly, and the thalami are fused in the midline.
- Alobar: there is an undivided and small forebrain with a dorsal sac that may contain some cortex. Severe facial defects usually coexist, such as cyclopia (single orbit with fused globes), cebocephaly (single nostril), and midline cleft lip.

Associated malformations such as congenital heart disease, scalp deficits, or polydactyly are common. Chromosomal anomalies may be present, and, on occasion, a complex syndromic disorder may occur. The diagnosis rests on a careful description of the external and internal morphology using MRI, followed by genetic assessment. Complications include hydrocephalus, endocrine deficits, epilepsy, and severe complex disability, usually with shortened life expectancy.

Disorders of Cortical Development

Malformations of the cerebral cortex are many and varied although relatively rare, with features depending on the stage of embryogenesis affected, and include lissencephaly/agyria (smooth cortex), pachygyria, (thickened cortex), and polymicrogyria (multiple small gyri).[19]

Identification of these features and their classification has been hugely advanced by MRI, which gives much better resolution of cerebral morphology than a CT scan. Genetic abnormalities have been identified for many of these malformations and can produce a multisystem syndrome. Known intrauterine insults in early pregnancy have been implicated in cases coming to autopsy. In survivors, clinical effects vary from asymptomatic to profound complex neurodisability. Learning disabilities, epilepsy, and focal neurologic deficits are common. Causes include genetic and environmental agents, and features include epilepsy, disorders of learning, motor dysfunction, and other system involvement. The severity likewise depends on the site and extent of the lesion.

Management of CP is symptomatic and multispecialty, with the child development team likely to be the key resource in the early years and many other specialities involved at times. In severely disabled children, the complications are increasingly difficult to treat because survival improves with better management of epilepsy, respiratory problems, and nutrition.

Progressive Neurologic Disorders

Brain Tumors

Brain and spinal tumors are the second most common type of tumor in childhood after leukemia, with location being equally divided between supratentorial and infratentorial areas (Table 22-4).[23] Pathologic classification is made according to cell of origin and by degree of malignancy from grade I (benign) to grade 4 (malignant).[24] Presentation will be determined by the location of the lesion and by the rate of growth and spread. Supratentorial lesions often produce focal neurologic signs that develop in a previously normal child and that increase in severity as the lesion expands and change in nature as adjacent areas of brain become involved by spread. If the lesion is rapidly expanding, and is accompanied by significant cerebral edema or causes obstruction to CSF drainage, the ICP will increase with the corresponding clinical features as already described. Ultimately, brainstem decompensation and death will ensue if the lesion is not treated. Very slow-growing lesions may produce little in the way of symptomatology even if ICP is high as the child adjusts to the gradual change. Very rapidly expanding tumors may produce few if any focal neurologic deficits, depending on the location of the tumor. In such situations, the clinical presentation will be dominated by symptoms of acutely rising ICP. Occasionally, hemorrhage may occur into the tumor, causing a dramatic progression of signs and mandating emergent treatment.

The diagnosis is usually confirmed using imaging techniques, ideally with MRI (if time allows), which can yield detailed information about the lesion and its characteristics, including the likely cell type. Tissue diagnosis via biopsy is always desirable, although this may not be possible when the tumor is situated in deep structures or in the brainstem. Microscopy of CSF may yield tumor cells and facilitate diagnosis. Image-guided biopsy may be possible and preferred for appropriately sited lesions.

Before surgery, cerebral edema should be treated with corticosteroids to reduce ICP, alleviate symptoms and signs, and enable correction of any fluid and electrolyte abnormalities. Seizures will require anticonvulsant therapy. Nutrition may be poor and necessitate aggressive management, enterally and parenterally. Operative intervention for raised ICP may require that CSF is diverted by shunting either internally or externally. Total resection of the tumor may be indicated depending on the tissue diagnosis and location, although the timing of the surgery may depend on whether the tumor should be first treated with radiation or chemotherapy. Aggressive surgery with the intent of completely resecting the tumor improves the prognosis in many tumor types but carries with it significant risks of residual neurologic deficits. Follow-up by the oncology team usually involves chemotherapy, often in multicenter trials, and may also include radiation therapy. The prognosis of CNS malignancy has improved dramatically with the combination of improved imaging, aggressive surgery, and evidence-based therapy.[25] Unfortunately, children who survive CNS tumors frequently have permanent neurologic deficits, epilepsy, learning disability, visual or hearing impairment, and growth and endocrine disorders. Close and long-term follow-up by specialist teams (e.g., late effects clinics) is required, along with careful emotional and social support for children and their families. In some benign and malignant tumors, genetic factors are implicated. These disorders require long-term specialist management for ongoing assessment of associated features and assessment and counseling by the medical genetics team. Examples of CNS tumors that may carry a genetic predisposition include lesions that occur in neurofibromatosis (schwannomas of the spinal cord, peripheral nerve tumors, skeletal deformities, carcinoid syndrome,

Table 22-4. Common Central Nervous System Tumors in Childhood

Tumor Type	Percentage of All Childhood CNS Tumors (%)	Clinical Features	Treatment	Prognosis/Survival
Medulloblastoma	14-20	Acute ataxia ↑ Intracranial pressure	Surgical excision + radiotherapy or chemotherapy in children <2 years old	75% at 5 years 50% at 10 years
Cerebellar astrocytoma (80% cystic)	15-20	Subacute-chronic ataxia Head tilt ± ↑ Intracranial pressure	Surgical excision	100% at 5 years, if totally excised
Posterior fossa ependymoma	6-10	Cranial nerve palsies Stiff neck ataxia ↑ Intracranial pressure	Surgical excision Radiotherapy	40% at 5 years but 14% if <5 years old
Brainstem glioma	6-16	Cranial nerve palsies Long tract signs (↑ intracranial pressure late)	(Stereotactic) biopsy if possible. Radiotherapy ± chemotherapy: ~age and cell type	Survival variable and depends on cell type
Craniopharyngioma	6-10	Endocrine disorders ↑ Intracranial pressure Visual impairment	Surgery Hormonal therapy	Survival variable
Visual pathway glioma	3-5	Proptosis, ↓ vision Associated disorders, e.g., neurofibromatosis type I	Controversial and individualized	Very variable
Pineal region tumors	<2	↑ Intracranial pressure Loss of upward gaze	Surgery ± radiotherapy	Variable
Hemisphere glioma	25-30	α location: ↑ intracranial pressure, seizures, focal neurologic deficit	Surgery ± radiotherapy ± chemotherapy	Depends on cell type
Meningioma	<2	↑ Intracranial pressure Seizures	Surgery	Variable
Ganglioma and dysembryoplastic neuroepithelial tumor (DNET)	1-5	Focal epilepsy	Surgery	Good May cure epilepsy
Primitive neuroepithelial tumor (PNET)	1-2	↑ Intracranial pressure, focal neurologic deficit	Surgery + radiotherapy	Poor
Intraventricular tumors Various cell type	5	↑ Intracranial pressure: hydrocephalus	Shunting and surgical excision	Variable
Basal ganglia tumors Various cell types	5	Hemiparesis; dystonia	Stereotactic biopsy Radiotherapy if malignant	Depends on cell type

multiple endocrine neoplasia including pheochromocytoma) and tuberous sclerosis (brain tumors, cardiac rhabdomyomas, renal abnormalities, hepatoma).

Tumors of the spinal cord are relatively rare in childhood. They may be either benign or malignant and sited within the cord (intramedullary) or outside (extramedullary). Symptoms and signs may initially be nonspecific and vague, especially in young children in whom detailed neurologic examination is difficult. This may lead to delay in diagnosis, with the risk of spinal cord compression, which is a neurosurgical emergency of at least equal urgency to that of the acute brain tumor. Delay in relief of compression may cause vascular compromise that may lead to total and irreversible paralysis of the limbs, bladder, and bowel with permanent severe disability. Diagnosis is best made by MRI of the cord, which provides details of the lesion and adjacent structures without the risk of further decompensation, a problem raised by the use of myelography in the past.[23] Treatment usually involves surgery to decompress the cord and excise

or biopsy the lesion. For intramedullary tumors, excision may be impossible and biopsy may risk further damage to the spinal cord. Cell type may be determined by CSF examination. Follow-up treatment with radiotherapy may be indicated. For children with established neurologic deficits, a program of rehabilitation will be necessary.

Metabolic Disease

Inborn errors of metabolism, which may affect carbohydrate, protein, or fat metabolism, are almost all genetic in origin. These metabolic diseases may cause a static encephalopathy but more often produce a progressive course with loss of physical and/or intellectual skills. Epilepsy, especially myoclonus, is common, as is loss of vision, neuropathy, deafness, or involvement of other organ systems (particularly cardiac). Major advances in the genetics of these diseases have been made with molecular defects identified in many of the disorders. The clinical manifestations of this group of diseases are numerous and varied.

Some are associated with intellectual deficits and some with physical deficits, of which systemic features may be prominent and neurologic signs are common (Table 22-5). Treatment is available for only a few of the diseases and consists primarily of dietary strategies, although occasionally pharmacologic treatments are used. Risks of general anesthesia usually reside in the problems posed by fasting and by the need to keep metabolism on an even keel at a time of stress to the body systems. Meticulous planning with the patient's metabolic specialist is essential for elective procedures, and in case of emergencies, children and parents should have written guidance to carry with them on what caregivers and clinicians should do and whom to call for assistance.

There are three main groups of neurometabolic diseases[26]:

1. Those in which an enzymatic defect is known
   a. Disorders of amino acid metabolism (e.g., phenylketonuria)
   b. Peroxisomal disorders (e.g., adrenoleukodystrophy)
   c. Lysosomal storage disorders (e.g., Tay-Sachs disease)
2. Those in which abnormal storage accumulates in CNS cells
   a. Lysosomal storage disorders
   b. Mucopolysaccharidoses
3. Those with no (as yet) recognized biochemical defect, a heterogeneous group that is shrinking as advances identify the biochemical defects
   a. Cockayne syndrome
   b. Pelizaeus-Merzbacher disease
   c. Neuronal ceroid lipofuscinosis

As can be seen there is overlap between groups, and the number of disorders in which the biochemical defect is still unknown is steadily shrinking. All of these disorders are rare; and, although some are treatable, most are relentlessly progressive with early death. Many show a steady decline with a gradual increase in symptomatology and loss of function or a stepwise deterioration with bouts of acute illness, leading to a sudden loss of function. Treatment started early, especially in the presymptomatic phase, may prevent neurologic complications. An example is phenylketonuria, a disorder of amino acid metabolism that is very common in many populations. It is screened for in the neonatal period, leading to introduction of a special diet in affected children. Those individuals who have good

Table 22-5. Neurometabolic Disorders

Lysosomal diseases
Mucolipidoses, sialidoses, disorders of glycoprotein metabolism
Peroxisomal disorders
Amino acid disorders
Organic acid disorders
Neurotransmitter disorders
Urea cycle disorders
Disorders of vitamin metabolism
Lactic acidosis
Respiratory chain disorders
Mitochondrial fatty acid β-oxidation defects
Disorders of cholesterol metabolism
Disorders of copper metabolism
Miscellaneous

dietary management throughout life may develop relatively few problems, although close monitoring by a specialist team of physicians and dieticians is essential to ensure metabolic stability.

The disorders that cause lactic acidosis together make up the most frequently occurring of these diseases, although it is becoming recognized that many individuals who harbor the genetic substrate for one of these disorders may not manifest it at all or may come to diagnosis very late in life.[27] The features of these diseases are extremely varied, and although the neuropathologic, biochemical, and imaging abnormalities are well recognized, a precise diagnosis may still be elusive and, unfortunately, treatments may be of questionable benefit to many children.

Neuromuscular Disorders

These are the disorders of the lower motor neuron and motor unit comprising the anterior horn cell in the spinal cord, motor nerve, neuromuscular junction, and the muscle fiber (Fig. 22-1).[28] The cardinal features are weakness of skeletal muscles that is proximal, distal, or generalized in distribution with hypotonia and reduced deep tendon reflexes. True fatigability is suggestive of a defect of the neuromuscular junction. Neuropathy is characterized by distal weakness and sensory deficit. Joint contracture scoliosis and respiratory and cardiac involvement are frequent complications, and some conditions are associated with cognitive deficits.

Disorders of the Anterior Horn Cell

Spinal Muscular Atrophies

The spinal muscular atrophies are a group of disorders in which there is progressive degeneration of the anterior horns of the spinal cord with death of motor neurons. They are inherited as an autosomal recessive trait. The most common types are associated with infancy and childhood and may be classified according to severity.[28] The diagnosis is a clinical one, but confirmation on molecular testing of the survival motor neuron gene (*SMN*) is now possible on a blood sample so that electrophysiology and muscle biopsy are no longer necessary.[29] A curative treatment is not yet available, but much can be done to improve duration and quality of life, especially in the mildly affected children.

Type I SMA (Werdnig-Hoffmann disease) manifests at or soon after birth in most cases. Occasionally, the diagnosis is delayed for several months. It is possible for the infant to appear neurologically normal at first, but the typical picture soon emerges. Parents who have had an affected child will often note the abnormal breathing pattern first as the intercostal muscles are affected and the respiratory pattern is diaphragmatic with a "bell-shaped" chest both clinically and on radiography. The infant is usually very alert and interactive but severely weak and floppy. There is good facial expression and normal eye movements, but the tongue fasciculates and the tendon reflexes are absent. There is no cardiac involvement. Management is essentially palliative with gentle physiotherapy to keep limbs flexible and care with feeding. Although most children do not survive the first year of life, mainly due to respiratory complications, some do, possibly owing to a slightly milder pattern of weakness, meticulous clinical management, devoted care, and a degree of

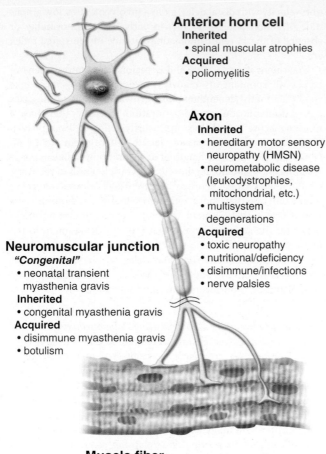

Anterior horn cell
Inherited
• spinal muscular atrophies
Acquired
• poliomyelitis

Axon
Inherited
• hereditary motor sensory
  neuropathy (HMSN)
• neurometabolic disease
  (leukodystrophies,
  mitochondrial, etc.)
• multisystem
  degenerations
Acquired
• toxic neuropathy
• nutritional/deficiency
• disimmune/infections
• nerve palsies

Neuromuscular junction
"Congenital"
• neonatal transient
  myasthenia gravis
Inherited
• congenital myasthenia gravis
Acquired
• disimmune myasthenia gravis
• botulism

Muscle fiber
Inherited
• congenital myopathies
• muscular dystrophies
• myotonias
• metabolic myopathies
Acquired
• disimmune myopathies (dermatomyositis)
• endocrine myopathies
• toxic e.g., drug-induced (steroid)

Figure 22-1. Diagram of a lower motor neuron. (Modified from Dubowitz V: Muscle Disorders in Childhood. Philadelphia, WB Saunders, 1978. Courtesy of Dr. A. Moosa.)

good luck in avoiding major respiratory infections. Noninvasive nocturnal ventilation is increasingly being utilized for these children, but invasive ventilation via a tracheostomy is not considered appropriate in most centers. This issue has provoked considerable debate in the literature.[30]

Type II SMA is an intermediate form and the most prevalent in that the weakness is milder and many children survive for years with meticulous multidisciplinary therapy, orthopedic and respiratory management, and care with nutrition. The clinical signs are very similar to those of type I SMA, and the children are bright, intelligent, and particularly verbal. Whereas type I infants never learn to sit unaided, in type II, independent sitting is usually achieved at some stage but these children never bear weight or walk. Respiratory infections are a particular problem, and noninvasive nocturnal respiratory support (bilateral or continuous positive airway pressure) with a face mask and portable

ventilator is well tolerated by children and parents alike. This improves well-being and enables remarkably full activity despite weakness.[31]

Joint contractures are almost inevitable, as is progressive scoliosis, which usually appears early in these children, with management being difficult in the very young child. Operative correction and stabilization with instrumentation is delayed as long as possible to prevent the complications of pubertal growth with a fixed spine, and children usually tolerate the procedure well if they are carefully prepared and managed.

Feeding difficulties occur in some children with type II SMA either due to weakness of bulbar musculature or as a complication of chronic nocturnal hypoventilation. Good nutrition is essential for health and supplementation, and gastrostomy feeding may be required.[32]

Type III SMA (Kugelberg-Welander disease) is a mild variant with similar signs of flaccid and areflexic weakness of lower more so than upper limbs, with proximal predominance. These children attain independent walking, although it may be later than normal and tenuous. There is often deterioration around the time of puberty when the growth spurt causes the previously precariously balanced muscle groups to become dysfunctional. Obesity and joint contracture are other adverse factors that may affect the situation. Aggressive measures to keep the child walking are often effective and delay or prevent scoliosis and lower limb contracture.[33] Respiratory support may be necessary for nocturnal hypoventilation. Prognosis for long-term survival is good.

Other SMA variants exist in childhood, with a rare type showing severe diaphragmatic involvement and respiratory failure in infancy (SMARD)[34]; others have additional features such as cerebellar atrophy, distal involvement, or additional myopathic features.

Poliomyelitis
Poliomyelitis is a viral infection of the CNS that causes a three-phase acute illness of which the third phase is one of acute flaccid/lower motor neuron paralysis. This is typically asymmetrical and may affect any muscle group. There is an association with local trauma so that cases with bulbar involvement have been described after tonsillectomy during the incubation period. The outcome may be localized, with part of a single limb being involved (usually a leg or part thereof), or there may be tetraparesis with involvement of respiratory muscles. Long-term treatment consists of orthotics and orthopedic surgery. In those patients with respiratory involvement, ventilation may be needed lifelong and in the past was usually implemented with a cuirass system. Fortunately this situation is now almost unheard of in the Western World as polio has now been almost completely eradicated by immunization.[35] Unfortunately, the infection is a lifelong disease with "post-polio syndrome" resulting in mild to severe disease progression later in life.

Axonal Disorders

Hereditary Motor Sensory Neuropathies
Hereditary neuropathies, although rare, are often symptomatic in childhood (e.g., Charcot-Marie-Tooth disease).[36] Diagnosis may be delayed because signs are mild and rather nonspecific, especially in the infant or young child whose cooperation for detailed neurologic examination is less than complete. Children will usually present with disorders of gait or foot deformity or

may come to the neurologist or geneticist via an affected parent. Clinical signs are usually confined to the lower limb in the early years and may lead to orthopedic intervention before diagnosis. In some neuropathies there is multisystem involvement, including cardiac, autonomic, and respiratory systems; and a complete preoperative assessment is essential in these children.[37]

Peripheral neuropathy is a component of various neurometabolic disorders in which there is involvement of other parts of the nervous system or of other organs. For example, in the leukodystrophies, demyelination affects central and peripheral axons, giving a clinical picture of combined upper and lower neuron features. There are a large number of these disorders, with variants causing presentation at all ages from birth to adulthood (e.g., mucopolysaccharidoses, sphingolipidoses, urea cycle disorders, organic and amino acid disorders). In the mitochondrial diseases, peripheral neuropathy is often found, along with a myriad of other features.[38]

Multisystem degenerations are often genetically determined disorders of the nervous system that rarely have onset in childhood.[37] Features may include dementia, epilepsy, extrapyramidal signs, brainstem dysfunction, vision and hearing impairment, anterior horn cell involvement, and peripheral neuropathy. They tend to have a progressive course.

Acquired Disorders of the Peripheral Nerves

Acquired disorders of the peripheral nerves are much less common in childhood than in adulthood. Acquired neuropathies are extremely rare in childhood; in clinical practice in the developed world those complicating metabolic or nutritional disorders and treatment for cancer are most common. In underdeveloped parts of the world nutritional deficiencies, especially of vitamins, are important (i.e., deficiencies of vitamins E, B_1, B_6, B_{12}, niacin, and thiamine). The neuropathic features may be overshadowed by the other features of the disease.

Acute Inflammatory Neuropathy/Acute Polyradiculitis: Guillain-Barré Syndrome

This acute demyelinating disorder causes progressive weakness usually 2 to 4 weeks after an illness with features of a viral infection or after immunization.[27] There are inflammatory lesions in the peripheral nerves typically associated with loss of myelin. In severe cases the axons are damaged, a feature that is also seen in some acute cases without significant demyelination. The precise pathologic process is yet to be delineated and various antibodies, immune complexes, and complement components have been found, suggesting heterogeneity of etiology. The disorder is rare in children younger than 3 years of age and the onset is usually sudden, although subacute presentations are seen. The first sign is weakness of the lower limbs, which characteristically ascends the body, next affecting the trunk, then the upper limbs, and, on occasion, the cranial nerves. It causes a flaccid paralysis, usually with sparing of sensory function but with pain a prominent feature and areflexia at all levels. Autonomic neuropathy may develop, causing instability of blood pressure and cardiac arrhythmias. Involvement of respiratory muscles may cause acute respiratory failure or apnea that necessitates tracheal intubation.

Diagnosis is made by the clinical picture and is reinforced by finding a raised protein level in the CSF despite normal cell count and abnormalities on nerve conduction studies. The latter may confirm demyelination by showing lowered nerve conduction velocity with distal delay, axonal involvement by low amplitude of action potentials, and, in early cases, abnormality or absence of the H reflex, indicating absence of the spinal reflex arc.

Treatment is supportive and occasionally requires intensive care until spontaneous recovery takes place. This may take weeks to months depending on severity and extent. Some cases have a dramatic and rapid deterioration, whereas others have a more subacute onset. Both are usually followed by a plateau phase that may be of variable length. There seems to be no consistent view that the length of deterioration or plateau phase is significant in predicting duration or completeness of recovery. Children with axonal neuropathies are usually slower to recover motor function than those with demyelination, and our impression is that early treatment with intravenous immunoglobulin may alter the course. There appears to be disagreement in the literature about differences between adults and children. Corticosteroids are ineffective and may delay recovery, and plasmapheresis is effective in adults and children. An alternative is the administration of intravenous immunoglobulin.[38]

Chronic Inflammatory Demyelinating Polyneuropathy

This disorder is extremely rare in childhood and is usually confined to older age groups. It is manifested in a subacute or relapsing/remitting pattern with prominent sensory involvement. Investigations are similar to those for acute Guillain-Barré syndrome, and treatment now relies on intravenous immunoglobulin therapy. Although this treatment may be effective in the short term, in many cases of recurrence the usual pattern is that of a chronic disabling and relapsing/remitting condition that does not threaten longevity but interferes significantly with the quality of life.[39]

Nerve Palsies

Like neuropathies, nerve palsies are uncommon in childhood.[36] The most common palsy encountered in children is neonatal/congenital facial nerve palsy. Cranial nerve palsies, especially those that involve the eye muscles, are usually related to intracranial disease such as raised ICP in children but may also be isolated findings that result from viral infections. In the latter instances, recovery is the norm.

Peripheral nerve palsies such as carpal tunnel syndrome have been reported in childhood.[40] It may complicate severe juvenile arthritis[41] or storage disorders such as mucopolysaccharidoses. Because symptoms may be difficult to elucidate from children at the best of times, palsies may be particularly difficult to detect in the severely learning disabled children. Specialist care may require routine assessment of nerve conduction and possible surgical decompression. Concern has been expressed regarding the emergence of carpal tunnel syndrome as a type of repetitive strain injury in children due to excessive use of video games.[42] Case reviews refer to other types of repetitive strain injury such as basketball training and skiing as etiologic factors.[43]

Disorders of the Neuromuscular Junction

Myasthenia Gravis

Myasthenia gravis is a disorder of the neuromuscular junction that is characterized by one of a number of lesions of acetylcholine-mediated transmission.[44]

Neonatal Transient Myasthenia Gravis

Neonatal myasthenia gravis is due to placental transfer of antibodies to acetylcholine receptors from an affected/previously affected mother. The infant may present with feeding difficulties or respiratory dysfunction.[45] Treatment, which involves anticholinesterase medications, must be tailored to the nature and severity of the weakness, with intensive support occasionally required. This form of myasthenia gravis is a transient disorder for which treatment is temporary and the risk of recurrence small. It should be anticipated in the offspring of any woman who has active myasthenia gravis or a history of the disorder, because cases have been described in infants of mothers in remission from myasthenia gravis.

Congenital Myasthenia Gravis

Congenital myasthenia gravis represents a number of genetically determined defects of the neuromuscular junction.[46] The defects are inherited disorders usually following an autosomal recessive inheritance pattern. Although extremely rare, congenital myasthenia gravis should be considered in the differential diagnosis of any infant who presents with weakness and hypotonia and who has a fluctuating degree of muscle weakness with a pattern of true muscle fatigue, that is, strength decreases with exercise. These children may characteristically be at their best in the morning or after a rest or nap and much weaker in the evening after a busy day. In small children it is difficult to test this clinically because cooperation is usually lacking for exercise testing. Even the simple clinical tests for muscle fatigue that are easy to perform in adults such as maintenance of upward gaze or repeated use of a limb muscle (e.g., squeezing a sphygmomanometer bulb) are often not possible in younger children. Diagnosis may be difficult because the classic features of myasthenia gravis, including responses to anticholinesterase medications, may be absent.[47] Molecular analysis in a specialist center should be sought.

Juvenile Myasthenia Gravis

Juvenile myasthenia gravis, like the adult version of the disease, is an immunologic disorder that may be associated with enlargement of the thymus gland and the presence of circulating anti–acetylcholine receptor antibodies. Occurring at any age, fatigable weakness suggests the diagnosis, which may be confirmed by electromyography and by anti–acetylcholine receptor antibody analysis. Treatment of myasthenia gravis varies with the type and biochemical characteristics. Careful titration of pyridostigmine is needed. The use of corticosteroids and surgical thymectomy are indicated for those patients with immunologic abnormalities.[48]

Botulism

The toxin of *Clostridium botulinum* produces a myasthenic-like syndrome that may occur through different mechanisms: (1) ingestion of food contaminated by *C. botulinum* toxin, including contaminated honey, and (2) wound infection by *C. botulinum*.

Features include blurring of vision, with ptosis, dilated and unresponsive pupils, cranial nerve palsies, limb paralysis with areflexia, feeding difficulty, and respiratory insufficiency. Diagnosis depends on clinical suspicion, identification of the toxin in residual food, and electromyography. Treatment is supportive, and recovery may take weeks to months.[49]

Disorders of Muscle Fibers

Congenital Myopathies

Congenital myopathies are rare disorders that demonstrate extreme variation in type and severity of features (Table 22-6).[50] They may present at any age but in many cases only become apparent in adulthood, making the designation "congenital" curious.[51] In infancy, the usual features are weakness and hypotonia—"the floppy baby."[52] Although these are inherited disorders there is often no family history, and because many are autosomal dominant or X-linked recessive, the "carrier" parent may have subclinical signs of a myopathy. Children usually present with ptosis, facial weakness, and limb weakness (proximal > distal), and there may be evidence of respiratory muscle weakness and cardiomyopathy. In some cases, the extraocular muscles may be affected with external ophthalmoplegia or joint contractures, including scoliosis. Infants often have characteristic facies, with a long narrow face, prominent ears, and narrow high-arched palate. Deep tendon reflexes are reduced or absent. Diagnosis is usually confirmed by characteristic findings on muscle biopsy. Molecular analysis is available for many of these myopathies in specialist laboratories.[53]

In parallel with the clinical features, the course of congenital myopathies is extremely variable. Many individuals are very mildly affected and, indeed, may only come to diagnosis if a more severely affected child is diagnosed. Thus, all parents, even those with no symptoms, must be carefully examined by a neurologist with an expertise in neuromuscular disease to detect very mild weakness of particular muscles. It may be helpful to perform a muscle biopsy in a parent who demonstrates weakness, and molecular testing should be used to confirm the diagnosis. For many children with congenital myopathy there is little or no deterioration in muscle strength with age, and numerous children actually improve over time with gradual improvement in muscle strength and reduction in symptoms. However, in some cases, weakness is severe and clinical complications including deglutition difficulties and respiratory failure limit survival, although the features are not specific to congenital myopathies.[54,55]

Support of respiration and nutrition may be necessary. Minimally invasive methods such as noninvasive nocturnal ventilation by face mask are indicated to assist with management at home. Regular passive movements and careful management of posture and positioning to prevent contractures, especially scoliosis, is essential. Meticulous care of skin, joints, bowels, and teeth help to avoid the need for more invasive management. A complete evaluation of cardiovascular and respiratory status is required before anesthesia and surgery.[56]

Table 22-6. Common Congenital Myopathies

Disorder	Genetics
Central core disease	19q13, ryanodine receptor
Multicore/mini-core disease	1p36, SEPN 1
Nemaline myopathy	2q21.2-q22, nebulin
Desmin myopathy	2q35
Myotubular/centronuclear myopathy	Xq27.3-q28, myotubularin

www.neuro.wustl.edu/neuromuscular/syncm.html.

Table 22-11. Antiepileptic Drugs

Drug	Seizure Type	Side Effects	Therapeutic Level
Phenobarbital	T-C	Somnolence, hyperactivity	10-40 mg/L
Phenytoin	Focal, T-C	Gum hypertrophy, skin, bones	15-20 mg/L
Carbamazepine	Focal; T-C	Rash, sleep	8-12 mg/L
Valproate	Most	Weight gain, tremor	None
Ethosuximide	Absence	Sleep, slow learning	?
Benzodiazepines			
Diazepam	Status epilepticus, GTC, myoclonic,	Respiratory depression, irritability, sedation,	
Lorazepam	spasms	increased secretions	
Clobazam			
Clonazepam			
Nitrazepam			
Vigabatrin	Spasms	Irritability, visual field defects	–
Lamotrigine	All	Rash, tremor, vomiting	–
Gabapentin	Focal	Behavior	–
Topiramate	? all	Mood, weight loss	–
Oxcarbazepine	Focal	Rash, hyponatremia	–
Levetiracetam	GTC	Mood, psychosis	–
Paraldehyde	Status epilepticus	Sedation	–
Tiagabine*	Focal	Sedation, behavior	–
Acetazolamide	Absence	Hypokalemia	(electrolytes)
Sulthiame*	Benign focal		–
Felbamate*	Myoclonic	Bone marrow suppression	–

*Not licensed as antiepileptic therapy for children in the United Kingdom.
GTC, generalized tonic-clonic; T-C, tonic-clonic.

although there are limitations for some drugs, especially in younger children. Not all of these drugs are available in all countries. The aim of the treatment is to eliminate all seizures with medications that produce no side effects, a situation that is not always achievable. Doses of the medications are determined on a body weight basis, taking into account possible drug interactions. Initially, we start with a low dose of the antiepileptic drug and increase the dose slowly to give the body systems time to become accustomed to the medication, so-called low and slow escalation. For children with epilepsy who are undergoing surgical procedures under anesthesia, the main problems are provocation or increased frequency of seizures. This may occur due to

- Medication being missed due to perioperative fasting
- Provocative anesthetic or premedication drugs
- Hypoxia during induction or maintenance of anesthesia
- Electrolyte disturbance especially hyponatremia
- The direct effect of neurosurgery on the brain
- Cerebrovascular instability
- A coincidental exacerbation of severe epilepsy

An important additional consideration is the presence of other disorders either related to the epilepsy or not that may introduce complicating factors of significance such as cardiorespiratory deficits, nutritional difficulties, and learning disabilities.[97]

Preparation for surgery should include a thorough review of the child's clinical status, including consultation with the physician who manages the child's epilepsy. For most minor elective procedures there is no need to miss or omit any medication in the perioperative period and parents should be advised to give regular medication as usual on the morning of surgery

Table 22-12. Perioperative Medication Management in Children with Epilepsy

Preoperative

Liaise with child's pediatrician/neurologist.

Clarify usual seizure type(s), frequency and trigger factors.

Review and document regular medication regimen (ideally twice daily).

Check antiepileptic drug level (phenobarbitone/phenytoin/carbamazepine only).

Review rescue medication regimen.

Check drug allergies/adverse reactions.

For Minor/Day Surgery

Schedule for early afternoon.

Allow usual morning medication.

Avoid prolonged fasting.

Aim for evening medication as usual.

For Major Surgery

Ensure regular medications up to fasting.

Use intravenous preparations of regular drugs if possible; same doses: twice or thrice daily.

- Phenytoin, phenobarbitone, valproate, benzodiazepine
- If regular drugs not possible, IV:
- Phenytoin IV load (15-18 mg/kg, max 1 g) then twice-daily maintenance level 15-20 mg/L
- Benzodiazepine IV as rescue

When enteral administration is possible, reestablish regular maintenance and wean IV phenytoin dose.

and anesthesia. Careful scheduling of the time of surgery may facilitate this because many children receive antiepileptic drugs on twice-daily regimens, with doses being given at 8 AM and 8 PM. If surgery is scheduled toward late morning or early afternoon, no medication need be missed. For children with complex epilepsy, such as those undergoing neurosurgery for the epilepsy itself, a careful preoperative assessment is imperative.[98]

In managing surgery and anesthesia in children with epilepsy the aim is to prevent seizures and enable smooth and effective treatment (Table 22-12).

Summary

Neurologic disease is common in childhood, with many severely disabled children living longer but with increasingly complex medical and social needs. The challenges for surgeons and anesthesiologists in treating such children include consent, complications of anesthesia, and issues related to long-term outcome. The key to effective management is good basic neurologic and pediatric care with careful preparation, including close liaison with parents and the child's usual clinicians.

Annotated References

Aicardi J: Diseases of the Nervous System in Childhood, 2nd ed. London, Mac Keith Press, 1998
This is a superb comprehensive text that is well illustrated and extensively referenced.
Alderson P, Sutcliffe K, Curtis K: Children as partners with adults in their medical care. Arch Dis Child 2006; 91:300-303. Epub 2006; Jan 6
This important paper is for any clinician undertaking interventions on children and young people.
Chinnery PF, Howell N, Andrews RM, Turnbull DM: Clinical mitochondrial genetics. J Med Genet 1999; 36:425-436
An excellent and understandable review of an extremely complex subject.
Dubowitz V: Muscle Disorders in Childhood. Philadelphia, WB Saunders, 1978
This is THE text for a basic understanding of the neuromuscular disorders in childhood. While not recent enough to cover molecular advances, its strength lies in the clear clinical description of the salient points of these disorders.

Emery AEH: The Muscular Dystrophies. Oxford, Oxford University Press, 2001
This book provides a supplementary and up-to-date text on the muscular dystrophies with review of molecular genetics and advances in management.
Klinger W, Lehmann-Horn F, Jurgat-Rott K: Complications of anaesthesia in neuromuscular disorders. Neuromuscul Disord 2005; 15:195-206
This article provides a good review of the topic for anesthesiologists.
Lyon G, Adams RD, Kolodny EH: Neurology of Hereditary Metabolic Diseases of Children, 2nd ed. New York, McGraw-Hill, 1996
A comprehensive text, it covers an extremely complex area of pediatrics. Although somewhat outdated by the more recent genetic advances, it gives the clinician an excellent framework by which to approach a child with a metabolic disorder by dealing with the presenting features of the various diseases.

References

Please see www.expertconsult.com

Pediatric Neurosurgical Anesthesia

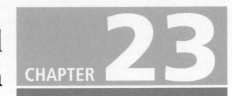

CHAPTER 23

Craig D. McClain, Sulpicio G. Soriano, and Mark A. Rockoff

CHILDREN REQUIRING NEUROSURGICAL PROCEDURES present special challenges to anesthesiologists. In addition to addressing problems common to general pediatric anesthesia practice, special considerations must be given to the effects of anesthesia on the developing central nervous system (CNS) of children with neurologic disease. In this chapter, we review the age-dependent physiology of the CNS as it relates to the anesthetic management of the child undergoing a neurosurgical procedure.

Pathophysiology

Intracranial Compartments

The skull can be compared to a rigid container with nearly incompressible contents. Under normal conditions the intracranial space is occupied by the brain and its interstitial fluid (80%), cerebrospinal fluid (CSF) (10%), and blood (10%). In pathologic states, space-occupying lesions such as edema, tumor, hematoma, or abscess will alter these relationships. The Monro-Kellie hypothesis, elaborated in the 19th century, states that the sum of all intracranial volumes is constant. Thus, an increase in volume of one compartment must be accompanied by an approximately equal decrease in volume of the other compartments, except when the cranium can expand to accommodate a larger volume. Neonates and infants are an exception to this rule because of their open fontanelles and nonfused sutures. Gradual increases in intracranial volume, such as a slow-growing

tumor or hydrocephalus, are compensated by the compliant nature of the fontanelles and sutures.[1] In the presence of open fontanelles or open cranial sutures, this pathologic process may be partially attenuated by increasing head circumference. It is important to note, however, that herniation can still occur in children with open fontanelles when large increases in intracranial pressure (ICP) develop acutely. Furthermore, in the nonacute situation, the brain can compensate for pathologic increases in intracranial volume by intracellular dehydration and reduction of interstitial fluid.[2-4]

Under normal conditions, CSF exists in dynamic equilibrium, with absorption balancing production. The rate of CSF production in adults is approximately 0.35 mL/min or 500 mL/day.[5] The average adult has 100 to 150 mL of CSF distributed throughout the brain and subarachnoid space. Thus, CSF is replaced several times each day. Children have correspondingly smaller volumes of CSF, but the rate of CSF production is similar to that of adults.[5,6]

Production of CSF is only slightly affected by alterations of ICP and is usually unchanged in children with hydrocephalus.[6] Some drugs, including acetazolamide, furosemide, and corticosteroids, are mildly effective in transiently decreasing CSF production.[1,7,8] There is an inverse relationship between the rate of CSF production and serum osmolality; an increase in serum osmolality causes a decrease in CSF production. Choroid plexus papillomas causing overproduction of CSF are rare but are more likely to occur during childhood.

509

Absorption of CSF is not well understood, but the arachnoid villi appear to be important sites for reabsorption of CSF into the venous system. One-way valves that appear to be open at about 5 mm Hg exist between the subarachnoid space and the sagittal sinus. Some reabsorption may also occur from the spinal subarachnoid space and the ependymal lining of the ventricles. Reabsorption increases with elevation of ICP. However, pathologic processes that obstruct arachnoid villi or interfere with CSF flow result in decreased CSF absorption. Such conditions include intracranial hemorrhage, infection, tumor, and congenital malformations.[9]

Translocation of CSF initially compensates for increases in intracranial volume and minimizes elevation of ICP. This translocation occurs through the foramen magnum to the distensible spinal subarachnoid space. A new equilibrium is then temporarily achieved by a decrease in the production of CSF or an increase in the rate of absorption. However, when intracranial volume surpasses these compensatory mechanisms, ICP rises precipitously, resulting in rapid clinical deterioration. Distortion of normal anatomy may obstruct CSF pathways and venous drainage, and herniation of brain tissue eventually occurs.

Intracranial Pressure

Increased ICP causes secondary brain injury by producing cerebral ischemia and, ultimately, herniation. Ischemia occurs when ICP increases and cerebral perfusion pressure (CPP) decreases. As cerebral blood flow (CBF) and the supply of nutrients are curtailed, cell damage and death occur, leading to increased intracellular and extracellular water and further increases in ICP. When ICP exceeds blood pressure, CPP decreases, the brain becomes ischemic, and cell death occurs (Fig. 23-1).[10]

Herniation Syndromes

Several herniation syndromes exist. The most common is *transtentorial* herniation in which the uncus of the temporal lobe is displaced from the supratentorial to the infratentorial space. Compression of the third cranial nerve and brainstem results in pathognomonic signs of pupillary dilatation, hemiparesis, and loss of consciousness. If this compression is not promptly relieved, apnea, bradycardia, and death occur.

In *cerebellar* herniation the cerebellar tonsils herniate through the foramen magnum from the posterior fossa to the cervical spinal space. This can lead to obstruction of CSF circulation and ultimately to hydrocephalus. Compression of the brainstem results in cardiorespiratory failure and death.

Signs of Increased Intracranial Pressure

In children, the clinical signs of increased ICP are highly variable. Papilledema, pupillary dilatation, hypertension, and bradycardia may be absent despite intracranial hypertension, or they may occur with normal ICP.[9,11] When associated with increased ICP, they are usually late and dangerous signs.[12] Chronic increases in ICP are often manifested by complaints of headache, irritability, and vomiting, particularly in the morning. Papilledema may not be present even in children dying as a result of intracranial hypertension.[13] A diminished level of consciousness and abnormal motor responses to painful stimuli are frequently associated with an increased ICP.[9] Computed tomography (CT) or magnetic resonance imaging (MRI) can reveal small or obliterated ventricles or basilar cisterns, hydrocephalus, intracranial masses, or midline shifts. Diffuse cerebral edema is

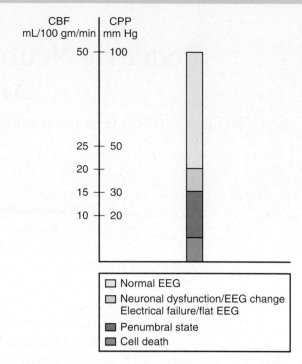

Figure 23-1. Cerebral blood flow (CBF), cerebral perfusion pressure (CPP), and brain ischemia. Changes in CBF and CPP affect neuronal synaptic function and cellular integrity. When CBF decreases to 15 to 20 mL/100 g/min there is distinct neuronal dysfunction on the electroencephalogram (EEG). At 15 mL/100 g/min the EEG is essentially flat and electrical activity ceases to function. At 6 to 15 mL/100 g/min a penumbral state occurs in which there is energy for cellular integrity but insufficient energy for synaptic function. Neuronal survival is unlikely if this low CBF is allowed to occur for more than an ill-defined but critical period of time. At less than 6 mL/100 g/min there is no energy for cellular membrane integrity. Infarction occurs at this stage unless reperfusion is accomplished immediately.

a common finding when increased ICP is associated with closed-head injury, encephalopathy, or encephalitis.

Monitoring Intracranial Pressure

Techniques to monitor ICP in adults have been successfully used in children.[14-16] Ventricular catheters are generally accepted as the most accurate and reliable means of measurement. They also permit removal of CSF for diagnostic or therapeutic indications. The major risks of intraventricular catheters are infection and hemorrhage that, although rare, may cause devastating complications. In addition, these catheters may be difficult to insert precisely in the conditions in which they are needed most, as in severe cerebral edema with small ventricles. In comparison with intraventricular catheters, subarachnoid bolts can be placed when the ventricles are obliterated. This procedure minimizes trauma to brain tissue and poses less risk of serious infection and hemorrhage. The major disadvantages are that subarachnoid bolts may underestimate ICP, particularly in areas distant from their insertion site, and they are difficult to stabilize in infants with a thin calvaria. Epidural monitors that do not require a fluid interface can be implanted outside the dura, thus avoiding the risks of CSF contamination and the limitations of fluid-dependent systems.[17,18] Most epidural systems correlate well with intraventricular measurements, but they cannot be recalibrated after insertion. Epidural monitors have also been secured noninvasively to the open anterior fontanelle of infants and appear to reflect changes in ICP. Fiberoptic catheters with self-contained transducers can also be used to measure ICP from intraventricular, subarachnoid, or intraparenchymal sites. These monitors avoid some of the problems of external fluid-filled transducers but, like epidural transducers, they cannot be recalibrated after insertion.

Normal values for ICP are generally accepted as less than 15 mm Hg. In full-term neonates, normal ICP is 2 to 6 mm Hg and is probably lower in preterm infants. Children with intra-cranial pathology but normal ICP occasionally exhibit pressure waves, which are considered abnormal.[9] In the presence of open fontanelles, ICP may remain normal despite a significant intra-cranial pathologic process; increasing head circumference may be the first clinical sign. Furthermore, bulging fontanelles may not develop, especially when the process evolves slowly.

Intracranial Compliance

The absolute value of ICP does not indicate how much compen-sation is possible. If ICP increases significantly, compensatory mechanisms have failed. However, pathologic states may be present despite an ICP within the normal range. Intracranial compliance (the change in pressure relative to a change in volume) is a valuable concept when applied to intracranial dynamics. Figure 23-2 presents a schematic relationship between the addition of volume to intracranial compartments and ICP. The actual shape of the curve depends on the time over which the volume increases and the relative size of the compartments. At normal intracranial volumes (point 1), ICP is low but compli-ance is high and remains so despite small increases in volume. When volume increases rapidly, compensatory abilities are sur-passed; further increases in volume are reflected as increases in pressure. This can occur when the actual ICP is still within normal limits but the compliance is low (point 2). When ICP is already high, further volume expansion results in rapid ICP elevation (point 3). In clinical practice, compliance can be evalu-ated with a ventriculostomy catheter or by observing the response of ICP to external stimulation, for instance, tracheal suction, coughing, and agitation.

Intracranial compliance is notably reduced in children com-pared with adults. Several physiologic and mechanical factors such as a greater ratio of brain water content, less CSF volume, and greater ratio of brain content to intracranial capacity all contribute to a relatively decreased intracranial compliance in

children.[2] Thus, children may be at increased risk of herniation compared with adults when similar relative increases in ICP have occurred. Infants, on the other hand, if faced with a slowly increasing ICP, may have a greater compliance due to their open fontanelles and sutures.

Cerebral Blood Volume and Cerebral Blood Flow

In addition to CSF, cerebral blood volume (CBV) represents another compartment in which compensatory mechanisms influence ICP. Although the CBV occupies only a small propor-tion (10%) of the intracranial space, changes related to dynamic blood volume occur, often initiated by anesthesia or intensive care procedures. As with other vascular beds, most intracranial blood is contained in the low-pressure, high-capacitance venous system. Increases in intracranial volume are initially met by decreases in CBV. This response is apparent in hydrocephalic infants in whom venous blood shifts from intracranial to extra-cranial vessels, producing distended scalp veins.[19]

In the normal adult, CBF is approximately 55 mL/100 g of brain tissue per minute.[20-22] This represents almost 15% of the cardiac output for an organ that accounts for only 2% of body weight. Estimates of CBF are less uniform in children. Normal CBF in healthy awake children is approximately 100 mL per 100 g of brain tissue per minute, which represents up to 25% of cardiac output.[23,24] CBF in neonates and preterm infants (approximately 40 mL/100 g/min) is less than in children and adults.[25,26] In infants, CBF is subject to modification by sleep states and feeding.[27]

CBF is regulated to meet the metabolic demands of the brain. In adults, the cerebral metabolic rate for oxygen ($CMRO_2$) is 3.5 to 4.5 mL O_2/100 g/min; in children, it is greater.[23] General anes-thesia reduces $CMRO_2$ as much as 50%.[28] The coupling of CBF and $CMRO_2$ is probably mediated by the effect of local hydrogen ion concentration on cerebral vessels. Conditions that cause acidosis (hypoxemia, hypercarbia, ischemia) dilate the cerebral vasculature, which augments both CBF and CBV. Similarly, a reduction in brain metabolism ($CMRO_2$) normally reduces CBF and CBV. When autoregulation is impaired, CBF is determined by factors other than metabolic demand. When CBF exceeds metabolic requirements, luxury perfusion or hyperemia is said to exist. Many pharmacologic agents act directly on the cerebral vasculature to alter CBF and CBV.

Cerebral Perfusion Pressure

CPP is a useful and practical estimate of the adequacy of the cerebral circulation because CBF is neither easily nor widely measured. CPP, defined as the pressure gradient across the brain, is the difference between the systemic mean arterial pres-sure (MAP) at the entrance to the brain and the mean exit pressure (central venous pressure [CVP]). When ICP is increased, it replaces CVP in the calculation of CPP. In supine children, mean CPP is the difference between the MAP and the mean ICP (CPP = MAP − ICP). If the brain and heart are posi-tioned at different heights, all pressures should be referenced at the level of the head (external auditory meatus).

Cerebrovascular Autoregulation

Effects of Blood Pressure

In adults, CBF remains relatively constant within a MAP range of 50 to 150 mm Hg (Fig. 23-3). Autoregulation enables brain

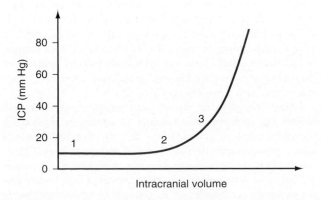

Figure 23-2. Idealized intracranial compliance curve (see text for details).

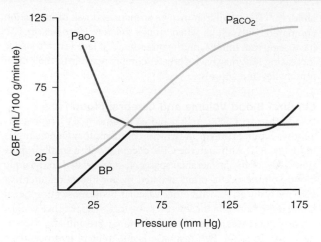

Figure 23-3. The effect of mean blood pressure, PaO_2, and $PaCO_2$ on cerebral blood flow (CBF) in the normal brain. (From Shapiro HM: Intracranial hypertension: therapeutic and anesthetic considerations. Anesthesiology 1975; 43:447.)

perfusion to remain stable despite moderate changes in MAP or ICP. Normally, when ICP and CVP are low, MAP approximates CPP. Beyond the range of autoregulation, CBF becomes pressure dependent. In chronic hypertensive cases, both the upper and lower limits of autoregulation are increased. Cerebral autoregulation can be abolished by acidosis, medications, tumor, cerebral edema, and vascular malformations, even at sites far removed from a discrete lesion.[20]

Autoregulation is partially mediated by myogenic control of arteriolar resistance. When CPP decreases, cerebral vessels dilate to maintain CBF, thereby increasing CBV. When CPP increases, cerebral vasoconstriction occurs, maintaining CBF with a reduced CBV. Outside the limits of autoregulation, CBF is passively dependent on the CPP. Small decreases in blood pressure may result in ischemia, and small increases in blood pressure will increase CBF and ICP. Abrupt increases in blood pressure can disrupt autoregulatory mechanisms and vasodilate blood vessels, increase CBF, and cause cerebral edema. The duration of this breakthrough and the rate at which normal autoregulation is re-established vary greatly.

The limits of autoregulation are not known for normal infants and children; autoregulation probably occurs at lower absolute values than in adults.[29] Although the lower limit of autoregulation in adults is approximately 50 mm Hg, this blood pressure is usually beyond that of the neonate. Intact autoregulatory mechanisms have been demonstrated within lower blood pressure ranges in newborn animals when compared with those in mature animals.[30] Cerebral autoregulation may also be abolished in critically ill humans.[31]

Effects of Oxygen

CBF is constant over a wide range of oxygen tensions. When the partial pressure of arterial O_2 (PaO_2) decreases to less than 50 mm Hg, CBF increases exponentially in adults (e.g., at a PaO_2 of 15 mm Hg, CBF increases fourfold (Fig. 23-3).[32] The resultant increase in CBV increases ICP when intracranial compliance is low; the lower limit for PaO_2 is probably less in neonates. Oxygen delivery is more important than the actual PaO_2. Evidence suggests that hyperoxia decreases CBF. Kety and Schmidt demonstrated a 10% decrease in CBF in adults breathing 100%

O_2, although decreases of 33% have been reported in neonates.[33,34]

Effects of Carbon Dioxide

The relationship between the arterial partial pressure of carbon dioxide ($PaCO_2$) and CBF is linear (Fig. 23-3). In adults, a 1-mm Hg increase in $PaCO_2$ increases CBF approximately 2 mL/100 g/min.[33] The direct effect of changes in $PaCO_2$ on CBF, and therefore of CBV, is the basis for the effect of hyperventilation to reduce ICP. Likewise, increases in $PaCO_2$ increase CBF, although the limits at which this occurs in neonates differ from those in adults. In both lambs and monkeys, CBF does not seem to change in response to decreased $PaCO_2$.[35] There are no data to suggest what the limits of $PaCO_2$ are in human infants and children. Similarly, there is little information about the extent and duration of cerebrovascular responsiveness to hyperventilation in brain-injured and critically ill children. Moderate hyperventilation is frequently utilized to reduce ICP acutely. However, recent reports have demonstrated worsening cerebral ischemia in children with compromised cerebral perfusion.[36-38]

Autoregulation of CBF is impaired in areas of damaged brain.[39] Blood vessels in an ischemic zone are subject to hypoxemia, hypercarbia, and acidosis, which are potent stimuli for vasodilation. These vessels develop maximally reduced cerebrovascular tone or vasomotor paralysis. Furthermore, small localized lesions may impair autoregulation in areas far removed from the site of injury.[20] The extent of autoregulatory impairment is variable in brain-damaged children. Techniques that measure global CBF may not detect localized changes. Although ICP may be initially normal, intracranial compliance is significantly reduced.

Anesthetic Management

Preoperative Evaluation

History

The preoperative evaluation of infants and children is discussed in Chapter 4. Children who are scheduled for neurosurgery may have been normal until the onset of their symptoms, be developmentally delayed from birth, or have impaired neuromuscular function. The anesthetic plan, including postoperative care, needs to consider the particular issues of each child and the disease state.

A history of food or drug allergies, eczema, or asthma may provide a warning of an adverse reaction to contrast agents frequently used in neuroradiologic procedures. Special attention should be given to symptoms of allergy to latex products, such as lip swelling after blowing up a toy balloon or tongue swelling after a rubber dam is inserted into the mouth by a dentist, because latex anaphylaxis has been reported in a number of these children who have undergone multiple operations, especially those with a meningomyelocele.[40]

Concurrent pediatric diseases and symptoms of neurologic lesions may influence the conduct of anesthesia. Protracted vomiting, enuresis, and anorexia due to intracranial lesions should prompt evaluation of hydration and electrolytes. Diabetes insipidus or inappropriate secretion of antidiuretic hormone are common. A history of the use of aspirin or aspirin-containing remedies for headaches or respiratory tract infections is information that is not usually forthcoming yet may have important implications for operative and postoperative bleeding. Corticosteroids are often initiated at the time of diagnosis of intracranial tumors; they need to be continued and a pulse dose administered during the perioperative period. Therapeutic levels of anticonvulsants should be verified preoperatively and maintained perioperatively. Children on long-term anticonvulsants may develop toxicity, especially if seizures are difficult to control; this is frequently manifest as abnormalities in hematologic or hepatic function or both. Children on chronic anticonvulsant therapy may also require increased amounts of sedatives, nondepolarizing muscle relaxants, and opioids because of enhanced metabolism of these drugs (see also Chapter 22).[41-43]

Physical Examination

The physical examination should encompass a brief neurologic evaluation, including level of consciousness, motor and sensory function, normal and pathologic reflexes, integrity of the cranial nerves, and signs and symptoms of intracranial hypertension. Examination of pupillary size and responsiveness can detect benign anisocoria. Preoperative respiratory assessment should specifically include the effects of motor weakness, impaired gag and swallowing mechanisms, and evidence of active pulmonary disease, such as aspiration pneumonia. Muscle atrophy and weakness should be noted because upregulation of acetylcholine receptors may precipitate sudden hyperkalemia after administration of succinylcholine and induce resistance to nondepolarizing muscle relaxants in the affected limbs.[44]

Laboratory and Radiologic Evaluation

In all but the most minor procedures, laboratory data should include a hematocrit determination. Blood typing and cross-matching should be performed for any major procedure. The need for additional studies, such as evaluation of coagulation parameters, serum electrolyte levels and osmolality, blood urea nitrogen and creatinine values, arterial blood gas analysis, chest radiography, or electrocardiography (ECG), is determined on an individual basis. Liver function tests and a hematologic profile should be obtained if not recently reviewed in children on long-term therapy with anticonvulsants. Specific neuroradiologic studies are usually obtained by the neurosurgeon and should also be reviewed by the anesthesiologist. For example, the anesthesiologist should know which children with a ventriculoperitoneal shunt have "slit ventricles," because these children have special risks in the perioperative period[45] (see later section on hydrocephalus). In addition, the amount of sedation necessary to perform radiologic studies may also be helpful in planning the induction of anesthesia. Preoperative neurophysiologic studies, including electroencephalography (EEG) and evoked potentials, may provide a baseline for comparison of intraoperative and postoperative evaluations.

Preoperative Discussions

Once a child has been fully assessed, it is important to discuss the case with the entire surgical team involved—the neurosurgeons, nurses, and, when appropriate, neurophysiologists. Each member of the team has concerns, such as positioning of the child during surgery, equipment required, and type of anesthetic technique to be used. Communication is important so that everyone understands what is planned.

It is also vital to have a thorough and candid discussion with the child's parents (and with the child if age appropriate). They should be able to confirm their understanding of the planned procedure, including the site of operation, and be aware, when applicable, of the specific needs for invasive monitoring, blood products, and postoperative intensive care. They should have an opportunity to have all their questions answered and understand the consent form they are asked to sign.

Premedication

Sedation is usually withheld from pediatric neurosurgical patients until they arrive in the preoperative area to allow titration of drug to desired effect while under direct supervision. Opioids are usually withheld preoperatively because they may cause nausea or respiratory depression, especially in children with increased ICP; sedatives alone are generally adequate to relieve anxiety.

Sedatives are administered in the parents' presence to facilitate a smooth separation and induction. Midazolam (0.5-1.0 mg/kg) may be given orally; it usually requires 10 to 20 minutes to take effect. Alternatively, an intravenous catheter can be inserted after application of EMLA cream. Incremental doses of intravenous midazolam (0.05-0.1 mg/kg) may then be carefully titrated. Another method is to administer barbiturates rectally (methohexital, 20-30 mg/kg, given as a 10% solution in sterile water or saline). Rectal barbiturates probably reduce ICP in a manner similar to intravenous barbiturates, provided that airway obstruction is avoided. Methohexital reduces the seizure threshold in children with psychomotor and temporal lobe epilepsy and is best avoided in these situations.[46] Thiopental administered via the rectum in the same dose is a reasonable alternative in these circumstances. The risk of severe respiratory depression may be increased in children with myelodysplasia who are given methohexital rectally; special caution should be exercised in this population.[47]

Monitoring

Minimal monitoring for pediatric neuroanesthesia requires a stethoscope (precordial or esophageal), electrocardiograph, pulse oximeter, sphygmomanometer, capnograph, and thermometer. Neuromuscular blockade monitoring is also important, but nerve stimulators may give misleading information about the extent of relaxation if applied to a denervated extremity. When paresis is present, nerve stimulation should be at a site of normal neurologic function. A precordial Doppler is recommended in children undergoing craniotomy, especially in the head up position, because the relatively large head size of children places them at increased risk for air emboli. Monitoring devices for ICP are used for the same indications as in adults. Intraoperative EEG and electrophysiologic monitoring require advanced coordination among the neurosurgeon, anesthesiologist, and neurophysiologist. Urinary output should be measured during prolonged procedures, in cases with anticipated large blood loss, and when diuretics or osmotic agents are administered.

In general, an arterial catheter is placed for craniotomies in which there is a potential for sudden and severe hemodynamic changes. *Small child size should not preclude the use of invasive monitoring and may actually be an indication for a more aggressive approach.* An increase in the paradoxical arterial pressure waveform with positive-pressure ventilation is often an excellent indication of intravascular volume deficiency and the need for fluid replacement (see Fig. 10-11). Intra-arterial catheters (22 to 24 gauge) can be placed percutaneously in the radial, dorsalis pedis, or posterior tibial arteries even in small infants; it is rarely necessary to resort to surgical cutdown. The arterial transducer should be zeroed at the level of the head if the head and heart positions differ so that CPP can be accurately assessed. The lateral corner of the eye or the external auditory meatus approximates the level of the foramen of Monro and either is a convenient landmark. In the first days of life, both the umbilical artery and the umbilical vein can be cannulated. These catheters should be discontinued as soon as alternative access is established because of the potential for serious complications.

Percutaneous central venous cannulation (external or internal jugular, femoral, or subclavian veins) using the Seldinger technique is possible even in the smallest infants (see Chapter 49). However, in children undergoing neurosurgical resections, consideration should be given to sites other than neck veins, such as the femoral vein, thereby avoiding the Trendelenburg position during catheter insertion and the risk of accidental carotid artery puncture and hematoma formation, which could compromise both CBF and intracranial venous drainage. If there is no issue with ICP, then the subclavian vein is a reasonable alternative. Cannulation of antecubital veins may also provide central venous access, but threading the catheter into the inlet of the right atrium may be technically difficult in small children. When rapid blood loss is a consideration in a small child in whom adequate peripheral venous access is difficult to obtain, a single-lumen, large-bore catheter is most commonly inserted in a femoral vein. Catheters inserted into the femoral veins are generally accessible to the anesthesiologist during most neurosurgical procedures. Multiple-lumen central venous catheters are inadequate for rapid blood transfusion. All central catheters should be removed as soon as possible after the procedure to minimize the risk of central venous thrombosis.

Induction

In the presence of intracranial hypertension, the primary goals during induction are to minimize severe increases in ICP and decreases in blood pressure. In general, most intravenous drugs decrease $CMRO_2$ and CBF, which consequently decreases ICP.[48] Barbiturates are often the induction agents of choice because they do not cause pain with injection in small intravenous catheters. Sodium thiopental (4-8 mg/kg) is most frequently used. Propofol (2-4 mg/kg) appears to have similar cerebral properties, plus an antiemetic effect; however, its antiemetic effect is usually not relevant for lengthy procedures. Etomidate, a possible neuroprotective agent, can also be used if hemodynamic stability is a concern.[49-51] Ketamine should be avoided because of its known ability to increase cerebral metabolism, CBF, and ICP. Sudden increases in ICP have been reported after ketamine administration, especially in infants and children with hydrocephalus.[52,53]

Other measures to reduce ICP during induction include controlled hyperventilation and administration of fentanyl and supplemental barbiturates before laryngoscopy and intubation. Lidocaine (1.0-1.5 mg/kg) has also been shown to limit the increase in ICP when administered intravenously just before laryngoscopy.[54] However, it is probably no more effective than additional barbiturate or opioid and may reduce the seizure threshold.

Oral midazolam is an effective anxiolytic without causing the same degree of sedation as methohexital and it is useful in children of all ages. Alternatively, rectal barbiturates are particularly useful in children younger than 5 years of age who resist separation from their parents. As soon as consciousness is blunted, an intravenous catheter is placed or an inhalation induction is performed.

Sevoflurane has replaced halothane for inhaled inductions because of its more rapid onset, child acceptability, and hemodynamic stability. In cases with increased ICP, not a "true" full stomach, and yet intravenous access is very difficult, inhalation of sevoflurane to light levels of anesthesia may be used to facilitate insertion of an intravenous catheter. Similar to isoflurane in its cerebral physiologic effects, sevoflurane with hyperventilation appears to blunt the increase in ICP secondary to cerebral vasodilatation from inhalational anesthetic agents alone.[55-57] Sevoflurane offers an additional advantage because it causes less myocardial depression compared with halothane.[58] However, sevoflurane has also been demonstrated occasionally to produce epileptiform activity as measured by EEG. This may occur even in children with no history of clinical seizure activity (see Chapter 6 for a more detailed discussion).[59]

A common problem is an uncooperative toddler who has an intracranial tumor and moderately decreased intracranial compliance yet is agitated and resistant to separation from parents. Some clinicians would argue that a crying, agitated child has demonstrated a tolerance to increased ICP and that an intravenous induction is safer. Fortunately (for the anesthesiologist, although not for the child), children who have severe intracranial hypertension generally have a decreased level of consciousness and it becomes easier to insert an intravenous catheter in those situations when it is most necessary.

Airway Management and Intubation

It is crucial that airway management be effective and smooth to avoid the ICP-increasing effects of hypoxemia, hypercarbia, and coughing. Opioid administration and supplemental barbiturates before intubation improve cerebral compliance and minimize increases in ICP caused by laryngoscopy and intubation.

Oral intubation is often preferred because it is expeditious and minimizes airway stimulation and duration of apnea; it certainly is the technique of choice when a rapid-sequence induction is indicated. When the airway is secured and an adequate depth of anesthesia is ensured, an oral endotracheal tube can be exchanged for a nasotracheal tube if necessary. Nasotracheal intubation offers the advantage of increased stability and increased comfort for children when postoperative intubation is necessary. Nasotracheal tubes are often used for children who will be in the prone position and whose airway will be inaccessible during the surgical procedure (e.g., a posterior fossa craniotomy).

Contraindications to nasal intubation include choanal stenosis, possible basilar skull fracture, trans-sphenoidal procedures, and sinusitis. If nasotracheal intubation is planned, it is advantageous to prepare the nares with topical vasoconstrictors, recognizing that systemic hypertension can occur in response to nasally administered vasoconstrictors. Placing a few drops of 0.25% phenylephrine (Neo-Synephrine) or oxymetazoline on cotton-tipped applicators and positioning them in the nares against the nasal mucosa will prevent overdosage and help to gauge the patency of the nasal passage when anesthesia has been induced. It may also be useful to use a red rubber catheter or a non-latex nasal trumpet to gently dilate the nares and minimize the risk of bleeding.[60] Whichever route is chosen for intubation, it is important to secure the endotracheal tube with liberal amounts of tincture of benzoin and waterproof tape; waterproof adhesive dressings can also protect the tape from surgical preparation solutions. Once the tube has been inserted into the nose and secured in position, the neck should be maximally flexed and bilateral air entry reassessed to determine if an endobronchial intubation might occur when the child is positioned in the prone position and the neck is flexed as per a post-fossa craniotomy. If an oral endotracheal tube is used, it should be placed on the side of the mouth that will be upward (generally ipsilateral to the side of the craniotomy) so that draining oral secretions will not loosen the tape.

In prolonged combined neurosurgical and craniofacial reconstructions, the endotracheal tube may be sutured to the nasal septum or wired to the teeth. A nasogastric or orogastric tube is inserted after intubation to decompress the stomach and evacuate gastric contents; leaving it open to gravity drainage during the case will prevent positive pressure from building up in the stomach should air leak around an uncuffed endotracheal tube. Finally, the child's eyes should be closed and covered with a large, clear, waterproof dressing. Placing lubricant in the eyes before this has not been shown to reduce the risk of corneal abrasions.[61] In children, application of lubricant to the eyes may actually increase the risk of corneal abrasions because children will often scratch their eyes in the postoperative period if their vision has been blurred by lubricating ointments.

Muscle Relaxants

Because of its rapid onset and brief duration of action, succinylcholine is frequently used to facilitate intubation in children with a full stomach. The intubating dose is 1 to 2 mg/kg given intravenously or 3 to 4 mg/kg intramuscularly.[62] In children it is safest to precede this with atropine (0.01-0.02 mg/kg), to prevent bradycardia. Succinylcholine does not significantly increase ICP in humans[63]; any effect may be minimized by pretreatment with a nondepolarizing muscle relaxant.[64] However, this may make succinylcholine less effective, even when the dose of succinylcholine is increased. Succinylcholine is contraindicated in those situations when it may induce life-threatening hyperkalemia in the presence of denervation injuries due to various causes, including severe head trauma, crush injury, burns, spinal cord dysfunction, encephalitis, multiple sclerosis, muscular dystrophies, stroke, or tetanus.[65]

Alternatively, nondepolarizing muscle relaxants such as rocuronium, pancuronium, cisatracurium, or vecuronium may be used, but all have a slower onset of action than succinylcholine. However, when rocuronium is administered in sufficiently large doses (1.2 mg/kg), the onset of action approaches that of succinylcholine.[66] If the neurosurgeon plans direct nerve stimulation, succinylcholine is best avoided in the event that pseudocholinesterase deficiency is present. Nondepolarizing muscle relaxants should not be given until recovery of neuromuscular function after succinylcholine. As noted earlier, the amount of most nondepolarizing muscle relaxants necessary to maintain paralysis is increased in children who are receiving chronic anticonvulsant medications, although cisatracurium, like atracurium, has not shown this tendency, probably because of its metabolism through Hoffman elimination.[67]

Positioning

Positioning is an especially important consideration in pediatric neuroanesthesia. Children with increased ICP should be transported to the preoperative holding area and operating room with the head elevated in the midline position to maximize cerebral venous drainage.

Once the child is in the operating room, the neurosurgeons and anesthesiologists all must have adequate access to the child. In infants and small children, slight displacement of the endotracheal tube can result in extubation or endobronchial intubation. During prolonged procedures, it is important for the anesthesiologist to be able to visually inspect the endotracheal tube and circuit connections and to suction the endotracheal tube when necessary. Using proper draping and a flashlight, one can usually create a "tunnel" to ensure access to the airway. It is also important to position the head to avoid soft tissue and ischemic nerve damage. Generally this is not a problem because most children are often placed in pins in a Mayfield head holder. The position of the nasotracheal tube exiting the nose should be examined to ensure that excess pressure is not applied to the alae nasae. The direction of the tube exiting the nasae should be adjusted to remove pressure and avoid the risk of ischemia, particularly for cases that will continue for several hours. Neonates and small infants have a thin calvaria, so head pinning systems are often avoided. Instead, there are a variety of non–pin-based headrests available for these children. Adequate padding should be used in such situations (Figs. 23-4 and 23-5). Extreme head flexion can cause brainstem compression in children with posterior fossa pathology, such as a mass lesion or Arnold-Chiari malformation. Extreme flexion can also cause high cervical spinal cord ischemia and endotracheal tube obstruction by kinking caudad to the carina or into the right main-stem bronchus (see earlier).[68]

Intravascular catheters should also be accessible for visual inspection because they may infiltrate, causing local soft tissue damage and extravascular administration of fluids, blood products, and medications. Furthermore, ischemic pressure necrosis of the ipsilateral hand or foot digits can occur as a result of a tourniquet effect of a name or allergy bracelet proximal to the intravenous site. The child's eyes should be closed and covered with a waterproof dressing. Additional protective padding such as gauze pads or foam can be placed over the face and eyes if necessary. Extremities should be secured in a neutral position (palm supinated or neutral to avoid ulnar nerve compression) and well padded. It is important to avoid stretching peripheral nerves and to prevent skin and soft tissue pressure injury owing to direct contact with surgical accessories such as instrument stands and grounding wires (see Fig. 23-5). It is also important to ensure that extremities that are not directly visible to the anesthesiologist (e.g., those on the opposite side of the operating room table) cannot fall off the table during surgery—even if the position of the table is changed. In older children and adolescents undergoing prolonged procedures, deep vein thrombosis prophylaxis should be considered using compression or pneumatic stockings.[69,70]

Prone Position

The prone position is commonly used for posterior fossa and spinal cord surgery. The torso is usually supported by padding under the chest and pelvis. It is important to ensure free abdom-

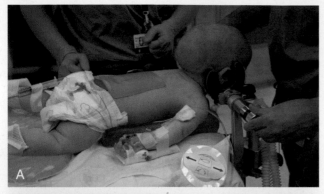

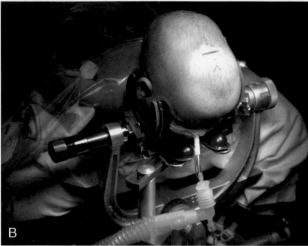

Figure 23-4. A, Child positioned prone before surgery. Extreme head extension was for correction of craniosynostosis, but the equipment for securing the head is the same as that used for a prone craniotomy. **B,** This particular frame uses gel pads to support the chin, ears, and forehead.

inal wall motion because increased intra-abdominal pressure may impair ventilation, cause vena cava compression, and increase epidural venous pressure and bleeding. This is achieved most easily by placing silicone rolls or rolled blankets laterally on each side of the child's chest running from the shoulders toward the pelvis. A separate silicone roll or rolled blanket under the pelvis may occasionally be necessary in larger children. It is important to be sure that these rolls do not press into the flexed hips or compress the femoral nerve or genitalia. Placing the rolls in this position should also allow a precordial Doppler monitor to be easily placed on the anterior chest without undue pressure.

There are several different positions for the head depending on the exact surgery. If the surgery is limited to the lower spine, the head may simply be rotated and supported by padding, with care taken to avoid direct pressure on the eyes and nose and to keep the ears flat. In contrast, for posterior fossa surgery, the head is often suspended in a horseshoe or in pins to maintain central alignment of the head and maximal flexion. For infants and toddlers, a cerebellar head frame is another alternative when the cranium is too thin for pins. In this situation, the child's forehead and cheeks rest on a well-padded head frame and the eyes are free in the center of a horseshoe-shaped

support. Most surgeons prefer head pins and a head frame for older children. One should ensure that the endotracheal tube is properly positioned (after taping) and does not migrate to a mainstem position during positioning prone. This can be confirmed while the child is still supine, by flexing the child's head onto the chest and auscultating the air entry bilaterally. Care should be taken to avoid pressure on the alae nasae from an upturned endotracheal or nasogastric tube as it exits the nose. Tape used to fix other tubes (gastric, esophageal) should not adhere to the tracheal tube tape so that accidental dislodgement of these tubes do not cause an extubation. The breathing circuit should be suspended from the operating table and all connections reinforced. An emergency plan should be formulated to turn the child supine should this suddenly become necessary.[71]

Significant airway edema may develop in a child who is in the prone position for an extended period of time. Oral airways are best avoided because they can cause significant edema of the tongue. Alternatively, a folded piece of gauze can be inserted between the jaws to prevent the tongue from extruding. Rarely, prophylactic postoperative intubation may be necessary if a great deal of facial swelling has developed during a prolonged surgery. Recently, postoperative vision loss has been linked with prolonged spine surgery in the prone position and blood loss.[72] Therefore, avoidance of direct pressure on the globe of the eyes, staged procedures to decrease the individual surgical time, and maintenance of stable hemodynamics should be ensured in prone children.[73]

Modified Lateral Position

Insertion or revision of ventriculoperitoneal shunts may require that the child be rotated from the supine to the semilateral position. This is achieved by placing a roll under the child's dependent axilla (to prevent a brachial plexus injury). The knees should be supported in a slightly flexed position and the heels padded. This position is also used for some temporal and parietal craniotomies.

Sitting Position

The sitting position is used less commonly in pediatric neurosurgical procedures today and is rarely used in children younger than 3 years of age. However, this position may be used for morbidly obese children who cannot tolerate the prone position due to excessive intrathoracic and abdominal pressures. When it is used, precautions to prevent hypotension and air embolism must be followed. Positioning should be undertaken gradually, with continuous monitoring. The lower extremities should be wrapped in elastic bandages. The head must be carefully flexed to avoid kinking the endotracheal tube, advancing it into a bronchial position, or compressing the chin on the chest (which can block venous and lymphatic drainage of the tongue). Extreme flexion can also result in brainstem or cervical spinal cord ischemia, or both. As in the prone position, nasotracheal tubes are often used because they are more secure. The child's upper extremities are supported in the child's lap. All pressure points and extremities must be well padded to prevent peripheral nerve (especially sciatic, brachial plexus, and peroneal) damage and pressure sores. Control levers to lower the head position should be easily accessible to the anesthesiologist and unencumbered by wires and drapes (see Fig. 23-5).

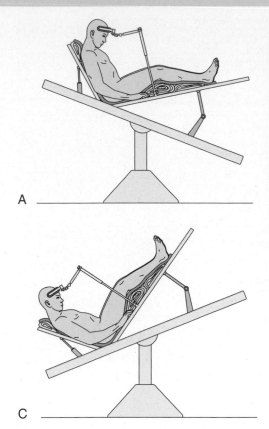

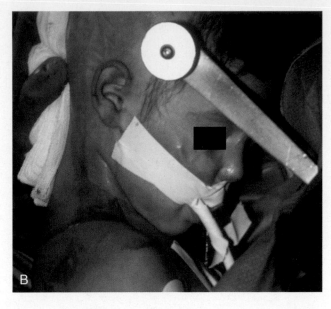

Figure 23-5. Resuscitation from the modified standard sitting position. Normal operative position (**A and B**) and resuscitation position (**C**). Note that the position can be expeditiously changed by one control of the operating table.

Local Anesthesia

Local anesthetic should be injected subcutaneously before skin incision to provide analgesia during incision and when epinephrine is included in the local anesthetic to reduce cutaneous blood loss. If 0.25% bupivacaine with 1:200,000 epinephrine is utilized, the dose should be limited to 0.5 to 1.0 mL/kg. This will deliver 1.25 to 2.5 mg/kg of bupivacaine and 2.5 to 5.0 µg/kg of epinephrine, both well within the safe range, even if some of the drug is accidentally administered intravenously. When greater volumes are required, the solution should be diluted with normal saline. This dilute solution is effective for vasoconstriction and to provide a prolonged sensory block postoperatively. Specific blocks of supraorbital and supratrochlear nerves can provide analgesia from the frontal area to the midcoronal portion of the occiput.[74] Blockade of the great occipital nerve will provide analgesia from the posterior of the occiput to the midcoronal area of the occiput, whereas block of the supraorbital will provide analgesia to the front of the occiput (see Figs. 42-13 and 42-14).[75,76]

Maintenance

General anesthesia is required for most therapeutic as well as many diagnostic procedures in neurosurgery. Ventilation is controlled whenever intracranial hypertension is a concern and in all infants. Although spontaneous ventilation provides another indication of brainstem function, its disadvantages (hypoventilation, increased potential for air embolism) are generally outweighed by the safety of controlled ventilation.

Maintenance of general anesthesia can be accomplished using inhalation anesthetics, intravenous infusions, or a combination of these. Anesthetics that decrease ICP and $CMRO_2$ and maintain CPP are most desirable (Table 23-1). The commonly used inhalational agents generally uncouple CBF and $CMRO_2$ such that CBF increases while $CMRO_2$ decreases. All potent inhalation agents are cerebral vasodilators (thus causing increases in both CBF and ICP). Low concentrations of isoflurane, sevoflurane, or desflurane, combined with mild hyperventilation, minimally affect CBF and ICP.[55,56,77] Isoflurane is often the inhalational agent of choice for maintenance of neuroanesthesia. At two times the minimal alveolar concentration (MAC), this dose of isoflurane induces a level of anesthesia that is associated with an isoelectric EEG while, unlike several other inhalational agents, still maintaining hemodynamic stability. Enflurane is no longer used and may be epileptogenic, especially when combined with hyperventilation.[78] Other studies have demonstrated a similar effect with sevoflurane and hyperventilation, but the clinical implications of this are yet to be defined.[79] All inhalational agents cause dose-dependent myocardial depression, some degree of peripheral vasodilatation, and systemic hypotension. These effects make their use in the sitting position more challenging.

There remains debate among practitioners regarding the routine use of nitrous oxide for intracranial neurosurgical procedures. Opponents cite the increased risk of postoperative nausea and vomiting (PONV) with nitrous oxide in a surgical population already at greater risk for PONV.[80] In contrast, proponents cite studies that failed to demonstrate an increased risk of PONV.[81] In addition, nitrous oxide increased CBF in humans in a dose-dependent fashion through cerebral vasodilatation.[82,83] This increase in CBF leads to an increase in ICP, which can be

Table 23-1. Neurophysiologic Effects of Common Anesthetic Agents

	MAP	CBF	CPP	ICP	CMRO$_2$	CSF Production	CSF Absorption	SSEP Amplitude	SSEP Latency
Nitrous oxide	∅-↓	↑↑↑	↓	↑↑↑	↓↑	↑↓	↑↓	↓	↑-∅
Inhalational Anesthetics									
Halothane	↓↓	↑↑↑	↑↑	↑↑	↓↓	↑↓	∅-↓	↓	↑
Enflurane	↓↓	↑↑	↑↑	↑↑	↓↓	↑	↓	↓	↑
Isoflurane	↓↓	↑	↑↑	↑	↓↓↓	↓↑	↑	↓	↑
Sevoflurane	↓↓	↑	↑	↑	↓↓↓	↑	↓	↓	↑
Desflurane	↓↓	↑	↑	↑	↓	↑↓	↑	↓	↑
Hypnotics									
Thiopental	↓↓	↓↓↓	↑↑↑	↓↓↓	↓↓↓	↑↓	↑	↓	↑
Propofol	↓↓↓	↓↓↓		↓↓	↓↓↓	↑↓	↑	↑	↑
Etomidate	∅-↓	↓↓↓	↑↑	↓↓↓	↓↓↓	↑↓	↑	↑	↑
Ketamine	↑↑	↑↑↑	↓	↑↑↑	↑	↑↓	↓	↑	∅
Benzodiazepine	∅-↓	↓↓	↑	∅-↓	↓↓		↑	↓	∅-↑
Opioids	∅-↓	↓	↑↓	∅-↓	↓	↑↓	↑	↓	↑
Droperidol	↓↓		↑	↓	∅-↓				

CBF, cerebral blood flow; CMRO$_2$, cerebral metabolic rate for oxygen; CPP, cerebral perfusion pressure; CSF, cerebrospinal fluid; ICP, intracranial pressure; MAP, mean arterial pressure; ∅, no change; SSEP, somatosensory evoked potential.

deleterious if the child already has reduced intracranial compliance.[84] Nitrous oxide can also affect somatosensory and motor evoked potentials, especially when concentrations in excess of 50% are used.[85-87] Finally, animal data have shown that nitrous oxide can counteract the protective effects of thiopental in a model of cerebral ischemia.[88]

Proponents of the use of nitrous oxide for intracranial procedures cite the long track record of safety. There are no outcome studies in humans showing a difference between using nitrous oxide or not. The combination of nitrous oxide, a low concentration of inhalational agent, and intravenous opioid, allow for a rapid emergence after intracranial procedures. It is often of great clinical interest to obtain a neurologic assessment immediately after the conclusion of an intracranial procedure. Studies have demonstrated the safety of using nitrous oxide, in a variety of combinations with other agents, during intracranial procedures.[89]

Nitrous oxide is relatively contraindicated, however, if the child has undergone a recent craniotomy (within the past few weeks) because air can remain in the head for prolonged periods after previous neurosurgery.[90] In this situation, high-dose opioids combined with an anxiolytic (benzodiazepine) or a greater concentration of inhalational agent in oxygen may be used initially and nitrous oxide added when the dura is opened to avoid the risk of a tension pneumocephalus.

Fentanyl is often administered as part of an opioid-based technique because it is easily titratable with minimal side effects. A common loading dose is 10 μg/kg, although it is best to give this amount in divided doses (part at induction and part before incision) because of the prolonged neurosurgical preparation. A dose of 2 μg/kg/hr is then usually adequate for maintenance, although some children, particularly those receiving chronic anticonvulsants, may require more

(>3 μg/kg/hr). The ultra-short-acting opioid remifentanil along with propofol may also be administered by continuous infusion (see Chapters 6 and 7). However, hypertension due to the onset of pain can rapidly develop when these infusions are discontinued unless long-acting opioids have been administered.[91] Dexmedetomidine is an α$_2$ agonist, sedative medication that has been used in children for neurophysiologic monitoring, for awake craniotomies, to facilitate smooth wake-ups after neurosurgical procedures, and for neuroprotection.[92-95]

Apoptotic Neurodegeneration

Several investigators have demonstrated that commonly used anesthesia drugs accelerate programmed cell death (apoptosis) in the CNS of immature rodents and rhesus monkeys.[96-98] This laboratory observation has provoked a heated debate on its relevance to anesthetizing neonates,[99-101] which has been extended to the lay press.[102] Although these experimental paradigms have yielded some surprising findings, extrapolating these data to the practice of anesthetizing human neonates is very questionable. Most, if not all, of the animal and in-vitro studies have significant limitations with respect to the experimental model, agent dosage or concentration, duration of exposure (both absolute and in comparison to human), lack of surgical stimulation, and developmental age and stage. There is no detectable clinical marker or syndrome associated with early anesthesia exposure in former neonates who have undergone surgery and anesthesia at birth or in the first several years of life during rapid brain growth (synaptogenesis). In the only primate study, the degree of apoptosis after 3 hours of a ketamine infusion was similar to control but significantly less than after a 24-hour infusion.[98] This is in the presence of blood concentrations of ketamine that are 10-fold to several hundred-fold greater than those reported after a single dose of ketamine in infants. This suggests that in this model, ketamine-associated neurodegeneration is a time-dependent, dose-dependent phenomenon whose limits have not been established. Despite the confounding effects on prematurity and coexisting congenital anomalies, clearly characterized syndromes have been associated with maternal consumption of alcohol and anticonvulsant drugs. Furthermore, discrepancies in neurocognitive outcomes exist.[97,103] Finally, most neonatal and infant surgery is urgent and anesthesia care is essential to proceed safely.

Blood and Fluid Management

Blood loss is difficult to estimate accurately during neurosurgery because most of the losses are absorbed by the operative drapes and the surgical field is difficult for the anesthesiologist to visualize. Accuracy can be improved if all suctioned blood is collected in calibrated containers visible to the anesthesiologist and an overhead camera provides a view of the operative field at all times. Blood loss is usually greatest at the beginning of surgery, when the scalp is incised. Although bleeding from bone is difficult to control, blood loss from the scalp can be decreased by the subcutaneous infiltration of dilute a local anesthetic and epinephrine solution before incision.

Fluid and blood product management is discussed in Chapters 8 and 10. Disruption of the blood-brain barrier by underlying pathologic processes, trauma, or surgery predisposes neurosurgical patients to cerebral edema, which may be exacerbated by excessive administration of intravenous fluids. Intravenous fluid management during neurosurgical anesthesia involves (1) cerebral perfusion, (2) cerebral edema, (3) water and sodium homeostasis, and (4) serum glucose concentration.

When large blood loss is expected and blood transfusion is very likely, it is prudent to commence blood transfusions at the beginning of surgery rather than to wait until the child becomes severely anemic. In such situations, blood replacement on a milliliter-for-milliliter basis is appropriate. In most cases, however, blood transfusions are not anticipated and attempts should be made to avoid administration of blood products with their associated risks. In such situations, crystalloid solutions are administered. Although the use of crystalloid or colloid solutions in children during neurosurgery is controversial, most investigators believe that osmotic pressure gradients are more important than oncotic pressure gradients when trying to minimize cerebral edema. Thus, unless indicated by a specific situation, crystalloid solutions are the preferred intravenous solutions for neurosurgery. Lactated Ringer's solution is not considered a truly isotonic solution, because its osmolality is 273 mOsm/L (normal: 285 to 290 mOsm/L). Normal saline, which is slightly hypertonic (308 mOsm/L), is the fluid of choice because reduction of serum osmolality is not desirable. However, rapid infusion of large volumes of normal saline has been associated with hyperchloremic acidosis.[104] Should there be large fluid requirements during surgery, alternating bags of lactated Ringer's solution with normal saline will minimize the risk of hypernatremia and acidosis and still avoid hypo-osmolality.

Inducing dehydration with osmotic and loop diuretics is a useful strategy to minimize cerebral edema and provide an optimal surgical field. However, hypotension and rebound effects may be associated with their use. Rapid administration of hypertonic solutions can cause profound but transient hypotension due to peripheral vasodilation.[105] Glucose-containing solutions are generally unnecessary during neurosurgical procedures because blood glucose levels are usually well-maintained even in small children in the absence of intravenous glucose administration during typical (balanced) neurosurgical anesthetics. However, glucose may be indicated when hypoglycemia is a concern, such as in diabetic children, children receiving hyperalimentation, preterm and full-term neonates, and malnourished or debilitated children. In these children, glucose solutions should be administered at or slightly below maintenance rates (by constant infusion pump) and serum glucose levels should be monitored periodically throughout surgery. The potential association of larger cerebral infarct size with hyperglycemia (blood glucose values in excess of 250 mg/dL) during ischemia is of particular concern.[106]

Meticulous management of fluids and blood products to minimize cerebral edema is a cornerstone of pediatric neuroanesthesia. Although cerebral hemorrhage is fortunately a rare event, when it does occur, it can be sudden and catastrophic. Therefore, all children should have secure, large-bore intravenous access and blood products should be available along with the means for warming the blood.

Temperature Control

Because the head accounts for a large proportion of an infant's body surface area, infants are particularly susceptible to heat loss during neurosurgical procedures (see Chapter 25). Special attention should be focused on maintaining normal temperature from the time the child is brought into the operating room, although moderate hypothermia during neurosurgery may be useful to decrease the $CMRO_2$. Ambient room temperature should be increased during positioning, preparation, and draping. Infrared warming lights may be helpful for infants, and warming blankets may be useful for infants weighing less than 10 kg. Heated or passive humidifiers can be used for anesthesia lasting more than 1 hour. Forced hot air warming mattresses remain the most effective means of maintaining body temperature.[107]

Venous Air Emboli

Venous air embolism (VAE) is a potential danger during intracranial procedures. The larger the pressure gradient between the operative site and the heart, the greater the potential for clinically significant entrainment of air into the central circulation.[108] For example, when the operative site is far above the heart (as in a seated craniotomy) or when the CVP is low (such as acute blood loss during craniofacial procedures), it creates an environment for a VAE. Intracranial procedures are particularly of concern because intracranial venous sinuses have dural attachments that impede their ability to collapse. Other potential air entry sites during neurosurgical procedures include bone, bridging veins, and spinal epidural veins. The sequence of events that should be followed when a VAE occurs is (1) to identify the problem, (2) to stop further air entrainment, and (3) to support the circulation.

When air enters the central circulation, it accumulates in either the right atrium or the right ventricular outflow tract. Cardiac output may be reduced depending on the size of the air lock. If enough air is entrained into the circulation, either the preload to the right ventricle decreases and the right side of the heart fails or the right-sided heart afterload increases acutely, which can lead to cor pulmonale, acutely decreasing left ventricular preload and, ultimately, resulting in cardiovascular collapse. Furthermore, intracardiac shunts such as a patent foramen ovale, atrial or ventricular septal defects, and other congenital cardiac defects may allow air to access the systemic circulation (including the coronaries and brain). The concern for VAE is even greater in infants and children because potential intracardiac shunts exist in many otherwise healthy infants and children. These may become clinically important if pulmonary hypertension develops acutely after a large air embolism. Some recommend preoperative echocardiographic screening for patent foramen ovale in any child being considered for a sitting craniotomy; others regard a patent foramen ovale to be an absolute contraindication to the sitting position.[109,110]

Although the incidence of VAE is greatest in the sitting position, the lateral, supine, and prone positions are not risk free. VAE have also been observed during craniotomy for craniosynostosis even when the operating room table is flat. The incidence of VAE in children undergoing suboccipital craniotomy in the sitting position is not significantly different from that in adults, but children appear to have a higher incidence of hypotension and a smaller likelihood of successful aspiration of central (intravascular) air.[111]

It is important to monitor for VAE due to the potential catastrophic complications of such an event. There are several modalities for detecting VAE, all with varying degrees of sensitivity. Many practitioners elect to employ several methods simultaneously.

Precordial Doppler ultrasonography is the earliest and most sensitive indicator of intravascular air (Fig. 23-6).[112] The precordial Doppler probe is usually placed over the fourth or fifth intercostal space at the right sternal border where it best monitors right-sided heart sounds. Appropriate Doppler positioning can be confirmed by listening for the characteristic change in sounds after rapid administration of a few milliliters of saline into a venous catheter. The precordial Doppler probe is particularly valuable because it is inexpensive, easy to use, benign, and noninvasive. Although echocardiography (transthoracic or

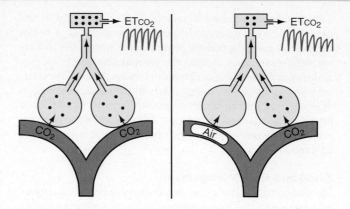

Figure 23-7. Mechanism of decreased end-tidal CO_2 after an air embolus. (Courtesy of Dr. J. Drummond.)

transesophageal) is the most specific method for detecting small air emboli, it is not easily used intraoperatively, especially in small infants and children.[109,113,114]

Monitoring end-tidal gas tensions is important during neurosurgical procedures. When VAE occurs, there is reflex pulmonary vasoconstriction and ventilation/perfusion mismatch caused by the air blocking passage of blood. This increases dead space ventilation and a sudden decrease in end-tidal CO_2 concentration. Thus, the end-tidal CO_2 concentration is useful in diagnosing VAE and can be used to monitor the severity and duration of air emboli (Fig. 23-7). An increase in end-tidal nitrogen concentration during continuous monitoring is a specific sign of air emboli. Although slightly more sensitive than a decrease in end-tidal CO_2, an increase in end-tidal nitrogen is not detected by most infrared analyzers in practice and is usually of such small magnitude that it may be difficult to detect.

Other less sensitive methods to detect VAE include ECG changes, changes in heart rate, decreases in systemic blood pressure, and increases in right atrial and pulmonary arterial pressures. Increases in right atrial and pulmonary artery pressures correlate with the size of emboli, but these delayed findings should not be relied on alone for monitoring and diagnosis.

On suspected or obvious diagnosis of VAE, immediate measures must be taken by both surgeons and anesthesiologists to prevent continued entrainment of air and consequent hemodynamic deterioration. The surgeon should immediately flood the field with saline and apply bone wax to exposed bone edges. The anesthesiologist should discontinue nitrous oxide and place the child in the Trendelenburg position. This will have the effect of increasing cerebral venous pressure and stopping entrainment of air, as well as augmenting the child's peripheral venous return and increasing systemic blood pressure. Some practitioners advocate occlusion of the internal jugular veins in an attempt to increase cerebral venous pressure, thereby making the pressure gradient less favorable for entrainment of air. This should be done with great care because occlusion of the carotid arteries can lead to cerebral ischemia. Attempts can be made to aspirate air through a central venous catheter if one is in place. The application of positive end-expiratory pressure increases CVP but also decreases cardiac filling pressure, cardiac output, and blood pressure; extreme increases in positive end-expiratory pressure are usually unwarranted. Vasopressors and fluid resuscitation may be required.

AIR EMBOLISM
Relative sensitivity

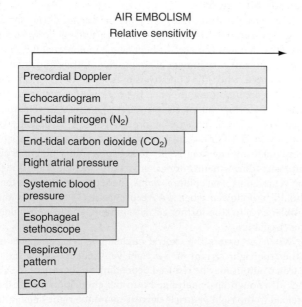

Precordial Doppler

Echocardiogram

End-tidal nitrogen (N_2)

End-tidal carbon dioxide (CO_2)

Right atrial pressure

Systemic blood pressure

Esophageal stethoscope

Respiratory pattern

ECG

Figure 23-6. Relative sensitivity of air embolism–monitoring modalities.

Aspiration of air from a central venous catheter is rarely successful unless massive amounts have been entrained. If small VAE are detected by other devices (e.g., Doppler, end-tidal CO_2), the value of aspirating through the central venous catheter is quite limited. When central venous pressure catheters are necessary, such as for a child in the sitting position or when massive blood loss is anticipated, an attempt should be made to place the tip at the junction of the superior vena cava and right atrium. This location provides the optimal location for aspiration of entrained air. More importantly, a central venous catheter is useful to estimate maintenance of circulating blood volume and to rapidly administer fluids and resuscitative medications when necessary. The position of a central venous catheter near the heart should be confirmed by radiograph, by transducing CVPs, or with the aid of ECG monitoring (biphasic p waves will develop in a lead at the tip of the catheter). For central venous catheters that will remain in situ in the postoperative period, their positions should be confirmed radiographically. Erosion of the catheter tip through the heart causing fatal pericardial tamponade has occurred after surgery in small children so soft silicone catheters are recommended.[115,116]

Once the child's condition has been stabilized, the procedure is resumed and a revised anesthetic plan is instituted. The decision to administer nitrous oxide after successful treatment of VAE is controversial. If reinstitution of nitrous oxide is associated with another decrease in end-tidal CO_2 concentration or clinical deterioration, then nitrous oxide should be discontinued. If no changes occur, clinicians may reinstitute nitrous oxide.

Emergence

Protecting the brain is a major strategy during neurosurgical procedures (Table 23-2). However, emergence and extubation should be smooth and controlled to prevent fluctuations in ICP and venous and arterial pressures.[117] To avoid vomiting during emergence, a multimodal antiemetic approach is often used. Despite this approach, the incidence of PONV is very high. This may be attributed to two factors: (1) blood in the CSF is a potent emetic and (2) opioids are often used to treat postoperative headache. Although ondansetron has not been shown to be effective for prophylaxis in children undergoing a craniotomy,[118] it may be combined with dexamethasone and used prophylactically.

Intravenous lidocaine (1.0-1.5 mg/kg) given before extubation may help to suppress coughing and straining on the endotracheal tube, although fentanyl appears to be equally effective and may even be less sedating. Labetalol, an α- and β-adrenergic blocking agent, can be administered incrementally for the control of blood pressure during the acute period of emergence, but this is rarely necessary in children who have received adequate doses of opioids during surgery. For adolescents, labetalol (up to 3 mg/kg total dose) may be necessary, but this usually does not have to be repeated in the postoperative period. Esmolol is also used by some practitioners and has been shown to be as effective as labetalol in controlling hypertension after intracranial surgery in adults.[119] However, esmolol should be used with caution in infants and smaller children because their cardiac output is dependent on heart rate. There are no studies evaluating the use of esmolol in children for such an application.

Table 23-2. Maneuvers of Neuroprotection

Goals	Avoid cerebral edema
	Avoid cerebral hypoxia
	Avoid cerebral hypoperfusion
	Avoid cerebral hypermetabolism
	Avoid neuronal membrane damage
Maneuver	
Head of bed at 30 degrees in midline	Increases cerebral venous drainage while maintaining CPP
Corticosteroids	May improve outcome in spinal cord injury
	Decrease vasogenic cerebral edema in children with tumors
	Stabilize neuronal membranes
	Free-radical scavengers
Controlled ventilation	Maintains $PaCO_2$ at normal to slightly low levels: prevents both cerebral vasodilation and increased ICP
Muscle paralysis	Avoids coughing, straining, child movement, and other causes of increased ICP
Ventricular drainage	Decreases ICP
Antihypertensives	Prevent further cerebral edema, ischemia, and/or cerebral hemorrhage
	Severe hypotension can significantly decrease CPP.
Anticonvulsants	Prevent seizure activity and increased ICP
Hypothermia	Decreases $CMRO_2$ and CMRglu consumption
Barbiturate coma	Membrane-stabilizing effect
	Decreases CBF and $CMRO_2$

CBF, cerebral blood flow; CMRglu, cerebral metabolic rate for glucose; $CMRO_2$, cerebral metabolic rate for oxygen; CPP, cerebral perfusion pressure; ICP, intracranial pressure; $PaCO_2$, partial pressure of arterial carbon dioxide.

As previously mentioned, dexmedetomidine may be useful in facilitating a smooth emergence while still allowing evaluation of the child's neurologic status.

Neuromuscular blockade should be pharmacologically reversed because even the slightest residual weakness is poorly tolerated and may complicate the neurologic examination. Adequate spontaneous ventilation and oxygenation and an awake mental status should be present before extubation. If postoperative intracranial hypertension is possible or if the child does not meet respiratory or neurologic criteria for extubation, the trachea should not be extubated. Sedation should be administered and the child transported to an intensive care unit.

It is desirable to have the child as fully alert as possible immediately after the operation to permit repeated neurologic examinations to assess recovery and to detect a deteriorating status. In unconscious children, ICP can be monitored invasively. CT scans are extremely helpful in evaluating the cause of an increased ICP or deteriorating mental status.

Pain is usually not severe after a craniotomy but can be treated with incremental doses of opioids. Ketorolac is best avoided in the early postoperative period because of its effects on platelet function. Acetaminophen may be administered either orally or rectally for mild pain and fever.[120]

Diabetes insipidus or inappropriate secretion of antidiuretic hormone may complicate postoperative fluid and electrolyte management, particularly when surgery is in the region of the hypothalamus and pituitary gland. Careful observation of fluid status and repeated laboratory evaluation of blood and urine osmolality and sodium are important in this situation. When diabetes insipidus occurs, it can be managed with a continuous infusion of dilute aqueous vasopressin (1-10 mU/kg/hr).[121] In such circumstances, large volumes of hypotonic intravenous solutions must be avoided, because they may rapidly decrease the serum sodium and osmolality. If normal saline is administered in strictly limited volumes, aqueous vasopressin can control the electrolyte and fluid balances of children with diabetes insipidus until they resume oral fluids. At that time, intranasal desmopressin (DDAVP) can be substituted. When diabetes insipidus develops after surgery in the pituitary region (e.g., during resection of a craniopharyngioma), it may only be transient. Therefore, it is important to assess the need for vasopressin repeatedly.

Portable EEGs and evoked auditory, somatosensory, and, less commonly, visual potentials may be helpful in assessing children who are deeply sedated or paralyzed. Observation in an intensive care unit capable of managing children is vital for the prevention or early detection and treatment of postoperative complications. CT and MRI are often performed 1 or 2 days after a craniotomy.

Special Situations

Trauma

Head Injury

Trauma is the primary cause of death in children, and head injuries produce the majority of the mortality and much of the morbidity in survivors.[122-124] Motor vehicle accidents continue to be the most frequent preventable cause of head injury, although domestic violence and sports are also common causes of trauma in children (see Fig. 39-10A-J). Assaults and suicide attempts have become increasingly common in adolescents.

Children with head trauma may have minimal neurologic abnormalities at the time of initial evaluation. However, increased ICP and neurologic deficits may progressively develop. These occur slowly because brain injuries occur in two stages. The primary insult that occurs at the time of impact results from the biomechanical forces that disrupt the cranium, neural tissue, and vasculature. The secondary insult is the parenchymal damage caused by pathologic sequelae subsequent to the primary insult. This can result from hypotension, hypoxia, cerebral edema, or intracranial hypertension. Whereas prevention of primary injuries must be addressed in a sociopolitical forum such as through seatbelt laws, sports injury prevention, and domestic violence legislation, anesthesiologists are instrumental in preventing or minimizing the secondary insult (see Chapter 39).

There are significant differences between children and adults in the pattern of CNS injuries. Although intracranial hematomas (epidural, subdural, or intraparenchymal) are common in adults, they are less frequent in children. In contrast, diffuse cerebral edema after blunt head trauma occurs more often in children than in adults.[125]

Scalp Injuries

One of the most common operative head injuries in children is the scalp laceration. Most of these can be managed in the emergency department, but more serious injuries may require the operating room to provide immobility and comfort. Children can lose a significant amount of blood from a scalp injury, because a larger fraction of the cardiac output perfuses the head compared with adults. Infants younger than 1 year of age may become hemodynamically unstable from blood loss from a subgaleal hematoma alone, as in a closed scalp injury, so hypovolemia should always be considered and treated before induction of anesthesia. Good intravenous access should be established and blood products should always be available. In addition, coexisting intracranial or other injuries need to be considered and a preoperative CT may be warranted.

Skull Fractures

Skull fractures are a common manifestation of head trauma in children. The vast majority are linear and do not require surgical treatment. These fractures are of concern primarily because the force required to produce them may damage the underlying brain and vasculature. A linear fracture over a major blood vessel (e.g., the middle meningeal artery) or a large dural sinus may result in intracranial hemorrhage. Fortunately, most children have an uneventful course after sustaining a simple skull fracture. A small minority develop a leptomeningeal cyst or growing fracture that eventually requires surgical treatment. Multiple skull fractures in the absence of documented major trauma should always raise the suspicion of child abuse.

Depressed skull fractures often require surgical repair. These may occur even in the absence of a scalp laceration. However, displacement of the inner table of the skull requires greater force than that needed to produce a simple linear fracture and has greater potential to damage underlying tissues. Approximately one third of all depressed fractures are uncomplicated, another one third are associated with dural lacerations, and the remaining one third are associated with cortical lacerations. The extent of cortical injury is the primary determinant of morbidity and mortality. Surgical débridement and elevation of the depressed bone are usually performed as soon as possible after the injury (Fig. 23-8A).

Basilar skull fractures are less common in children. Despite the force needed to produce these fractures, they have an excellent prognosis and rarely require surgical intervention. However, the possibility of a basilar skull fracture should be considered when caring for children with altered mental status, seizures, or associated trauma requiring surgery. Findings include periorbital ecchymoses ("raccoon eyes"), retroauricular ecchymosis (Battle's sign) (see Fig. 39-10J), hemotympanum, clear rhinorrhea, or otorrhea. Unless absolutely necessary (e.g., in mandibular wiring), nasotracheal intubation or passage of a nasogastric tube is best avoided because these tubes have inadvertently traversed these skull fractures and entered the cranium.[126-128] Complications of basilar skull fracture include meningitis from a CSF leak, cranial nerve damage, and anosmia.

Epidural Hematoma

Epidural hematomas most commonly develop in the temporoparietal region due to arterial bleeding from a severed middle meningeal artery. They can also develop in the posterior fossa as a result of bleeding from a venous sinus. Epidural hematomas are not necessarily associated with an overlying skull fracture. The classic natural history in adults is a "lucid interval" between

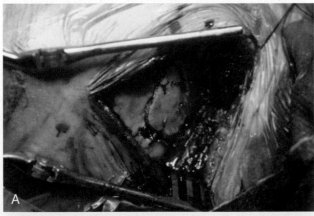

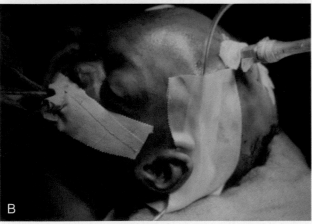

Figure 23-8. A, Depressed skull fracture requiring surgical intervention. **B,** Children with severe head trauma (in this case a shaken baby) may present with marked increases in ICP.

the initial loss of consciousness and subsequent neurologic deterioration. Infants and children may not demonstrate an altered mental status in the early stages after the injury. However, as the hematoma expands, it can lead to a loss of consciousness, hemiparesis, and pupillary dilatation. This deterioration can be quite rapid once a mass effect occurs. Treatment is prompt surgical evacuation because delays are associated with increased morbidity. Medical therapy directed at decreasing ICP should be instituted as soon as a diagnosis is suspected (see Fig. 23-8B). Children generally recover well after these hemorrhages, although morbidity is usually a reflection of underlying brain injury.

Subdural Hematoma

Subdural hematomas are usually associated with cortical damage resulting from either direct parenchymal contusion or laceration of venous blood vessels. Acute subdural hematomas are almost always traumatic and are frequently a result of abuse (shaking of small children, particularly those younger than 1 year of age). The shaken baby syndrome, a well-known entity, occurs when an infant is shaken so vigorously that significant neuronal disruption occurs, as well as tears in the cortical bridging veins that cause subdural hematomas.[129-131] These infants suffer significant brain damage complicated by episodes of apnea and further hypoxic insult.

Subdural hematomas also occasionally occur secondary to birth trauma within the first hours of life. Vitamin K deficiency, congenital coagulopathies, and disseminated intravascular coagulation are all considerations in these children. Great force is required to produce a subdural hematoma, whether by direct impact, laceration of blood vessels, or traumatic separation of the brain and overlying dura. Aggressive resuscitation and medical management are instituted simultaneously with preparation for surgical evacuation. Cerebral edema, uncontrolled intracranial hypertension, and persistent neurologic deficits often characterize the postoperative course. Chronic subdural hematomas or effusions may also develop in infancy, although these children do not usually present with acute symptoms. They are often diagnosed when the child is noted to be irritable and vomiting or develops an increase in head circumference. Chronic subdural hematomas can increase in size, causing slow but significant increases in ICP. Although a craniotomy is sometimes performed, most children undergo some form of hematoma drainage or shunting procedure as definitive treatment.

Intracerebral Hematoma

Intracerebral hematomas are fortunately rare but have a poor prognosis. Deep parenchymal hematomas are most often extensions of cortical contusions in a child with severe neurologic injury. Rarely, a localized hematoma may be appropriate for surgical evacuation to decompress the brain. In general, however, intraparenchymal hematomas are not evacuated for fear of damaging viable brain tissue. Anticonvulsants are usually administered prophylactically, and it is safest in the initial period after injury to avoid any medications that interfere with coagulation (e.g., ketorolac or heparin).

Spinal Injury

Although isolated cervical spine injuries are uncommon in children, those with severe head trauma should always be managed as if they have a cervical spine injury as well.[132,133] Different causes of spinal injuries are associated with specific age groups.

Motor vehicle accidents produce the largest number of injuries in older children and adolescents, whereas birth injuries and falls are the most common cause in infants and young children.[134] Spinal cord injury itself may be caused by a variety of forces, including hyperflexion, hyperextension, rotation, vertical compression, flexion rotation, and shearing. The injury may involve bony, ligamentous, cartilaginous, vascular, or neural components of the spine or adjacent structures. The biomechanics and functional anatomy of the pediatric spine also vary depending on the age of the child. Older children and teenagers are more likely to sustain injuries in the thoracolumbar region of the spine, whereas infants and younger children are more likely to suffer injuries in the high cervical region, particularly in the atlantoaxial region. The cervical spine is at greater risk in the infant and younger child because of the relatively weak and flexible neck muscles that support a proportionally large and heavy head, with the atlanto-occipital area acting as a pivot point. Atlanto-occipital dislocations are generally the most devastating neurologic injuries, leaving children neurologically devastated but not necessarily dead.

As with brain injury, spinal cord injury occurs in two phases. The primary insult results from biomechanical forces and bony fragments directly impacting the spinal cord. The secondary insult results from the pathologic sequelae of the primary insult: edema and ischemia due to cortical compression, hypotension, and/or hypoxia. Inappropriate manipulation of a child with an unstable fracture can exacerbate both primary and secondary injuries. Anesthesiologists who provide care for a child with a potential cervical spine injury should be aware that spinal cord injuries in children commonly occur without actual evidence of spinal bone fractures on plain cervical radiographs. These injuries are known as SCIWORA (spinal cord injuries without radiologic abnormality).[135] Injuries to the cervical spine in particular are often difficult to recognize but may be identified by odontoid displacement or prevertebral swelling on radiograph. As a result, CT is frequently indicated when a spinal injury is initially suspected in a child with trauma. Once a child with a potential spine injury is determined to be medically stable, these studies should be obtained as soon as possible. However, the child's airway and cardiorespiratory function must be continuously and closely monitored until a spinal cord injury can be ruled out. Sometimes, as with brain injury, there can be a delay in the onset of neurologic deficits with SCIWORA injuries.[136]

Respiratory failure is the most common cause of death after isolated cervical spine injury. Impaired respiratory function is a major cause of morbidity. The level of injury determines the degree of impairment. The phrenic nerve originates primarily from C4 but receives contributions of fibers from C3 and C5. Lesions at C5 leave partial diaphragmatic innervation but impair abdominal and intercostal accessory muscles. Lesions between C6 and T7 preserve diaphragmatic innervation but diminish accessory muscle function.

Children with a cervical spine injury may rapidly develop respiratory failure due to decreased vital capacity, increased dead space, retention of secretions, and respiratory muscle fatigue. Resultant hypercarbia and hypoxia aggravate the secondary injury to both brain and spinal cord. Respiratory status may be further impaired by associated trauma to the chest causing pulmonary contusion or pneumothorax or by aspiration of gastric contents.

Prompt airway management is critical to avoid hypoxia, ensure adequate respiratory mechanics, preserve neural function, and prevent extension of spinal injury. The head and neck must be immediately immobilized; restraint of the extremities may also be required. During airway manipulation, an assistant should maintain the head and neck in a neutral position (see Figs. 39-6 and 39-7). Various endotracheal tubes and laryngoscope blades should be available, as well as equipment and personnel for an emergency tracheostomy. Insertion of a laryngeal mask airway may be lifesaving until a more secure airway can be achieved with fiberoptic or other means.[137-142] Small fiberoptic bronchoscopes are available (2.2 mm diameter) that can fit through infant-sized endotracheal tubes. Retrograde intubation using a guidewire introduced through the cricothyroid membrane may be useful in older children or adolescents (see Chapter 12). However, an unstable infant or child whose airway cannot be secured by conventional means is probably best managed by an emergency tracheostomy. As a temporizing measure, a cricothyroidotomy can be performed (see Fig. 12-27).[143] This permits oxygenation (although inadequate ventilation) until personnel and equipment for tracheostomy are assembled.

Hemodynamic instability may also be a problem due to hypovolemia from other injuries or severe head trauma. Other sites of bleeding such as long bone fractures and abdominal trauma should be ruled out. Children with spinal shock exhibit loss of vasomotor tone or loss of normal neurocardiac function with associated bradycardia and decreased myocardial contractility. Intravenous fluids and vasopressors may be necessary for management.

Although there are currently few data regarding children, corticosteroids are usually administered to children with spinal injuries as soon as possible after the initial trauma in the hopes of reducing the neurologic injury. The most commonly used drug is methylprednisolone, 30 mg/kg, administered over the first 15 minutes, followed by an infusion of 5.4 mg/kg/hr for the following 23 hours.[144,145] Methylprednisolone is believed to be effective via multiple mechanisms, including improved spinal blood flow, inhibition of the arachidonic acid cascade, and modulation of the local immune response.[146] In addition, some evidence suggests that GM_1-ganglioside, with or without methylprednisolone, may be advantageous in decreasing demyelination and promoting neurologic recovery if administered soon after a spinal injury.[147-153]

If the spinal cord injury is greater than 24 hours old, succinylcholine should not be administered because it can result in massive hyperkalemia.[154] In addition, physiologic changes may occur due to autonomic hyperreflexia, which frequently develops after cervical or high thoracic spinal lesions. This autonomic hyperreflexia is capable of producing severe, even life-threatening, vasomotor instability with hypertension and arrhythmias.[155,156]

Craniotomy

Tumors

Brain tumors are the most common solid tumors in children, exceeded only by the leukemias as the most common pediatric malignancy.[157] There are 1500 to 2000 new brain tumors diagnosed annually in children in the United States. Unlike those in adults, the majority of brain tumors in children are infratentorial, in the posterior fossa. These include medulloblastomas, cerebellar astrocytomas, brainstem gliomas, and ependymomas of the fourth ventricle. Because posterior fossa tumors usually obstruct CSF flow, increased ICP occurs early. Presenting signs and symptoms include early morning vomiting and irritability or lethargy. Cranial nerve palsies and ataxia are also common findings, with respiratory and cardiac irregularities usually occurring late. Sedation or general anesthesia may be required for radiologic evaluation or radiation therapy.

Surgical resection of a posterior fossa tumor presents a number of anesthetic challenges. Children are usually positioned prone, although the lateral or sitting positions are utilized by some neurosurgeons. In any case, the head will be flexed and the position and patency of the endotracheal tube must be meticulously ensured. A nasotracheal tube is often preferred when the child is prone. In the event that the endotracheal tube does become dislodged when the child is in a head holder and prone, successful emergent airway management has been described utilizing a laryngeal mask airway.[158]

Arrhythmias and acute blood pressure changes may occur during surgical exploration, especially when the brainstem is manipulated. Consequently, the electrocardiogram and arterial waveform should be monitored. Altered respiratory control is generally masked by muscle relaxants and mechanical ventilation. Even when ICP is only marginally increased, intracranial compliance is presumed to have decreased. This warrants precautions against further increases in ICP. If ICP is markedly increased or acutely worsens, a ventricular catheter may be inserted before the tumor is resected. VAE is a potentially serious complication that is not eliminated by repositioning to the prone or lateral position because head-up gradients of 10 to 20 degrees are frequently used to improve cerebral venous drainage. In infants and toddlers, large head size relative to body size accentuates this problem.

Supratentorial tumors in the midbrain include craniopharyngiomas, optic gliomas, pituitary adenomas, and hypothalamic tumors and account for approximately 15% of intracranial tumors. Hypothalamic tumors (hamartomas, gliomas, and teratomas) frequently present with precocious puberty in children who are large for their chronologic age. Craniopharyngiomas are the most common perisellar tumors in children and adolescents and may be associated with hypothalamic and pituitary dysfunction. Symptoms often include growth failure, visual impairment, and endocrine abnormalities.

Signs and symptoms of hypothyroidism should be sought and thyroid function tests measured. Corticosteroid replacement (dexamethasone or hydrocortisone) is generally administered because the integrity of the hypothalamic-pituitary-adrenal axis may be uncertain. In addition, diabetes insipidus occurs preoperatively and is a common postoperative problem. The history usually reveals this condition preoperatively, especially if attention is focused on nocturnal drinking and enuresis. Evaluation of serum electrolytes and osmolality, urine specific gravity, and urine output are helpful because hypernatremia and hyperosmolality, along with dilute urine, are typical findings. If diabetes insipidus does not exist preoperatively, it usually does not develop until the postoperative period because there is an adequate reserve of antidiuretic hormone in the posterior pituitary gland capable of functioning for many hours, even when the hypothalamic-pituitary stalk is damaged intraoperatively.

Postoperative diabetes insipidus is marked by a sudden large increase in dilute urine output associated with an increasing serum sodium concentration and osmolality. Protocols have been developed to guide both intraoperative as well as postoperative management of diabetes insipidus (see earlier and Chapter 8).[121] Return of antidiuretic hormone activity a few days postoperatively may cause a marked decrease in urinary output, water intoxication, seizures, and cerebral edema if it is not recognized and fluid administration is not adjusted appropriately.

Transsphenoidal surgery is generally performed only in adolescents and older children with pituitary adenomas. However, it should be treated like other midbrain tumors in terms of monitoring and vascular access. Children are usually intubated orally to give the surgeon optimal access to the nasopharynx, and preparations for an emergent craniotomy should be anticipated in case unexpected massive bleeding develops. Because nasal packs are inserted at the end of surgery, children should be fully awake before tracheal extubation.

Gliomas of the optic pathways occur with increased frequency in children with neurofibromatosis. Presenting symptoms include visual changes and proptosis; increased ICP and hypothalamic dysfunction are usually late findings. There are two main forms of neurofibromatosis: type 1, also known as peripheral or von Recklinghausen neurofibromatosis, and type 2, also known as central or bilateral acoustic neurofibromatosis. Type 1 neurofibromatosis is associated with other tumors, including pheochromocytomas, neuroblastomas, leukemia, sarcomas, and Wilms tumors. Neurofibromas tend to be highly vascular, and thus the anesthesiologist should be prepared for significant blood loss.

Approximately 25% of intracranial tumors in children involve the cerebral hemispheres. These are primarily astrocytomas, oligodendrogliomas, ependymomas, and glioblastomas. Neurologic symptoms are more likely to include a seizure disorder or focal deficits. Succinylcholine should be avoided if motor weakness is present because it can cause sudden severe hyperkalemia. Nondepolarizing muscle relaxants and opioids may be metabolized more rapidly than usual in children who are receiving chronic anticonvulsants. Choroid plexus papillomas are rare but occur most often in children younger than 3 years of age. They usually arise from the choroid plexus of the lateral ventricle and produce early hydrocephalus as a result of increased production of CSF and obstruction of CSF flow. Hydrocephalus usually resolves with surgical resection. When lesions lie near the motor or sensory strip, a special type of somatosensory evoked potential monitoring called "phase reversal" may also be used to delineate these locations.[159] If cortical stimulation is planned to help identify motor areas, muscle relaxants must be permitted to wear off. Nitrous oxide (less than 50%), propofol, isoflurane (less than 0.5 MAC), and opioids are usually sufficient to prevent the children from moving during these periods. Dexmedetomidine may be a useful adjunct to augment sedation.

Stereotactic biopsies or craniotomies present special concerns regarding airway accessibility. Newer head frames are available that have adjustable anterior positions so that the airway is readily accessible (Fig. 23-9, see website). It is more comfortable and less distressing for the child to be anesthetized before the head frame is applied, even though this means the anesthesiologist must induce anesthesia in the radiology suite and then transport the child from the CT scanner to the operating room. The wrench that is used to apply (and remove) the head frame should be taped to the frame itself so that it is always readily available should emergent removal of the head frame become necessary.

Vascular Anomalies

Arteriovenous Malformations

Arteriovenous malformations consist of large arterial feeding vessels, dilated communicating vessels, and large draining veins carrying arterialized blood. Large malformations, especially those involving the posterior cerebral artery and vein of Galen, may manifest as congestive heart failure (high-output heart failure, often with pulmonary hypertension) in the neonate. The prognosis for these types of arteriovenous malformations is generally quite poor. Saccular dilation of the vein of Galen may manifest later in infancy or childhood as hydrocephalus secondary to obstruction of the aqueduct of Sylvius. Malformations not large enough to produce congestive heart failure usually remain clinically silent unless they cause seizures or a stroke or until the acute rupture of a communicating vessel results in subarachnoid or intracerebral hemorrhage.[160] Intracranial hemorrhages are the most common presentation in this population, with an associated mortality of 25%.

Treatment usually consists of embolization or radiation of deep malformations, surgical excision (usually of the more superficial ones), or a combination of these modalities. Anesthetic management for elective embolic procedures usually involves a standard general anesthetic with muscle relaxants and secure intravenous access. Moderate hyperventilation may actually enhance visualization of abnormal blood vessels that do not respond with vasoconstriction. The anesthesiologist should be knowledgeable about the types of embolic agents that will be used and their potential complications. Anticonvulsant therapy is routine. Neonates in cardiac failure may be receiving several inotropic agents. Bleeding, especially from the femoral arterial puncture site (which cannot always be visualized), should always be a consideration. Fluid overload can occur due to the large amount of contrast agents administered, especially in a young infant who may already be in high-output cardiac failure. One should always be prepared for the possibility of an emergency craniotomy should a vessel rupture.

Aneurysms

Intracranial aneurysms are most often due to a congenital malformation in an arterial wall. Children with coarctation of the aorta or polycystic kidney disease have an increased incidence of these aneurysms. They usually remain asymptomatic during childhood; most ruptures that occur in childhood are fatal. Symptoms of subarachnoid or intracerebral hemorrhage frequently appear suddenly in a previously healthy young adult. When technically feasible, surgical ligation or clipping constitutes the treatment of choice.[161]

Anesthesia for surgical resection of vascular malformations and aneurysms in children presents unique challenges, especially if the diagnosis has been preceded by an intracranial hemorrhage. These are some of the few situations in pediatric neuroanesthesia in which deep preoperative sedation may be beneficial to avoid sudden hypertensive episodes. Blood products should be in the operating room and verified before the start of the procedure. An adequate depth of anesthesia should be ensured before any invasive maneuver to prevent precipitous hypertension. Adequate venous access to respond to a sudden and massive blood loss is crucial but can wait until after induc-

tion of anesthesia. A blood warming device, such as a rapid transfusion device, should be immediately available.

Controlled hypotension may also be valuable in some situations for brief periods of time to reduce tension in the abnormal blood vessels and improve the safety of surgical manipulation.[162] It is not clear, however, whether the benefits of controlled hypotension are worth the risks, especially in small children (see Chapter 10). Controlled hypotension should not be used in the presence of increased ICP because of the risk of decreasing CPP with resulting ischemia and further increased ICP. Controlled hypotension may be induced with potent inhalation anesthetics combined with vasodilators (nitroprusside or nitroglycerin) when necessary. Intermediate-acting adrenergic antagonists (labetalol, esmolol) are also effective. Remifentanil infusions have also been used to provide a moderate degree of control hypotension. Although the absolute limits of acceptable hypotension are unknown, a mean blood pressure greater than 40 mm Hg (for infants) and 50 mm Hg (for older children) generally appears safe. At the conclusion of the procedure the blood pressure is returned to normal, but before closing the dura, the operative site should be inspected for bleeding.

Hemodynamic stability is also important during emergence to avoid bucking, coughing, straining, and hypertension during extubation. Excessive hypertension should be avoided to prevent postoperative bleeding, although in most cases of aneurysm clipping, a slightly increased blood pressure may be desirable postoperatively to minimize the risk of vasospasm. Postoperatively, after resection of an arteriovenous malformation, there can be serious complications due to cerebral edema with increased ICP or hemorrhage. This is generally called normal perfusion pressure breakthrough and is believed to be caused by hyperemia of the areas surrounding the previous arteriovenous malformation site where vessels suffer from continued vasomotor paralysis and cannot vasoconstrict. Treatment is controversial but generally involves therapy for increased ICP (diuretics, moderate hyperventilation, head elevation) in addition to judicious use of moderate hypotension (while maintaining CPP) and moderate hypothermia. When surgery is completed, it is particularly important that children are able to cooperate with a neurologic examination and that there is careful control of blood pressure in the intensive care unit.

Moyamoya Disease

Moyamoya disease is an anomaly that results in progressive and life-threatening occlusion of intracranial vessels, primarily the internal carotid arteries near the circle of Willis.[163] An abnormal vascular network of collaterals develops at the base of the brain giving rise to the Japanese name (translated roughly as "puff of smoke") associated with the angiographic appearance of this condition (Fig. 23-10A). In the congenital form, the dysplastic process may involve systemic (especially renal) arteries as well. The acquired variety may be associated with meningitis, neurofibromatosis, chronic inflammation, connective tissue diseases, certain hematologic disorders, Down syndrome, or prior intracranial radiation. For reasons that are unknown, this disease appears to be more common in children of Japanese ancestry. Associated intracranial aneurysms are rare in children but may occur in more than 10% of adult patients. Abnormal electrocardiographic findings have also been described with this syndrome in adults. Moyamoya disease usually manifests as transient ischemic attacks progressing to strokes and fixed

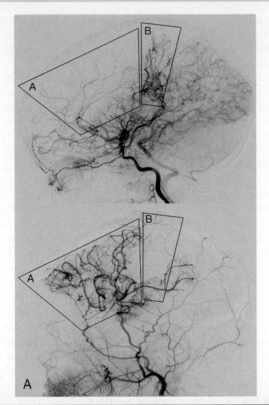

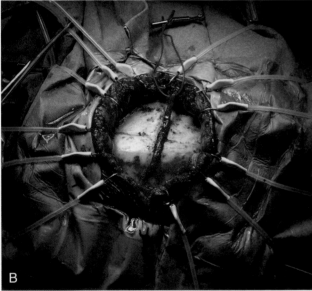

Figure 23-10. Moyamoya disease. **A,** The top angiogram represents the pattern of arterial filling after injection of the internal carotid artery in a child with moyamoya disease before pial synangiosis. The area represented by A shows poor filling from the middle cerebral artery as a result of the disease process. The area represented by B shows the characteristic "hazy" collaterals" or moyamoya vessels. The bottom angiogram is from the same child after pial synangiosis. This angiogram was obtained after injection of the superficial temporal artery, which now shows good filling in the middle cerebral artery distribution in A. The area B does not fill from the middle cerebral artery. **B,** Pial synangiosis. The superficial temporal artery is prepared to be sutured to the pia of the cerebral cortex. After the craniotomy is completed, this artery can then be sewn directly onto the underlying pia mater. The result of this procedure is improvement of blood flow to ischemic areas of the cerebral cortex.

neurologic deficits in children. The attacks may be precipitated by hyperventilation.[164] There is a high morbidity and mortality rate if the condition is left untreated. Medical management consists of antiplatelet therapy, such as aspirin or calcium channel blockers. The most common surgical operation for correction in children is pial synangiosis, which involves suturing a scalp artery (usually the superficial temporal artery) onto the pial surface of the brain to enhance revascularization (Fig. 23-10B).[165]

Careful and continuous monitoring of end-tidal CO_2 concentration is essential to anesthetic management.[166] Children with moyamoya disease have reduced hemispheric blood flow in both hemispheres, and hyperventilation may also further reduce regional blood flow and cause significant EEG and neurologic changes.[167] Thus, it is crucial that normocapnia be maintained throughout the procedure. In effect, this may be one of the only conditions in pediatric neuroanesthesia in which mild hyperventilation is inappropriate.[168] Adequate hydration and maintenance of baseline blood pressure are also extremely important. The majority of these children have an intravenous catheter inserted the night before surgery and are given one and a half times maintenance fluids to avoid dehydration during the perioperative period. There may be benefit in EEG monitoring during these procedures to detect and potentially treat ischemia that appears to be a result of cerebral vasoconstriction in response to direct surgical manipulation of the brain itself. Normothermia is maintained, particularly at the end of the procedure, to avoid postoperative shivering and stress response. As in most neurosurgical procedures, a smooth extubation without hypertension or crying is desirable. Although very little literature exists regarding intraoperative and postoperative complications during moyamoya surgery, it appears that most complications (strokes) occur postoperatively and are associated with dehydration and crying (hyperventilation) episodes.[169]

Seizure Surgery

Epilepsy is one of the most common neurologic disorders of childhood. Despite the development of new drugs and regimens, the prevalence of pharmacologically intractable seizures is still high. Advances in neuroimaging and EEG provide epileptologists anatomic targets that mediate some medically intractable seizure disorders. Recent advances in pediatric neurosurgery have exploited these technologies and dramatically improved the outcome in infants and children.[170]

Children presenting for surgical management of seizures also take anticonvulsant medications. Several of these medications have serious potential side effects. These generally manifest as abnormalities of hematologic function (particularly valproic acid and carbamazepine) such as abnormal coagulation, depression of red or white blood cell production, or decreased platelet counts. Other problems may arise from altered hepatic function. Specific anticonvulsant levels should be determined preoperatively to detect subtherapeutic or toxic concentrations. It is also worth noting that many anticonvulsants enhance metabolism of nondepolarizing muscle relaxants and opioids, thereby leading to an increase (up to 50%) in the amount of these drugs needed during a surgical procedure. The preoperative evaluation should also detect underlying conditions that are causing the seizures, as well as disabilities that can result from progressive neurologic dysfunction.

One of the major surgical concerns during resection of seizure foci is to avoid harming brain tissue that controls vital functions, such as motion, sensation, speech, and memory, especially if a seizure focus is adjacent to cortical areas controlling these functions. Cooperative adolescents and adults can assist in determination of the limits of safe cortical resection if they can be continually assessed during the surgical procedure. Thus, the technique of "awake" craniotomy is often performed in carefully selected children. The concept of "awake" craniotomy actually encompasses a wide variety of techniques whose common goal is to allow intraoperative assessment and feedback to determine if eloquent cortex is at risk during resection.

Some practitioners will perform the entire procedure including line placement, infiltration of local anesthetic, skull and dural opening, and resection with the child completely awake or with minimal sedation. This particular approach requires an extremely motivated child. A variation on this technique utilizes short-acting sedatives and analgesics, such as propofol and fentanyl, titrated to induce unconsciousness but maintain spontaneous ventilation for instillation of local anesthetics, insertion of monitoring catheters, placement of head pins, and skull opening.[171] Subsequently, children can be allowed to awaken during surgical resection. They can then have sedatives and opioids reinstituted for the craniotomy closure.

Alternatively, some anesthesiologists utilize the asleep-awake-asleep technique. Basically this consists of inducing general anesthesia and maintaining airway control with a supraglottic device (i.e., a laryngeal mask airway). General anesthesia is maintained for line placement, placement of head pins, and skull and dural opening. The child is then awakened, the supraglottic airway is removed, and the surgeons then proceed with resection. At the conclusion of the resection, general anesthesia is once again induced and the supraglottic airway reinserted for closure of the dura, skull, and skin. There are several disadvantages to the asleep-awake-asleep approach. One of the major concerns when employing this approach is airway management during emergence and induction while the child is in head pins. Should the child cough or buck while immobilized, cervical spine injuries or scalp lacerations can occur. Additionally, brain swelling is a real concern in a child who is breathing spontaneously under general anesthesia with an inhalational anesthetic and possibly nitrous oxide.

Regardless of the technique chosen, it is important for the anesthesiologist to have an in-depth discussion with the child with respect to intraoperative needs and expectations. The preoperative period is the time to decide whether the child is a candidate for an "awake" craniotomy. There are no randomized controlled trials comparing the safety or effectiveness of the techniques just described.

Younger children (<10 years) or uncooperative children of any age generally will not tolerate this approach and will require general anesthesia throughout. In such circumstances, intraoperative electrophysiologic studies, such as somatosensory evoked potentials, EEG, and motor stimulation, may be used to help localize and determine the function of the site of planned resection. If EEG studies are to be performed, a nitrous oxide/opioid technique enables all potent inhalational agents that depress cerebral electrical activity to be eliminated by the time of study. If direct cortical motor stimulation is planned, muscle relaxants must be permitted to wear off as well. Occasionally, a seizure focus is difficult to identify intraoperatively. In these situations, hyperventilation or methohexital (in small doses, 0.25-0.5 mg/kg) may be helpful in lowering the seizure threshold and producing EEG seizure activity.[172,173]

In some children, the site of origin of generalized seizures is difficult to determine. When this occurs, evaluation with intracranial EEG monitoring ("grids and strips") may be accomplished by direct electrocorticography (Fig. 23-11, see website). These leads are placed on the surface of the cortex after a craniotomy under general anesthesia. Intraoperative EEG monitoring is limited during these procedures merely to ensure that all leads are functional; the actual monitoring for seizures takes place over the next several days to see if a "focus" can be identified that is amenable to resection. These children need to be observed carefully in the postoperative period, because complications can develop from having intracranial electrodes in place. Air frequently persists in the skull for up to 3 weeks after a craniotomy,[90] so these children should not have nitrous oxide administered for their subsequent procedure (to resect a seizure focus and/or remove the electrocorticography leads) until their dura has been opened to prevent the development of tension pneumocephalus. We have found it is helpful to insert a peripheral intravenous central catheter (PICC line) in children who are initially undergoing these procedures because intravenous antibiotic therapy is administered while the electrodes are in place (usually about 1 week) and this avoids the need for multiple peripheral intravenous catheter insertions.

When a focal resection is not possible, a lobectomy or corpus callosotomy may be attempted. It should be noted, however, that children undergoing this latter procedure are often somnolent for the first few postoperative days, especially if a "complete" callosotomy is performed. This also occurs in children who have undergone insertion of multiple subdural grids and strips. Occasionally, small children will undergo a hemispherectomy because their seizures are attributed to an abnormal hemisphere that is usually already severely dysfunctional, as when a hemiparesis is already present. These can be very challenging cases for the anesthesiologist because much blood can be lost (from one half to multiples of the estimated blood volume).[174] This procedure is usually performed when children are very young (to permit the other hemisphere to "take over" function of both sides); thus, ensuring adequate intravenous access can be challenging. Frequently, a large-bore catheter inserted into a femoral vein is helpful in these cases to facilitate rapid replacement of blood, crystalloid solutions, and medications. Arterial pressure monitoring is routine for such cases. Many practitioners also utilize central venous pressure monitoring for these procedures.

One advance in the treatment of epilepsy has been the development of the vagal nerve stimulator. Although the exact mechanism of how it functions is not understood at this time, it appears to inhibit seizure activity at brainstem or cortical levels.[175,176] It is becoming a popular form of treatment because it has shown benefit with minimal side effects in many children who are disabled by intractable seizures. Large, randomized trials are currently underway to determine the overall efficacy of this treatment. There are few published series of vagal nerve stimulation in children but it is estimated that there is a 60% to 70% improvement in seizure control in children receiving vagal nerve stimulation, with the best results in those with drop attacks.[177,178]

The vagal nerve stimulator device is a programmable stimulator similar to a cardiac pacemaker placed subcutaneously under the left anterior chest wall. Bipolar platinum stimulating electrode coils, which are implanted around the left vagus nerve, are connected to the generator via subcutaneously tunneled wires. The procedure usually takes about 2 hours. The device automatically activates for up to 30 seconds every 5 minutes. Although stimulation of the vagal nerve in this manner may affect vocal cord function, sudden bradycardia or other side effects are uncommon.[179] When children with vagal nerve stimulators return for subsequent surgeries, it may be appropriate to deactivate the stimulator while the child is under general anesthesia to prevent vocal cord motion.

Hydrocephalus

Hydrocephalus is a condition involving a mismatch of CSF production and absorption resulting in an increased intracranial CSF volume. It can be caused by a variety of pathologic processes, including arachnoid cysts (Fig. 23-12). Except for rare instances of excess CSF production, such as in choroid plexus

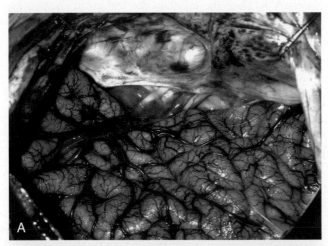

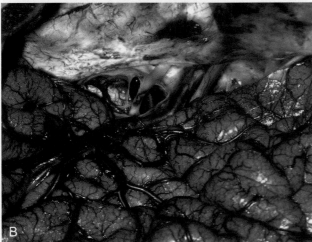

Figure 23-12. Arachnoid cyst. Arachnoid cysts can cause hydrocephalus in children. **A,** Before decompression, the mass effect is obvious. **B,** After fenestration of the cyst, cerebrospinal fluid has a path of egress from the inside of the cyst to the normal cerebrospinal fluid circulation. Thus, the mass effect is resolved.

papillomas, the majority of cases of hydrocephalus are secondary to some type of obstruction or inability to absorb CSF appropriately. Commonly, this is a result of hemorrhage (neonatal intraventricular or subarachnoid), congenital problems (aqueductal stenosis), trauma, infection, or tumors (especially in the posterior fossa). Hydrocephalus can be classified as nonobstructive/communicating or obstructive/noncommunicating based on the ability of CSF to flow around the spinal cord in its usual manner.

Intracranial hypertension or a decrease in intracranial compliance almost always accompanies untreated hydrocephalus in children. How much intracranial compliance exists and how acutely hydrocephalus develops are both factors in how severe the signs and symptoms of hydrocephalus will be. In the young infant, if hydrocephalus develops slowly, the skull will expand and the cerebral cortical mantle will stretch until massive craniomegaly (often with irreversible neurologic damage) occurs. However, if the cranial bones are fused or the cranium cannot expand fast enough, neurologic signs and symptoms rapidly become apparent. The child may become progressively more lethargic and develop vomiting, cranial nerve dysfunction ("setting sun" sign), bradycardia, and, ultimately, brain herniation and death.

Unless the etiology of the hydrocephalus can be definitively treated, treatment entails surgical placement of an extracranial shunt. Most shunts transport CSF from the lateral ventricles to the peritoneal cavity (ventriculoperitoneal shunts). Occasionally the distal end of the shunt must be placed in the right atrium or pleural cavity, usually owing to problems with the ability of the peritoneal cavity to absorb CSF. Newer shunt systems with "programmable" valves are being tried to reduce the need for shunt revisions.[180]

The use of a percutaneous flexible neuroendoscope through a burr hole in the skull has provided an alternative to extracranial shunt placement.[181] During these procedures, a ventriculostomy may be made to bypass an obstruction (e.g., aqueductal stenosis) by forming a communicating hole from one area of CSF flow to another using a blunt probe inserted through the neuroendoscope. Common locations for a ventriculostomy are through the septum pellucidum (so the lateral ventricles can communicate) or through the floor of the third ventricle into the adjacent CSF cisterns. Complications such as damage to the basilar artery or its branches or neural injuries can be life-threatening when they occur, and the anesthesiologist should be prepared for an emergency craniotomy during these procedures.

The anesthetic plan in a child with hydrocephalus should be directed at controlling ICP and relieving the obstruction as soon as possible. In the presence of increased ICP, these children are often at risk for vomiting and pulmonary aspiration, in which case a rapid-sequence induction and tracheal intubation with cricoid pressure should be performed. Ketamine is a particularly dangerous anesthetic to use in these situations because it can lead to sudden massive intracranial hypertension. Therefore, barbiturates are generally used for induction. Hydrocephalus often produces large dilated scalp veins in infants, and these can be used for induction of anesthesia if necessary. If intravenous access cannot be established, then an inhalation induction with sevoflurane and gentle cricoid pressure may be an alternative, though less desirable, method of induction.[182] This method results in venodilation and generally facilitates establishment of intravenous access. Once an intravenous catheter is inserted, the child may be paralyzed, the lungs hyperventilated, the trachea intubated, the inhalation agent decreased or discontinued, and the remainder of the anesthetic maintained with a balanced nitrous oxide/opioid technique or low concentrations of isoflurane. The possibility of VAE during placement of the distal end of a ventriculoatrial shunt should always be kept in mind. Postoperatively, children should be observed carefully because an altered mental status and recent peritoneal incision place them at greater risk for pulmonary aspiration once feeding begins.

There are a few special situations involving shunts with which anesthesiologists should be familiar. Children who develop a shunt infection usually have their entire shunt system removed and external ventricular drainage established. They return to the operating room for insertion of a new shunt several days after their infection has been treated with antibiotics. While an external drain is in place, one must be careful not to dislodge the ventricular tubing. In addition, the height of the drainage bag should not be significantly changed in relation to the child's head to avoid sudden changes in ICP. For example, suddenly lowering an open drainage bag can siphon CSF rapidly from the head, resulting in collapse of the ventricles and rupture of cortical veins. When transporting children with CSF drainage, or when moving them from a stretcher to an operating room table, it is best to close off the ventriculostomy tubing during these brief periods.

Anesthesiologists should also be aware of a special condition known as slit ventricle syndrome (Fig. 23-13). This situation develops in 5% to 10% of children with CSF shunts and is associated with overdrainage of CSF and small, "slit-like," lateral ventricular spaces. Children with this condition do not have the usual amount of intracranial CSF to compensate for alterations in brain or intracranial blood volume. Thus, special attention should be paid to children in whom CT scans indicate the presence of this condition. In particular, it is probably safest to avoid the administration of excess or hypotonic intravenous solutions in these situations in the intraoperative and postoperative periods to minimize the potential for brain swelling. Some of these children cannot seem to accommodate to situations that otherwise healthy children would easily tolerate. Episodes of postoperative cerebral herniation have been reported after uneventful surgical procedures.[45]

Congenital Anomalies

Congenital anomalies of the CNS generally occur as midline defects. This dysraphism may occur anywhere along the neural axis, involving the head (encephalocele) or spine (meningomyelocele) (Fig. 23-14). The defect may be relatively minor and affect only superficial bony and membranous structures or may include a large segment of malformed neural tissue.

Encephalocele

Encephaloceles can occur anywhere from the occiput to the frontal area. They can even appear as nasal "polyps" if they protrude through the cribriform plate. Rarely, they are filled with so much CSF that the defect can be nearly as large as the head itself. Large defects may present challenges to endotracheal intubation. Blood loss can be severe, especially if venous sinuses are involved. Adequate intravenous access should be ensured and blood products readily available. If hemodynamic instability is anticipated, an arterial catheter may be indicated.

Myelodysplasia

Defects in the spine are known as spina bifida. Meningoceles are lesions containing CSF without spinal tissue. When neural tissue is also present within the lesion, the defect is called a meningomyelocele. Open neural tissue is known as rachischisis. Hydrocephalus is usually present when paralysis occurs below the lesion and is often associated with an Arnold-Chiari malformation (see later).

Most children with a meningomyelocele present for primary closure within the first 48 hours of life to minimize the risk of infection. Many are now scheduled electively before birth for repair because the defect is usually apparent on prenatal ultrasonography. Many neurosurgeons prefer to insert a ventriculoperitoneal shunt at the time of initial surgery. Alternatively, a shunt may be inserted a few days later or even occasionally deferred if there is no evidence of hydrocephalus at birth. A major anesthetic consideration is positioning the neonate for induction at surgery. In most cases, tracheal intubation can be performed with the infant in the supine position and the uninvolved portion of the child's back supported with towels (or a "donut" ring) so there is no direct pressure on the meningomyelocele. For very large defects, it is occasionally necessary to place the infant in the left lateral position for induction and tracheal intubation. Succinylcholine is rarely needed for tracheal intubation, although it is not associated with hyperkalemia because the defect develops early in gestation not associated with muscle denervation.[183] Airway management, mask fit, and intubation may be difficult in infants with massive hydrocephalus or very large defects. In such cases, awake intubation after preoxygenation and administration of atropine may occasionally be the safest alternative. Blood loss may be considerable during repair of a meningomyelocele when large amounts of skin are to be undermined to cover the defect.

Children with myelodysplasia are at high risk of developing a sensitivity (and possibly anaphylaxis) to latex.[40] This is likely a result of repeated exposures to latex products encountered during repeated bladder catheterizations and multiple (usually >5) surgical procedures where latex gloves have been in contact with large mucosal surfaces. Therefore, these children are best managed in a latex-free environment from birth to minimize the chances for sensitization.[184] Latex should be at the top of the list should signs and symptoms of anaphylaxis develop during surgery. During an acute reaction, all latex-containing objects including gloves, tape, elastic bands, catheters, and so on, should be removed immediately. Latex anaphylaxis should be treated with intravenous epinephrine in a dose of 1 to 10 μg/kg as required. Many hospitals have replaced most or all of their latex-containing supplies with non-latex alternatives. Children who develop latex allergy exhibit cross-reactivity with some antibiotics[185,186] and foods (including tropical fruits such as avocado, kiwi, and banana as well as tomatoes and potatoes).

Postoperatively, respiratory status should be carefully assessed. Pulse oximetry is valuable during recovery from anesthesia because breathing difficulties may occur after a tight skin closure and the ventilatory responses to hypoxia and hypercarbia may be diminished or absent when a Chiari malformation coexists.[187] Intrauterine surgery is currently being investigated as a way of diminishing the degree of damage caused by myelodysplasia.[188,189]

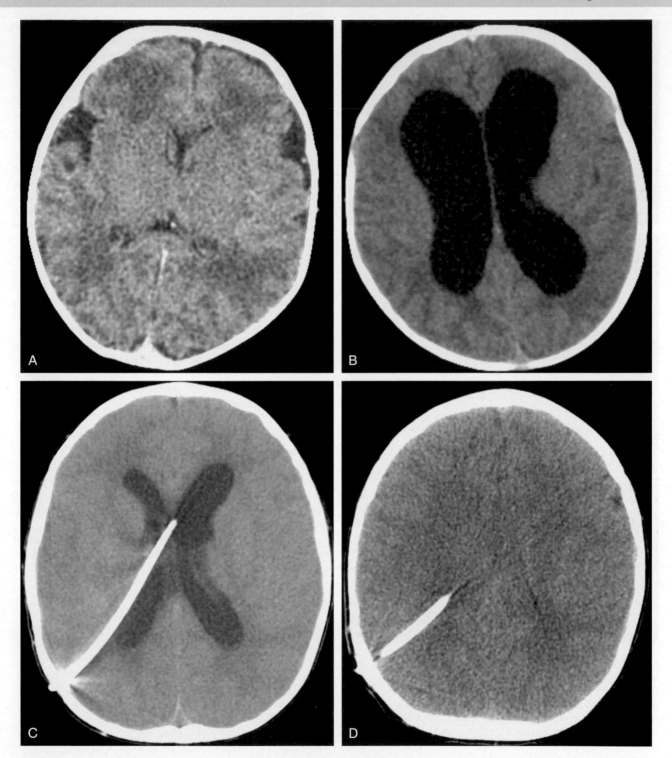

Figure 23-13. CT scans in children with (**A**) normal-sized ventricles, (**B**) untreated hydrocephalus, (**C**) hydrocephalus treated with a ventricular shunt, and (**D**) hydrocephalus treated with a ventricular shunt resulting in slit ventricles. (Courtesy of Ellen Grant, MD.)

Chiari Malformations

There are several types of Chiari malformations (Table 23-3). The Arnold-Chiari malformation (type II) almost always coexists in children with myelodysplasia. This defect consists of a bony abnormality in the posterior fossa and upper cervical spine with caudal displacement of the cerebellar vermis, fourth ventricle, and lower brainstem below the plane of the foramen magnum. Medullary cervical cord compression can occur (Figs. 23-15 and 23-16). Vocal cord paralysis with stridor and respiratory distress, apnea, abnormal swallowing and pulmonary aspi-

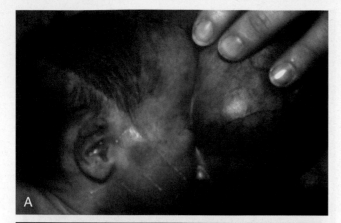

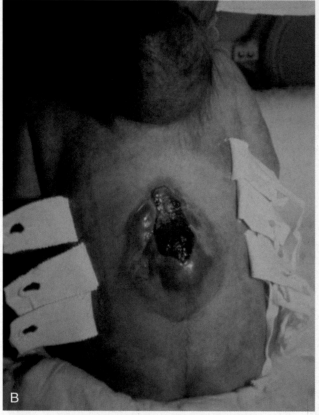

Figure 23-14. A, An infant with an anterior encephalocele. **B,** An infant with both a posterior encephalocele and myelomeningocele defects. Note the large exposed surface areas that make this child prone to dehydration. Difficulty may be encountered in positioning for induction of anesthesia, and significant loss of blood and cerebrospinal fluid during surgical correction should be anticipated.

ration, opisthotonos, and cranial nerve deficits may be associated with the Arnold-Chiari malformation and usually manifest during infancy. Children with vocal cord paralysis or a diminished gag reflex may require tracheostomy and gastrostomy to secure the airway and minimize chronic aspiration. Children of any age may have abnormal responses to hypoxia and hypercarbia because of cranial nerve and brainstem dysfunction.[187,190] Extreme head flexion may cause brainstem compression in otherwise asymptomatic children.

Chiari malformations (type I) can occur in healthy children without myelodysplasia. These defects involve caudal displacement of the cerebellar tonsils below the foramen magnum, but children generally have much milder symptoms, sometimes presenting only with headache or neck pain.[191] Surgical treatment usually involves a decompressive suboccipital craniectomy with cervical laminectomies.

Other Spinal Defects

Other spinal anomalies (lipomeningoceles, lipomyelomeningoceles, diastematomyelias, and dermoid tracts) may manifest as tethered cords. Skin defects, generally over the lower lumbar region, may occur as dural sinus tracks or lipomeningoceles. Hair tufts, skin dimples, or fatty pads may all be associated with spinal defects. Sometimes these anomalies manifest when toilet training or ambulation is noted to be abnormal or later in childhood when children complain of back pain. Children who have had a meningomyelocele repaired after birth may also develop an ascending neurologic deficit from a tethered spinal cord during growth. Early detection of a tethered cord is now easily diagnosed with MRI. Prophylactic surgical untethering is common. Anesthetic management for surgical release of a tethered cord usually entails monitoring the innervation of the lower extremities and bowel and bladder with nerve stimulators and rectal electromyelograms or manometry. Thus, muscle relaxants must be avoided or permitted to dissipate before intraoperative assessment.

Neuroradiologic Procedures

A wide variety of neuroradiologic procedures are performed in children. These procedures require immobilization and relief of the child's anxiety. Anesthetic considerations for neurodiagnostic procedures (e.g., CT, MRI) are discussed elsewhere in this book (see Chapter 46), but certain therapeutic neuroradiologic procedures are discussed here.

Embolization of arterial malformations or aneurysms can be performed during angiography. The anesthesiologist should be

Table 23-3. Types of Chiari Malformations

Type I	Caudal displacement of cerebellar tonsils below the plane of the foramen magnum
Type II (Arnold-Chiari; associated with myelomeningocele)	Caudal displacement of the cerebellar vermis, fourth ventricle, and the lower brainstem below the plane of the foramen magnum. Dysplastic brainstem with characteristic "kink," elongation of the fourth ventricle, "beaking" of the quadrigeminal plate, hypoplastic tentorium with small posterior fossa, polymicrogyria, enlargement of the massa intermedia
Type III	Caudal displacement of the cerebellum and brainstem into a high cervical meningocele
Type IV	Cerebellar hypoplasia

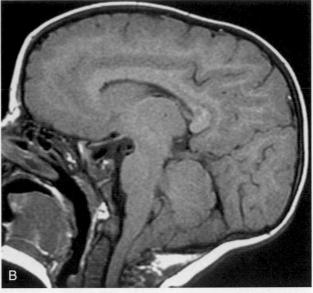

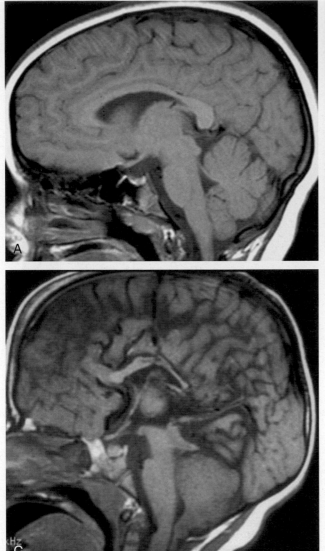

Figure 23-15. A, Sagittal T1-weighted MR image of a normal child. **B,** Sagittal T1-weighted MR image of a child with a Chiari I malformation. The type I Chiari malformation consists of caudal displacement of the cerebellar tonsils at least 5 mm into the upper cervical spinal canal and there may be no clinical symptoms. **C,** Sagittal T1-weighted MR image of a child with a type II Chiari malformation that is the combination of caudal displacement of the cerebellar tonsils and additional brain anomalies in combination with a meningomyelocele deformity. (Courtesy of Ellen Grant, MD.)

aware of the embolic material being injected (e.g., coils, glue, alcohol) because complications can develop. Stereotactic head frames may also be placed before the procedures to help to localize the surgery or radiation therapy. Anesthesia should be induced before the head frame is applied, not only for the child's comfort but also to ensure the airway can be secured with an endotracheal tube. A modified head frame (see Fig. 23-9) with a moveable piece over the face has been developed. It is safer than the conventional "rigid" stereotactic head frame, which often protrudes over the child's nose or mouth.[192] Anesthesia is maintained after the initial radiologic procedures are performed, keeping the child asleep in the recovery room if necessary, until transport to the operating room for surgery or radiosurgery is completed and the head frame is removed.

To improve intraoperative navigation during intracranial procedures, the concept of intraoperative MRI was introduced in the mid 1990s. Currently, that technology has advanced to include a variety of operating room suite designs that include MRI machines (Fig. 23-17, see website). These procedures present special challenges for both neurosurgeons and anesthesiologists.[193-196] As with anesthetics for diagnostic MRI scans, special monitors, infusion pumps and an MRI-safe or conditional anesthesia machine are required. However, it is much more challenging to do surgical procedures in this environment, especially because these procedures may take many hours, they may be associated with blood loss, and access to the child is severely limited. Some monitoring equipment found in conventional operating rooms (e.g., precordial Doppler ultrasonography, core temperature probes, fluid warmers) are not as yet MRI safe or conditional. Nevertheless, numerous neurosurgical procedures have been safely performed in children in these MRI operating rooms and the equipment for these procedures is rapidly evolving.

Acknowledgment

We wish to thank Veronica Miller, MD and Elizabeth A. Eldredge, MD for their prior contributions to this chapter.

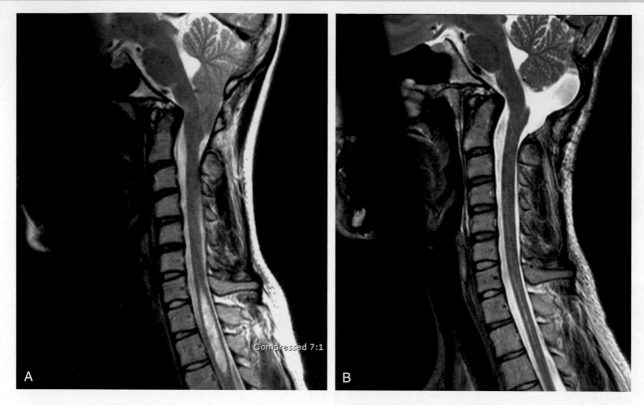

Figure 23-16. This pair of images show the posterior fossa in a child with a Chiari II malformation both before and after posterior fossa decompression. **A,** Note the downward herniation of the cerebellar tonsils. **B,** Resolution of cerebellar tonsillar herniation after posterior fossa decompression.

Annotated References

Coles JP, Fryer TD, Coleman MR, et al: Hyperventilation following head injury: effect on ischemic burden and cerebral oxidative metabolism. Crit Care Med 2007; 35:568-578.

This article demonstrates the detrimental effect hyperventilation has on brain tissue at risk after head injury. This article is important because it refutes often taught dogma regarding routine hyperventilation especially after a traumatic brain injury. This article and several others on the same subject should give the anesthesiologist pause when hyperventilating children with intracranial pathology.

Jevtovic-Todorovic V, Hartman RE, Izumi Y, et al: Early exposure to common anesthetic agents causes widespread neurodegeneration in the developing rat brain and persistent learning deficits. J Neurosci 2003;23:876-82.

This is an extremely important paper regarding the current controversies surrounding the use of common anesthetic agents in neonates. This paper presents compelling animal data that commonly used anesthetic agents such as isoflurane cause histologic evidence of neurodegeneration as well as behavioral problems with cognition. This is one of the references commonly cited when this discussion arises. However, it should be noted that no human data regarding this issue yet exist; therefore extrapolating these data to the practice of anesthetizing human neonates is very questionable.

Lassen NA, Christensen MS: Physiology of cerebral blood flow. Br J Anaesth 1976;48:719-734.

This is a very nice review article discussing the various physiologic mechanisms of control of cerebral blood flow.

Pollack IF: Brain tumors in children. N Engl J Med 1994;331:1500-1507.

Although this review is from the 1990s, it provides a comprehensive overview of the epidemiology of pediatric brain tumors as well as treatment approaches. A knowledge of different treatment approaches to different histologic types of tumors will inform the anesthesiologist as to the extent of the process behind the procedure and how aggressive the surgery needs to be to achieve a desired outcome.

Reasoner DK, Todd MM, Scamman FL, et al: The incidence of pneumocephalus after supratentorial craniotomy: Observations on the disappearance of intracranial air. Anesthesiology 1994;80:1008-1012.

This is a well conceived study that evaluates the length of time pneumocephalus persists after supratentorial craniotomy. The take home message is that air persists in the head for several weeks after craniotomy and care should be taken not to exacerbate the situation during subsequent administration of anesthetics. Nitrous oxide should be avoided in these children as tension pneumocephalus could develop.

References

Please see www.expertconsult.com

Essentials of Endocrinology

Elliot J. Krane, Erinn T. Rhodes, E. Kirk Neely, Joseph I. Wolfsdorf, and Carolyn I. Chi

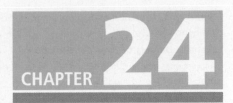

CHAPTER 24

Diabetes Mellitus*

The incidence of both type 1 and type 2 diabetes mellitus in children is increasing worldwide.[1-6] Together with the advent of continuous insulin delivery devices and long- and rapid-acting insulin analogues, perioperative management of blood glucose concentrations for children with diabetes has become increasingly complex. Anesthesiologists must carefully consider the pathophysiology of the disease as well as each child's specific diabetes treatment regimen, glycemic control, intended surgery, and anticipated postoperative course when devising an appropriate perioperative management plan. Standardized algorithms for perioperative diabetes management improve care[7-9] without significantly increasing costs[9]; several guidelines and studies of perioperative management of children with diabetes are available in the literature and examples are included.[10-14]

Classification and Epidemiology in Children

The most common forms of diabetes are type 1 and type 2 diabetes.[15,16] Type 1 diabetes results from the destruction of pan-

creatic beta cells, usually via an immune-mediated process that leads to an absolute deficiency of insulin.[16] In contrast, type 2 diabetes, which was previously considered a disorder that afflicted primarily middle-aged and elderly adults, results from a combination of insulin resistance and a relative deficiency of insulin.[15,16] Children with type 2 diabetes are typically overweight and frequently have a family history of type 2 diabetes in a first- or second-degree relative.[15] However, the increasing prevalence of obesity in children[17] has made distinction between type 1 and type 2 diabetes, at times, rather difficult. Children with phenotypic characteristics of type 2 diabetes have been noted to have pancreatic autoimmunity,[18,19] and an increasing number of children with diabetes who require exogenous insulin at diagnosis are overweight.[20] Other less common forms of diabetes may be encountered in children (Table 24-1). Additional modifications to the perioperative treatment regimen may be necessary when diabetes is associated with genetic syndromes and/or other endocrinopathies, such as adrenal insufficiency (see later).

Although the worldwide incidence of type 1 diabetes is highly variable,[21] the incidence appears to be increasing in almost all populations throughout the world.[4] In the United States, data from the early 1990s suggested an annual incidence of type 1 diabetes in children 14 years of age or younger of 11.7 to 17.8

*Adapted from Rhodes E, Ferrari L, Wolfsdorf J. Perioperative management of pediatric surgical patients with diabetes mellitus. Anesth Analg 2005; 101:986-999.

Table 24-1. Classification of Less Common Forms of Diabetes Mellitus

Genetic Defects of Beta Cell Function

Monogenic diabetes (formerly referred to as maturity-onset diabetes of the young [MODY])

Permanent neonatal diabetes

Mitochondrial disorders

Disease of the Exocrine Pancreas

Cystic fibrosis–related diabetes

Drug-Induced Diabetes

Steroids

Chemotherapeutic agents

Genetic Syndromes

Prader-Willi syndrome

Down syndrome

Turner syndrome

Wolfram syndrome

Endocrinopathies

Autoimmune polyglandular syndrome

Cushing syndrome

Adapted from Rhodes ET, Ferrari LR, Wolfsdorf JI: Perioperative management of pediatric surgical patients with diabetes mellitus. Anesth Analg 2005; 101:986-999.

per 100,000.[20] The epidemic of obesity has also contributed to a progressive increase in the incidence and prevalence of type 2 diabetes in U.S. children.[1,22] In the National Health and Nutrition Examination Survey (1999-2002), 4,370 U.S. adolescents (aged 12 to 19 years) self-reported diabetes, which was 0.5% (95% confidence interval [CI], 0.24%-0.76%) of the sample. Among these, 71% (95% CI, 56%-86%) were categorized as having type 1 diabetes and 29% (95% CI, 14%-44%) as having type 2 diabetes, the latter being equivalent to 39,005 adolescents.[22] Similar increases in the incidence and prevalence of type 2 diabetes have been noted in other parts of the world.[2,3,5,6,23-26]

General Management Principles

Understanding both the pharmacokinetic and pharmacodynamic properties of different insulin preparations and antihyperglycemic medications is critical to developing an appropriate perioperative plan.

Type 1 diabetes always requires treatment with insulin. However, an increasing number of insulin preparations (Table 24-2) as well as delivery systems are available. Conventional insulin regimens typically require two to three injections of insulin per day. They incorporate a combination of an intermediate-acting insulin (e.g., NPH) and/or a long-acting insulin (e.g., insulin detemir [Levemir] or insulin glargine [Lantus]) for basal coverage with a short- or rapid-acting insulin (e.g., Regular, insulin aspart [NovoLog], insulin lispro [Humalog], or insulin glulisine [Apidra]) to provide prandial glycemic coverage. Other intermediate- and long-acting insulins previously used in such regimens included Lente and Ultralente but, as of 2006, these preparations are no longer available in the United States. More intensive insulin regimens, which include at least three injections per day, are also being used with greater frequency. Such regimens typically utilize insulin glargine, a long-acting insulin, which provides a relatively constant 24-hour basal concentration of circulating insulin without a pronounced peak so as to emulate basal insulin secretion,[27] in conjunction with rapid-acting insulin administered with food. Some studies have demonstrated superior glycemic control with such regimens as compared with regimens utilizing NPH insulin and Regular insulin,[28] although the ideal insulin regimen for children with type 1 diabetes remains controversial.[29] The newer long-acting

Table 24-2. Insulin Preparations Classified According to Their Pharmacodynamic Profiles*

	Onset (hours)	Peak (hours)	Duration (hours)
Rapid-Acting[†]			
Insulin lispro (Humalog)[‡]	0.25-0.5	0.5-2.5	≤5
Insulin aspart (Novolog)[‡]	<0.25	1-3	3-5
Insulin glulisine (Apidra)[‡]	<0.25	0.5-1.5	3-5
Short-Acting[†]			
Regular (soluble)	0.5-1	2-4	5-8
Intermediate and Long-Acting[†]			
NPH (isophane)	1-2	2-8	14-24
Insulin glargine (Lantus)[‡]	2-4	Peakless	20-24
Insulin detemir (Levemir)[‡]	1-2	3-9	Up to 24

*Times of onset, peak, and duration of action vary within and between patients and are affected by numerous factors, including dosage, site, depth of injection, dilution, temperature, and other factors.

[†]Premixed combinations of intermediate-acting and either rapid- or short-acting insulins are available whose pharmacodynamic profiles have a bimodal pattern reflecting the two insulin components.

[‡]Insulin analogue developed by modifying the amino acid sequence of the human insulin molecule.

NPH, neutral protamine Hagedorn.

Adapted from Rhodes ET, Ferrari LR, Wolfsdorf JI: Perioperative management of pediatric surgical patients with diabetes mellitus. Anesth Analg 2005; 101:986-999.

insulin, insulin detemir (Levemir), may also be used in intensive insulin regimens and has demonstrated more predictable glucose-lowering effects than both NPH insulin[30-32] and insulin glargine.[30]

Intensive management of type 1 diabetes with insulin pumps in children is also increasingly common.[33,34] The insulin pump is a device that administers a continuous subcutaneous infusion of insulin (typically a rapid-acting insulin such as insulin lispro or insulin aspart) at a basal rate that is supplemented by additional bolus doses of insulin that are given with meals and snacks and to correct hyperglycemia. In appropriately selected children such management has demonstrated superiority over injection regimens.[35-38] Standard insulin preparations are U100, meaning that there are 100 units of insulin per milliliter. However, very young patients with type 1 diabetes may, on occasion, require diluted insulin (e.g., U10 with 10 units of insulin/mL) to achieve accurate dosing of very small doses of insulin.[39] Families of toddlers with type 1 diabetes should be specifically questioned about their use of diluted insulin.

Most children with type 2 diabetes are managed with insulin and/or oral metformin, the only oral agent approved for use in diabetic children in the United States.[40,41] Metformin's primary action is to decrease hepatic glucose production and, secondarily, to increase insulin sensitivity in peripheral tissues. Occasionally, other oral agents including sulfonylureas, which promote insulin secretion, and thiazolidinediones, which increase insulin sensitivity in muscle and adipose tissue, are used in adolescents.[40,42] Nutritional therapy is always included in the management of children with type 2 diabetes. Studies such as the Treatment Options for Type 2 Diabetes in Adolescents and Youth (TODAY) trial[43] are evaluating the optimal treatment for type 2 diabetes in children, although the final results are pending.

Newer medications and delivery systems introduced to manage adults with diabetes may eventually become available for use in children. Incretins, including glucose-dependent insulinotropic polypeptide (GIP) and glucagon-like peptide-1 (GLP-1), are gastrointestinal hormones released after eating that stimulate insulin secretion and are necessary for normal glucose tolerance.[44,45] GLP-1 acts through a G protein–coupled receptor (GLP-1-R) to promote glucose-dependent insulin secretion, suppression of glucagon secretion, slowing of gastric emptying, and reduction in food intake.[44] Exenatide (Byetta) is a GLP-1 receptor agonist that is approved for use in adults with type 2 diabetes as an adjunctive therapy for those taking metformin and/or a sulfonylurea.[46] Inhibitors of dipeptidyl peptidase-IV (DPP-IV), the enzyme that degrades GLP-1, are also under development[47] with the first, sitagliptin (Januvia), released in 2006. Pramlintide acetate (Symlin) is a synthetic amylin receptor agonist that can be used as an adjunct to insulin therapy in adults with type 1 or type 2 diabetes.[48-51] Amylin is a 37-amino acid polypeptide islet hormone co-secreted with insulin from beta islet cells.[44] Stimulation of the amylin receptor may be effective in the treatment of diabetes via three physiologic mechanisms: delayed gastric emptying, inhibition of glucagon secretion, and modulation of satiety.[44] Finally, an inhaled preparation of insulin (Exubera Inhalation Powder) has been used in adult patients with type 1 diabetes together with a long-acting injected insulin for basal coverage[52] and as either monotherapy for type 2 diabetes patients or in conjunction with a long-acting injected insulin or an oral medication.[53-55] However, after 2007, it was no longer actively marketed in the United States. Long-term studies of inhaled insulin in patients younger than 18 years of age have not been conducted.

Metabolic Response to Surgery

Trauma of any kind, and surgery in particular, causes a complex neuroendocrine stress response including suppression of insulin secretion and increased production of counterregulatory hormones (frequently called "stress hormones" in the anesthesiology literature), particularly cortisol and catecholamines.[56,57] Insulin is the primary anabolic hormone that promotes glucose uptake in muscle and adipose tissue while suppressing glucose production (glycogenolysis and gluconeogenesis) by the liver.[58] The counterregulatory hormones, including epinephrine, glucagon, cortisol, and growth hormone, have the opposite effects, resulting in resistance to insulin in multiple peripheral tissues, such as liver and muscle.[59-61] The counterregulatory hormones increase blood glucose concentration by stimulating glycogenolysis and gluconeogenesis in the liver, by increasing lipolysis and ketogenesis, and by inhibiting glucose uptake and utilization in muscle and fat. Glucagon, secreted by alpha islet cells in the pancreas, suppresses insulin secretion while stimulating hepatic glycogenolysis, gluconeogenesis, and ketogenesis.[58,59] Epinephrine, which acts via β_2- and α_2-adrenergic receptors, stimulates glucagon production, increases glycogenolysis and gluconeogenesis, stimulates lipolysis, limits insulin secretion, and limits glucose utilization in insulin-sensitive tissues.[58] Cortisol stimulates gluconeogenesis, proteolysis, and lipolysis and decreases glucose utilization.[59,62] Finally, growth hormone augments glucose production, decreases glucose utilization, and accelerates lipolysis.[63] Proinflammatory cytokines may further stimulate secretion of counterregulatory hormones and alter insulin receptor signaling.[61] These changes increase catabolism, as evidenced by increased hepatic glucose production and breakdown of protein and fat. In the diabetic patient with absolute or relative insulin deficiency, the enhanced catabolism stimulated by surgical trauma can lead to marked hyperglycemia and even diabetic ketoacidosis.[64] These metabolic effects may be exacerbated by a prolonged fast before and during surgery.

Metabolic Response to Anesthesia

Although adequate analgesia is essential to minimize the neuroendocrine stress response to surgery, some anesthetic agents may also independently contribute to perioperative hyperglycemia.[10,65] Studies have demonstrated that inhalational anesthetics, such as isoflurane, may cause hyperglycemia by inhibiting insulin secretion.[66,67] The hyperglycemia results from both impaired glucose uptake and increased glucose production.[65] In contrast, epidural analgesia with local anesthesia has been shown to prevent this hyperglycemic effect[68,69] through an inhibitory effect on endogenous glucose production.[65] Similarly, intravenous anesthesia with opioids mitigates the hyperglycemic response of surgery[65,70,71] through its apparent neutral effect on endogenous glucose production but decrease in glucose clearance.[65] Although these differences are important to consider, the metabolic effects of the anesthesia are relatively minor compared with the direct effects of surgery.[10]

Adverse Consequences of Hyperglycemia

Hyperglycemia can impair wound healing by hindering collagen production, which may decrease the tensile strength of the surgical wound.[72] Hyperglycemia may also have adverse effects on neutrophil function, including decreased chemotaxis, phagocytosis, and bactericidal killing.[73-76] Evidence from controlled experimental studies in rabbits demonstrated that these effects may be reversed, in part, by glycemia-independent effects of insulin.[77] However, the overall benefits of intensive insulin therapy, including a reduction in mortality, were derived mainly from maintenance of normoglycemia, whereas glycemia-independent actions of insulin exert only minor, organ-specific effects.[77]

Clinical studies in humans have not consistently supported the relationship between perioperative glycemic control and short-term risk of infection or morbidity.[78,79] In 411 adults with diabetes undergoing coronary artery surgery, postoperative hyperglycemia was an independent predictor of short-term infectious complications.[80] In adult diabetic patients undergoing open-heart surgery, maintaining a postoperative mean blood glucose concentration less than 200 mg/dL significantly reduced the incidence of deep wound infections.[81] In critically ill adult patients treated in intensive care units (ICUs), intensive glycemic control with insulin significantly reduced overall morbidity and mortality.[82,83] These interventions have also been shown to be cost saving.[84] In children, a study of 184 infants younger than 1 year of age who underwent cardiac surgery requiring cardiopulmonary bypass showed the duration and magnitude of postoperative hyperglycemia were associated with an increased incidence of adverse outcomes, including infection and death.[85] The duration of hyperglycemia was also associated with an increased duration of hospital stay, of cardiac ICU stay, and of mechanical ventilation.[85] Other studies of critically ill children managed in pediatric ICUs have demonstrated similar findings.[86,87] Such studies support the generally accepted recommendation that during the perioperative period, blood glucose concentrations should be maintained close to normal values.[59]

Preoperative Assessment

When feasible, children with diabetes should not undergo elective surgery until they are metabolically stable (Fig. 24-1, box 4), that is, there is no evidence of ketonuria, serum electrolytes are normal, and the HbA1c value is close to or within the ideal range for the child's age. Although there is no consensus regarding the ideal metabolic targets for control of diabetes in children,[88] the American Diabetes Association recommends an HbA1c in a range of 7.5% to 8.5% for children younger than age 6 years; less than 8% for children age 6 to 12 years; and less than 7.5% for age 13 years or older with a more stringent target of less than 7% to be considered in this age group for children in whom this can be achieved without excessive hypoglycemia[89] as well as for those with type 2 diabetes.[15] The preoperative consultation to assess the adequacy of metabolic control should be scheduled at least 10 days before the procedure (see Fig. 24-1, box 3), and surgery should be delayed, if possible, if the metabolic control is poor. Both the endocrinology and anesthesiology services should participate in this assessment. Whenever possible, surgery for children with diabetes should be scheduled as the first case in the morning so that prolonged fasting is avoided and diabetes treatment regimens may be most easily adjusted.

Children who present for emergent surgery, for example, due to trauma or acute surgical conditions, require a multidisciplinary preoperative assessment with collaborative involvement of both the endocrinology and anesthesiology services. However, in these situations surgery often cannot be delayed even if metabolic control is poor, as in the case of a patient requiring emergent surgery who presents in diabetic ketoacidosis. This has implications for the intraoperative management of such children as described later under "Special Surgical Situations."

Preoperative Management

The regimen for managing diabetes before, during, and after a surgical or diagnostic procedure that requires the child to fast should aim to maintain near-normoglycemia, that is, blood glucose level of 100 to 200 mg/dL. In this blood glucose range there will be a reduced risk of osmotic diuresis, dehydration, electrolyte imbalance, metabolic acidosis, infection, and hypoglycemia in the sedated child who may be unaware of hypoglycemia or unable to communicate with staff.[90] The child need not be admitted before the day of surgery but rather early on the same morning as the surgery or procedure. Children should be instructed regarding modifying their diabetes regimen before and for the day of surgery. On admission to the hospital, metabolic control of their diabetes should be assessed, including a preoperative determination of glucose concentration. On the morning of surgery, no rapid- or short-acting acting insulin is administered *unless* the blood glucose level is more than 250 mg/dL. However, admission to the hospital before *major* surgical procedures in children[10] and for adults has been recommended by some if preoperative metabolic control needs to be optimized.[59] If the surgery must be delayed for any reason, frequent blood glucose monitoring is mandatory to prevent perioperative hypoglycemia or hyperglycemia.

If the blood glucose is more than 250 mg/dL, a conservative dose of rapid-acting insulin (e.g., insulin lispro or insulin aspart) or short-acting insulin (Regular) is administered to restore near-normoglycemia. This is achieved using the child's usual sliding scale, or a "correction factor." The insulin "correction factor" is the decrease in the blood glucose concentration expected after administering 1 unit of rapid-acting or short-acting insulin. This can be calculated using the "1500 rule:" divide 1500 by the child's usual total daily dose (TDD) of insulin. For example, if a child typically takes 30 units of insulin daily, this child's "correction factor" would be $1500 \div 30 = 50$. Therefore, 1 unit of rapid-acting or short-acting insulin would be expected to decrease the child's blood glucose concentration by approximately 50 mg/dL. Various correction factors have been described including a "1500 rule" for short-acting insulin (Regular) and an "1800 rule" for rapid-acting insulin, such as insulin lispro.[91] For simplicity and because of insulin resistance stimulated by surgical stress, the "1500 rule" is appropriate in this setting even with the use of a rapid-acting insulin. To then calculate an appropriate corrective dose of insulin to restore near-normoglycemia, the anesthesiologist should aim for a target blood glucose concentration of 150 mg/dL.

The "correction factor" rather than a sliding scale is used to manage a child with hyperglycemia and restore the blood glucose concentration to 150 mg/dL. For example, if the child has a correction factor of 1 unit of rapid-acting or short-acting insulin to reduce the blood glucose concentration by about 50 mg/dL, and the current blood glucose value is 300 mg/dL, to reduce the blood glucose concentration from 300 mg/dL to 150 mg/dL, a total dose of $(300 - 150)/50$ or 3 units of insulin would be required. This dose may be administered subcutaneously for those taking rapid-acting insulin or intravenously for

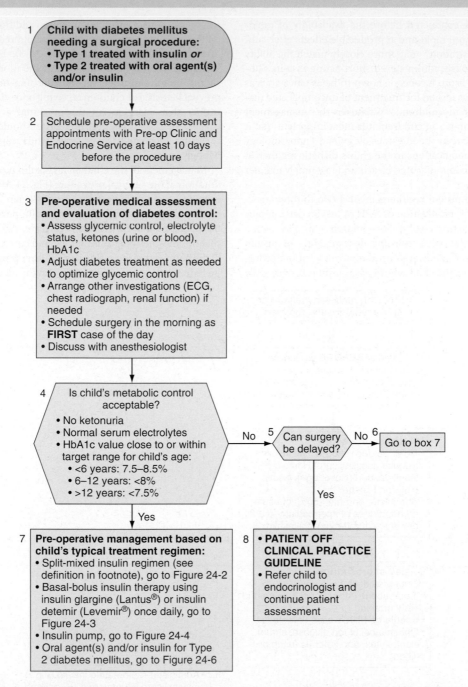

Figure 24-1. Clinical practice guideline for perioperative management of diabetes mellitus. Split-mixed insulin regimen refers to a regimen combining multiple daily injections of intermediate- or long-acting insulins (e.g., NPH or insulin detemir [Levemir]) and multiple injections of rapid- or short-acting insulins (Regular, insulin lispro [Humalog], insulin aspart [NovoLog], or insulin glulisine [Apidra]). (Modified from Rhodes ET, Ferrari LR, Wolfsdorf JI: Perioperative management of pediatric surgical patients with diabetes mellitus. Anesth Analg 2005; 101:986-999.)

those taking short-acting insulin (Regular) and who will be managed with an intravenous insulin infusion during the procedure. For children with type 2 diabetes who do *not* require insulin (but who are, by definition, insulin resistant), an insulin dose of 0.1 unit/kg of rapid-acting insulin may be administered subcutaneously to correct a blood glucose concentration greater than 250 mg/dL.

More detailed preoperative recommendations must be based on the individual child's baseline treatment regimen. For most

children with diabetes undergoing minor outpatient surgical procedures, insulin can still be provided perioperatively with subcutaneous injections. In adults, especially those with type 2 diabetes, this practice is commonly,[90] although not universally, preferred.[92] Others routinely recommend insulin infusions even for minor outpatient surgical procedures in children.[10] Several reports suggest that better glycemic control can be achieved in the perioperative period with a continuous intravenous infusion rather than subcutaneous insulin administration.[12,93,94] However, these studies were conducted before the availability of rapid-acting insulins whose rapid and reproducible effects after subcutaneous administration[95] may more closely match the ability to titrate intravenously administered short-acting insulin. Subcutaneous insulin lispro has been shown to be as efficacious as Regular intravenous insulin for treatment of uncomplicated diabetic ketoacidosis in children.[96] Whatever the management strategy for the diabetes in children, it is most important that it is coordinated between the anesthesiology and endocrinology services and the modifications to the child's diabetic regimen at home needs to be communicated clearly and in a timely manner to the family.

The split-mixed insulin regimens involve two to three injections per day with a combination of NPH or insulin detemir plus a rapid- or short-acting insulin. For children who take such a regimen, 50% of the usual morning dose of NPH or insulin detemir should be administered on the morning of the procedure (Fig. 24-2). For the child whose basal insulin is once-daily

insulin glargine or insulin detemir, no additional insulin is given on the morning of the surgery if the child received a dose in the evening of the previous day (Fig. 24-3). However, if insulin glargine is typically administered in the morning, the full dose should be administered on the morning of the procedure to prevent ketosis. For children receiving once-daily insulin detemir (rather than glargine) in the morning, a modest reduction to 75% of the usual morning dose should be administered to ensure adequate basal coverage while minimizing the risk of hypoglycemia.

Management of the child on an insulin pump depends on the duration of the surgical procedure (Fig. 24-4). Those undergoing minor procedures expected to last less than 2 hours in duration can usually continue to use their insulin pump with their usual basal rate for that time of day. However, this approach requires that the anesthesiologist is familiar and comfortable with the use of the pump in the operating room. Other protocols, for example, include transitioning those with insulin pumps to intravenous

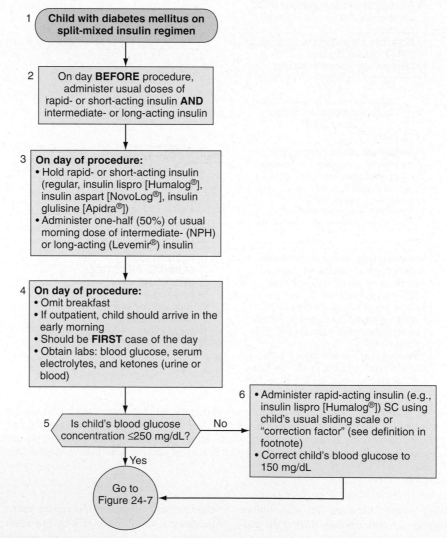

Figure 24-2. Preoperative management for children with diabetes mellitus on split-mixed insulin regimens. The calculation for insulin correction factor is as follows:
1. Divide 1500 by child's total daily dose (TDD).
2. If daily dose varies (i.e., use of sliding scales), use the *average* daily dose in the past week to determine TDD.
3. Example: if TDD = 50 units, then insulin correction factor is 1 unit insulin lispro (Humalog) to lower blood glucose by 30 mg/dL.
(Modified from Rhodes ET, Ferrari LR, Wolfsdorf JI: Perioperative management of pediatric surgical patients with diabetes mellitus. Anesth Analg 2005; 101:986-999.)

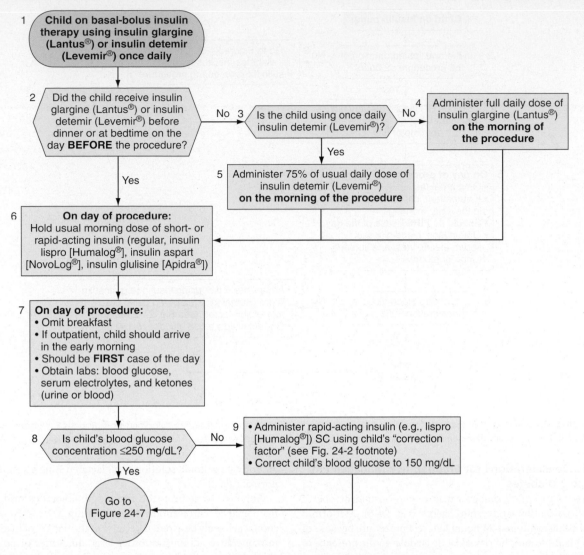

Figure 24-3. Preoperative management for children with diabetes mellitus on once-daily insulin glargine [Lantus] or insulin detemir [Levemir] regimens. Note that insulin glargine [Lantus] and insulin detemir [Levemir] should not be mixed with any other insulin. (Modified from Rhodes ET, Ferrari LR, Wolfsdorf JI: Perioperative management of pediatric surgical patients with diabetes mellitus. Anesth Analg 2005; 101:986-999.)

insulin infusions or subcutaneous insulin glargine.[59] For procedures greater than 2 hours in duration, children should be transitioned to an intravenous insulin infusion, as described in the next section.

Major Surgery and Intravenous Insulin Infusions

For children requiring major surgery, especially procedures anticipated to last for more than 2 hours, intravenous insulin infusion is the preferred perioperative diabetes management plan (Fig. 24-5). Studies in children[12] and adults[7] have demonstrated that glycemic control with infusions of intravenous insulin is superior compared with subcutaneous injections. These children should receive their usual doses of insulin on the day before the procedure. On the morning of the procedure, an intravenous infusion of 10% dextrose in half-normal saline should be started at a maintenance rate and an intravenous insulin infusion should also be provided to accommodate the dextrose infusion to maintain blood glucose in the target range

of 100 to 200 mg/dL (see Fig. 24-5). The maintenance rate for intravenous fluids in a child depends on body size and can be calculated either based on body weight (4 mL/kg/hr for the first 10 kg body weight, 2 mL/kg/hr for 11 to 20 kg, and then 1 mL/kg/hr for each kg over 20 kg) or body surface area (1.5 L/m[2]/day). Because prepubertal children are relatively more sensitive to insulin than pubertal adolescents,[97] the insulin dose for children varies with age. In prepubertal children with type 1 diabetes, after the remission (honeymoon) period, the insulin requirement is typically 0.6 to 0.8 unit/kg/day, whereas in adolescents, the requirement is 1 to 1.5 units/kg/day.[98,99] Children with type 2 diabetes may require even greater doses of insulin because of their insulin resistance. With intravenous insulin, a suitable ratio of insulin to dextrose for prepubertal children is typically 1 unit per 5 g of intravenous dextrose and for adolescents (>12 years of age) 1 unit per 3 g of intravenous dextrose. Only Regular insulin should be used for intravenous infusions.

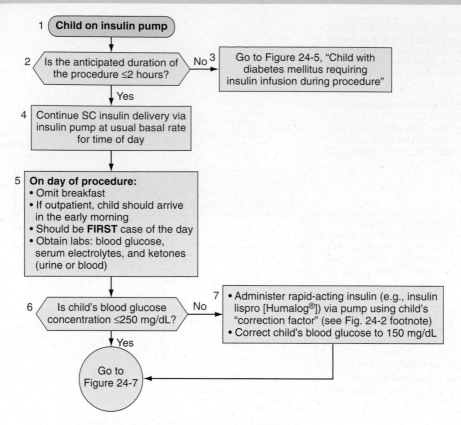

Figure 24-4. Preoperative management for children with diabetes mellitus on an insulin pump. (Modified from Rhodes ET, Ferrari LR, Wolfsdorf JI: Perioperative management of pediatric surgical patients with diabetes mellitus. Anesth Analg 2005; 101:986-999.)

Special Considerations for Preoperative Management of Type 2 Diabetes

Children with type 2 diabetes may require insulin or one of several oral antihyperglycemic agents (Fig. 24-6). Metformin should be discontinued 24 hours before a procedure because of its long half-life and the risk of lactic acidosis in the presence of dehydration, hypoxemia, or poor tissue perfusion.[100] Other oral agents, such as sulfonylureas and thiazolidinediones, may be discontinued on the morning of the procedure. Figure 24-6 outlines additional recommendations for children with type 2 diabetes who utilize split-mixed insulin, a common insulin regimen for type 2 diabetic patients. Alternatively, if a child with type 2 diabetes is treated with once-daily insulin glargine, adjustments as in Figure 24-3 will be necessary. Adjustments for other insulin regimens in type 2 diabetes should be determined in consultation with an endocrinologist or diabetologist.

Intraoperative Management

The insulin and fluid regimen during and after surgery depends on the duration of the procedure. If the procedure is likely to be brief (e.g., ≤1 hour) and one can reasonably anticipate that the child will be able to drink soon after the procedure, it may not be necessary to start a glucose-containing intravenous infusion. If the duration of fasting is likely to be more prolonged, an intravenous infusion should be started at a maintenance rate as described earlier (Fig. 24-7). Intraoperative maintenance fluid should then be replaced with a glucose-containing solution. However, replacement of insensible losses and intravascular volume owing to blood or other body fluid should be with an appropriate isotonic solution (e.g., lactated Ringer's solution or normal saline).

Although some protocols include potassium chloride in the maintenance intravenous fluid solution,[10,59,90] this practice should generally be avoided because of the danger of inadvertent intraoperative administration of large quantities of potassium chloride during fluid resuscitation. Children undergoing a brief procedure with a normal serum concentration of potassium and diabetes under good metabolic control have a low risk of hypokalemia. Those undergoing more prolonged surgeries or emergent surgeries during which metabolic decompensation is more likely require intraoperative assessment of electrolytes and appropriate adjustment of the electrolyte composition of their intravenous solution. *In all cases, blood glucose concentrations should be measured hourly and either insulin or dextrose adjusted, as necessary, to maintain blood glucose in the target range of 100 to 200 mg/dL (see Fig. 24-7).*

Postoperative Management

As soon as the child is able to resume drinking and eating normally, the usual diabetes regimen, including insulin and/or oral agents, may be reinstituted and the dextrose infusion discontinued, if applicable (Fig. 24-8). One exception to this approach is for children with type 2 diabetes who take metformin; in these children, metformin should be held for 48 hours and renal function must be within normal limits before reinstituting that medication. For children who are unable to eat or drink, intravenous dextrose and electrolyte solution should be continued until oral intake is restored. An infusion of intravenous short-acting insulin (Regular) or intermittent subcutaneous rapid-

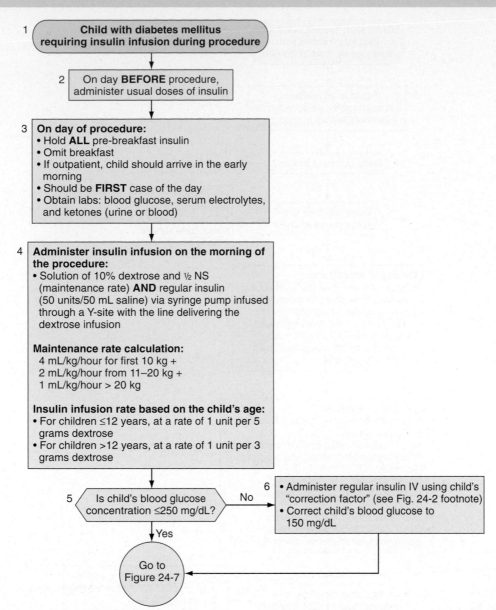

1 Child with diabetes mellitus requiring insulin infusion during procedure

2 On day **BEFORE** procedure, administer usual doses of insulin

3 **On day of procedure:**
- Hold **ALL** pre-breakfast insulin
- Omit breakfast
- If outpatient, child should arrive in the early morning
- Should be **FIRST** case of the day
- Obtain labs: blood glucose, serum electrolytes, and ketones (urine or blood)

4 **Administer insulin infusion on the morning of the procedure:**
- Solution of 10% dextrose and ½ NS (maintenance rate) **AND** regular insulin (50 units/50 mL saline) via syringe pump infused through a Y-site with the line delivering the dextrose infusion

Maintenance rate calculation:
4 mL/kg/hour for first 10 kg +
2 mL/kg/hour from 11–20 kg +
1 mL/kg/hour > 20 kg

Insulin infusion rate based on the child's age:
- For children ≤12 years, at a rate of 1 unit per 5 grams dextrose
- For children >12 years, at a rate of 1 unit per 3 grams dextrose

5 Is child's blood glucose concentration ≤250 mg/dL?

No → 6
- Administer regular insulin IV using child's "correction factor" (see Fig. 24-2 footnote)
- Correct child's blood glucose to 150 mg/dL

Yes

Go to Figure 24-7

Figure 24-5. Preoperative management for children with diabetes mellitus who require insulin infusions during surgery. (Modified from Rhodes ET, Ferrari LR, Wolfsdorf JI: Perioperative management of pediatric surgical patients with diabetes mellitus. Anesth Analg 2005; 101:986-999.)

acting insulin should be administered to maintain blood glucose in the target range of 100 to 200 mg/dL. Frequent blood glucose monitoring as well as monitoring blood or urine ketones is essential because of the variable effects of surgical trauma, inactivity, pain, anxiety, nausea and/or vomiting with poor oral intake, medications, and postoperative infection. At the time of discharge from the hospital, children and their family or care providers should be given appropriate guidelines regarding these issues. Those who are admitted to the hospital overnight after surgery should be managed in consultation with the endocrinology service, if possible, to coordinate appropriate scheduling and subsequent dosing of insulin.

Special Surgical Situations
Diabetic children who need urgent surgery must be fully assessed clinically and biochemically. Frequently, the problem necessitat-

ing surgery may have led to metabolic decompensation that must first be corrected and stabilized, unless the need for surgery is immediate. These children are often dehydrated; and, in such a setting, rehydration in addition to insulin administration is critical in addressing the metabolic derangements and restoring normal glomerular filtration rate and renal function. In most cases, these children require emergent surgery that should be managed with an intravenous infusion of insulin as described earlier (see Fig. 24-5). Children with diabetic ketoacidosis require close collaboration between the anesthesiology and endocrinology services.

Diabetes Insipidus

Children undergoing neurosurgical procedures for tumors in or near the pituitary gland, especially craniopharyngioma, often

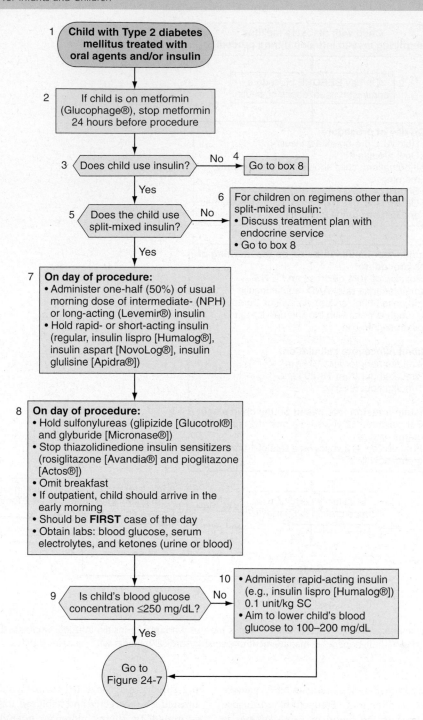

Figure 24-6. Preoperative management for type 2 diabetes children on oral agents and/or insulin. (Modified from Rhodes ET, Ferrari LR, Wolfsdorf JI: Perioperative management of pediatric surgical patients with diabetes mellitus. Anesth Analg 2005; 101:986-999.)

require management of diabetes insipidus (DI), as do children with known DI who require anesthesia for surgical or radiologic procedures. The perioperative management of these children is frequently complicated by either overhydration or underhydration and electrolyte disturbances.

DI is caused by a deficiency of the antidiuretic hormone arginine vasopressin, which acts on the distal tubule and collecting duct of the kidney to promote reabsorption of water. Central

(hypothalamic, neurogenic or vasopressin-sensitive) DI can be caused by disorders of vasopressin gene structure; accidental or surgical trauma to vasopressin neurons; congenital anatomic hypothalamic or pituitary defects; neoplasms; infiltrative, autoimmune, and infectious diseases affecting vasopressin neurons or fiber tracts; and increased metabolism of vasopressin. The etiology is unknown in approximately 50% of children with central DI.

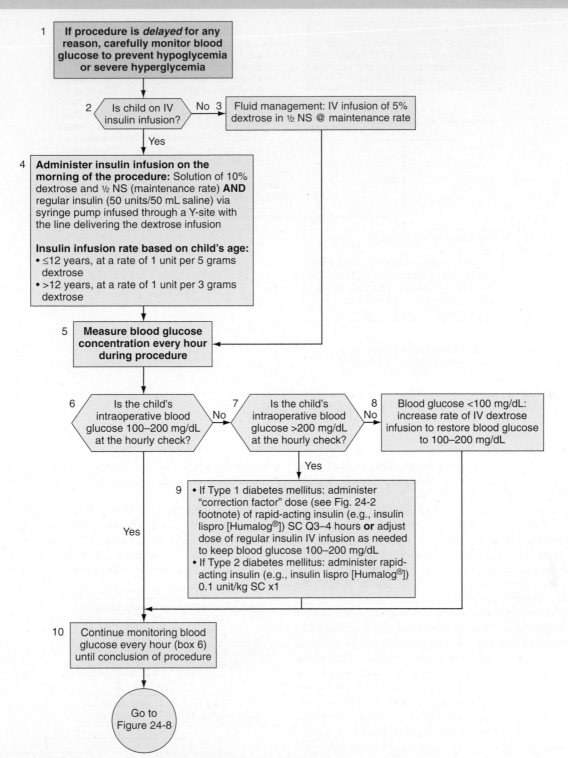

Figure 24-7. Diabetes mellitus: intraoperative management. The management goal for the diabetic child is near-normoglycemia (100-200 mg/dL). Maintenance fluid rate calculation is 4 mL/kg/hr for the first 10 kg of body weight, 2 mL/kg/hour for body weight between 11 and 20 kg, and 1 mL/kg/hr for every kg of body weight over 20 kg. (Modified from Rhodes ET, Ferrari LR, Wolfsdorf JI: Perioperative management of pediatric surgical patients with diabetes mellitus. Anesth Analg 2005; 101:986-999.)

Diagnosis of Neurosurgical Diabetes Insipidus: The Triple-Phase Response

It is important to distinguish polyuria caused by the onset of acute post-surgical central DI from polyuria resulting from diuresis of fluids given during surgery. In both cases, children may have a high volume (exceeding 200 mL/m²/hr) of dilute urine. Serum osmolality will be high in DI but will be normal in the child excreting excess salt and fluid. The normal child who excretes excess salt and water has a moderate to high urine osmolality. A meticulous examination of the intraoperative and

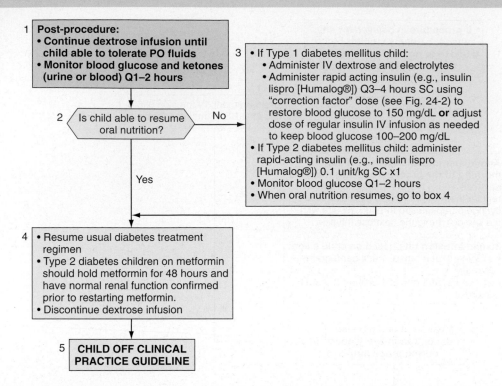

Figure 24-8. Diabetes mellitus: postoperative management. (Modified from Rhodes ET, Ferrari LR, Wolfsdorf JI: Perioperative management of pediatric surgical patients with diabetes mellitus. Anesth Analg 2005; 101:986-999.)

postoperative records and careful bedside assessment of volume status (jugular venous distention, capillary refill) will generally distinguish between these two entities.

Of special interest is the triphasic pattern of vasopressin secretion, often, but not always, observed after neurosurgical procedures that interfere with the supraoptic-hypophyseal tract.[101] After surgery, an initial phase of transient DI may be observed, lasting between 12 hours and 2 days. This may be due to local edema that interferes with normal vasopressin secretion. If significant vasopressin-secreting cell damage has occurred, release of stored vasopressin from damaged neurons leads to a second phase that involves water retention, caused by the syndrome of inappropriate antidiuretic hormone secretion (SIADH), which may last up to 10 days. Finally, a third phase, permanent neurogenic DI, may follow if more than 90% of vasopressin cells are destroyed. Pronounced SIADH in the second phase generally portends permanent DI in the final phase of the triple response. In children with both vasopressin and cortisol deficiency (e.g., in combined anterior and posterior hypopituitarism after neurosurgical treatment of craniopharyngioma), symptoms of DI may be masked because cortisol deficiency impairs renal free water clearance. Institution of glucocorticoid therapy may precipitate polyuria, leading to the diagnosis of DI (Fig. 24-9).

Perioperative Management of Minor Procedures

Children with preexisting DI who are scheduled for a minor procedure, that is, a procedure without significant blood loss and not followed by a period of further fasting or fluid shifts (e.g., myringotomy, radiologic imaging, peripheral orthopedic procedures) are treated differently from those undergoing a

more major procedure associated with blood loss or fluid shifts and delayed postoperative resumption of fluid intake (see Fig. 24-9).

Children undergoing minor procedures under anesthesia should receive their usual morning dose of desamino-8-D-arginine vasopressin (DDAVP), hereafter referred to as desmopressin (Table 24-3). The anesthetic technique is tailored to the procedure (e.g., intravenous sedation for MRI, general endotra-

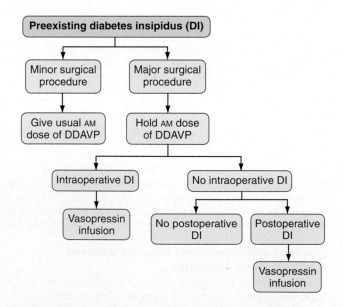

Figure 24-9. Perioperative management of diabetes insipidus. DDAVP, 1-deamino(8-D-arginine) vasopressin.

Table 24-3. Medications for Management of Central Diabetes Insipidus

Desmopressin acetate (100-, 200-µg tablets; rhinal tube 10 µg/0.1 mL; nasal spray 10 µg/0.1 mL: delivers 0.1 mL/spray)

Oral	Dose: 100-400 µg q12 hr
	Oral doses are 10-20 times intranasal doses of desmopressin
	Onset of action: ~15-30 min
	Duration: 8-12 hr
	May develop tachyphylaxis
Intranasal	Dose: ~10-20 µg/dose q12-24 hr
	Onset of action: 5-15 min
	Duration: 8-12 hr

Vasopressin (Pitressin) (20 units/mL; 0.5-mL, 1-mL, and 10-mL vials; conversion: 1 unit = 2.5 µg)

Intravenous	Dose: 1.5 mU/kg/hr
	Onset of action: minutes
	Half life: 5-10 min

cheal anesthesia for tonsillectomy). Arterial and urinary catheters are not required, and recovery takes place in the postanesthesia care unit (PACU). Once the morning dose of desmopressin has been administered, intraoperative and postoperative fluids should be restricted to the rate of 1 L/m²/24 hr, that is, to match insensible free water losses. Oral fluids may be offered once the child is awake. Although modern PACU policies often no longer require successful fluid intake before discharging the ambulatory patient, discharging the child with DI should be delayed until the child is able to take *ad libitum* oral fluids without vomiting. Subsequent doses of desmopressin are administered according to the child's usual preoperative schedule.

Perioperative Management of Major Procedures

A major surgical procedure is defined as an operation associated with the potential for significant blood loss, intraoperative or postoperative hemodynamic, neurologic, respiratory instability, entry into a body cavity (e.g., craniotomy, abdominal surgery, thoracic surgery), craniofacial or airway surgery, major orthopedic surgery (e.g., spine surgery, tumor resection or amputation, major osteotomies), and/or surgery followed by delayed resumption of *ad libitum* fluid intake. The child with DI should be scheduled as the first case of the day. On the day before the procedure the child treated with desmopressin should receive the usual morning dose but only 50% of the usual evening or bedtime dose (see Fig. 24-9). On the morning of the procedure, desmopressin is withheld. The child undergoing a major procedure should receive general anesthesia with conventional monitoring as well as insertion of arterial and urinary catheters and after surgery is admitted to the ICU. A central venous catheter for monitoring central venous pressure, although not indicated solely for the management of DI, is frequently useful in the postoperative period.

At the start of the procedure, an infusion of aqueous vasopressin (20 U/1000 mL to yield a final concentration of 20 mU/mL) should be started at 1.5 mU/kg/hr. Intravenous fluids should total 1 L/m²/24 hr to approximate insensible losses and obligate urine output using normal saline with 5% dextrose. Additional intravenous saline, isotonic fluid, or blood products may be given, as needed, to correct blood and surgical fluid loss, to correct third space fluid loss, and to maintain hemodynamic stability. Urine output should not be corrected in the child receiving a vasopressin infusion.

New Perioperative Diagnosis

The new diagnosis of intraoperative or postoperative DI is based on clinical and laboratory findings, including serum sodium level greater than 145 mmol/L, polyuria (>4 mL/kg/hr) for 30 minutes or more, increased plasma osmolality (>300 mOsm/kg) in association with hypotonic urine (<300 mOsm/kg), and after excluding the presence of glucosuria, diuretic, or mannitol administration as possible causes of polyuria.

When DI occurs, an infusion of aqueous vasopressin (20 U/1000 mL) is initiated at 1.5 mU/kg/hr and the dose is doubled after 15 to 30 minutes if the child does not respond, until urine output decreases to less than 2 mL/kg/hr. Once a urine output of less than 2 mL/kg/hr is achieved, the vasopressin infusion is maintained at a constant rate.

Intravenous desmopressin should *not* be used in the acute management of postoperative central DI because it offers no advantage over aqueous vasopressin and because its long half-life (8-12 hours) compared with that of vasopressin (5-10 minutes) increases the risk of water intoxication and precludes dose titration.

Postoperative Management

The child with DI should be cared for in an ICU after major surgery. Fluid input and output, serum electrolytes, and osmolality are monitored closely (hourly if necessary) in the intraoperative and postoperative periods. Until stability is achieved, it is important to have a urinary catheter in place to distinguish postoperative urinary retention from oliguria. The vasopressin infusion initiated intraoperatively is continued in the ICU. Fluid administration is *not* adjusted according to urine output; however, fluid deficits are replaced and blood pressure supported until antidiuresis is clearly established. Total (oral and IV) maintenance fluids should not exceed insensible plus obligatory urinary losses of 1 L/m²/24 hr. In the postoperative period, appropriate maintenance fluid is generally 5% dextrose in half-normal saline with 0 to 40 mEq/L of potassium chloride (depending on the serum potassium concentration). Blood loss should be replaced with normal saline, 5% albumin, or blood products, as appropriate.

Aqueous vasopressin at a dose of 1.5 mU/kg/hr results in a supranormal blood vasopressin concentration of approximately 10 pg/mL, twice that needed for full antidiuretic activity.[102] The effect of vasopressin is maximal within 2 hours of starting an infusion.[102] After hypothalamic (but not transsphenoidal) surgery, higher initial concentrations of vasopressin are occasionally required to treat acute DI. This may be attributable to the release of a substance related to vasopressin from the damaged hypothalamoneurohypophyseal system, which acts as an antagonist to normal vasopressin activity.[103] Much higher rates of vasopressin infusions, resulting in plasma concentrations above 1000 pg/mL, should be avoided because they may cause cutaneous necrosis,[104] rhabdomyolysis,[104,105] and cardiac rhythm disturbances.[106]

Post–Intensive Care Unit Management

Children treated with vasopressin for post-neurosurgical DI should be switched from intravenous to oral fluid intake at the earliest opportunity because thirst sensation, if intact, will better regulate blood osmolality. Once oral intake has been resumed without nausea and vomiting (often by the morning of the day after surgery), the vasopressin infusion should be stopped; all intravenous infusions should be stopped to avoid iatrogenic fluid overload, and oral fluids are permitted *ad libitum*. Desmopressin is reinstituted (nasally or orally) in the child with preexisting DI or begun in the child who has new-onset DI (see Table 24-3).

Syndrome of Inappropriate Antidiuretic Hormone Secretion

SIADH is characterized by hypotonic hyponatremia, urine osmolality in excess of plasma osmolality, natriuresis in the absence of edema and volume depletion, and normal renal and normal adrenal function.[107] The dilutional hyponatremia of SIADH develops due to persistent detectable or increased plasma arginine vasopressin (AVP; also known as antidiuretic hormone [ADH]) concentrations in the presence of continued fluid intake. Chronic hyponatremia, however, is the result of a combination of water retention and sodium excretion.[108] The major causes of SIADH are neurologic diseases, neoplasia, lung diseases, and drugs (Table 24-4).[109] Inappropriate infusion of hypotonic fluids in the postoperative period is among the most common causes.[110] The clinical manifestations are principally neuromuscular (headache, nausea, vomiting, muscle cramps, lethargy, restlessness, disorientation, and depressed reflexes). The severity of symptoms is related to both the absolute serum sodium concentration (most patients with serum sodium greater than 125 mEq/L are asymptomatic) and its rate of decrease, especially if greater than 0.5 mEq/L/hr.

Although ADH secretion impairs water excretion, the mechanisms that regulate volume (renin-angiotensin-aldosterone system and atrial natriuretic peptide) are intact. Volume expansion activates natriuretic mechanisms (decreased proximal sodium reabsorption and decreased aldosterone production), resulting in sodium and water excretion and the restoration of near-euvolemia. With *chronic* SIADH, sodium loss is a more prominent feature than is water retention. Severe hyponatremia increases cell size due to entry of water into the cell along its osmotic gradient and may be associated with loss of intracellular potassium and other solutes in an attempt to restore cell volume.

Perioperative Management

Many of the causes of SIADH are transient and resolve as the underlying condition is corrected. Treatment of chronic SIADH consists of water restriction; that is, fluid intake is restricted to less than or equal to 1 L/m²/24 hr. Unless sodium intake is adequate, water restriction can lead to volume depletion in children with a sodium deficit. In asymptomatic chronic (>3 days) dilutional hyponatremia and in chronic SIADH, specific therapy may not be required.

Hypertonic (3%) saline should be used with caution in children. Rapid correction of chronic hyponatremia can lead to serious, permanent, and even fatal neurologic complications

Table 24-4. Causes of SIADH

Central Nervous System Disturbances
Head injury
Brain tumor
Subarachnoid hemorrhage
Stroke
Infection (meningitis, encephalitis)
Acute psychosis

Drugs
Vasopressin, desmopressin
Carbamazepine, oxcarbamazepine
Cyclophosphamide
Vinca alkaloids
Cisplatin
Phenothiazines
Serotonin uptake inhibitors (e.g., fluoxetine, sertraline)
Tricyclic antidepressants
Monoamine oxidase inhibitors
Methylenedioxymethamphetamine ("ecstasy")
Nicotine

Major Surgery
Major abdominal or thoracic surgery
Pituitary surgery
Pain
Severe nausea

Pulmonary Disease
Pneumonia, tuberculosis
Asthma
Atelectasis
Pneumothorax
Positive-pressure ventilation

Neoplasia
Carcinoma of lung (e.g., small cell carcinoma)
Leukemia
Thymoma
Lymphoma
Other tumors

Infection
Human immunodeficiency virus

Hereditary SIADH
Functional mutations in the vasopressin-2 receptor

from osmotic demyelination (central pontine myelinolysis).[111] Only children with neurologic symptoms attributable to acute hyponatremia of less than 3 days' duration (e.g., altered level of consciousness, coma, or seizures) require rapid initial correction. The rate of increase of serum sodium concentration should not exceed 0.5 mEq/L/hr (or 8-10 mEq/L/24 hr).[112,113] The saline infusion should stop when the absolute concentration of serum sodium reaches 120 to 125 mEq/L. Hypertonic saline is usually combined with furosemide to limit treatment-induced expansion of the extracellular fluid volume.[113] Thereafter, treatment should consist of fluid restriction.

Thyroid Disorders

Thyroid hormones play an important role in metabolic processes, growth, and development in children.[114] The thyroid gland develops from the embryonic pharyngeal floor and descends along the thyroglossal duct to its final position in the anterior neck. Thyroid hormone production is controlled by the hypothalamic-pituitary-thyroid axis. Although thyroxine (T_4) is the predominant circulating thyroid hormone, triiodothyronine (T_3) is the most active thyroid metabolite and is primarily formed by peripheral conversion from T_4. Serum T_3 and T_4 concentrations in turn regulate hypothalamic thyroid-releasing hormone (TRH) and pituitary thyroid-stimulating hormone (TSH) secretion via negative feedback. Thyroid hormones are transported in the blood by carrier proteins, including thyroxine-binding globulin (TBG), prealbumin, and albumin. Protein-bound T_4 and T_3 are not biologically active. Only 0.03% of circulating T_4 and 0.3% of T_3 are unbound and active.[115,116]

Hypothyroidism

Classification and Epidemiology

Hypothyroidism, the most common thyroid disorder in children, can range from subclinical to overt disease. In subclinical hypothyroidism, children maintain a normal thyroxine level by increasing TSH levels. Over time, however, thyroid function can decompensate despite increased stimulation and progresses to thyroid hormone deficiency.[117-119] Iodine deficiency continues to be the foremost cause of hypothyroidism worldwide.[120] However, in the United States and other regions in which the intake of iodine is adequate, autoimmune thyroid disease is the most common cause of hypothyroidism.[118] Other less frequent causes of hypothyroidism include secondary and tertiary processes resulting from pituitary or hypothalamic insufficiency, respectively, which are relevant in many surgical situations, especially tumors of the central nervous system (CNS).

Biochemical Tests of Thyroid Function

In general, measurement of serum TSH and either total T_4 or free T_4 suffices for assessment of thyroid normalcy. However, several conditions exist in which thyroid hormone levels appear abnormal yet the individual is clinically euthyroid. These conditions may lead to erroneous diagnosis and inappropriate treatment for hypothyroidism or hyperthyroidism. TSH is the most sensitive test for diagnosing primary thyroid disorders and generally precedes noticeable changes in total T_4 and T_3 levels. Thyroid function can also be assessed by measurement of unbound or free T_4 along with thyroid hormone-binding proteins (TBG). When total T_4 levels are reduced but free T_4 and TSH values are normal, TBG deficiency is the most likely diagnosis. No treatment is required for TBG deficiency because individuals are fundamentally euthyroid. Likewise, medical intervention is unnecessary for familial dysalbuminemic hyperthyroxinemia, which manifests with increased total T_4 levels but normal free T_4 and TSH values.[121]

Importantly, if the hypothalamic-pituitary axis is not intact, TSH becomes a useless measurement of thyroid function. Therefore, in cases of secondary/tertiary (central) thyroid disorders, diagnosis and treatment is based solely on peripheral thyroid hormone levels and clinical signs. During times of stress or acute illness, increased conversion of T_3 to a metabolically inactive form, reverse T_3, occurs. In addition, T_4 and TSH values may both be reduced, reflecting a decreased metabolic state. Individuals are considered euthyroid based on nonelevated TSH values but the differential diagnosis includes central hypothyroidism, a distinction that often cannot be made by laboratory evaluation. However, controversy still exists in regard to possible benefits of using T_4 or T_3 to treat euthyroid sick syndrome, in which there are abnormal thyroid tests in the setting of a nonthyroidal illness such as during a critical illness. Typically, children with euthyroid sick syndrome have a low thyroxine level with a normal or low-normal TSH level, indicating a decreased metabolic state.[122-125]

Clinical Manifestations

Because thyroid hormone affects all metabolically active cells, hormone deficiency leads to a wide array of systemic abnormalities. Classic signs and symptoms of hypothyroidism in children include short stature due to a decline in growth rate, fatigue, cold intolerance, weight gain, dry skin, hair loss, constipation, hoarse voice, and coarse facial features. Myxedema coma is a severe manifestation of hypothyroidism that can occur in profoundly hypothyroid individuals exposed to an external stress such as infection, surgery, hypnotics, or cold temperature. Myxedema coma can result in severe life-threatening heart failure or coma[126,127] and should be considered in any postoperative child with unexplained cardiovascular dysfunction, difficulty weaning from ventilatory support, or delirium.[90] Other medical conditions associated with hypothyroidism include anemia, hyperlipidemia, and pubertal disorders.

Neonatal Hypothyroidism

Congenital hypothyroidism remains the most frequent cause of preventable mental retardation. Thyroid dysgenesis or agenesis accounts for the majority of cases, whereas a smaller percentage is due to thyroid dyshormonogenesis and secondary/tertiary hypothyroidism.[128] Because neonates do not exhibit the classic signs or symptoms of hypothyroidism, testing for congenital hypothyroidism occurs with the neonatal screen. Usually based on TSH thresholds, the neonatal screen detects only primary thyroid deficiency and not the central hypothyroidism that accompanies hypopituitarism or CNS anomalies, such as septo-optic dysplasia. Early detection and implementation of thyroid replacement are essential to avoid permanent neurologic sequelae. In general, affected children who receive adequate thyroid replacement starting in the neonatal period lead normal lives.

Treatment

The goal of thyroid replacement is to normalize the TSH and T_4 levels and consequently reverse the metabolic derangements caused by hypothyroidism. In general, daily levothyroxine (LT_4) replacement leads to normalization in T_4 levels within a week but equilibration of TSH occurs more slowly, over 4 to 6 weeks.[129] The appropriate starting LT_4 dose varies with age and disease state. For neonates, the starting dose is 10 to 15 µg/kg/day, which is much greater than the conventional replacement dose of 2 to 4 µg/kg/day in children and adolescents.[130] In healthy children with acute hypothyroidism, full LT_4 replacement can be started immediately. However, in symptomatic children with chronic hypothyroidism, potential problems with pseudotumor cerebri or slipped capital femoral epiphysis may develop if they are started on full LT$_4$ doses. Therefore, treatment should begin at one fourth of the expected dose with slow titration every 4 to 6 weeks.[131,132] After dose stabilization, children and adolescents should continue to have regular clinical examinations and TSH monitoring owing to increased dose requirements during puberty and pregnancy.[133,134] Thyroid replacement can be given parenterally if needed. The intravenous dose of LT$_4$ is 50% less than the oral dose, and should be given once daily.

Preoperative Management

Because thyroid hormones play a critical role in regulating metabolism, children should be clinically and biochemically euthyroid before any type of elective surgery. Several case studies have shown decreased cardiac function, diminished breathing capacity, and increased sensitivity to anesthetic agents with moderate to severe hypothyroidism.[135-137] Children with known hypothyroidism should have documented normal thyroid function tests before surgery. For individuals with undiagnosed hypothyroidism, a detailed history should be obtained in regard to previous thyroid disorders, head and neck radiation, radioactive iodine therapy, thyroid surgery, and family history of thyroid disease.[138] In addition, children with autoimmune disorders, type 1 diabetes mellitus, celiac disease, and children with particular genetic syndromes, such as trisomy 21 and Turner syndrome, are at increased risk for developing autoimmune thyroiditis and should be screened if symptomatic.[139-141]

Children with subclinical or mild hypothyroidism often must undergo urgent surgery without delay. Thyroid replacement can be started and continued with the same regimen as described in the outpatient setting. But for children with moderate to severe hypothyroidism, surgery should be postponed if possible until thyroid hormone levels normalize on replacement therapy. However, if urgent surgery is required, perioperative treatment with intravenous thyroxine with or without glucocorticoids should be given to prevent myxedema coma.[90,138] An exception to this strategy applies to the child who is scheduled for cardiovascular surgery or cardiac catheterization in which thyroid replacement could precipitate or worsen unstable coronary syndromes. Several studies in adults reported no adverse outcomes in cardiac patients undergoing surgery without thyroid replacement.[90,138,142] Therefore, thyroid replacement could be initiated postoperatively in children with cardiovascular disease undergoing cardiac surgery or cardiac evaluation.

Hyperthyroidism

Classification and Epidemiology

Hyperthyroidism is a condition caused by excess circulating thyroid hormones resulting in an increase in metabolic activity of various peripheral tissues in the body. Almost all children with hyperthyroidism have suppressed serum TSH concentrations due to negative feedback by high T$_4$ and T$_3$ concentrations. Hyperthyroidism can be either overt or subclinical.[143] Overt hyperthyroidism is characterized by both clinical and biochemical manifestations of the disease. In subclinical hyperthyroidism, children are asymptomatic but exhibit the biochemical abnormality of a suppressed TSH level.

Hyperthyroidism occurs less frequently in children than hypothyroidism and is nearly always caused by Graves disease. Other causes of childhood thyrotoxicosis include autoimmune thyroiditis (Hashimoto thyroiditis), infections of the thyroid

gland, autonomously functioning thyroid nodules, iodine-induced hyperthyroidism, McCune-Albright syndrome, TSH-producing pituitary adenomas, and thyroid hormone ingestion.[144] A rare thyroid disorder that mimics hyperthyroidism is thyroid hormone resistance. However, unlike other causes of childhood thyrotoxicosis, thyroid hormone resistance should not be treated with antithyroid medications.[145,146]

Graves Disease

Graves disease, an autoimmune disorder, is the most common cause of childhood hyperthyroidism. The pathophysiology of Graves disease involves thyroid-stimulating immunoglobulins that bind to the TSH receptor, causing hyperstimulation of the thyroid gland. Most children with Graves disease have a diffuse goiter, and some develop autoimmune ophthalmopathy and myxedema. Because few children with Graves disease enter spontaneous remission, treatment of hyperthyroidism is required. Current treatment options include antithyroid medications (methimazole or propylthiouracil), surgical removal of the thyroid gland, or radioactive iodine.[147,148] Although virtually all children go into remission during therapy with antithyroid drugs, side effects are common (see later) and the majority of children treated for 2 to 3 years relapse shortly after discontinuation of therapy.[149,150] Radioactive ablation is usually definitive and carries less risk than surgery.[151]

Thyroiditis

The term *thyroiditis* is used to describe a group of heterogeneous disorders that result in inflammation of the thyroid gland with subsequent release of preformed thyroid hormone. Transient hyperthyroidism can result from the initial inflammatory process, but symptoms generally last only a few weeks until stored thyroid hormone concentrations are exhausted. Some children will develop hypothyroidism after the recovery phase due to lymphocytic infiltration of the gland and destruction of thyroid tissue. Treatment with antithyroid drugs is generally not indicated for transient hyperthyroidism, but for symptomatic children, β blockers should be used during the thyrotoxic phase to control symptoms.[152]

Thyroiditis can also manifest as painful inflammation of the gland and fever owing to bacterial or viral infection. *Haemophilus influenzae,* group A streptococci, and *Staphylococcus* are the most frequent causes of acute thyroiditis, which can be associated with thyrocutaneous fistulas.[153] Viral infections of the thyroid gland are less severe and result in subacute thyroiditis.[154] Owing to the difficulty in distinguishing bacterial from viral infections, all cases of infectious thyroiditis are treated with antibiotics.

Clinical Manifestations

Most of the symptoms that children experience are the same regardless of the cause of hyperthyroidism. Classic signs and symptoms of hyperthyroidism include goiter, tachycardia/palpitations, tremors, brisk reflexes, heat intolerance, dyspnea, insomnia, diarrhea, nervousness, and weight loss despite a normal or increased appetite. Many children with hyperthyroidism have poor school performance and are initially mistakenly diagnosed with attention-deficit hyperactivity disorder. Other medical conditions associated with long-standing hyperthyroidism include osteoporosis and irregular menses.[155]

As stated previously, individuals with Graves disease may develop additional autoimmune manifestations such as ophthalmopathy and pretibial myxedema. Eye involvement in Graves disease is characterized by inflammation of the extraocular muscles, connective tissue, and orbital fat, which results in proptosis, restricted eye movement, and periorbital edema.[156,157] Children with Graves ophthalmopathy may complain of eye irritation or dryness due to lid retraction. If left untreated, corneal ulceration may develop and lead to irreversible eye damage, including blindness. Unfortunately, ophthalmopathy usually persists in spite of treatment of the hyperthyroidism.[147,158]

Treatment

Antithyroid medications remain the first-line of treatment for many physicians because one third of children go into remission after several years of drug therapy.[149,159] Long-term remission rates are greater in pubertal children than prepubertal children. Other favorable prognostic indicators include a small thyroid gland and normal levels of TSH receptor antibodies at the time of diagnosis.[160,161] Thionamides (methimazole or propylthiouracil) are the mainstay of antithyroid therapy. Minor adverse effects occur in 25% of children treated with thionamides and include increases in liver enzymes, neutropenia, rash, and lymphadenopathy. Serious adverse effects, such as agranulocytosis and liver failure, are rare, occurring in up to 0.5% to 1% of individuals.[162]

Perioperative Management

For children who relapse after antithyroid drug therapy or who require immediate definitive therapy, radioactive iodine is a safe and effective alternative to thyroidectomy. Treatment consists of ^{131}I uptake in the thyroid gland, which leads to cell destruction by internal radiation. Several longitudinal studies have shown that children are not at increased risk for developing thyroid cancer if appropriate doses of radioiodine are used.[163,164] In cases in which radioactive iodine is contraindicated, surgical removal of the entire thyroid gland can also cure the hyperthyroid state. Children should be euthyroid or slightly hypothyroid before surgery to avoid precipitation of thyroid storm. In addition, because of potential serious complications from neck surgery, only surgeons with expertise in performing thyroidectomies in children should perform the surgery.[165]

In special circumstances, perioperative rapid control of hyperthyroidism can be achieved by using large doses of iodine (Lugol solution or saturated potassium iodine), which inhibit thyroid hormone synthesis. The effect is short-lived due to eventual escape from the Wolff-Chaikoff effect; and, therefore, addition of a thionamide is necessary for long-term treatment. Rarely, untreated hyperthyroidism can lead to thyroid storm, a potentially lethal complication. Thyroid storm may be difficult to differentiate from an acute malignant hyperthermic reaction. Thyroid storm produces less severe acidosis, no increase in creatine phosphokinase, and no response to dantrolene. However, thyroid storm responds to symptomatic treatment including parenteral β blockers and propylthiouracil, the latter per nasogastric tube. If left untreated, the mortality rate due to thyroid storm ranges from 20% to 30%.[166] Various external factors such as surgery, infection, or stress are predisposing factors for onset of thyroid storm. Because of the dramatically increased metabolic state, acute management of hyperthyroidism and targeted symptomatic treatment is essential to avoid death.[126,144,167] A multidrug approach is necessary to (1) halt production and release of thyroid hormone, (2) prevent conversion of T_4 to T_3, (3) antagonize the peripheral (adrenergic) effects of thyroid hormone, and (4) control systemic disturbances with supportive therapy (Table 24-5).[126,147,162,168-170]

Parathyroid and Calcium Disorders

Physiology of Calcium Homeostasis

The four parathyroid glands are usually present in pairs at the superior and inferior poles of the thyroid gland, with the inferior pair occasionally ectopic elsewhere in the neck or chest. Parathyroid hormone (PTH) is released from secretory granules in

---

Table 24-5. Management of Hyperthyroid Crisis

Drug Class	Recommended Drug	Starting Dose	Mechanism of Action
Iodine	Potassium iodide (SSKI)	3-5 drops by mouth q6 hr	Blocks release of thyroid hormone from gland
	Lugol solution	4-8 drops by mouth q6-8 hr	Blocks release of thyroid hormone from gland
β Blockers	Propranolol	Infant: 2 mg/kg/day by mouth divided q8-12 hr Child: 10-40 mg by mouth q6-8 hr	β-adrenergic blockade; decreased T_4 to T_3 conversion
	Esmolol	100-200 μg/kg/min IV infusion	β-adrenergic blockade
Thionamide	Propylthiouracil	5-10 mg/kg/day by mouth divided q8 hr	Inhibits new hormone synthesis; decreases T_4 to T_3 conversion
	Methimazole	0.4 mg/kg/day by mouth divided q8-12 hr	Inhibits new hormone synthesis
Supportive treatment	Intravenous fluid	20-40 mL/kg normal saline	Replacement of increased insensible losses due to fever, diaphoresis, vomiting, and diarrhea
	Cooling blankets, ice packs		Reduce fever
	Acetaminophen	15 mg/kg/dose by mouth q4-6 hr or 40 mg/kg per rectum loading dose then 20 mg/kg/dose q6 hr	
	Hydrocortisone	Adult: 100 mg IV q8 hr (no pediatric dose recommended)	Decreases T_4 to T_3 conversion; enhances vasomotor stability

response to a decrease in serum ionized calcium; it is inhibited by hyperphosphatemia, profound hypomagnesemia or hypermagnesemia, or increased $1,25(OH)_2$-vitamin D (calcitriol). The calcium-sensing receptor (CaR) in the parathyroid mediates PTH release and also directly regulates calcium reabsorption in the distal tubule. Inactivating CaR mutations establish a greater serum calcium set point in familial hypocalciuric hypercalcemia, now a relatively common and incidental diagnosis that is benign unless homozygotic, whereas activating mutations result in autosomal dominant hypocalcemia with hypercalciuria.[171,172]

PTH has three primary modes of increasing serum calcium: (1) calcium reabsorption and concomitant phosphaturia in the distal tubule; (2) upregulation of osteoclast-mediated calcium and phosphate release from bone; and (3) renal conversion of 25-OH-vitamin D to the active metabolite, $1,25(OH)_2$-vitamin D (calcitriol). In turn, calcitriol has direct calcium-releasing effects on bone and, most importantly, increases absorption of calcium and phosphate from the gut. Calcitonin is secreted by the thyroid C cells and has calcium-lowering properties via its own G protein–coupled receptor, but its physiologic role is uncertain at this time.

Hypocalcemia

Neonatal Hypocalcemia

Neonatal hypocalcemia is common but usually transient, owing to prematurity, maternal diabetes, maternal hyperparathyroidism, excessive diuretic use or phosphate load, and transient neonatal hypoparathyroidism.[173] Neonatal hypocalcemia requires exclusion of velocardiofacial syndrome (VCF/DiGeorge/Shprintzen), which often has an associated congenital cardiac left-sided lesion, by cytogenetic screening at 22q11.[174-176] The hypocalcemia of VCF is due to an incomplete hypoparathyroidism that tends to normalize eventually but may recur. Low PTH, or PTH resistance (pseudohypoparathyroidism), causes hyperphosphatemia beyond the already high neonatal normal range, whereas vitamin D deficiency or resistance is associated with low to normal serum P levels. Maternal 25OH-vitamin D deficiency is another common cause of early or late infantile hypocalcemia in the United States, regardless of the infant's dietary intake.[177,178] Childhood hypocalcemia with low PTH may be the first endocrine sign of polyglandular autoimmune disease type I, now called autoimmune polyendocrinopathy-candidiasis-ectodermal dystrophy (APECED).[179]

Childhood Hypocalcemia

Persistent hypocalcemia in children can have many manifestations, including poor feeding, tetany, seizures, laryngospasm, paresthesias, and muscle cramping. Initial evaluation of hypocalcemia, regardless of age, generally includes serum calcium, phosphate, magnesium, alkaline phosphatase, creatinine, PTH, 25OH-vitamin D, and $1,25(OH)_2$-vitamin D, plus urine calcium and phosphate. Therapy for acute hypocalcemia includes parenteral calcium, followed by oral replacement and 25OH-vitamin D if low,[178] and calcitriol as a substitute for PTH, because PTH itself, an anabolic bone agent in adults,[180] is contraindicated in children owing to concerns about its possible role in osteosarcoma.

Perioperative Management

Hypocalcemia is most frequently managed by intravenous infusion of calcium in the form of 10% calcium chloride, or 10% calcium gluconate, and with frequent measurement of serum ionized calcium levels to guide therapy (see Chapter 10). Calcium salts release free calcium ions and as such should be given via a central venous catheter because their hypertonicity and the high concentration of ionized calcium will produce intense local vasoconstriction that may lead to necrosis of the skin and subcutaneous tissues and possible gangrene of the affected limb if administered via a peripheral intravenous cannula that becomes interstitial. In the postoperative period after the child is tolerating oral intake, intravenous calcium supplementation may be converted to oral supplementation.

Hypercalcemia

Hyperparathyroidism (HPT) is less common in children than in adults.[181] In most cases of HPT in children an adenoma is present that is unresponsive to the increased serum calcium level. Other causes of HPT may occur in children as well, including generalized parathyroid hyperplasia, and, infrequently, parathyroid carcinoma.[182]

Parathyroid hyperplasia occurs in familial forms of HPT, including multiple endocrine neoplasia type 1 (MEN 1), in which HPT is a nearly universal manifestation of the mutation of the menin gene; the hyperparathyroid abnormality occurs more commonly and earlier in presentation than the associated pancreatic, pituitary, and gastrointestinal neuroendocrine tumors associated with MEN 1.[183,184] HPT is a less common manifestation in MEN 2A, in which medullary thyroid carcinoma and pheochromocytoma occur due to the rearranged proto-oncogene mutation.[185] Secondary HPT with relatively normal calcium levels is a common pediatric phenomenon that accompanies renal failure, renal tubular acidosis, and hypophosphatemic rickets.[186] When hypercalcemia is present, the differential diagnosis includes Williams syndrome, vitamin A intoxication, vitamin D excess, and conversion to $1,25(OH)_2$-vitamin D in granulomatous disorders and infantile subcutaneous fat necrosis.[187] Solid tumors may secrete high levels of parathyroid hormone–related protein (PTHrP). Tumors such as leukemias, lymphomas, and others may release excess cytokines and osteoclast-activating factors, with the hypercalcemia leading to the tumor diagnosis.[188,189]

Signs and symptoms of hypercalcemia are usually nonspecific, such as nausea and vomiting. Initial laboratory evaluation of hypercalcemia matches the list for hypocalcemia given earlier.[190]

Evaluation of unexplained hypercalcemia includes measurement of PTHrP for malignancy and of parental calcium levels for familial hypocalciuric hypercalcemia (FHH), additional hormones or genetic testing for MEN syndromes, tumor markers and bone marrow biopsy, and relevant imaging. When HPT is found, ultrasonography is a helpful step in assessing the parathyroid glands, but MRI or technetium-sestamibi scan is more precise, or intraoperative measurement of PTH can be provided for tumor localization.

Perioperative Management

Management of acute hypercalcemia begins with isotonic rehydration and administration of furosemide to induce calciuria. Treatment then proceeds to administration of calcitonin, to which tachyphylaxis may occur within 1 or 2 days, or to glucocorticoids. In the absence of a definitive therapy, such as surgical excision of the pathologic source of PTH, chronic hypercalcemia is responsive to bisphosphonates, such as pamidronate, which can be given by infusion every 3 months.[191,192] Acute management after parathyroidectomy requires careful monitoring and replacement of calcium and possibly the use of calcitriol for persistent hypocalcemia. In isolated parathyroid hyperplasia, MEN, or secondary HPT, surgeons may elect to leave a portion of one gland in the forearm to avoid permanent hypoparathyroidism and its management problems.

Adrenal Endocrinopathies

Physiology

Adrenal steroidogenesis begins with cholesterol as precursor and results in three types of steroid: mineralocorticoid, glucocorticoid, and sex steroid (androgen precursors).[193] Most of the enzymes involved in adrenal (or gonadal) steroidogenesis are cytochrome P450s. The adrenal cortex comprises three zones: the outer zona glomerulosa exclusively synthesizes mineralocorticoids, owing to localized expression of CYP11B2, whereas the zona fasciculata and reticularis synthesize glucocorticoid and androgens owing to localized expression of CYP17.[194] Cortisol, the end-product of the glucocorticoid pathway, is the primary regulator of the hypothalamic-pituitary-adrenal (HPA) axis, in which hypothalamic corticotropin-releasing hormone regulates pituitary adrenocorticotropic hormone (ACTH) secretion and downstream adrenal production of all three categories of steroid. ACTH release follows a diurnal pattern with a peak at 4 to 8 AM, and, most importantly, markedly increases in response to trauma, acute illness, high fever, and hypoglycemia.

Mineralocorticoid production is controlled independently by the renin-angiotensin system, in which angiotensinogen secreted by the liver is cleaved by renin to angiotensin I, which is converted to angiotensin II.[195] The mineralocorticoid pathway is clearly responsive to ACTH as well, as demonstrated by rises in all mineralocorticoid precursors and the end-product aldosterone within minutes of exogenous ACTH stimulation. Strictly speaking, hypopituitarism does not lead to mineralocorticoid deficiency because of this independent stimulation by an intact renin-angiotensin system. Nevertheless, apparent manifestations of mineralocorticoid deficiency, such as hyponatremia, hyperkalemia, and hypotension, are consequences of failure of the adrenal to release adequate glucocorticoid, which has mineralocorticoid properties, particularly inotropic activity.[196] This essential aspect of glucocorticoid activity is the most lethal potential consequence of both primary adrenal insufficiency and hypothalamic-pituitary deficiency and requires the utmost caution on the part of pediatrician, endocrinologist, surgeon, or anesthesiologist. When any question regarding adequacy of the HPA arises, it is prudent to provide exogenous glucocorticoid, particularly perioperatively.[197]

Causes of Adrenal Insufficiency

Primary adrenal insufficiency is suspected from features such as weight loss, nausea and vomiting, poor appetite, and, specifically, the characteristic hyperpigmentation secondary to melanocyte-stimulating hormone (MSH) receptor cross-stimulation by the extraordinarily high levels of ACTH.[198] Primary adrenal insufficiency is rarer in countries with advanced health care systems now that infectious diseases, such as tuberculosis, are

less prevalent, but adrenal hemorrhage still causes adrenal failure.[199] Autoimmune adrenal insufficiency, sometimes as part of polyendocrinopathies, is now the most common cause and includes both glucocorticoid and mineralocorticoid deficiency. Glucocorticoid deficiency with or without mineralocorticoid loss is integral to congenital adrenal hyperplasia (CAH).[200] Rare congenital disorders causing adrenal insufficiency include adrenoleukodystrophy,[201] congenital adrenal hypoplasia, X-linked adrenal hypoplasia congenita, and ACTH receptor defects.[202]

Congenital or acquired lesions of the hypothalamus or pituitary may lead to ACTH deficiency. In general, these lesions cause other pituitary deficiencies, particularly growth hormone (GH) or TSH insufficiency; isolated ACTH deficiency is rare. Both GH and ACTH deficiency are manifested by hypoglycemia in infancy. CNS malformations leading to ACTH deficiency usually will be detectable by MRI. A notable CNS anomaly with hypopituitarism is septo-optic dysplasia,[203-205] with an assortment of midline defects and optic nerve hypoplasia, but isolated pituitary agenesis or hypoplasia is more common. Acquired lesions leading to hypopituitarism include hydrocephalus, meningitis, infiltrative disorders,[206] and tumors such as craniopharyngioma or histiocytosis.[207] Tumor resection, especially craniopharyngioma resection, cranial irradiation, and chemotherapy can lead to multiple pituitary deficiencies, often evolving over many years.[208]

Testing for Adrenal Insufficiency

Cortisol levels follow a diurnal pattern, with peak levels due to an ACTH surge in the early morning and trough levels later in the day. Although a morning serum cortisol less than 5 ng/dL is low and suggestive of adrenal insufficiency, interpretation of a random cortisol level is fraught with problems. A low level at any other time of day is uninformative, and obtaining it to test for adrenal failure is pointless. In contrast, laboratory confirmation of primary mineralocorticoid deficiency by random serum sample is straightforward; it will demonstrate low aldosterone despite markedly increased renin.

Primary adrenal insufficiency may be effectively assessed in two ways,[209] either by measurement of serum ACTH or by stimulating the adrenal with exogenous ACTH (cosyntropin [Cortrosyn], the biologically active 1-24 fragment of ACTH). Markedly increased random serum ACTH is definitive for primary adrenal insufficiency, but levels can be moderately increased by the stress of phlebotomy itself. Therefore, blood for serum ACTH levels should be aspirated from an indwelling catheter to avoid false-positive values.

Hypothalamic-pituitary insufficiency is more difficult to assess. The complete absence of ACTH levels, as in the obvious case of pituitary ablation or destruction, leads eventually to adrenal atrophy and complete unresponsiveness to Cortrosyn stimulation, a finding that necessitates maintenance glucocorticoid replacement. However, adequate response to Cortrosyn implies only tonic ACTH secretion and does not guarantee the ability to generate a normal surge of ACTH during stress. As a consequence, any patient with a CNS lesion that might cause hypothalamic-pituitary-adrenal (HPA) deficiency should receive stress doses of glucocorticoid (see later). In practical terms, a post-Cortrosyn cortisol value of 10 to 20 ng/dL in an at-risk child suggests the need for stress coverage, whereas a value less than 10 ng/dL indicates long-term replacement.[209,210] As an alternative to the Cortrosyn test, metyrapone tests the adequacy of ACTH release in response to a temporary block in the 11β-hydroxylation step in the glucocorticoid pathway; failure to increase the precursor 11-deoxycortisol implies HPA insufficiency. However, this test is not widely performed in children.

Perioperative Management of Adrenal Insufficiency

Glucocorticoid Dosing

Endogenous cortisol secretion is 10 to 12 mg/m^2/day. Accordingly, a replacement dose of hydrocortisone depends on age and body size but might be 5.0 to 7.5 mg three times a day orally for an adolescent with chronic adrenal insufficiency. No dose monitoring is required, but the child's growth rate should be tracked according to age. With concomitant or isolated mineralocorticoid deficiency, replacement utilizes fludrocortisone (Florinef) at an approximate dose of 0.1 mg orally per day, independent of body size, with intermittent monitoring of blood pressure and renin levels. When the goal of glucocorticoid therapy is suppression of ACTH, as in congenital adrenal hyperplasia, the hydrocortisone dose is generally 15 to 20 mg/m^2, with routine monitoring of serum levels of 17-hydroxyprogesterone or other androgens such as dehydroepiandrosterone (DHEA) or testosterone. Alternatives to hydrocortisone include prednisone, which is four to five times more potent than hydrocortisone, and dexamethasone, which is 20 times more potent but has no mineralocorticoid activity and carries much more significant risk of adverse effects such as aseptic necrosis of the femoral head and, therefore, should not be used for chronic routine replacement therapy. Single-dose use of dexamethasone has not been associated with aseptic necrosis of the femoral head.

Conventional stress glucocorticoid coverage is 3 to 10 times the replacement dose, depending on the severity of illness or trauma, although this practice is not evidence based.[211] Therefore, with little risk associated with the transient use of excess glucocorticoid, for children who are on oral replacement therapy we recommend exogenous steroid replacement using three to five times their outpatient steroid oral maintenance dose for routine illness or fever and five to ten times their outpatient steroid oral maintenance dose after major surgery, during critical illness, or in major emergencies. For children who require stress glucocorticoid coverage but who do not take outpatient steroids, or who are unable to take medications by mouth, we recommend steroid replacement using parenteral cortisol (Solu-Cortef) at a dose of 0.5 mg/kg/day every 12 hours for routine illness or fever and 0.5 to 1 mg/kg every 6 hours for perioperative, intensive care, or emergency department indications for up to 72 hours.[212]

Iatrogenic Adrenal Suppression and Tapering

Exogenous glucocorticoids are used chronically in high doses for control of autoimmune disorders, suppression of transplant rejection, and control of inflammatory processes. Iatrogenic adrenal suppression depends on the duration and dose of glucocorticoid used. Periods of high-dose steroids up to 7 to 10 days do not suppress the HPA. Adrenally suppressive treatments lasting 3 to 6 weeks require a taper over 1 to 2 weeks to allow recovery of the HPA. Long-term high-dose treatment may require up to 6 to 9 months for complete return of HPA function and necessitates a taper during that period. At the termination of the taper, a repeat Cortrosyn stimulation test should be performed, and any repeat trauma or illness during the taper requires short-term stress coverage.

The glucocorticoid taper has two meanings. The tempo of therapeutic glucocorticoid tapers of prednisone by gastroenterologists, rheumatologists, nephrologists, and oncologists, and of dexamethasone by surgeons, is entirely dependent on their assessment of the immune or inflammatory process. As long as the glucocorticoid dose is in excess of the replacement dose, and regardless of the dose, the HPA continues to be suppressed. It is only when the steroid dose is tapered down to the daily replacement dose (approximately 10 mg/m^2 hydrocortisone, 2 mg/m^2 prednisone, or 0.5 mg/m^2 dexamethasone) that the endocrine taper begins. At that point, the prednisone should be switched to hydrocortisone for ease of starting a gradual taper from replacement therapy to lower doses while the HPA is reestablished. In the perioperative period, steroid coverage should be administered if there is any concern of the integrity of the HPA during any steroid taper.

Hypercortisolism (Cushing Syndrome)

Excess cortisol, whether exogenous or endogenous, results in muscle wasting, truncal obesity, moon facies, hyperglycemia, osteopenia, and growth deceleration.[213,214] Iatrogenic hypercortisolism is extremely common in pediatrics,[215] whereas Cushing disease or syndrome is rare.[216] Cushing disease refers to an ACTH-secreting pituitary adenoma that does not occur until adolescence. Cushing syndrome refers to other conditions of excess glucocorticoid, including ectopic ACTH-secreting tumors[217] and adrenal tumors secreting high levels of cortisol.[218] If hypercortisolism is detected in a younger child, one must consider an adrenal tumor as the most likely cause until proven otherwise. These tumors, which may be adenomas or carcinomas, can secrete any combination of steroids, although they commonly secrete virilizing hormones.[219] A unilateral tumor secreting glucocorticoids will likely cause HPA suppression, requiring careful tapering with hydrocortisone to reestablish normal cortisol production in the contralateral adrenal gland.[220]

In a child with signs of hypercortisolism (not simply obesity), the screening test is typically an overnight dexamethasone suppression test or measurement of 24-hour urinary free cortisol and salivary testing.[221] As soon as these confirm the diagnosis, additional adrenal steroids should be measured and an adrenal computed tomographic scan or magnetic resonance image obtained. In an adolescent with pure glucocorticoid effects and suspicious results of corticotropin-releasing hormone stimulation test or longer dexamethasone suppression test,[222] pituitary magnetic resonance imaging is warranted.[223] Because pituitary adenomas can be very small, occasionally bilateral petrosal sinus sampling is performed to help locate the adenoma.[224]

Perioperative Management of Hypercortisolism

Therapy for Cushing disease or Cushing syndrome is surgical.[225,226] There are no specific anesthetic considerations except the supportive management of secondary manifestations such as obesity and its attendant airway concerns, hypertension, and skin and bone fragility.

Annotated References

American Diabetes Association: Type 2 diabetes in children and adolescents. Diabetes Care 2000; 23:381-389

This consensus statement from the American Diabetes Association reviews the classification of diabetes in children, epidemiology of type 2 diabetes in U.S. children, along with recommendations for screening, treatment, and prevention of type 2 diabetes in children and adolescents.

Andersen LJ, Andersen JL, Schutten HJ, et al: Antidiuretic effect of subnormal levels of arginine vasopressin in normal humans. Am J Physiol 1990; 259:R53-R60

The renal response to 120-minute infusions of arginine vasopressin (AVP) was investigated in healthy volunteers undergoing water diuresis induced by an oral water load. The human kidney is sensitive to changes in the rate of secretion of AVP of less than 1 pg/min/kg and maximal change occurs after 1 to 2 hours of constant infusion. It is estimated that the rate of infusion of AVP required to produce isosmolar urine during overhydration is approximately 3 pg/min/kg.

Baylis PH: The syndrome of inappropriate antidiuretic hormone secretion. Int J Biochem Cell Biol 2003; 35:1495-1499

The author reviews the cardinal diagnostic criteria, clinical features, and pathophysiology of SIADH, which develops due to persistent detectable or elevated plasma arginine vasopressin concentrations in the presence of continued fluid intake. Inappropriate infusion of hypotonic fluids in the postoperative state is a common cause. For symptomatic patients with chronic SIADH, the mainstay of therapy is fluid restriction.

LaFranchi S: Congenital hypothyroidism: etiologies, diagnosis, and management. Thyroid 1999; 9:735-740

LaFranchi thoroughly reviews and discusses thyroid development and hypothyroidism in this article. He includes both embryologic and molecular defects of hypothyroidism.

Rhodes ET, Ferrari LR, Wolfsdorf JI: Perioperative management of pediatric surgical patients with diabetes mellitus. Anesth Analg 2005; 101:986-999

The authors review the fundamental pathophysiology and perioperative management of type 1 and type 2 diabetes mellitus in children who are surgical patients.

Rivkees SA: The treatment of Graves' disease in children. J Pediatr Endocrinol Metab 2006; 19:1095-1111

This article reviews the pathophysiology of hyperthyroidism with particular focus on Graves disease. Rivkees outlines current treatment options of hyperthyroidism including medical, surgical, and radioactive iodine ablation.

Sarlis NJ, Gourgiotis L: Thyroid emergencies. Rev Endocr Metab Disord 2003; 4:129-136

A concise review article on the presentation and management of extreme thyroid disorders, myxedema coma, and thyrotoxic storm.

Seckl JR, Dunger DB, Lightman SL: Neurohypophyseal peptide function during early postoperative diabetes insipidus. Brain 1987; 110 (Pt 3):737-746

Neurohypophyseal function, including serial measurements of plasma and urinary vasopressin (AVP) and the AVP prohormone/carrier peptide neurophysin I concentrations, was investigated in 11 children undergoing pituitary or suprasellar surgery. The authors conclude that early postoperative diabetes insipidus is not due to decreased levels of circulating AVP but may be related to the release of biologically inactive precursors from the damaged neurohypophysis. These may lead to renal refractoriness to AVP.

Silverstein J, Klingensmith G, Copeland K, et al: Care of children and adolescents with type 1 diabetes: a statement of the American Diabetes Association. Diabetes Care 2005; 28:186-212

This statement provides a comprehensive review of the diagnosis of diabetes, management of type 1 diabetes, and acute and chronic complications of type 1 diabetes.

Sterns RH, Riggs JE, Schochet SS Jr: Osmotic demyelination syndrome following correction of hyponatremia. N Engl J Med 1986; 314:1535-1542

This is a description of eight patients who developed a neurologic syndrome with clinical or pathologic findings typical of central pontine myelinolysis, which developed after they presented with severe hyponatremia. Each patient's condition worsened after relatively rapid correction of hyponatremia (>12 mmol of sodium per liter per day). The data suggest that the neurologic sequelae were associated with correction of hyponatremia by more than 12 mmol/L/day. When correction proceeded more slowly, patients had uneventful recoveries. Osmotic demyelination syndrome is a preventable complication of overly rapid correction of chronic hyponatremia.

Wolfsdorf J, Glaser N, Sperling MA: Diabetic ketoacidosis in infants, children, and adolescents: a consensus statement from the American Diabetes Association. Diabetes Care 2006; 29:1150-1159

The authors review the pathophysiology of diabetic ketoacidosis in childhood and discuss currently recommended treatment protocols. Current concepts regarding cerebral edema are presented, as are strategies for prediction and prevention of diabetic ketoacidosis.

References

Please see www.expertconsult.com

Thermal Regulation

Igor Luginbuehl and Bruno Bissonnette

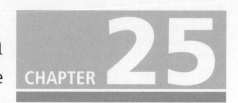

HUMANS MAINTAIN A CONSTANT body core temperature independent of changes in ambient temperature (within a limited range) and are therefore considered homeothermic organisms. Thermodynamically, the human body can be considered a three-compartment model that consists of a central (core), a peripheral, and a shell compartment. The central compartment consists of the vessel-rich group of organs (brain, heart, lungs, liver, kidneys, and endocrine glands). The peripheral compartment consists of the musculoskeletal system, which acts as a dynamic buffer between the central and the shell compartment in the thermoregulatory system. The shell compartment consists of the skin, which acts as a barrier between the body and the environment. Under normal conditions, the central temperature is maintained within a narrow range of $37 \pm 0.2°C$. Within this narrow range, referred to as the interthreshold range, no thermodynamic efforts are expended to control the body temperature and, strictly taken, the human body behaves poikilothermically. Despite a circadian rhythm in body temperature, the central temperature is very tightly controlled and regulated by a sophisticated and highly effective system that balances heat production and heat loss. Regardless of the efficiency of this regulatory system, however, it may easily be overwhelmed in daily life by external factors (e.g., extreme heat or cold), particularly if there is inadequate protection against these extremes (e.g., a lack of warm clothes in cold temperatures and not seeking shade in the summer heat).

Both anesthesia and surgery can significantly attenuate normal thermoregulation and result in cellular and tissue dysfunction. This explains not only the need for tight temperature regulation but also the need to closely monitor perioperative temperature and institute appropriate measures to avoid large swings in body temperature.

The definition of hypothermia is variable, although most accept a core temperature of less than 36.1°C (97°F) as being hypothermic. Hypothermia may be subdivided into three categories according to severity: mild (33.9°-36.0°C [93.0°-96.8°F]), moderate (32.2°-33.8°C [89.9°-92.8°F]), or severe (below 32.2°C [89.9°F]).

Unfortunately, hypothermia continues to complicate general anesthesia in children of all ages and has been accepted as a natural consequence of anesthesia and surgery. This observation led Pickering to issue his famous statement: "The most effective means of cooling a man is to give him an anesthetic."[1]

Temperature Monitoring

Temperature is most commonly measured in degrees Celsius (or centigrade), although in some regions temperature continues to be measured in degrees Fahrenheit. Kelvin is the temperature unit used in the Système Internationale that includes absolute zero temperature. The following formulas can be used to convert from one unit to the other:

$$°Celsius = 0.56 \times (°Fahrenheit - 32)$$

$$°Fahrenheit = (1.8 \times °Celsius) + 32$$

$$Kelvin = (273 + °Celsius)$$

Regarding temperature monitoring, the guidelines of the American Society of Anesthesiologists state that "every patient receiving anesthesia shall have temperature monitored when clinically significant changes in body temperature are intended, anticipated or suspected".* Temperature monitoring requires an appropriate site to measure the temperature and an accurate sensor. Today, the most common thermometers used in clinical practice are thermistors and thermocouples. The thermistor-type thermometer is based on an exponential, temperature-dependent change in the electrical resistance of a semiconductor resistor, which consists of a tiny drop of metal (e.g., copper, nickel, manganese, or cobalt). The change in resistance is used to measure temperature. The thermocouple thermometers employ two different metals, often copper and constantan (a copper-nickel-manganese-iron alloy), to sense the temperature. The principle behind thermocouples is the Seebeck effect, which depends on the fact that a small electrical current is generated at the junction between two different metals (of the thermoelectric series) that are exposed to a temperature gradient. The magnitude of this current is a measure of the temperature. Both, thermocouple and thermistor probes are inexpensive and sufficiently accurate for clinical purposes, which explains their wide usage in daily practice.

Depending on the site where it is measured, body temperature varies widely. While the central tissues maintain a constant temperature (core temperature) because of their high blood flow, the peripheral tissues usually maintain a significantly reduced and less homogeneous temperature. The temperature in the central and peripheral compartments may differ by several degrees within small measurable distances of each other.[2]

Core temperature is of the greatest clinical interest because it is the key thermoregulatory controller in the body. However, the definition of core temperature is far from straightforward. Although Benzinger suggested that the core temperature reflects the temperature of the hypothalamus and that tympanic temperature reliably reflects that temperature,[3] there is no physiologic evidence to suggest that the hypothalamic temperature precisely represents the core temperature. Core temperature may be measured at a number of sites within the body, including tympanic membrane, nasopharynx, distal esophagus, the pulmonary artery, and, with some limitations, bladder and rectum. Although these sites usually provide similar readings in awake as well as anesthetized humans undergoing noncardiac surgery,[4] they may actually represent different temperatures under certain conditions and the physiologic and clinical implications of these differences may vary.

The precision and accuracy of temperature measurements at different sites within the body have been evaluated,[3,4] and each site has its advantages and disadvantages. The ideal site for monitoring temperature should reflect the core temperature and should be associated with minimal or no morbidity. The tympanic membrane is often considered the most ideal site to monitor core temperature. When taking a tympanic membrane temperature, it is not necessary for the temperature probe to directly contact the membrane to achieve an accurate reading. In fact, to measure the tympanic membrane temperature, the external auditory canal must simply be sealed by the probe, thereby allowing the temperature of the air column trapped between the probe and the tympanic membrane to equilibrate. In some clinical scenarios, however, tympanic membrane temperature may not be accurate. For example, during the early

postcardiac surgery period, the tympanic membrane temperatures in infants and children do not correlate closely with the brain temperature[5] and, therefore, may not accurately reflect the core body temperature.[6] As a result of difficulties associated with obtaining appropriate-sized thermistors and based on reports of tympanic membrane perforation, the clinical use of tympanic membrane temperature monitoring has waned.

Monitoring the nasopharyngeal temperature provides a good estimate of the hypothalamic temperature and accurately reflects core body temperature if it is placed in the proper location, that is, the tip of the temperature probe should be positioned in the posterior nasopharynx in close proximity to the soft palate. However, if nasopharyngeal temperature is monitored in combination with an uncuffed endotracheal tube with a moderate to large air leak, then the large gas leak may be sufficient to cool the temperature probe, leading to an underestimation of core temperature. Slight and self-limiting bleeding from the nose is a common problem associated with nasopharyngeal temperature probes (especially in children with large adenoids), and its preclusion during mask anesthesia has limited its routine use. In contrast, monitoring the temperature in the oropharynx is considered to be less accurate than nasopharyngeal temperature[4] and is not recommended for monitoring core temperature during anesthesia and surgery.

Esophageal temperature probes are often combined with esophageal stethoscopes, making the esophagus a particularly appealing site to monitor temperature in children. However, the thin tissue planes between the trachea and the esophagus in infants, children, or cachectic adult patients affords limited thermal insulation between the tracheobronchial tree and the esophagus. Consequently, the respiratory gas flow may significantly perturb the temperature readings,[7] particularly when the inspiratory flow is great and there is a large temperature gradient between the respiratory gases and the body temperature. To accurately measure the core temperature at the esophageal site, it is important to position the tip of the temperature probe in the distal third of the esophagus, where the heart sounds are loudest.[7,8] This position is easily identified by auscultating the heart sounds through the esophageal stethoscope part of the combined probe as the stethoscope is passed through the esophagus. In children in whom the trachea has been intubated, the temperature from a probe in the esophagus is a more accurate measure of the core temperature than a probe in the rectum and more practical than the tympanic membrane temperature.

Axillary temperature remains the most widely used and most convenient site for monitoring temperature in children. However, the axillary site is a notoriously unreliable site to measure the core temperature because the probes are often misplaced within the axilla leading to erroneous temperature measurements. The axillary temperature may underestimate the core temperature if the room temperature is low or if room temperature intravenous fluids are infused at high flow rates, particularly in small children when the intravenous is infusing in the same extremity as the axillary temperature is monitored. In contrast, we have documented unusually high axillary temperatures when the tip of the probe senses the hot air from a forced warm air device. One study demonstrated that the axillary site may be as accurate for core temperature estimation as the tympanic membrane, esophageal, and rectal temperature sites.[7] The accuracy of the axillary probe depends on carefully

*http://www.asahq.org/publicationsAndServices/standards/02.pdf

positioning the tip of the probe close to the axillary artery while maintaining the arm tightly adducted.[7]

The rectal site, which is easy to access and associated with minimal morbidity, can also provide accurate core temperature measurements.[7] However, these measurements may be inaccurate if the probe becomes embedded in feces or is exposed to cool venous blood return from the legs or if readings become influenced by the proximity of the probe to an open abdominal cavity during laparotomy or the bladder while it is irrigated with either cold or warm fluids. Contraindications to the use of a rectal probe includes imperforate anus, and relative contraindications include inflammatory bowel disease, rectal tumors, neutropenia or thrombocytopenia, coagulopathy, and circumstances in which the bowel or bladder is being irrigated.

The least invasive site to monitor temperature is the skin surface. This site is a highly unreliable measure of the core temperature and varies dramatically depending on the part of the body where the skin temperature is measured.[7,9]

Bladder temperature is one of the most accurate sites for measuring core temperature; it is considered as accurate as pulmonary artery temperature provided that urine output is large.[10] With minimal or normal urine output, bladder temperature is a poor reflection of the core temperature.

A pulmonary artery catheter with a distal-tip thermistor accurately reflects pulmonary blood temperature, but its use in children is limited.

Physiology of Thermal Regulation

The human body tolerates cold temperatures with a threefold greater margin than hot temperatures. This is based on clinical studies of humans surviving temperatures as low as 13.7°C (56.6°F) but succumbing from sustained core temperatures as high as only 40.5°C to 43°C (104.9° to 109.4°F).[11] The thermoregulatory system depends on a negative feedback loop to maintain the body temperature within narrow limits, similar to other control systems in the body. Afferent impulses from temperature-sensitive cells in the brain, spinal cord, central core tissues (i.e., brain, heart, lungs, liver, kidneys, and endocrine glands),

respiratory tract, gastrointestinal tract, and skin are integrated in the hypothalamus, the body's thermoregulatory center. The afferent thermal input is processed in three stages: (1) afferent thermal sensing, (2) central regulation, and (3) efferent response.

Afferent Thermal Input

Ambient temperature is sensed by anatomically distinct warm and cold receptors in the periphery of the body. Warm receptors outnumber cold receptors by 10-fold, reflecting the greater importance of detecting and correcting an increase in body temperature than a decrease in body temperature. Thermosensitive receptors are also located in the brain and the spinal cord and in close proximity to the great vessels, the viscera, and the abdominal wall. Afferent nerves transmit temperature impulses from these receptors centrally through anatomically different nerve fibers, at a velocity that is more related to the intensity of the stimulus and the rate of temperature change than to the type of nerve fiber.

A-delta fibers transmit thermal impulses from cold-sensitive receptors to the preoptic area of the hypothalamus, whereas unmyelinated C fibers transmit impulses from the peripheral warm receptors. These same C fibers are also involved in detecting and conveying nociceptive impulses, which explains why intense heat is indistinguishable from severe pain.[12,13] Most afferent thermal impulses are transmitted along the spinothalamic tracts in the anterior spinal cord.

Central Regulation

Afferent thermal impulses are processed in the preoptic area of the anterior hypothalamus, whereas the efferent pathways to the effectors are controlled by the posterior hypothalamus. The central temperature at which a particular regulatory effector is triggered is called its threshold (Fig. 25-1). To maintain the body temperature, the hypothalamus initiates efferent responses whenever the integrated input from all sources exceeds the given thresholds. The hypothalamus orchestrates the mechanisms involved in heat generation and dissipation to maintain body temperature within the narrow limits of the interthreshold range.

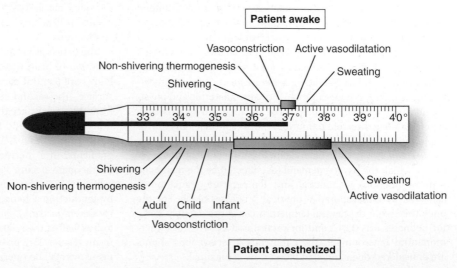

Figure 25-1. Illustration of the thermoregulatory thresholds and gains for awake and anesthetized infants, children, and adults in relation to the central (core) temperature. The distance between the edge of the thermometer and each effector response represents the maximal intensity of each response. The slopes of the lines (positive values for awake and negative values for anesthetized) between the thermometer and the response represent the gains of the responses. The threshold is defined as the corresponding core temperature that triggers a response. The sensitivity of the thermoregulatory system describes the range between the first cold response (vasoconstriction) and the first warm response (sweating), which is known as the interthreshold range.

The difference between the lowest temperature at which warm responses are triggered and the highest temperature at which cold responses are triggered indicates the thermal sensitivity of the system. The interthreshold range (i.e., the temperature range over which no thermoregulatory responses occur) changes from approximately 0.4°C in the awake state to up to 3.5°C under general anesthesia.

Efferent Response

Mean body temperature (MBT) is a physiologically weighted average temperature reflecting the thermoregulatory importance of various tissues but in particular of the central compartment. In unanesthetized subjects, the mean body temperature can be calculated as:

$$MBT = 0.85 \text{ (central T)} + 0.15 \text{ (skin T)}$$

where T denotes the temperature measured in °C.[14-16]

Skin temperature is the most important parameter that triggers behavioral changes to increases or decreases in core temperature outside the thermoneutral range, although the thermal input from the skin contributes only 20% to the thermoregulatory autonomic response.[17,18] This autonomic response, however, depends equally on the afferent input from the compartments that comprise the central core.[19-22] The thermoregulatory effectors adjust their own threshold and gain to meet physiologic needs. Behavioral changes associated with environmental temperatures outside the thermoneutral range (ambient temperature at 28°C for an unclothed adult) are the most important thermoregulatory effectors in humans (e.g., heating the home, looking for shelter, putting on a jacket) and are considered much more efficient than all the other autonomic responses combined.

Thermal Regulation in Infancy

Preterm and full-term neonates and infants who are small for gestational age have both a large skin-surface area compared to body mass ratio (normal skin-surface to body mass ratio in a term neonate is ~1; in the adult ~0.40) and increased thermal conductance (thin layer of subcutaneous fat). Furthermore, evaporative heat loss is greater in infants as a result of reduced keratin content in the infant's skin. In a similar environment, infants lose proportionately more heat through their skin than adults. In contrast to adults, the capabilities and the functional range of the neonatal thermoregulatory system are very limited and easily overwhelmed by environmental factors. The lower ambient temperature limit of thermal regulation in adults is 0°C, whereas in neonates it is 22°C. The combination of increased heat loss and diminished efficacy of the thermoregulatory response with reduced ability to generate heat markedly predisposes the infant to hypothermia. The same anatomic and physiologic characteristics that predispose the infant to hypothermia also facilitate a threefold to fourfold more rapid rate of rewarming in infants and children compared with adults.[23]

Thermoneutrality has been defined as the ambient temperature at which the oxygen demand (as reflected by the metabolic heat production) is minimal and temperature regulation is achieved by nonevaporative physical processes alone. For the unclothed adult the neutral temperature is approximately 28°C, for neonates it is 32°C, and for preterms it is 34°C. In a thermoneutral environment, the cutaneous arteriovenous shunts are considered open and skin blood flow is maximal.

In general, maintaining the core temperature in a cool environment leads to increased oxygen consumption and metabolic acidosis may develop. However, oxygen consumption in a full-term neonate does not correlate with a decreased rectal temperature but rather correlates directly with the skin-to-environment temperature gradient.[24] Oxygen consumption is minimal with skin-to-environment temperature gradients of 2°C to 4°C. Therefore, at environmental temperatures between 32°C and 34°C and an abdominal skin surface temperature of 36°C, the resting neonate is in a state of minimal oxygen consumption (i.e., the thermoneutral state). Given the significance of the skin-to-environment temperature gradient, normal rectal temperature in this age group is not necessarily associated with a state of minimal oxygen consumption.

In view of the limited ability of the neonate to thermoregulate, the head is of particular importance because it comprises up to 20% of the total body surface area and is the source for the greatest regional heat flux.[25] Furthermore, the thin skull bones, often sparse scalp hair, and the close proximity of the highly perfused brain (with core temperature) to the skin surface further favor a large caloric heat loss from the head. Facial cooling may increase oxygen requirements by up to 23% in the full term and 36% in the preterm infant,[26] which substantiates the practice of covering the infant's head to minimize heat loss.

Thermoregulatory vasoconstriction and vasodilatation are most likely established during the first day of life in both the preterm and the full-term neonate.[27] Vasoconstriction results in decreased cutaneous blood flow and an increased effect of tissue insulation; this results in an overall reduction in conductive and convective heat loss. In neonates who are small for gestational age, a slightly lower skin-surface area-to-volume ratio and an increased motor tone offer some (although minimal) protection when compared with the preterm infant with respect to heat loss or transfer. In addition to the physical limitations of heat conservation in infants and children, exposing the visceral surfaces of abdomen and chest during surgery may further increase evaporative heat and fluid losses.

Heat Loss Mechanisms

The ability of controlled dissipation and production of heat is a fundamental requirement for an organism to be homeothermic. Heat loss is a two-step process that ultimately results in heat loss via radiation, convection, evaporation, and conduction.

The first step in the heat dissipation process is internal redistribution of heat, which refers to the transfer of heat from the body core (central compartment) to the periphery and the skin surface. The second step in the process is the transfer of heat from the skin surface to the environment. Physiologic manipulation of regional blood flow and changes in the thermal conductance properties of the insulating tissue can influence both gradients. In a thermoneutral environment, total heat loss by the neonate occurs via four mechanisms with about 39% by radiation, 34% by convection, 24% by evaporation, and 3% by conduction. Changes in the environment (e.g., the air and/or room temperature) can affect the overall magnitude of the heat loss as well as the relative contributions of each of these mechanisms. Figure 25-2 provides an overview of the heat loss mechanisms within the operating room environment.

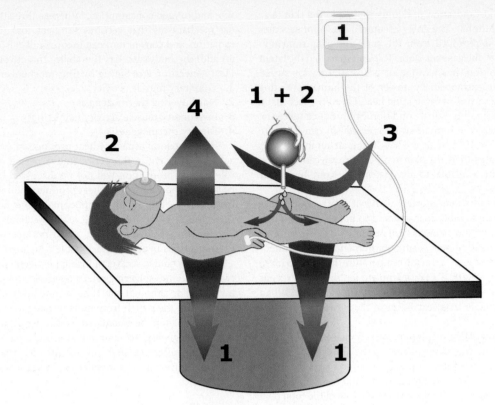

Figure 25-2. Schematic presentation of the four mechanisms contributing to perioperative hypothermia: (1) conduction, (2) evaporation, (3) convection, and (4) radiation. (Modified from Bissonnette B, Dalens B: Pediatric Anesthesia, Practice and Principles. New York, McGraw-Hill, 2002, p 175.)

Radiation

The transfer of energy between two objects that are not in direct contact but that differ in temperature is known as radiation (e.g., radiation is the mechanism by which the sun warms the earth). The emitted radiation carries energy in the infrared light spectrum from the warmer to the cooler object, thereby cooling the warmer object while warming the cooler object. Given the larger skin-surface area-to-volume ratios in neonates and infants compared with older children, radiation heat loss is proportionally greater in the former. In both, the awake and the anesthetized state, radiation is the most important mechanism of heat transfer in the neonate.

Heat exchange by radiation is based on the Stefan-Boltzmann law of radiation:

$$H = esA\ (T_1^4 - T_0^4)$$

where H is the energy transferred in Joules per second; e is the emissivity (0-1, human body is approximately 0.7); s is the Stefan-Boltzmann constant, 5.67×10^{-8} (Joules/s·m²·k⁴); A is the surface area (m²); and T is the temperature of the two bodies (K).

Using this equation with a body surface area for a neonate of 0.25 m², increasing the room (wall) temperature from 21°C to 30°C decreases the radiation heat loss by 63%, from 17.5 J/sec to 6.5 J/s. As the example illustrates, the radiant heat loss can be substantively reduced by increasing the room temperature, which diminishes the temperature gradient between the neonate and the walls and objects within the operating room. A thin cover can further dramatically reduce the losses by radiant energy transfer (see later).

Convection

Convective heat loss is the transfer of heat from a body to moving molecules such as air or liquid. The thin air layer adjacent to the skin is heated by conduction from the body but carries the heat away from the body in the ambient air currents. This leads to a convective heat loss. Changes in body posture and minute ventilation may affect convective heat loss, and the amount of heat loss by convection depends on the skin surface area, the air flow velocity, and the temperature difference between the air and the skin surface. Outdoors, convective heat loss may be experienced as the "wind chill factor."

Evaporation

Evaporative heat loss is the vaporization of water from the body or a mucosal surface, which uses the latent heat of vaporization of water as its source. Evaporative heat loss occurs through the skin and the respiratory tract. Under conditions of thermoneutrality, evaporation accounts for 10% to 25% of total heat loss. Physical factors that affect the evaporative heat loss include relative humidity of the ambient air, velocity of air flow, and lung minute ventilation. The difference in the vapor pressure is the driving force for water to evaporate from the body surface to the environment. Several factors contribute to the evaporative heat loss, including (1) sweat (sensible water loss); (2) insensible water loss from the skin, respiratory tract, and open surgical wounds; and (3) evaporation of liquids applied to the skin (e.g., antibacterial solutions). The energy required to evaporate water from a surface is removed from the surface during transition from the liquid to the gaseous state. This energy, called the latent heat of vaporization, has a value of 2.5×10^6 J/kg for sweat, emphasizing the extraordinary power of the human sweating mechanism as a means of dissipating heat. Given the fact that a healthy adult in good physical condition can produce up to 2 L of sweat per hour, the human sweat mechanism can dissipate approximately 5×10^6 J/hr or 1.4 kW. If the air temperature is equal to or greater than the skin temperature, sweating is the only mechanism available to dissipate heat from metabolic production.

Physiologic factors that interfere with evaporative heat losses relate to the infant's ability to sweat and to increase the minute ventilation. Despite the propensity of neonates to lose heat, they are capable of sweating in a warm environment. Full-term neonates begin to sweat at a rectal temperature between 37.5°C (99.5°F) and 37.9°C (100.2°F) or if ambient temperature exceeds 35°C (95.0°F). Preterm infants with a gestational age less than 30 weeks are unable to sweat because their sweat glands are immature.

Humidification of dry, inspired respiratory gases by evaporating water from the tracheobronchial epithelium results in only a small heat loss. In adults, humidification accounts for 5% to 10% of the total heat loss during anesthesia and surgery and total insensible losses account for approximately 25% of the total heat dissipated.[28] As a result of their greater minute ventilation per kilogram, the respiratory heat loss in children may account for up to 33% of the total heat loss, which increases further with the inhalation of cool, dry air as opposed to warm, moisturized air.[7,29] However, evaporative heat loss from a large surgical incision may equal all other sources of intraoperative heat loss combined.[30] Wet skin or contacting the child with wet drapes may result in hypothermia due to increased heat loss from evaporation.

Conduction

Conduction refers to heat transfer between two surfaces that are in direct contact. The amount of heat transferred depends on the temperature gradient between two objects, the surface area in contact, and the conductive heat transfer coefficient of the materials. During surgery, relatively little heat is lost to the environment via conduction because children are commonly well insulated from surrounding objects. However, conduction heat loss may occur through less obvious mechanisms such as cool irrigation solutions and intravenous fluids, which have the potential to significantly reduce body temperature. Covering infants with disposable drapes decreases the cutaneous heat loss by 29%.[24] The physiologic factors that control conductive heat loss in the neonate include the blood flow in the skin and the thickness of the subcutaneous tissue (insulation). Therefore, preheating the operating room table/sheets and covering the child with drapes will reduce the conductive heat loss.

Heat Generation

Maintaining a constant body temperature (i.e., homeothermia) requires not only the ability to dissipate heat in a warm environment, but also the ability to generate heat in a cool environment. In the latter scenario, generating heat increases the metabolic rate and oxygen consumption. Whereas three of the four physical mechanisms that account for heat loss (i.e., conduction, radiation, and convection) can theoretically also passively warm a child, the body also has the ability to actively produce heat. Heat generation is achieved by four mechanisms:

1. Voluntary muscle activity
2. Nonshivering thermogenesis
3. Involuntary muscle activity (shivering)
4. Dietary thermogenesis

The behavioral aspect of heat production (voluntary muscle activity) is absent in the perioperative period and therefore its role in heat production will not be discussed here. Of the two remaining mechanisms for heat production, nonshivering thermogenesis is the major component in the neonate, whereas shivering thermogenesis is the main mechanism for heat production in the adult. The contribution of nonshivering thermogenesis in adults is debatable (see later).[31]

The time course and relationship between nonshivering thermogenesis and shivering thermogenesis in infants has been investigated, although the time of and developmental factors that control the switch from nonshivering to shivering thermogenesis remain to be elucidated. The contribution of nonshivering thermogenesis to maintain the body temperature rapidly diminishes after the first year of life, whereas the contribution of shivering thermogenesis increases dramatically in importance.

Nonshivering Thermogenesis

Nonshivering thermogenesis is defined as an increase in metabolic heat production (above the basal metabolism) that is not associated with muscle activity. It refers mainly to the increased metabolism of brown fat, but to a lesser degree can also be detected in skeletal muscles, liver, brain, and white fat. Differentiation of brown fat in the human fetus occurs between 26 and 30 weeks of gestational age. It comprises only 2% to 6% of the infant's total body weight and is present in six main areas: between the scapulae, in large deposits in the axillae, in medium sized masses in the mediastinum, around the internal mammary vessels in the mediastinum, and around the adrenal glands or kidneys and in small masses around blood vessels in the neck.

Brown fat is highly vascularized and richly innervated with primarily β-sympathetic nerve fibers that are responsible for the uncoupling of oxidative phosphorylation.[32,33] The brown color of this fat is caused by the abundance of mitochondria in the cytoplasm of its multinucleated cells. These mitochondria are tightly packed with cristae and have a high content of respiratory chain components.[34] They are unique in their ability to uncouple oxidative phosphorylation, resulting in heat production instead of generating adenosine triphosphate. The activation of brown fat metabolism results in an increased proportion of the cardiac output (up to 25%) being diverted through the brown fat, thereby facilitating the direct warming of the blood. Inhalational anesthetics attenuate nonshivering thermogenesis as soon as 5 minutes after starting halothane, isoflurane, or enflurane or 50% nitrous oxide, but this effect wanes within approximately 15 minutes of discontinuing the anesthetic.[35] During general anesthesia in children, neither mild core hypothermia nor cold exposure may trigger nonshivering thermogenesis.[36] Nonshivering thermogenesis is also reduced in infants anesthetized with fentanyl and propofol.[36]

In contrast, awake preterm and full-term neonates and infants can double their metabolic heat production during cold exposure.[37-39] Clinically significant nonshivering thermogenesis is possible within hours of birth[40] and may persist up to the age of 2 years. Although it is the main source of thermoregulatory heat production in infants, one should keep in mind that its effects are limited and do not compensate for the inability of neonates and infants to effectively reduce heat loss by cutaneous vasoconstriction or to increase heat production by shivering.

Nonshivering thermogenesis seems to be quite variable in adults but does not appear to be functional or relevant.[41] Adults seem to have the potential to regenerate brown fat tissue under certain conditions (e.g., high and sustained sympathetic stimulation [pheochromocytoma] or marked cold acclimatization).[42-44]

Shivering Thermogenesis

As the infant and child mature, shivering thermogenesis assumes a more prominent role in thermoregulation. However, shivering is triggered only after all the other mechanisms such as behavioral responses, nonshivering thermogenesis (both ineffective under anesthesia), and maximal vasoconstriction have failed to maintain body temperature within the interthreshold range.[45,46] Shivering has not been regarded as a mechanism by which neonates and infants can maintain body temperature, presumably because the musculoskeletal system is immature and the muscle mass is limited, thus rendering muscle activity not very effective in cold defense. However, evidence has documented that shivering does occur in neonates at rectal temperatures of 35.0°C (95.0°F) to 35.3°C (95.5°F).[47] In general, however, neonates do not shiver; and if they do, it is of minor importance for thermoregulation.

Shivering, which is characterized by involuntary, irregular muscular activity that begins in the muscles of the upper body, can briefly increase metabolic heat production by up to sixfold,[48] but can sustain the increased production by only a twofold increase.[49] As a result of the increased muscle activity, oxygen consumption and carbon dioxide production increase proportionally by up to 400% to 600% for a brief period.[3,48-50] In healthy children, the increase in oxygen consumption results in an increase in cardiac output without evidence of hemodynamic compromise. However, in children with preexisting limited hemodynamic and coronary reserves, this increase in oxygen consumption can decrease mixed venous oxygen content that, under a less than perfect ventilation-perfusion ratio, may decrease arterial oxygen content and, consequently, decrease tissue oxygen delivery. An inverse correlation has been demonstrated between intraoperative temperature and postoperative oxygen consumption,[51] as well as between different anesthetics and postoperative oxygen consumption.

Shivering is not only an unpleasant experience for the child in the postoperative period but it can also increase intraocular and intracranial pressure.[52,53] The incidence of postoperative shivering is inversely related to the core temperature, but shivering has also been reported in children who were maintained strictly normothermic during isoflurane or desflurane anesthesia, suggesting that shivering may, in part, be triggered by nonthermoregulatory mechanisms such as pain.[54,55] Inhibiting shivering with meperidine in unanesthetized, actively cooled volunteers results in a more than threefold greater and more than fourfold prolonged core temperature afterdrop and a 37% decreased rewarming rate when compared with the shivering control group.[56] (Afterdrop refers to a decrease in core temperature caused by cold blood returning from the cold periphery.) The effectiveness of meperidine, along with clonidine and doxapram, to attenuate shivering after anesthesia has been well established.[57]

Dietary Thermogenesis

Stimulation of energy expenditure and thermogenesis by certain nutrients (i.e., proteins and amino acids) is well known.[58-63] Despite muscle paralysis and decreased metabolic rate during general anesthesia, an infusion of small amounts of amino acids may increase heat generation during anesthesia up to fivefold when compared with awake adults.[64] Although effective, the exact mechanism underlying this form of thermogenesis has not been fully elucidated. However, it seems that stimulation of cellular amino acid oxidation is crucial.

The Effects of Anesthesia on Thermoregulation

Thermoregulation and General Anesthesia

Anesthetics have the potential to interfere with thermoregulation at both peripheral and central receptor sites. In adults, general anesthesia decreases the thermoregulatory threshold temperature that triggers a response to hypothermia by approximately 2.5°C and increases the threshold temperature initiating a response by approximately 1.3°C.[65] Anesthesia also expands the interthreshold range (see Fig. 25-1), which widens the temperature range over which there is no active thermoregulatory response. Within this range, children are poikilothermic and their body temperature changes passively in proportion to the difference between metabolic heat production and heat loss to the environment. Vasoconstriction and nonshivering thermogenesis are the only thermoregulatory responses that are functional in an anesthetized, paralyzed, hypothermic infant or child. Children who become mildly hypothermic during surgery (e.g., a central body temperature around 34.5°C [94.1°F]) demonstrate profound peripheral vasoconstriction, which can easily be verified using skin-surface temperature gradients (e.g., forearm versus fingertip skin temperature), laser Doppler flowmeter, volume plethysmography, and other techniques.[65-67] The maximal intensity of peripheral vasoconstriction under anesthesia is similar to that in awake volunteers, indicating that the gain of the response is preserved, although at a markedly reduced threshold temperature. The only exception to this effect is desflurane, which not only reduces the threshold temperature for vasoconstriction but also reduces its gain.[68] The temperature at which vasoconstriction and nonshivering thermogenesis are triggered is the lower thermoregulatory threshold for the specific anesthetic agent at a specific concentration or dose.

Thermoregulation and Regional Anesthesia

Central thermoregulation remains intact during regional anesthesia, thus providing some protection against hypothermia. However, regional anesthesia interferes with thermal sensation (afferent and efferent pathways) in the blocked area, resulting in inhibition of cutaneous vasoconstriction and shivering in the anesthetized area with internal redistribution of body heat and increased heat loss to the environment, all of which contribute to intraoperative hypothermia. In many respects, the factors that cause intraoperative hypothermia during neuraxial anesthesia and general anesthesia are similar. As in the case of general anesthesia, the redistribution of body heat from core to peripheral compartments during a neuraxial block accounts for 89% of the initial (first hour) decrease in core temperature. During the subsequent 2 hours, redistribution accounts for 62% of the decrease in the core temperature.[69,70] The extent of this redistribution and, therefore, the decrease in core temperature depends on the inhibition of peripheral vasoconstriction rather than centrally mediated effects. Because neuraxial anesthesia usually affects a major part of the body mass, it may cause a dramatic decrease in core temperature. Heat production during regional anesthesia is only minimally decreased.[71] However, in contrast to general anesthesia, neuraxial anesthesia may prevent equilibration of heat loss and heat generation, in part, because peripheral vasoconstriction is completely inhibited by the neuraxial blockade. In addition, regional anesthesia may alter or even block the afferent thermal impulses to the hypothalamus from a major part of the body with the number of dermatomes blocked being directly proportional to the inhibition of central thermoregulation.[72-74] Heat loss may therefore continue until sympathetic function and consequently vasoconstriction are restored. Under these circumstances, hypothermia may become even more severe than under general anesthesia. Although the peripheral blood vessels that are unaffected by the regional anesthetic are maximally vasoconstricted, a further decrease in core temperature is difficult to prevent because the body mass unaffected by the block level is commonly much smaller than that part affected by the block.

Once the patient's core temperature reaches the shivering threshold, shivering begins. However, neuraxial blockade reduces the gain of shivering by more than 60%, predominantly by a failure of the upper body muscles to compensate for the lower body paralysis.[75] Recovery to normal body temperature after regional anesthesia may be prolonged.[76] In contrast to the thermoregulatory effects of regional anesthesia in adults, a caudal block placed in a child anesthetized with halothane does not significantly affect the threshold temperature for vasoconstriction (35.7°C [96.3°F] without caudal block versus 35.9°C [96.6°F] with a block).[77]

In a survey, the authors determined that only one third of clinicians monitor the child's temperature during regional anesthesia.[78] This practice is not to be condoned. Temperature should be monitored in most children, including those with regional blocks, because significant hypothermia commonly occurs and will remain undetected and untreated if it is not measured.

Anesthesia and Hypothermia

General anesthesia decreases the temperature threshold at which the body initiates a thermoregulatory response to cold stress. Mild intraoperative hypothermia (33.9°-36°C [93.0°-96.8°F]) unfortunately is all too common. It results from a combination of events

- A 30% reduction in the metabolic heat generation during anesthesia[78]
- Increased exposure to the environment
- Anesthesia-induced central inhibition of thermoregulation[79,80]
- Internal redistribution of heat[71]

Hypothermia has a typical profile during general anesthesia and usually develops in three phases: (1) internal redistribution of heat, (2) thermal imbalance, and (3) thermal steady-state (plateau or rewarming phase).

Internal Redistribution

To simplify our understanding of the internal redistribution concept, it is useful to consider the human body divided into three compartments—the central (or core), peripheral, and skin (or "shell") compartments. At rest, the central compartment in an awake adult accounts for approximately 66% of the body mass. During general anesthesia, this compartment expands to about 71% of the body mass.[81] The vessel-rich group of organs, which are part of the central compartment and receive approximately 75% of the cardiac output, represent approximately 10% of the body weight in adults and as much as 22% in neonates. The peripheral compartment comprises the remainder of the body mass and acts as a dynamic buffer to accommodate any changes in core temperature by vasodilatation or vasoconstriction.

Finally, the skin compartment is almost virtual and represents the barrier between the first two compartments and the environment. After induction of anesthesia, peripheral vasodilatation increases the size of the central compartment, thus forcing it to redistribute its heat over a larger volume. Furthermore, the decrease in metabolic heat production caused by anesthesia reduces the amount of energy available to compensate for the enlargement of this compartment. The concept of internal redistribution of heat refers not to the loss of heat to the environment but rather to a measurable decrease in core temperature with a complementary increase in the temperature of the peripheral and skin compartments.

With induction of anesthesia, the core temperature decreases rapidly, by 0.5°C to 1.5°C within the first hour of anesthesia. Although this process results in a reduced core temperature, the total-body heat content decreases only slightly, because heat is mainly redistributed and not dissipated. This redistribution of heat accounts for 81% of the core temperature decrease in the first hour of anesthesia, whereas the remainder is the result of an anesthesia-induced reduction in metabolism and increased total body heat loss. For the subsequent 2 hours of anesthesia, the impact of redistribution on total heat loss diminishes to approximately 43%.[70] Accordingly, by using a vasoconstrictor such as phenylephrine, the magnitude of hypothermia caused by redistribution can be decreased.[82]

The internal redistribution shrinks the peripheral compartment while it expands the central compartment, which explains not only the decrease in core temperature (the same amount of heat is now distributed to a larger volume), but also the increase in temperature of the peripheral and skin compartments. This is reflected by a more than fourfold increase in the perfusion of forearms and particularly legs after induction of anesthesia and a forearm-fingertip and/or calf-toe temperature gradient that may exceed 8°C.[70]

Thermal Imbalance

A combination of reduced heat production and increased heat loss to the environment leads to thermal imbalance. In this second phase of the hypothermic response, which lasts 2 to 3 hours, body heat is lost to the environment. This response results in a linear decrease in mean body temperature (typically

0.5°-1.0°C/hr). Anesthesia contributes to the decreased heat production by limiting muscular activity, reducing the metabolic rate, and eliminating the work of breathing.[8,83] Heat loss to the environment is a function of the temperature gradient between the skin and ambient structures (i.e., air, walls, and ceiling). As the gradient between the skin and ambient structures decreases (i.e., the child becomes more hypothermic), the heat loss from the body decreases passively (see also "Heat Loss Mechanisms").

Thermal Steady State (Plateau or Rewarming)

The third phase of the hypothermic response to anesthesia in adults consists of a thermal steady-state plateau, during which metabolic heat dissipation to the environment equals heat production and the core temperature remains constant. This plateau occurs between 34.5°C (94.1°F) and 35.5°C (95.5°F). To maintain the core temperature, the child must either increase heat production and/or decrease heat loss to prevent further decreases in temperature.

In contrast to adults, this third phase of the hypothermic response in infants and small children is a rewarming phase rather than a plateau phase. As mentioned, general anesthesia decreases heat production by inhibiting muscular activity and nonshivering thermogenesis and reducing metabolic heat generation. The only possible explanation for this rewarming phase is the development of intense vasoconstriction within the peripheral and central compartments that shrinks the central compartment. The amount of metabolic heat produced is distributed within an even smaller central compartment volume that increases the core temperature.

In contrast to adults, the intraoperative thermoregulatory response in infants is not effective enough to increase the core temperature in low ambient temperatures. With either active or passive rewarming, however, significant physiologic stress is imparted to the infant. Passive surface rewarming (by warm blankets, bundling, or other measures) turns the skin cold receptors off. If the normal core temperature is not reached or maintained by passive surface rewarming, hypothermia may result in hypoventilation or even apnea, relative anesthetic overdose (reduced minimal alveolar concentration at lower temperatures), and, finally, metabolic acidosis. The increased oxygen demand to maintain the normal core temperature in the anesthetized infant may create or exacerbate a preexisting cardiopulmonary insufficiency. The release of norepinephrine to trigger vasoconstriction may contribute to the development of acidosis and hypoxia, thereby increasing right-to-left pulmonary shunting. Sustained pulmonary artery hypertension and right-to-left pulmonary shunting could lead to a vicious cycle.

Anesthesia and Hyperthermia

As in the case of hypothermia, hyperthermia triggers important physiologic thermoregulatory responses that involve thresholds and gains. The threshold represents the central temperature at which a particular regulatory effector is activated, whereas the gain quantifies the intensity of the response (see Fig. 25-1). The effector mechanisms for hyperthermia are well preserved during anesthesia as central core temperature increases. Under controlled hyperthermia (i.e., increased central temperature), the efferent responses of awake subjects are also preserved in anesthetized subjects.[84] However, the efferent response threshold is shifted to greater temperatures, thereby creating an expansion of the interthreshold range, which corresponds to the difference between the normal central temperature and the first efferent response triggered by the hypothalamus. In a healthy, awake human, the variability of the system (interthreshold range) is only 0.4°C. Within this range, the individual is poikilothermic, that is, changes in the central temperature do not trigger thermoregulatory effector responses. The interesting aspect to the interthreshold range pertains to the difference between the magnitude of the variability before triggering a response during hypothermia compared with that during hyperthermia. The poikilothermic range during hypothermia in the anesthetized child may be as great as 2.5°C to 3.5°C, whereas the threshold for active vasodilatation and sweating during hyperthermia is only 1.0°C to 1.4°C greater in anesthetized than in awake adults.[84] This observation suggests that the human physiology mounts a more aggressive response to the threat of hyperthermia than it does for hypothermia. Thus, hyperthermia appears to be far more dangerous than a comparable degree of hypothermia.[84]

The efferent responses during hyperthermic stress are limited to two mechanisms, active vasodilatation and sweating. The vasodilatation triggered by a warm stress is not simply the absence of vasoconstriction but rather an active and effective vasodilatation that increases the dissipation of heat.[85] The observation that active cutaneous vasodilatation occurs in infants who are anesthetized, although difficult to quantify (skin flushing), suggests that the thermoregulatory response to hyperthermia is most likely preserved.

Sweating is an increase in the evaporative cutaneous heat loss during episodes of heat stress. Sweating increases the heat loss to the environment by up to fivefold, making it proportionally more effective than all of the cold defense mechanisms combined.[86] In adult volunteers, sweating remains a functional mechanism for heat loss even during isoflurane anesthesia.[87]

One of the clinical limitations in the utilization of induced hyperthermia to increase cutaneous blood flow is the efficiency of the sweating mechanism. Despite an active transfer of about 50 W across the patient's skin via convection and radiation,[88] central temperature remained relatively constant or even decreased. Although shivering can double the heat production, sweating can dissipate more than 10 times the amount of the normal basal heat production.

Strategies to Prevent Hypothermia

Heat loss in neonates and infants can be attributed to several causes, including the exposure of body cavities during major surgery to low environmental temperatures and humidity,[89] the infusion of cold fluids, and ventilation of the lungs with cold and dry gases, in combination with the infant's physical characteristics of the large body surface area-to-volume ratio and the thin insulating tissue layer. All of these factors increase the risk that an infant or child may become hypothermic during anesthesia and surgery. Nonetheless, hypothermia must not be considered an inevitable consequence of surgery.

While hypothermia may be protective in a small subgroup of patients with certain ischemic conditions,[90] for the vast majority of patients the adverse effects of hypothermia far outweigh the few benefits. A study of 200 adult patients undergoing colorectal surgery demonstrated that patients who were allowed to become hypothermic (34.7° ± 0.6°C) during the procedure experienced a threefold greater rate of postoperative surgical wound infection than the group that was actively warmed to keep the body temperature normal (36.6° ± 0.5°C).[91] Furthermore, both the time to suture removal and the time to discharge from the hospital in the normothermia group were less than in the hypothermia group. Vasoconstriction triggered by hypothermia may decrease the tissue oxygen partial pressure, which in turn could lead to increased wound infections and delayed wound healing. Hypothermia has also been shown to reduce chemotaxis and phagocytosis of granulocytes, natural killer cell cytotoxicity, migration of macrophages, and synthesis of immunoglobulins and thereby to directly affect the immune response.[92-95]

Hypothermia significantly affects the coagulation cascade by prolonging the prothrombin time and partial thromboplastin time and inhibiting platelet function, which prolongs the bleeding time.[96] Platelet dysfunction is completely reversible once the child has rewarmed. Blood loss in patients undergoing hip arthroplasty was significantly greater in the hypothermia group (core temperature 35° ± 0.5°C) than it was in the normothermia group (core temperature 36.6° ± 0.4°C).[97] Similar results have been confirmed by others.[98]

Myocardial ischemia and PaO_2 values below 80 mm Hg are more common in hypothermic when compared with normothermic adult patients during the first 24 hours after lower extremity surgery with either epidural or general anesthesia.[99] Due to the absence of coronary artery disease, these data may not be of great relevance to children but demonstrate the potential impact of hypothermia.

Hypothermia also decreases drug metabolism, often resulting in a prolonged duration of action. Enzyme activity for all metabolic pathways in the body decrease approximately twofold for every 10°C reduction (Q_{10}) (or 20% per °C decrease) in body temperature according to the Arrhenius equation.

In summary, avoiding hypothermia in infants and children is crucial and not only requires meticulous attention to prevent heat losses, but also a basic knowledge of thermal physiology. Radiant heaters are very effective for reducing heat loss during induction of anesthesia (reduced cutaneous heat loss ~77%) until the child is prepared and draped, which decreases cutaneous heat loss by 29%.[24] Prolonged use of radiant heaters, however, may increase insensible water losses. Also, radiant heaters should be kept at least 90 cm away from the patient to avoid skin burns. Reports concerning the use of reflective blankets in adults are conflicting, and information about their use in infants and children is sparse. Nevertheless, we recommend keeping uninvolved skin areas covered. Of special interest in this regard is the head, which comprises up to 20% of the total skin surface area in a neonate and also shows the highest regional heat flux.[25] Facial cooling may increase oxygen requirements by up to 23% in the term neonate and 36% in the preterm neonate.[26] The practice of covering the head with only a plastic bag easily and significantly reduces radiant, convective, and evaporative heat losses. In general, the percentage of covered skin surface area is more important than the choice of insulating material used or the specific skin region covered.[100]

In adults, the use of skin-surface warming devices before induction of anesthesia reduces the magnitude of heat loss from internal redistribution.[101] Aggressive skin-surface warming will vasodilate peripheral blood vessels, resulting in increased peripheral temperature to values that approach those of the central compartment. This will lead to an overall increased mean body temperature because skin-surface warming will reduce the amount of energy transferred from the central to the peripheral compartment after induction of anesthesia. A variety of passive and active skin-surface warmers are available, including circulating hot water blankets and convective forced-air heaters, which blow warm air through a disposable blanket to raise the ambient temperature of the layer immediately adjacent to the patient.[102-104] New systems simulating water immersion by a special garment and using computer-guided feedback algorithms to achieve a preset body temperature are available and seem to perform well in children.[105]

Convective forced-air warmers are by far the most effective devices to maintain the temperature and increase the temperature of cold children.[97] Not only do they maintain normal body temperature, but they also efficiently rewarm an already hypothermic child.[104,106-108] Warming mattresses primarily reduce conductive heat loss, which is the smallest mechanism of heat loss. Set at 40°C and covered with two layers of cotton blankets, they effectively conserve heat.[109] This measure is especially significant for infants whose surface area is less than 0.5 m² (~10 kg). In older children and adults, however, only a small fraction of the skin surface area is in contact with the heating mattress, which renders it relatively ineffective.

Rapid infusion of cold (1°-6°C) intravenous fluids is an effective technique to induce hypothermia or if given inadvertently to induce unexpected hypothermia. The administration of 1 L of an ice-cold solution to an adult will decrease the core temperature by approximately 1.7°C, or as much as 3°C depending on the circumstances.[110,111] If significant amounts of fluids are given to a child, it is advisable to prewarm all of the fluids, including blood products. However, the length and the type of the infusion tubing used must be carefully evaluated[112,113] because significant heat loss may occur during transit of the fluids between the warming device and the child (see Chapters 8, 10, and 53).[114,115] A recent study demonstrated that a conservative fluid management (1 mL/kg/hr of crystalloid solution warmed to 37°C) in children 1 to 3 years old maintained core temperature more effectively than did aggressive fluid replacement (10 mL/kg/hr) with the same, warmed solution.[116] However, with the widespread use of forced air warmers, the clinical relevance of this difference is diminished.

Convective and evaporative heat losses via the respiratory tract can be minimized using heated and humidified inspiratory gases. Airway humidification in children whose tracheas have been intubated reduces heat loss,[117,118] increases tracheal mucus flow,[119] and prevents tracheal damage from dry inspired gases.[120] Furthermore, maintaining a relative humidity of at least 50% (easily obtained with heat and moisture exchanging filters) preserves normal respiratory tract ciliary function and helps to prevent bronchospasm.[119,121,122] However, recent evidence suggests that these filters do not meet the minimum absolute humidity recommended of 30 to 33 mg H_2O/L for adequate humidity in infants and children.[123]

Airway humidification is even more effective at maintaining normothermia in children than adults because of the greater minute ventilation per kilogram body weight in children.[29,124] Several strategies have been investigated to maintain airway humidification. First, although heat and moisture exchanging filters are less effective than active humidifiers (especially during the first hour of anesthesia) to heat and humidify the fresh gas, they do provide a reasonable, simple, small and inexpensive alternative.[123,124] These filters will (falsely) increase the esophageal temperature by about 0.35°C above tympanic temperature or mean body temperature.[7] Second, the recent shift in practice from Mapleson D or F circuits to circle circuits in neonates, infants, and children has increased the effect of intrinsic humidification of the fresh gas flow by virtue of recycling expired gas and the reaction between carbon dioxide and carbon dioxide absorbent.[125]

Low fresh gas flows (0.6 L/min) increase the absolute humidity of inspired gases in children,[126] but they do not increase the relative humidity above the 50% threshold to prevent mucociliary dysfunction in infants.[127] Although the efficiency of heat and moisture exchanging filters is significantly less than that of active humidifiers (in terms of humidification and temperature conservation) and they fail to achieve the relative humidity required to preserve mucociliary function, they are still widely used and considered superior to no airway humidification. In most cases, small children are ventilated with intermittent positive-pressure ventilation during anesthesia, but one has to be aware of the fact that a heat and moisture exchanging filter increases the resistance in the breathing circuit and may increase the work of breathing during spontaneous respirations.

Particular care must be given to maintaining thermal homeostasis during transportation of the infant. All efforts to maintain intraoperative normothermia can be undone during even a brief transport to either the postanesthesia care unit or the intensive care unit if careful attention to heat conservation is overlooked during transport. For neonates, it is therefore important that the incubator is prewarmed before the transport to and from the operating room and that older infants and children should at least be covered with a warmed blanket during transport.

Strategies to Treat Hyperthermia

As described earlier, hyperthermia is better naturally defended by the body than hypothermia, but excessive hyperthermia is detrimental owing to the increased oxygen consumption and carbon dioxide production. Temperature increases during anesthesia are either iatrogenic or disease based. In most instances, aggressive external heat preservation strategies such as a warm operating room, warm blankets, plastic wrap, a hat, forced warm air mattress, warming blankets, warming lights, and heat and moisture exchanging filters increase the body temperature, particularly in smaller infants and children. In this scenario, hyperthermia is easily corrected by resetting the forced air warmer temperature to "ambient," removing the covers or plastic wrap, or exposing more skin to ambient air. Rarely must ice packs be applied to the head and neck to cool the child. However, if the increase in temperature is not stopped or reversed with these simple measures, then consideration should be given to other possible disease-based causes. The most common cause of pyrexia is an underlying viral or bacterial infection; a physical examination and review of the child's history will generally clarify this as a cause for the hyperthermia and appropriate treatment (taking a blood culture, starting antibiotics, administration of rectal acetaminophen) should be initiated. The differential diagnosis of fever and tachycardia without excessive carbon dioxide production in children with unknown mechanisms includes arthrogryposis multiplex congenita, osteogenesis imperfecta, and children with central nervous system abnormalities (Riley-Day syndrome). Other pathologic causes of hyperthermia such as thyroid storm, pheochromocytoma, neuroleptic malignant syndrome, monoamine oxidase inhibitors and meperidine and cocaine toxicity may be more difficult to diagnose and treat. The most worrisome cause, however, is an increase in body temperature that is accompanied by an increase in metabolic rate as evidenced by excessive carbon dioxide production. When the increase in carbon dioxide tension is not easily controlled, this suggests a diagnosis of malignant hyperthermia. This warrants immediate and aggressive investigation and treatment (see Chapter 41).

Annotated References

Beilin B, Shavit Y, Razumovsky J, et al: Effects of mild perioperative hypothermia on cellular immune responses. Anesthesiology 1998; 89:1133-1140

This study in 60 patients undergoing abdominal surgery showed that already mild perioperative hypothermia (by 1°C) can result in suppressed mitogen-induced activation of lymphocytes and decreased production of certain cytokines, IL-1b and IL-2. It was concluded that this might contribute to a higher rate of perioperative infections.

Frank SM, Nguyen JM, Garcia CM, Barnes RA: Temperature monitoring practices during regional anesthesia. Anesth Analg 1999; 88:373-377

This study shows that temperature monitoring is often not measured during regional anesthesia at all or that inappropriate monitoring sites are used. Significant hypothermia may thus not be noticed and go untreated.

Kurz A, Sessler DI, Lenhardt R: Perioperative normothermia to reduce the incidence of surgical-wound infection and shorten hospitalization. Study of Wound Infection and Temperature Group. N Engl J Med 1996; 334:1209-1121

This study in 200 adult patients undergoing colorectal surgery demonstrated that hypothermia by itself may affect wound healing and increase the risk of infections when compared with patients who were kept normothermic.

Schmied H, Kurz A, Sessler DI, et al: Mild hypothermia increases blood loss and transfusion requirements during total hip arthroplasty. Lancet 1996; 347:289-292

In 60 adult patients undergoing hip arthroplasty, the authors demonstrated that maintenance of normothermia reduces perioperative blood loss and allogeneic blood requirements significantly. They concluded that the typical drop in core temperature in these patients may augment blood loss by approximately 500 mL.

References

Please see www.expertconsult.com

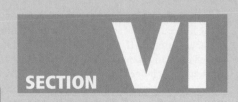

Essentials of Nephrology

Delbert Wigfall, John Foreman, and Allison Kinder Ross

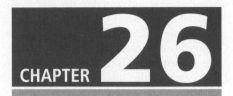

THE PERIOPERATIVE PERIOD IN a child with renal disease presents the anesthesia practitioner with challenges due to the need for vigilance regarding fluid homeostasis, acid-base balance, electrolyte management, choice of anesthetics, and awareness of potential complications. To keep a fine balance, particularly in the neonate and younger child, knowledge of the excretory and volume maintenance functions of the kidney is imperative. If not managed correctly, perioperative renal dysfunction can lead to multiorgan system compromise and significant morbidity. The anesthesia provider must therefore understand renal physiology, the appropriate preoperative preparation of the renal patient, intraoperative management, and postoperative care of a child with respect to renal function and the multiple roles of the kidneys.

Renal Physiology

The basic function of the kidney is to maintain body water and electrolyte homeostasis. The first step in this process is the production of the glomerular filtrate from the renal plasma. The glomerular filtration rate (GFR) is dependent on renal plasma flow, which in turn is dependent on blood pressure and circulating volume. The kidneys receive 20% to 30% of the cardiac output, and this is maintained over a wide range of blood pressures through changes in renal vascular resistance. Numerous hormones play a role in this autoregulation, including vasodilators (prostaglandins E and I_2, dopamine, and nitric oxide) and vasoconstrictors (angiotensin II, thromboxane, adrenergic stimulation, and endothelin). Congestive heart failure and volume contraction severely limit the kidney's ability to maintain autoregulation in the presence of changes in blood pressure.

In neonates, when renal blood flow is adjusted for body surface area it doubles during the first 2 weeks of postnatal life and continues to increase until it reaches adult values by the age of 2 years (see Fig. 6-7).[1,2] This is due to both an increase in cardiac output and a decrease in renal vascular resistance. Paralleling these changes in renal blood flow, the GFR, when adjusted for body surface area also doubles over the first 2 weeks of postnatal life and continues to rise until it reaches adult values by the age of 1 to 2 years. The initial GFR and the rate of rise correlate directly with gestational age at birth. For example, the GFR of an infant of 28 weeks' gestation is half that of a full-term infant.

An estimate of GFR can be made from the serum creatinine level and the height of the child according to the following formula[3,4]:

$$\text{GFR (mL/min/1.73 m}^2) = \text{height (cm)} \times \text{k /serum creatinine}$$

where k = 0.45 for infants, 0.55 for children, and 0.7 for adolescent boys.

Fluids and Electrolytes

One of the major roles of the kidney is to regulate total body sodium balance and maintain a normal extracellular and circulating volume.[5] The adult kidney filters 25,000 mEq of sodium a day yet excretes less than 1% through extremely efficient reabsorption mechanisms along the nephron. The proximal tubule reabsorbs 50% to 70%, the ascending limb of the loop of Henle reabsorbs about 25%, and the distal nephron accounts for 10% of the filtered load of sodium. A number of hormones, including renin, angiotensin II, aldosterone, and atrial natriuretic peptide, as well as changes in circulating volume, play a role in maintaining sodium balance.[6]

Serum osmolality is tightly regulated through changes in arginine vasopressin (AVP) release and the appreciation of thirst.[7-9] AVP, also called *antidiuretic hormone*, is synthesized in the hypothalamus and stored in the posterior pituitary, where it is released in response to an increasing plasma osmolality. AVP is also released in response to a decreased circulating volume or hypotension, including those responses to nausea, vomiting, and possibly opioids. AVP binds to receptors in the collecting duct, making the tubule permeable to water and leading to increased water reabsorption and concentrated urine. Neonates are much less able to conserve or excrete water as compared with older children, rendering the fluid management and volume issues important tasks of the pediatric anesthesiologist in this young age group.[10]

The regulation of serum potassium is managed by the kidney and dependent on the level of plasma aldosterone. Aldosterone binds to receptors on cells in the distal nephron, increasing their secretion of potassium in the urine. Neonates are much less efficient at excreting potassium loads compared with adults, and the normal range of serum potassium concentrations is therefore greater in neonates.[11] See Table 26-1 for normal potassium values in varying ages. In addition, potassium regulation is highly affected by the acid-base status, with potassium being excreted in the presence of alkalosis and excretion being depressed during an acidotic state. Causes of hyperkalemia and hypokalemia are presented in Tables 26-2 and 26-3, respectively.

Acid-Base Balance

The kidney is partially responsible for the day-to-day regulation of acid-base balance and the response to the stress of illness. The kidney reclaims virtually all of the filtered bicarbonate in the proximal tubule. The kidney also regenerates the bicarbonate lost in the neutralization of acid generated by the normal combustion of food, especially protein, and the formation of bone. New bicarbonate is generated by the cells of the distal nephron by decomposition of H_2CO_3 formed from H_2O and CO_2 by carbonic anhydrase. The H^+ generated from the decomposition of this H_2CO_3 is pumped into the lumen of the collecting duct, where it combines with either HPO_4^{2-} or NH_3 generated by the catabolism of amino acids, mainly glutamine, in the tubule cells.

Infants, especially neonates, maintain slightly reduced values of pH (7.37) and plasma bicarbonate (22 mEq/L) when compared with older children and adults (pH, 7.39; HCO_3^-, 24 to 28 mEq/L).[12] Neonates can maintain acid-base homeostasis but are limited in the ability to respond to an acid load.[13] This is

Table 26-2. Causes of Hyperkalemia

Transcellular Shifts
Acidosis
β Blockers
Insulin deficiency
Burns
Tumor lysis syndrome
Rhabdomyolysis

Decreased Excretion
Renal failure
Potassium-sparing diuretics
Cyclosporine
Nonsteroidal anti-inflammatory drugs
Angiotensin-converting enzyme inhibitors
Mineralocorticoid deficiency
Adrenal insufficiency
Congenital adrenal hyperplasia
Hyporeninemic hypoaldosteronism
Primary mineralocorticoid deficiency
Mineralocorticoid resistance
Prematurity
Obstructive uropathy
Pseudohypoaldosteronism

Increased Intake
Potassium supplements
Blood transfusions
Potassium-containing antibiotics

Table 26-3. Causes of Hypokalemia

Transcellular Shift
Insulin
β Agonists

Increased Excretion
Vomiting
Diarrhea
Nasogastric suction
Laxatives
Diuretics
Cisplatin
Amphotericin B
Renal tubular acidosis
Bartter syndrome
Corticosteroids

Decreased Intake
Malnutrition
Anorexia nervosa

Table 26-1. Normal Values of Serum Potassium

Age	Serum Potassium Range (mEq/L)
0-1 month	4.0-6.0
1 month-2 years	4.0-5.5
2-17 years	3.8-5.0
>18 years	3.2-4.8

especially true for preterm infants. This lower plasma HCO_3^- in infants appears to be the result of a reduced "threshold" or the plasma concentration at which HCO_3^- no longer is completely reabsorbed by the kidney.

Disease States

The differences in children from adults regarding renal disease may be significant. Adult renal disease is often a result of long-standing diabetes mellitus or hypertension with associated cardiovascular compromise. Children may also have renal failure secondary to diseases such as sickle cell anemia or systemic lupus erythematosus, but cardiovascular compromise is less common and there are differences in management.

Acute Renal Failure

Acute renal failure (ARF) or acute renal insufficiency can be defined as an abrupt deterioration in the kidney's ability to clear nitrogenous wastes, such as urea and creatinine. Concomitantly, there is a loss of ability to handle appropriately the excretion of other solutes and maintain normal water balance. This leads to the clinical picture of edema, hypertension, hyperkalemia, and uremia that often ensues in children with ARF.

The term *acute renal failure* is often incorrectly used interchangeably with *acute tubular necrosis*, which usually refers to a rapid deterioration in renal function occurring minutes to days after an ischemic or nephrotoxic event. Although acute tubular necrosis is an important cause of ARF, it is not the sole cause and the terms are not synonymous.

Etiology and Pathophysiology

To understand the treatment of ARF, it is important to understand its causes and pathophysiology. The causes of ARF are varied but overall can be classified as follows (Table 26-4):

- *Prerenal:* implies poor renal perfusion
- *Renal:* implies intrinsic renal disease or damage
- *Postrenal:* implies an obstruction to urine excretion

Prerenal insults are a common cause of ARF, accounting for up to 70% of all cases. Prerenal failure usually results from extracellular fluid loss, such as from gastroenteritis, burns, hemorrhage, or excessive diuresis. It also can be seen in the setting of cardiac failure or sepsis. The common feature of these conditions is diminished renal perfusion. In response to the reduction in flow there is a compensatory increase in afferent tone, with a reduction in glomerular filtration and an increase in salt and water retention. The net effect of these events is a drastic reduction in urine volume, often resulting in oliguria. If the underlying problem is recognized and treated aggressively, progressive renal insufficiency may be averted. Nonsteroidal anti-inflammatory drugs, angiotensin-converting enzyme (ACE) inhibitors,

Table 26-4. Etiology of Acute Renal Failure

Prerenal	Renal	Postrenal
Hypovolemia	Acute glomerulonephritis	Obstruction
Volume loss	Postinfectious	Intrinsic (papillary necrosis secondary
Gastrointestinal, renal losses	Membranoproliferative glomerulonephritis	to diabetes, sickle cell disease, or
Sequestration (burns, postoperative)	Rapidly progressive glomerulonephritis	analgesic nephropathy)
Hypotension	Glomerulonephritis secondary to systemic	Intrarenal abnormalities, ureteral
Shock	disease (e.g., HUS, DIC, SLE)	obstruction, obstruction of the
Vasodilators	Acute interstitial nephritis	bladder or urethra
Decreased effective blood flow	Drug-induced hypersensitivity (penicillin)	Extrinsic (tumor compression,
Low cardiac output	Infections	lymphadenopathy)
Cirrhosis	Tubular disease	
Nephrotic syndrome	ATN (ischemic, nephrotoxic)	
Renal hypoperfusion	Intratubular obstruction (uric acid, oxalate)	
Use of ACE inhibitors	Cortical necrosis	
Nonsteroidal anti-inflammatory drugs	Gram-negative sepsis	
Hepatorenal syndrome	Hemorrhage	
Vascular occlusion	Shock	
Thromboembolic phenomenon	Acute renal failure	
Aortic dissection	Toxins	
Renal vein thrombosis (dehydration,	Organic solvents	
hypercoagulable state, neoplasm)	Heavy metals	
	Insecticides	
	Other: hemoglobin, myoglobin	
	Chronic renal failure	
	Chronic interstitial nephritis	
	Chronic glomerulonephritis	
	Chronic glomerulosclerosis	
	Nephrocalcinosis	
	Obstructive uropathy	
	Hypertension	

ACE, angiotensin-converting enzyme; ATN, acute tubular necrosis; DIC, disseminated intravascular coagulation; HUS, hemolytic-uremic syndrome; SLE, systemic lupus erythematosus.

and angiotensin receptor blockers will aggravate prerenal azotemia by further reducing glomerular capillary pressure and GFR.[14]

ARF resulting from parenchymal disease or injury accounts for 20% to 30% of cases of abrupt renal insufficiency. Common causes in infants are birth asphyxia, sepsis, and cardiac surgery. Important causes of ARF in older children are trauma, sepsis, and the hemolytic-uremic syndrome. Prolonged prerenal azotemia may result in overt renal injury. Similarly, intrarenal obstruction to blood flow from thrombi or vasculitis may cause renal failure. Drugs such as aminoglycosides or amphotericin B or other nephrotoxins, including radiocontrast agents, may induce ARF through tubular injury or cause interstitial injury as a result of allergic reactions, as can be seen with penicillins. Acute glomerulonephritis is another cause of acute renal failure in children. Rarely, pyelonephritis can lead to acute renal failure.

The remaining causes of ARF are the result of obstruction to urine flow. These conditions, as a group, account for less than 10% of all cases of ARF and must lead to obstruction of both kidneys. Complete cessation of urine may be a clue to a postrenal cause. The obstruction can occur within the collecting system of the kidney (intrarenal), in the ureter, or in the urethra (extrarenal). Intrarenal obstruction may be seen with the tumor lysis syndrome with deposition of uric acid crystals or from medications such as acyclovir and cidofovir. Extrarenal obstruction can be caused by stones or from external compression secondary to lymph nodes or tumor. As with other forms of ARF, prompt recognition and appropriate intervention to relieve an obstruction may prevent a permanent decline in renal function.

The exact pathophysiology of ARF remains unclear, but a number of factors have been identified.[15] There is a profound vasoconstriction in the initial phase of ARF that plays a role in the reduced GFR (Fig. 26-1). A number of factors have been implicated in the increased vasoconstriction, including increased activity of the renin-angiotensin and the adrenergic systems and endothelial dysfunction with increased endothelin release and decreased nitric oxide synthesis. However, therapeutic interventions to increase vasodilatation, such as prostaglandin and dopamine infusions, ACE inhibitors, calcium-channel blockers, and endothelin receptor antagonists have not led to significant improvements in established ARF.[16]

Another factor in ARF is renal tubule cell injury as a direct result of a nephrotoxic agent or from ischemia (Fig. 26-2). Cellular injury leads to sloughing of the brush border, swelling, mitochondrial condensation, disruption of cellular architecture, and loss of adhesion to the basement membrane with shedding of cells into the tubular lumen.[17] These changes, occurring within minutes of an ischemic event, play a role in the decreased GFR by obstructing the lumen of the tubule.[15] In addition, these cellular changes allow the filtrate to leak back into the peritubular blood, reducing the excretion of solutes and the effective GFR.

A number of these cell derangements in ARF, such as a decline in ATP levels,[18] cell membrane injury by reactive oxygen molecules,[19] and increased intracellular calcium levels from changes in membrane phospholipids metabolism, lead to cell death. Reactive oxygen molecules also stimulate the production of cytokines and chemokines that play a role in cell injury and vasoconstriction.

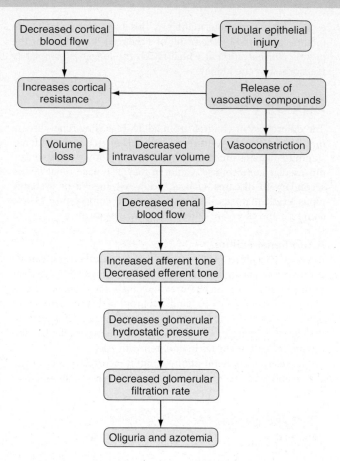

Figure 26-1. Hemodynamic factors in the pathogenesis of acute renal failure.

Infiltrating neutrophils, recruited during reperfusion injury after renal ischemia, also play a role in the parenchymal damage.[20] Reperfusion injury increases intracellular adhesion molecule 1 (ICAM 1) on endothelial cells promoting the adhesion on circulating neutrophils and eventual infiltration of them into the parenchyma. There neutrophils release reactive oxygen molecules, elastases, proteases, and other enzymes that lead to further tissue injury.

Diagnostic Procedures

A thorough history and physical examination will yield important clues to the possible etiology of acute renal failure. The initial laboratory assessment of a child with ARF should include the measurement of serum urea, creatinine, electrolytes, and a urinalysis. Prerenal azotemia is typically associated with a ratio of blood urea nitrogen (BUN) to creatinine that is usually greater than 20. In cases of renal parenchymal dysfunction this ratio is approximately 10. Hematuria and proteinuria are seen in all causes of ARF, but the presence of cellular casts, especially RBC casts, in the urinary sediment suggests glomerulonephritis. Granular casts may be seen in prerenal azotemia.

One test to distinguish prerenal azotemia from established renal failure from ischemia or nephrotoxins is the fractional excretion of sodium (FE_{Na}). The FE_{Na} is calculated using the following equation:

$$FE_{Na} = \frac{U_{Na} \times S_{Cr}}{S_{Na} \times U_{Cr}} \times 100\%$$

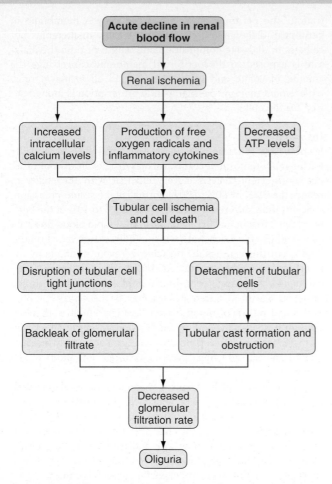

Figure 26-2. Influences of specific injury to the nephron in the pathogenesis of acute renal failure.

where U_{Na} and S_{Na} are urine and serum sodium concentrations and U_{Cr} and S_{Cr} are the urine and serum creatinine concentrations. In prerenal azotemia, the FE_{Na} is usually less than 1% for adults and children and less than 2.5% for infants. In established ARF from ischemia and nephrotoxins, but not acute glomerulonephritis, the FE_{Na} is usually increased above 1%. Diuretics confound the interpretation of this test.

The initial radiologic assessment of children with ARF is ultrasonography. The renal ultrasound does not depend on renal function and can define renal anatomy, changes in parenchymal density, and the possible presence of obstruction by demonstrating dilatation of the urinary tract. Doppler interrogation of the renal vessels provides information on vascular flow. Further radiographic studies, such as voiding cystourethrography, nuclear renal flow scanning, and abdominal CT may be indicated in selected children.

Therapeutic Interventions

Therapeutic interventions in children with ARF should be aimed at the underlying cause and at improving renal function and urine flow. Children with ARF secondary to hypovolemia should be fluid resuscitated with at least 20 mL/kg over 30 to 60 minutes of normal saline or lactated Ringer's solution. If significant hypotension is present, an alternative choice would be a colloid-containing solution. Children with oliguria secondary to hypo-

volemia usually respond within 4 to 6 hours with increased urine output. Although there are anecdotal reports supporting low dose dopamine in ARF, clinical trials have not shown a benefit of dopamine in preventing or improving ARF.[21]

Diuretics have been commonly used to treat oliguric ARF. There are several theoretic reasons why mannitol, furosemide, or other loop diuretics might ameliorate ARF. Diuretics may convert oliguric ARF to nonoliguric ARF. Diuretics may help flush tubular obstructions (casts) and reestablish urine flow. Loop diuretics decrease energy-driven transport in the loop of Henle, and this may protect cells in a region of decreased perfusion. However, neither mannitol nor loop diuretics can predictably convert an oliguric patient with ARF to a polyuric patient. Diuretics have not been shown in clinical studies to influence renal recovery, need for dialysis, or survival in patients with ARF.[22,23] Diuretics should only be used after the circulating volume has been adequately restored and stopped if there is no early response.

Dopamine has been widely used to prevent and manage ARF. Dopamine in low doses, 0.5 to 2.0 µg/kg/min, increases renal plasma flow, GFR, and renal sodium excretion through activation of dopaminergic receptors. Infusion rates above 3 µg/kg/min stimulate α-adrenergic receptors on systemic arterial resistance vasculature, resulting in vasoconstriction; cardiac β_1-adrenergic receptors, resulting in increased cardiac contractility, heart rate, and cardiac index; and β_2-adrenergic receptors on systemic arterial resistance vasculature, resulting in vasodilatation. In a meta-analysis of 24 studies and 854 patients, dopamine did not prevent renal failure, alter the need for dialysis, or change the mortality rate.[24] In a randomized clinical trial of low-dose dopamine in 328 critically ill patients, dopamine did not change the duration or severity of the acute renal failure, need for dialysis, or mortality.[25] From these data, the routine use of low-dose dopamine in patients with ARF cannot be supported.

Several other agents that were useful in experimental models of ARF have been tried, but without clinical success. Atrial natriuretic peptide was shown to increase GFR in animal models of ARF by increasing renal perfusion pressure and sodium excretion. Initial studies demonstrated a benefit in patients with ARF,[26] especially oliguric ARF,[27] but a later study of 222 patients with oliguric ARF revealed no statistical difference between patients treated with atrial natriuretic peptide and placebo with respect to need for dialysis or mortality.[28] Insulin-like growth factor-1 was also beneficial in animal models of ARF, presumably by potentiating cell regeneration. However, in a multicenter, placebo-controlled trial in 72 patients with ARF, insulin-like growth factor-1 did not hasten recovery, decrease the need for dialysis, or alter mortality.[29] Thyroxine was also shown to shorten the course of experimental acute renal failure but had no effect on the length of renal failure in patients and increased mortality.[30]

In patients with severe ARF, renal replacement therapy through dialysis is life sustaining. The generally accepted indications for initiation of dialytic therapy are persistent hyperkalemia, volume overload refractory to diuretics, severe metabolic acidosis, and overt signs and symptoms of uremia such as pericarditis and encephalopathy. Many nephrologists advocate for initiation of dialysis if the BUN value approaches 100 mg/dL or even earlier, especially in the oliguric patient, although this has not proven to alter outcome. A recent retrospective study comparing initiation of dialysis early (BUN <60 mg/dL) versus late (BUN >60 mg/dL) in 100 adult patients improved survival.[31] However, the timing of the initiation of dialysis remains an unresolved question.

There are three modalities of renal replacement for the support of critically ill children or adults: hemodialysis, peritoneal dialysis, and a variation of continuous replacement therapies, such as venovenous hemofiltration (CVVH), hemodialysis (CVVHD), and hemodiafiltration (CVVHDF). To date no form of replacement therapy has been shown to be clearly superior to the others. However, in the individual child one form may be more practical than the others. Hemodialysis is technically more difficult than peritoneal dialysis in the infant and hemodynamically unstable child. Continuous replacement therapies appear to cause less hemodynamic instability compared with hemodialysis yet offer more predictable solute and fluid removal than peritoneal dialysis. Both hemodialysis and continuous replacement therapies require large-bore vascular access to achieve the high blood flow rates necessary for these modalities.

Although the modalities differ technically, all are based on the same principles (Fig. 26-3). The aim of all renal replacement therapies is to promote the removal of nitrogenous wastes (urea), excess fluid, and excess solute (especially potassium). This is achieved by exposing blood to a salt solution (dialysate), with the two separated by a semipermeable membrane. The movement of solute occurs both by diffusion (with solute moving across the membrane in response to a concentration gradient) and ultrafiltration (osmotic or hydrostatic pressures). The rate of removal of water and solute waste is dependent on membrane characteristics (pore size and selectivity), diffusion, and ultrafiltration.[32]

The actual permeability characteristics and surface areas are known for specific dialyzers used in hemodialysis and hemofil-

tration. The peritoneum serves as the dialysis membrane in peritoneal dialysis and remains physically unalterable, but changes in dialysate composition and length of time the dialysate is exposed to the peritoneal membrane can change the amount of solute and water removed. In all forms of renal replacement therapy, the therapeutic prescription is individualized for the child.

Hemodialysis

Hemodialysis is not only useful for ARF but is the best modality for the rapid removal of toxins, such as drug overdoses or other ingestions. Hemodialysis is very efficient with the ability to reduce the BUN by 60% to 70%, normalize the serum potassium concentration, and remove fluid equal to 5% to 10% of the body weight in 3 to 4 hours. To accomplish this, rapid blood flows are necessary (5-10 mL/kg/min), which requires large vessel venous access, but this can usually be achieved even in infants by the insertion of a double-lumen catheter into the subclavian, internal jugular, or femoral vein. In small infants two single-lumen catheters placed in different sites may be necessary for both access and return of blood. Rarely, a single-lumen catheter is used for both outflow and return of blood. Modern hemodialysis machines have microprocessors that can accurately measure fluid removal, allowing precise volumes of fluid to be removed.

Hemodialysis usually requires systemic anticoagulation with heparin, the effectiveness of which can be monitored by the activated clotting time. Hemodialysis can be done without the use of an anticoagulant in the child at significant risk of bleeding by using a rapid blood flow rate and frequent rinsing of the blood circuit with saline. However, clotting of the circuit with subsequent loss of the extracorporeal blood is common.

In addition to the risk of bleeding, hemodialysis is associated with several other complications. The most common side effect is hypotension, which is usually related to aggressive volume removal but can be due to sepsis or the release of cytokine and autokine from blood passage over the hemodialysis filter surface. Muscle cramps, headache, nausea, and vomiting are also common complaints. A more serious complication of hemodialysis is the disequilibrium syndrome that is related to rapid removal of solute from the bloodstream with slow equilibration with the tissues, particularly in the brain. This can cause cerebral edema, manifested by headache, obtundation, seizures, or even coma. The disequilibrium syndrome is usually seen in new children undergoing dialysis for the first time. This can be avoided by short, frequent dialysis sessions initially, especially if the BUN value is quite high. Infection of the dialysis catheter is another common problem and can be minimized with sterile central line technique.

Peritoneal Dialysis

Peritoneal dialysis has a long history as a renal replacement therapy in children.[33] It is relatively simple and easily performed even in small infants. While not as efficient as hemodialysis, because it is done continuously, solute and water balance can be controlled in most children. It is also much less likely than hemodialysis to cause hemodynamic instability. Peritoneal dialysis involves the instillation of dialysate fluid into the peritoneum for a set period of time, which is then drained and replaced with fresh dialysate. This cycling removes waste products by diffusion and water by ultrafiltration as a consequence of a high

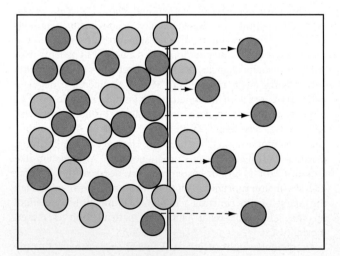

Figure 26-3. Principles of dialysis. Solute (*pink circles*) moves from the blood to the dialysate (*dashed arrows*) in response to a concentration gradient (diffusion). There is an obligate passive movement of water (*blue circles*) to attempt to maintain appropriate osmolarity. This flux of solute and water (ultrafiltration) may be enhanced by increased osmotic pressure (i.e., glucose in peritoneal dialysis fluid) or by increased hydrostatic pressure (created mechanically as transmembrane pressure in hemodialysis).

glucose concentration in the dialysate. The efficacy of peritoneal dialysis is dependent on the volume instilled and the number of cycles/day. Most children with acute renal failure can be managed with 1- to 2-hour cycles of 15- to 30-mL/kg dwell volumes. Children with chronic renal failure are managed with longer cycle times and larger dwell volumes. Fluid removal can be varied by changing the concentration of glucose in the dialysate. Short-term peritoneal dialysis can be accomplished with a nontunneled catheter, but dialysis that is to continue beyond 3 to 5 days is best done with a subcutaneously tunneled cuffed catheter to minimize the risk of peritonitis.

The principal complications of peritoneal dialysis are infection and mechanical problems related to the catheter. Not uncommonly there will be poor flow from the catheter, usually from fibrin occlusion of the catheter or from omentum or bowel. The catheter may leak at its point of insertion. Hernias, especially inguinal hernias in boys, may develop as a consequence of the increased abdominal pressure from the infused dialysate. Mild hyponatremia may develop in infants because of the relative low sodium concentration (130 mEq/L) in commercial dialysate. Less common but serious complications include bowel injury and intra-abdominal hemorrhage from catheter insertion and peritonitis.

Chronic Renal Failure

The loss of functioning renal mass results in a compensatory increase in filtration by the remaining renal tissue.[34] For example, after a unilateral nephrectomy, there is a demonstrable increase in the GFR and evidence of contralateral renal hypertrophy within the first 48 hours. By 2 to 4 weeks, the GFR has returned to 80% of normal and there is no clinical evidence of renal dysfunction. With the loss of 50% to 75% of renal mass there is an increase in the residual function to 50% to 80% of normal and often little evidence of clinical renal insufficiency. When the residual renal function falls to 30% to 50% of normal, the term *chronic renal insufficiency* applies. At this point, acute illness and other stress states may result in acidosis, hyperkalemia, and dehydration. It is only when the residual function falls to less than 30% of normal that the term *chronic renal failure* is used. At this point, electrolyte abnormalities begin to appear and, more importantly, there is limited ability of the kidney to adjust to variations in fluid and electrolyte homeostasis. The term *uremia* refers to the symptoms of anorexia, nausea, lethargy, and somnolence that develop as a result of chronic renal failure. Uremia ultimately results in death unless dialysis therapy or renal transplantation is performed. The performance of dialysis or renal transplantation is referred to as end-stage renal disease care.

Despite losses of up to 90% of renal function, sodium homeostasis usually is well maintained in chronic renal failure. In the presence of large decreases in the GFR, the kidney maintains a normal serum sodium by increasing the FE_{Na} from less than 1% up to 25% to 30%, largely through decreases in distal tubular reabsorption. Some of the hormonal factors involved in this adaptation include aldosterone, atrial natriuretic factor, and a poorly characterized natriuretic hormone that inhibits Na^+-K^+ ATPase. With chronic renal failure, the ability of the kidney to handle a wide range of sodium intake, from 1 to 250 mEq/m²/day, is lost. Instead, the kidney may be able to handle an intake of only 50 to 100 mEq/m²/day. It may be possible to decrease this obligatory excretion of sodium to 5 to 20 mEq/m²/day, but

only after weeks of decreasing the sodium intake slowly. Certain children with renal disease, especially those with obstructive uropathy or tubulointerstitial disease, may be unable to adjust to a decreased sodium intake and display a "salt-losing" nephropathy. These children are prone to dehydration with salt restriction and may need salt supplementation for normal growth. In others, a regular diet may lead to sodium retention, volume overload, and hypertension. Sodium intake must be individualized to fit the limitations of each child.

Water balance also is affected by chronic renal failure. There is an obligatory total osmolar excretion that limits the ability of the kidney to excrete free water. In addition, the concentrating ability of the kidney is affected, limiting its ability to make a maximally concentrated or dilute urine. These limitations may result in both water retention and hyponatremia or dehydration if water is administered in amounts exceeding the kidney's capabilities. These limitations must be considered in the treatment of children with chronic renal failure in such clinical situations as the time before surgery when free access to water is restricted.

In the presence of chronic renal failure, normal serum potassium levels usually are maintained until the GFR is less than 10% of normal. Potassium excretion in normal and uremic states is maintained by potassium secretion in the distal nephron. In response to an increase in potassium intake or loss of renal mass there is an increase in Na^+-K^+ ATPase in the remaining collecting tubules that seems to be partly responsible for augmented excretion of potassium per nephron. Excretion of potassium at a rate sixfold greater than normal and 1.5 times the filtered potassium load can be demonstrated in renal tubules from uremic animals. Partial adaptation can occur in the absence of aldosterone, but aldosterone plays an important role in the maintenance of normal potassium homeostasis. This is demonstrated by the presence of hyperkalemia in children with hyporeninemic hypoaldosteronism or in those treated with the aldosterone antagonist spironolactone.

The colon normally is responsible for the excretion of less than 13% of dietary potassium. In the presence of chronic renal failure this can be increased to 50% by the activation of colonic Na^+-K^+ ATPase. Aldosterone plays a role in this augmentation of colonic Na^+-K^+ ATPase. An additional mechanism that plays an essential role in the adaptation to an acute potassium load is the redistribution of potassium from the extracellular to the intracellular compartment, which is dependent on insulin, β-adrenergic catecholamines, aldosterone, and pH. Despite the presence of total-body potassium depletion in uremia, there is impaired uptake of potassium into the cells. This contributes to the intolerance of an acute potassium load in uremia despite the ability to excrete a potassium load.

Hyperkalemia is a major problem in chronic renal failure.[35] In contrast, significant hypokalemia is unusual in the absence of potassium restriction, alkalosis, or diuretic therapy. Hyperkalemia can result from an extrinsic potassium load, but it also can be caused by fasting or acidosis, in which case the source of the potassium is the intracellular compartment. This can be a particular problem when a child is fasted before surgery and can be ameliorated by an infusion of glucose and insulin. Drugs that can cause hyperkalemia in renal failure include spironolactone, β-adrenergic blockers, and ACE inhibitors. When clinically significant hyperkalemia develops in a child with chronic renal failure, it is treated best initially by stabilizing the myocardium with calcium gluconate and redistributing the potassium into the intracellular compartment with insulin and glucose. More definitive correction of hyperkalemia is accomplished by removing potassium from the body using dialysis or Kayexalate. Nebulized albuterol at eight times the normal asthma dose also has been found to be effective in stimulating potassium redistribution, whereas $NaHCO_3$ administration has not.

Metabolic acidosis commonly is present with chronic renal failure.[36] The metabolic acidosis is associated with a normal anion gap in moderate renal insufficiency, but with severe renal insufficiency there is retention of phosphate, sulfate, and organic acids, resulting in an elevated anion gap. The primary cause of metabolic acidosis in chronic renal failure is inability of the remaining proximal renal tubules to increase ammonium formation to keep pace with the loss of renal mass. The kidney becomes unable to generate the 1 to 3 mEq/kg/day of new bicarbonate that is necessary to compensate for that lost to buffer endogenous acid production. Previous studies have suggested a major role for decreased reabsorption of bicarbonate by the proximal renal tubule in chronic renal failure. Although this may occur in the presence of volume overload, severe secondary hyperparathyroidism, and disorders such as Fanconi syndrome, it is not a major mechanism causing acidosis in chronic renal failure. Except for severe phosphate depletion, decreased excretion of phosphate as a titratable acid normally does not contribute to metabolic acidosis.

One of the earliest manifestations of chronic renal failure is secondary hyperparathyroidism.[37] Secondary hyperparathyroidism resulting from inadequate formation of 1,25-$(OH)_2$ vitamin D develops in moderate renal insufficiency in the presence of normal serum concentrations of calcium and phosphorus. With more severe renal insufficiency, overt hypocalcemia and hyperphosphatemia often develop. Hypocalcemia is caused by decreased calcium absorption from the gastrointestinal tract as a result of true deficiency of 1,25-$(OH)_2$ vitamin D. In addition, diminished release of calcium from bone occurs as a result of resistance to the action of parathyroid hormone, and calcium and phosphate are deposited in soft tissues as a consequence of hyperphosphatemia.

The kidney plays a key role in the maintenance of normal phosphate homeostasis by regulating its excretion. In the presence of a normal GFR, the kidney excretes 5% to 15% of the filtered load of phosphate, whereas in chronic renal failure the kidney can increase the fractional excretion of phosphate to 60% to 80%. Through this adaptation, the kidneys in chronic renal failure are able to maintain phosphate balance but at an increased serum phosphate level. However, they have no reserve with which to increase phosphate excretion in response to a phosphate load. In children with chronic renal failure, a large phosphate load, such as can occur with the administration of a phosphate-containing enema, can lead to life-threatening hyperphosphatemia and hypocalcemia.

Hematologic Problems

One of the most common manifestations of chronic renal failure is anemia. The anemia of chronic renal failure results from impaired erythropoiesis, hemolysis, and bleeding. Of these, impaired erythropoiesis is most important and usually the result of a deficiency of erythropoietin production. Erythropoietin is synthesized and secreted by peritubular cells in the renal cortex in response to decreased tissue oxygenation. It acts on receptors on the erythroid burst-forming units and erythroid colony-forming units. With loss of renal mass, erythropoietin secretion does not respond adequately to hypoxia, and anemia results. With the advent of recombinant human erythropoietin therapy, children with chronic renal failure are now routinely treated with erythropoietin.[38,39] Current recommendations are to treat children with chronic renal failure in whom the hematocrit is less than 30%, starting at a dosage of 50 to 150 units/kg intravenously three times a week. When a target hematocrit of 36% is reached, a maintenance dosage of about 75 units/kg is instituted. Subcutaneous administration of erythropoietin has been found to be more effective on a per-unit basis, can be given only once a week, and obviates the need for intravenous injections. Dosages of greater than 150 units/kg increase the hematocrit faster than lesser dosages, but both therapies take 4 to 8 weeks to reach target hematocrit values of 33% to 36%. The most common cause for failure of erythropoietin is concurrent iron deficiency. Current recommendations are to maintain serum ferritin levels above 250 ng/mL and transferrin saturation above 25%. Other causes for failure of erythropoietin to increase or maintain the hematocrit are occult infections, hemolysis, aluminum overload, severe hyperparathyroidism, or occult bleeding. Complications of erythropoietin therapy include worsening of hypertension and a possible increased incidence of thrombosis of polytetrafluoroethylene vascular grafts.

The other major hematologic problem in chronic renal failure is bleeding. This is a classic and lethal complication in children with terminal uremia and results from platelet dysfunction in the presence of a normal coagulation profile and normal platelet counts. The best indicator of platelet dysfunction in children with chronic renal failure is a prolonged bleeding time. The platelet dysfunction is the result of poorly described abnormalities attributed to the uremic environment, and platelet transfusions are ineffective. Dialysis improves the platelet dysfunction, as does improvement in the hematocrit with transfusion or erythropoietin therapy. Desmopressin (1-deamino-8-D-arginine vasopressin, DDAVP) has been shown to be effective preoperatively in improving the bleeding time in children with uremia when it is administered at an intravenous dosage of 0.3 μg/kg.

Cardiovascular Complications

Hypertension is one of the most common complications of chronic renal failure and contributes significantly to the morbidity and mortality of these children. The cause is multifactorial and includes volume overload and hormonal abnormalities, such as increased secretion of renin, that result from the underlying renal disorder. In children receiving dialysis, volume overload is the result of inadequate removal of volume by the process of ultrafiltration during dialysis. The goal of ultrafiltration is to remove sufficient salt and water to achieve the "dry weight" that is appropriate for each child. The dry weight is that weight at which the child has no signs of volume overload but below which the child has hypotension. The initial response to volume overload is to increase the cardiac output. Later, the cardiac output returns to normal but the peripheral resistance becomes elevated because of peripheral vasoconstriction, resulting in hypertension. These children may have no other signs of volume overload, such as edema, but with a reduction in total body salt and water content, the blood pressure can be controlled with little or no antihypertensive medication.

In other children, intrinsic renal abnormalities play a primary role in hypertension. In these patients, bilateral nephrectomy may be necessary to control severe refractory hypertension, although it usually can be controlled with oral antihypertensive agents. Of the mechanisms that cause hypertension in these children, increased renin secretion is the best understood. Renin activates the formation of angiotensin I, which, when converted to angiotensin II, is a powerful vasoconstrictor. Children with renin-dependent hypertension respond poorly to control of blood pressure by salt and water removal alone but respond well to ACE inhibitors such as captopril.

Cardiovascular disease is the most common cause of death in patients receiving long-term dialysis, including children.[40] Patients with chronic renal failure can have abnormalities of the pericardium, myocardium, cardiac valves, and coronary arteries. Another cardiac manifestation, pericarditis, has long been recognized as a complication of uremia. Whereas it once was considered a sign of the terminal phase of uremia, it now is present in 15% of children receiving dialysis and can be symptomatic or clinically silent. In nondialyzed uremic patients with pericarditis, intensive dialysis often results in its resolution within about 2 weeks. In certain patients, surgical procedures such as pericardiocentesis, pericardial drainage with a catheter or through a pericardial window, and even pericardiectomy are required.

Left ventricular failure also is a common complication of chronic renal failure. In older patients, coronary artery disease may lead to myocardial dysfunction, severely limiting cardiac output. Volume overload and hypertension, which increase preload and afterload, respectively, are important causes of heart failure. With proper fluid management and antihypertensive medication, these abnormalities can be controlled. Anemia is another contributing factor that can be controlled with the use of erythropoietin therapy. Finally, an array of metabolic abnormalities associated with chronic renal failure, such as secondary hyperparathyroidism, electrolyte and acid-base imbalances, and the accumulation of nonspecific uremic toxins, all contribute to abnormal myocardial function.

Causes of Chronic Renal Failure

The causes of chronic renal insufficiency and failure can be summarized relative to age (Table 26-5). Chronic renal failure that is commonly encountered in early infancy results largely from congenital anomalies or perinatal asphyxia. Later in childhood, renal failure may result from dysplasia, or acquired lesions, whereas those affected in adolescence may have deterioration of function related to acquired disease, manifestation of inherited disease, or secondary lesions resulting from other illnesses (e.g., systemic lupus erythematosus or sickle cell disease) or their treatments.

Preoperative Preparation of the Child with Renal Dysfunction

The preoperative preparation of the renal patient is dependent on the type of renal disease and the presence of hypertension. Renal diseases that may affect the choice of anesthetic agents include renal failure, nephrotic syndrome, and tubular disorders. In children with known renal disease, careful delineation of the type of renal disease and a knowledge of the child's medications should be reviewed at the time of the preoperative visit to anticipate potential problems during the procedure. Identification of patients with occult renal disease can be difficult. Clues to the presence of renal disease include the presence of edema, hypertension, failure to thrive, anemia, and rickets.

Children with tubular disorders, obstructive uropathy, or hypoplastic/dysplastic kidneys may have fixed polyuria and are at risk for dehydration if they are made NPO for long periods of time. Following the ASA guidelines and allowing liberal clear fluids up until 2 hours before the procedure may avoid potential dehydration as well as alleviate anxiety in a fasting child. Alternatively, for the in-house patient, maintenance intravenous fluids should be continued while the child is NPO.

Perioperative renal dysfunction may occur in children with normal renal function when subjected to perioperative insults such as hypoperfusion from hypotension and/or hypovolemia. Preexisting renal insufficiency compounds this risk, and precautions to preserve renal perfusion must be taken.[41] Associated risk factors include hypovolemia leading to vasoconstriction, nephrotoxic agents such as contrast media, embolic events in cases involving cross clamping, renal ischemia, and inflammation. Perioperative renal failure is associated with mortality rates of 60% to 90%, and therefore care to avoid contributing factors to preexisting dysfunction is imperative.[42,43]

Table 26-5. Causes of Chronic Renal Failure

Infancy	Childhood	Adolescence
Congenital anomalies	Dysplasia	Focal segmental glomerulosclerosis
Prune-belly syndrome	Agenesis	Membranoproliferative glomerulonephritis
Congenital obstruction	Autosomal dominant polycystic kidney	Secondary glomerulonephritis
Posterior urethral valves	disease	Systemic lupus erythematosus
Multicystic dysplasia	Reflux nephropathy	Sickle cell disease
Agenesis	Obstruction	HIV-associated nephropathy
Autosomal recessive polycystic kidney disease	Focal segmental glomerulosclerosis	Diabetes mellitus
Reflux nephropathy	Membranoproliferative glomerulonephritis	Vasculitis
		Hemolytic-uremic syndrome
		Henoch-Schönlein purpura
		Interstitial nephritis
		Malignancy

Preoperative Laboratory Evaluation

A number of preoperative laboratory tests should be assessed before surgery in a child with renal compromise. This allows the practitioner to determine the severity of the presenting disease and provides a baseline that may be compared with intraoperative and postoperative laboratory values to ensure proper protective renal care.

Children with known renal failure, especially those with a significant reduction in function, should have their serum electrolytes, calcium, and hemoglobin measured within 24 hours of the procedure, and on the morning of the procedure if known lability exists. Abnormal potassium levels often present in children with renal failure, and acceptable limits depend on the status of the child and the trends in the potassium. Chronic hypokalemic or hyperkalemic states are less likely to have cardiac effects than acute changes. Acute hypokalemia reduces the arrhythmia threshold and increases cardiac excitability. Acute hyperkalemia may result in life-threatening arrhythmias from electrical conduction suppression. Therefore, a child with chronic renal failure who typically lives with potassium levels in the 5.5- to 6.0-mEq/L range does not need correction for the hyperkalemia, whereas a child with an acute increase to a potassium value above 5.5 mEq/L requires intervention before the surgical procedure and anesthetic. Existing acidosis must be taken into consideration in determining total body potassium levels, with the understanding that acute acidosis promotes extracellular hyperkalemia at a rate of 0.5 mEq/L for every decrease in pH of 0.1 unit. Hypomagnesemia likewise predisposes a child to the risks of supraventricular and ventricular arrhythmias and should be corrected preoperatively. Hypermagnesemia or hypophosphatemia may cause muscle weakness and potentiate the action of muscle relaxants. Administration of calcium is helpful in treating hyperkalemia or hypermagnesemia.

Hemoglobin, hematocrit, and platelet counts should be part of the preoperative evaluation. Anemia is a common finding in children with renal disease, and morbidity and mortality are associated with hemoglobin values less than 11 g/dL in adult patients with renal failure.[44] This relationship was based on the effect of anemia on the incidence of left ventricular hypertrophy (LVH) and associated morbidity and may be less of a concern in the pediatric population. Recombinant erythropoietin reduces the risks of cardiac compromise from LVH by increasing the hemoglobin to normal values.[45,46] Although these large studies in adults have shown efficacy, the use of erythropoietin to increase the hemoglobin in children with chronic renal failure has only been demonstrated to be effective in older children.[47] Blood transfusion is generally not indicated if the hematocrit is more than 25%.

Platelet counts, although typically normal in children with renal failure, are not predictive of platelet dysfunction. The best indicator of platelet dysfunction in children with chronic renal failure is a prolonged bleeding time. Signs of coagulopathy such as petechiae should alert the practitioner of abnormal platelet function and will not necessarily improve with platelet transfusion. Dialysis improves the platelet dysfunction, as does improvement in the hematocrit with transfusion or erythropoietin therapy. Desmopressin can improve the bleeding time in children with uremia and will minimize hypotension when given 1 hour before surgery. The infusion dose is 0.3 μg/kg desmopressin intravenously over 15 to 20 minutes. This will release endothelial von Willebrand factor/factor VIII complex and improve platelet function for 6 to 12 hours. Cryoprecipitate is an alternative and should be used in those children who have received desmopressin and continue to have coagulopathy.

A preoperative urinalysis can be useful in identifying children with unknown renal disease, although a normal result does not always exclude the possibility that a child has significant renal disease.

Depending on the degree of renal failure and suspected cardiac involvement, additional testing including electrocardiogram, chest radiograph, and echocardiogram should be considered. These tests will help the practitioner determine evidence of LVH, arrhythmias, and presence or absence of pericardial effusions.

Perioperative Dialysis

Dialysis in the child with renal failure is implemented to avoid hyperkalemia and pulmonary edema. On the other hand, excessive dialysis may lead to electrolyte abnormalities and hypovolemia, so the timing of this therapy or need for the therapy should be discussed with the child's nephrologist. Ideally, renal failure patients on *intermittent* hemodialysis should be dialyzed the day before surgery to optimize their fluid and electrolyte status and minimize problems with acute fluid shifts with hypotension, hypokalemia, and anticoagulation that may occur if hemodialysis occurs the day of surgery. Children on peritoneal dialysis can be dialyzed up until the day of surgery. Peritoneal dialysis should be resumed with the consideration that the child's pulmonary function must be able to tolerate the increased abdominal distention. Consultation with the child's nephrologist before the surgical procedure is useful to optimize the child's clinical status before the procedure and to arrange the appropriate timing of the peritoneal dialysis.

Medications

Children with renal failure are often on a myriad of medications, including antihypertensives. Proceeding with elective surgery with moderate hypertension may be acceptable, but severe or labile hypertension should be controlled before surgery. Anesthetic induction typically results in a hypotensive episode in children with chronic hypertension. In adults, it has been shown that there is a time relationship for hypotension in those patients who take ACE inhibitors for blood pressure control.[48] Moderate hypotension was more frequent in those patients who discontinued their ACE inhibitor within 10 hours of their anesthetic induction compared with those patients who had not taken their medication for more than 10 hours before induction. There was no significant difference between the two groups with regard to severe hypotension, use of vasopressors, or postoperative complications. There seems to be a pendulum swing that has occurred in the past 10 years where instead of diuretics and antihypertensives being typically withheld before surgery, children are instructed to remain on their medications. In general, children should take their usual doses of antihypertensive medications and immunosuppressive agents, particularly if they are on chronic corticosteroid therapy. Most other medications can be safely held until they can be resumed postoperatively.

If treating acute hypertension before an urgent procedure, clonidine is an effective antihypertensive agent. Because of the risk of rebound hypertension on discontinuation, oral therapy should be started as soon as the child can tolerate oral intake, or, alternatively, a transdermal clonidine patch may be applied to avoid postoperative rebound hypertension.

Intraoperative Management

Special Considerations

Children with chronic renal failure frequently require surgery but have several problems that complicate the required anesthesia.[49,50] These problems stem mainly from fluid and electrolyte abnormalities, complications of chronic renal failure such as anemia and hypertension, and differences in the pharmacokinetics of anesthetic agents in renal failure.

In addition to routine monitoring, consideration should be given as to the absolute need for arterial lines that may affect future shunt sites, careful positioning in children with renal osteodystrophy, and careful antiseptic techniques for line placements due to increased risks of infection. In addition, careful preparation of the room temperature and application of a warming blanket are necessary to avoid hypothermia. An arterial line may be useful to assess the labile blood pressures that are likely to occur during induction and to rebound during surgical stimulation and emergence. An arterial or central line also allows the ability to check laboratory values during prolonged procedures, those with anticipated fluid shifts, or in the severely affected renal patient. In particular, serum potassium concentrations must be monitored and corrected to avoid arrhythmias or conduction problems.

Fluids and Blood Products

Fluid delivery in the operating room is challenging in the child with significant renal disease. On the one hand, the child with renal failure and history of hypertension is prone to periods of hypotension and blood pressure lability and will require some degree of fluid resuscitation for stability. On the other hand, these same children may have hypoalbuminemia with low oncotic pressure that puts them at risk for pulmonary edema. Ideally, if the child is euvolemic, standard fluid therapy based on typical surgical fluid management may ensue. Normal saline is preferable to the use of lactated Ringer's solution due to the increased potassium load that may be found in the latter in children at risk for hyperkalemia.

Hemoglobin levels should also be followed because bleeding is a common complication in children with significant renal failure. This is a classic and lethal complication in children with terminal uremia and results from platelet dysfunction in the presence of a normal coagulation profile and normal platelet counts. Blood and component therapy may be used in accordance with surgical losses and to keep hemoglobins greater than 11 g/dL. Other components to alleviate surgical oozing or occult bleeding may be given based on clinical need because coagulation studies may not be true indicators of coagulation status in these children with platelet dysfunction.

Anesthetic Agents

The pharmacokinetics and, therefore, pharmacodynamics of anesthetic agents and perioperative medications may be altered in children with significant renal failure. The medications most likely to be affected are those that are dependent on renal excretion, such as the lipid-insoluble, highly ionized agents. Because of this, it is evident that agents that depend primarily on renal

excretion for elimination should have reduced dosing. Examples of commonly used perioperative medications that primarily depend on renal elimination are the penicillins, cephalosporins, aminoglycosides, vancomycin, and digoxin. Anesthetic agents need to be considered on an individual basis depending on the circumstances and child. For example, agents that are delivered as a single bolus have a duration of action that is more dependent on redistribution rather than elimination. Additionally, agents that are only partially dependent on renal elimination should not have a prolonged duration when delivered as a bolus or short-term infusion. There are many anesthetic agents that are partially dependent on renal elimination and they include pancuronium, vecuronium, atropine, glycopyrrolate, and neostigmine. The vasoactive agents milrinone and amrinone are also in this group. Long-acting agents and infusions must be used with caution in renal failure patients owing to the risk of accumulation of the drug.

Because uremic children are more susceptible to excessive sedation, premedication should be kept to a minimum in children with severe renal disease. However, in the anxious child, a short-acting anxiolytic such as midazolam may be used with caution; certainly if the child is encephalopathic, no premedicant should be used.

The induction of anesthesia may be carried out safely as long as the child has been made euvolemic and the pharmacokinetics and pharmacodynamics of the induction agent are taken into consideration. Anesthetic agents may be affected by the presence of anemia, acidosis, and altered drug binding due to hypoproteinemia in children with renal disease. In addition, the presence of certain antihypertensives such as ACE inhibitors, particularly in combination with diuretics, may lead to profound hypotension.[51]

Propofol induction doses using the bispectral index and clinical signs to indicate a state of hypnosis in adult patients with renal failure were significantly greater than in children without renal disease.[52] This was presumably from the larger volume of distribution found in renal failure patients and was consistent with earlier studies on thiopental.[53] Another contributing factor was the presence of anemia, which may indirectly cause a greater plasma volume and greater cardiac output. When propofol is delivered as an infusion, no significant differences in pharmacokinetic or pharmacodynamic parameters have been observed.[54]

There are insufficient data on inhaled agents being used for induction in children with renal impairment and their effects. For maintenance anesthesia in adults, desflurane and isoflurane do not further impair renal function in patients with preexisting renal disease.[55] Sevoflurane at low flows is associated with increased circuit concentrations of compound A, which has been shown to be nephrotoxic in rats.[56,57] In adult patients with normal renal function, low-flow sevoflurane anesthesia has been associated with mild transient proteinuria but no changes in BUN, creatinine, or creatinine clearance.[58] In adults with renal insufficiency, low-flow sevoflurane has been shown to be as safe as low-flow isoflurane in terms of kidney function.[57]

Muscle relaxants have evolved over the years and allow for the practitioner to have a choice of agents in the child with renal disease. Children with chronic renal failure may have existing autonomic neuropathy and associated delayed gastric emptying that puts them at risk for aspiration. This, along with renal implications, should be kept in mind when determining the

General Abdominal and Urologic Surgery

CHAPTER 27

Per-Arne Lönnqvist and Jerrold Lerman

ABDOMINAL SURGERY AND UROLOGIC interventions after the infancy period make up a large fraction of anesthetic practice for the pediatric anesthesiologist. Although the physiology of the young child is approaching that of adults, meticulous attention is still necessary regarding a number of the issues relevant to the situation in neonates and infants, such as airway management, thermoregulation, and fluid balance. The focus in this chapter is on general issues related to abdominal and urologic surgery, particularly those affecting this age group; management of infants for pyloromyotomy and other neonatal abdominal procedures is discussed in Chapter 36.

Abdominal Surgery

When anesthetizing infants and children for abdominal surgery, the following issues must be included in the development of a specific anesthetic prescription before bringing them to the operating room:

1. "The full stomach"—the risk for vomiting or regurgitation during induction of anesthesia. Is this an upper or lower abdominal obstruction with vomiting?
2. Fluid balance—the risk for dehydration and hypovolemia secondary to third space losses or preoperative bowel preparation. Has the child been adequately volume resuscitated?
3. The potential presence of strangulated or ischemic bowel. Is there the potential for hemodynamic instability and metabolic acidosis due to vasoactive substances?
4. Presence of concomitant septicemia. Does the child have a disseminated coagulopathy or hemodynamic instability secondary to generalized sepsis?
5. Presence of abdominal compartment syndrome. Is intraabdominal organ function, in particular renal and hepatic function, impaired secondary to increased intra-abdominal pressure?
6. Will the child require transfusion of blood products? Has blood been sent to the blood bank for blood typing and crossmatch?
7. What options are available for postoperative pain management?

"The Full Stomach": The Risk for Pulmonary Aspiration of Gastric Contents

A large number of abdominal surgeries are performed as emergency procedures. Consequently, all of these children should be regarded as being at risk for vomiting and/or regurgitation during induction of anesthesia and possible pulmonary aspiration of gastric contents. Because most young children generally do not tolerate a nasogastric tube being inserted, one must assume the presence of significant volumes of gastric contents if evidence of bowel stasis is present. Even after adhering to normal fasting times, the stomach in a child with an acute abdomen must be assumed to contain substantial residual volumes. Because one cannot rely on normal fasting guidelines to empty the stomach when a gastrointestinal pathologic process exists, delaying the surgical procedure is unlikely to empty the stomach. Our experience has been that the fullness of the stomach relates to time of last food intake before the development of the pathologic condition. If bowel sounds are present, then the stomach may empty with a delay of 4 to 6 hours. Alternately, if bowel sounds are absent and the child is vomiting or is nauseated, then postponing surgery will not change anything. Currently, there is no easy and reliable method to determine gastric residual volumes in children preoperatively. However, because many children undergo abdominal ultrasonography and/or CT as presurgical investigations, one will often have the opportunity to also visualize the stomach and thereby estimate the volume of the gastric contents. The lack of visual contents at these investigations cannot be seen as a guarantee against the risk for vomiting or regurgitation, but a positive finding will provide important information for the anesthesiologist.

Indications for Preoperative Nasogastric Tube Placement

Although there are no published guidelines on this subject, it is reasonable to insert a nasogastric tube preoperatively to allow drainage of gastrointestinal contents in cases of documented bowel obstruction (e.g., ileus, strangulated bowel, pyloric obstruction) or in other cases when aspiration is judged to be an overt risk. The discomfort of inserting a nasogastric tube in a child may be extreme, but this discomfort must be balanced against the risk of aspiration. Insertion of a nasogastric tube may allow emptying of gastric contents and reduce the incidence of active vomiting in these children. In the remaining cases, the placement of a nasogastric tube can wait until after tracheal intubation.

Rapid-Sequence Induction

Rapid-sequence induction (RSI) is the preferred and recommended approach to securing the airway in the presence of a full stomach. This approach is intended to minimize the risk of aspiration during induction of anesthesia in children with clear evidence of upper gastrointestinal obstruction, that is, those who are actively vomiting. In infants and toddlers this technique is not as easily practiced as it is in older children and adults. First, a moderate head-up tilt of the operating table does not provide the same hydrostatic barrier against regurgitation due to the small size of the child.[1] Second, preoxygenation is sometimes difficult to perform due to poor acceptance of the face mask. Third, external cricoid pressure can distort the view during laryngoscopy, if not performed properly.[2,3] Furthermore, the use of RSI exposes the child to the risks involved with the use of succinylcholine, although high-dose rocuronium is a reasonable alternative.[4,5] On occasion, venous access has proved difficult, thus precluding establishment of a peripheral venous access preoperatively.

Although the incidence of aspiration in children (birth to 9 years of age) (8/10,000)[6] is greater than it is in adults (3/10,000), the risk remains relatively small and, thus, the routine use of RSI has been challenged.[2] A survey of clinical practice among British anesthesiologists showed that use of RSI with succinylcholine and cricoid pressure varied with the child's age, the procedure, and the training of the anesthesiologist. RSI was modified more frequently for infants, particularly by more recently trained consultants. For example, cricoid pressure was used in 96% of school-age children undergoing RSI but in only 50% of infants undergoing pyloromyotomy. In addition, RSI was used by 86% of anesthesiologists in children undergoing appendectomy but only 60% of children with forearm fractures. Many did not routinely use RSI but instead used either an intravenous induction including the use of nondepolarizing muscle relaxants or an inhalational induction with sevoflurane.[7,8] It is also important to appreciate that the superiority of RSI over other induction techniques in children who are at risk for regurgitation and aspiration is not evidence based.[9] Despite recent recommendations that RSI is the preferred technique to protect the airway when there is a risk of aspiration, exceptions to this rule are widespread. It should be noted that delayed recognition of esophageal intubation is associated with both RSI and the use of cricoid pressure in children, particularly infants younger than 1 year of age. It is unclear if expired CO_2 monitoring was routinely used in this cohort.[10] Currently, many recommend the RSI technique to secure the airway in children who are at risk for aspiration, although awake intubations in neonates and simple intravenous inductions with rapid-acting anesthetic medications are reasonable alternatives (see also discussions of RSI in Chapters 37 and 39).

Fluid Balance

Many acute abdominal emergencies are associated with pronounced disturbances in the fluid balance, mainly in the form of dehydration, electrolyte losses, third space fluid shifts, and hypovolemia. Adequate correction of these problems is mandatory in most instances before proceeding with anesthesia and surgery. Thus, adequate rehydration, correction of electrolyte status, and hypovolemia should occur before induction of anesthesia. However, when a large fraction of the bowel becomes strangulated, when a delay may lead to major bowel resection with subsequent chronic nutritional problems, correction of the existing fluid deficits must be performed simultaneously with rapid induction of anesthesia, even if this will increase overall risk. Even in some elective cases (e.g., bowel resection due to inflammatory bowel disease) fluid and electrolyte balance should be the focus of special interest because the child may not be fully compensated at the time of surgery.

Potential Presence of Strangulated or Ischemic Bowel

If the bowel is suspected of being ischemic and/or necrotic, then anesthesia and surgery become more urgent. For example, if true volvulus is suspected, immediate action is necessary; otherwise the child is at risk for massive bowel resection with subsequent short bowel syndrome, a condition associated with serious life-long medical problems. Even if such children may be far from optimized, anesthesia must be induced and maintained simultaneously with correction of dehydration/hypovolemia and electrolyte imbalance. The situation is obviously different in children with an incarcerated inguinal hernia, but still undue delay of surgery should be avoided.

Furthermore, translocation of bacteria from the intestinal tract and subsequent septicemia are possible (see later) and the ischemic bowel may release various mediators that can cause severe hemodynamic instability. Thus, in a case in which a substantial part of the bowel may be ischemic, the anesthesiologist needs to be prepared to treat hemodynamic instability by appropriate volume replacement and administration of inotropic/vasoactive medications. It should be noted that such hemodynamic instability might be acutely worsened when reperfusion of the bowel is established or with simple opening of the abdomen that alters venous return to the heart.

Presence of Concomitant Septicemia

Children with acute intra-abdominal disease should always be regarded as being at risk for bacterial translocation with subsequent septicemia. Children with overt sepsis are usually not difficult to identify and may already be admitted to the pediatric intensive care unit. However, incipient or early sepsis is often subtle. Thus, signs of sepsis should be actively sought. If septicemia is present or suspected, appropriate intravenous antibiotics should be administered without delay, most definitely before anesthesia and surgery.

Septic or pre-septic children can be extremely unstable hemodynamically, and their lungs may be difficult to ventilate due to established or developing acute lung injury. Thus, the anesthesiologist needs to be prepared to provide invasive monitoring (arterial and central venous pressures) as well as the means to administer inotropic/vasoactive drugs; an anesthetic machine capable of providing advanced respiratory support is also very useful in these cases.

Presence of Abdominal Compartment Syndrome

More significant acute intra-abdominal disease processes may give rise to a situation with seriously increased intra-abdominal pressure. If the abdominal pressure increases above the capillary perfusion pressure of the intra-abdominal organs, a situation comparable to a muscular compartment syndrome can occur. Thus, organ perfusion will become insufficient and ischemia and even necrosis may develop. The most commonly affected organs in this situation are the bowels, kidneys, and liver. Abdominal compartment syndrome occurs less frequently in children than it does in adults.[11] Causes include abdominal trauma,[12,13] burns,[14] extracorporeal membrane oxygenation,[15] closure of gastroschisis or omphalocoele,[16] critically ill children in the pediatric intensive care unit,[17] and a variety of intra-abdominal diagnoses such as necrotizing enterocolitis, Hirschsprung's enterocolitis, perforated bowel, diaphragmatic hernia, and Wilms' tumor.[18,19]

Insufficient perfusion of the bowel may cause an ileus, translocation of bacteria, lactate accumulation, and production of various mediators that will cause hemodynamic instability. Increased abdominal pressure can reduce liver blood flow that will affect liver function, mainly manifested as an inability to metabolize lactate, a delay in drug metabolism, and, in severe cases, impaired synthesis of coagulation factors. Because the pressure is also transmitted to the retroperitoneal space, renal function may be affected, resulting in oliguria or anuria.[20] Furthermore, owing to cranial displacement and splinting of the diaphragm, ventilation can be seriously compromised.

If acute intra-abdominal compartment syndrome is suspected, then the intra-abdominal pressure should be measured to determine if it exceeds the critical threshold of 20 to 25 mm Hg; some centers consider vesicular pressures greater than 10 to 12 mm Hg to be consistent with this diagnosis.[21,22] These pressures can be measured either via the nasogastric tube or via the bladder (Foley) catheter.[23] Intra-abdominal compartment syndrome is diagnosed when the triad of (1) massive abdominal distention, (2) increased bladder pressures and increased peak inspiratory airway pressures, and (3) evidence of renal and/or cardiac dysfunction is present.[24-26]

Children with acute intra-abdominal compartment syndrome can become extremely hemodynamically unstable during surgery. Although decompression of the abdomen by a laparotomy will immediately normalize the intra-abdominal pressure, reperfusion of the ischemic tissues almost always releases a host of biologically active substances that will cause serious hypotension and that may also precipitate acute renal failure. Thus, as in the case of sepsis, the anesthesiologist must be fully prepared to address these challenges by having blood products in the operating room and vasopressors available before induction of anesthesia. Some children will require a patch abdominoplasty as a temporizing measure with later closure.[25,27]

Preoperative Laboratory Testing and Investigations

Most minor elective cases (e.g., umbilical or inguinal hernia repair) do not require any further preoperative work-up apart from a basic history and physical examination. More extensive elective cases may merit specific laboratory testing, such as basic hematology screening and electrolyte status. In the typical case of an appendectomy, testing for C-reactive protein and obtaining a white blood cell count may be helpful to confirm the diagnosis.[28,29]

In more critically ill children, preoperative laboratory testing is strongly advisable. Liver and renal function tests, coagulation profile, serum albumin concentration, and blood type and crossmatch should be determined. In children who are septic or who have an acute intra-abdominal compartment syndrome, a preoperative chest radiograph will provide the anesthesiologist with important preoperative information regarding the severity of pulmonary compromise and the need for positive end-expiratory pressure or other ventilation strategies. If there is any evidence of cardiac dysfunction, an echocardiogram might be of value to ascertain both cardiac contractility and volume status.

Monitoring Requirements

Routine elective cases rarely require more than standard monitoring equipment (see Chapters 49 and 53). In children undergoing major intra-abdominal procedures, invasive blood pressure monitoring may be considered appropriate. The sickest children may require the insertion of a multiple-lumen central venous line to administer inotropic/vasoactive drugs as well as to measure central venous pressure. In select children, transesophageal echocardiographic or transesophageal Doppler evaluation may provide valuable intraoperative information regarding the child's volume status as well as cardiac contractility.[30-35] In the past, the role of echocardiography or of Doppler imaging has been primarily limited to scientific investigation,[36-38] but the use of this technology is increasing in the critical care unit and operating room settings.[32,39-41] Further studies are needed to confirm their efficacy in the pediatric setting.[41] If available, the spirometry module of the anesthetic machine should be used to follow pulmonary mechanics and to aid in the optimization of ventilation. The placement of a urinary (Foley) catheter is particularly helpful in almost any type of intra-abdominal surgery. For children, a urometer (i.e., a graduated collection receptacle), which provides an accurate measure of the urine output, should be used instead of a collection bag. The measurement of hourly urine output safeguards against the development of hypovolemia and possible prerenal azotemia. See the later section on laparoscopy for the changes in urine output with increased intra-abdominal pressure.

The continuous measurement of intra-abdominal pressure is important in laparoscopic surgery, although for neonatal surgery such as omphalocele or gastroschisis it will not provide any useful information as long as the abdomen is still open. Measuring the intra-abdominal pressure at the end of surgery will provide very useful information on whether it is reasonable to close the abdomen or leave it open (see Chapter 36).

Urologic Surgery

With the exception of acute drainage of urinary obstruction (i.e., ultrasound-guided nephrostomy or cystostomy procedures) and torsion of the testes, most pediatric urologic cases are elective surgeries. In the vast majority of cases, these children are otherwise healthy or are in a stable medical condition that does not merit any more complex medical work-up apart from taking a careful history and performing a physical examination as well as checking the patient's medical record. However, in certain circumstances, further actions are necessary to ensure that the child is medically optimized to be able to provide the best anesthetic care.

Special Conditions to Consider During Preoperative Assessment

Reduced Renal Function
Children with chronic renal disease may have impaired renal function; and in the most severe cases, the child may already require dialysis. In these cases, it is vital to ascertain the degree of renal impairment, which is best done by preoperative consultation with the child's nephrologist. Furthermore, apart from basic blood tests, preoperative assessment of the serum creatinine, blood urea nitrogen, sodium, and potassium values are essential. Because reduced renal function may also affect coagulation, especially platelet function, a coagulation panel is often warranted. Another consideration for children with reduced renal function is the issue of possible overhydration/hypervolemia. Apart from clinical signs associated with this condition, easy ways of obtaining a good indication of the child's volume status is weighing the child and comparing that with the child's "normal weight" according to the parents or to recent values in the medical record. If the cardiac or volume status remains in doubt, an echocardiographic examination will provide objective evidence. Furthermore, children with chronic renal insufficiency may demonstrate impaired left ventricular function even before they require dialysis so a preoperative echocardiogram may also be indicated to determine the severity of cardiac impairment.[42-46] In cases in which overhydration/hypervolemia is present, this should be treated before any elective surgical procedure. If the child requires dialysis, hemodialysis or peritoneal dialysis can be performed up to the day before surgery (see Chapter 26) to optimize the child for anesthesia and surgery while allowing sufficient time for body fluids to equilibrate post dialysis. It is best to avoid dialysis within 12 hours of anesthesia for these reasons. Dialysis will correct hyperkalemia and intravascular volume status and positively influence platelet function; this treatment may also result in a hypovolemic state. Post-dialysis laboratory indices for electrolytes (serum potassium), hemoglobin/hematocrit, and renal function (creatinine and blood urea nitrogen) should be obtained.

Hypertension
Hypertension is a common concomitant condition in adults with renal insufficiency but it is rare in children. However, some children with urologic problems may develop significant hypertension because of disturbances in the renal renin-angiotensin system. As in adults, it is important that hypertension is controlled before induction of anesthesia. In contrast to adults, hypervolemia is an important cause of hypertension in these children and should be considered and treated preoperatively. Some children with long-term renal failure may also present with a pericardial effusion or cardiac dysfunction (see earlier); the evaluation of these children will also be enhanced with a preoperative echocardiogram.

With respect to antihypertensive medications, children are often treated with the same categories of medications as adults. These medications should be continued up to and including the morning of surgery to maintain intraoperative and postoperative hemodynamic stability. However, this does not apply to angiotensin-converting enzyme (ACE) inhibitors[47] because these drugs are known to cause pronounced intraoperative hypotension if they are not discontinued at least 1 day before surgery.[48,49] Because therapy-resistant renal hypertension is an indication for nephrectomy in some children, one should be prepared to treat wide fluctuations in blood pressure, including severe hypertension during the first stage of the operation as well as quite serious hypotension when the kidney that was responsible for the hypertension is removed. Thus, long-acting antihypertensive agents are best avoided during the early stages of these surgeries.

Corticosteroid Medication
Some children with renal disease are chronically treated with corticosteroids as part of their medical management (e.g., children who have undergone previous renal transplant surgery). In such cases, supplemental doses of parenteral corticosteroids during surgery as well as during the immediate postoperative period are indicated. Corticosteroid supplementation is necessary until the child resumes his or her normal corticosteroid medication by the enteral route. In more complex situations, consultation with a pediatric nephrologist or endocrinologist is advised to optimize corticosteroid supplementation, but in more straightforward cases a dose of 2.5 mg/kg of hydrocortisone two to three times a day intravenously is usually adequate (see Chapter 24).

Infection or Sepsis
Obstructive urinary tract disease or chronic renal insufficiency increases the risk for urinary tract infections. If treated properly, the infection is usually well controlled and should not interfere with the anesthetic. However, in children who demonstrate

overt signs of systemic illness or septicemia, the anesthetic and postoperative course may be stormy.

Monitoring Requirements

The vast majority of urologic procedures in children are of a minor or moderate magnitude (e.g., circumcision, orchidopexy, pyeloplasty, and ureter neoimplantation) and require only standard noninvasive monitoring. For major surgical interventions, as well as in cases with concomitant problems (e.g., decreased renal function, significant hypertension, associated cardiac dysfunction, sepsis), invasive monitoring is often indicated (i.e., invasive blood pressure monitoring, central venous access for pressure measurements and administration of vasoactive drugs). If central venous access is deemed to be necessary, the coagulation status of the child should be evaluated because platelet function may be substantially compromised. In cases in which a coagulopathy is present or is suspected on clinical grounds, ultrasound guidance is very helpful in securing central venous access with less potential for unintended puncture of a major vessel (see Chapter 49).

In the unstable child, even more complex monitoring (e.g., esophageal Doppler monitoring or transesophageal echocardiography) should be considered.

Monitoring the urine output is important, although the volume of the urine may not reflect renal function. During surgeries that involve the bladder or in those children who are anuric, urine output will not be available for part or all of the surgery. Hence, indices of fluid status and perfusion other than urine output must be considered: in the infant, systolic blood pressure is a reliable index of volume status and perfusion, whereas in the older child, central venous pressure and invasive arterial pressure measuring should be considered.

Choice of Anesthetic

For the anesthetic management of elective or acutely ill children, the anesthesiologist may use his or her personal preference regarding the choice of anesthetic technique. However, airway management associated with intra-abdominal surgery does merit attention. Even when the child is not at an increased risk of regurgitation and aspiration, the risk of regurgitation can be increased if the surgeon manipulates the bowels, when the child is positioned head down, and if gas is insufflated into the abdomen as in laparoscopic procedures. The ProSeal laryngeal mask airway (LMA North America, Inc., San Diego, CA) has been compared with endotracheal intubation in one pediatric series. Peak inspiratory pressures increased in both groups during pneumoperitoneum, but ventilatory parameters did not differ significantly.[50] The authors argued that with the better laryngeal seal compared with a traditional laryngeal mask airway,[51] this device provided "comparable ventilatory efficiency" to the endotracheal tube. However, we caution against overenthusiastic use of the laryngeal mask airway and instead recommend endotracheal intubation as the standard in the majority of these cases. In critically ill and unstable children, it is not possible to recommend specific anesthetic regimens but a high-dose opioid-based anesthetic, similar to that used in cardiac anesthesia (i.e., fentanyl 25-50 µg/kg), or a ketamine infusion-based anesthetic may be considered to maintain circulatory homeostasis.

Regional anesthetic techniques may be useful adjuncts in children undergoing both minor and major abdominal surgery. However, in critically unstable or septic children, the use of epidural anesthesia should be very carefully considered owing to the risk of the hemodynamic instability that can accompany sympathetic blockade as well as to the risk of epidural abscess formation. For children who have had a laparoscopic procedure, simple local infiltration of the port insertion sites combined with low-dose opioid, diclofenac, or acetaminophen will provide adequate postoperative analgesia, whereas those who have had an open procedure will require intravenous opioids (see Chapter 44).[52]

Laparoscopic Surgery

Although laparoscopic surgery was introduced more than 80 years ago, its popularity in pediatric surgery has been notable only in the past 10 to 15 years. To a large extent, this has been directly attributed to improved technology in the optics and miniaturization of the instruments required for such surgery in neonates, infants, and children. Laparoscopic surgery involves the creation of three to four small incisions (1.0 to 1.5 cm) to accommodate the instruments. Laparoscopic surgery is associated with more rapid emergence from anesthesia and faster ambulation and discharge from hospital than open surgery. An increasing number of general and urologic surgical procedures are now performed using either laparoscopic or robotic techniques in children of all ages, including neonates.[53-59] The spectrum of procedures performed using the laparoscopic techniques ranges from diagnostic procedures such as exploration of undescended testicles and hernias to staging cancer to surgical excision of an acute appendix, gallbladder, or Meckel's diverticulum. More sophisticated laparoscopic techniques have enabled the performance of complex surgical procedures, including Nissen fundoplication, colectomy, pyeloplasty, bowel pull-through, and removal of large organs, including kidney and spleen.[60-63]

Laparoscopic surgery requires the insufflation of gas into the abdominal cavity to facilitate visualization of the intra-abdominal organs. Carbon dioxide is the preferred gas because it does not support combustion, is rapidly cleared from the peritoneal cavity at the end of surgery, and does not expand bubbles or spaces.[61,64] The major disadvantage of CO_2 is that it is rapidly absorbed from the peritoneum (in infants > adults). Usually the $Paco_2$ increases 25% to 50 mm Hg after abdominal insufflation.[61] If surgery is more than 1 hour long, hypercapnia can occur, necessitating an increase in minute ventilation of 50% to 75%.[61] Dramatic increases in $Paco_2$ may initiate a sympathetic response with increases in heart rate and blood pressure, may cause an increase in cerebral blood flow, and may precipitate ventricular arrhythmias. The hypercarbia may also trigger spontaneous breathing efforts that could interfere with the conduct of surgery. Fortunately, current ether anesthetics do not sensitize the myocardium to CO_2 as does halothane, making arrhythmias uncommon. Intravascular embolization of CO_2 may occur, resulting in sudden cardiovascular collapse: precordial Doppler evaluation and monitoring of end-tidal nitrogen concentrations are effective for diagnosing such an event, but a sudden decrease in end-tidal CO_2 may not occur. In contrast to CO_2, insufflation of oxygen, air, or nitrous oxide is contraindicated in the presence of cautery because they all support combustion. Because nitrous oxide expands gas-filled cavities, its use during laparoscopic surgery may expand the lumen of the bowel and obscure the view of the surgical site; thus its use for insufflation or for the conduct of anesthesia is not recommended. Helium is an alternative gas, but it is more expensive and it can cause serious sequelae if embolized into the vascular system because of its minimal solubility in blood (blood/gas solubility is 0.007).[64]

Irrespective of the gas used, when laparoscopic surgery is planned for the abdomen, the stomach must be decompressed to enhance the view of the upper abdominal contents and the bladder should be emptied to enhance the view of the lower abdominal contents. Decompressing the stomach is usually achieved by passing an orogastric tube after tracheal intubation. A nasogastric tube is often inserted and usually remains in situ until several days after surgery.

Pulmonary Effects

The intra-abdominal pressure created by the pneumoperitoneum usually ranges from 6 to 20 mm Hg. The greater this pressure, the greater the cardiorespiratory effects, particularly if the intra-abdominal pressure is increased more than marginally. The respiratory manifestations of increased intra-abdominal pressure include cephalad displacement of the diaphragm, decreased excursion of the diaphragm, and decreases in pulmonary and thoracic compliance, vital capacity, functional residual capacity, and closing volume.[65] Cephalad displacement of the diaphragm shifts ventilation to the nondependent parts of the lungs, creating ventilation/perfusion mismatch. With a small functional residual capacity in children, cephalad displacement of the diaphragm further compresses the lungs, causing collapse of the small airways, ventilation/perfusion mismatch, and possibly hypoxemia. These physiologic effects are compounded by the gas being used as well as body position (i.e., extreme head-up or head-down positions).[66-68] Inspired oxygen concentrations in excess of 30% may be required, together with a small amount of positive end-expiratory pressure to restore adequate oxygenation. One study found that the difference between the end-tidal and arterial CO_2 ($Paco_2$-$ETco_2$ gradient) before and after pneumoperitoneum increased from a mean of 5.7 mm Hg to 13.4 mm Hg, suggesting that the $ETco_2$ may not reliably reflect the $PaCO_2$.[69] However, the opposite results have also been reported when CO_2 was used to create the pneumoperitoneum. In this case, the $ETco_2$ exceeded the $Paco_2$ by up to about 9 mm Hg.[70] It also appears that the $ETco_2$ increases more rapidly in younger children, although it is unclear whether this is due to an increased absorption of CO_2 or to a greater metabolic rate in the younger age group.[71]

Several studies have also reported the changes in pulmonary mechanics after pneumoperitoneum. Insufflating the abdomen increases the peak inspiratory pressures by 27% and decreases the compliance by about 39%.[72] Positioning the child head down (i.e., Trendelenburg position) decreases compliance by 17%, and adding on a pneumoperitoneum decreases compliance 27%, with peak inflation pressures increasing 19% and 32%, respectively.[73]

Carbon dioxide is the gas most frequently used to insufflate the abdomen because it will be rapidly absorbed, thereby reducing the severity of a pulmonary gas embolism. In addition to the mechanical effects on respirations leading to mild to moderate hypercarbia, CO_2 will also be absorbed via the peritoneum itself, thereby further increasing the CO_2 load to the child. Advanced mass spectrometry studies have demonstrated that 10% to 20% of exhaled CO_2 after 10 minutes of pneumoperitoneum is derived from exogenous CO_2.[74] To offset the increased CO_2 load and the mechanical effects on respirations, alveolar minute ventilation must be increased by 25% to 30% under normal circum-

stances.[66] The need to further adjust minute ventilation can be caused by cranial displacement and splinting of the diaphragm if abdominal pressures are increased excessively and/or if the child is placed in a head-down position. Thus, in rare instances it may be a considerable challenge to adequately ventilate some children whose surgery is performed laparoscopically. The combination of increased intra-abdominal pressure and a cranially displaced diaphragm increases the risk of atelectasis. To reduce this risk, we recommend using a cuffed tracheal tube, volume-controlled ventilation mode, and a small amount of positive end-expiratory pressure.

Management of the airway during laparoscopic surgery requires tracheal intubation. Ventilation must be controlled to offset the decrease in pulmonary compliance and the increase in $Paco_2$. The combination of a pneumoperitoneum and Trendelenburg position may, however, displace the tip of the endotracheal tube in a rostral direction, possibly leading to an endobronchial intubation. Depending on the size of the child, the tip of the tube can migrate between 1.2 and 2.7 cm.[75] A persistent 5% reduction in oxygen saturation has been shown to be associated with partial or intermittent endobronchial intubation.[76] If the child has a mature tracheotomy, the extent of the air leak around the tracheotomy must be assessed before undertaking laparoscopic surgery. If the leak is sufficiently large, then the increased intra-abdominal pressure may prevent adequate ventilation during surgery. In such a situation, the tracheotomy should be replaced with an armored (cuffed) tracheotomy tube during surgery. If the air leak around the tracheotomy is insignificant, then ventilation should be adequate in the presence of increased intra-abdominal pressure during laparoscopic surgery. Excessive intra-abdominal pressure may cause gas to tract across the diaphragm causing a pneumomediastinum or pneumothorax. This is more common in hiatal hernia surgery and Nissen fundoplication, during which dissection of the esophagus may create passages for gas to traverse the diaphragm. Pneumomediastinum should be suspected if subcutaneous emphysema begins to appear. If surgery creates a transdiaphragmatic passage for CO_2 to accumulate in the pleural space, the resulting pneumothorax may produce cardiorespiratory manifestations. A chest radiograph should be obtained if subcutaneous emphysema appears during or after surgery or if there is a high index of suspicion that a pneumothorax has formed.

Pulmonary function appears to be restored more readily after laparoscopic than open surgery.[61] Although data in children are scant, evidence from the adult literature suggests that this is the case. Finally, gasless laparoscopy is possible, but this requires lifting the anterior abdominal wall to create a normal pressure intra-abdominal tent.[64] With this technique, the absence of a pneumoperitoneum decreases the physiologic effects of the laparoscopic surgery and sequelae from gas insufflation.

Cardiovascular Effects

A pneumoperitoneum can also adversely affect cardiovascular indices.[64,77] Three major factors contribute to the cardiovascular changes: intra-abdominal pressure, position (i.e., steep head-up or reverse Trendelenburg), and absorbed CO_2. In neonatal pigs, cardiac index decreased as intra-abdominal pressure exceeded 20 mm Hg; that is, at 20 mm Hg, cardiac index decreased 55%. The major effect of the pneumoperitoneum is to increase afterload and decrease cardiac output. Systemic vascular resistance may increase 65%, pulmonary vascular resistance may increase

90%, and cardiac output may decrease 20% to 30%.[78] The effect of intra-abdominal pressure on venous return and, therefore, cardiac output depends on the magnitude of the pressure in the abdominal cavity: when intra-abdominal pressure is greater than 15 mm Hg, the inferior vena cava is compressed, decreasing venous return and cardiac output, whereas when it is less than or equal to 15 mm Hg, blood is squeezed out of the splanchnic circulation, increasing venous return and attenuating the effect on cardiac output. Other studies in children suggest that at intra-abdominal pressures greater than 12 mm Hg, cardiac function in terms of myocardial contractility may be mildly depressed[79] and venous return decreased.[66] In two such studies, one using echocardiography and one using impedance cardiography, intra-abdominal pressures of 12 mm Hg decreased the cardiac index 13%.[80,81] These decreases in cardiac index returned to postinduction values when the abdomen was desufflated. When simple standard indices of cardiovascular responses were measured, intra-abdominal pressures less than or equal to 10 mm Hg yielded no significant changes during laparoscopic Nissen fundoplication.[82] If intra-abdominal pressures are maintained at less than or equal to 10 mm Hg, then the impact on hemodynamics should be clinically insignificant because venous return is enhanced due to displacement of blood from the splanchnic bed and afterload is not increased.[66]

An intra-abdominal pressure of 12 mm Hg has been associated with transient left ventricular septal wall hypokinesia.[71] An echocardiographic study in children with an intra-abdominal pressure of less than or equal to 10 mm Hg during laparoscopy reported increases in left ventricular end-diastolic volume, left ventricular end-systolic volume, and left ventricular wall stress, suggesting that the intra-abdominal pressure alters both preload and afterload.[83]

Position during laparoscopic surgery in children may exaggerate these cardiovascular changes. For Nissen fundoplication, steep head-up position (25 to 30 degrees) is often used. This degree of head-up position exceeds that used for laparoscopic gallbladder surgery (15 to 20 degrees). The head-up position reduces venous return, and a steep head-up position decreases venous return even further. A study of laparoscopic surgery for Nissen fundoplication in adult pigs reported increased pleural and mediastinal pressures that reduced cardiac output episodically at intra-abdominal pressures of 15 mm Hg.[84] These decreases in cardiac output were manifested by episodes of hypotension and hypoxia. In one study, children positioned in the steep head-up position developed transient hypotension and bradycardia that were reversed immediately with fluid loading and atropine.[85]

Pneumoperitoneum markedly decreases intraoperative urine output, particularly in infants younger than 1 year of age.[86] Whether the oliguria is the result of a decreased perfusion from the increased intra-abdominal pressure or decreased cardiac output is unclear.

To minimize the cardiovascular effects of laparoscopic surgery, it is imperative to continuously monitor intra-abdominal pressures throughout the procedure to avoid excessive pressures. Some recommend maximum intra-abdominal pressures during laparoscopy of 6 to 8 mm Hg,[87] but most suggest a range of 10 to 12 mm Hg. Based on the current literature, the net cardiovascular effects of insufflating the abdomen to pressures less than or equal to 12 mm Hg combined with steep head-up position are likely to be small if adequate hydration is maintained and bradycardia is avoided.[85] If pressures greater than 15 mm Hg are required for surgery, then an open laparotomy should be considered to eliminate the risks of adverse cardiopulmonary and renal manifestations.

Neurologic Effects

Laparoscopic surgery must be carefully evaluated if planned for a child with raised intracranial pressure or a ventriculoperitoneal shunt. The combination of increased intra-abdominal pressure, increased systemic vascular resistance, increased $Paco_2$ tension, and Trendelenburg position (as in lower abdominal surgery) may markedly increase intracranial pressure. Patency of a ventriculoperitoneal shunt should be evaluated before the procedure to prevent sudden increases in intracranial pressure during the procedure. Some advocate externalizing the shunt, clamping the distal end of the shunt before surgery, or monitoring intracranial pressure to prevent/detect increases in intracranial pressure and retraction of abdominal tissue in the shunt during the laparoscopic surgery. Children with reduced brain compliance may sustain marked increases in intracranial pressure if the intra-abdominal pressure is sufficient to attenuate the drainage of cerebrospinal fluid into the abdominal cavity. In one study, intracranial pressure increased from 7.6 to 21.4 mm Hg with a 25% decrease in perfusion pressure, when intra-abdominal pressures of 25 mm Hg were used for surgery. In two children with Chiari malformations, intra-abdominal pressures of 10 mm Hg or less in functioning shunts developed a 100% increase in intracranial pressure from 12 to 25 mm Hg, necessitating the removal of cerebrospinal fluid to restore the intracranial pressure and prevent sequelae.[88] In a retrospective review of 18 children with ventriculoperitoneal shunts who underwent laparoscopic surgery, there was no evidence of increased intracranial pressure as suggested by bradycardia and hypertension when the intra-abdominal pressure was maintained at 16 mm Hg for approximately 3 hours.[89] There is no single strategy to manage children with ventriculoperitoneal shunts during laparoscopic surgery. However, careful assessment of shunt function and consultation among the general surgeon, neurosurgeon, and anesthesiologist would seem prudent.

Renal Function and Fluid Requirements

Increased intra-abdominal pressure decreases renal blood flow, renal function (creatinine clearance and glomerular filtration rate), and urine output.[90,91] The mechanism for these changes has been attributed in part to decreased stroke volume, but cellular responses including nitric oxide and endothelin-1 effects have been considered. Renal tubular injury does not appear to play any role in renal dysfunction changes associated with increased intra-abdominal pressure.[92] In a study of adult donor nephrectomy patients, an overnight infusion of fluids followed by a colloid bolus immediately before the pneumoperitoneum attenuated the hemodynamic effects and reduced the magnitude of changes in creatinine clearance associated with increased intra-abdominal pressure.[93]

Fluid administration during laparoscopic surgery should be carefully monitored. Open abdominal surgeries may require 10 to 15 mL/kg/hr to account for third space fluid losses. During laparoscopic surgery, however, these fluid requirements are reduced because there are no insensible fluid losses and limited manipulation of the bowels is required. Care must be taken to avoid fluid overload during these surgeries. Urine output is often used as an index of preload in children undergoing abdominal surgery. However, during laparoscopic surgery in children, 88% of infants (<1 year of age) and 33% of children develop anuria or oliguria that completely resolves within several hours of desufflation.[94] Transient oliguria in children after laparoscopic surgery should not be viewed as a harbinger of impending renal dysfunction.

Pain Management

Postoperative pain after open general and urologic surgeries is primarily required to manage the pain from the skin and muscle incisions. With the small incisions used during laparoscopic surgery, perioperative pain is expected to be less than with open surgery. Laparoscopic surgery for a number of conditions (e.g., hernia, appendectomy) in children is associated with less pain than after open surgery.[95-97] Pain after laparoscopic surgery arises from several sites, including the incision sites, residual gas in the abdomen, referred pain from the diaphragm, and stretch on nerves from odd positioning. During laparoscopic surgery, surgeons infiltrate local anesthetic around the incision sites to prevent postoperative incisional pain. Some children do develop pain after laparoscopic surgery, including back and shoulder pain. In these instances, multimodal pain therapy including acetaminophen, nonsteroidal anti-inflammatory agents, and, less commonly, opioids is effective.[62,64] In one study, children required no supplementary analgesics for the first 24 hours after surgery.[85]

Specific Conditions and Surgery

Circumcision

Circumcision is performed in neonates, infants, children, and adults under local, regional, or general anesthesia. The indications for circumcision include phimosis, recurrent balanitis, or parental preference. The classic circumcision involves cutting the foreskin and cauterizing and suturing the skin edges. The duration of surgery is usually less than 1 hour. The type of anesthetic and airway management do not significantly affect perioperative outcome. The most common complication arising from circumcision is bleeding.

In infants and children, circumcision is performed under general anesthesia. Multimodal pain therapy includes acetaminophen 30 to 40 mg/kg rectally, parenteral opioids (i.e., morphine 0.05-0.1 mg/kg), and/or local anesthetic without epinephrine (dorsal penile block, caudal block, subcutaneous ring block, and topical EMLA) (see Chapter 42).[98] In a comparison of a subcutaneous ring block of the penis with a subpubic penile block both without epinephrine, the latter provided better analgesia.[99] When caudal block is compared with penile block and parenteral analgesics, a Cochrane review issued a limited analysis due to the paucity of studies. However, it was reported that rescue analgesia was reduced with caudal blocks compared with parenteral analgesics and nausea and vomiting was reduced compared with parenteral analgesics.[100]

Hypospadias and Chordee

This congenital malformation occurs in 1:250 liveborn males. It often occurs in isolation, without other congenital anomalies. Hypospadias refers to a malposition of the meatus of the urethra: rather than opening at the distal tip of the penis, the urethra opens along the undersurface of the penis anywhere from just proximal to the glans to the scrotum. The majority of hypospadias defects are distal, occurring near the glans of the penis. Associated with hypospadias is a 15% to 50% incidence of curvature of the penis or chordee; a minority (8%) of males with hypospadias have an undescended testis.

Surgery is undertaken with an expected duration between 1 and 4 hours depending on the severity of the hypospadias. It is important to establish an understanding with the urologist of the type of regional block that will suit the extent of surgery: those requiring a minor hypospadias repair (single-stage procedure, i.e., MAGPI [meatal advancement and glanduloplasty technique], Mathieu, or other) may be managed with a face mask, laryngeal mask airway, or tracheal tube; the anesthetic is at the discretion of the anesthesiologist; the children are outpatients and receive either a penile block or a single-shot caudal block. Those with a more extensive hypospadias who require a more involved surgery will undergo surgery of greater duration necessitating either a laryngeal mask airway or a tracheal tube and a general anesthetic and will require admission to a hospital for one to two nights together with a strategy for continuous postoperative analgesia. For the latter, either a caudal catheter may be inserted or a lumbar epidural anesthetic can be used in older children during surgery to reduce the anesthetic requirements and postoperatively for analgesia. If opioids are avoided, a caudal/epidural block is not associated with delayed micturition after the urinary catheter has been removed.[101]

The anesthetic care that is required for infants and children with hypospadias is routine and includes the use of a forced-air heating mattress. However, in the presence of minimal tissue exposure during surgery, the use of such a heater may cause overheating and hyperthermia. Temperature should be monitored in these young children; and at the first signs of a rapidly increasing temperature, the temperature of the heater should be reduced to ambient or 32°C.

Cryptorchidism and Hernias: Inguinal and Umbilical

These surgeries together with hydrocele repair are common outpatient procedures. *Orchidopexy* refers to securing an undescended testis that remains in the inguinal canal or less commonly within the abdominal cavity in the scrotum. Approximately 33% of preterm infant males are born with one undescended testis, whereas only 3% of full-term males are similarly afflicted. Although the incidence of undescended testis decreases to 1.0% by 3 months of age, the incidence remains at 1% thereafter. Cryptorchidism usually occurs in isolation, although it is associated with a number of conditions including Prader-Willi syndrome, Noonan's syndrome, and cloacal exstrophy.

Undescended testes are categorized based on physical examination to include testes that are truly undescended, those that are ectopic, and those that are retractile. The retractile are not true undescended testis because they can be massaged into the scrotum and require no treatment. In the case of the true undescended testis, the testis must be found and fixed within the scrotal sac to ensure viability of the testis. Failure to bring the testis out of the inguinal canal or abdomen may result in atrophy of the testis, torsion of the testis, testicular cancer, and hernias.

An *inguinal hernia* in a child is a congenital failure of the processus vaginalis to obliterate. In this case, a loop of bowel protrudes beyond the internal ring, causing a bulge in the inguinal region or scrotum. These protuberances may appear periodically with complete resolution in the interim. However, on occasion, a loop of bowel does not reduce spontaneously and remains trapped in the canal, necessitating a visit to the emergency department. A surgeon is often required to manually reduce the trapped bowel. In these cases, the hernia repair is then scheduled as an urgent or elective surgery, depending on whether there is suspicion of ongoing ischemia to the bowel. In some cases, the entrapped bowel cannot be reduced and an incarcerated hernia or obstructed bowel is diagnosed. Incarcerated hernias and bowel obstructions are surgical emergencies that presume that the child has a full stomach. A general anesthetic and muscle relaxation are required to reduce the bowel that is strangled. At the time of open reduction, if the bowel does not appear to have adequate perfusion, a segment of the ischemic/necrotic bowel may have to be resected.

An umbilical hernia is a 1- to 5-cm defect in the anterior abdominal wall with intermittent protuberance of bowel through the defect. This defect occurs in 15% of children, more commonly in children of African descent than in Caucasian children and equally in males and females.[102] It occurs in preterm and low birth weight infants. If the defect is small, then an LMA may be sufficient to manage the airway, whereas if the defect is large, tracheal intubation may be required. For this defect, relaxation may be required when the surgeon attempts to close the umbilical defect. Although there are many techniques to resolve this issue, it is our experience that an intravenous bolus of propofol (1-2 mg/kg) provides adequate relaxation to reduce the defect.

Management of cryptorchidism and inguinal hernia requires general anesthesia (face mask, laryngeal mask airway, or tracheal tube) and an adequate pain management strategy. Multimodal pain therapy as described earlier is reasonable together with a regional block. Anesthetic complications are common when inexperienced anesthesiologists anesthetize children for such surgery. When the surgeon pulls on the foreskin, hernia sac, or testis during surgery, laryngospasm may occur if the depth of anesthesia is inadequate. Anesthesia can be deepened most rapidly by an intravenous bolus of propofol, although some increase the inspired concentration of inhalational anesthetic. For both orchidopexy and inguinal hernia surgery, a regional block should be administered: either an ilioinguinal, iliohypogastric, and scrotal block or a caudal/epidural block.

Torsion of the Testes

Presentation of a male with sudden onset of acute scrotal pain in the absence of trauma requires immediate investigation and possible surgery to preserve a potentially viable testis. The differential diagnosis of acute onset of pain includes torsion of the testicular appendix, torsion of the spermatic cord, epididymitis, and incarcerated hernia. If confirmed by Doppler ultrasonography or suspected on clinical grounds, the majority of the testes can be saved if surgery is performed within 6 hours of the onset of pain.[103] The salvage rate decreases to 50% if surgery is undertaken between 6 and 12 hours.

Children with suspected acute testicular torsion are assumed to have a full stomach and require RSI and tracheal intubation. Although pain at the time of induction of anesthesia may be intense, when the torsion is relieved, the pain abates. Hence, at the conclusion of surgery, many of these children no longer have substantive pain that warrants treatment.

Posterior Urethral Valves

This diagnosis often made antenatally is manifested by bladder distention, megaureters, and hydronephrosis. In utero, decompression of the urogenital system may be achieved by a vesicoamniotic shunt. Although some recommend that an intervention should be undertaken as quickly as possible to minimize the impact on renal function, evidence suggests that early intervention makes no difference in outcome because renal damage may have already occurred in utero.[104,105]

Postnatally, a lack of or decrease in urine output, urinary retention, or a poor urine stream may be the only indications of the presence of these valves.[106] These children can have associated renal insufficiency due to congenital renal dysplasia and postnatal urethral valve obstruction. Because of the impairment of the renal concentrating mechanism, these infants often present with abnormally high urine output. Consequently, careful monitoring of the urine output and fluid replacement is required. Primary valve ablation is required to decompress the urogenital system. A good predictor of renal function as an adult is the serum creatinine concentration at 1 year of age.

Usually these infants present after having fasted for elective surgery. A general anesthetic is administered with management of the general anesthetic and airway up to the discretion of the anesthesiologist. There are few special considerations required.

Prune Belly Syndrome

Prune belly syndrome is a disorder that occurs predominantly in males (97% of cases) with an incidence of 1:40,000 births. Presentation abnormalities ranges from stillborn to a full-term neonate with involvement of the abdomen, lungs, cryptorchidism, and urologic anomalies.[107] Other associated organ involvement includes orthopedic in 50% (congenital hip dislocation and scoliosis), gastrointestinal in 30% (malrotation and volvulus), and congenital heart disease in 10% (tetralogy of Fallot and ventricular septal defect), trisomy 18 (alternately known as Edward's syndrome), and trisomy 21.[108]

In utero, the child's abdomen often swells with fluid (in the presence of oligohydramnios) that is resorbed by birth, leaving the characteristic wrinkled redundant abdominal wall. The pathophysiology of this syndrome is unclear, but it has been suggested that a urethral obstruction in utero leads to dilatation of the urethra (megaurethra is a common finding) combined with bladder distention and ascites, which causes distention of the abdomen in utero. This ultimately leads to vesicoureteral reflux and ureteral dilatation in 80% of children.

Abdominal overdistention in utero results in weak rectus abdominis muscles that limit expiration and the ability to cough. As a result, some of these children suffer from chronic aspiration, pneumonia, and death. Some have suggested that aggressive intervention to correct the weak rectus muscles by plication and muscle transfer may improve respiratory function.[108] However, this view is not shared by many who prefer to observe the child for signs of regurgitation and aspiration before intervening. Controlling the type of feeds, preventing gastrointestinal reflux disease, and using antibiotics to treat pneumonia permit the child to grow. Constipation is a frequent problem that arises from an inability to increase intra-abdominal pressure during defecation. To prevent constipation and the possibility of abdominal distention in these children, stool softeners are generally prescribed. Should surgery be contemplated, pneumonia must be aggressively treated and cleared. Moreover, if feeding is problematic, it is best to avoid placement of a percutaneous endoscopic gastroscopy tube because abdominal wall surgery will be much more difficult.

These children often require urologic surgery to correct vesicoureteral reflux and orchidopexy. Urethral obstruction may be due to the angulation of the urethra within the prostate.

Trisomy 18, the second most common autosomal trisomy, occurs in 1 in 7,000 live births. It is associated with prune belly syndrome. Approximately 80% of these infants are female. It is characterized by severe neurologic developmental problems (including microcephaly), micro/retrognathia, microstomia, auricular abnormalities, and others. In fact, 95% die in utero with only 5% to 10% surviving 1 year after birth and 1% reaching 10 years. Mortality results from cardiac anomalies (90% of affected children will have ventricular septal defect, valvular heart defects, atrial septal defect, hypoplastic left heart syndrome, tetralogy of Fallot, and others), renal anomalies, failure to thrive, and apnea. Other findings include pulmonary hypoplasia and gastrointestinal anomalies (including prune belly syndrome, omphalocele, ileal atresias, and esophageal atresia).

General anesthesia with tracheal intubation is required for most surgeries in these children. Because of the variability in the strength of the abdominal musculature, controlled ventilation is recommended. While the trachea is intubated, it is prudent to suction the lungs to assess the extent of pulmonary infection. It may be wise to minimize the use of muscle relaxants and limit their use within the last hour of surgery, to maximize the probability of extubating the trachea.

Ureteral Reimplantation

Vesicoureteral reflux is a congenital disorder affecting 0.5% to 2% of children, in which urine passes retrograde up the ureter. Depending on the severity of the reflux, recurrent episodes of pyelonephritis may occur, leading to renal scarring and impaired renal function. The pathology is believed to be due to an abnormal insertion of the ureter into the bladder and its failure to close when the bladder fills or contracts. A voiding cystourethrogram is required to assess the severity of the reflux.

Mild forms of vesicoureteral reflux are managed with daily antibiotics until the child outgrows the reflux. However, more severe forms of the disease or those who develop kidney infections despite antibiotic therapy require a surgical intervention. The classic surgical approach is an open surgery in which the affected ureters are reimplanted into the bladder wall, re-creating a normal muscle flap valve.[109] This involves a lower abdominal incision and 3 to 4 hours of surgery. Postoperatively, the pain is often intense, necessitating 2 to 3 days of a continuous infusion of local anesthetic via an indwelling caudal or epidural catheter.

More recently, laparoscopic techniques have been developed with and without robotic control, for reimplantation of the ureters.[109] Preliminary evidence suggests a high success rate (>90%) for this technique,[110] although the time for the surgery is more than twice the open technique and more complications were identified in children with small bladders.

Surgical alternatives in the past 20 years have spawned a number of compounds for injection into the terminal submucosal tract of the ureter by passing a 23-gauge needle through a specially designed small cystoscope. Initially, polytetrafluoro-ethylene (Teflon) was injected endoscopically, but the material has been refined in the past 20 years, resulting in a safer, more durable product that is a dextranomer/hyaluronic acid (Deflux). In this way, the surgeons create a swelling just inferior to the opening of the ureter into the bladder that prevents reflux of urine. The technique is successful in 80% of cases with one injection and in more than 90% with two injections. The endoscopic procedure is brief (usually 15-30 minutes), requires general anesthesia, avoids an incision, and can be performed as an outpatient. The benefit of such an approach is the avoidance of an abdominal incision, the elimination of postoperative pain, and the shift of this surgery to an ambulatory procedure. However, the results of this procedure continue to be monitored because the long-term outcome and sequelae have not been determined.

Pyeloplasty

Pyeloplasty is performed to decompress the renal pelvis either due to intrinsic (congenital) or extrinsic (major vessel) compression of the ureter. A distended renal pelvis is often diagnosed antenatally and, in some instances, decompressed in utero with a percutaneous nephrostomy. The ureteric narrowing often occurs at the ureteropelvic junction as the ureter exits the renal pelvis. Surgery involves dismembering the ureter at the renal pelvis, reshaping it, and then reinserting it into the kidney. Such surgery is often performed in the lateral or prone positions, with the table jack-knifed with a success rate of approximately 95%. Duration of surgery is about 2 hours. Dissection is often retroperitoneal, but the incision is placed immediately below the rib cage. This procedure has been performed laparoscopically and with the use of robotics.

The anesthetic considerations include the prone or lateral child, postoperative pain, and adequate fluid resuscitation. Intravenous access should be established in an upper extremity to maintain adequate atrial filling pressures. If the table is jack-knifed, it is very important to measure the child's blood pressure before and after the table is jack-knifed because venous return may be severely embarrassed in the jack-knife position. The laparoscopic approach to pyeloplasty is a new application of minimally invasive surgery in children. In renal surgery, CO_2 is insufflated in the retroperitoneal space to allow for surgical access.[111] Because of the anatomic differences between the retroperitoneal and intraperitoneal spaces, greater pressures are needed to provide adequate surgical visibility in the former. A mean retroperitoneal pressure of 12 mm Hg increases $ETCO_2$ and peak inspiratory pressures and decreases blood pressure.[112] Early evidence indicates that laparoscopic surgery yields similar outcomes as the open approach, although the duration of surgery is approximately one third greater.[113,114] In part, this has been attributed to the learning curve with this technique. Some evidence suggests that the laparoscopic approach decreases the hospital length of stay and may decrease postoperative pain.[114] See later in the chapter for a discussion of postoperative pain management.

Nephrectomy

Indications for nephrectomy and partial nephrectomy in children include nonfunctioning kidney, dysplastic kidney, urolithiasis, Wilm's or other tumor, end-stage renal failure (pretransplantation or to control hypertension), hemolytic-uremic syndrome, and polycystic disease.

Pectus Excavatum

Although this is a deformity of the chest wall, pediatric surgeons most often carry out the corrective procedure. Correction of the pectus excavatum by the classic approach involves an open procedure with fracture of the sternum, removal of many costal cartilages, and lifting of the sternum anteriorly with fixation using one or two stainless steel bars. In recent years, a less invasive technique, the Nuss procedure was introduced.[115,116] Initially this was a blind technique whereby a U-shaped bar was blindly passed through the thorax hugging the undersurface of the sternum. Once across the chest, the bar is flipped, which in the process pushes the sternum anteriorly without fracturing the sternum and thus avoiding creating a flail chest by the removal of the costal cartilages. This procedure has since been modified whereby the bar is passed through the thorax under direct vision using thoroscopy to reduce possible perforation to major structures (e.g., the heart or lungs)[117-119] which has been reported with the blind procedure. Although the risk of this complication is reduced when the Nuss procedure is performed under direct vision, it may still occur.[120-122] Both approaches will cause significant postoperative pain, which may be treated with patient-controlled analgesia, a thoracic epidural catheter, or a lumbar epidural catheter and epidural morphine (see Chapters 42 and 44).[123] Because these procedures are generally performed in teenagers, the thoracic epidural is preferably placed with the teenager awake but sedated. Compliance with inserting the epidural catheter awake may be difficult in more immature teenagers. It is unclear whether the thoracic epidural provides improved analgesia compared with standard patient-controlled analgesia for this procedure.[124] It should be noted that these children will return for removal of the pectus bar after several years. Occasionally, the bar has become adherent to the pericardium or lung, resulting in a severe, sudden and catastrophic rupture of a major vessel or chamber in the heart at the time of removal of the bar.[125] It would be prudent to establish ample intravenous access to massively resuscitate and transfuse fluids to these children should a catastrophe occur.

Nissen Fundoplication

This surgery is indicated for children with documented gastric fluid reflux that failed medical management. It involves mobilizing the muscles around the esophagus and suturing them tightly around the esophagus at the level of the lower esophageal sphincter. This surgery requires general anesthesia and tracheal intubation and is usually performed laparoscopically (see earlier).

Children who require a Nissen fundoplication often have a cerebral neurologic injury (i.e., cerebral palsy) that causes esophageal dysmotility. This dysmotility heralds esophageal reflux that may cause aspiration pneumonia. If medical and gastric tube therapies fail, a Nissen fundoplication should be considered. The anesthetic considerations are few because this surgery is not associated with postoperative pain, large fluid shifts, or large blood loss. Anesthesia contributes immensely to this surgery by simply positioning a bougie within the esophagus for the duration of surgery. The bougie allows the surgeons to gauge how tight to tie the muscles around the esophagus because without the bougie the muscles around the esophagus may be overtightened, causing an esophageal obstruction. Care must be taken so as to not dislodge the endotracheal tube. At the end of the procedure it is common for the surgeon to request insufflation of 50 to 60 mL of air via a gastric tube and syringe so as to ensure that there are no leaks in the stomach as a result of the procedure. At the end of surgery, these children emerge from anesthesia and their tracheas are extubated.

Two series of children who have undergone laparoscopic Nissen fundoplication demonstrate that this surgery can be performed in less than 1 hour in experienced hands, the complication rate is about 10%, the hospital stay is about 1.6 days, and postoperative pain is easily managed.[126,127]

Postoperative Analgesia

Open abdominal and urologic surgery offers exceptional opportunities to provide excellent intraoperative and postoperative analgesia using a number of regional anesthetic techniques. Single administration epidural/caudal anesthesia as well as continuous epidural and patient-controlled epidural analgesia are commonly utilized.[128,129] Epidural analgesia has proven of particular benefit in association with Nissen fundoplication surgery, with reduction of morbidity as well as cost savings for the hospital.[130] One surgery whose postoperative pain control has been difficult and not well managed was open pyeloplasty. However, strategies such as epidural and caudal anesthesia are effective and detailed elsewhere (see Chapters 42 to 44). If regional techniques cannot be used, then pain should be controlled with an appropriate systemic alternative, that is, continuous morphine infusions or patient-controlled analgesia. Another effective and versatile alternative to both ilioinguinal-iliohypogastric nerve blocks as well as caudal or epidural blockade in children undergoing unilateral abdominal and urologic surgery is the paravertebral block, particularly if there is concern for a bleeding diathesis (see Chapter 42).

Annotated References

McNeely JK, Farber NE, Rusy LM, Hoffman GM: Epidural analgesia improves outcome following pediatric fundoplication: a retrospective analysis. Reg Anesth 1997; 22:16-23

Despite the retrospective character of this study it represents the best current evidence of the benefits of the use of epidural anesthesia in pediatric anesthesia because it shows significant improvement in hard outcome end points and not only in a surrogate end point such as better pain relief.

Naja ZM, Raf M, El Rajab M, et al: A comparison of nerve stimulator–guided paravertebral block and ilioinguinal nerve block for analgesia after inguinal herniorrhaphy in children. Anaesthesia 2006; 61:1064-1068

First ever prospective randomized controlled trial in children comparing paravertebral blockade to ilioinguinal nerve block for hernia repair, showing paravertebral block to be a superior alternative.

Pacilli M, Pierro A, Kingsley C, et al: Absorption of carbon dioxide during laparoscopy in children measured using a novel mass spectrometric technique. Br J Anaesth 2006; 97:215-219

Shows with very high precision the contribution of intra-abdominal CO_2 insufflation to exhaled/end-tidal CO_2 readings.

Suominen PK, Pakarinen MP, Rautiainen P, et al: Comparison of direct and intravesical measurement of intraabdominal pressure in children. J Pediatr Surg 2006; 41:1381-1385

Provides important data that show that intravesical pressure measurements very accurately reflect directly measured intra-abdominal pressure.

References

Please see www.expertconsult.com

Essentials of Hepatology

Marcus R. Rivera, Robert H. Squires, Jr., and Peter J. Davis

 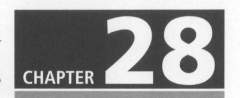

Anatomy

The liver and biliary tree develop from the endoderm of the dorsal foregut during the late third to the early fourth week of gestation. By the sixth week of gestation, it is capable of hematopoiesis, its main function in fetal life, and represents 10% of the fetal weight by 9 weeks gestation. The fetal liver is relatively inactive with respect to glycolysis, bile acid synthesis, and metabolic waste processing because the maternal liver is responsible for these functions through the fetoplacental circulation.

At the time of delivery, the liver weighs 120 to 160 g, or approximately 4% of the infant body weight, and is not yet structurally mature. Peripheral branches of the intrahepatic biliary system require an additional 4 to 8 weeks after birth before they develop into identifiable portal ducts. The liver is divided into eight structurally independent segments containing a hepatic artery, portal vein, hepatic vein, and bile duct. Segment 1 is the caudate lobe. Segments 2 and 3 form the left lateral segment; and with segment 4, the left lobe of the liver is defined. Segments 5, 6, 7, and 8 constitute the right lobe of the liver. A unique feature of the liver is its dual blood supply, with venous blood being derived from the spleen and intestines through the portal vein and arterial (oxygenated) blood being derived from the hepatic artery. Approximately 30% of the hepatic blood flow reaches the liver through the hepatic artery and the balance (70%) reaches it via the portal vein. Both large vessels enter the liver via the porta hepatis, which is located on the inferior surface of the liver. As soon as the blood passes through the liver it is returned to the venous circulation via the left and right hepatic veins, which coalesce and join the inferior vena cava below the level of the atrium. At any given time, the liver contains approximately 13% of the circulating blood volume. Fetal hepatic circulation differs significantly from that of postnatal life. The ductus venosus, a venous connection between the umbilical vein and inferior vena cava, is one of three essential shunts present in fetal life. Its purpose is to shunt oxygenated blood around the immature liver to enter the right atrium, with flow controlled by a sphincter mechanism. Functional closure of the ductus begins immediately after birth when the pressure in the umbilical vein decreases. Complete functional closure is achieved in 95% of infants by 2 weeks of age, with anatomic closure occurring shortly thereafter. Rarely, the ductus may remain patent, which is known as congenital portosystemic venous shunt. It can manifest as hepatic dysfunction and possibly encephalopathy, with closure resulting in reversal of symptoms.

The structural unit of the liver parenchyma is the lobule, a wheel-like structure with the hub being the central vein that is bordered by portal tracts that contain the triad of a bile duct and tributaries of the portal vein and hepatic artery. Blood from the portal venule and hepatic arteriole leave the portal tract and bathe hepatocytes through fenestrated capillaries that terminate at the central vein of the hepatic lobule. Bile flows in the opposite direction through a canalicular matrix that then enters the bile ductule contained in the portal tract. The functional unit of the liver is the hepatic acinus, which is centered around the portal track and extends in three concentric zones (zones of Rappaport) outward to the central vein (Fig. 28-1). It is perfused by afferent blood vessels extending radially through zones of decreasing oxygen and nutrient content. The more central zones (zones 1 and 2) are most active in oxidative processes, whereas the distal zone, zone 3 (which is closer to the central vein), is more dependent on glycolysis and more susceptible to ischemic and toxic injury.

Principles of Hepatic Drug Metabolism

Lipid solubility is an important and desired feature of most administered drugs that allows for the passive diffusion across cellular membranes. Lipophilic drugs are also difficult to excrete. They have a propensity to accumulate in the body's fat stores and are bound to proteins in plasma, thereby limiting renal excretion. Renal and biliary excretion of lipid-soluble compounds can result in their reabsorption across their respective membranes. Thus, a major role of the liver is to transform

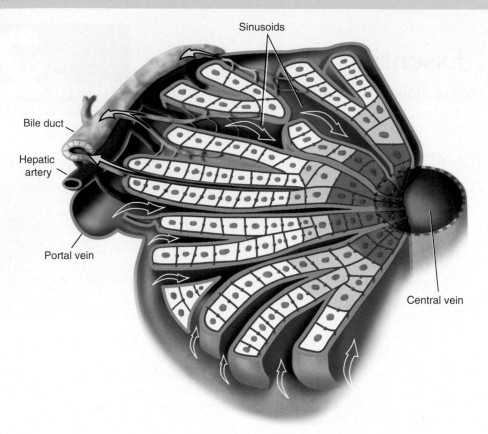

Figure 28-1. Blood flows from the hepatic arteries and portal vein along sinusoids toward the central vein. The hepatic triad consists of the bile duct, a branch of the portal vein, and the hepatic artery, with zone 1 (*white*) surrounding the triad, followed by zone 2 (*pink*) and zone 3 (*red*). Cytochrome P-450 expression is higher in zone 3 with more extensive drug metabolism. (From Oinonen T, Lindros KO: Zonation of hepatic cytochrome P-450 expression and regulation. Biochem J 1998; 329:17-35.)

lipid-soluble drugs into water-soluble compounds that become easily excreted metabolites. An interesting example of the need for this biotransformation is the anesthetic compound thiopental, which if not transformed into its less lipophilic counterpart would have a plasma half-life of approximately 25 years.[1] The primary family of liver enzymes assigned the task of metabolizing these exogenous substances is the cytochrome P-450 (CYP-450) family.

The primary reactions involved in the drug biotransformation and metabolism are hydroxylation and conjugation. Hydroxylation prepares the metabolite for conjugation. Thus, the process has been divided into two designated phases: phase I, primarily hydroxylation, and phase II, conjugation. The majority of the phase I reactions involve the large family of enzymes of cytochrome P-450. These enzymes were first thought to be chemically similar to mitochondrial cytochromes, with the "P" designation given for "pigment," because these enzymes were red (owing to the presence of heme). They are the biggest contributor to the red-brown coloration of the microsomes and readily absorb light at the 450-nm wavelength, hence the term P-450.[2]

The cytochrome P-450 enzymes likely evolved as a mechanism by which the host was able to protect itself from toxins ingested from the environment. Originally, the P-450 superfamily was thought to consist of hundreds, possibly thousands, of different specific enzymes. On the contrary, recent work has shown that there are relatively few enzymes. The majority of the enzymes involved in hepatic drug metabolism may be divided into three distinct families, known as CYP1, CYP2, and CYP3. Each family is further divided into subfamilies, designated with capital letters, and then numbered again in the order in which they were discovered. It is also known that the P-450 enzymes are generally conserved across species. However, the regulation and catalytic activity of these enzymes vary in different species, thus making laboratory analysis of drug metabolism difficult.[2]

There is a wide range of variability in the enzymatic activity across all cytochrome P-450 enzymes. Both genetic and nongenetic factors can influence the activity of the enzymes, either singly or in concert, in metabolizing drugs. Approximately 5% of caucasians lack CYP2D6 activity and are described as "poor metabolizers," resulting in an enhanced effect of certain drugs that require the enzyme for efficient metabolism, such as haloperidol and metoprolol. In contrast, codeine is metabolized to morphine by CYP2D6 and a deficiency of CYP2D6 results in little or no analgesia from codeine.

Nongenetic factors also greatly influence the activity of the cytochrome P-450s, including concomitant disease states, diminished nutritional states, and exposure to certain pharmacologic and naturally occurring compounds. Many drugs can inhibit or stimulate the enzyme system (Table 28-1). Inhibition

Table 28-1. Major Human Liver Cytochrome P-450s

P-450	Substrate	Inhibitors	Inducers
CYP1A2	Caffeine Clozapine Estradiol Theophylline	Fluvoxamine Furafylline	Omeprazole Tobacco smoke
CYP2A6	Halothane Nicotine	Methoxasalen	
CYP2C8	Rosiglitazone Taxol		Phenytoin Rifampin
CYP2C9	Diclofenac Ibuprofen Tolbutamide Warfarin	Sulfaphenazole	Rifampin Secobarbital
CYP2C19	Omeprazole	Fluvoxamine Ketoconazole	
CYP2D6	Codeine Chlorpromazine Desipramine Dextromethorphan Encainide Haloperidol Metoprolol	Fluoxetine Quinidine	
CYP2E1	Acetaminophen Halothane	Disulfiram	Ethanol Isoniazid
CYP3A4	Cyclosporin A Estradiol Indinavir Lovastatin Midazolam Nifedipine Quinidine Docetaxel	Delavirdine Erythromycin Grapefruit juice Ketoconazole Ritonavir Troleandomycin	Carbamazepine Phenobarbital Phenytoin Rifampin St. John's wort Troglitazone

Adapted from Watkins PB: The role of cytochrome P450s in drug-induced liver disease. In Kaplowitz N, Deleve LD (eds): Drug-Induced Liver Disease. New York, Marcel Dekker, 2003, pp 15-33.

of the cytochrome P-450s is accomplished by a simple mechanism of competition for the same enzyme. Factors that determine whether the competing drugs will yield a clinically significant interaction include (1) the relative amount of the specific cytochrome P-450, (2) the concentrations of each drug, (3) the degree of pharmacologically active metabolite generated through this system, (4) the importance of the enzyme in elimination of the drugs, and (5) the therapeutic index of the drugs.[2] Induction of cytochrome P-450s commonly results from increased transcription of the specific gene. Rifampin and phenytoin induce CYP3A4 through the cytosolic receptor human pregnenolone-X receptor (hPXR) or the steroid xenobiotic receptor (SXR).[3] The inducer compounds bind the receptor, translocate it into the nucleus, and subsequently bind to regulator elements of the CYP3A4 gene, leading to increased transcription. It is unclear whether this same receptor is also involved in the inductive effects of rifampin on CYP2C8 and CYP2C9. The process of induction not only leads to toxic levels of inter-

mediates, as is the case with children receiving cyclosporin A and erythromycin, but subtherapeutic levels of cyclosporine in transplant patients.[4]

Cytochrome P-450 Activity

The superfamily of cytochrome P-450 enzymes is further divided into subfamilies based on sequence homology, with all members demonstrating broad substrate specificities. Each enzyme, however, does have more discrete specificities, with both inducible and constitutive forms present. The CYP3A subfamily is the most abundant group of cytochromes involved in the metabolism of a large number of xenobiotics. There are three identified isoforms within this family. CYP3A4 is the most abundant single enzyme in the human liver, accounting for the metabolism of approximately 50% of the clinically used pharmaceuticals.[5] CYP3A5 is more commonly found in the kidneys and lungs and to a lesser degree in the liver. The third isoform, CYP3A7, is the predominant form in the prenatal liver but is replaced after birth by CYP3A4. Because of the extent of its involvement in hepatic biotransformation, the CYP3A family of enzymes has been used to study and estimate hepatic drug clearance in various age groups. Both gender differences and age differences exist when analyzing cytochrome P-450–mediated drug biotransformation.

During the neonatal period, the liver is immature in its ability to metabolize and clear xenobiotics. Factors believed to affect clearance of medications include hepatic blood flow and the developmental status of hepatic transport and enzyme systems. Size simply does not account for this observed degree of immaturity, because the fetal and neonatal liver account for a greater percentage of body weight than the adult counterpart (3.6% of body weight vs. 2.4% in adults).[6] The neonatal liver contains approximately 20% fewer hepatocytes than adult livers, and the cells are nearly half the size of adult hepatocytes. These structural features may play some role in the functional deficiencies exhibited by infant livers. Cellular growth and hypertrophy of the liver continue at a rapid pace into young adulthood.

Hepatic developmental changes occur throughout gestation. Hepatic hematopoiesis develops in utero at 5 to 6 weeks gestation, followed closely by protein synthesis.[7] The ability to metabolize carbohydrates and lipids begins by 10 weeks gestation, followed closely by the development of drug metabolizing systems of both phase I reactions and phase II reactions (glucuronide, sulfate, and glutathione conjugation, and acetylation).

Changes in the distribution and activity of the cytochrome P-450 enzyme systems also occur with hepatic growth and maturation. The CYP3A family is homogeneously distributed across the liver parenchyma. However, during postnatal growth, expression of the CYP3A protein shifts toward the centrilobular region of the acinus. Furthermore, by adulthood, expression of CYP2A becomes increasingly limited to the midzonal and centrilobular hepatocytes, with sparse expression in the periportal regions.[8] Other examples of developmental changes in the cytochrome P-450 system involve the CYP2C and CYP3A3/4 systems. The CYP2C subfamily has negligible expression in the fetus but has significant, increased expression in the first few weeks of life.[9] Lacroix and associates demonstrated decreased levels of CYP3A3/4 mRNA levels in fetuses and infants compared with adults.[10] Changes in activity of the various CYP enzyme families and the subfamilies have been correlated with drug clearance. Specifically, midazolam clearance correlates with changes in CYP3A4 activity (decreased clearance in fetal and neonatal livers with increase to adult values [400-500 mL/hr/kg] by 3 months of age).[11,12] The opposite holds for CYP3A7, whose activity peaks at about 1 week post partum and steadily diminishes during the first year of life, finally reaching adult levels of approximately 10% that of fetal livers.

Phase II Reactions

Hepatic biotransformation also involves the phase II reactions of conjugation. Conjugation decreases the lipid solubility of compounds and facilitates their excretion.[13] Conjugation reactions include sulfation, glucuronidation, methylation, glutathione conjugation, and acetylation. Development of these systems is enzyme specific, but the overall activity of enzymes involved in these processes appear to be decreased in infants when compared with adults.[14]

Glucuronidation is catalyzed by the uridine 5′-diphosphate (UDP)-glucuronosyltransferase (UGT), with more than 18 members constituting two families: UGT1A and UGT2B. Separate genes give rise to the various members of the UGT2 family, whereas alternative splicing of a single gene transcript leads to the diverse nature of the UGT1A family.[15] UGT enzymes are responsible for the metabolism of several drugs and drug metabolites, including phenols, estrogens, and opioids. As with the enzymes of the CYP 450 system, individual enzymes demonstrate substrate specificity and can act in concert to metabolize single compounds. The ontogeny of the family of UGT enzymes is poorly described. Glucuronidation is limited in infants, leading, in part, to the risk of toxic drug accumulation in this population.[16] Studies have shown low levels of hepatic UGT enzymes during both fetal and early postnatal development. By approximately 3 months of age, infants have reduced levels of the full range of enzymes, estimated at 25% of adult levels.[17] Clearance of morphine, demonstrated by in-vivo pharmacokinetics, is decreased in infants, supporting the finding of immature UGT pathways.

UGT1A, whose postulated substrates include bilirubin and ethinylestradiol, shows decreased activity in the fetus, with rapid increase in activity and protein levels until adult levels are reached at 3 to 6 months.[18] UGT1A6, having acetaminophen and naproxen as substrates, has been shown to have 10% of adult activity in the fetus and neonate, with only 50% activity levels at 6 months of age.[16] Another important UGT enzyme is UGT 2B7, which is, in part, responsible for the metabolism of nonsteroidal anti-inflammatory drugs, naloxone, codeine, and lorazepam. Fetal activity approaches 10% to 20% of adult levels, with a rapid increase to adult levels by 2 months of age.[19]

Sulfate conjugation is accomplished by sulfotransferases, a family of cytosolic enzymes that are divided into two categories: catechol and phenol sulfotransferase. These enzymes conjugate inorganic sulfate from 3′-phosphoadenosine-5′-sulfophosphate (PAPS) with compounds containing functional hydroxyl groups.[13] The catechol transferases develop earlier in fetal life than the phenol counterparts and appear to exhibit decreased activity in the developing neonate. Whereas specific sulfotransferase substrates remain to be identified, the activity of these enzymes is increased in fetuses and neonates and theorized to be an efficient pathway in this age group. Because it has been shown that UGT and sulfotransferases have overlapping specificity, and because the UGT pathway is deficient in neonates compared with adults, sulfation is the predominant pathway for detoxification and homeostasis.

Glutathione S-transferases (GSTs) act to conjugate glutathione with a broad spectrum of lipophilic and electrophilic compounds. The family of GSTs is composed of up to five different groups in various classes designated μ, α, θ, and π, believed to arise from at least three different genetic loci.[20] Tissue-specific expression of these enzymes has been demonstrated, with the liver expressing the greatest amount of protein. Variable time-dependent expression has also been shown, because α- and π-class GSTs are greatly expressed between 16 and 24 weeks gestation, whereas only α-class enzymes predominate in the neonate and adult liver.[21] The hepatic π-class enzymes disappear from their hepatocellular location by 6 months of age and can be found only in the epithelial cells of the biliary canaliculi.

Unfortunately, the variability of the developmental expression of this class of enzymes makes understanding their clinical implications difficult.[21] What has been suggested by the limited data available is that the developmental pattern appears well developed in the infant and, as is the case with the other enzymes systems, very substrate dependent.

Acetylation phase II reactions are catalyzed by *N*-acetyltransferases, which act to transfer an acetyl group from acetyl-CoA to one of their substrates (e.g., *p*-aminobenzoic acid, *p*-aminosalicylic acid, and procainamide). Two genes, *NAT1* and *NAT2*, have been identified and yield two specific enzymes with different allelic forms. Despite sharing approximately 87% sequence homology, these enzymes exhibit different substrate specificity.[22] They are cytosolic enzymes involved in the biotransformation of several drugs and the bioactivation of several human carcinogens. Only NAT2 has exhibited polymorphisms that divide patients into slow and rapid acetylators. While NAT1 has been found in a multitude of tissues, NAT2 is located primarily in the liver. NAT1 is present in fetal tissues, whereas NAT2 appears at 1 year of age and, as such, extrahepatic sources account for the majority of *N*-acetyltransferase substrate metabolism in this age group. The rate of maturation is variable and, in part, is related to their status as slow versus rapid acetylators. Infants younger than 1 year of age are, for the most part, slow acetylators, followed by age-dependent alterations leading to each individual's targeted acetylator status.[23] Individuals who are genetically rapid acetylators will become fast acetylators by 2 to 4 years of age. Although specific data regarding the ontogenesis of these enzymes and their specific substrates is scant, it appears that the process of acetylation is limited in infants and does not reach adult levels until 1 to 2 years of age.

Anesthetic Agents

The discovery of the clinical benefit of ether and chloroform in the 1840s marked the beginning of the modern era of anesthesia, despite ether's initial discovery dating back to 1275 by Spanish chemist Raymundus Lullius. Ether was first synthesized in 1540 by a German chemist Valerius Cordus around the time that its hypnotic effects had been recorded. The use of ether as a surgical anesthetic was not identified until 1842, when Dr. Crawford Williamson Long used it as the anesthetic to remove a tumor from the neck of a patient. More widespread acceptance of ether, however, did not occur until 1846, following a successful demonstration by Drs. William T. G. Morton and John Collins Warren at Massachusetts General Hospital.[24] Both ether and chloroform remained the most popular anesthetics well into the 20th century, despite notable problems with their use. Chloroform is known to depress the cardiac and respiratory systems, has an arrhythmogenic effect, and is significantly nephrotoxic and hepatotoxic, causing cellular necrosis in both organs. Newer volatile anesthetics were developed in the 20th century to circumvent these unwanted effects.

Halothane was first introduced in the 1950s and shown to be nonirritating, rapid acting, and potent, as well as easy to administer compared with ether and chloroform.[25] Suckling first synthesized it in 1951, and it was used clinically by Johnstone in 1956. Several studies have shown an association between exposure to halothane and development of severe liver injury, prompting its replacement with newer, less hepatotoxic agents, such as enflurane, isoflurane, desflurane, and sevoflurane.

Inhalation Anesthetic Metabolism

The volatile anesthetics are poorly metabolized in humans, with only about 20% of inhaled halothane undergoing biotransformation. Both distinct oxidative and reductive pathways are involved in its metabolism, a process catalyzed by the CYP450 enzymes. The reductive pathway, accomplished by a variety of CYP enzymes, is the lesser utilized of the two, occurring more commonly at low oxygen tensions. Through this pathway, an electron is inserted to create a trifluorochlorobromoethyl radical as the initial step in metabolism. The major pathway of metabolism of halothane is the oxidative route, by which an oxygen species is inserted into the compound, leading to debromination and producing trifluoroacetyl chloride, the reactive intermediate.[26] This compound can undergo further glutathione conjugation and covalent binding to lipids and proteins or interact with water to yield the urinary metabolite trifluoracetate. While several enzymes accomplish the reductive step, the oxidative pathway is preferentially catalyzed by CYP2E1.[27]

The other inhaled volatile anesthetics are metabolized to a lesser degree than halothane and do not undergo the reductive process. Both enflurane and isoflurane are metabolized by CYP2E1, with 2% to 4% metabolism of enflurane and 0.2% for isoflurane.[28] Enflurane undergoes glucuronide conjugation before being excreted in the urine or binds covalently to liver proteins.[29] Isoflurane, on the other hand, is excreted as inorganic fluoride and trifluoracetic acid, following oxidative metabolism in the liver.[30] Desflurane is the least metabolized of the volatile anesthetics—0.02%, approximately 10% the rate of isoflurane.[31] Both are metabolized in the liver along similar paths because the urinary metabolite for desflurane, trifluoroacetic acid, is the same as for isoflurane.

Only 2% to 5% of inhaled sevoflurane is metabolized in humans, through the hepatic CYP2E1, just as the other anesthetics.[32] Oxidation of sevoflurane generates an intermediate known as formyl fluoride, a highly reactive species believed to generate liver protein adducts. Both carbon dioxide and inorganic fluoride are released through this oxidative mechanism, with the final product being hexafluoroisopropanol, which undergoes glucuronide conjugation and is further excreted in the urine.[33]

Neuromuscular Blocking Drugs

Neuromuscular blockade causing muscle paralysis is achieved by a variety of different mechanisms and essentially by two different classes of compounds: depolarizing and nondepolarizing neuromuscular blockers. Both groups act at the acetylcholine receptor; however, they differ significantly in the manner in which they are metabolized. Liver disease, such as is seen in children with cirrhosis or hepatitis, can significantly affect the action of this class of compounds.[34]

The only depolarizing agent still in use is short-acting suxamethonium (succinylcholine), having been largely replaced by the nondepolarizing variety.[35] Succinylcholine is hydrolyzed by plasma cholinesterases (pseudocholinesterase), which are a group of proteins synthesized by the liver and only by functioning hepatocytes. It has been shown that 0% of this medication is excreted through the biliary or renal system, as it is completely metabolized by these circulating proteins.[36] There is a direct correlation between the level of circulating cholinesterases and the degree of liver disease. Enzyme activity is decreased in those with liver disease[37] and varies widely with the age of the child.

Nondepolarizing muscle relaxants are divided into two groups: aminosteroids and benzyl isoquinolinium diesters. The first group consists of pipecuronium bromide, pancuronium, vecuronium, and rocuronium bromide. The latter group contains doxacurium chloride, atracurium, and cisatracurium besylate. Although there is little effect on their pharmacokinetics from age (outside the neonatal period) or gender or even anesthetic technique (as is the case with inhalation anesthetics), the concomitant presence of renal and/or hepatic disease plays a significant role in their safety and efficacy.[34] Hepatic elimination, although minimal in this class of compounds, is dependent on protein binding, hepatic blood flow, and drug extraction. The volume of drug distribution is increased in hepatic disease, leading to both a slower onset and prolonged effect. In children with cholestatic liver disease, such as biliary atresia, Alagille syndrome, and the group of diseases known as progressive familial intrahepatic cholestasis, uptake of these compounds by the liver is decreased, which decreases plasma clearance and prolongs their effects.[38,39] Approximately 75% of the administered dose of these medications is bound to plasma proteins, with the majority to albumin. Despite this, children with liver disease and a correspondingly low albumin level are at minimal risk of adverse effects from this group of drugs.[40] As a rule, the pharmacokinetics of this class of compounds is generally minimally affected by the concomitant presence of mild hepatic dysfunction, with the exception of vecuronium and rocuronium. Rocuronium is an analogue of vecuronium, with a more rapid onset of action. Compared with the other members of this group, which largely undergo renal excretion, rocuronium appears to be minimally cleared through the kidney, at 12% to 22% of the administered dose.[41] In the presence of hepatic disease, the volume of distribution of rocuronium increased by 33% versus healthy controls.[42] Another study demonstrated that the clearance was decreased by 28% in cirrhotic patients versus healthy adults, while three separate studies observed a β-elimination half-life ($T^{1}/_{2}β$) increase between 46% and 74%.[43] The receptor sensitivity, as measured by the EC_{50} remained unchanged between the two groups.[43] Another study examined the pharmacokinetics of rocuronium during three phases of liver transplantation[44]; the extent of drug clearance was only slightly reduced in the diseased native liver when compared with both the functioning allograft and healthy individuals. The investigators concluded that the degree of hepatic dysfunction exerts little influence in hepatic drug elimination.[44] Another study examined the infusion requirements of rocuronium during the three phases of hepatic transplantation.[45] They concluded that reduced infusion requirements may be an indicator of graft dysfunction and that this was due to changes in the pharmacodynamics associated with liver dysfunction. The increased volume of distribution of rocuronium in patients with liver disease is believed to lead to its extended effect, especially in instances of prolonged drug exposure during lengthy surgical procedures.[45]

The role of hepatic elimination of the second class of neuromuscular blockers, benzyl isoquinolinium, is yet to be determined but hepatic dysfunction has been noted to affect their efficacy. Doxacurium, despite high concentration in biliary secretions, does not exhibit altered pharmacokinetics in the presence of hepatocellular injury. It has been noted that recovery parameters are prolonged in this group.[46] Mivacurium (no longer available in the United States), which exists as three stereoisomers, *cis-cis*, *cis-trans*, and *trans-trans*, shows variable negative effects when administered to patients with liver disease. Both the *trans-trans* and *cis-trans* have a decrease in clearance when compared with healthy controls.[47] The clearance of the third isomer is unchanged in liver disease. Prolonged recovery was also noted, secondary to a decrease in plasma cholinesterases found with significant liver disease.[47] Cisatracurium has been shown to have decreased clearance compared with healthy individuals, with no delay in recovery and minimal delay in onset of action. Children with liver disease, regardless of cause, generally tolerate this class of compounds, with no observed toxicity.[48]

Sedatives, Opioids, and Liver Disease

The commonly used sedatives midazolam, propofol, and ketamine all undergo hepatic metabolism, via both oxidation and conjugation. These compounds are all lipid soluble and their effects are altered by liver disease.[49] Midazolam has a high clearance rate that is, in part, dependent on hepatic blood flow. In children with cirrhosis, the clearance of midazolam is halved with a corresponding doubling of the half-life compared with healthy controls.[50] Also, because 95% to 97% is bound to albumin, diseases decreasing the level of albumin will lead to an increased free fraction of drug and a greater effect pharmacodynamically.[51,52] Propofol is eliminated primarily in the urine (>88%), and hepatocellular injury does not alter its pharmacokinetics.[53] Ketamine is also highly lipophilic and undergoes metabolism in the liver. However, unlike the others just mentioned, it does so via methylation and its clearance is minimally affected by liver dysfunction.[54]

Opioid effects are a direct result of their binding to specific receptors. The more opioid that binds to the receptors due to a greater concentration available at the target, the greater the corresponding effect. Hepatic clearance and protein binding are two methods by which this concentration can be altered.[55] The major metabolic pathway for opioids is via oxidation in the liver, with morphine, buprenorphine, and remifentanil being exceptions. The first two undergo glucuronidation, whereas the latter is metabolized via ester hydrolysis. The ability of the diseased liver to oxidize these compounds is diminished, leading to increased oral bioavailability secondary to decreased first-pass metabolism and decreased drug clearance. Interestingly, the clearance of morphine, despite being metabolized by glucuronidation, is also negatively affected by the presence of cirrhosis.[56] Clearance of drugs that are highly extracted by the liver, such as meperidine, is dependent on hepatic blood flow.[57,58] Clearance is a function of hepatic blood flow (Q_H) and the extraction ratio (E_H), describing the ability of the liver to efficiently remove the drug. This clearance is described by

$$CL_H = Q_H \times E_H$$

In situations in which E_H is greater than 0.7, as with meperidine, lidocaine, and pentazocine, CL_H approaches Q_H.

Conditions that alter hepatic blood flow, such as cirrhosis, portal vein thrombosis, and portacaval shunting, will significantly alter the clearance of these drugs. On the other end of spectrum, drugs with low E_H, such as methadone and naproxen, are not dependent on hepatic blood flow. The metabolic activity of the liver and the plasma protein-binding fraction affect the clearance to a greater degree. The hepatic clearance of these drugs is described by

$$CL_H = CL_{INT} \times f_u$$

where f_u is the fraction of unbound drug and CL_{INT} describes the metabolic activity. When the f_u is low, as with methadone (<0.1), the clearance is mainly affected by reduced enzyme capacity.[55]

The analgesic effect of codeine, obtained after its demethylation to morphine, is reduced in the presence of liver disease. Liver disease can affect glucuronidation and thereby decrease clearance and prolong the half-life of morphine.[59] Alfentanil has been shown to have decreased protein binding and reduced clearance in the presence of hepatic dysfunction,[60,61] whereas methadone has a prolonged half-life and increased volume of distribution in severe dysfunction.[62] Fentanyl, remifentanil, and sufentanil appear to have unaffected pharmacokinetics in the presence of significant hepatic dysfunction.[63-65] Because the degree of dysfunction exhibits interindividual variability, the level of adverse events of these medications is also variable. Careful use in and monitoring of children with liver disease is required when administering opioids.

Anesthetic Effects on Normal Hepatic Cellular Functions

Carbohydrates

Carbohydrates account for the majority of the energy sources ingested by humans. The primary monosaccharides are glucose, fructose, and galactose, with glucose being the most important because both fructose and galactose are converted into glucose for use. The rate and degree of glucose metabolism is influenced by the availability of the substrate, the rate of entry into cells, and the ability of the target organ to convert glucose into energy or synthesize it into fats. In healthy individuals, hepatic glucose production accounts for the majority of whole-body glucose production and is narrowly regulated both directly and indirectly by insulin.[66] Insulin directly inhibits gluconeogenesis and glycogenolysis by binding to insulin receptors in the liver, thereby diminishing hepatic glucose production, as demonstrated in the liver-specific insulin receptor knockout (LIRKO) mouse.[67] Of the glucose available to the liver, about 50% undergoes glycolysis and is converted to energy. Thirty to 40 percent is converted to fat for storage, and 10% to 20% is shunted to glycogen.[68] Studies have shown that anesthetics inhibit glucose uptake by hepatocytes, an action now termed the *anti-insulin effect of anesthesia.* Although all inhaled anesthetics exhibit this tendency, halothane had the greatest impact on serum glucose, with isoflurane and sevoflurane having lesser effects.[69,70] Anesthetic concentrations of 1 and 2 MAC can inhibit glucose uptake by as much as 50%. The combined effects of anesthetics and stress from surgery or trauma increase serum glucose concentrations.

Gluconeogenesis requires functional mitochondria and is a process that generates glucose from lactate and pyruvate. Gluconeogenesis is the major pathway of reducing lactate. It is also a sensitive measure and indication of anesthetic-induced metabolic alterations. Halothane decreases gluconeogenesis in the isolated perfused rat liver[71]; in adults, exposure to halothane, through increased oxygen extraction from the splanchnic vasculature, has demonstrated that there is an increase in oxygen consumption and that release of hepatic glucose is decreased. Using a constant amino acid infusion in fasting individuals with and without exposure to halothane, the same investigators noted that halothane inhibited gluconeogenesis.[72]

Protein Synthesis

The impact of anesthesia and surgery on protein synthesis and metabolism is poorly understood. Albumin, a large, soluble, single polypeptide protein with a molecular weight of 66 kD, is an important protein synthesized by the liver. Six to 12 g is produced per day and can be increased twofold to threefold depending on the individual's needs. Albumin functions as a binding and transport protein and maintains colloid oncotic pressure. Albumin plasma levels are a simple assessment of hepatic function. Any action that injures the liver, either through ischemia or toxin-mediated damage, will negatively impact the synthesis of albumin and other proteins. Diethyl ether causes reversible inhibition of protein synthesis in rat hepatocytes,[73] whereas halothane and enflurane block protein synthesis in a dose-dependent manner.[74] Other investigators have shown that halothane, sevoflurane, and enflurane inhibit protein synthesis and secretion and that this may be an early indicator of hepatic cytotoxic injury. In fact, the hepatic protein synthesis rate has been utilized as a predictor of viability in liver transplantation.[75]

Bilirubin Metabolism

Bilirubin is the end product of heme metabolism, which results from erythrocyte destruction and release of heme. Heme is converted to unconjugated bilirubin via macrophages in the spleen and bone marrow and transported to the liver bound to plasma albumin, for further conjugation and excretion. Uptake of unconjugated bilirubin is a carrier-mediated process, which exhibits saturation effects in that this carrier is also shared by bile acids and bacterial endotoxins. The liver conjugates it to glucuronate, taurine, and, to a lesser extent, glucose via glucuronosyltransferase, thereby converting it to a water-soluble compound that is excreted in the bile. Secretion of bilirubin across the canalicular space is the rate-limiting step in bilirubin metabolism and involves an active transport against a concentration gradient. Secretion is ordinarily not affected by hepatic disease. Injury to the liver can lead to elevations of both conjugated and/or unconjugated bilirubin, evidenced clinically as jaundice. Unconjugated bilirubin, given its lipophilic status, can easily diffuse across the blood-brain barrier and cause irreversible brain injury, known as kernicterus.

Engelking and colleagues looked at bile excretion and serum bilirubin levels in horses that were exposed to halothane for 2 hours. Under constant bile acid infusion, to maintain steady-state bile flow, they noted that halothane caused a 138% increase in excretion and a 16% serum bilirubin concentration reduction. They concluded that exposure to the anesthetic did not alter bile flow and that hepatic injury due to halothane occurred via a different mechanism.[76]

Hepatotoxicity

A consensus definition of liver injury as it pertains to hepatotoxic drugs was outlined in 1989 by a panel of 12 European and

a 1-year-old child with hepatoblastoma. This child survived 13 months.

Despite the initial success of the first pediatric liver transplant, the 1-year survival rate in subsequent transplant patients remained less than 50%. In 1979, with the introduction of cyclosporine, the 1-year patient survival increased to 70%.[3,4] In 1989, FK-506 (tacrolimus) was introduced and replaced cyclosporine[5] and the 1-year survival further increased to approximately 80%.

Demographics and Epidemiology

The number of liver transplants performed in the United States has increased steadily between 1988 and 2005, from 1,713 transplants to 6,444, mostly in adults. The annual number of pediatric liver transplants increased from 509 in 1990 to 587 in 2000, where it remains. This is only a 10% to 11% increase, compared with the 169% increase in adult liver transplants (2,177 in 1990 to 5,875), according to the United Network for Organ Sharing (UNOS) Scientific Registry as of 2005. The indications for liver transplantation are listed in Table 29-1 (see website). In children, the most common cause for liver transplantation is cholestatic liver disease secondary to biliary atresia, particularly in infants (50%),[6] although cholestatic liver disease secondary to total parenteral nutrition has become more common, accounting for approximately 5% of pediatric liver transplants. After cholestatic liver disease, metabolic disorders and acute hepatic failure are the next most common causes for pediatric liver transplantation. In the past, the most common metabolic disorders in decreasing frequency were α_1-antitrypsin deficiency, tyrosinemia, Wilson disease, oxalosis, and glycogen storage diseases. Currently, a greater percentage of transplants for metabolic disorders are being performed for maple syrup urine disease and cystic fibrosis (UNOS/OPTN.org).

The cause of acute or fulminant hepatic failure in the majority of children is not known. Acetaminophen is the most common cause of drug/toxin-induced liver failure.[7] Viral agents are the second leading cause of acute hepatic failure, and toxins are a distant third.

Indications for liver transplantation in children include the presence of an underlying primary liver pathologic process, with acute or chronic liver failure caused by cholestatic liver disease, metabolic disorders, tumors, toxins, cirrhosis, and other derangements (e.g., Budd-Chiari syndrome) (see Table 29-1 on website). There are few absolute contraindications to pediatric liver transplantation. Children with neoplastic processes such as hepatocellular carcinoma and infectious processes such as human immunodeficiency virus infection undergo transplantation. However, those with acute infections from bacterial or fungal agents, metastatic neoplasm, or disease processes that are considered an immediate threat to life (severe cardiopulmonary disease, sepsis/septic shock) are generally not accepted for transplantation.

Allocation of the available livers to the appropriate recipients has been a challenge. Initially, liver transplant candidates were prioritized based on geographic location and medical condition as defined by the Child-Turcotte-Pugh (CTP) score. Children were ranked as status 1, 2a, 2b, or 3. Status 1 children received the highest priority and were defined by the presence of acute liver failure of less than 6 weeks or a failed liver transplant within 1 week. Status 2a, 2b, and 3 were defined by their CTP score and time on the wait list.[8] Efforts by the UNOS/Organ Procure-

ment and Transplantation Network (OPTN) Liver Disease Severity Scale (LDSS) committee to identify predictors of mortality in patients with chronic liver disease resulted in the Model for End-Stage Liver Disease (MELD) and the Pediatric End-Stage Liver Disease (PELD) severity scores. The PELD score incorporates variables for age, growth failure, serum albumin, bilirubin, and international normalized ratio (INR) (Table 29-2, see website). Serum creatinine is incorporated in the MELD score because it predicts mortality for adult patients waiting for liver transplantation. This value may predict survival after liver transplantation but it does not predict mortality in the child awaiting liver transplantation.[9]

The allocation of deceased liver donors has changed with the new MELD/PELD policy. Before this policy, organs from donors younger than 18 years old were distributed only to pediatric recipients. With the new policy, the donor graft is first allocated to a status 1 pediatric recipient in the local region. If none is available, it is offered to the next status 1 adult in the region. If no status 1 adult is available, the liver is made available to pediatric patients with more than a 50% risk of mortality. Adults with mortality risk greater than 50% are next, and then all pediatric patients are offered the graft over all other adult candidates. If there are no appropriate pediatric recipients in the region, the donor organ is offered to the national pool.[10] Early analysis of pre- and post-MELD/PELD data indicates that access to donor livers has not decreased with the new system (in fact, it may have increased) and mortality while waiting for a transplant has decreased, especially in children younger than 2 years old. It is not clear yet whether the PELD scoring system has affected survival in children. For children with scores less than 10, there may not be a survival benefit. However, other outcomes such as improved growth and cognitive function need to be evaluated.[11]

Pathophysiology of Liver Disease

The liver is the only organ that can regenerate itself when damaged. The stigmata and multiorgan involvement from endstage liver disease arise from the loss of hepatocytes, which results in fibrosis that, in turn, leads to decreased synthetic function and portal hypertension. This cellular dysfunction is manifested by coagulopathy, hypocholesterolemia, hypoalbuminemia, and encephalopathy. Attempts at cellular regeneration result in fibrosis and destruction of the portal triad with increased resistance to liver blood flow that causes portal hypertension. Portal hypertension is manifested by varices (esophageal, bowel), hemorrhoids, ascites, spontaneous bacterial peritonitis, splenomegaly with thrombocytopenia, and hepatic encephalopathy.

Cardiac Manifestations

Cardiac disturbances occur because of altered physiology, congenital heart defects, and toxic side effects. A hyperdynamic circulation secondary to vasodilation with a compensatory increase in cardiac output characterizes the altered cardiac physiology from liver disease, which likely results from vasoactive mediators. These mediators or gut-derived "humoral factors" (nitric oxide [NO], tumor necrosis factor [TNF]-α, endocannabinoids) enter the systemic circulation through portosystemic collaterals and bypass the hepatic detoxification that usually occurs.[12] Shunting also occurs at the level of the skin and the lungs. Mixed venous saturation increases in children with liver disease. Poor oxygen extraction likely explains the increased mixed venous saturation.

Cardiomyopathy associated with portal hypertension is well characterized in adults but not in children. However, children with liver disease can develop a cardiomyopathy for other reasons. Inborn errors of metabolism,[13] including Wilson disease, oxalosis, glycogen storage disease type III, and Gaucher disease as well as other syndromes are associated with cardiomyopathies and cardiac anomalies. Tacrolimus and cyclosporin A have also been associated with hypertrophic cardiomyopathy in animal studies and in pediatric liver transplant recipients.[14-16] Echocardiographic assessment of cardiac function is generally well preserved in children receiving tacrolimus, although subtle cardiovascular changes that predispose a small percentage of children to develop hypertrophic cardiomyopathy have been reported.[17] Alagille disease is commonly associated with pulmonary stenosis, coarctation, tetralogy of Fallot, and atrial and ventricular septal defects.

QT prolongation has also been described in adult patients with alcoholic liver disease and may be associated with sudden cardiac death.[18] A decrease in K^+ currents in cardiomyocytes in rats with cirrhosis may provide a possible mechanism for the QT prolongation. Children with liver failure may also have an increase in QT interval (QTc > 450 msec in 18% of children with liver disease), possibly increasing the risk for ventricular arrhythmias. However, they do appear to be transient and reversible with liver transplantation.[19] Nonselective β blockade has also been shown to reduce the QT prolongation, but it is unclear if this reduces the risk of arrhythmias or improves survival.[20] Although QT prolongation may be fairly common in children with liver disease, more recent data do not suggest that it predicts decreased survival.[21]

Pulmonary Manifestations

Hallmarks of the pulmonary manifestations of liver disease are hypoxia and pulmonary hypertension. Hypoxia is secondary to hepatopulmonary syndrome and ventilation/perfusion mismatch from atelectasis due to tense ascites, hepatosplenomegaly, and/or pleural effusions. Hepatopulmonary syndrome is characterized by hypoxia from intrapulmonary arteriovenous shunting and intrapulmonary vascular dilatation.[22] The diagnosis is predicated on either arterial hypoxia ($PaO_2 < 70$ mm Hg) or an alveolar-arterial gradient greater than 20 mm Hg in the setting of pulmonary vascular dilatation. Intrapulmonary vascular dilatation can best be demonstrated on echocardiography or lung perfusion scan with macroaggregated albumin.[23] Hepatopulmonary syndrome occurs in 15% to 20% of adults with cirrhosis[24] and in 0.5% to 20% of infants and children as young as 6 months of age.[25] It appears to be more prevalent in those with biliary atresia and polysplenia syndrome.[25,26] Treatment of hypoxia is long-term supplemental oxygen. Definitive treatment is liver transplantation. In a case series of seven children with hepatopulmonary syndrome who were successfully transplanted, all recovered from their hepatopulmonary syndrome postoperatively, with their hypoxia resolving within an average of 24 weeks.[27]

Portopulmonary hypertension (PPH) is defined by the World Health Organization (WHO) as pulmonary artery hypertension (pulmonary systolic pressure ≥25 mm Hg) in the setting of normal pulmonary capillary wedge pressure and portal hypertension.[28] The incidence of PPH is 0.2% to 0.7% in adults with cirrhosis and 3% to 9% of adults who present for liver transplantation.[29] The number of children with PPH is not known, but occurrences are limited to case reports and one case series. The signs and symptoms of PPH on presentation include a new heart murmur, dyspnea, and syncope. Echocardiography can diagnose pulmonary hypertension in children and adults with PPH.[30] The severity of PPH predicts mortality. In a retrospective review, mild PPH did not increase mortality in adults who underwent orthotopic liver transplantation (OLT). In contrast, moderate PPH (pulmonary artery pressure [PAP]) = 35 to 45 mm Hg) increased the mortality to 50% in those who underwent OLT and severe PPH (PAP > 50 mm Hg) increased it to 100%.[31]

There are no recommendations for the management of children with PPH. Early identification is essential, and this may be achieved by performing echocardiography in all children who present for liver transplantation. If it is present, cardiac catheterization should be performed to confirm the diagnosis, measure the PAPs, and assess the response to NO and epoprostenol. Children who respond to medical management may be candidates for liver transplantation.[32] Otherwise, severe PPH is generally a contraindication for liver transplantation because of the increased risk of mortality.

Neurologic Manifestations

Hepatic encephalopathy is a significant neurologic complication of liver disease that is classified as either acute (seen in fulminant hepatic failure) or chronic (seen in chronic cirrhosis or chronic portal hypertension). The classification of the severity of acute and chronic hepatic encephalopathy is similar and is shown in Table 29-3 (West Haven Staging of Hepatic Encephalopathy). The pathophysiology is not entirely known, but cerebral edema appears to be a feature of both forms. The cerebral edema is more severe in acute hepatic encephalopathy and can cause increased intracranial pressure (ICP). Ammonia has been repeatedly implicated in the pathogenesis. It is postulated to cause astrocytes to swell, leading to low-grade cerebral edema.[33,34] The two major sources of ammonia in humans are from catabolism of endogenous protein and gastrointestinal absorption. Bacterial breakdown of nitrogen-containing products in the gut results in ammonia formation, which is then absorbed into the portal circulation. Factors that can increase blood ammonia levels and exacerbate the signs and symptoms of hepatic encephalopathy include increased catabolism from infection, increased gut absorption from high protein diets, constipation, and

Table 29-3. West Haven Staging Classification of the Severity of Acute and Chronic Hepatic Encephalopathy

Grade	Description
0	Detectable only by neuropsychological testing
1	Lack of awareness, euphoria, or anxiety; shortened attention span; impaired addition and subtraction
2	Lethargy, minimal disorientation to time, personality change, inappropriate behavior
3	Somnolence but responsive to verbal stimuli, confusion, gross disorientation, bizarre behavior
4	Comatose

An important issue that is rarely communicated to the ward team when the child is admitted for surgery is that all preoperative intravenous access should be placed in the lower extremities. This ensures that none of the veins that the anesthesiologist will require intraoperatively (i.e., those originating in the upper extremities or neck) will be compromised preoperatively.

A key portion of the preoperative evaluation is the preparation of the child and the family for the anticipated risks, benefits, and clinical course. Informed consent should include a discussion about the use of blood products and risks associated with prolonged positioning (peripheral nerve injury, occipital alopecia). Specifically, the child will likely remain anesthetized, intubated, and mechanically ventilated in the immediate postoperative period and may have significant facial and extremity edema. Likewise, informing the family about the potential number and location of the intravascular catheters and their associated risks can be helpful in preparing them to see their child postoperatively.

Intraoperative Care

Appropriate intraoperative care requires an understanding of the surgical and anesthetic issues. Several factors affect the child's physiology, including the underlying pathophysiology of liver disease, surgery, and response to anesthetics. In general, the surgical approach for OLT in children is similar to that in adults. The most significant difference is the reduced size of the recipient. The obstacles imposed by the size of the child include a smaller blood volume, more challenging vascular access, size restriction of donor graft, venovenous bypass, and incidence of surgical complications such as hepatic artery thrombosis.

During the preoperative assessment, children older than age 1 year will likely be anxious. They should be premedicated, for example, with oral midazolam. Those who are encephalopathic, however, should not be premedicated.

Most children are considered to have a full stomach because of delayed gastric emptying from ascites, gastrointestinal bleeding, hepatic encephalopathy, and the nonelective nature of most transplants. The exception may be the child who presents for an "elective" transplant without any stigmata of portal hypertension (e.g., Crigler-Najjar syndrome). Those considered to have a full stomach should receive a rapid-sequence intravenous induction. Induction agents should be tailored to meet the needs of the child, but etomidate (0.2-0.3 mg/kg), sodium thiopental (4-6 mg/kg), propofol (2-4 mg/kg), and ketamine (2 mg/kg) are all suitable choices. Appropriate muscle relaxants for rapid-sequence induction include succinylcholine and high-dose rocuronium because of their rapid onset. Children who are not at risk for aspiration can have an inhalation induction with sevoflurane and nitrous oxide. The use of nitrous oxide is not recommended after induction because it may increase the risk of bowel distention and expansion of gas emboli.

The trachea should be secured with a cuffed or uncuffed endotracheal tube. If the tracheal tube is uncuffed, the leak should be 15 to 20 cm H_2O peak inflation pressure or greater. Some children may require high inspiratory pressures to achieve adequate ventilation in the perioperative period because of atelectasis from pleural effusions and ascites, surgical retractors placed on the abdominal and chest wall, and a tight abdominal closure. PEEP should be used during all liver transplantations.

Anesthesia is typically maintained with an inhalational agent, an opioid, and a muscle relaxant. Isoflurane, sevoflurane, or desflurane may be used because they are readily available, undergo minimal hepatic metabolism, and appear to have minimal adverse effects on the liver, although all three have been associated with isolated case reports of hepatotoxicity.[51-53] Propofol may also be used, particularly if the child is susceptible to malignant hyperthermia. Even though the primary metabolic pathway for propofol is hepatic, there appears to be extrahepatic metabolism in the lung, kidney, and intestine.[54,55] However, when used for a prolonged period, the pharmacokinetics of propofol switch from a short-acting to long-acting anesthetic and the risk of propofol infusion syndrome becomes a substantive concern (see Chapter 6). Neuromuscular blockade can be maintained with any nondepolarizing muscle relaxant. Pancuronium may have the advantages of tachycardia, prolonged duration of action, and low cost. The disadvantage of pancuronium, rocuronium, and vecuronium is their partial hepatic metabolism, but this can be overcome with appropriate monitoring and dose adjustments. Dose requirements of continuous infusions of rocuronium, vecuronium, and pancuronium are reduced during the anhepatic phase of transplantation but return to initial values after reperfusion.[56] There is no change in the dose requirements of atracurium during the anhepatic phase.[57] Atracurium or cisatracurium may be ideal in children with combined hepatic and renal insufficiency because they are cleared by Hoffman elimination and do not rely on hepatic or renal function.

The liver metabolizes all opioids, with the exception of remifentanil, which is metabolized by plasma and tissue esterases. The metabolic pathway for most opioids is oxidation, although morphine undergoes glucuronidation.[58] There is evidence that the elimination half-life and clearance of alfentanil and fentanyl are not dramatically altered in those with cholestatic and cirrhotic liver disease.[59,60] Fentanyl, sufentanil, alfentanil, and morphine have all been used during liver transplantation. Fentanyl is commonly selected and is usually administered as a bolus during induction (2-10 µg/kg) and maintained as an infusion throughout the anesthetic and the immediate postoperative period (2-5 µg/kg/hr).

Vascular access is important for resuscitation and monitoring. At least two peripheral upper extremity intravenous catheters should be placed together with a central venous line for resuscitation. The central venous line can also be used to monitor trends in central venous pressure and to measure superior vena cava oxygen saturation (a surrogate marker for $S\bar{v}O_2$). Larger children tolerate rapid infusion catheters placed in upper extremities. Blood loss during the surgery can be significant with estimates between 0.5 to 25 blood volumes (mean: ~4 blood volumes).[46] Fluid warmers and infusion devices (see Chapters 10 and 53) need to be available to facilitate resuscitation if significant hemorrhage occurs. The Level 1 Rapid Infuser has been associated with massive air emboli, and all air needs to be removed from the infusion bags before using the device.[61] More recent models of the Level 1 Rapid Infuser come with optional air detection, which may reduce the risk of air emboli. The Rapid Infusion System (RIS-Hemonetics) is no longer manufactured, but it was not routinely used in smaller recipients. The Belmont FMS is the replacement. Its maximum capacity of infusion is one half the capacity of the RIS but greater than the capacity of Level 1. The choice of resuscitation fluids should be limited to 0.9% normal saline and Plasmalyte. Lactated Ringer's is not recommended because the lactate will accumulate unmetabolized during the anhepatic stage. Many children with liver disease are hypoalbuminemic, and the use of 5% albumin is appropriate.

Standard monitoring should include an electrocardiogram, pulse oximetry (×2), noninvasive blood pressure, invasive arterial blood pressure, central venous pressure, and temperature. Other high technology monitoring that is commonly employed in adult liver transplantation includes transesophageal echocardiography (TEE), continuous cardiac output (CCO) catheter, bispectral index (BIS), venovenous bypass (VVBP), and more than one arterial catheter. In infants and children there are limitations to these monitors because of their size. A United States–based utilization survey found that TEE, CCO, BIS, and VVBP are used in 0%, 7.7%, 15.4%, and 7.7% of pediatric transplant centers, respectively.[62]

Hematologic and electrolyte changes are common during liver transplantation, and measurements of arterial blood gases, sodium, potassium, calcium, magnesium, hemoglobin, platelets, and coagulation parameters (PT, PTT, fibrinogen, and D-dimers) need to be performed frequently throughout the procedure. Most centers use either portable devices or an operating room laboratory. Assessment of coagulation variables can be obtained with thromboelastography. Although TEE is an effective clinical tool to assess dynamic clotting parameters, only 28% of pediatric transplant centers use this procedure routinely[62] (Fig. 29-1, see website).

Positioning is critical to prevent soft tissue and peripheral nerve injuries. All of the extremities should be padded, and all cables and wires need to be wrapped and protected from the skin. The head should be turned and repositioned periodically to prevent pressure sores and alopecia. Sponge crate pads are very effective to prevent pressure sores under the torso. To minimize the risk of peripheral neuropathy, the upper extremities should be abducted 90 degrees or less and positioned supine (palms up) or in the neutral position. The wrist should not be hyperextended for the arterial catheter.

Surgical Technique

The surgical approach to OLT is divided into four stages: hepatectomy, anhepatic, reperfusion, and biliary reconstruction.

Hepatectomy (Stage 1)

The initial description of OLT is referred to as the "classic" technique. In the "classic" approach the liver is dissected to its vascular supply and the suprahepatic and infrahepatic vena cava are clamped along with the portal vein and hepatic artery. The liver is removed en bloc (Fig. 29-2). The disadvantage of this approach is that the vena cava is cross clamped, thus reducing preload. The piggyback technique is the preferred approach for pediatric transplants because there is more flexibility with the organ size and it requires only partial clamping of the vena cava.[63] The liver is dissected away from the inferior vena cava, the short hepatic veins, portal vein, and left, right, and middle hepatic veins. The infrahepatic vena cava of the donor is oversewn, and the suprahepatic vena cava is anastomosed to the native hepatic veins (Figs. 29-3 and 29-4). This requires only partial clamping of the inferior vena cava. A portocaval shunt can be established for children who do not tolerate clamping of the portal vein. Typically, these recipients have not developed collateral flow secondary to portal hypertension (e.g., maple syrup urine disease).

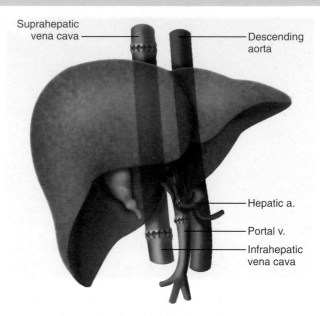

Figure 29-2. The classic approach for orthotopic liver transplantation. The suture lines are visible at the suprahepatic and infrahepatic anastomoses. (Starzl TE, Iwatsuki S, VanTheil DH, et al. Evolution of liver transplantation. Hepatology 1982; 2:614-636.)

There are several physiologic considerations that take place during the hepatic dissection that affect the anesthetic management. Hypotension is common and can occur for a variety of reasons. These include changes to the cardiovascular, hematologic, and metabolic systems. The most common cause of hypotension includes hypovolemia secondary to hemorrhage and third space volume losses. Resuscitation with citrated blood products can result in hypocalcemia, and surgical manipulation

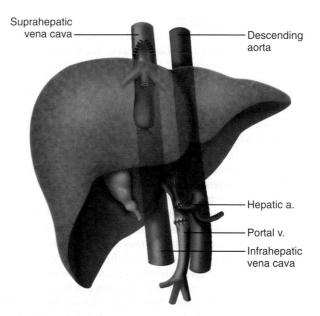

Figure 29-3. The piggyback technique preserves the inferior vena cava. This is the view of the liver graft after the recipient's hepatic confluence is anastomosed to the donor's IVC (the infrahepatic IVC of the donor is ligated). (From Tzakis A, Todo S, Starzl TE: Orthotopic liver transplantation with preservation of the inferior vena cava. Ann Surg 1989; 210:649-652.)

emia persists and is generally related to immunosuppression medications.[123] The incidence of diabetes requiring insulin treatment is 2.6%. Tacrolimus use and African-American race are the two major risk factors for insulin-dependent diabetes.[135]

Anemia is common both before and after transplantation. Anemia is due to a decrease in erythropoietin production and iron deficiency. In post-transplant patients, calcineurin inhibitors, especially tacrolimus, are additional risk factors for anemia.[136] In children who require dialysis for the first time, anemia was associated with a greater risk of death and prolonged hospitalization.[102] Treatment of anemia slows the progression of renal disease in adults.[137] In children with chronic renal failure, a hematocrit less than 33% is a risk factor for progression to end-stage renal disease.[104] Anemia may be associated with LVH in children[126,130] and adults with chronic renal disease. Erythropoietin has been shown to improve LVH.[138]

Preoperative Evaluation

Immediately before transplantation, the child's condition should be stable and fluid or electrolyte imbalances should be corrected. It is important to assess the urine output (anuric, polyuric) so that appropriate intraoperative fluid replacement can be administered before unclamping the blood vessels of the donor organ. Active infection is a contraindication for transplantation. Any concurrent systemic disorders should be optimized. Finally, the NPO status of the child should be ascertained; many who present for cadaveric transplantation have a full stomach.

Surgical Technique

The surgical techniques used in the pediatric recipient differ from those used in the adult and depend on the child's size and underlying preexisting abnormalities, as well as the approach to the transplant (intraperitoneal or extraperitoneal). The extraperitoneal approach may be more technically difficult in smaller children. Removal of native tissue, either concurrently or (ideally) previously, occurred in 23% of children registered in the NAPRTCS database.[104] Preservation of urine-producing native kidneys may be desirable to prevent fluid overload during dialysis, especially for small children.[139]

Native nephrectomy may be required for polycystic kidney disease, uncontrollable hypertension, urinary tract infection, or nephrotic syndrome.[139-142] Nephrectomy for severe nephrosis may be necessary to resolve associated hypoalbuminemia, malnutrition, and hypercoagulability. Ideally, native nephrectomy is performed before transplant.[141-143] Native nephrectomy performed at the time of transplant increases operative time and cadaveric graft ischemic time[139] and has also been shown to be a risk factor for acute tubular necrosis in the grafted organ.[104]

Children Weighing More Than 20 kg

In larger children, the surgical approach is similar to that in the adult transplant patient; the kidney is placed in the iliac fossa, and the vascular anastomoses are to the common iliac vein and artery.[140,141] In larger children, the external iliac vessels may be used.[141] An extraperitoneal approach has the advantage of increased ease of future graft biopsy and ability to resume peritoneal dialysis in case of delayed graft failure.[139]

Children Weighing Less Than 20 kg

If renal transplantation in smaller children were restricted to size-compatible organs, then the surgical approach would be similar to that of the larger patient. However, a 1992 NAPRTCS

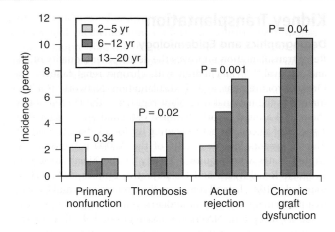

Figure 29-7. Causes of graft loss-relationship with recipient age. (Hwang AH, Cho YW, Cicciarelli J, et al: Risk factors for short- and long-term survival of primary cadaveric renal allografts in pediatric recipients: a UNOS analysis. Transplantation 2005; 80:466-70.)

report noted an increased loss of cadaveric grafts from pediatric donors. These pediatric donor organs had a higher rate of graft thrombosis and primary nonfunction (Fig. 29-7,) as well as a greater risk for acute rejection (Fig. 29-8, see website).[144,145] Consequently, the use of cadaveric pediatric donors has declined. In addition, the ability to transplant an adult-sized kidney into a small child permits the use of living-related donation (Fig. 29-9), with its improved graft and patient survival rates (Figs. 29-10 and 29-11, see website).[104]

For these reasons, the surgical technique for renal transplantation in the infant and small child has been modified to accommodate the adult-sized kidney. The use of a size-discrepant organ precludes the traditional approach. As Starzl and associates[146] describe, "the adult organ almost completely fills a child's right paravertebral gutter, extending from the undersurface of the liver to the pelvis." Typically, a midline incision from pubis to xiphoid is used and the cecum and right colon are mobilized.[140,143,146,147] An alternate approach is a right lower quadrant

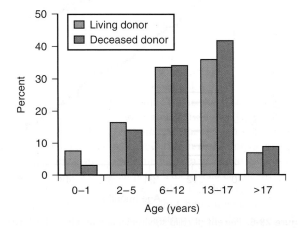

Figure 29-9. Age at transplant and donor source. (From NAPRTCS Annual Report. 2006. Accessed September 18, 2006, at www. naprtcs.org.)

incision, dissecting extraperitoneally.[141,148] Depending on the size of the recipient's vessels, the donor organ anastomoses may be made to the common iliac artery and vein or directly to the aorta and vena cava.[140,141,143,146,147]

In addition to difficulties in surgical technique, adult organs in pediatric recipients present physiologic challenges. The adult-sized organ sequesters a disproportionate amount of the infant's blood volume and cardiac output.[139,140,149] In one study that involved nine infant recipients of adult-sized kidneys, pre-transplant, early post-transplant, and late post-transplant blood flows were determined in both the infant's aorta and the adult graft.[150] Pre-transplant graft flow was approximately 618 mL/min, whereas 8 to 12 days post transplant, graft flow had decreased to 385 mL/min, despite aortic blood flow increasing from 331 mL/min to 761 mL/min. A further decrease was observed at 4 to 6 months, with aortic blood flow at 665 mL/min and graft flow at 296 mL/min. At 4 months, the graft size had decreased by 26%. Even with excellent conditions, optimal hydration, and a doubling of aortic blood-flow, these adult grafts are still underperfused both during transplant and in the late post-transplant period. In addition, the transplanted kidney is vulnerable to further reductions of flow from gastrointestinal illness, poor oral intake, or hypotension during nontransplant surgery.[145] This may explain why early graft loss in these smaller children is either from primary nonfunction or thrombosis (Fig. 29-7).[151]

Anesthetic Approach

Peri-induction

A living donor renal transplantation is an elective procedure whose only time constraints involve coordination with the donor harvest team, whereas in a cadaveric transplant any delay could potentially increase donor organ cold ischemic time. As such, most recipients of living donor kidneys will arrive in the operating room with an intravenous line, have been properly fasted (empty stomach), have had completed blood work, and have immunosuppressant induction treatment underway. Conversely, recipients of cadaveric kidneys may have full stomachs, have pending blood work, and may have immunosuppressant induction medications ordered but not yet given. An acceptable electrolyte panel, assurance that any crossmatching is underway, and confirmation with the treatment team regarding type of immunosuppressant induction (and premedicant) planned is necessary. In particular, it is important to confirm that any immunosuppressant induction drug and its premedicant (if any) is ordered and will be immediately available when the child arrives in the operating room.

Immunosuppressant Induction Therapy

Children may receive immunotherapy perioperatively to assist the development of immunotolerance[152] of the implanted graft and potentially to delay the administration of the nephrotoxic calcineurin inhibitors (Table 29-9, see website).[139,140] Antilymphocyte antibodies include muronab-CD3 (OKT3), alemtuzumab (Campath), antithymocyte globulin (equine) (Atgam), and antithymocyte globulin (Thymoglobulin). The infusion of these agents causes a cytokine response. This cytokine response can include fever, chills, rigors, and malaise that should be pretreated with acetaminophen, corticosteroids, and diphenhydramine.[152,153] Anti–interleukin-2 antibodies include basiliximab (Simulect), and daclizumab (Zenapax).

These medications do not cause a cytokine response. Side effects from anti–interleukin-2 antibodies are comparable to placebo except for an acute hypersensitivity reaction that can occur with basiliximab.[152]

Depending on the child, premedication may be administered to facilitate separation from the family. The cytokine effects of the antilymphocyte induction drugs can be unpleasant and can erode the coping mechanisms of any child or teenager. In children with a suspected full stomach, a rapid-sequence induction can be performed. Succinylcholine may be used in the absence of contraindications such as hyperkalemia; alternatively, high-dose rocuronium (1.2 mg/kg) may be substituted. In children with an empty stomach, an inhalational, intravenous, or combination technique may be used. Drug choices should avoid medications primarily metabolized or excreted by the kidney. One should not assume immediate resumption of renal function by the new graft. Because renal failure affects both protein binding and volume of distribution, anesthetic agents and adjuncts should be titrated to effect. Preferential use should be made of medications that undergo organ-independent elimination (cisatracurium, remifentanil) or do not rely exclusively on the kidney for metabolism (propofol) or whose renally excreted metabolites are inactive (midazolam, fentanyl). Regarding medications with renally excreted metabolites that are active (morphine), these agents should be used cautiously and titrated to effect. Medications with renally excreted metabolites that are toxic (i.e., meperidine) should be avoided.

Monitors and Vascular Access

Standard monitors, including core temperature, should be used. The need for vascular access should reflect third-spacing requirements and the potential for brisk blood loss inherent in a long intra-abdominal procedure in which the surgeon will be directly accessing large vessels. Urine output may not reflect intravascular volume status secondary to native renal dysfunction and discontinuity between the grafted organ and the Foley catheter or to polyuria in the reperfused graft.[139,140] Smaller children have the most severe fluid shifts and are the most vulnerable to graft hypoperfusion. Therefore, central venous and arterial catheters to monitor intraoperative and postoperative pressures may be indicated.[139-141,149,154] In larger children for whom assessment and maintenance of intravascular volume is more reliable, a central venous catheter may not be necessary in the presence of adequate peripheral access.[141] Children who have a large-bore hemodialysis catheter in situ may be accessed to monitor central venous pressure but only after the high-concentration heparin has been removed from the catheter.

Maintenance and Reperfusion

The anesthetic management plan should take into account hemodynamic conditions necessary for adequate perfusion of the donor organ. Combined general-regional techniques have been used but have been associated with larger intraoperative fluid requirements and the need for intravenous opioid supplementation in about half the children.[154] A hypnotic agent supplemented with an opioid to minimize negative inotropy is appropriate, and avoiding nitrous oxide in a long intra-abdominal case is prudent. Sevoflurane has been associated with the production of inorganic fluoride and compound A (see Chapter 6). Although no negative outcome data exist for the use of this agent in human renal transplant recipients, case numbers are insufficient to demonstrate its safety in this population.

have been reports of neonatal transplants crossing the ABO barrier.[172-174] Donor-to-recipient weight ratios up to 3.0 have been used successfully. In a comparison with more equally matched donor-recipient weight ratios, children who received hearts from oversized donors had no differences in ICU ventilator days, fractional shortening as assessed by echocardiography, ability to close the chest, or duration of inotropic support.[175] In contrast to the use of oversized donor organs, undersized donor organs were associated with an increased rate of donor organ failure. Recipient PVR is a major determinant for appropriate donor selection, and larger donor hearts should be considered for those with increased PVR to permit the right ventricle to compensate for the increased afterload.[176] Myocardial preservation of the donor organ is aimed at minimizing the ischemia time. Ischemic times of 6 hours were thought to be ideal, but pediatric allograft ischemic times may be extended to 8 hours with little adverse consequence.[177,178]

Preoperative Evaluation

A comprehensive, multidisciplinary evaluation of a potential cardiac allograft recipient is required to determine the recipient's suitability for transplantation. This evaluation includes an assessment of the child's underlying cardiopulmonary, hepatic, renal, neurologic, infectious disease, and immune system status, as well as socioeconomic and psychosocial function (Table 29-10).

Assessment of cardiopulmonary function usually begins with a thorough history with attention to exercise tolerance, oxygen requirements, and need for diuretics and inotropic support. Examination of the electrocardiogram (ECG), chest radiographs, echocardiograms, and Holter monitors may be helpful in the discovery of pleural or pericardial effusions, conduction disturbances, cardiac function, and arrhythmias. Radionuclide angiography may be useful in defining systemic ventricular dysfunction in children with complex cardiac morphology. The pre-transplant assessment ultimately includes cardiac catheterization with angiography. The anatomy and hemodynamics of the recipient must be carefully delineated because this influences anesthetic management and surgical donor harvesting and recipient transplant technique. For instance, in children with unrepaired HLHS, the donor harvest team has to harvest a large segment of donor aorta to facilitate reconstruction of the recipient aorta. The anesthetic management of this child before bypass must account for the possibility of pulmonary overcirculation. Determination of the Pulmonary Vascular Resistance Index (PVRI), transpulmonary gradient (TPG), and reactivity of the pulmonary vascular bed to pharmacologic manipulation is crucial to the assessment of suitability for cardiac transplant.

$$PVRI \ (units/m^2) = PAP \ (mm \ Hg) - PAWP \ (mm \ Hg)/CI$$
$$(L/min/m^2)$$

$$TPG \ (mm \ Hg) = PAP \ (mm \ Hg) - PAWP \ (mm \ Hg)$$

where PAP is the mean pulmonary artery pressure, PAWP is the mean pulmonary artery wedge pressure, and CI is the cardiac index.

A PVRI greater than 6 to 10 Wood units/m^2 or a TPG in excess of 15 mm Hg can lead to acute right ventricular graft failure, although the upper limit of PVR associated with successful cardiac transplantation has not been established in children. An endomyocardial biopsy can identify acute myocarditis and

Table 29-10. Routine Precardiac Transplant Evaluation

History and Physical Examination

Age, height, weight, body surface area

Diagnoses

Medical history

Medications

Allergies

Immunization record

Laboratory Data

Liver and kidney function studies

Urinalysis

Glomerular filtration rate

Prothrombin time/partial thromboplastin time/INR, platelet count

Complete blood cell count with differential

PPD skin test

Serologies for HIV, hepatitis, cytomegalovirus, Epstein-Barr virus, toxoplasmosis, syphilis

ABO type

Panel reactive antibody

Cardiomyopathy Work-up

Thyroid function studies

Blood lactate, pyruvate, ammonia, acyl carnitine

Urine organic acids, acyl carnitine

Skeletal muscle biopsy

Karyotype

Cardiopulmonary Data

Electrocardiogram

Chest radiograph

Echocardiogram

Radionuclide angiography

Cardiac catheterization

Endomyocardial biopsy

Pulmonary function studies

Oxygen consumption

Psychosocial Evaluation

History of abuse or neglect

Parental substance abuse

Long-term supportive care and reliability of caregivers

Possible relocation

Other Consultations as Needed

Dental services

Social services

Other

INR, international normalized ratio; PPD, purified protein derivative.
Adapted from Boucek MM, Shaddy RE: Pediatric heart transplantation. In Allen HD, Gutgesell HP, Clark EB, et al (eds): Moss and Adams' Heart Disease in Infants, Children, and Adolescents Including the Fetus and Young Adult, 6th ed. Philadelphia, Lippincott Williams & Wilkins, 2001, pp 295-407.

myocardial infiltrates. Pulmonary function studies may be useful in older children with chronic lung disease.

Laboratory evaluation should include serum electrolytes, complete blood cell count with differential, coagulation profile, viral titers for possible latent viral infections such as cytomegalovirus (CMV) and EBV, and metabolic or genetic work-ups. Donor matching is based on ABO typing, although successful transplantation of ABO-incompatible hearts in infants has increased the potential donor pool for children who are in critical need.[179,180] ABO-incompatible hearts are possible because of the immaturity of the infant immune system and the lack of production of ABO antibodies during the first 3 to 6 months of life. The use of triple-volume exchange transfusions also minimizes the potential reaction to maternally transmitted preformed ABO antibodies. The recipient's blood is also screened for antibodies against sera of random blood donors and, if reactive, a serum crossmatch with the donor may be performed. Panel reactive antibodies are preformed circulating HLA alloantibodies that, in high titers, are associated with diminished graft survival.[181-183] These antibodies arise from the use of homologous blood products, and blood products should be avoided if at all possible in the pre-transplant period. Treatments to reduce panel reactive antibodies may include intravenous immunoglobulin, cyclophosphamide, and plasmapheresis.[184] Although human leukocyte antigen (HLA) compatibility may improve graft survival, HLA matching is not routinely performed, owing to time constraints and limited availability of donor organs.

The mean time from listing for transplant to actual surgery is about 3 months but varies with the child's age, blood group, and list status. UNOS has developed allocation procedures that give priority to the most urgently ill children. Status 1 children have a projected life expectancy of less than 6 months, and status 2 children have a projected life expectancy of more than six months. Status 1 children generally require mechanical or pharmacologic support to sustain life, and most require support in ICUs. These children are further subdivided into 1A and 1B, where 1A is reserved for those with a projected life expectancy of less than 1 month. Physicians of status 1A children must recertify every 7 to 14 days if their patients do not require mechanical support for acute hemodynamic decompensation and even those who require mechanical support are only guaranteed 30 days until physician recertification becomes necessary. Approximately 20% of children with cardiomyopathy and 30% of those with end-stage congenital heart disease die while waiting for a donor heart.[185-187] Medical stabilization frequently includes the use of diuretics, inotropic agents, arrhythmia therapy, oxygen or subatmospheric oxygen, and mechanical ventilation if warranted. Studies of β-blockade therapy (carvedilol) have shown promise in children with dilated cardiomyopathy and chronic heart failure.[188,189] Those with severe chamber enlargement, arrhythmias and low cardiac output may require systemic anticoagulation to prevent thrombus formation and systemic embolization. Implantable defibrillators have been effective in children large enough for these devices, and biventricular pacing is showing promise as well.[190,191]

Children with end-stage myocardial failure will require mechanical circulatory support as a bridge to transplantation. Extracorporeal membrane oxygenation (ECMO) has been used for up to 1200 hours as a bridge to cardiac transplantation.[192]

Newer ventricular assist devices show more promise and applicability to a broad range of children for a much more prolonged period of support (see Chapter 19).[193-196] Renal failure that requires dialysis reduces survival.[197] Sepsis, neurologic injury, and bleeding are also serious complications of mechanical circulatory support.

Congenital heart disease is the primary indication for cardiac transplantation in infants younger than 1 year of age, and many of these recipients will have HLHS. The patency of the ductus arteriosus must be maintained with prostaglandin E_1 initially as a continuous infusion and perhaps by stenting the ductus in the catheterization laboratory later if a suitable donor organ is not found. Alteration of flow across the atrial septal defect can be addressed as well by the interventional cardiologist. If the balance between systemic and pulmonary blood flow cannot be managed medically, pulmonary artery banding may be necessary to reduce pulmonary overcirculation while waiting for a donor organ.

Surgical Technique

The original orthotopic technique devised by Lower and Shumway in adults was popular for many years in pediatric cases where the anatomy was straightforward.[198] This technique avoided individual systemic and pulmonary venous anastomoses by leaving a large cuff of right and left atrial recipient tissue behind and anastomosing the donor right and left atria to these cuffs. The resulting atrial chambers were a combination of donor and recipient atria that contracted asynchronously. Because the atrial contribution to cardiac output may be augmented with total cardiac transplantation, most centers have converted to the "bicaval" technique with a modification to utilize the standard left atrial anastomosis.[199-202] This technique improves sinus node function, causes less tricuspid regurgitation, and improves exercise tolerance.[203,204]

Cardiac transplantation in children with congenital heart disease may require surgery of greater complexity involving reconstruction of the great vessels or alterations in venous anastomoses. It is important that the donor harvesting team understand the recipient's anatomy and the potential harvest needs that may require large portions of aorta, pulmonary arteries, and venae cavae. In children with HLHS who require aortic arch reconstruction, deep hypothermic circulatory arrest may be necessary.[205-207]

The recipient is placed on cardiopulmonary bypass (CPB) after median sternotomy with aortic and bicaval cannulation. Cannulation may be modified depending on the cardiac anatomy encountered. The aorta is cross clamped, and both the aorta and the pulmonary artery are divided at the level of their semilunar valves. The superior and inferior vena cavae are transected, preserving a cuff of atrial tissue on each to facilitate the anastomoses. The interatrial groove is prepared, and an encircling left atriotomy is performed and the recipient heart is removed from the field. The donor organ is prepared and brought to the field. The left atrial anastomosis is completed first; and while iced saline is bathing the interior and exterior of the heart, the aortic anastomosis is completed. A vent is left in the left ventricular cavity for decompression and evacuation of air as the caval anastomoses are completed while the child is rewarming. The cross clamp is removed, and the donor heart is reperfused while the pulmonary arterial anastomosis is completed. Ventilation is resumed, and the child is liberated from CPB after return of cardiac function is documented by transesophageal echocardiography. Epicardial pacing wires are placed, mediastinal drainage tubes are positioned, and the chest is closed.

Intraoperative Problems and Management

Some children listed for cardiac transplantation may be hemodynamically stable and living at home. In these children, preoperative fasting may be an issue. The anesthesiologist must carefully assess the relative risks of a full stomach compared with the potential complications associated with an unexpected difficult airway in a child undergoing a rapid-sequence induction. Several hours may lapse between the call to mobilize the team and the actual surgery, but therapy to modify gastric pH and volume and the application of cricoid pressure may be warranted. It is equally likely that the pediatric recipient is hospitalized and requires a host of treatments designed to promote hemodynamic stability while a donor organ is sought. These children have minimal cardiovascular reserve. Anesthetic agents, positive-pressure ventilation, and surgical stress frequently result in hemodynamic instability. Anesthetic preparation should include the immediate availability of a variety of medications for the perioperative manipulation of myocardial function and hemodynamics. Vasoactive drugs and inotropic agents such as epinephrine, phenylephrine, dopamine, dobutamine, isoproterenol, milrinone, nitroprusside, and nitroglycerin should be readily available. For children with underlying congenital heart disease, the anesthesiologist needs to understand the child's underlying pathophysiology. The anesthetic management before CPB is similar to that for nontransplant cardiac surgery. For children with end-stage myocardial dysfunction, the sympathetic nervous system is chronically activated with downregulation of the cardiac β_1 receptors and an impaired response to β agonists.[208] Reduced renal perfusion stimulates the renin-angiotensin system, leading to increases in vasoconstriction, venoconstriction, and increased intravascular volume. These compensatory changes further aggravate the congestive heart failure by increasing preload and afterload. A dysfunctional, dilated myocardium is very sensitive to changes in preload, afterload, heart rate, and contractility. Both systolic and diastolic myocardial function is impaired, and a high mean atrial pressure is needed to ensure adequate ventricular filling volume. Increasing heart rate results in a decreased diastolic filling time and, therefore, a diminution in stroke volume as a result of the poor systolic and diastolic ventricular function, atrial pressure increase, and atrial enlargement. There is a loss of preload reserve. Cardiac output then becomes more heart rate dependent, and a decrease in heart rate results in a decreased cardiac output. Furthermore, small increases in afterload result in an increased end-systolic volume, decreased stroke output, and a further decrease in cardiac output. Dysrhythmias are poorly tolerated in these children.

Coordination of the arrival of the child to the operating room with the donor team ensures the briefest possible ischemic time for the donor organ. Premedication is best administered under monitored conditions. If the child was receiving supplemental oxygen, it should be continued during the preinduction period. Before induction, monitoring devices such as a precordial stethoscope, electrocardiogram, noninvasive blood pressure cuff, and pulse oximeter are applied. Meticulous airway management is critical because hypoxemia and hypercarbia may alter

PVR and further depress cardiac output. A wide variety of anesthetic agents have been used depending on the nature of the cardiac disease and the risk of pulmonary aspiration. After induction, invasive monitoring does not differ from that used during routine pediatric cardiac open-heart surgery. Some centers avoid right internal jugular vein cannulation because that vessel may be repeatedly accessed for post-transplant endomyocardial biopsy. TEE is useful to assess graft function, mechanical issues, and pulmonary hypertension. In children, TEE has been shown to be a more sensitive monitor for changes in cardiac function than hemodynamic changes.[209,210] Many experienced centers do not use pulmonary artery catheters routinely because the value of the information gained does not warrant the additional risk. In children who have undergone multiple cardiac operations, the potential risks of reoperation should be addressed and include the need for adequate-sized vascular catheters, the availability of blood products in the operating room, the preparation for alternate cannulation sites, and the use of antifibrinolytics such as aprotinin. Aprotinin has been shown to diminish blood loss in children during heart transplantation if they have had a previous median sternotomy.[211] The use of ultrafiltration during CPB may be beneficial by removing free water, hemoconcentrating the red blood cells and coagulation factors, and modulating the inflammatory response.[212-216]

Anesthesia is generally maintained with opioids, benzodiazepines, isoflurane, and a nondepolarizing muscle relaxant. In children with congenital heart disease, this anesthetic technique preserves cardiac output better than some inhalational agents, provided the heart rate is maintained.[217] In the preparation for termination of CPB, it is critical that the hemodynamics are optimized. A stable cardiac rhythm and acceptable heart rate are desirable. Chronotropic support using intravenous therapy with β-adrenergic agents such as isoproterenol and epinephrine or the use of epicardial pacing may be needed to maintain an appropriate heart rate between 120 and 150 beats per minute. The denervated transplanted heart does not respond in the normal fashion to hypotension. Medications with indirect cardiac effects such as atropine, glycopyrrolate, or ephedrine will likewise be ineffective. Direct-acting medications such as dopamine, dobutamine, epinephrine, or isoproterenol are required if inotropic or chronotropic support is needed. Some children benefit from vasodilator infusions to improve left ventricular stroke volume and cardiac output.[218] The use of inotropic agents to separate from CPB and provide early postoperative stability is common, and the choices are based largely on the perceived balances between pulmonary and systemic vascular resistance and myocardial dysfunction to blood pressure and cardiac output. Ventilation should be managed to ensure mild respiratory alkalosis and adequate oxygenation. Factors that potentially increase PVR such as hypothermia, acidosis, hypercarbia, hypoxemia, increased adrenergic tone secondary to light anesthesia, and polycythemia should be eliminated. Children with increased PAP before bypass show a greater response to ventilatory changes than those without increased PAP. In addition, children with congenital heart disease and associated pulmonary hypertension may develop severe pulmonary hypertension in response to hypoxemia.[219-221] The narrow range of afterload that the donor right ventricle is capable of handling is critical; if success in managing the pulmonary hypertension with conservative methods fails, more aggressive pharmacotherapy is warranted. The use of prostaglandin, prostacyclin, nitroglycerin, high-dose milrinone, calcium-channel blockers, sildenafil, and inhaled nitric oxide (iNO) have all been effective in treating pulmonary hypertension in children.[222-234] In extreme cases, mechanical assist devices or ECMO have been used.[235,236]

Dysrhythmias may be common in the post-bypass period, and, depending on the technique of implantation, there may be two independent P waves on the electrocardiogram, one from the recipient sinoatrial node and the other from the donor sinoatrial node. It is only the donor sinoatrial node that transmits impulses to the atrioventricular node and thus to the ventricle. The most common dysrhythmias are junctional rhythms, underscoring the utility of direct-acting β agonists and epicardial atrioventricular sequential pacing. This denervated state results in the loss of the baroreceptor reflex, forcing cardiac output to become primarily dependent on venous return and circulating catecholamines and thus unable to respond acutely to changes in the circulating blood volume and blood pressure.[237,238]

After separation from CPB, hemodynamic stabilization, and control of surgical bleeding, protamine sulfate is administered slowly to reverse anticoagulation. Risk factors for hypotension in children after protamine administration post bypass include female sex, greater protamine doses, and less heparin doses.[239] Transfusion of blood products should be guided by the balance of the need weighed against the associated risks of administration. There may be significant acid-base and electrolyte disturbances associated with large volume transfusions. These disturbances may be decreased by washing the cells before transfusion.[240,241] Donor blood should be screened for CMV and, ideally, CMV-negative recipients should receive blood screened negative for CMV.[242] Leukocyte reduction by filtration may be associated with a diminished risk of exposure to CMV through transfusion.[243,244] Another concern associated with transfusion in cardiac transplant recipients is the risk of transfusion-associated graft-versus-host disease (TAGVHD). This results from active T lymphocytes in the transfused blood of a recipient who is unable to reject them, such as a neonate, those undergoing chemotherapy, and the otherwise immunocompromised child.[245,246] To limit the risk of TAGVHD in cardiac transplant recipients, some centers routinely gamma irradiate cellular blood products before administration. At recommended doses, gamma irradiation has an insignificant effect on platelet, red cell, or granulocyte function but it may increase the potassium concentrations.[242,247]

Transport of the child from the operating room proceeds as in any other open-heart procedure. In selected recipients with excellent allograft function and hemodynamics, extubation of the trachea is possible in the operating room or within a few hours of arrival in the ICU. It is important that these children are comfortable but otherwise ventilating adequately to prevent atelectasis, hypoxemia, or hypercarbia that may increase PAP and thus strain the donor right ventricle. Newer agents such as dexmedetomidine may facilitate early extubation in these children.[248] Other children may require sedation and mechanical ventilation due to hemodynamic instability or due to delayed sternal closure, particularly if a large donor-to-recipient mismatch is present.

Immediate Postoperative Management

Early postoperative management consists primarily in maintaining hemodynamic stability. Infusions and volume needs are adjusted to maintain an optimal balance of preload, afterload, cardiac output, and peripheral perfusion. Attention should be directed toward maintaining normal acid-base and electrolyte balance. In some children, pulmonary hypertension remains a serious concern and management of sedation, ventilation, inotrope infusions, and pulmonary vasodilator administration is required to optimize right ventricular function. Ventilation modes may need to be adjusted to lower the mean intrathoracic (airway) pressure. Renal dysfunction continues to be a major source of morbidity and mortality after cardiac transplantation.[164] Decreased perioperative renal function can occur in as many as 20% of children after cardiac transplantation.[249,250] A peritoneal dialysis catheter placed at the time of cardiac transplant can be used to reduce ascites and improve ventilatory mechanics in those with right-sided heart dysfunction and in the treatment of renal insufficiency. Arrhythmias in the postoperative period may herald rejection.

Immunosuppression begins with corticosteroids administered before removal of the aortic cross clamp and continues into the postoperative period. Immunosuppression induction continues postoperatively with infusions of antibodies to reduce early rejection and to diminish dose requirements of corticosteroids and calcineurins. T-cell–depleting antibodies include polyclonal rabbit antithymocyte globulin (thymoglobulin), equine ATGAM, and monoclonal muronab-CD3 (OKT3). Interleukin-2 blockers (basiliximab and daclizumab) may also be used for induction. Maintenance therapy is guided largely by institutional experience and the recipient's clinical profile. The goal of maintenance therapy is to prevent acute and chronic rejection while minimizing the adverse effects of immunosuppression. All maintenance regimens involve a calcineurin inhibitor along with antiproliferative agents, or sirolimus. Corticosteroids may also be used, although most centers limit or avoid their long-term use. Calcineurin inhibitors include cyclosporine and tacrolimus. Antiproliferative agents include azathioprine and mycophenolate mofetil (CellCept). Sirolimus (rapamycin) is a macrolide antibiotic that acts synergistically with the calcineurin inhibitors and can be used to reduce the dose of cyclosporine or tacrolimus. Sirolimus may also inhibit the process of coronary arteriopathy.[251]

First-line therapy for acute rejection is high-dose corticosteroids. Other agents, including monoclonal and polyclonal anti–T-lymphocyte antibodies, are reserved for refractory or recurrent severe acute rejection or rejection with severe hemodynamic compromise. Recurrent moderate rejection is usually controlled with modulation of the maintenance therapy dosing.[252]

In spite of the remarkable improvements in immunosuppression and patient selection, acute and chronic rejection remain the major cause of death after pediatric cardiac transplantation (Tables 29-11 and 29-12, see website).[253,254] Monitoring and diagnosis of allograft rejection remain a challenge. Some studies suggest that transplant before 1 year of age offers protection from episodes of acute rejection and significantly greater freedom from rejection and time to first rejection.[255] Rejection surveillance in children includes three levels of detection. The clinical assessment includes nursing and parental accounts of changes in the child's activity and appetite, nausea, emesis, malaise, resting heart rate 15 to 20 beats per minute above normal, and presence of ectopy. Echocardiography has become very important in the postoperative follow-up, especially in neonates. These studies are performed frequently, especially in the first months after the transplant. Acute changes in left ventricular end-diastolic dimension, posterior wall thickness, and shortening fraction are potential signs of acute rejection.[256] Endomyocardial biopsy remains the standard in the diagnosis of acute cardiac allograft rejection. It provides tissue for both precise documentation of the presence or absence of rejection and allows more accurate titration of immunosuppression to avoid the adverse effects of increased use of immunosuppression based on clinical and noninvasive examinations only. Biopsy specimens are also analyzed for signs of humoral and vascular rejection. The biopsy specimen is examined for evidence of lymphocytic accumulations in the graft interstitium and perivascular tissue and in severe forms of cellular rejection, myocardial necrosis, and polymorphonuclear cell infiltrates. Over time, it is also possible to develop chronic rejection, which is primarily a vasculopathy that involves vascular inflammation with binding of IgG and/or IgM and complement. This produces a diffuse and concentric stenosis affecting the mid and distal coronary arteries and is often asymptomatic. Although annual coronary angiography is recommended, accelerated graft arteriosclerosis is underestimated angiographically.

New techniques are being developed to identify early evidence of rejection. Serum vascular endothelial growth factor may be a marker for cellular rejection.[257] Vascular endothelial growth factor is an established angiogenesis factor and is expressed in allografts undergoing rejection, but its function in the rejection process has not been defined. The possibility also exists for the detection of graft rejection by the examination of the characteristic gene expression patterns in peripheral blood mononuclear cells of heart transplant recipients.[258]

Long-Term Outcome and Quality of Life

Over 300 pediatric heart transplants are performed annually, giving a total of more than 5,000 worldwide since 1982.[164] Approximately 50% of the recipients do not require hospitalization in the first year after transplantation and, by 3 years, more than 70% are free from hospitalization.[164] One year after transplant 93% of survivors are without functional limitations. This increases to 95% by 5 years after transplant (Figs. 29-16 and 29-17, see website; Table 29-13).[164] The prevalence of post-

Table 29-13. Post–Heart Transplant Morbidity for Pediatric Patients: Cumulative Prevalence in Survivors within 1 Year Post Transplant (Follow-ups: April 1994–June 2004)

Outcome	Morbidity within 1 Year (%)	Total No. with Known Response
Hypertension	46.7	2184
Renal dysfunction	5.8	2183
Abnormal creatinine <2.5 mg/dL	3.8	
Creatinine >2.5 mg/dL	1.3	
Chronic dialysis	0.6	
Renal transplant	0.0	
Hyperlipidemia	10.1	2285
Diabetes	3.2	2188
Coronary artery vasculopathy	2.5	1996

From Boucek MM, Edwards LB, Keck BM, et al: Registry of the International Society for Heart and Lung Transplantation: eighth official pediatric report—2005. J Heart Lung Transplant 2005; 24:968-982.

transplant morbidities for 5-year transplant survivors is as follows: hypertension (61%), hyperlipidemia (21%), coronary vasculopathy (11%), renal dysfunction (9%), and diabetes mellitus (5%) (Table 29-14, see website).[164] At one center, 13% of pediatric cardiac recipients returned to the operating rooms for noncardiac procedures.[259] Preoperative evaluation requires an understanding of the unique features associated with the transplanted heart, such as its denervation, risk of vasculopathy (coronary artery disease), and arrhythmias. The interaction of the immunosuppressive regimens with anesthetic agents and their association with hypertension and renal dysfunction are additional considerations. Medication and monitoring choice should be tailored to the individual needs of the child to minimize anesthetic morbidity. Most medically stable cardiac transplant patients can undergo routine noncardiac surgical procedures in a similar fashion to nontransplanted children. It is important to remember that reflex mechanisms are impaired in the denervated heart and changes as a result of light anesthesia, hypovolemia, or contractility will be delayed until circulating catecholamines can influence the cardiac β receptors directly.[260,261] As cardiac transplant patients live longer, the risks of coronary vasculopathy increase, with coronary ischemia becoming a major concern. Therefore, attention to the maintenance of coronary perfusion is paramount. As in all immunocompromised patients, these children are vulnerable to infection, and strict adherence to aseptic and sterile technique is mandatory.

Heart-Lung and Lung Transplantation

Demographics and Epidemiology

Pediatric heart-lung transplants and, even more so, lung transplants, unavailable just a generation ago, are now relatively commonplace at a number of pediatric specialty hospitals. The first successful heart-lung transplant was performed at the Children's Hospital of Pittsburgh in 1985. The first adult lung transplant recipient survived for 18 days in 1962, but it was not until advances in surgical technique and immunosuppressive therapy in the early 1980s that the modern era of lung transplant was ushered in. Subsequently, heart-lung and lung transplantation have become well-accepted treatments for both adults and children with end-stage cardiopulmonary and pulmonary disease. There have been 950 pediatric lung transplants through 2004, with an additional 447 heart-lung transplants.[262] Management of the heart-lung transplant patient shares many similarities with that of the lung transplant patient, including many of the underlying disease processes. Nonetheless, the number of heart-lung transplants continues to decrease annually, from a zenith of 17 in the late 1990s to 9 in 2001. This decrease may be related to a decrease in suitable donors, but, more likely, it is due to an increasing awareness that right ventricular dysfunction, even long standing in the presence of significant pulmonary hypertension, exhibits reversibility after lung transplant, making heart-lung transplants less necessary than previously thought. The number of centers that perform heart-lung transplants and the total number of heart-lung transplants both hover around 10 per year. These children (heart-lung transplant and lung transplant patients) with end-stage pulmonary and cardiopulmonary disease frequently undergo a variety of interventions before and after transplant and require special anesthetic considerations.

Donor identification and management are more selective for heart-lung and lung transplant candidates than for isolated heart transplants. For instance, the thoracic capacity of the donor should be smaller than that of the recipient or the transplanted lungs will be at an increased risk for postoperative atelectasis and infections.[263] Donor supply remains the largest obstacle in transplantation, with as many as one third of all children on the waiting list dying before receiving lung transplantation.[264,265] The average waiting time for cadaveric lungs is 20 months for adolescents and 6 to 12 months for children younger than 2 years old. As experience in pediatric lung transplantation increases, it is likely that accepted indications for transplantation will increase as well. In that eventuality, the time spent on the waiting list is likely to grow, as there is no indication that the donor pool is increasing. A variety of strategies have been undertaken to increase the size of the donor pool, including television, radio, and print advertisements, the opportunity to declare oneself a potential donor when one obtains a driver's license, and in some states such as Pennsylvania having laws that require nurses to ask patients' family members whether they will consent for donation in the event of the patient's death.

Persons in some countries have a long-standing reluctance to donate organs. In the case of some countries such as Japan there are religious as well as legal barriers. In other instances, these barriers can be dismantled by education, but more often it takes a dramatic event to engender a societal change. Nicholas Green, a 7-year-old American boy, was vacationing in Italy in 1999 when he was shot in the head by a random act of violence and subsequently declared brain dead. His parents elected to donate his organs. Seven Italian citizens received his organs. In the wake of the publicity of the shooting and subsequent organ donation, Italian signed organ donation cards quadrupled, while actual donations tripled. Donor's families may also gain some solace. Green's father stated: *"There is some consolation with the process. It puts something on the other side of the balance. It will never bring my son back, but it can help somewhat with the grief."*[266]

Pathophysiology of the Disease

The indication for heart-lung and lung transplantation is severe end-stage pulmonary disease for which there is no other medical treatment and a life expectancy less than 18 months. The listing criteria includes considerations of the functional status of the child, the hemodynamic parameters, and the natural history of the underlying disease (e.g., children with pulmonary hypertension may progress to end-stage pulmonary disease rapidly). Most pediatric lung transplant patients are 11 to 17 years of age, with a smaller subset of children younger than 2 years old.[267] The most common underlying disease in elder pediatric lung transplantation is cystic fibrosis, accounting for nearly half of all pediatric lung transplants. Ninety-five percent of children with cystic fibrosis will eventually succumb from pulmonary issues. Factors associated with the less than 50% expected 12 month survival in cystic fibrosis patients include an FEV_1 less than 30%, a PaO_2 less than 55 mm Hg, or a $PaCO_2$ greater than 50 mm Hg.[268] Pulmonary vascular disease accounts for nearly 25% of the remaining transplants. Infants who require transplantation most often have a variety of relatively rare diseases such as surfactant B deficiency, primary alveolar proteinosis, or pulmonary vascular disease.[269] These infants are frequently severely ill at the time of their transplants: either their airways are intubated and they are mechanically supported for oxygenation and ventilation or they are dependent on ECMO. Independent risks for mortality after lung transplant include repeat transplant, mechanical ventilation at transplant,[270] and congenital heart disease.[271,272] At one time it was thought that prior thoracic surgery was a contraindication for lung transplantation. As experience has grown, this is not considered a contraindication and, in fact, a significant number of children who receive lung transplantation have had previous thoracic surgery for congenital heart disease. Today, the primary contraindications to lung transplantation surgery are active malignant disease within the prior 2 years (which may be unmasked by the immunosuppressive therapy required in transplantation), significant active infectious processes (including human immunodeficiency virus infection and hepatitis B and C), significant coexisting cardiac, hepatic, or renal disease (although these children may be candidates for multiple organ transplants), collagen vascular disease, major irreversible neurologic injury, and personal or family history of poor medical compliance or severe psychiatric illness that would preclude the child from effective post-transplant care. Relative contraindications include significant musculoskeletal disease, invasive ventilation, colonization with atypical mycobacteria or fungi, poor nutritional status (body mass index at either extreme), and inability to reduce dependency on corticosteroids. A lung allocation score is calculated for each child 12 years or older on the waiting list. The variables considered in calculating the individual child's score include age, underlying illness, forced vital capacity, functional status, and need for supplemental oxygen.[273] UNOS also includes ABO compatibility and distance between the donor and the recipient in its considerations for organ allocation.

The care of the donor is critical. First, the donor must meet criteria for brain death and the donor's lungs should have been ventilated less than 5 days to decrease the risk of lung injury, particularly ventilator-associated pneumonia. The donor should be free of active infection and tracheal secretions. The donor should have a PaO_2 greater than 300 mm Hg at an FIO_2 1.0 or greater than 100 mm Hg at an FIO_2 of 0.4 with an inflation pressure less than 30 cm H_2O with tidal volumes of 15 mL/kg and a PEEP of 4. The donor may need significant inotropic or pressor support to maintain hemodynamics. The donor may have diabetes insipidus with the requirement of desmopressin to maintain an adequate fluid balance and prevent excess lung water. In general, if a child is known to be a candidate for lung donation, the donor should remain euvolemic to slightly hypovolemic, as the hemodynamics allow, with central venous pressures maintained in the 8- to 10-mm Hg range. On occasion, this places the physicians who wish to utilize the donor kidneys at odds with those who wish to utilize the heart and lungs. In such a situation, the goal is to meet the desires of all within reason so that as many of the potential organs may be utilized as possible. When the lungs are harvested they are perfused with a preservative solution and prostaglandins, which reduce the incidence of graft failures. The lungs are inflated and the trachea is stapled shut, thereby maintaining an inflated position. The organs are then transported to the recipient at a temperature of 4° C. Ischemic times should be less than 8 hours, with less than 3 to 4 hours being ideal.

Another avenue being explored to increase the availability of organs suitable for lung transplant is the non–heart-beating-donor (NHBD).[274] Kidneys,[275] livers,[276] and other tissues have been utilized successfully from NHBDs. NHBDs may prove to be an as yet untapped resource and facilitate an expansion of pediatric lung transplantation. A system in Madrid, Spain has been developed that allows out-of-hospital emergency services personnel and transplant teams to initiate a protocol to harvest organs from NHBDs. They reported success in two patients who were discharged to home after receiving lung transplants from an NHBD.[277] NHBDs are generally younger than traditional donors.

An additional resource of lung tissue is that of a living-related donor with transplantation of adult lobes into the child.[278,279] Living-related transplants overcome some of the difficulties inherent in attempting to predict the clinical course of the underlying disease by being able to electively schedule the transplant. The inherent size mismatch also limits the use of this technique to children 5 years and older. Typically, the left lower lobe is harvested from one donor while the right lower lobe is harvested from another donor. The technique is similar to that of a lobectomy, however, the techniques require an appropriate length of bronchus and adequate vascular pedicles which is a drawback in that donor morbidity may reach as great as two thirds for the donors.[280]

Preoperative Evaluation

Children who are listed for lung transplantation undergo an extensive work-up. Commonly they will have chest radiographs, pulmonary function tests, arterial blood gas analysis, a complete metabolic panel, an electrocardiogram, and an echocardiogram. Should these children have pulmonary hypertension and/or associated cardiac defects, they also will have a cardiac catheterization. The catheterization will define the child's anatomy and allow measurement of PVR.

When the decision is made to proceed with transplant, the donor team is notified. There is a desire to have as short an ischemic time (the time from when the donor lungs are explanted to when they are implanted into the recipient) as possible. Prolonged ischemic times have been implicated in increasing the risk of bronchiolitis obliterans, a major source of morbidity in the post-transplant period. In light of this desire to proceed expeditiously, it is common that the anesthesiologist has a limited amount of time in which to collate all these data and perform the preoperative evaluation. One also may take advantage of what time is available to optimize the child preoperatively with inhaled bronchodilators and possibly chest physiotherapy. In the midst of this flurry of activity to facilitate an expeditious start to the procedure it is very important to recall that the child has likely been looking forward to this day for a long while. Even though the child may be excited, he or she also is often fearful. The cautious use of premedication may be considered to allay these anxieties. More commonly utilized options include midazolam, ketamine, or dexmedetomidine, which is an α_1-agonist sedative with minimal depression of respiratory drive.

Surgical Technique

Children most commonly receive bilateral lung transplants.[281,282] To facilitate this, most pediatric lung transplants are performed via a bilateral anterolateral trans-sternal "clamshell" incision. As much dissection as possible is carried out before CPB. The anastomosis itself comprises two bronchial anastomoses rather than one tracheal anastomosis. Tracheal anastomoses produce less satisfactory results than bilateral bronchial reanastomoses and have largely fallen out of favor. Bilateral bronchial anastomoses produce better outcomes without the risk of tracheal stenosis. Each bronchus is anastomosed with either an end-to-end anastomosis or the technique that is now increasing in popularity, telescoping anastomosis, in which the larger bronchus is telescoped several centimeters over the smaller bronchus portion with peribronchial tissue being wrapped around the junction to ensure blood supply because the bronchial blood supply is not reestablished. If the end-to-end anastomosis technique is used, the traditional approach includes an omental wrap around the suture line. Once the bronchus is reanastomosed, the pulmonary artery is reanastomosed. The donor lung includes an atrial cuff, which is sutured directly to the left atrium of the recipient. The use of the donor cuff avoids stenosing the pulmonary vein. While donor lungs are selected to be a size match, occasionally the lungs are too large for the recipient and cannot be used without incurring significant areas of atelectasis. If it is deemed that the lungs are too large, volume reduction may be undertaken to remove areas that are prone to atelectasis.

Single-lung transplants are infrequently performed in children. They are specifically avoided in children with cystic fibrosis to avoid soiling from the remaining diseased lung. If a single-lung transplant is performed in a child without cystic fibrosis, the side chosen to transplant is the most diseased side, preserving the best lung in situ. Additionally, if emphysematous changes are present, the most emphysematous lung is removed to decrease the risk of compression of the donor lung. Single-lung transplants are most often performed without CPB. Single-lung ventilation is established and a thoracotomy is performed, exposing the bronchus and vessels. A test occlusion by the surgeon of the pulmonary artery is then performed to evaluate the ability of the child to withstand the procedure without CPB. Presuming the child tolerates the test clamp, surgery proceeds with the removal of the native lung. The donor lung is anastomosed by first connecting the pulmonary vein atrial flap to the native left atrium, then by reanastomosing the pulmonary artery. As in the technique for sequential bilateral lung transplants previously described, the smaller of the two bronchial ends is telescoped into the other, with an overlap of one cartilage ring. The lung is then gently inflated. Air within the lung vasculature is vented via the pulmonary artery or the atrial cuff with the left atrium partially occluded. Once de-airing is accomplished, ventilation and perfusion are both established.

Intraoperative Problems and Management

Children for lung and heart-lung transplant are often critically ill. Cystic fibrosis patients are often quite compromised when they arrive for transplant and frequently unable to comfortably lie down due to excess secretions. Those with pulmonary fibrosis or end-stage chronic obstructive pulmonary disease may be marginally hypoxic and hypercarbic at baseline with increased PAPs and right-sided heart dysfunction. If premedication is necessary, caution must be exercised to not decrease respiratory drive, possibly precipitating worsening hypoxemia, hypercarbia, and right-sided heart failure.

Pretransplant patients commonly have a "full stomach" because of the short interval between their notification of impending transplant and the timing of the transplant itself. In such circumstances, a rapid-sequence or modified rapid-sequence induction may be considered; however, if possible, the best route is likely one of a gentle induction. The choice of induction agents is broad and must take into account comorbid illnesses, such as significant right-sided heart dysfunction or other congenital anomalies in addition to the end-stage pulmonary disease. A one-size-fits-all anesthetic technique is not appropriate for heart-lung and lung transplants. Once standard monitors have been applied, an intravenous or inhalational induction may be performed either alone or in combination with opioids or benzodiazepines. Much of the peri-transplant anesthetic considerations focus on optimizing the PVR. Increases in PVR may cause acute right ventricular failure with reduced cardiac output. Right-sided pressures can increase such that they cause significant right-to-left shunting through intracardiac lesions and result in desaturation. Heart-lung transplants are generally reserved for those children with the worst pulmonary hypertension and right-sided heart dysfunction. Ketamine does not appear to significantly alter PVR in infants[283] and may be considered as a first-choice drug.[284-286] Given the desire to rapidly intubate and control the airway, a relatively rapid-onset neuromuscular blocking agent, such as high-dose rocuronium, is most commonly given. Initial ventilator settings must take into account the underlying disease process. For example, fibrotic lungs may be better served by smaller tidal volumes, with a faster rate allowing for a decreased peak inspiratory pressure while preserving minute ventilation. On the other hand, severe obstructive disease may best be served by a slower pattern, with an expiratory time long enough not to induce dynamic hyperinflation (auto-PEEP). PEEP may be beneficial to improve oxygenation and ventilation and decrease atelectasis. Nonetheless, both dynamic hyperinflation and PEEP may compromise the hemodynamics by increasing intrathoracic pressure and thus decreasing venous return, particularly in relatively hypovolemic children. Should hemodynamic collapse occur with the institution of ventilation in a child with severe obstructive lung disease, dynamic hyperinflation should be immediately considered among the possible causes. Rapid treatment is provided by disconnecting the child from the ventilator circuit and allowing the child to freely exhale. When ventilation is reinstituted, care must be taken to allow an adequate expiratory time.

Maintenance of the anesthetic is most commonly opioid based and supplemented with inhalational anesthesia to ensure amnesia. Pure inhaled anesthetic–based techniques are less common owing to their cardiovascular depression and vasodilation. Furthermore, inhalational anesthetics blunt hypoxic pulmonary vasoconstriction, making it more difficult to maintain adequate oxygenation should lung transplantation off CPB be preferred. Nitrous oxide is avoided owing to its propensity to increase PVR[287-289] and to expand small air bubbles, which may be in the microcirculation of the transplanted lung on reimplantation. Consideration may also be given to regional anesthesia techniques. Because of concerns regarding the use of CPB for these procedures and the need for systemic heparinization, epidural thoracic catheters used for postoperative pain control are generally placed postoperatively when the child's coagulation profile has become normal.

The vast majority of lung transplants in children are performed with the assistance of CPB compared with adult lung transplants, which commonly do not use CPB. There are several reasons for this differing practice. Children with cystic fibrosis have a significant risk of cross contamination of the donor lung during a bilateral sequential lung transplant. This risk of soilage is minimized by the simultaneous removal of both lungs. Additionally, many children are too small to accommodate a double-lumen tube. Furthermore, children with pulmonary hypertension are frequently too unstable to tolerate single-lung ventilation. CPB alleviates these issues and allows the surgeon a quiet field with good exposure and predictable hemodynamics, thus speeding the time for anastomosis and decreasing the overall ischemic time.

If the child undergoes either single-lung transplant or sequential bilateral lung transplant off pump, continual vigilance and reassessment of the child's condition is required. These are extremely ill children undergoing dramatic perturbations to their homeostasis. Single-lung ventilation often precipitates hypoxemia and hypercarbia. The combination of the increased afterload on the right side of the heart by the clamping of the pulmonary artery along with hypercarbia and hypoxemic-induced pulmonary hypertension in the contralateral lung may precipitate right-sided heart failure. Attempts to diminish the pulmonary hypertension should be undertaken, including the use of pulmonary vascular dilators and inotropes such as milrinone, prostaglandins, or NO together with maintaining an adequate right-sided filling pressure. Nonetheless, continued right-sided heart failure may necessitate CPB. If the child can tolerate clamping of the pulmonary artery, it is typical that the gas exchange improves as shunting through the nonventilated lung is stopped and the perfusion/ventilation mismatch is diminished.

Bilateral sequential lung transplants performed on CPB are not associated with these problems. Nonetheless, CPB does not come without cost. Gas exchange may worsen due to reperfusion injury and pulmonary edema with the concomitant decrease in lung compliance. Inflammatory mediators are liberated, and the complement cascade is initiated, perhaps contributing to reperfusion injury in the transplanted lungs. The systemic heparinization required for CPB further increases the risk for perioperative bleeding and the need for transfusion of blood products. Packed red blood cells, platelets, and clotting factors are typically required. The need for clotting factors may be mitigated, in part, with the addition of fibrinolytics.

Given that lung transplantation in children is usually performed on CPB, obviating the need to perform single-lung ventilation, airway management of the child is accomplished with a single-lumen endotracheal tube. Cuffed endotracheal tubes are typically chosen for the ability to provide a better tracheal fit and allow for the potential need to ventilate the lungs with relatively high pressures both before and after transplant with fewer concerns regarding excessive air leak. In the rare circumstance in which lung transplantation is performed without CPB, single-lung ventilation will be required. Double-lumen tubes may be utilized in older children (see Chapter 13). If a double-lumen tube is utilized, it is exchanged for a single-lumen endotracheal tube at the conclusion of the operation, unless there is a need to continue with differential lung ventilation or there is a concern about lung soilage. In small children, either a bronchial blocker or selective intubation of a single bronchus may be considered. These choices, however, preclude the ability to suction the nonventilated lung. Once the child has been intubated, additional invasive monitoring is placed. This typically includes an arterial catheter and a central venous catheter along with two large-bore intravenous lines. In some centers it is customary to place a pulmonary artery catheter in addition to or in place of the percutaneous central venous line. Occasionally, the surgeon will place a right atrial line. If a pulmonary artery catheter is placed, it must be withdrawn into the main pulmonary artery before pneumonectomy. Position can be confirmed by palpation. A TEE probe is then placed to assist in evaluation of residual cardiac abnormalities and cardiac performance, particularly right ventricular performance, both before and after transplant while weaning from CPB.[290]

Perioperative bleeding is common, both in the operating room after coming off CPB and in the immediate postoperative period. Extensive pulmonary to systemic collaterals, coagulopathies due to hepatic dysfunction, and significant adhesions from prior surgeries or cystic fibrosis may make the surgical dissection difficult and precipitate blood loss. Aprotinin has been effective in reducing bleeding in children with previous thoracic surgery.[291] Aprotinin may reduce the inflammatory mediators responsible for reperfusion injury. Repeated use of aprotinin, however, carries with it a risk of anaphylaxis. There has not been a long-term prospective outcome study in which significant renal dysfunction was associated with the use of aprotinin in children.[292]

During CPB the child is typically cooled to 32°C. Cystic fibrosis patients are colonized with bacteria; thus, the tracheal stump is irrigated with antibiotic solution after the native lungs are removed so as to reduce contamination of the transplanted lungs. Despite best efforts, occasionally these children develop sepsis or a syndrome similar to septic shock due to liberation of bacteria and toxic mediators during the removal of the native lungs. Such children require intensive therapy and most often do poorly.

Once the first lung has been implanted, a small amount of blood is allowed to eject into the pulmonary artery while the second lung is being anastomosed, reducing ischemic time for the first lung. After the second lung is implanted, the lungs are ventilated to remove all areas of atelectasis. Post-transplant ventilation strategy limits tidal volumes to maintain peak inspiratory pressures less than 35 cm H_2O and PEEP in the range of 5 to 10 cm H_2O. Before termination of CPB, it is typical to augment myocardial performance with inotropic support. Occasionally, a combination of inotropes, dilators, or pressors may be required. Some centers also routinely utilize NO and/or prostaglandin E_1 to reduce PVR, whereas other centers reserve their use only if pulmonary hypertension becomes a problem. A fiberoptic bronchoscopy may be performed to assess the bronchial anastomotic sites in the operating room or along with a lung perfusion scan performed within the first 24 hours postoperatively.

In the heart-lung transplant patient, weaning from CPB is analogous to that for cardiac transplantation. However, there remains the need to support the denervated heart with adequate fluids and inotropy. Maintaining adequate fluid status in these children may require more effort owing to the increased bleeding as compared to heart transplant patients. Extensive collaterals and bronchial circulation have often developed in these children.

The onset of acute graft dysfunction can manifest as persistent hypoxemia after weaning from CPB. Although this may be attributable to relatively reversible causes such as inadequate ventilation, atelectasis, or right ventricular dysfunction with right-to-left shunting, a more ominous problem however may be reperfusion injury. Free radicals and inflammatory mediators are readily produced by the lung during both the ischemic time as well as during reperfusion. Reperfusion injury is correlated with longer ischemic times. Reperfusion injury manifests as hypoxemia in the presence of adequate ventilation and no other clear etiology for the hypoxemia. Pink frothy secretions are often noted in the endotracheal tube. Prostaglandin E_1 may, in the presence of reperfusion injury, reduce reperfusion injury risk and symptoms. Ventilation strategy aims to maintain adequate oxygenation and ventilation with PEEP and as low peak inspiratory pressures as possible. FIO_2 is aimed to keep PaO_2 less than 120 mm Hg to avoid oxygen toxicity. NO is also gaining favor in this setting. Although it has not been shown that prophylactic NO will prevent reperfusion injury, NO improves oxygenation and hemodynamics in the presence of reperfusion injury with hypoxemia and increased pulmonary and right-sided heart pressures when used in the dose range of 20 to 60 parts per million.[293,294] Another option may be inhaled prostacyclin, which has been demonstrated to be safe and useful in the treatment of pulmonary hypertension and reperfusion injury.[295] Nonetheless, on occasion, all these measures remain inadequate. In this event, ECMO should be instituted to allow the donor lungs time to recover.[296]

Immediate Postoperative Management

The immediate postoperative care of the child is individualized based on the child's age, pre-transplant diagnosis, and pre-transplant comorbid conditions. The older cystic fibrosis patients require mechanical ventilation for several days.[297] After extubation, these children may still require some supplemental oxygen for exercise therapy. Non–cystic fibrosis infants and children, typically more acutely ill before transplant, require an average of more than 3 weeks of mechanical ventilation and average nearly 2 months of critical care stay.[298] These younger transplant patients are smaller, have an increased incidence of airway complications, and may suffer from associated congenital cardiac defects. Children with significant pre-transplant pulmonary hypertension often manifest significant hemodynamic instability postoperatively. In anticipation for this, these children remain sedated, intubated, and frequently paralyzed for the first several postoperative days.

Post-transplant children require aggressive chest physiotherapy to avoid lung congestion that could lead to infection and respiratory failure. The child's cough reflex is absent, mucociliary transport is disrupted across the bronchial suture line, and frequent endotracheal suctioning is mandatory. Therapeutic bronchoscopy for pulmonary toilet may also be required. In addition to the pulmonary considerations, surgical sites, catheters, and drains, these children are often predisposed to infection owing to an underlying poor nutritional status, especially when combined with their post-transplant immunosuppressive regimen. Prophylactic antibiotics are given, including antiviral and antifungal agents, particularly if underlying fungal infection or viral infection (e.g., CMV) is present in either the donor or recipient.

Postoperative pain control is critical to ensure effective pulmonary toilet. It is most readily obtained with judicious use of opioids, with consideration of patient-controlled analgesia in those children deemed able to use such a device. Regional anesthesia may also be utilized, but because of the systemic heparinization for CPB many practitioners are reluctant to place a catheter before CPB. If regional anesthesia is desired, a thoracic epidural catheter may be placed postoperatively when the coagulation status of the child has normalized. Dexmedetomidine may also be considered. Dexmedetomidine decreases opioid use by 50% in postoperative children and provides arousable sedation with minimal effect on respiratory drive.

Long-Term Issues

Immunosuppressive drugs are used in greater doses in lung transplant and heart-lung transplant children than in other organ transplants owing to the large endothelial surface in the lungs and the resulting large number of immunologically active cells that predispose to major histocompatibility class antigens and an extreme lymphocyte-directed host response. Induction immunosuppression is used in more than one half of the heart-lung and lung transplant centers.[299] Most transplant centers use a continuing multiple-drug immunosuppressive regimen.[300] Bearing in mind the side effect profiles and efficacy of immunosuppression, the International Pediatric Lung Transplant Collaborative has recommended that tacrolimus, mycophenolate mofetil, and prednisone form the mainstay of immunosuppressive therapy. The most widely used regimens rely on a calcineurin phosphatase inhibitor coupled with a cell cycle inhibitor and a corticosteroid. The most commonly used calcineurin inhibitors are cyclosporine and tacrolimus. Both work similarly, and both have significant side effect profiles. Neither appears to be superior in preventing bronchiolitis obliterans. The major side effects of tacrolimus include hyperglycemia, alopecia, worsening renal function, and possibly an increased risk of PTLD. Cyclosporine's major side effects include hypercholesterolemia, hirsutism, gingival hyperplasia, and hypertension. Cyclosporine may prolong the neuromuscular blockade of atracurium and vecuronium.[301] Cyclosporine blood levels must be monitored closely, particularly in cystic fibrosis patients, who are prone to variable intestinal absorption. Increased concentrations of cyclosporine have been implicated in central nervous system side effects such as seizures, headaches, and even strokes.[302,303] Corticosteroids are included in nearly all lung transplant programs. Over time, the corticosteroid dose is weaned to prevent complications from chronic use such as hyperglycemia and osteoporosis, yet at 1 year and 5 years, nearly all lung transplant patients remain on a dose of prednisone. Cell cycle inhibitors are used in addition to the calcineurin inhibitors and corticosteroids. Mycophenolate use is increasing, but as yet there has not been clearly demonstrated a benefit over azathioprine. Additionally, azathioprine may prolong neuromuscular blockade of succinylcholine.[304] Sirolimus acts by blocking interleukin-2– induced T-cell proliferation. Its role as a primary medication is limited by its hindrance of wound healing, potentially contributing to a dehiscence. It may be used as rescue therapy in children with bronchiolitis obliterans with mature suture lines.

More than one third of children on chronic immunosuppression develop hypertension during the first post-transplant year and 75% do so by 5 years. Additionally, a significant number of these children, particularly those receiving tacrolimus, develop chronic renal insufficiency with decreasing creatinine clearance, with some requiring dialysis and renal transplantation.

Post-transplant airway complications may be devastating. Whereas life-threatening bronchial dehiscence is uncommon, bronchial stenosis and tracheomalacia remain problematic.[305,306] Bronchial stenosis is thought to be related to relative ischemia at the anastomotic site, recurrent infections, and possibly high-dose corticosteroid therapy. Initial treatment of stenosis is

balloon dilation; however, up to 50% of the children with bronchial stenosis will require placement of bronchial stents. In younger children, dynamic obstruction may be a complication that makes extubation of the trachea difficult. This dynamic airway obstruction usually is self-limited, improves over time, and does not require intervention.

Post-transplant children are followed closely with pulmonary function tests for signs of rejection, infection, and/or bronchiolitis obliterans. The choice of anesthetic for post-transplant patients must be individualized based on the child's coexisting disease, underlying right-sided heart dysfunction, the child's ability to handle secretions, and the need for endotracheal intubation. Flexible fiberoptic bronchoscopies with bronchioalveolar lavage and transbronchial biopsies are the most common indications for anesthesia in these children.[307] Bronchoscopies are performed at regular intervals, typically every 3 months, to evaluate even very early pathologic changes. Flexible fiberoptic bronchoscopies are most frequently performed under general anesthesia in children. The laryngeal mask airway is the preferred manner in which to manage the airway; it allows the bronchoscopist to use a large fiberoptic bronchoscope, facilitating improved view, improved suctioning, and therefore easier bronchoalveolar lavage, together with enhancing the ability to obtain adequate transbronchial biopsies.[308] Acute rejection is common in the first several weeks to months after transplant. Although acute rejection is often asymptomatic, fever and dyspnea may be present. Radiographic findings may include infiltrates and pleural effusions. Pulmonary function tests may demonstrate a decreased FEV_1 and forced vital capacity. Diagnosis is confirmed by bronchoscopy, bronchioalveolar lavage, and transtracheal biopsy. Acute rejection is graded on a scale of A0 to A4. Grades A2 and greater are treated with increased immunosuppression. The major manifestation of chronic rejection, bronchiolitis obliterans, remains the bane of the lung transplant surgeons, occurring in greater than 50% of all post–lung transplant patients within 5 years of transplant. Bronchiolitis obliterans is the leading cause of death after the first post-transplant year. It manifests as progressive deterioration of exercise tolerance and deterioration in airflow and is characterized by fibrosis of small airways and thickening of blood vessels. Bronchiolitis obliterans is diagnosed by a decrease in FEV_1 compared with the immediately previous FEV_1. Known risk factors include prolonged ischemic time of the donor lung, more than two rejection episodes, and age older than 3 years.[309] There is no reliable treatment. A variety of immunosuppressive medications have been used with variable results. The primary treatment is immunosuppressive prevention of acute rejection and prompt treatment of CMV infection. In severe instances, retransplantation is the only treatment option.

Post-transplant vascular complications are uncommon, but when they do occur they are most commonly due to mechanical obstruction to blood flow secondary to redundant tissue in either the pulmonary artery or at the cuff of the atrial tissue impeding venous return. Vascular complications may be difficult to distinguish from reperfusion injury, presenting as elevated right-sided and pulmonary artery pressures with pink frothy secretions in the endotracheal tube. Pulmonary arterial or venous stenosis may be diagnosed in the operating room or at the bedside in the critical care unit with a TEE. If there are still questions regarding the diagnosis, cardiac catheterization may be required. Depending on the findings, the children are treated with a stent placed during cardiac catheterization or they may require reoperation to alleviate the stenosis. Furthermore, lymphatics are not reanastomosed after lung transplantation, resulting in the loss of lymphatic drainage. This loss of lymphatics increases the risk for pulmonary edema in the postoperative period. The increased parenchymal water and increased vascular filling further serve to decrease the compliance of the post-transplant lungs.[310]

The post-transplant donor lungs are denervated. Although this produces minimal effect on airway reflexes, mucociliary transport, and bronchial reactivity,[311] the larger effect is the loss of stimuli to the respiratory drive center with a loss of coordination of the respiratory accessory muscles that may be apparent to visual observation. Additionally, in the early post-transplant period, episodes of bradycardia occur; whereas in the later periods, there is an increase in sympathetic tone and in heart rate.[312]

Phrenic, recurrent laryngeal and vagus nerve injuries are common after lung transplant.[313] While phrenic nerve injury is typically transient, the resulting diaphragmatic paralysis may result in prolonged need for mechanical ventilation or even consideration of placement of a diaphragmatic pacer. Recurrent laryngeal nerve injury may occur in up to 1 of every 10 pediatric lung transplant patients. The left recurrent laryngeal nerve is most often involved, effecting a left vocal cord paralysis, from which most children recover.[314]

Gastroesophageal reflux disease is a considerable problem for post–lung transplant patients, with some centers reporting a significant number who ultimately require a Nissen fundoplication. This reflux and gastroparesis may be precipitated by vagal nerve injury. Recurrent aspiration pneumonias contribute to the failure of the transplanted lungs, whereas delayed gastric emptying results in unreliable absorption of immunosuppressive drugs. Children with cystic fibrosis in particular have a high incidence of intestinal obstruction after lung transplants. These children may require gastrostomy, jejunostomy, or other procedures for ileus. As many as 1 in 10 cystic fibrosis patients have intestinal obstruction after lung transplantation.[315]

Post–lung transplant graft rejections are common. Older children average 10 times more episodes of rejection than infants,[316,317] likely owing to the infant's more immature immune system. The signs and symptoms of rejection are nonspecific. Any diminished clinical measure is generally aggressively investigated to rule out rejection. If rejection is confirmed, aggressive treatment with immunosuppressive therapy is instituted.

CMV infection is one of the most common infections in the post-transplant child. CMV infections may manifest as mild symptoms but may progress to pneumonitis, gastrointestinal symptoms, or even a sepsis syndrome with multiorgan failure. CMV infection has been associated with both acute cellular rejection and chronic rejection.[318] *Pseudomonas aeruginosa* or fungal organisms may also be noted. Aggressive treatment is warranted.

Additionally, a number of malignancies have been reported in the post–lung transplant child at greater rates than their age-matched counterparts and may be attributed to immunosuppressive therapy. PTLD has a greater incidence in lung and heart-lung transplant children than in other solid organ transplant patients, perhaps owing to the higher level of immunosuppression required. Even in this group of children, the cystic fibrosis subgroup of transplant patients has an even greater incidence of PTLD. Mortality has been reported to be more than 60% for those afflicted, with a number of the deaths attributed to graft failure as a result of the treatment of PTLD by decreasing immunosuppressive therapy. As many as 25% of cystic fibrosis patients may suffer from PTLD. PTLD is, in most cases, associated with EBV infection, either as a reactivation of the virus with immunosuppression or with new infection acquired from the donor lung. EBV occurs uncommonly in children who are seropositive for EBV before transplant, whereas in those who are seronegative EBV-associated disease occurs in one in five children. The diagnosis of PTLD is made by the symptoms, evidence of lymphoproliferation on biopsy, and EBV DNA or RNA in the sampled tissue. PTLD manifests as a variety of nonspecific symptoms, including a mononucleosis-type syndrome. The most common symptoms include elevated temperature, lymphadenopathy, and gastrointestinal symptoms. Most PTLD occurs in the first year after transplant.

The treatment of PTLD is reduction or withdrawal of immunosuppressive therapy,[319] which may double survival rates.[320] Unfortunately, reduction or withdrawal of immunosuppressive therapy places these children at risk for graft failure. Additional treatments that have been demonstrated to be effective include localized excision of the lesion, antiviral therapy,[321] monoclonal antibodies,[322] interferon,[323,324] immunoglobulin, and cytotoxic T lymphocytes.[325] Chemotherapy does not appear to offer an advantage and may worsen survival.[326] Dysrhythmias may also occur after lung transplant but are relatively uncommon and typically do not require treatment. Atrial dysrhythmias associated with extensive left atrial suture lines were among the first dysrhythmias to be described.[327,328] However, the types of dysrhythmias after lung transplant surgery include functional escape rhythm, nonsustained ventricular tachycardia, accelerated junctional rhythm, sinus bradycardia, nonsustained supraventricular tachycardia, ectopic atrial tachycardia, and second-degree heart block. The incidence of the dysrhythmias is small (<5%) without apparent sustained supraventricular tachycardia, atrial flutter, atrial fibrillation, or complete heart block. Treatment is not usually required.[329]

Postoperative lung transplant children are below their contemporaries insofar as height and weight are concerned for their age, with the overall growth rate only two thirds of the predicted value. It appears, based on pulmonary function tests, radiographic studies, and histologic examination that the transplanted lung or lungs grow in the recipient appropriate for the recipient's height and weight. Functional reserve capacity,[330] and airway size[331] and absolute number of alveoli increase as height and weight grow in a manner comparable to their normal counterparts. Furthermore, recipients of mature living-related lobar lungs also grow. Transplanted mature lung lobes expand and fill the entire chest. In these mature lung lobes, however, while the airways appear to grow in size the alveoli appear to become distended rather than increasing in absolute number.

Just over 50% of the transplant children will survive 5 years. This follows 1-year and 3-year survival rates of three fourths and two thirds of the children, respectively. Infants have a particularly high death rate of 25%. Those with significant pre-transplant pulmonary hypertension and those receiving re-transplants also have a greater than average death rate. More than one half of early (first month) deaths in all ages are due to primary graft failure. The principal culprits in later deaths are infection, bronchiolitis obliterans, and malignancies. The leading cause of death from 1 month through 1 year is non-CMV infections. The leading cause of death from 1 to 3 years is bronchiolitis obliterans, followed by non-CMV infections. After 3 years, bronchiolitis obliterans is the leading cause of death. The majority of malignancies are from PTLD. In those children who do survive, more than three fourths of them have minimal limitation on activity at 1, 3, and 5 years after transplant, respectively.

Acknowledgment

We wish to thank Drs. Erich A. Everts, Jr, Marla S. Gendelman, and Mateen Raazi for their prior contributions to this chapter.

Annotated References

Aggarwal S, Kang Y, Freeman JA, et al: Postreperfusion syndrome: cardiovascular collapse following hepatic reperfusion during liver transplantation. Transplant Proc 1987; 19(Suppl 3):54-55
A classic paper describing the hemodynamic instability after reperfusion of the liver during transplantation
Bailey LL: Heart transplantation techniques in complex congenital heart disease. J Heart Lung Transplant 1993; 12(6 pt 2):S168-S175
An excellent discussion of transplantation techniques in children with complex congenital heart defects
Beebe DS, Belani KG, Mergens P, et al: Anesthetic management of infants receiving an adult kidney transplant. Anesth Analg 1991; 73:725-730
Description of intraoperative management of renal transplantation in infants
Sweet SC: Pediatric lung transplantation update 2003. Pediatr Clin North Am 2003; 50:1393-1417
A discussion of the current status of pediatric lung transplantation, including indications, outcomes, and complications
West LJ, Pollock-Barziv SM, Dipchand AI, et al: ABO-Incompatible heart transplantation in infants. N Engl J Med 2001; 344:793-800
A discussion of ABO-incompatible heart transplantation in infants

References

Please see www.expertconsult.com

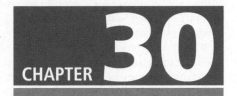

Other Surgeries

SECTION VII

Orthopedic and Spine Surgery

Niall Wilton and Brian Anderson

CHAPTER 30

ANESTHESIA FOR ORTHOPEDIC AND spinal surgery provides a multitude of challenges. Children often present with concomitant diseases that affect cardiovascular and respiratory function. The ability to maintain a clear airway during anesthesia is not straightforward in some of these children (e.g., those with arthrogryposis multiplex congenita).[1] Operating times can be protracted. Significant blood loss can occur and requires strate-gies for blood product management and transfusion reduction (see Chapter 10). Major trauma causing orthopedic injuries invariably involves other organ systems that may adversely interact with or compromise anesthetic management (see Chapter 39). The risks of aspiration of gastric contents into the lungs and the requisite fasting times, after even minor trauma involving an isolated forearm fracture, continue to be debated.

Fat embolus is uncommon in children with fractures of the long bones but should be sought in any child with hypoxia and altered consciousness.[2] Tumor surgery may be complicated by chemotherapy, altered drug disposition, or bone grafting considerations akin to plastic and reconstructive surgery (see Chapter 33).

Children with chronic illnesses present repeatedly for surgical or diagnostic procedures. A single bad experience can blight attitudes to anesthesia for a considerable time. These children should be managed with sensitivity and compassion. Positioning children on the operating table involves care, especially in those with limb deformities and contractures. Padding, pillows, and special frames are required to protect against damage from inadvertent pressure ischemia while achieving the best posture for surgery. Plaster application, particularly around the hip, should allow for bowel and bladder function, avoid skin breakdown due to pressure or friction, and allow access to epidural catheters. The postoperative management of casts on peripheral limbs must account for the possibility of compartment syndromes attributable to restrictive casts or compartment pathology. Regional techniques should not mask pressure effects under plaster casts or compartment syndrome, although epidural blocks may be ineffective against the discomfort of pressure.[3,4] Intraoperative temperature regulation (see Chapter 25) may be affected by tourniquet application owing to a combination of decreased heat loss from the ischemic limb and reduced heat transfer from the central to ischemic peripheral compartment. Some disease processes are associated with altered temperature regulation (e.g., osteogenesis imperfecta, arthrogryposis multiplex congenita). The use of radiology is common during orthopedic surgery, and precautions against radiation exposure during bony manipulations should not be neglected by the anesthesiologist.

Regional anesthesia (see Chapter 42) reduces anesthesia requirements intraoperatively and provides analgesia postoperatively. The use of ultrasound techniques to locate neural tissue improves success and reduces local anesthetic doses (see Chapters 42 and 43).[5,6] The recent introduction of ultrasound techniques has heralded a rapidly increasing use of peripheral nerve blockade rather than central blockade for unilateral lower limb surgery. Acetaminophen (paracetamol) and NSAIDs are the most common analgesics prescribed to children for moderate pain. The regular administration of acetaminophen and NSAIDs decreases the amount of systemic opioids administered,[7] but NSAIDs decrease osteogenic activity and may increase the incidence of nonunion after spinal fusion.[8,9] Intravenous administration of acetaminophen improves the early effectiveness of this drug before the child is able to tolerate oral intake, but this formulation is not available in all countries.[10] Long-term pain associated with limb-lengthening techniques (e.g., Ilizarov frame) may require oral opioids after hospital discharge.

Scoliosis Surgery

Children presenting for scoliosis surgery represent a spectrum from the uncomplicated adolescent to severely compromised children with neuromuscular disease, respiratory failure, and cardiac problems. The age range at presentation varies from infancy to young adulthood, and anesthetic approaches need to be tailored for each individual child.

Terminology, History, and Surgical Development

Hindu literature (3500-1800 BC) describes Lord Krishna curing a woman whose back was "deformed in three places."[11] The words "scoliosis" (crooked), "kyphosis" (humpbacked), and "lordosis" (bent backward) originated with the Greek physician Galen. *Scoliosis* is a lateral deviation of the normal vertical line of the spine, which when measured by x-ray, is greater than 10 degrees. There is a lateral curvature of the spine with rotation of the vertebrae within the curve. *Lordosis* refers to an anterior angulation of the spine in the sagittal plane, and *kyphosis* refers to a posterior angulation of the spine as evaluated on a side view of the spine. Curves may be simple or complex, flexible or rigid, and structural or nonstructural. Primary curves are the earliest to appear and occur most frequently in the thoracic and lumbar regions. Secondary (or compensatory) curves can develop above or below the primary curve and evolve to maintain normal body alignment. The varying combinations of curve types result in different pathophysiologic consequences.

The magnitude of the scoliosis curve is most commonly measured using the Cobb method.[12] Measurement is made from an anteroposterior radiograph and requires accurate identification of the upper and lower end vertebrae involved with the curve. These are the vertebrae that tilt most severely toward the concavity of the curve. The Cobb method of angle measurement is shown in Figure 30-1.

Hippocrates (circa 400 BC) developed treatments that relied primarily on manipulation and traction, using an elaborate traction table called a scamnum.[13] Nonsurgical treatments for spinal deformities persisted until 1839 when a surgical treatment in the form of a subcutaneous tenotomy and myotomy was described by the French surgeon Jules Guerin.[14] Posterior spinal fusion appears to have been first described by Russell Hibbs for tuberculous spinal deformity in 1911.[15] The original spinal instrumentation system was the Harrington rod system.[16] Modification of this technique allowing segmental fixation of the rods, and early mobilization followed.[17] These systems treated

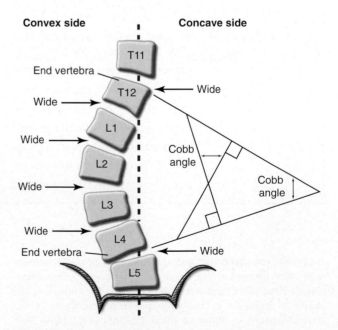

Figure 30-1. Diagram of anteroposterior spinal radiograph showing Cobb method of scoliosis curve measurement.

the lateral curve but did not allow for correction of the axial rotation. Subsequent developments allowed both via cantilever maneuvers using Cotrel-Dubousset instrumentation.[18] Pedicle screws rather than hooks were the next advance. These were initially used with lumber curves as a distal anchor and were found to enhance correction and stabilization, even when used with hooks for the more proximal curves (hybrid constructs).[19] Pedicle screw instrumentation techniques for total curve correction have been a recent development and have been shown to offer better curve correction than hook techniques[20] and the hybrid pedicle screw/hook technique.[21]

Classification

Classification of scoliosis deformities is imperfect because the systems used are clinically rather than etiologically based. Most classifications are surgically based and relate to surgical decision-making. Curves can be described on the basis of age at onset, associated pathology, and anatomic configurations of the curve (e.g., single, double, or triple curves; amount of pelvic tilt; curve flexibility, as well as systems based on three-dimensional analysis).[22] From an anesthetic perspective, a classification that gives some idea of the risk of adverse outcome, in particular respiratory failure, would be of clinical benefit. Children with scoliosis of early onset (<5 years) or with independent cardiac or pulmonary disease appear to be at increased risk of respiratory failure, whereas children with idiopathic scoliosis in whom the curve develops at adolescence appear to have minimal risk.[23] A classification adapted from that proposed by the Scoliosis Research Society in 1973 remains relevant to anesthesiologists (Table 30-1).[24]

Pathophysiology and Natural History

Vertebral rotation and rib cage deformity usually accompany any lateral curvature. With progression of the curve, the vertebral bodies in the area of the primary curve rotate toward the convex aspect of the curve and the spinous process rotates to the concave side. This vertebral rotation can be determined by measurement of the position of the pedicles from the midline (Moes method).[25] The vertebral bodies and the discs develop a wedge-shaped appearance with the apex of the wedge toward the concave side. On the convex side of the curve the ribs are pushed posteriorly, which narrows the thoracic cavity and causes the characteristic hump. On the concave side the same rotation forces the ribs laterally, with consequent crowding toward their lateral margins (Fig. 30-2). These changes result in an increasing restrictive lung defect. Exactly when this becomes a problem depends on the child's accompanying pathology. The thoracic and lumbar regions are the most common sites of the primary curve. In children in whom the primary curve is in the lumbar region, the rotation of the vertebral bodies and spinous processes should be taken into consideration when a spinal or epidural drug is to be administered.

The physical distortion in the thorax results in restriction of lung volumes and function. Ventilation depends on the mobility of the thoracic cage, the volume of each hemithorax, and the muscle power and elastic forces required to move the thorax. Children with idiopathic scoliosis with a mild decrease in vital capacity (VC) also have reduced forced expired volume at 1 second (FEV$_1$), gas transfer factor, and maximum static expiratory airway pressures (PEmax) (see Chapter 11). The predominant deformity of lateral flexion and vertebral rotation results in

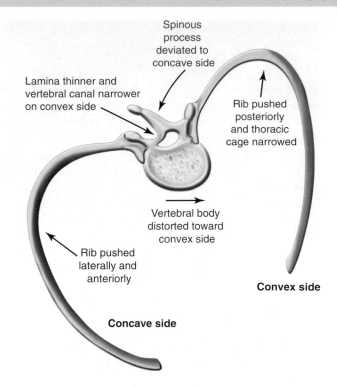

Figure 30-2. Characteristic distortion of vertebra and ribs in thoracic scoliosis. (Modified from Kleim HA: Scoliosis. Ciba Foundation Symposium, Summit, NJ, Ciba, 1978, vol 1, p 609 and Gregory GA [ed]: Anesthesia for orthopaedic surgery. In Paediatric Anesthesia, 3rd ed. Edinburgh, Churchill Livingstone, 1994.)

the lung on the concave side being able to achieve a near-normal end-expiratory position but not end-inspiratory position, whereas the lung on the convex side achieves a normal end-inspiratory position but cannot reach a normal end-expiratory position. The concave side will contribute less than normal at total lung capacity (TLC), resulting in a decrease in PEmax. Similarly, because the convex side does not reach a normal end-expiratory position, the intercostal muscles and hemidiaphragm will be less efficient, resulting in a reduced maximum static inspiratory airway pressure (PImax), although this reduction may not be quite so marked.[26] The main effect of scoliosis on respiratory function is thought to be mechanical, with the anatomic changes in the chest wall causing impaired movement and reduced compliance. Potential long-term respiratory problems when these defects are left untreated include hypoxemia, hypercarbia, recurrent lung infections, and pulmonary hypertension.

Idiopathic Scoliosis

Although adolescent idiopathic scoliosis is relatively common, severe morbidity, and even mortality is only seen in children with early onset (infantile or juvenile) idiopathic scoliosis.[27] Respiratory deterioration alone is seldom the reason for surgery in children who develop scoliosis after the age of 5 years.[23] This is probably because most of the multiplication, division, and development of alveoli in the lungs have occurred by this age.[28,29]

The scoliosis evolves during periods of development and physical growth, and curve progression occurs during growth spurts. This is not the case in children with neuromuscular

cord stimulation is achieved electrically and can be applied using electrodes placed either outside or inside the spinal cord rostral to the area of interest. Single stimuli rather than brief pulse trains are commonly used for spinal cord stimulation.[74]

Responses can be recorded anywhere distal to the area of interest. These have included the lower lumbar epidural space (epidural MEP), peripheral nerve (neurogenic MEP), and peripheral muscles using compound muscle action potential (CMAP) (see Fig. 30-7B).[75] Each recording site has its limitations regarding the accuracy of the information displayed and the susceptibility to anesthetic drug interference. Epidural MEPs are the least affected by muscle relaxants, but they only monitor conduction in the (cortico)spinal tract and provide no information about the anterior horn gray matter.[76] They have a much slower response to acute spinal cord ischemia when compared with myogenic responses (CMAP).[77] Neurogenic MEPs are also resistant to anesthetic interference but appear not to accurately measure motor conduction. Most of the spinally elicited peripheral nerve responses seen with neurogenic MEPs have been shown to occur via the dorsal columns in a retrograde fashion and are sensory rather than motor.[78] Furthermore, anterior spinal cord injury has occurred with normal neurogenic MEPs.[79] CMAPs after transcranial stimulation are believed to be exclusively generated via motor tract conduction and unlike epidural MEPs include the ischemia-sensitive anterior horn alpha motor neurons.[75] These responses are very sensitive to anesthetic agents. A total intravenous anesthetic (TIVA) ± <0.5% MAC isoflurane may be requested. The responses obtained with CMAP after spinal cord stimulation also appear to contain signals that include transmission via the dorsal columns and may represent a mixed response.[80]

One outstanding problem with MEP monitoring is deciding when and how much change in the signal is significant and indicative of spinal cord ischemia. Some centers use the same criteria they have adopted for SSEP monitoring, whereas others require a greater degree of change, such as a 75% decrease in amplitude.[81] More recently, an amplitude decrease of 80% at one of six sites using transcranial myogenic MEP monitoring was demonstrated to have a sensitivity of 1.0 and a specificity of 0.91 when used as the sole monitor during spine surgery.[82] An alternative technique of measuring MEP has been described whereby a minimum threshold for producing a response is established and a significant increase in that threshold is used to indicate a problem.[83] Supportive data for this technique are lacking.

Whether MEP monitoring should replace SSEP monitoring, or whether the two should be used together, is a source of controversy at the time of writing. There is some evidence that the dorsal columns may be injured without involvement of the motor tract.[84] Occasionally, adverse changes in SSEP occur without changes in MEP but the association with neurologic deficit is unclear.[74]

Preoperative Assessment and Postoperative Planning

Respiratory Assessment and Planning for Postoperative Ventilatory Support

The preoperative pulmonary assessment should identify those children at increased risk from short-term postoperative pulmonary complications as well as long-term respiratory failure (or

failure to wean from a ventilator). Rigid statements regarding either issue are difficult because different surgical approaches, child and institutional variabilities, and author interest has resulted in heterogeneous reporting. Children with idiopathic scoliosis tend to have less decrease in pulmonary function with correspondingly low complication rates, so most studies have been directed at nonidiopathic children.[56] The rate of postoperative pulmonary complications correlates broadly with the decrease in VC.[39,85,86] VC less than 30% to 35% of predicted indicates marginal respiratory reserve and a level at which complications and a need for postoperative respiratory support are likely. Many children with these low vital capacities are unable to cough effectively, rendering them prone to postoperative atelectasis, pneumonia, and respiratory failure.

Studies involving a mixed population with a VC less than 40% (but with few neuromuscular patients) suggest that although short- and mid-term pulmonary complications occur, these children can be successfully managed to achieve discharge to home, although some will require prolonged postoperative ventilation.[87,88] Modest numbers of children with a VC less than 25% predicted are described in these studies and do not appear to have a higher complication rate than those with greater VC. Anterior or combined approaches increase the likelihood of respiratory complications, particularly due to pleural effusion.[87,88]

Children with neuromuscular scoliosis are at particular risk for postoperative ventilation that is often prolonged.[39,86] These children may also have abnormalities in the central control of breathing and impaired airway defense mechanisms. Impaired coordination of laryngeal and pharyngeal muscles may result in impaired swallowing and inadequate cough with increased risk of aspiration. Initial work suggested that as the VC decreased to less than 35% predicted, most children would need a brief period of postoperative ventilation.[84] Recent studies suggest that scoliosis surgery can be successfully undertaken in children with a VC of less than 35% predicted, often with no more than 24 hours of planned ventilation, followed by a period of noninvasive ventilation (e.g., bilevel positive airway pressure [BiPAP]).[39,89,90] The overall complication rate is similar whether the FVC is more or less than 30%, with an average hospital stay of approximately 3 weeks.[90] Again, the successful management of children with an FVC of less than 25% predicted is described. With the known changes in VC after surgery, it would seem reasonable to anticipate using noninvasive ventilator support for up to a week after spine stabilization surgery in these children. Children with neuromuscular scoliosis and early-onset respiratory failure requiring nocturnal noninvasive ventilation (BiPAP) have successfully undergone scoliosis surgery. A small group of children with a mean FVC of 20% predicted has been successfully managed with a short period of postoperative ventilation and transitioned to BiPAP within 48 hours without any respiratory complications.[91]

Whether a child should be denied surgery requires consideration of individual patient factors. The successful management of a few children with a VC of 15% to 20% predicted have been described, but the numbers are small.[87-90] Although the risk of an unsuccessful outcome will increase at this level, individual circumstances may justify that risk.

Cardiovascular Assessment

Muscle disorders may affect the myocardium as well as the skeletal system. Children with DMD develop a cardiomyopathy that may be difficult to evaluate because the child is wheelchair bound. Sinus tachycardia is an early manifestation, and evidence of decreased cardiac function increases in frequency and severity from early adolescence.[92] Over 90% of adolescents with DMD have subclinical or clinical cardiac involvement.[93] Echocardiography is an essential part of the evaluation of any wheelchair-bound child presenting for scoliosis surgery.

Postoperative Pain Management

Scoliosis surgery is associated with severe pain that lasts for at least 3 days.[94] Analgesia minimizes postoperative respiratory complications by allowing deep breathing, chest physiotherapy, early ambulation, and rehabilitation. The two broad approaches to postoperative pain management are either systemic or epidural analgesics. A multimodal approach is likely to be most effective.

Intraoperative intrathecal morphine has been demonstrated to provide potent analgesia during the first 24 hours after spinal fusion in children.[95] Intrathecal morphine also decreases the amount of remifentanil required intraoperatively and so may minimize the development of acute opioid tolerance that may be seen after the use of high-dose remifentanil infusions.[96,97]

Nonsteroidal Anti-inflammatory Drugs

NSAIDs, but not acetaminophen, impair fracture healing in animal models.[98] Cyclooxygenase-2 activity plays an important role in bone healing, and the use of NSAIDs decreases osteogenic activity that may increase the incidence of nonunion after spinal fusion.[8,9] The effect on osteogenic activity is dose dependent and reversible.[99] Similar effects have not been demonstrated in humans. Nonetheless, based on animal evidence, NSAIDs should be used with caution and in consultation with the surgeon during the first 3 to 5 days after scoliosis surgery.[100]

Systemic Analgesics

Morphine is the mainstay of systemic analgesic regimens. Morphine infusions of 20 to 40 µg/kg/hr are required during the first 48 hours after surgery. Achieving a balance of effective analgesia while avoiding incapacitating sedation can be difficult in children with neurodevelopmental delay. Regular evaluation of these children is important if complications are to be avoided. Patient-controlled analgesia (PCA) is appropriate for children older than the age of 6 to 7 years and can be used with a typical bolus dose of 20 µg/kg and a lockout interval of 5 to 10 minutes. The use of a background morphine infusion may be effective in some children, although its inclusion is controversial.[101,102] Our preference is to add a night-time background infusion at 5- to 10-µg/kg/hr but to use PCA alone during the day (see Chapter 44). Nurse- and parent-controlled analgesia have also been shown to be effective if the child is too young or unable to use PCA.[103] A low-dose ketamine infusion (0.05-0.2 mg/kg/hr) has been used as an adjunct to morphine infusions or PCA, although its role is debated[104-109]; its use is generally reserved for those with morphine-resistant pain. Ketamine may be initiated intraoperatively (an infusion of 5 µg/kg/min, decreasing to 2 µg/kg/min at the end of surgery) as part of the anesthetic technique to minimize the hyperalgesia reported after high-dose remifentanil infusions.[110,111] If added to PCA, the optimal combination of morphine/ketamine is 1:1.[107]

Epidural Analgesia

Continuous epidural analgesia, using both single- and double-catheter techniques, may provide effective analgesia after spine surgery. The single-catheter technique using bupivacaine-fentanyl and sited at T6-T7 for children undergoing a mean 12-level scoliosis surgery correction has been reported to provide similar analgesia to PCA. Bowel sounds returned earlier in the epidural group, but liquid intake and hospitalization were similar.[112] Similar results were reported with a bupivacaine-morphine combination in children undergoing 10-level spinal fusions. Full diet and discharge from hospital were achieved half a day earlier with the epidural technique than with PCA.[113] A retrospective review of more than 600 patients treated with either epidural analgesia or PCA for postscoliosis analgesia, in which an average number of segments fused was 8.5, confirmed the effectiveness of epidural analgesia.[114] In that study a bupivacaine-hydromorphone epidural combination was used and although pain management was effective, more complications occurred in the epidural group. Respiratory depression and transient neurologic changes were the most common complications observed. Thirteen percent of adolescants with an epidural catheter required discontinuation of the epidural, most commonly for inadequate pain relief.[114] Patient-controlled epidural analgesia (PCEA) has been successfully used in children older than age 5 years for orthopedic surgery and thoracotomies but experience after scoliosis surgery is limited.[115]

Double epidural techniques comprise an upper catheter positioned in the upper or mid thoracic segments and a lower catheter at the mid lumbar level. Initial reports of this technique involved a ropivacaine-hydromorphone mixture with catheters that were in situ for 5 postoperative days without adverse effects.[116,117] Ropivacaine, 0.3% 10 mL/hr, for nine-segment scoliosis surgery improved pain scores both at rest and with movement compared with a morphine infusion. Bowel activity returned earlier, and a decreased incidence of postoperative nausea and vomiting was observed in the epidural group.[118]

Anesthetic and Intraoperative Management

Positioning and Related Issues

It is essential that the child is positioned so that extreme pressure points are avoided, the limb positions are adjusted to prevent nerve injury, and the abdomen is free, to minimize venous congestion. This is usually achieved by the use of the Relton-Hall frame or a variant.[119] The frame comprises four well-padded supports arranged into V-shaped pairs with the upper pads supporting the thoracic cage and the lower pair supporting the anterolateral aspects of the pelvic girdle at the anterior iliac crests. The arms should not be abducted or extended greater than 90 degrees from their natural position, and the weight of the arms should be evenly distributed across the forearm to avoid pressure on the ulnar nerve at the elbow. This can present quite a challenge in children with severe deformities, and creative positioning may be required. In some centers, the nipples are covered with Tegaderm (3M, St. Paul, MN) and positioned free of direct pressure. It is also essential that the head is maintained in a neutral position and that pressure is evenly distributed between the forehead and face, avoiding direct pressure on the eyeballs. Care must be taken to avoid

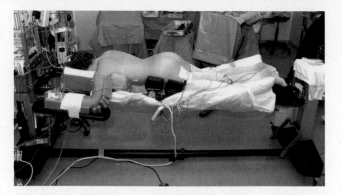

Figure 30-8. Positioning on the OSI Jackson frame showing protected pressure points and underframe forced air warming blanket.

any direct pressure on the knees, with distribution of the child's weight spread throughout the lower limb (Fig. 30-8). Reston (3M, St. Paul, MN) may be used to pad the pelvic brim and knees.

Not all spinal tables and frames affect cardiac function in the same way. There is some evidence that the Jackson spine table or longitudinal bolsters have minimal effects on cardiac function, whereas Wilson, Siemens, and Andrews frames may negatively impact cardiac function.[120]

Postoperative visual loss is an uncommon, unpredictable, but devastating complication associated with spinal surgery. The incidence may be as great as 0.2% of cases; and although most of the reports involve adult patients, older children are not immune.[121,122] The most common cause is ischemic optic neuropathy, but the etiology remains obscure. Prolonged operating time (>6 hours) and increased or uncontrolled blood loss are a feature of most of the reports.[123-126] The phenomenon is unrelated to pressure on the globe and usually occurs without evidence of any other ischemia-related complications.[126] There are no data to support controlled hypotension or hemodilution as contributory factors despite occasional "expert" opinions to the contrary.[123,126,127]

Temperature Regulation

The long preparation time and exposure of an undraped child on the spinal frame render children susceptible to hypothermia. Hypothermia is associated with hemodynamic instability and increased blood loss.[128] A threefold increase in surgical wound infection occurs with a 2°C decrease in core temperature.[129] Efforts should be made to increase the ambient temperature in the operating room while the child is prepared for surgery. Subsequent hypothermia will be minimized if the room temperature is maintained at 24°C during this period rather than 18 to 21°C as is often encountered during surgery.[130] Once the child has cooled during preparation and positioning, it may take several hours before the core temperature begins to return toward normal. Even with forced air warming systems, it is often difficult to restore normothermia because only a small amount of the child's body is exposed to these devices. It may be possible to position a warming blanket underneath the frame so that warming from below as well as from above occurs (see Fig. 30-8).

Patient Monitoring

Patient monitoring needs to be tailored to the individual case, but, at a minimum, hemoglobin oxygen saturation, end-tidal CO_2, systemic blood pressure, electrocardiographic findings, core temperature, and urine output should be recorded. In most cases invasive arterial and central venous pressures are monitored because of large blood losses, fluid shifts, and the risk of cardiovascular instability. Direct pressure by the surgeon during either dissection or curve correction may compromise cardiac function or filling. Central venous pressure is an accurate and valid measurement in the prone position, providing the zero is adjusted for the child's position on the spinal frame. Children with a significant kyphotic component are at increased risk of venous air embolism and should be monitored for this possibility. Depth of anesthesia monitoring should be considered, particularly when MEP monitoring limits the concentrations of anesthetic drugs. Care should be taken with positioning the head because pressure on the forehead by the sensor while the child is in the prone position for many hours can cause erythema, localized swelling, and possible tissue necrosis. Contact dermatitis from the adhesive has also been reported.[131] Transesophageal echocardiography can be useful for determining ventricular filling and function when hemodynamic compromise is identified or suspected preoperatively.

Minimizing Blood Loss and Decreasing Transfusion Requirements

Scoliosis surgery involves exposure of a large wound over a considerable period of time. Positioning the child with the abdomen free to avoid venous compression is important to control and minimize blood loss. Increased intra-abdominal pressure attributable to positioning can double intraoperative blood loss.[132]

The reported estimated blood loss (EBL) for this type of surgery varies from institution to institution and from one surgical technique to another. Posterior spinal fusion procedures tend to lose more blood than anterior procedures. This loss is probably due to the greater number of vertebral levels fused with the posterior approach. Blood loss increases as the number of vertebrae included in the fusion increases. The EBL is 750 to 1500 mL in children with idiopathic scoliosis, which equates to 60 to 150 mL per vertebral segment fused. The blood loss is significantly greater in children with cerebral palsy—1300 to 2200 mL—which equates to 100 to 190 mL per level. Children with DMD have the greatest EBL of 2500 to 4000 mL, which equates to an EBL of 200 to 280 mL per vertebral level.[133]

Children with neuromuscular scoliosis demonstrate a prolonged prothrombin time and a decrease in factor VII activity intraoperatively, suggesting that consumption of clotting factors as well as dilution of clotting factors enhances the blood loss.[134] It has been postulated that children with DMD lack dystrophin in all muscle types and that the poor vascular smooth muscle vasoconstrictor response may be a factor in the increased blood loss.[135] Hypothermia exacerbates blood loss by decreasing platelet function, decreasing coagulation factor activity, and slowing vasoconstriction.[128]

Hypotensive Techniques

Controlled hypotension has been used to minimize blood loss during scoliosis surgery. A greater than 50% decrease in blood loss with a decreased need for blood replacement, as well as a reduced operating time, was demonstrated in early studies. Ganglion-blocking agents (pentolinium and trimethaphan) have been superseded by β blockers, direct arterial vasodilators, calcium-channel blockers, and α 2 agonists. Evidence from studies in which sodium nitroprusside and trimethaphan were compared suggests that the mean arterial pressure and not cardiac output determines intraoperative blood loss.[136] On the other hand, a study in which a β blocker and nitroprusside were compared suggests that a slower heart rate and hence cardiac output is associated with reduced blood loss.[137] A target mean arterial pressure (MAP) of 50 to 65 mm Hg has been recommended. Although this appears to be safe from published data and knowledge of the autoregulation of cerebral and spinal cord blood flow, there is no doubt that the margin of safety for cerebral and spinal cord ischemia is reduced by controlled hypotension. This is of particular concern when this target MAP is used in long operations, with the potential for periods of hypovolemic hypotension in addition to drug-induced (controlled) hypotension.[138] From this stems concern that low MAP may be associated with cerebral ischemia, spinal cord ischemia, and end-organ failure.[139] The incidence of these feared complications is fortunately very low with or without the use of controlled hypotension. Renal function appears well preserved even when hypotensive anesthesia is used during scoliosis surgery, but hypotension may cause decreased SSEPs used as a monitor and indicator of spinal cord function.[140,141] Because of these concerns and the concomitant use of hemodilution, less extreme degrees of hypotension are usually employed today. This can often be achieved without the use of specific vasoactive drugs. In most cases, adequate hypotension can be achieved using a remifentanil infusion titrated to the desired blood pressure without concerns of prolonged blood pressure or sedation effects.[142]

Clonidine is a useful adjunct for reducing blood pressure in children.[143] We have found that using an anesthetic combination of less than 1 MAC of inhalation agent plus remifentanil with clonidine (2 μg/kg) results in controlled hypotension in most children without the need for any additional agents.

Although not considered a hypotensive agent, intrathecal morphine decreases blood loss and may facilitate blood pressure control, particularly with a remifentanil infusion. At an analgesic dose of 5 μg/kg, a decrease in EBL from 41 to 14 mL/kg occurred.[95] Again, using this technique, blood pressure control can often be achieved without any additional agents.

Nicardipine has been used to produce hypotension in children undergoing spinal surgery and is associated with less blood loss at the same mean arterial pressure when compared with sodium nitroprusside.[144,145] A slower return to baseline blood pressure (27 vs. 7 minutes) is the problem with this drug and may be the reason it is not widely used. If a hypotensive technique is to be used, then invasive arterial and central venous pressure catheters are essential for the safe conduct of anesthesia (see Chapter 10).

Hemodilution

Decreasing the hemoglobin concentration by removing red cells and replacing the volume with a combination of crystalloid and albumin means that for a given volume loss there is less red cell loss (see Chapter 10). The decreased metabolic rate during anesthesia implies that oxygen delivery can be maintained with a lower hemoglobin concentration providing normovolemia is maintained. In many cases, deciding on the degree of hemodilu-

tion and establishing a threshold for transfusion is difficult. Many clinicians use a hematocrit below 20% to 25% (hemoglobin of 7 to 8 g/dL) as the trigger for transfusion. At this hemoglobin concentration, tachycardia and hemodynamic instability frequently first appear. More extreme degrees of hemodilution have been described, but the decrease in oxygen-carrying capacity reduces the margin of safety to prevent cerebral and spinal cord ischemia. Myocardial ischemia becomes a risk at hemoglobin concentrations less than 5 g/dL.[146] Cyanosis cannot occur at these levels because 5 g/dL of desaturated hemoglobin is required for cyanosis to be observed. Many children demonstrate tachycardia and circulatory instability at a hemoglobin in excess of this level, so extreme hemodilution techniques such as these are reserved for Jehovah's Witnesses and those who are opposed to blood transfusion. In one report, children were hemodiluted during scoliosis surgery to a hemoglobin concentration of 3 g/dL in the absence of any preexisting cardiac disease.[147] Presumably, adequate oxygen transport was achieved by an increase in oxygen extraction and an increase in cardiac output. Cardiac output increased by over 30% with only a modest increase in heart rate and decrease in blood pressure.[147] Although no cerebral sequelae were reported, *this degree of extreme hemodilution is not recommended.*

Hemodilution modeling in adult patients has suggested that as many as 5 units of blood need to be removed before there is a decrease in transfusion requirements.[148] This is significantly greater than the usual 2 to 3 units removed in most adult-sized children. Despite these theoretical concerns, a relatively conservative hemodilution strategy is commonly and readily employed in children with idiopathic scoliosis. Reduction to an initial hematocrit of 30% has been shown to be effective in reducing and minimizing transfusion requirements.[149] These numbers must be tailored for each child because a unit of blood in a 35-kg child is a much larger fraction of the circulating blood volume than in a 70-kg child.

Autologous Pre-donation

Alternately, several other preoperative strategies may be used, including pre-donation of blood and preoperative red cell augmentation. In the latter case, sequestration of several units of blood after induction of anesthesia but before surgery can be achieved provided the child's hemoglobin concentration has been increased to 16 to 18 g/dL preoperatively with parenteral erythropoietin, oral iron, and vitamin C (see Chapter 10). Sequestration of several units of blood can be achieved (and returned to the circulation as needed) without decreasing the hemoglobin concentration to values that put the brain, spinal cord, and heart at risk for adverse sequelae.

Antifibrinolytic Agents

The use of synthetic antifibrinolytic agents to decrease perioperative blood loss after scoliosis surgery has produced mixed results. It should be emphasized that for an antifibrinolytic to be most effective an effective plasma concentration should be established before skin incision. ε-Aminocaproic acid (EACA) has been shown to decrease the EBL by 25% during the perioperative period,[150] mainly attributable to decreasing postoperative suction drainage.[151] In contrast, tranexamic acid, 10 mg/kg followed by an infusion of 1 mg/kg/hr, failed to significantly decrease blood loss in a small sample.[152] High-dose tranexamic acid (100 mg/kg loading dose followed by an infusion of 10 mg/kg/hr) did decrease blood loss by 40% but did not affect transfusion requirements. Post hoc analysis in children with secondary (neuromuscular) scoliosis showed significant reduction in both blood loss and transfusion requiremnts.[153] Aprotinin,* in a dose approximating the full dose "Hammersmith" regimen in adults (240 mg/m^2 loading dose followed by an infusion of 56 mg/m^2/hr for children with body surface area (BSA) $<1 \text{ m}^2$ or 280 mg loading dose followed by an infusion of 70 mg/hr for BSA $>1 \text{ m}^2$) has been associated with a 40% decrease in blood loss, which equated to a decrease from 76 to 38 mL per vertebral level fused. This decrease in blood loss with aprotinin also resulted in fewer units of blood transfused (2.2 [control] vs. 1.1 units [aprotinin]).[154] In adult patients undergoing complex spine surgery, using approximately one half "Hammersmith" dose, aprotinin effectively reduced the blood loss, blood component therapy after surgery, and was associated with a decrease in respiratory morbidity. This was not observed in patients treated with EACA.[155] Aprotinin may not be indicated for all children because it is expensive and carries allergic risks, but it may be appropriate for those at risk for postoperative pulmonary complications and for those undergoing complex curve corrections.

Desmopressin probably has no beneficial effect on decreasing blood loss associated with spinal surgery. Initial beneficial results[156] have not been reproduced in children with idiopathic scoliosis[157,158] or in those with neuromuscular scoliosis.[159,160]

Intraoperative Salvage of Shed Blood

Decisions concerning the use of intraoperative salvage of shed blood (cell saver) are dependent on the anticipated blood loss, size of the child, and use of other methods to minimize blood transfusion, such as pre-donation and hemodilution (see Chapter 10). The addition of a cell saver was found to be beneficial in less than 5% of adolescents with idiopathic scoliosis involved with either an autologous pre-donation program and/or modest intraoperative hemodilution.[149] The technique is beneficial in children with a smaller body weight and greater anticipated blood loss such as children with neuromuscular scoliosis undergoing extensive spinal fusion.[161,162]

Managing Blood Loss

Using autologous blood requires an organized schedule of donation with or without the administration of erythropoietin.[163,164] This may be the safest and most effective method of avoiding or minimizing the use of allogenic blood products in this group of children.[165] A pre-donation program was effective in minimizing blood exposure in idiopathic adolescents undergoing surgical correction for their scoliosis; a mean of 3.7 units of blood was donated by each child before surgery, and 97% of adolescents avoided the use of allogeneic blood during and after surgery.[163]

Measurement of blood loss during scoliosis surgery is difficult. Accuracy is lost as measurements embrace blood suctioned from the operative field that includes irrigation fluid, weighing or estimating blood collected on swabs and sponges, approximations of blood on drapes and gowns, as well as consideration of evaporation from the wound.

The decision when to administer blood component therapy (i.e., non–red cell blood components) is often based on clinical

*Aprotinin has recently been removed from all hospital pharmacies and warehouses and is not available for purchase in the United States. It is available as an investigational drug only under certain guidelines. Please see http://www.fda.gov/CDER/DRUG/infopage/aprotinin/default.htm

judgment. Dilutional thrombocytopenia would be expected only after several blood volumes have been lost and depends on the initial platelet count before surgery (see Chapter 10). Platelet concentrations should be measured after loss of one blood volume and at periodic intervals after this. Dilution of coagulation factors may also lead to surgical bleeding when packed red blood cells only are used to replace blood loss. Prolongation of prothrombin time and activated partial thromboplastin time may occur when the blood loss exceeds one blood volume and should be checked at this time. These coagulation tests are not usually associated with increased bleeding until values are greater than 1.5 times mean control values, at which time increased surgical bleeding can be effectively treated with fresh frozen plasma.[166] Platelet counts after one blood volume loss, whether associated with normal or abnormal clotting, were within the normal range.[166] Blood component therapy should probably be based on abnormal clotting tests, uncontrolled bleeding, or the absence of normal clotting in the surgical field. It is preferable to intervene with blood component therapy before uncontrolled bleeding develops. If pooled blood in a dependent part of the operative field fails to show evidence of clotting, it is time to transfuse with blood components starting with fresh frozen plasma and only administering platelets if this is not effective.[166]

Recombinant factor VIIa may be a useful therapy for children with a dilutional coagulopathy and who do not respond to blood component replacement therapy. Successful use has been described in two children with neuromuscular scoliosis, but its use for this indication remains unapproved.[167]

Anesthetic Agents: Effect on SSEP and MEP

Spinal cord monitoring is an integral part of providing care for children undergoing scoliosis surgery. Knowledge of the effects of drugs on evoked potentials is pivotal for developing a successful anesthetic regimen. Anesthetic agents produce their effects by either directly inhibiting synaptic pathways or indirectly changing the balance of inhibitory and excitatory influences.[168,169] In general terms, the greater the number of synapses and the more complex the neuronal pathway being monitored, the greater the potential impact from anesthetic agents. Most anesthetic agents depress the amplitude and increase the latency of both the SSEP and MEP. For this reason, cortical SSEPs are more sensitive than spinal cord or brainstem-measured SSEPs. MEPs are susceptible to anesthetic agents at three sites: the motor cortex, the anterior horn cell, and the neuromuscular junction. Consequently, transcranial stimulation with peripheral muscle detection (using CMAP) is most susceptible to anesthetic interference. Although inhalational anesthetics and most intravenous anesthetics markedly depress SSEP and MEP, ketamine and etomidate appear to enhance the amplitudes of both, possibly by attenuating inhibition.[169]

Inhalational Anesthetics

The inhalational anesthetics cause dose-dependent depression of the SSEP and MEP; myogenic MEP is affected to a greater degree than SSEP. This means that while inhalation agents can be used during SSEP monitoring, they often need to be used in subanesthetic doses during MEP monitoring. Adequate cortical SSEPs and subcortical SSEPs can be measured with up to 1 MAC of isoflurane, sevoflurane, and desflurane, although some increase in latency and decrease in amplitude may be detected.[170,171] It is important to maintain constant end-tidal concentrations throughout the anesthetic once baseline measurements have been established. The concentrations of these anesthetics that allow adequate monitoring are significantly lower than was possible with halothane.[172]

Myogenic MEPs (CMAPs) are only recordable at low concentrations of inhalation anesthetics. The exact concentration depends on the system being used and is greatly influenced by the number of pulses in the stimulus. Single-pulse transcranial stimuli may be inhibited by end-tidal concentrations as low as 0.2 MAC and abolished by end-tidal concentrations as low as 0.5 MAC.[173-175] This suppression can be partially overcome by using higher-intensity stimuli with multiple-pulse stimulation of up to six pulses per stimulus. An increasing number of children lose recordable myogenic MEPs, even when multiple-pulse stimuli are used as the concentration of inhalational anesthetic exceeds 0.5 MAC. At end-tidal concentrations in excess of 0.75% isoflurane, monitoring conditions may become unacceptable.[176-180] Stimulus intensity as well as pulse train frequency is probably a factor in determining successful myogenic MEPs with inhalational anesthetics. Using direct stimulation of the cortex during craniotomy, CMAP was easily recordable at 1 MAC of both isoflurane and sevoflurane.[181] Similar results have been demonstrated with sevoflurane using transcranial stimulation.[182,197] Information regarding desflurane is limited; although it causes a dose-dependent depression, myogenic MEPs have been successfully recorded at 0.5 MAC.[180,183] With the use of a multiple-pulse stimulation technique, intraoperative recording of MEPs was equally successful during desflurane or propofol anesthesia.[184] In contrast to its effects on SSEPs, halothane depresses myogenic MEPs to a lesser extent than the newer inhalational anesthetics.[182]

Nitrous Oxide

Nitrous oxide reduces the amplitude of the cortical SSEP, but comparisons with other inhalational anesthetics are limited. Nitrous oxide, 0.5 MAC, depresses SSEPs to a greater extent than isoflurane at a similar MAC.[185] Similarly, nitrous oxide, 66%, depressed SSEPs to a greater extent than propofol 6 mg/kg/hr (100 μg/kg/min).[186] Nitrous oxide also depresses myogenic MEPs.[171] The effect relative to inhalational anesthetics is difficult to determine. Nitrous oxide appears to affect CMAP amplitude to a lesser extent than isoflurane.[187] Multiple-pulse stimulus techniques can partially reverse nitrous oxide–induced depression of amplitude. Compared with a propofol infusion designed to maintain a target concentration of 3 μg/mL, 50% nitrous oxide decreased CMAPs with both single and paired stimuli to a lesser extent.[188] When 60% nitrous was added to low-dose propofol infusion at a target concentration of 1 μg/mL, adequated CMAPs were obtained using multiple-pulse transcranial stimulation.[189] Conversely, the addition of nitrous oxide to a variety of different total intravenous techniques significantly depressed the CMAP such that some were not recordable.[190]

With the widespread availability of remifentanil and the variable but mostly negative effects of nitrous oxide on SSEP and MEP signals, it would seem that nitrous oxide is best avoided when spinal cord monitoring is used.

Propofol

Propofol produces a decrease in amplitude of the cortical SSEP, but adequate signals can be recorded, even in the presence of nitrous oxide, at doses used for anesthesia (6 mg/kg/hr).[191] Pro-

pofol better preserves cortical SSEP amplitude and provides a deeper level of hypnosis as measured by processed electroencephalographic values than combinations of low-dose isoflurane/N₂O or low-dose isoflurane or sevoflurane alone.[192-194]

Propofol depresses the amplitude of myogenic MEPs. In addition to its cortical effect, it also suppresses activation of the alpha motor neuron at the level of the spinal gray matter.[195,196] Low-dose propofol infusions have become popular as part of the anesthetic technique with MEP monitoring owing to the rapid improvement of signals when the drug is terminated and because multiple-pulse stimulation techniques can improve the response amplitude.[177,178] Propofol, even in combination with nitrous oxide, depresses multiple-pulse transcranial CMAP less than isoflurane.[177] Propofol, 5 mg/kg/hr, combined with 66% nitrous oxide produced satisfactory CMAP recordings in 75% of patients when a four-pulse stimulation sequence was used. In contrast, no recordings were possible with 1 MAC isoflurane.[178] The infusion rates or target concentrations that allow acceptable myogenic MEP recordings vary considerably and reflect different adjuvants (e.g., opioids, ketamine, and nitrous oxide), degrees of neuromuscular blockade, and transcranial pulse rates. Propofol at a target of 4 μg/mL or at an infusion rate of 6 mg/kg/hr produces acceptable signals with multiple-pulse stimuli.[198,199]

α₂-Adrenoreceptor Agonists: Clonidine and Dexmedetomidine

The cerebral effects of the α₂ agonists appear to be mainly at the locus coeruleus rather than by the more generalized inhibition of synaptic pathways, as in the case of general anesthetics.[200] Clonidine at intravenous doses of 2 to 5 μg/kg had minimal effects on cortical SSEPs when added to isoflurane.[201-203] In view of its lack of effect on SSEPs and its anesthetic sparing properties with both inhalational agents and propofol,[203-205] it seems reasonable to consider clonidine at a dose of 2 to 4 μg/kg as part of an anesthetic technique. Dexmedetomidine appears to have similar beneficial properties on SSEPs.[206,207] There are no published studies on the effects of clonidine or dexmedetomidine on MEPs, but one might speculate that they would improve signal recordings of MEPs by allowing lower concentrations of inhalational anesthetics or propofol.

Opioids

Alfentanil, fentanyl, sufentanil, and remifentanil produce minimal effects on SSEP and MEP signal recording.[208,209] Dose-dependent depression of CMAP does occur at doses of opioids that far exceed those used in clinical anesthesia.[210,211] Comparison of alfentanil, fentanyl, and sufentanil at doses sufficient to suppress noxious stimuli suggested that sufentanil exerted the least effect.[210] A similar study including remifentanil showed that this drug had the least depressive effects, with CMAPs measurable at infusion rates of 0.6 μg/kg/min.[211] It is likely that larger doses can be used if clinically indicated.

Ketamine and Etomidate

Ketamine enhances cortical SSEP amplitude and has a minimal effect on subcortical and peripheral SSEP responses.[212] It also produces minimal effects on the myogenic MEP responses, either as a bolus of 0.5 mg/kg[213] or when used in moderate doses (1-4 mg/kg/hr) as a supplement to a nitrous oxide/opioid anesthesia.[213,214] Experimental evidence suggests S(+)-ketamine modulates CMAP by a peripheral mechanism at or distal to the spinal alpha motor neuron.[215]

Etomidate, although capable of inducing general anesthesia, behaves more like ketamine in its effect on evoked potentials. It improves the quality of SSEPs and enhances the amplitude of MEPs.[216] It produces minimal changes in MEPs when compared with barbiturates or propofol.[195] Etomidate infusions (10-35 μg/kg/min) produce adequate MEP monitoring signals.[213,217] Concerns regarding adrenocortical depression with etomidate infusions remain and limit its widespread use.[218] Bolus doses of etomidate however, can transiently depress MEPs.[213]

Midazolam

Intravenous midazolam (0.2 mg/kg) decreases the SSEP amplitude by 60%.[219] This does not seem to occur with subcortical SSEPs, in which a slight increase in latency but no change in amplitude has been demonstrated.[220] Although midazolam (0.5 mg/kg) caused marked depression of MEP in monkeys that persisted during awakening,[221] this does not hold true in human studies. MEP amplitude was not affected by a midazolam-ketamine infusion technique, in comparison with propofol-ketamine or propofol-alfentanil techniques.[190] Midazolam did not suppress myogenic MEP, even at doses sufficient to produce anesthesia[211]; effects were similar to those with etomidate.[211]

Neuromuscular Blockade

Neuromuscular blocking drugs (NMBDs) exert little or no effect on the SSEP. They prevent or limit recording of CMAP during myogenic MEP recording because of their effects on the neuromuscular junction. Partial neuromuscular blockade, however, is commonly used during MEP monitoring because it improves conditions for surgery by providing adequate muscle relaxation when retraction of the tissues is required and limits any child movement during the stimulus generation. Partial muscle relaxation may also reduce noise caused by spontaneous muscle movement. It is important that constant neuromuscular blockade is maintained during the procedure. Many centers avoid neuromuscular blockade after intubation, the initial incision, and muscle dissection.

Two methods have been used to assess the degree of neuromuscular blockade for MEP monitoring. One is measurement of the amplitude of the CMAP produced by single supramaximal stimulation (T1) before use of an NMBD. When T1 is maintained between 20% and 50% of the baseline level, reproducible CMAP responses can be obtained with a degree of muscular blockade that allows surgery.[217,222] The other technique is to adjust the neuromuscular blockade based on the train-of-four responses. Comparison of the fourth twitch (T4) with that of first twitch (T1) suggests acceptable CMAP monitoring is possible when two of the four twitches remain (see Fig. 6-26).[222-224] Neuromuscular blockade should be evaluated in the specific muscle groups that are used for electrophysiologic monitoring because different muscle groups have different sensitivities to the NMBDs. Children with preoperative neuromuscular dysfunction tend to demonstrate greater reduction after partial neuromuscular blockade than children with normal preoperative motor function. It is appropriate to avoid neuromuscular blockade in most of these children.[217]

Choosing the Optimal Combination of Anesthetic Drugs and Techniques

There is no one anesthetic technique suitable for evoked potential monitoring that is applicable to all children. The choice of anesthesia will depend on the child's pathology and the choice of electrophysiologic monitoring planned during the operation. A marked increase in the use of MEPs and advances in MEP techniques have occurred in recent years. CMAP appear to provide the most useful data for minimizing the risk of spinal cord injury.

The key to success is to use a technique that allows a stable concentration of the "hypnotic" component of anesthesia. There is probably no difference between the inhalational anesthetics (<1 MAC) and propofol (<6 mg/kg/hr). Concentrations of the inhalational anesthetics approaching 1 MAC are now compatible with multiple-pulse MEP monitoring systems that did not appear possible several years ago. Short-acting medications offer greater flexibility should the monitored signals deteriorate. The use of a remifentanil infusion allows a rapidly titratable "analgesic" component with minimal effect on spinal cord monitoring. Clonidine may be used to decrease the concentration of "hypnotic" drugs during SSEP monitoring and possibly during MEP monitoring. Ketamine may be added as an adjunct to improve MEP monitoring because it better preserves the MEP signals and also allows a reduced dose of other "hypnotic" agents to be used. If a processed electroencephalographic monitor is used to determine anesthetic depth, then the addition of ketamine may confound the processed electroencephalographic monitor reading (by increasing it).[225,226] This occurs despite a deepening in the level of hypnosis.[225] NMBD improves the SSEP monitoring and may be used in conjunction with MEP monitoring within the confines described earlier. However, even in children with idiopathic scoliosis, adequate operating conditions after the initial muscle dissection can be produced in the absence of neuromuscular blockade. In the absence of muscle relaxation, muscle contractions including the masseter muscles will occur during stimulation. In this situation, it would be prudent to insert a bite block to prevent obstructing the tracheal tube or to intubate the child nasally.

Tourniquet

The tourniquet has been used since Roman times to control bleeding during amputation.[227]

Indications

The arterial tourniquet is used during orthopedic procedures to reduce blood loss and provide good operating conditions, for intravenous regional blockade and sympathectomy, and for isolated limb perfusion in the management of localized malignancy.[228]

Design

The word "tourniquet" is derived from the French verb tourner, meaning "to turn," referring to the twisting or screwing action applied to the constricting bandage to tighten it. Von Esmarch introduced the use of a flat rubber bandage wrapped repeatedly around a limb in 1873.[227] Although this rubber bandage is still used to render a limb bloodless, the pneumatic tourniquet, introduced by Cushing in 1904, has replaced the rubber bandage to maintain ischemia. Compressed gas (nitrogen or air) is used for inflation. The target pressure is preset and compensatory feedback mechanisms maintain that pressure during inflation. Curved and wider tourniquet cuffs, designed to fit conical limbs, are associated with lower arterial occlusion pressures than standard cuffs.[229] A soft dressing applied to the limb before tourniquet application helps prevent wrinkles and blisters that may occur when the skin is pinched.[230] Adequate exsanguination can also be achieved by elevation of the arm at 90 degrees or the leg at 45 degrees for 5 minutes.[231,232]

Physiology

Ischemia

Ischemia leads to tissue hypoxia and acidosis. The severity and consequences of the associated changes (e.g., increased capillary permeability, coagulation alteration, and cell membrane sodium pump activity) vary depending on the tissue type, duration of ischemia, and collateral circulation. Muscle is more susceptible to ischemic damage than nerves. Histologic changes are more pronounced in muscle beneath the tourniquet compared with muscle distal to the tourniquet.

Reperfusion

Reperfusion removes toxic metabolites and restores energy supplies. There is a sudden release of lactic acid, creatine phosphokinase, potassium (peak increase 0.32 mEq/L), and carbon dioxide (peak increase 0.8-18 mm Hg) when the cuff is deflated suddenly. Metabolic changes are greater after a longer period of ischemia but return to baseline within 30 minutes. Muscle damage may result in the release of myoglobin that can collect in the collecting tubules of the kidney, precipitating renal failure. Systemic effects after deflation of the tourniquet include a shift of blood volume back into the limb with a transient decrease in blood pressure that is exacerbated by a postischemic reactive hyperemia in the limb. CO_2 release generates a transient increased minute volume. The rapid increase in CO_2 is also associated with a transient (8-10 minute) increase in cerebral blood volume that may affect children with raised intracranial pressure.[228]

Increased microvascular permeability of muscle and nerve tissue occurs with tourniquet release after 2 to 4 hours of ischemia. Interstitial and intracellular edema as well as capillary occlusion secondary to endothelial edema and leukocyte aggregates may take months to resolve.

Ischemic Conditioning

Short periods of ischemia followed by reperfusion render muscle more resistant to subsequent ischemia. Such ischemic preconditioning improves skeletal muscle force, contractility, and performance and decreases fatigue of skeletal muscle. This preconditioning may enable prolongation of orthopedic and reconstructive procedures.[233]

Complications

Local

Muscle Damage

Histologic changes in the muscle beneath the tourniquet are present after 2 hours of tourniquet time (at 200 mm Hg, 26.7 kPa), but similar changes can occur after 4 hours of tourniquet in the distal ischemic muscle. Direct pressure and mechanical deformation contribute to increased severity of muscle damage under the cuff.[228] These changes include an increase in the number of inflammatory cells in the perifascicular space, focal fiber necrosis, and signs of hyaline degeneration.

The combination of muscle ischemia, edema, and microvascular congestion contributes to "post-tourniquet syndrome": edema, stiffness, pallor, weakness without paralysis, and subjective numbness of the extremity without objective anesthesia. The common use of postoperative casts may conceal the true incidence of this syndrome. Recovery usually occurs over 7 days.[234]

Nerve Damage

Direct compression under the cuff rather than ischemia is thought to cause nerve injuries. Sheer forces that are maximal at the upper and lower edges of the tourniquet cause the most damage. These forces are greater with the Esmarch bandage than with the pneumatic tourniquet. The incidence is greater in the upper limb (1/11,000) than in the lower limb (1/250,000), with the radial nerve being the most vulnerable nerve in the upper extremity and the sciatic nerve in the lower extremity.[235]

Vascular Damage

Arterial injury is uncommon in children. It is an injury of adults with atheromatous vessels, and the tourniquet should be avoided in those patients with absent distal pulses, poor capillary return, a calcified femoropopliteal system, or a history of vascular surgery on the involved limb.[236]

Skin Safety

Pressure necrosis and friction burns may occur with poorly applied tourniquets, and some form of skin protection should be used routinely.[237] Chemical burns may result from antiseptic skin preparations that seep beneath the tourniquet and are then retained and compressed against the skin.

Tourniquet Pain

The tourniquet causes a vague dull ache that becomes intolerable after approximately 30 minutes.[238] This pain is associated with an increase in both heart rate and blood pressure that is not ameliorated by general anesthesia and neuraxial blockade.[239] This pain is transmitted by unmyelinated C-fibers. These fibers are normally inhibited by fast pain impulses transmitted by myelinated A-delta fibers, but mechanical compression causes reduced transmission in these larger fibers.[239]

Systemic

Temperature Regulation

The combination of decreased heat loss from the ischemic limb and reduced heat transfer from the central to ischemic peripheral compartment increases core body temperature.[240,241] The temperature increase is greater with bilateral tourniquets compared with a unilateral tourniquet.[241] Children requiring intraoperative tourniquets should not be aggressively warmed during surgery.[241] Redistribution of body heat and the efflux of hypothermic venous blood from the ischemic area into the systemic circulation after deflation of the tourniquet decreases the core body temperature, which may switch off thermoregulatory vasodilation and cause a decrease in skin-surface temperature.[242]

Deep Vein Thrombosis and Emboli

The incidence of emboli after release of the tourniquet in children is uncertain. The tourniquet appears to have no influence on deep venous thromboembolism formation, but release of the tourniquet may be associated with an increased risk of embolism in adults. Some authors have suggested that heparin be used during total joint arthroplasty in adults to prevent emboli formation,[243] although this practice is not routine in children. Some surgeons will use such therapy in adolescents.

Sickle Cell Disease

Hypoxia, acidosis, and circulatory stasis all contribute to the sickling of sickle cells in susceptible individuals. However, several institutions routinely use tourniquets in children with sickle cell disease while maintaining acid-base status and oxygenation throughout the procedure.[244,245] Each case must be assessed individually for the balance between the advantages of a bloodless field and the risks of precipitating sickling crises (see Chapter 9).

Drug Effects

Antibiotics given after the tourniquet is inflated will not produce effective blood and tissue concentrations of antibiotics in the ischemic limb. Inflation of the tourniquet should be delayed at least 5 minutes after administration of the antibiotics.[246,247] Medications administered before inflation of the tourniquet may be sequestered in the ischemic limb and then re-released into the systemic circulation when the tourniquet is deflated. The antibiotic effect will depend on the amount of antibiotic sequestered, the tissue binding, and the concentration-response relationship for the antibiotic, although the impact is minimal for most medications used in anesthesia. Volume of distribution may be reduced if the drug is administered after tourniquet inflation, but the plasma clearance remains unaffected.

Recommended Cuff Pressures

Tourniquets should generally remain inflated less than 2 hours, with most authors suggesting a maximal time of 1.5 to 2 hours. Techniques such as hourly release of the tourniquet for 10 minutes, cooling of the affected limb, and alternating dual cuffs may reduce the risk of injury.[248] Both nerve and muscle injuries that occur beneath the tourniquet cuff are related to the pneumatic pressure. Consequently, the lowest possible pressure that maintains ischemic conditions should be sought. Hypotensive anesthetic techniques have been used in adults to reduce the need for high cuff inflation pressures,[249] but there seems to be little need for this in children. One author has suggested that pediatric occlusion pressures should be measured by Doppler imaging and the tourniquet pressure set at 50 mm Hg above this value. The maximum mean pressures recommended for the upper and lower extremities are 173.4 ± 11.6 mm Hg (range: 155-190 mm Hg) and 176.7 ± 28.7 mm Hg (range: 140-250 mm Hg), respectively.[250] Wider cuffs exert less force per unit area and reduce the risk of local sequelae. Recommendations for adults suggest that the cuff should exceed the circumference of the extremity by 7 to 15 cm. This is difficult to achieve in infants in whom the proximal limb length is proportionally shorter than adults and wide cuffs would impinge on the surgical field.

Acute Bone and Joint Infections

The mainstays of management for osteomyelitis and septic arthritis are antibiotics and surgical drainage. The incidence of these infections is increasing, particularly in immunocompromised children with human immunodeficiency virus (HIV) infection. Tuberculosis remains a scourge in many developing countries. Mortality rates for both hospital-acquired staphylococcal disease in compromised children[251] and community-acquired disease in healthy children[252,253] range from 8% to 47% in those presenting with severe sepsis.[254] *Mycobacterium* and *Staphylococcus* organisms resistant to conventional antibiotics increase morbidity and mortality.

Pathophysiology

Staphylococcus aureus is the most common pathogen. Osteomyelitis develops after a bacteremia mostly in prepubertal children. Normal bone is highly resistant to infection, but *S. aureus* adheres to bone by expressing receptors for components of bone matrix, and the expression of collagen-binding adhesin permits the attachment to cartilage.[255] Once the microorganisms adhere to bone they express phenotypic resistance to antimicrobial treatment.[255]

The metaphyseal region around the growth plate is the predominant area of infection. Sluggish blood flow in the metaphysis predisposes to bacterial infection, and endothelial gaps in developing vessels allow bacteria to escape into the metaphysis. Subsequent abscesses may decompress into the joint or subperiosteally. Infection may involve adjacent tissue planes, and hematogenous spread causes multiple pathologic processes beyond the primary site of infection.

Septic arthritis is more common in neonates because transphyseal vessels link the metaphysics and epiphysis. Growth plate and epiphyseal destruction may both occur in this age group. Articular cartilage damage is attributable to the release of proteolytic enzymes from both the pathogen and activated neutrophils.

Clinical Presentation

The majority of children with staphylococcal disease present with musculoskeletal symptoms and fever, but those with disseminated disease can present critically ill (4%-10%) with severe sepsis and lung disease.[252,253] There is often a history of trauma.[252,253] It can be difficult to diagnose extracutaneous foci. One study[251] reported that 50% of extracutaneous foci of staphylococcal infection were not detected on hospital admission, and one third of these lesions were noted for the first time at autopsy. An absolute polymorphonuclear cell count of greater than $10,000/mm^3$ or an absolute bandform count of greater than $500/mm^3$, or both, correlates with the presence of one or more inadequately treated sites of staphylococcal infection.[251] Tuberculosis is the great mimic and must always be suspected in endemic areas.

Diagnosis is confirmed by blood, bone, or joint aspirate culture. Radiologic procedures (plain radiographs, computed tomography, magnetic resonance imaging, radionuclide scans) are often required to identify foci, and the anesthesiologist is often requested to provide sedation/analgesia.

Treatment Options

Antibiotic therapy is the mainstay of treatment. Initial antibiotic choice is dictated by age, local pathogen, and sensitivity profiles. Antibiotic treatment should be extended to cover gram-negative enterococci in neonates and streptococci in older children. *Haemophilus influenzae* remains a pathogen in unvaccinated regions. Surgical decompression of acute osteomyelitis that is responding poorly to antimicrobial therapy may release intramedullary or subperiosteal pus and lead to clinical improvement. Pus within fascial planes also requires release. Venous thrombosis attributable to pus in soft tissue planes around major joints was associated with a high mortality in one series.[252] Determining and eradicating the primary focus improves both mortality and recurrence rates.[256] An aggressive search for foci and surgical drainage of infective foci is required.

Highly active antiretroviral therapy (HAART) has positively altered the mortality rates in HIV-infected children. However, acute bone and joint infections still occur[257] and these drugs have the potential to cause significant morbidity secondary to changes in fat distribution, lipid profiles, glucose, homeostasis, and bone turnover.[258] Infarction may replace infection as the major cause of morbidity and mortality from HIV.[258] It is uncertain that HAART should be continued during acute osteomyelitis. Worsening cell-mediated immune function may occur during tuberculosis treatment if HAART is continued.[259] The combination of HIV infection and tuberculosis is potentially lethal in children, and antituberculous treatment is continued for 12 to 18 months.

Anesthesia Considerations

Anesthesiology services are commonly required for sedation during diagnostic investigation, anesthesia for surgical exploration and release of pus or fixation of pathologic fractures, management of pulmonary complications (intercostal chest drain insertion, pleurodesis), central venous cannulation for long-term antibiotic treatment and analgesic modalities.

Children with disseminated staphylococcal disease may be critically ill with multisystem disease and require fluid volume augmentation, inotrope support, positive-pressure ventilation, extracorporeal renal support, and coagulation factor replacement. Others may appear clinically stable before anesthetic induction; the assessment of hypovolemia in children is subject to moderate to poor inter-rater agreement.[260] Intravenous access and rehydration are required before beginning anesthesia to avoid a precipitous blood pressure drop immediately after induction. Bacteremic showering during manipulation and drainage of pus causes further decompensation. Excessive bleeding due to altered coagulation status should also be anticipated.

The presence of a septic arthritis in the shoulder or neck may cause cervical ligamentous laxity predisposing to C1/C2 subluxation during intubation.[261] Pneumatoceles from staphylococcal pneumonia can rupture during positive-pressure ventilation. A spontaneous breathing mode, however, may be difficult to achieve because of laryngospasm, breath holding, increased secretions, and bronchospasm. The use of NMBDs and positive-pressure ventilation in these children with a low threshold to introduce inotropes to support the cardiovascular system is an easier option. Vigilance is required for the presence of an acute pneumothorax.

Myocarditis, pericarditis, and pericardial effusions compromise myocardial function; one author reported a 12% prevalence of infective endocarditis in children with hospital-acquired *S. aureus* bacteremia. This prevalence of infective endocarditis was frequently associated with congenital heart disease and multiple blood cultures.[262] The incidence of infective endocarditis among those children with community-acquired disease without preexisting cardiac abnormalities was low,[252] suggesting that echocardiography could be reserved for children with preexisting cardiac disease, suspicious clinical findings, those whose temperature fails to settle, or those who have prolonged bacteremia without an obvious source of infection.

Pain Management

Morphine and acetaminophen are the analgesics commonly used for postoperative pain management. The use of tramadol in children is increasing as our understanding of the pharmacokinetics of this medication increases.[263,264] The low incidence of respiratory depression and constipation, fewer controls on use, and similar frequency of nausea and vomiting (10%-40%) compared with opioids make tramadol an attractive alternative.[265-267] NSAIDs are relatively contraindicated in the presence of coagulation disorders, altered renal function, and cyclooxygenase-2–mediated inhibition of osteogenesis.

The performance of regional blockade in children with acute bone or joint infection is controversial. There are no studies addressing the risk/benefit ratios of regional techniques in this population. It would seem reasonable to use these techniques only after 24 hours of appropriate antibiotic therapy in apyrexial children who show no signs of a coagulopathy.

Common Syndromes

Children with some specific conditions present repeatedly for orthopedic procedures. It is worthwhile maintaining a database for these children detailing their anesthetic management. In addition, there should be 24-hour access to standard texts concerning anesthesia and uncommon pediatric diseases.

Cerebral Palsy

Clinical Features

Cerebral palsy is an umbrella term that describes a group of nonprogressive, but often changing, motor impairment syndromes secondary to lesions or anomalies in the brain that occur during the early stages of its development.[268] It is the leading cause of motor disability during childhood, with a prevalence of approximately 2 per 1000 live births in developed countries.[269] Disorders include cognitive impairment, sensory loss (vision and hearing), seizures, and communication and behavioral disturbances. Systemic disorders resulting from cerebral palsy affect the gastrointestinal, respiratory, urinary tract and orthopedic systems. Cerebral palsy is divided into three broad categories: spastic (70%), dyskinetic (10%), and ataxic (10%) (see Chapter 22).[268] Those children suffering from spastic cerebral palsy commonly present for orthopedic procedures because of the development of contractures at major peripheral joints.[270,271] Functional improvement after surgery in children with spastic diplegia and spastic hemiplegia is better than for those suffering spastic quadriplegia.[270]

Orthopedic Considerations

Orthopedic manipulations form only part of treatments designed to either improve performance or improve the ease of care. Management includes orthopedic surgery, physical and occupational therapy, recreational therapy, orthotics, and assistive devices improve functional outcomes. Medical modalities such as intramuscular injections of botulinum toxin, and intrathecal administration of baclofen via an implanted pump may also be of benefit.[272] Selective dorsal rhizotomy has also been used to control spasticity.[273,274] The indications and timing of surgical interventions vary. Gait analysis increases the age of the first orthopedic surgical procedure, and treatment with botulinum toxin type A delays and reduces the frequency of surgical procedures on the lower extremities.[275,276] Bone and soft tissue surgical procedures are designed to lengthen or weaken spastic muscles to give opposing muscles a chance to attain muscle balance.

Anesthetic Considerations

Children presenting for orthopedic surgery often have previous experience of operating rooms. These children should be handled with sensitivity because communication disorders and sensory deficits may mask mild or normal intellect. They may be accompanied by their parent or a caregiver and/or be premedicated before induction of anesthesia. If there is a communication problem, then the parent or caregiver should be present before and after anesthesia.[270,277] Medical conditions (seizure control, respiratory function, gastroesophageal reflux) should be optimized preoperatively. Contracture deformities, spinal deformities, decubitus ulceration, and skin infection must be considered when positioning the child for anesthesia and surgery. Poor nutritional status affects postoperative wound healing and the risk of infection. Concurrent medications may influence the anesthetic considerations: cisapride for gastroesophageal reflux is associated with prolonged QT interval, sodium valproate can cause platelet dysfunction and affect drug metabolism, and anticonvulsant use increases resistance to NMBDs.[278] A history of latex allergy should be sought because of exposure to latex allergens from an early age.[279]

Intravenous access may be difficult. Drooling, a decreased ability to swallow secretions, and gastroesophageal reflux may dissuade some against an inhalational induction, but there is no evidence that rapid sequence induction is safer. Succinylcholine use is not associated with hyperkalemia because the muscles of these patients have never been denervated. Noncommunicative/nonverbal children with cerebral palsy require less propofol to obtain the same bispectral index values (i.e., 35-45) than do otherwise healthy children.[280] The MAC of halothane is 20% less in children suffering from cerebral palsy, whether or not they take anticonvulsant drugs (MAC, 0.62 and 0.71, respectively).[281] Intraoperative hypothermia is common in those children with disordered temperature regulation secondary to hypothalamic dysfunction, reduced muscle bulk, and fat deposits. Thermal homeostasis should be managed aggressively from the moment the child enters the operating room. Extensive plaster casting is an important component of bone and soft tissue surgical procedures. These casts may conceal blood loss, and limb swelling within the cast may contribute to compartment syndromes. Plaster jackets and hip spicas have been associated with mesenteric occlusion and acute gastric dilatation. Pain and spasm are regular features postoperatively. Epidural analgesia is particularly valuable when major orthopedic procedures are performed.[270] Occasionally, two epidurals at different spinal sites may be required for multilevel surgery. Systemic benzodiazepines, baclofen, dantrolene, and clonidine have been used to reduce muscle spasms. Selective dorsal rhizotomy is associated with severe pain, muscle spasms, and dysesthesia. Epidural and intrathecal morphine have been used to control this pain. Intravenous morphine and midazolam has also been successfully used.[282] Oral benzodiazepines may be required to reduce the incidence and severity of muscle spasms but should be used with caution if combined with opioid analgesia.

Pain assessment is difficult in these children, but there are a number of scoring systems available (see Chapter 44).[283,284] The opinions of parents and caregivers are extremely valuable in the assessment of pain and discrimination from other factors such as irritability on anesthetic emergence, poor positioning, a full bladder, or nausea.

Spina Bifida

Spina bifida is characterized by developmental abnormalities of the vertebrae and spinal cord that may be associated with changes in the cerebrum, brainstem, and peripheral nerves. The failure of fusion of the vertebral arches is commonly known as spina bifida. *Spina bifida occulta* refers to spina bifida that occurs when skin and soft tissues cover the defect. *Spina bifida aperta* is used to describe those lesions where the defect communicates with the outside as either a meningocele or a myelomeningocele (incidence 1:1,000 live births) (see also Chapter 23). The myelomeningocele sac contains nerve roots that do not function below the level of the lesion.

Clinical Features

Nerve root dysfunction results in muscle paralysis as well as a neurogenic bowel and bladder. The majority (80%) of children develop hydrocephalus consequent to aqueductal stenosis (Arnold-Chiari type II malformation). Skeletal abnormalities such as clubfoot and congenital dislocation of the hip are common. Scoliosis may be due to either congenital vertebral abnormalities or, more commonly, abnormal neuromuscular control. Epilepsy and learning disorders can also occur, but most children have normal intelligence.

Orthopedic Considerations

Denervation causes muscle imbalance that results in abnormalities at the hip, knee, and foot. The aims of surgery are to reduce flexor posture at the hip and knee and plantigrade feet. Clubfeet, hip subluxation, and scoliosis are common presentations for orthopedic correction.

Anesthetic Considerations

The potential for infection of the central nervous system dictates early closure of the sac within the first few days of life. Subsequent surgical procedures and urinary catheterizations set the stage for sensitivity to latex.[285] Primary prophylaxis (avoiding all latex materials and a latex-free operating room) is recommended for prevention of latex allergy and anaphylaxis.[286]

Preoperative assessment should include motor and sensory deficits, respiratory and renal function, and functioning of the ventriculoperitoneal shunt, if present. Positioning on the operating table may require additional pillows for support of limbs with contractures. As a result of hypoesthesia in the lower extremities, intravenous cannulae can be inserted painlessly. However, venous access is usually poor in the lower extremities because of their limited use. The risk of endobronchial intubation is increased because of a short trachea (36%).[287] Kyphoscoliosis may distort tracheal anatomy. Renal dysfunction may dictate choice of NMBD and avoidance of NSAIDs. Succinylcholine does not cause hyperkalemia.[288] A reduced hypercapnic ventilation response means that these children should be closely observed in the recovery period.

Osteogenesis Imperfecta

Osteogenesis imperfecta was believed to have afflicted Ivar the Boneless (Ivar Ragnarsson), a Viking chieftain who led a successful invasion of the East Anglia region of England in AD 865. He is reported to have had legs as soft as cartilage so that he was unable to walk and had to be carried on a shield. Ivar's name is also associated with an early form of thoracoplasty. When the King of Northumbria, Aelle, was captured a few years later, he was subjected to the horrific "blood eagle" ordeal by the Vikings. His ribs were torn out and folded back to form the shape of an eagle's wings and his lungs were removed.

Clinical Features

Osteogenesis imperfecta (OI) is a genetically determined disorder of connective tissue that is characterized by bone fragility. The disease state encompasses a phenotypically and genotypically heterogeneous group of inherited disorders that result from mutations in the genes that code for type I collagen.[289] The disorder is manifest in tissues in which the principal matrix protein is type I collagen (mainly bone, dentin, sclerae, and ligaments). Musculoskeletal manifestations are variable in severity along a continuum ranging from perinatal lethal forms with crumpled bones to moderate forms with deformity and propensity for fracture to clinically silent forms with subtle osteopenia and no deformity.[289] Classification (types I-IV) is based on the timing of fractures or on multiple clinical, genetic, and radiologic features. Type I is the most common (1:30,000 live births) and, together with type IV, has autosomal dominant inheritance patterns. These children have the classic triad of blue sclerae, multiple fractures, and conductive hearing loss in adolescence. Bowing of the lower limbs, genu valgum, flat feet, and scoliosis develop with age. Type IV is characterized by osteoporosis, leading to bone fragility without many of the other features of type I. Types II and III are more severe forms of OI and have autosomal recessive inheritance patterns. Molecular genetic studies have identified more than 150 mutations of the *COL1A1* and *COL1A2* genes, which encode for type I procollagen.[289]

Orthopedic Considerations

The goals of treatment of OI are to maximize function, minimize deformity and disability, maintain comfort, achieve relative independence in activities of daily living, and enhance social integration. Physiotherapy, rehabilitation, and orthopedic surgery are the mainstay of treatment in moderate to severe forms of OI. Medical treatment with the antiresorptive bisphosphonates (e.g., pamidronate) can decrease pain, lower fracture incidence, and improve mobility. Initial investigations have demonstrated an acceptable safety profile for pamidronate. Currently, there is a lack of long-term follow-up data, which will be necessary for the development of responsible guidelines for therapy.[290] Medical therapies other than bisphosphonates, such as growth hormone and parathyroid hormone, currently contribute only a minor role. Gene-based therapy currently remains in the early stages of preclinical research.[291,292]

Operative intervention is indicated for recurrent fractures or deformity that impairs function.[289] Fractures in mild to moderately severe cases of OI type I are treated using the same methods as for children without OI. Realignment of deformed bones that are fracturing frequently followed by external or internal support is commonly performed. It is important in selecting various modes of treatment to consider the natural history of the particular type of OI and to set realistic goals.[293-297]

Anesthetic Considerations

In common with other children suffering chronic disability, these children are veterans to the operating room. Chronic pain from frequent fractures complicates handling. Deafness may hinder communication. Preoperative assessment centers on the chest wall deformity because this determines the severity of restrictive lung disease and subsequent cardiovascular compromise. Neck mobility, mouth opening, and dentition should also be assessed.

There is a risk of further fractures with positioning, tourniquet application, airway handing, and even use of a blood pressure cuff. Invasive pressure monitoring may be less traumatic than a blood pressure cuff for some children. If noninvasive blood pressure monitoring is used, less frequent monitoring of the blood pressure is recommended if possible. A laryngeal mask airway may avoid pressure from face masks. An individual history may help determine the risk-benefit ratio for each child. Succinylcholine has the theoretical potential to cause fasciculation-induced fractures.

Abnormal temperature homeostasis may result in intraoperative hyperthermia that may be severe and accompanied by tachycardia and metabolic acidosis. This response differs from that of malignant hyperthermia in that there is an absence of respiratory acidosis and muscle rigidity.[298] Surface cooling is usually effective in restoring thermal homeostasis.

Duchenne Muscular Dystrophy

Clinical Features

Duchenne muscular dystrophy is the most common of the progressive muscular dystrophies. It is an X-linked recessive disorder with an incidence of 3:10,000 births (see Chapter 22). The DMD gene (*Xp21*) codes for a large sarcolemmal membrane protein (dystrophin)-associated muscle cell membrane integrity. Dystrophin is missing or nonfunctional in DMD children. Children usually present before school age with a waddling gait and go on to develop a lumbar lordosis and difficulty climbing stairs. Children use their arms to assist standing up, owing to proximal weakness of the hip girdle. Distal muscles, such as the calves, appear hypertrophied. The disease process is progressive with increasing muscle weakness with age: often these children become wheelchair bound by 10 to 11 years of age. Respiratory weakness, often exacerbated by scoliosis and by difficulty swallowing secretions due to pharyngeal involvement, can progress to a terminal pneumonia in late teenage years.[299]

Most clinicians regard DMD as a static disease, but this could not be farther from the truth. In early childhood, skeletal muscle is constantly catabolized and unstable. The use of membrane destabilizing medications such as succinylcholine and potent inhalational anesthetics (halothane in particular) in these young children can result in hyperkalemia, rhabdomyolysis, and cardiac arrest (see later). However, once the children reach adolescence, the bulk of the skeletal muscle catabolism has arrested and membrane-destabilizing medications are left with no substrate. Indeed, at The Hospital for Sick Children in Toronto, both succinylcholine and potent inhalational anesthetics were used in adolescents with DMD who were undergoing scoliosis surgery and instrumentation without sequelae. In contrast, cardiac and smooth muscle consequences of DMD are minor and insignificant in childhood but may become life-threatening during adolescence and adulthood (see later). It is imperative to appreciate the developmental nature of DMD and to recognize the risks that may be associated with the use of succinylcholine and inhalational anesthetics in this group of children.

DMD can affect cardiac and smooth muscle as well as skeletal muscle. Right ventricular function may be compromised by nocturnal oxygen desaturation and sleep apnea contributing to pulmonary hypertension. Sinus tachycardia and arrhythmias may occur at an early age, but clinically apparent cardiomyopathy usually does not develop before 10 years of age. One third of children have a degree of intellectual impairment.

Clinical suspicion of DMD should arise in male preschool-aged children with delayed walking ability and serum creatine phosphokinase concentration measured as a screening tool. Corticosteroids are increasingly used for the management of DMD; it is believed that they increase muscle mass by decreasing protein breakdown.[300]

Becker muscular dystrophy (BMD) is a milder form of DMD with onset around puberty or later in the teenage years. Clinical expression is variable, but even adolescents presenting with mild or subclinical weakness can develop a cardiomyopathy with age progression. Death secondary to cardiac or respiratory failure does not usually occur until the fourth or fifth decade. Improvements in respiratory care have resulted in dilated cardiomyopathy as being the major cause of death.[301] This autosomal recessive myopathy is also due to mutations of dystrophin with a deletion of exons 11 to 13 in the *Xp21* gene.[302] Dystrophin exerts its effect at the voltage-gated chloride channel (CLCN1). Genetic analysis is an essential step in confirming the diagnosis. Additional electromyographic procedures may be of diagnostic value even when muscle biopsy may reveal no evidence of dystrophy.

Two thirds of children with mild or subclinical BMD have evidence of right ventricular dilatation and one third have evidence of LV dysfunction.[303] A thorough cardiac evaluation (similar to DMD) is recommended before scoliosis surgery.[301] Hyperthermia plus heart failure, mimicking malignant hyperthermia and hyperkalemia with rhabdomyolysis after inhalational agents, have both been reported with BMD.[304,305] Despite these reports, the relationship between BMD and malignant hyperthermia remains unclear.

Orthopedic Considerations

Orthopedic surgery is indicated to improve or maintain ambulation and standing. Early treatment of contractures of the hips and the lower limbs prevents severe contractures and delays the progression of scoliosis.[306] Techniques designed to improve deformities and permit early postoperative mobilization include subcutaneous release of contracted tendons and percutaneous removal of cancellous bone with corrective manipulation of the feet. Maintenance of the upright posture extends the ability of these children to attend to their tasks of daily living.[307] Spinal deformities attributable to muscle imbalance or a collapsing spine are corrected to improve or maintain sitting posture. Spinal fusion may also decrease the rate of deterioration of respiratory function, although this has been questioned.[308]

Anesthetic Considerations

Respiratory and cardiovascular compromise dominates preoperative assessment. Deformities and contractures of limb joints hinder vascular access, regional anesthetic techniques, and positioning on the operating table. Hypertrophy of the tongue may cause difficulty during intubation. Gastric motility is delayed with prolonged gastric emptying times.[309] Tracheobronchial tree compression has been described in a child positioned prone for spinal instrumentation.[310] These children have a tendency to

greater blood loss during surgery. The precise etiology remains unclear but may be because fat and connective tissue have replaced muscle or because of abnormalities in the blood vessels.[135]

Nondepolarizing NMBDs have a slow onset of action and prolonged duration of action.[311-313] All NMBDs should be monitored with a peripheral nerve stimulator.[314] *Succinylcholine is contraindicated in these children because of the risk of hyperkalemia, muscle rigidity, rhabdomyolysis, myoglobinuria, arrhythmias, and cardiac arrest.* There is no clear link between DMD and malignant hyperthermia.[315,316] The predominant candidate gene for malignant hyperthermia is located on the long arm of chromosome 19, whereas the gene for DMD is located on the short arm of the X chromosome.[317] Although volatile anesthetic agents continue to be used in young children with DMD, rhabdomyolysis and hyperkalemia have been reported in the recovery room after halothane, isoflurane, desflurane, and sevoflurane anesthesia.[318-322] *Potent inhalational anesthetics should be avoided in young children with DMD and supplanted with alternative anesthetics that do not trigger rhabdomyolysis and hyperkalemia.*[323]

Regional techniques such as epidurals may be technically more difficult due to kyphoscoliosis and obesity. The use of ultrasound-guided peripheral nerve blockade can improve the quality and reduce complications of neuronal blockade.[6] Opioids are not contraindicated in the postoperative period but should be used with caution in children with respiratory compromise. Tramadol is an effective alternative. Noninvasive ventilation support using bilateral or continuous airway pressure is sometimes required after major surgery or in those already receiving this treatment overnight.

Arthrogryposis Multiplex Congenita

Clinical Features

Arthrogryposis multiplex congenita is a syndrome of multiple persistent limb contractures often accompanied by associated anomalies, including cleft palate, genitourinary defects, gastroschisis, and cardiac defects.[324] The incidence is 1 in 3000 births. Joint contractures are present at birth and are a result of immobility in utero, commonly related to a neurogenic abnormality or myopathy.[325] These children have been likened to a "thin, wooden doll" because muscles connected with affected joints are atrophic and replaced by fibrous tissue and fat.[326] The temporomandibular joint may also be involved, causing restricted jaw opening and micrognathia. Scoliosis commonly develops. Restrictive lung disease, rib cage deformities, and pulmonary hypoplasia predispose to recurrent chest infections.

Orthopedic Considerations

The aims of surgery are to improve function. The majority of surgery involves the soft tissues, tendons, and osteotomies of the lower limbs and hips.[327] Upper limb surgery is less common. The extension contracture of the elbow joint makes it impossible to reach the mouth or to perform hygienic necessities. Improvement in passive elbow flexion by capsulotomy or in active flexion by triceps transfer can increase independence and personal hygiene. When both arms are involved, consideration may be given to have one arm in flexion for reaching the head and mouth passively or even actively and one arm in extension for basic hygiene cares.[328]

Anesthetic Considerations

Arthrogryposis multiplex congenita is commonly associated with other syndromes that may complicate anesthesia.[324,329] Venous cannulation is difficult because veins tend to be small and fragile. The concavity of joints is difficult to access. Care must be taken with positioning on the operating table and protecting skin overlying bony joints to prevent pathologic fractures. These children should be evaluated for a difficult airway because of temporomandibular joint limitation and micrognathia.[330-332] Fusion or underdevelopment of the first and second cervical vertebrae may further complicate laryngoscopy and tracheal intubation. Tracheal intubation may become progressively more difficult with age. During infancy, however, evaluating mouth opening may be difficult; it may be necessary to insert a tongue blade into the mouth to determine whether the mandible can be distracted from the maxilla. Succinylcholine has been used without incident in these children, although teleologically the use of a depolarizing muscle relaxant in the presence of anterior horn cell disease is contentious. The response to nondepolarizing NMBDs should be monitored.

Hyperthermia and persistent tachycardia have both been reported during general anesthesia.[324,333-335] These signs occur irrespective of the anesthetic agent and are not associated with malignant hyperthermia. In this case, hyperthermia responds to simple cooling techniques.

Pulmonary dysfunction and an increased sensitivity to opioids dictate suitable monitoring postoperatively. Regional techniques may be difficult in the presence of contractures but, if successful, offer both intraoperative and postoperative analgesia.[326] Success can be improved using ultrasound-guided techniques.

Annotated References

Harper CM, Ambler G, Edge G: The prognostic value of preoperative predicted forced vital capacity in corrective spinal surgery for Duchenne's muscular dystrophy. Anaesthesia 2004; 59:1160-1162

Performing scoliosis surgery on DMD children with an FVC of 30% has been questioned owing to the high incidence of postoperative pulmonary complications. This simple clinical paper demonstrated that with careful attention to detail, children with an FVC less than 30% can undergo scoliosis surgery with results similar to those with an FVC greater than 30%. Early extubation followed by the use of noninvasive ventilation was identified as playing a key role in reducing respiratory complications.

Murray DJ, Pennell BJ, Weinstein SL, Olson JD: Packed red cells in acute blood loss: dilutional coagulopathy as a cause of surgical bleeding. Anesth Analg 1995; 80:336-342

In this interesting paper the authors identify coagulation factor dilution rather than thrombocytopenia as the cause of increased surgical bleeding when packed red cells are required for massive blood loss during scoliosis surgery. An increase in prothrombin time and particularly activated partial thromboplastin time was the most common hemostatic abnormality rather than thrombocytopenia. Clinically, increased bleeding was identified by recurrent bleeding from wound margins after initial hemostasis without a change in blood pressure and decreased clot formation in blood pooled in the surgical field. In most children both the clinical bleeding and hemostatic abnormalities were successfully treated by fresh frozen plasma alone (10 mL/kg).

Nolan J, Chalkiadis GA, Low J, et al: Anaesthesia and pain management in cerebral palsy. Anaesthesia 2000; 55:32-41

Children with cerebral palsy frequently present for a variety of orthopedic procedures. This well-written review from a large children's hospital details the many issues and concerns involved with anesthetizing and caring for these patients postoperatively.

Reinacher PC, Priebe HJ, Blumrich W, et al: The effects of stimulation pattern and sevoflurane concentration on intraoperative motor-evoked potentials. Anesth Analg 2006; 102:888-895

Scheufler KM, Reinacher PC, Blumrich W, et al: The modifying effects of stimulation pattern and propofol plasma concentration on motor-evoked potentials. Anesth Analg 2005; 100:440-447

The authors of this pair of complicated but interesting articles investigated the influence of both anesthetic agent concentration (sevoflurane and propofol) and stimulation pattern on intraoperative motor evoked potentials (MEPs). Although conducted in children undergoing craniotomy, the finding that the MEP characteristics were more dependent on stimulation pattern than anesthetic agent concentration is important for spinal surgery. Their finding that using a train of three or more stimuli (MEP recording was possible at 1 MAC sevoflurane or with propofol TCI at 6 μg/mL) demonstrates that with modern monitoring systems anesthetic concentrations of these agents can be used for spinal surgery while preserving MEPs.

Yemen TA, McClain C: Muscular dystrophy, anesthesia and the safety of inhalational agents revisited again. Paediatr Anaesth 2006; 16:105-108

In this thought-provoking editorial, the authors discuss the risk of rhabdomyolysis in patients with DMD. The essence of the paper challenges us to reevaluate our approach to patient safety based on an increasing number of case reports (but in the absence of "scientific evidence") linking rhabdomyolysis to inhalational agents in this group of patients.

Yuan N, Fraire JA, Margetis MM, et al: The effect of scoliosis surgery on lung function in the immediate postoperative period. Spine 2005; 30:2182-2185

This study clearly demonstrated the dramatic decrease in pulmonary function in the days after scoliosis surgery, readily explaining why children are at risk from pulmonary complications during this period. Pulmonary function tests (FEV_1, FVC, FEV_1/FVC, and $FEF_{25-75\%}$) were measured daily for 10 days after scoliosis repair. PFTs decreased by up to 60% after surgery with a nadir at 3 days. The FEV_1 and FVC were still only at 60% of the preoperative values on the 10th postoperative day.

References

Please see www.expertconsult.com

Otorhinolaryngologic Procedures

CHAPTER 31

Raafat S. Hannallah, Karen A. Brown, and
Susan T. Verghese

Anesthesia for Otologic Procedures
Myringotomy and Ventilating Tube Insertion
Middle Ear and Mastoid Surgery
Cochlear Implants
Anesthesia for Rhinologic Procedures
Adenotonsillectomy
Preoperative Evaluation
Anesthetic Management and Postoperative
Considerations
Discharge Policy for Ambulatory
Adenotonsillectomy

Post-tonsillectomy Bleeding
Peritonsillar Abscess
Anesthesia for Endoscopy
Diagnostic Laryngoscopy and Bronchoscopy
Croup
Acute Epiglottitis
Obstructive Laryngeal Papillomatosis
Aspirated Foreign Bodies
Tracheostomy
Laryngotracheal Reconstruction
Airway Trauma

OTORHINOLARYNGOLOGIC PROCEDURES REPRESENT A large segment of elective pediatric surgery. Anesthetic management of these children is provided by both pediatric and general anesthesiologists. Many work in the anesthesia care team mode. Today, a majority of these children undergo surgery and anesthesia outside the traditional hospital environment, such as ambulatory surgery centers and office practices. Additionally, anesthesiologists are often consulted to help in the management of potentially life-threatening pediatric otolaryngologic emergencies. These include airway obstruction in children suffering from acute epiglottitis, croup, foreign body aspiration, and airway trauma.[1] In both the elective and emergent scenarios, it is essential that the pathophysiology of these conditions be fully understood and the anesthetic plan be discussed in advance with the surgeon who will frequently be sharing the airway with the anesthesiologist. This ensures safe anesthetic management and ideal conditions for both children and surgeons.

Anesthesia for Otologic Procedures

Myringotomy and Ventilating Tube Insertion

Chronic serous otitis media is common in young children. It can lead to hearing loss and formation of cholesteatoma. When conservative medical management fails, surgical drainage of accumulated fluid in the middle ear is indicated. Myringotomy creates an opening in the tympanic membrane through which fluid can drain. It may be performed alone; however, when the

incision heals, the drainage path is occluded. Therefore, it is frequently accompanied by placement of a ventilation tube. A small plastic tube (a variation of the grommet or the T-tube) inserted in the tympanic membrane serves as a stent for the ostium and allows for continued drainage of the middle ear until the tubes are naturally extruded in 6 months to a year or surgically removed at an appropriate time.

Children with cleft palate have a high frequency of middle ear disease compared with the noncleft population because of associated abnormalities of the cartilage and muscles surrounding the eustachian tubes. Surgical drainage and ventilation tube insertion is a standard treatment of chronic otitis media in these children. This is usually performed at the time of the surgical repair of the cleft.

Almost all young children require general anesthesia for tympanotomy tube placement, although an occasional older child may tolerate topical anesthesia. This may be accomplished by iontophoresis or instillation of EMLA cream, which is allowed to sit in the ear canal for an hour and is then suctioned out before the procedure.

Myringotomy with tube insertion is a very brief operation, and anesthesia is usually accomplished as an ambulatory procedure with a potent inhalational agent (usually sevoflurane), oxygen, and nitrous oxide administered by face mask. An oropharyngeal airway may assist in maintaining a patent airway and reduces head movement during spontaneous respirations. This minimizes movement as viewed through the surgeon's

657

microscope. Gentle manual assistance of ventilation can also help reduce head movement. Occasionally, a laryngeal mask airway (LMA) may be used in children in whom the procedure is expected to be prolonged (e.g., children with Down syndrome who often have narrow ear canals). Most children can be managed safely without intravenous access, but it is reasonable to have an intravenous setup ready for use should the need arise. Some children with severe underlying medical or surgical conditions will require intravenous access despite the anticipated brief duration of the procedure. Although premedication is often omitted because the duration of action of most sedative premedicants outlasts the duration of this brief surgical procedure, an anxious child may still benefit from a sedative premedication.

In some instances, it is desirable to remove a retained tympanostomy tube. This can be easily done in the surgeon's office without anesthesia. Some particularly stiff-flanged grommet tubes will require a general anesthetic for removal. If the incision does not heal spontaneously, a paper patch or fat graft may be required to stimulate healing of the tympanic membrane. The anesthetic would be the same as that for the tube placement, except that nitrous oxide is best avoided to minimize the chance of graft dislodgment (see later discussion).

When halothane is used, discomfort after myringotomy and tube insertion is usually minimal. Administration of acetaminophen, either via the oral route preoperatively or the rectal route immediately after induction, provides adequate postoperative analgesia. The recommended oral dose of acetaminophen is 10 to 20 mg/kg, but the initial rectal dose that is required to achieve analgesic blood levels is greater (30 to 40 mg/kg).[2-4] Unfortunately, the onset time of rectal acetaminophen is 60 to 90 minutes and the peak effect is not reached until 2 or 3 hours, whereas oral acetaminophen is very rapidly absorbed. Consequently, the oral route is preferred for this procedure.

Preschool-aged children who receive unsupplemented sevoflurane anesthesia for myringotomy and tube insertion may exhibit emergence delirium and postoperative agitation. Although pain may be partially responsible for this response, the etiology is not totally clear. Because the procedure is so brief and intravenous access is not usually established, the use of intranasal fentanyl in a dose of 1 to 2 μg/kg has been found to be effective in providing analgesia and in preventing emergence agitation in this population.[5,6] The only significant side effect is a 12% incidence of vomiting when early oral fluid administration is attempted.[5] Other authors have reported the use of sedatives and/or analgesic drugs to modify that response. Intravenous ketorolac (1 mg/kg) and nasal butorphanol (25 μg/kg) have been shown to reduce rescue analgesic requirements in these children.[7,8] Some practitioners prefer to use more soluble anesthetics such as isoflurane for anesthesia maintenance to possibly reduce the incidence of agitation after myringotomy and tube insertion.

Children with chronic otitis frequently have persistent rhinorrhea and suffer recurrent upper respiratory tract infection (see Chapter 11). Eradication of middle ear congestion and fluid drainage often resolves the concomitant symptoms. No significant differences in perioperative complications between asymptomatic children and children with mild upper respiratory tract infections have been found. In general, morbidity is not increased in children who present for minor surgery with acute uncomplicated upper respiratory tract infection provided they do not require tracheal intubation.[9,10] Canceling this surgery because of rhinorrhea or recurrent mild respiratory symptoms is not usually justified. It is, however, recommended that children with respiratory symptoms have oxygen saturation measured before induction of general anesthesia and that supplemental oxygen is administered postoperatively to those children who have oxygen saturation less than 93%.[11]

Middle Ear and Mastoid Surgery

Tympanoplasty and mastoidectomy are two of the most common major ear operations performed on children. Anesthesia usually consists of an inhalational anesthetic and intravenous opioids. Surgical identification and preservation of the facial nerve are necessary because of its proximity to the surgical field. The nerve can be identified and its function verified by means of electrical stimulation. Therefore, neuromuscular blocking agents are usually avoided in these children. If a muscle relaxant must be used, a smaller dose should be given to facilitate tracheal intubation; and if a muscle relaxant is used for maintenance, suppression of the twitch response should not exceed 70%.

To gain access to the surgical site, the child's head is sometimes positioned on a headrest, which may be positioned below the operating table. In addition, extreme degrees of lateral rotation may be required. The anesthesiologist and surgeon must be extremely vigilant to ensure that nerves, muscles, and bony structures are not injured by the extreme positioning. Extreme tension should not be placed on the heads of the sternocleidomastoid muscle, and this limits the safe degree of lateral head rotation. Sometimes tilting the operating room table to the side will minimize the need for extreme rotation of the child's head (e.g., Down syndrome). The laxity of the ligaments of the cervical spine as well as immaturity of the odontoid process in children makes them especially prone to C1-C2 subluxation. Fifteen to 31 percent of children with Down syndrome or achondroplasia may have atlantoaxial instability.[12-15] Care in anteroposterior positioning can avoid injury in this area. The positioning of the operating room table to allow access to the respective middle ear and accommodate all the extra surgical equipment can pose a challenge. Depending on the room configuration, the table may be rotated 90 or even 180 degrees away from the anesthesia machine (Fig. 31-1). The resultant limited access to the airway mandates extreme care in securing the tracheal tube and the use of extra-long breathing circuits. Draping must allow immediate access should that be required.

Bleeding must be kept to a minimum during surgery on the small structures of the middle ear. Relative hypotension (i.e., mean arterial pressure ≤25% less than baseline) may help to reduce bleeding. Concentrated epinephrine solution, 1:8000, is frequently applied to the tympanic membrane to vasoconstrict the blood vessels. Close attention should be paid to the dose of injected epinephrine to avoid arrhythmias and wide variations in blood pressure. The maximum dosage of epinephrine is 10 μg/kg, which may be repeated after 30 minutes.

The middle ear and sinuses are air-filled, nondistensible cavities. An increase in the volume of gas within these cavities increases the pressure within the cavities. Nitrous oxide diffuses along a concentration gradient into air-filled middle ear spaces more rapidly than nitrogen moves out because nitrous oxide is 34 times more soluble than nitrogen in the blood. The middle ear is vented through the opening of the eustachian tube. Normal passive venting of the eustachian tube occurs at 20 to

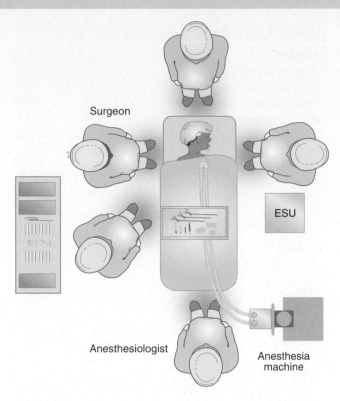

Figure 31-1. An operating room table turned 180 degrees may limit access to the patient during ear surgery. ESU, electrosurgical unit.

Labels on figure: Surgeon, ESU, Anesthesiologist, Anesthesia machine

30 cm H_2O pressure. It has been shown that use of nitrous oxide increases the pressures such that they exceed the ability of the eustachian tube to vent the middle ear within 5 minutes, leading to pressure buildup.[16] If eustachian tube function is interfered with during the surgical procedure, then pressure in the middle ear can increase further. Venting of the middle ear occurs intermittently, leading to constant changes in middle ear pressure, which in turn cause movement of the tympanic membrane.[17] During procedures in which the tympanic membrane is replaced or a perforation is patched, nitrous oxide should be discontinued or, if this is not possible, limited to a maximum of 50% before the application of the tympanic membrane graft to reduce the potential for pressure-related displacement.[18] The omission of nitrous oxide does not significantly increase the requirements (minimal alveolar concentration) for the less soluble inhaled anesthetics, desflurane, or sevoflurane in children.[19] After nitrous oxide is discontinued, it is quickly reabsorbed, creating a void in the middle ear, with resulting negative pressure. This negative pressure may result in serous otitis, disarticulation of the ossicles in the middle ear (especially the stapes), and hearing impairment, which may last up to 6 weeks postoperatively. The use of nitrous oxide may increase the incidence of postoperative nausea and vomiting (PONV), as a direct result of negative middle ear pressure during recovery. The negative pressure created by the reabsorption of nitrous oxide stimulates the vestibular system by producing traction on the round window. Although all children have the potential for PONV, older children seem to be at greater risk.[20] Prophylactic administration of antiemetics (usually dexamethasone and ondansetron) is usually warranted in these children. Local infiltration of the great auric-

ular nerve can provide pain relief equivalent to that of opioids and may reduce the incidence of opioid-induced vomiting.[21]

A smooth quiet emergence is desirable in these children. Deep tracheal extubation can be accomplished if the child is allowed to breathe spontaneously during the last 15 to 20 minutes of surgery and if opioids are titrated to produce regular slow respirations. Gentle suctioning of the oropharynx and possibly the use of intravenous lidocaine (1-1.5 mg/kg) in children older than 1 year of age can minimize or even prevent coughing after the tracheal tube is removed.

Cochlear Implants

In recent years, the indications for cochlear implants have broadened and continue to be in a state of evolution. With the application of universal neonatal hearing screening programs, a large pool of newly identified hearing-impaired infants has been identified. The benefits of early intervention with cochlear implants are being explored. Younger children with severe to profound hearing loss will better their auditory, speech, and language skills and more can be easily mainstreamed with their age-appropriate hearing peers when they receive an implant early in life. Experience has shown that cochlear implant surgery is safe in infants older than 6 months of age provided that special attention is paid to the physiologic and anatomic differences present in this age group. Surgery requires meticulous care with hemostasis, soft tissue dissection, and bone drilling because bleeding from marrow can be difficult to control. Availability of skilled postoperative nursing and a pediatric intensive care unit is also essential.[22] Postoperative fitting of the externally worn speech processor is very important for successful use of the cochlear implant. However, especially in infants and young children, this fitting process can be difficult because of limited communication capabilities. The use of intraoperatively obtained stapedius reflex thresholds has been proposed for postoperative speech processor fitting, but the influence of anesthetics on threshold values needs to be taken into account. More reliable threshold values can be obtained by adjusting the dosage of hypnotics to achieve a lighter level of hypnosis during stapedius reflex measurement.[23] In most children, increasing the concentration of inhalational anesthetics increases the stapedius reflex threshold. As always, appropriate communication with the surgeon will help ensure a successful outcome.

Anesthesia for Rhinologic Procedures

Chronic sinusitis in children can be caused by resistant bacteria and is usually treated with broad-spectrum antibiotics. In some children with obstructive adenoid pads, adenoidectomy will improve the signs and symptoms of sinusitis. Functional endoscopic sinus surgery using sharp biting instruments and/or a microdébrider has become the primary method of surgical therapy for chronic sinusitis.[24] Current techniques aim to leave the mucosa in this area intact to prevent scarring in the frontal recess. Although sometimes controversial, there is no evidence at present that functional endoscopic sinus surgery affects facial growth in children. Of interest to the anesthesiologist is that many of the children who require functional endoscopic sinus surgery have coexisting medical problems, such as asthma and cystic fibrosis. These conditions must be optimized before surgery (see Chapter 11).

Anesthetic management of these children usually requires tracheal intubation to secure the airway. The use of an oral preformed tracheal tube (e.g., the Ring-Adair-Elwyn [RAE] tube) allows secure fixation to the mandible and unobstructed access to the maxilla and sinuses. The use of a cuffed tracheal tube is particularly advantageous to eliminate a gas leak that could fog up the endoscopic instruments. A throat pack is frequently inserted to absorb blood in the oropharynx and limit the gas escaping around an uncuffed tube. It is vital that the pack is removed before tracheal extubation. Occasionally, an LMA may be used to facilitate a quick "second look."

Because bleeding is inevitable with this surgery and it can interfere with the visualization, packing the nasal cavity with a vasoconstricting solution is frequently performed before surgery commences. The most commonly used topical vasoconstrictors are oxymetazoline 0.025% to 0.05%, phenylephrine 0.25% to 1%, and cocaine 4% to 10%. It is important for the anesthesiologist to be aware of the type and dose of the vasoconstrictor used and that no more than the maximum effective dose is applied. Application of topical phenylephrine or other potent vasoconstrictors to the mucous membrane or raw surgical site can cause severe hypertension, reflex bradycardia, and even cardiac arrest.[25] Hypertension that is induced by topically applied vasoconstrictors often resolves spontaneously and may not require aggressive treatment. The use of β blockers or calcium-channel blockers to control blood pressure in these circumstances can depress cardiac output and lead to pulmonary edema and cardiac arrest.[25] It is recommended that in children the initial topical dose of phenylephrine should not exceed 20 μg/kg.[25]

Corticosteroids such as intravenous dexamethasone (0.25-0.5 mg/kg) are usually administered to reduce swelling and scarring. Frequently, the surgeon will want to leave an absorbable stenting material such as MeroGel at the end of surgery. Unfortunately, this will interfere with nasal breathing and will increase the incidence of emergence agitation. An anesthetic technique that ensures adequate analgesia and rapid return of consciousness at the end of surgery is therefore desirable. One of us (RSH) has found that a combination of desflurane, fentanyl, and low-dose propofol works well. A sensory block of the infraorbital nerve can also be performed by use of an intraoral route or extraoral route to provide analgesia.[26]

Adenotonsillectomy

Adenotonsillectomy is one of the oldest and most commonly performed pediatric surgical procedures worldwide. More selective indications, however, have dramatically reduced the annual caseload.[27,28] Chronic or recurrent tonsillitis and obstructive adenotonsillar hyperplasia are the major indications for surgical removal, although other indications do exist (Table 31-1).[29,30] Surgical treatment is required when tonsillitis recurs despite adequate medical therapy or when it is associated with peritonsillar abscess or acute airway obstruction. Halitosis, persistent pharyngitis, and cervical adenitis may accompany chronic tonsillitis. Tonsillar hyperplasia may lead to chronic airway obstruction, resulting in sleep apnea, carbon dioxide (CO_2) retention, cor pulmonale, failure to thrive, swallowing disorders, and speech abnormalities (Fig. 31-2). Many of these adverse effects are reversible with surgical excision of the tonsils. Children with cardiac valvular disease may be at risk for endocarditis due to recurrent streptococcal bacteremia secondary to infected tonsils (see Chapter 14).

Table 31-1. Indications for Adenotonsillectomy

Infection
Acute tonsillitis or adenoiditis

Recurrent tonsillitis or adenoiditis

Chronic tonsillitis or adenoiditis

Peritonsillar abscess

Halitosis

Obstruction
Nasal airway (adenoids)

Pharyngeal airway (tonsils)

Sleep apnea

Cyanosis

Failure to thrive

Cor pulmonale due to airway obstruction

Mass Lesion
Tonsillar/adenoidal

Benign

Malignant

Adenoidectomy is usually performed in conjunction with tonsillectomy; however, in some situations only adenoidectomy is performed. Indications for adenoidectomy alone include chronic or recurrent purulent adenoiditis (despite adequate medical therapy), recurrent otitis media with effusion secondary to adenoidal hyperplasia, and chronic sinusitis. Advanced degrees of adenoidal hyperplasia may lead to nasopharyngeal obstruction, obligate mouth breathing, poor feeding resulting in failure to thrive, speech disorders, and sleep disturbances. Long-standing nasal obstruction can result in orofacial abnormalities with a narrowing of the upper airway and dental abnormalities, which may be avoided by removal of hypertrophied adenoid tissue.

Surgical techniques for adenotonsillectomy vary and include guillotine and snare techniques, cold and hot knife dissection, suction, ultrasound coblation, and unipolar and bipolar

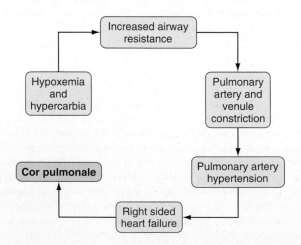

Figure 31-2. Patients with chronic tonsillar hypertrophy may have long-standing hypoxemia and hypercarbia, which can lead to cor pulmonale.

electrocautery techniques. A major advantage of the electrocautery dissection technique is a reduction in the incidence of intraoperative blood loss as well as postoperative primary and secondary hemorrhage. A major disadvantage is greater pain and poor oral intake postoperatively.[31-35]

The mortality associated with adenotonsillectomy is estimated to be 1 per 16,000 to 1 per 35,000 procedures.[36,37] Hospital-based reviews of anesthetic mortality continue to list adenotonsillectomy as a surgical procedure associated with perioperative cardiac arrest and death.[38,39] Surgical complications after adenotonsillectomy are rare but include uvular amputation, uvular edema, velopharyngeal insufficiency, and nasopharyngeal stenosis. Atlantoaxial subluxation manifesting as neck pain and torticollis, mandibular subluxation and condylar fracture, cervical adenitis, and cervical osteomyelitis have been reported.[37,40]

Throat pain, otalgia, emesis, poor oral intake, and dehydration are common morbidities. Respiratory morbidity after adenotonsillectomy in the otherwise healthy child affects less than 1%[41-43] but has assumed a greater importance since obstructive breathing has replaced infection and halitosis as the most common indication for adenotonsillectomy.

Age has a major influence on post-adenotonsillectomy complications. Secondary post-adenotonsillectomy hemorrhage is more common in children older than the age of 10 years.[44,45] Young age is a risk factor for both poor oral intake and respiratory complications. The majority of children younger than age 3 years experience airway problems after adenotonsillectomy for obstructive breathing.[46,47]

Preoperative Evaluation

The general health of the child and the indications for surgery must be reviewed. Upper respiratory tract infections are frequent in these children and can interfere with the timing of adenotonsillectomy because the risk of respiratory morbidity and hemorrhage is increased.[37,41,48,49] A history of bleeding tendencies requires investigation. Medications that interfere with coagulation include aspirin, nonsteroidal anti-inflammatory drugs, and valproic acid. Discontinuation of these drugs preoperatively is sometimes problematic, and preoperative consultation with neurology, cardiology and hematology may be indicated.

A careful cardiorespiratory history and physical examination is essential. Children with chronic tonsillar hypertrophy may have long-standing hypoxemia and hypercarbia, which can lead to cor pulmonale (see Fig. 31-2). The oropharynx should be evaluated and the tonsillar size classified (Fig. 31-3).[50] In some centers, a complete blood cell count is required before adenotonsillectomy. There is no evidence to routinely perform preoperative coagulation studies unless it is indicated by history.[51,52]

Special Considerations for the Child with Obstructive Sleep Apnea

The single most important task during the preoperative evaluation of the child for adenotonsillectomy is to distinguish the child with obstructive sleep apnea (OSA) from the child with obstructive breathing, because the child with OSA is at greater risk to develop severe perioperative respiratory complications, possibly including death, after adenotonsillectomy.[53-56]

OSA is the extreme limit of the spectrum of sleep-disordered breathing. This spectrum, which ranges from normal respiration to OSA, includes primary snoring, upper airway resistance syndrome (UARS), obstructive hypopnea, and OSA. At the most extreme form of sleep-disordered breathing, OSA, clinical signs of partial or complete upper airway obstruction must be present during sleep as well as some degree of hypercarbia and/or hypoxemia.[57] Although it is important to recognize the significance of OSA in children who are scheduled for adenotonsillectomy, children who do not meet the criteria for OSA but who have less severe forms of sleep-disordered breathing such as UARS or obstructive hypopnea may also be at increased risk for morbidity after surgery. The latter requires further investigation before guidelines for risk assessment are published.

A high index of suspicion is required to identify the child with OSA on clinical criteria. There is a greater incidence of OSA in Asian and African-American populations.[58,59] In addition, African-American children desaturate more profoundly during sleep-related obstructive airway events than caucasian and Hispanic children[60]; the reasons for this apparent difference are unclear.

Anatomic features including increased nasal resistance may underlie the pathogenesis of OSA; common medical conditions and syndromes that predispose to the development of OSA are listed in Table 31-2. Infants suffering acute life-threatening events have a greater incidence of OSA in childhood and adolescence.[61-63]

The obstructive events that characterize OSA result in recurrent episodes of hypoxia, hypercarbia, and sleep disruption, a trilogy that has been linked to the development of medical

Table 31-2. Medical Conditions in Children That Predispose to Development of Obstructive Sleep Apnea

Craniofacial Syndromes
Crouzon syndrome
Apert's syndrome
Pfeiffer syndrome
Treacher Collins syndrome
Pierre Robin sequence
Goldenhar's syndrome
Larsen's syndrome
Disorders of Cranial Base
Arnold-Chiari malformation
Achondroplasia
Syringobulbia
Neuromuscular Disorders
Cerebral palsy
Trisomy 21
Infiltrative Disorders
Mucopolysaccharidoses
Acromegaly
Obesity
Prader-Willi syndrome
Temporomandibular Joint Ankylosis

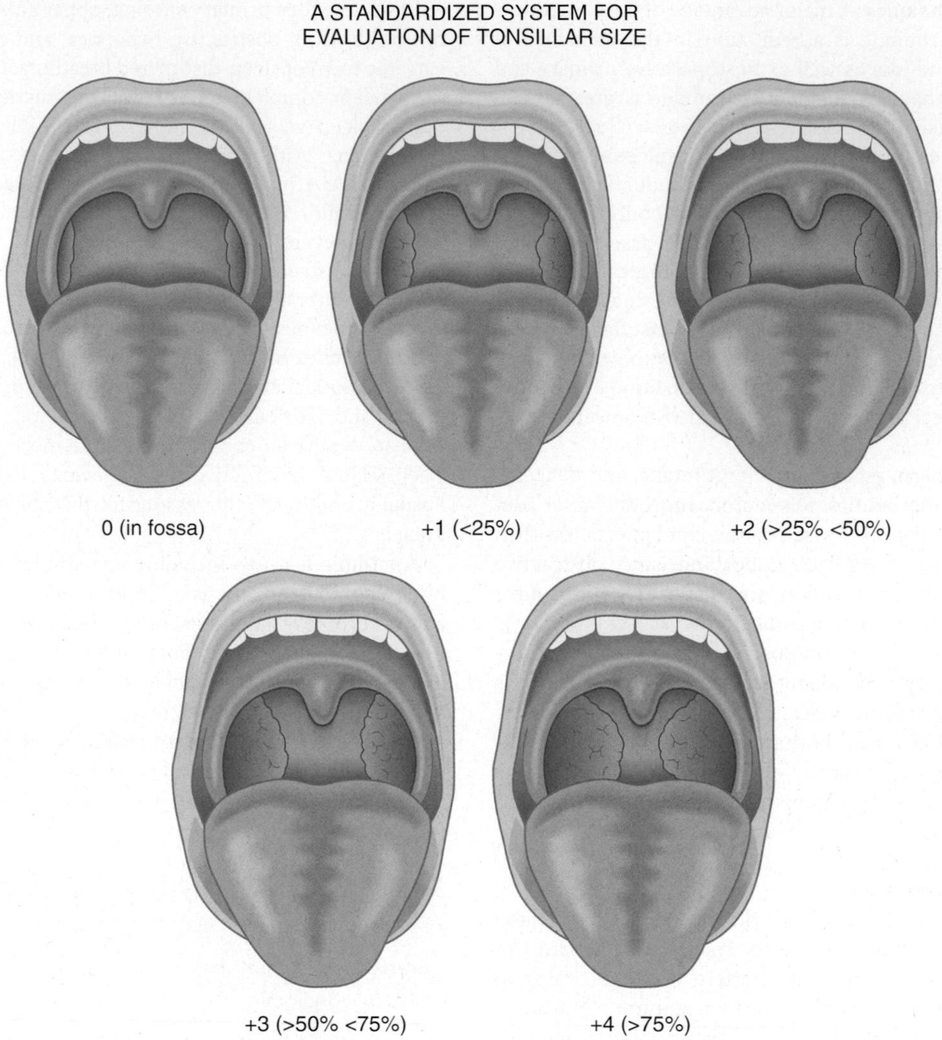

A STANDARDIZED SYSTEM FOR
EVALUATION OF TONSILLAR SIZE

0 (in fossa)   +1 (<25%)   +2 (>25% <50%)

+3 (>50% <75%)   +4 (>75%)

Figure 31-3. Classifying tonsil size may be helpful in evaluating the degree of airway obstruction. Patients classified as +3 or greater (i.e., having more than 50% of the pharyngeal area occupied by hypertrophied tonsils) are at an increased risk of developing airway obstruction during anesthetic induction. (Modified from Brodsky L: Modern assessment of tonsils and adenoids. Pediatr Clin North Am 1989; 36:1551-1569; illustration by Jon S. Krasner.)

sequelae that accompany severe OSA. Because adenotonsillectomy is very often the initial treatment for the majority of children, these children may present with a spectrum of disease affecting multiple organ systems. Failure to thrive is common. Cardiovascular abnormalities including ventricular dysfunction, a depressed ventricular ejection fraction, right ventricular hypertrophy, and pulmonary hypertension may be present.[64-67] Repeated infections affecting the lower respiratory tract have been linked to chronic aspiration.[68]

The severity of OSA is assessed by the frequency and severity of the obstructive respiratory events during sleep. Both vary with sleep stage and occur most often during active rapid eye movement (REM) sleep. The frequency and severity of obstructive events worsen after midnight, a finding that may reflect the greater proportion of REM sleep in the latter part of the night and fatigue of the upper airway musculature.[69-71]

Apneas are classified as central, obstructive, and mixed. Central apnea occurs when there is no apparent respiratory effort. Obstructive apnea is associated with apparent, often vigorous, inspiratory efforts that are ineffective due to lack of upper airway patency. A mixed obstructive apnea is diagnosed when both central and obstructive apnea occur without interruption by effective respirations. The presence of sleep-disordered breathing is documented by polysomnography and is quantitated by the frequency of obstructive events and by desaturation indices. The polysomnogram simultaneously records the electroencephalogram, electromyogram, electrocardiogram, pulse oximetry, airflow, and thoracic and abdominal movement during sleep. To date, there is no consensus on the criteria for diagnosing OSA in children.[66] A common definition of an obstructive apnea in children is an obstructive effort that includes more than two obstructive breaths, regardless of the duration of the apnea.[69] An obstructive apnea index of 1 is the cutoff for normality in children.[72] *Hypopnea* is defined as a reduction in airflow of more than 50%.[69] The apnea hypopnea index (AHI) is the summation of the number of obstructive apnea and hypopnea events and is analogous to the respiratory disturbance index (RDI). A common definition of desaturation is a 4% decrease in oxygen saturation from baseline. The saturation nadir is the lowest saturation recorded during the sleep study. A saturation nadir of 92% is the cutoff for normality in children.[72,73]

The severity of OSA predicts the nature of perioperative respiratory complications (Table 31-3). An RDI of greater than 20 events per hour is associated with breath holding during induction, whereas an RDI greater than 30 is associated with laryngospasm and desaturation during emergence.[74] Ten obstructive events per hour during the polysomnogram is the threshold for postoperative severe respiratory complications.[54] A saturation nadir less than 80% is associated with a greater incidence of respiratory morbidity after adenotonsillectomy compared with a saturation nadir greater than 80%.[53,56]

The RDI and AHI correlate inversely with the saturation nadir,[75,76] making simplified testing with continuous pulse oximetry a meaningful metric. The McGill oximetry score has been shown to correlate with the risk of respiratory complications after adenotonsillectomy in children (Fig. 31-4). Twenty-four percent of children with a McGill oximetry score of 4 experienced major postoperative respiratory complications.[76]

Children with severe OSA may require additional preoperative testing before adenotonsillectomy. A capillary blood gas sample drawn in the morning can be evaluated for an increased concentration of bicarbonate, suggestive of CO_2 retention during sleep. When indicated, a preoperative electrocardiogram or echocardiogram may provide evidence of right ventricular hypertrophy and/or pulmonary hypertension. A chest radiograph may suggest lower airways disease or cardiomegaly.

Anesthesia consultation to plan the perioperative care of children with severe OSA is important. Young children with profound desaturation during sleep and CO_2 retention may require admission to the pediatric intensive care unit for optimization before and/or management after adenotonsillectomy.[27,77] Urgent adenotonsillectomy is associated with significant respiratory morbidity after surgery.[55,78] On occasion, adenotonsillar hypertrophy may progress to compromise the upper airway during wakefulness. In some instances the anesthetic considerations for the obstructed and difficult airways may overlap.

Anesthetic Management and Postoperative Considerations

The anesthetic goals for adenotonsillectomy are (1) to provide a smooth atraumatic induction; (2) to provide the surgeon with optimal operating conditions; (3) to establish intravenous access for volume expansion and medications as indicated; and (4) to provide rapid emergence so that the child is awake and able to protect the recently instrumented airway. The need for a premedication is determined during the preanesthetic evaluation. *Children with symptoms of sleep-disordered breathing who require premedication should be closely observed and monitored with oximetry after administration of sedative medications depending on the accuracy of the diagnosis of OSA.*[79] *Premedication with short-acting drugs and/or those that can be antagonized is advised (see further).*

The anesthetic techniques for adenotonsillectomy are varied and include the choice of an inhalational or intravenous technique, the choice of an endotracheal tube (ETT) or an LMA, and the choice of spontaneous or controlled ventilation. Of the currently available inhalational agents, sevoflurane provides a smooth induction of anesthesia and desflurane provides a rapid emergence and recovery when the latter is used during the maintenance of anesthesia.[80,81] The rapid return of airway reflexes is particularly important when the dose of opioids must be titrated after extubation.

Children who are scheduled for adenotonsillectomy have a high incidence of airway reactivity and laryngospasm. This will influence the choice of airway management. Placement of an ETT with a leak at 20 cm of H_2O (the leak increases with neck extension and insertion of the mouth gag) is generally sufficient to prevent soiling of the trachea during the surgery yet reduces the incidence of post-extubation croup. More recently, the use of cuffed ETTs is becoming common.[82] A cuffed tube prevents an air leak and the bubbling of gases through the oropharyngeal secretions and blood that can interfere with surgery. It also minimizes pollution by anesthetic gases and decreases the need for multiple laryngoscopies and tube changes to select the appropriate size. A cuff design that is high compliance, short, and close to the tip of the tube may be advantageous.[83]

Blood and secretions may be present in the oropharynx at the conclusion of surgery and should be carefully suctioned before emergence from anesthesia. Emptying the stomach with an orogastric tube, a maneuver usually performed by the surgeon under direct vision after completion of surgery, may reduce the incidence of emesis.

Table 31-3. Clinical Diagnostic Criteria for Pediatric Obstructive Sleep Apnea Syndrome

1. Predisposing physical characteristics
   a. Body mass index greater than 95th percentile for age and gender
   b. Craniofacial abnormalities affecting the airway
   c. Anatomic nasal obstruction
   d. Tonsils nearly touching or touching in the midline
2. History of apparent airway obstruction during sleep (*two or more of the following*)
   a. Loud snoring (loud enough to be heard through a closed door)
   b. Frequent snoring
   c. Observed pauses in breathing during sleep
   d. Frequent arousals from sleep
   e. Intermittent vocalization during sleep
   f. Parental report of restless sleep, difficulty breathing, or struggling respiratory efforts during sleep
3. Somnolence (*one or more of the following*)
   a. Parent or teacher comments that the child appears sleepy during the day, is easily distracted, is overly aggressive, or has difficulty concentrating
   b. Child often is difficult to arouse at the usual awakening time

Note: If signs and symptoms in at least two categories are present there is a significant probability of moderate OSA. If severe abnormalities are present, children should be treated as having severe OSA.
Adapted from Table 1 in Practice Guidelines for the Perioperative Management of Patients with Obstructive Sleep Apnea: A report by the American Society of Anesthesiologists Task Force on Perioperative Management of Patients with Obstructive Sleep Apnea. Anesthesiology 2006; 104:1081-1093.

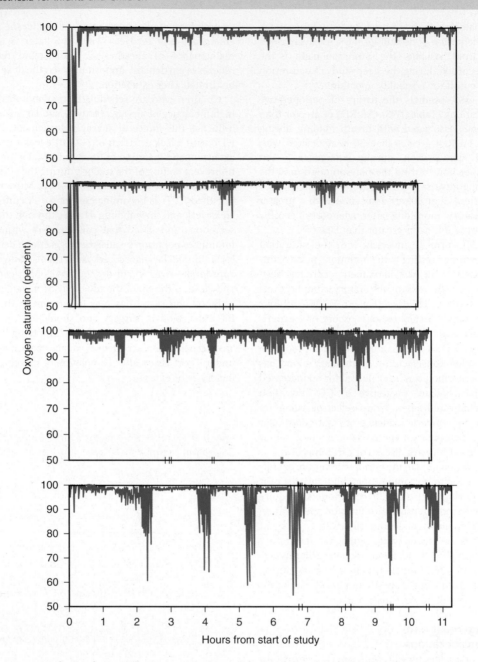

Figure 31-4. Representative figures for McGill oximetry scores 1 to 4 (*top to bottom*). McGill oximetry scores 2 to 4 are abnormal in that they all show at least three clusters of desaturation. The severity of the saturation nadir determines the score such that McGill 2, 3, and 4 correspond to saturation nadirs <90%, <85%, and <80%, respectively. (From Nixon GM, Kermack AS, Davis GM, et al: Planning adenotonsillectomy in children with obstructive sleep apnea: the role of overnight oximetry. Pediatrics 2004; 113:e19-e25.)

It is preferable to wait until the child is fully awake and able to clear blood and secretions from the oropharynx before removing the ETT. A common practice is to position the child in the lateral position (known as the "tonsil" or "recovery" position) with the head slightly down at the time of extubation to permit blood and secretions to pool in the dependent cheek rather than accumulate at the laryngeal inlet. Intact airway and pharyngeal reflexes are of utmost importance in preventing aspiration, laryngospasm, and airway obstruction.[84] After surgery, the child should remain in the tonsil position and be transported to the recovery room for careful observation and monitoring.

The use of the LMA for adenotonsillectomy was described in 1990, but it was not until the widespread availability of a model with a flexible spiral-metallic reinforced shaft that it was widely utilized.[85,86] The wide, rigid tube of the original model did not fit under the mouth gag and was easily compressed or dislodged during full mouth opening. The newer, flexible model has a soft, reinforced shaft, which easily fits under the mouth gag without becoming dislodged or compressed. Adequate surgical access can be achieved and the airways are reasonably well protected from exposure to blood during the surgery.[87,88]

Insertion of an LMA is possible after either the intravenous administration of up to 3.5 mg/kg propofol or when sufficient depth of anesthesia is achieved with an inhalational anesthetic.[89] It has been recommended that the LMA be used only in spontaneously breathing children and that positive-pressure ventilation be avoided, although gentle assisted ventilation is both safe and effective if peak inspiratory pressure is less than or equal to 20 cm H_2O.[83] The leak fraction produced during ventilation with the LMA increases with increasing airway pressure. The frequency of gastric insufflation ranges from 2% at a peak inspiratory pressure of 15 cm H_2O to 35% at 30 cm H_2O in adults.[90] Positive-pressure ventilation of the lungs via the LMA is usually adequate if both the airway resistance and pulmonary compliance are normal, but gas may be insufflated into the stomach if increased ventilatory pressures are needed. This may increase the risk of regurgitation of gastric contents. Insertion of the LMA may be difficult in the presence of tonsillar enlargement.[91] Maneuvers to overcome this difficulty include increased head extension, lateral insertion of the mask, anterior displacement of the tongue, pressure on the tip of the LMA using the index finger as it negotiates the pharyngeal curve, or use of the laryngoscope if all else fails. The LMA is not dislodged when the neck is placed in extreme extension, assuming that good position and adequate ventilation were present before the neck was extended.[92] Advantages of the LMA over traditional endotracheal intubation include a decrease in the incidence of postoperative stridor and laryngospasm and an increase in immediate postoperative oxygen saturation.[93] Recovery may be improved overall with fewer episodes of airway obstruction reported by some investigators.[87] In spite of the theoretical advantages, there is no evidence that the LMA decreases morbidity when compared with a tracheal tube for adenotonsillectomy. The LMA is most useful in children who can tolerate spontaneous respirations. If the child is breathing spontaneously at a regular rate and depth, the LMA may be removed before the child emerges from anesthesia, provided comorbid conditions, including OSA, obesity, or a difficult airway, are not present. The oropharynx should be gently suctioned with a soft flexible catheter, the LMA removed, and the respirations assisted with 100% oxygen delivered by mask. It may be distressing for young children to awaken with the LMA still in place. Although the LMA is an appropriate substitute for the oral airway in the adult population, the same is not true for children. If the practitioner wishes to remove the LMA when the child has emerged from anesthesia, it should be removed as soon as consciousness has returned.

Analgesic Management

Surgical technique has a major impact on the analgesic requirements after adenotonsillectomy because electrocautery techniques are associated with greater pain, presumably owing to increased thermal injury.[31,32,94] Opioids have been the mainstay to secure analgesia. However, because opioids increase the incidence of emesis and respiratory morbidity, the use of opioid-sparing adjuncts has been advocated and include dexamethasone, acetaminophen, and nonsteroidal anti-inflammatory drugs (NSAIDs).

A single intraoperative dose of dexamethasone reduces post-adenotonsillectomy pain and edema when electrocautery has been used. Large doses are traditionally used, especially in children with OSA. Dexamethasone (1 mg/kg) administration is associated with reduced parental and physician rated pain scores after adenotonsillectomy (Table 31-4).[32] Although the minimum morphine-sparing dose for dexamethasone is reported to be 0.5 mg/kg,[95] a recent study found no difference between 0.0625 and 1.0 mg/kg in the incidence of postoperative vomiting, pain scores, time to first liquid, and time to first analgesics.[96] Single doses of dexamethasone have never been associated with aseptic necrosis of the hip or other steroid-induced complications.

The routine use of NSAIDs for adenotonsillectomy remains controversial because of the potential for post-adenotonsillectomy hemorrhage. A meta-analysis of seven randomized controlled trials (505 children) on the effects of NSAIDs on bleeding risk after tonsillectomy reported the number needed to harm in terms of reoperation for hemostasis to be 29.[97] NSAIDs were associated with a greater risk of both postoperative bleeding that required treatment and reoperation for hemostasis. The Cochrane Collaboration assessed the effect of NSAIDs on bleeding after pediatric tonsillectomy in 13 trials (955 children) and did not report any increase in bleeding that required reoperation for hemostasis.[98] An audit of more than 4800 pediatric tonsillectomies in which the NSAIDs diclofenac and ibuprofen were routinely used reported a primary hemorrhage rate of 0.9%.[45] Because the effects of ketorolac on platelet function are reversible, the effect is dependent on the presence of ketorolac within the body.[99] Thus, unlike aspirin, this effect is short lived. However, we recommend administering NSAIDs only after consulting with the surgeon and, if in agreement, administering them after hemostasis is achieved.[100] Acetaminophen is commonly used as a component of multimodal analgesic approach in these children. Intravenous acetaminophen is now available in some countries and has the theoretical advantage of greater predictability compared with the oral and rectal routes. However, recent studies suggest that the duration of analgesia after 15 mg/kg of acetaminophen given intravenously is less than after 40 mg/kg given rectally.[101]

Infiltration of local anesthetics into the tonsillar fossa during tonsillectomy is sometimes reported to decrease postoperative pain, but the pain relief is transient (Fig. 31-5, see website).[102] In

Table 31-4. Effect of Single Intraoperative Dose of Dexamethasone on Postoperative Pain in Pediatric Tonsillectomy or Adenotonsillectomy: A Comparison of Randomized, Double-Blinded Studies

Source	No. of Children	Dexamethasone Dose	Electrocautery Technique	Effect on Pain
Catlin and Grimes[203]	25	8 mg/m²	No	No difference
Ohlms et al.[204]	69	0.5 mg/kg	No	No difference
Tom et al.[205]	58	1.0 mg/kg	Yes	Reduced
April et al.[206]	80	1.0 mg/kg	Yes	No difference
Hanasono et al.[32]	219	1.0 mg/kg	Yes	Reduced

Adapted from Hanasono MM, Lalakea ML, Mikulec AA, et al: Perioperative steroids in tonsillectomy using electrocautery and sharp dissection techniques. Arch Otolaryngol Head Neck Surg 2004; 130:917-921.

addition, serious life-threatening complications have been reported after local anesthetic infiltration in the tonsillar fossa, including intracranial hemorrhage, bulbar paralysis, deep cervical abscess, cervical osteomyelitis, medullopontine infarct, and cardiac arrest. The risks associated with injection of local anesthesia in the tonsillar fossa may outweigh its potential benefits.[103,104]

Postoperative Nausea and Vomiting

Emesis and poor oral intake are common comorbid conditions after adenotonsillectomy. Propofol and ondansetron are widely used to reduce the incidence of post-adenotonsillectomy emesis. Opioids increase the incidence of PONV, with two thirds of children experiencing PONV.[28,45,105] Post-discharge vomiting can continue for days in some children. One study has shown that at-home use of oral ondansetron disintegrating tablets may prevent emesis during the first 3 days after adenotonsillectomy.[106] A single intraoperative dose of dexamethasone reduces the incidence of emesis during the first 24 hours after adenotonsillectomy. The number needed to treat was only four children, which means that the use of dexamethasone in four children undergoing adenotonsillectomy results in one less child experiencing PONV. In addition, children who received dexamethasone were more likely to advance to a soft diet on postoperative day one than those receiving placebo with a number

needed to treat of 5. Given the antiemetic and possible morphine-sparing advantages of a single dose of dexamethasone and its low cost and safety profile, the evidence suggests that routine use of dexamethasone reduces morbidity after adenotonsillectomy in children.[32,107] Although the literature supports the effectiveness of a single dose of dexamethasone, the smallest effective dose remains somewhat unclear. One study suggested an intravenous dose of 0.15 mg/kg,[108] whereas another reported no difference in postoperative vomiting, pain scores, time to first liquid, and time to first analgesics between doses of 0.0625 and 1.0 mg/kg (Fig. 31-6).[96]

Special Considerations for Children with OSA

Children with OSA who require premedication should be closely observed because transient desaturation has been reported in 3% of children with sleep or clinical diagnoses of OSA who received 0.5 mg/kg oral midazolam.[79]

Induction of Anesthesia

Compared with children undergoing adenotonsillectomy for chronic tonsillitis, those whose indication was OSA experienced more respiratory complications during induction of anesthesia.[74] The vulnerability of the upper airway musculature described for halothane[109] has subsequently been reported for most anesthetic agents, resulting in a graded reduction in airway

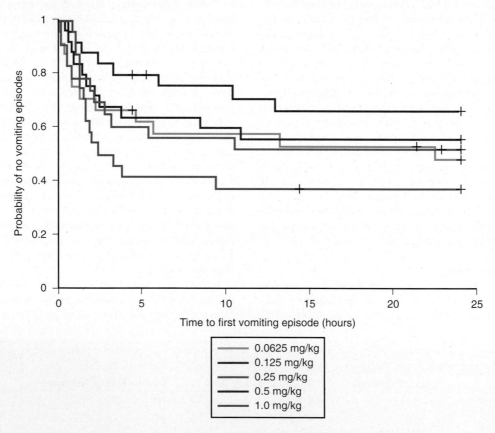

Figure 31-6. No dose escalation response to dexamethasone to prevent vomiting in children undergoing tonsillectomy. Time-to-event analysis for first vomiting episode was performed; tick marks indicate time of censoring for patients who did not have complete follow-up ($N = 13$). No significant difference was found between dose levels, $P = .28$ (Cox Proportional Hazard Likelihood Ratio Test). (Redrawn with permission from Kim MS, Coté CJ, Cristoloveanu C, et al: There is no dose-escalation response to dexamethasone (0.0625-1.0 mg/kg) in pediatric tonsillectomy or adenotonsillectomy patients for preventing vomiting, reducing pain, shortening time to first liquid intake, or the incidence of voice change. Anesth Analg 2007; 104:1052-1058.)

caliber with increasing anesthetic concentration.[110-112] The level of airway obstruction occurs in the upper two thirds of the pharyngeal airway, and the smallest pharyngeal dimension is in the area of overlap between the adenoids and tonsils.[113] During induction of anesthesia, early pharyngeal airway obstruction may require a jaw thrust maneuver, insertion of an oral or naso-pharyngeal airway, and the application of continuous positive airway pressure (CPAP). Propofol-associated loss in airway caliber is reversed with the application of CPAP,[114] which acts as a pneumatic splint to increase the caliber of the pharyngeal airway.[115] Of equal importance, CPAP increases longitudinal tension on the pharyngeal airway, thereby decreasing the collapsibility of the upper airway (see Fig. 12-10), and increases lung volumes.[116,117] Small increments in CPAP between 5 and 10 cm H_2O increase the dimension of the pharyngeal airway dramatically (Fig. 31-7).[118,119] The closing pressure of the pharynx increases with OSA severity such that greater levels of CPAP are required in children with severe OSA compared with those with mild OSA. It is prudent to consider securing intravenous access before induction of anesthesia in children with severe OSA to expedite administration of muscle relaxants or intravenous agents should pharyngeal obstruction or laryngospasm occur during induction of anesthesia. The small oropharynx and adenotonsillar hypertrophy associated with severe OSA may increase the difficulty in properly inserting an LMA.

Analgesic Management in Children with OSA
Severe OSA is characterized by recurrent episodes of hypoxia and hypercarbia during sleep. In animal models, exposure to intermittent hypoxia during development affects the opioid system, resulting in an increase in the density of μ opioid receptors in the respiratory-related areas of the brainstem. The cellular mechanism whereby this increased density is achieved has

yet to be elucidated, but it may represent an adaptive response to the effects of recurrent intermittent hypoxia that allows μ opioid respiratory effects to predominate.[120-123]

For children with severe OSA, the severity of the nocturnal desaturation correlates with the sensitivity to exogenously administered opioids (Fig. 31-8).[124-126] The morphine dose required to achieve a uniform analgesic endpoint was less in children with OSA whose preoperative saturation nadir during sleep was less (Fig. 31-9).[125] Young age was also associated with an increased sensitivity to opioids. *An unforeseen risk of opioid use in children with severe OSA is that smaller than expected doses of opioids may produce exaggerated respiratory depression in these children.* Forty-six percent of children with severe OSA who were anesthetized with halothane experienced apnea after a uniform dose of fentanyl, compared with 4% of controls.[127] This increased sensitivity to the respiratory depressant effects of fentanyl in children with OSA is supported by the exaggerated respiratory depression to subsequent administration of a uniform dose of fentanyl in developing rat pups exposed to intermittent hypoxia.[128] Hence, the use of spontaneous respiration during maintenance of anesthesia enables an assessment of the response to small challenges of opioid analgesics. In this manner, the anesthesiologist can assess the sensitivity of the child with OSA to opioids. Controlling respiration precludes such an evaluation.

Sleep fragmentation blunts the arousal response to acute airway occlusion during sleep.[129,130] In addition, exposure to intermittent hypoxia during development is associated with an increase in the arousal latency to hypoxia.[131-133] Morphine acting at the level of the basal forebrain blunts arousal.[134] If the increased sensitivity to both the analgesic and respiratory effects of exogenously administered opioids reported in children with OSA extends to arousal mechanisms, the use of opioids in children

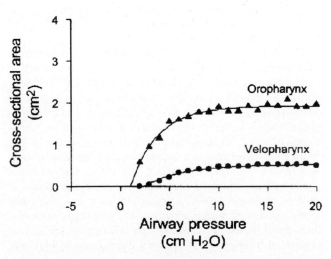

Figure 31-7. The relationship between airway pressure and the cross-sectional area of the pharynx. Maximal airway dimension is achieved between 15 and 20 cm H_2O. At lower airway pressures, around 5 cm H_2O, small increments in airway pressure make a large difference in airway caliber. (From Isono S, Tanaka A, Nishino T: Dynamic interaction between the tongue and soft palate during obstructive apnea in anesthetized patients with sleep-disordered breathing. J Appl Physiology 2003; 95:2257-2264.)

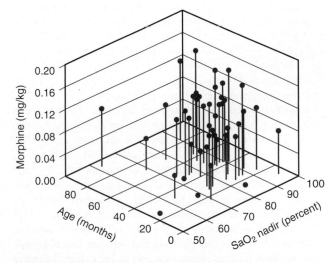

Figure 31-8. Relationship between morphine requirement, age, and the preoperative saturation nadir in 46 children who were otherwise well. The lengths of the stems supporting the 46 dots are proportional to the morphine dose. The stems in the foreground are shorter than those in the background, indicating a significant correlation between the three variables. (From Brown KA, Laferrière A, Moss IR: Recurrent hypoxemia in young children with obstructive sleep apnea is associated with reduced opioid requirements for analgesia. Anesthesiology 2004; 100:806-810.)

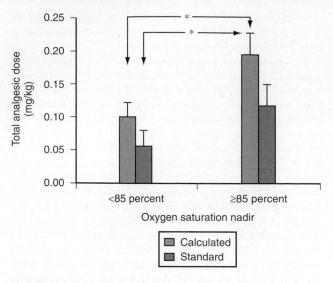

Figure 31-9. The morphine dosage required to achieve a uniform analgesic endpoint in children with obstructive sleep apnea (OSA) whose preoperative saturation nadir was less that 85% is one half that required in children whose saturation nadir was greater than 85%. (From Brown KA, Laferrière A, Lakheeram I, Moss IR: Recurrent hypoxemia in children is associated with increased analgesic sensitivity to opiates. Anesthesiology 2006; 105:665-669.)

with severe OSA may further impair arousal mechanisms. Guidelines for the perioperative management of OSA assign a greater risk score if opioids are used for postoperative analgesic regimens in children with OSA.[73] Although these guidelines suggest that the use of low-potency oral opioid analgesia carries a reduced perioperative risk, the use of codeine, a "low-risk" oral opioid commonly used in the ambulatory setting, may also be problematic in children with OSA. Codeine is metabolized by the cytochrome P450 debrisoquine 4-hydroxylase (CYP2D6) to its active analgesic metabolites. The CYP2D6 gene displays polymorphism including gene duplication (ultra-rapid metabolizers) and inactive genes. Gene duplication may lead to ultra-rapid metabolism, which for prodrugs such as codeine might yield a 50% greater fraction of morphine and its glucuronides compared with extensive metabolizers.[135] Respiratory arrest after codeine has been reported in both adults and children who demonstrate ultra-rapid metabolism of codeine.[136,137] Whereas the ultra-rapid metabolizing genotype is present in 3% of Caucasians, it is present in 10 to 30% of Arabian and Northeast African populations. In contrast, almost 10% of children lack CYP2D6, rendering codeine an ineffective analgesic. Given the broad variability in codeine metabolism and our lack of knowledge of which polymorphism is carried by each child, the use of codeine and the dose prescribed for children with OSA must be very carefully considered.

Neural Blockade

Blockade of neural input to the upper airway dilator musculature in children with OSA is also problematic. Serious life-threatening complications, including severe upper airway obstruction and pulmonary edema, have been reported after local anesthetics have been infiltrated in the tonsillar fossa to prevent pain after adenotonsillectomy in children with OSA. The pharynx in children with OSA is not only smaller in size[113,138] but also more collapsible even during wakefulness compared with those children who do not have OSA.[139-141] Topical anesthesia applied to the mucosa of the pharynx of children with OSA reduces the caliber of the pharynx compared with control subjects.[142]

Extubation Strategy and Management of the Postoperative Period in Children with OSA

Extubation of the trachea is usually performed when the child is fully awake. Techniques that involve minimal stimulation of the airway have been suggested.[84] Although a minority of children receive muscle relaxants for adenotonsillectomy, residual neuromuscular blockade in the recovery room will selectively depress the function of the upper airway dilators relative to the diaphragm, promoting collapse of the pharyngeal airway.[143] Full antagonism of neuromuscular blockade is strongly recommended before extubating the tracheas of children with OSA.[73] Antagonism of neuromuscular blockade with atropine and neostigmine after tonsillectomy has been associated with less PONV than antagonism with glycopyrrolate and neostigmine.[144]

Several other factors may increase the risk of respiratory difficulties after adenotonsillectomy in children with OSA. Otherwise healthy children with severe OSA whose adenotonsillectomy is performed in the morning are less likely to desaturate when managed in a postanesthesia care unit setting than those whose surgery is performed in the afternoon.[145] In addition, meticulous attention to the position of the head and neck is required during recovery from anesthesia, because hypercarbia and a loss of lung volume (functional lung capacity) both promote collapse of the pharyngeal airway.[117,146,147] Extension of the cervical spine, the sniffing position, the lateral recovery position, and mouth opening with anterior advancement of the mandible all increase the dimension of the pharynx[148-152] and reduce the risk of upper airway obstruction.

Two drugs, atropine and naloxone, have the potential to augment the function of the upper airway. Atropine administered after induction of anesthesia decreased the risk of post-adenotonsillectomy respiratory complications.[55] Of possible relevance is the report that muscarinic blockade of the hypoglossal nucleus in the rat model enhances activity of the genioglossus muscle.[147] The µ opioid stimulation depresses the activity of the pharyngeal dilator muscles, including the genioglossus muscle.[121,153-155] Given the increased sensitivity to both analgesic and respiratory effects of exogenously administered opioids in children with severe OSA, a similar sensitivity may also apply to the respiratory-related activity of the pharyngeal musculature. Small doses of naloxone may alleviate upper airway obstruction after adenotonsillectomy if exogenous opioids have been administered.

The severity of OSA is a predictor of the outcome after adenotonsillectomy; for example, a preoperative RDI above 19 may predict an RDI in excess of 5 in long-term follow-up.[75] Children with OSA continue to demonstrate obstructive apnea and desaturation during sleep on the first night after adenotonsillectomy, with the frequency of the obstructive events and the severity of desaturation usually greater in those children with severe OSA (Fig. 31-10).[156,157]

Measures to support airway patency in the postoperative period have included insertion of nasal airways, administration of CPAP, reintubation, ventilation, and the administration of bronchodilators, racemic epinephrine, and heliox. Bilevel positive airway pressure (BiPAP) may be useful in children with preexisting neurologic disorders.[158] However, nasal secretions may be copious after adenotonsillectomy, limiting the efficacy of nasal CPAP postoperatively. Children with complex medical diseases who are critically dependent on the function of upper airway musculature may benefit from delayed extubation. Acute relief of chronic upper airway obstruction favors the exudation of intravascular fluid into the pulmonary interstitium and noncardiogenic pulmonary edema, which may present preoperatively, intraoperatively, and postoperatively. Supportive measures include the administration of oxygen, endotracheal intubation, mechanical ventilation with positive end-expiratory pressure, and administration of furosemide.[159-161]

Discharge Policy for Ambulatory Adenotonsillectomy

Children younger than 3 years of age and those with complex medical disorders are not candidates for adenotonsillectomy as outpatients.[29,162] *Although children undergoing adenotonsillectomy for obstructive breathing without apnea may undergo ambulatory surgery, those with OSA should not.* A diagnosis of OSA doubles the likelihood of respiratory complications after adenotonsillectomy from 10% in otherwise healthy children to 20% in those with OSA.[28]

The majority of children who are scheduled for adenotonsillectomy have symptoms of obstructive breathing,[33,163,164] yet only 55% with clinical criteria suggestive of OSA subsequently meet sleep laboratory criteria for OSA.[165] Sleep screening of children undergoing routine adenotonsillectomy for chronic

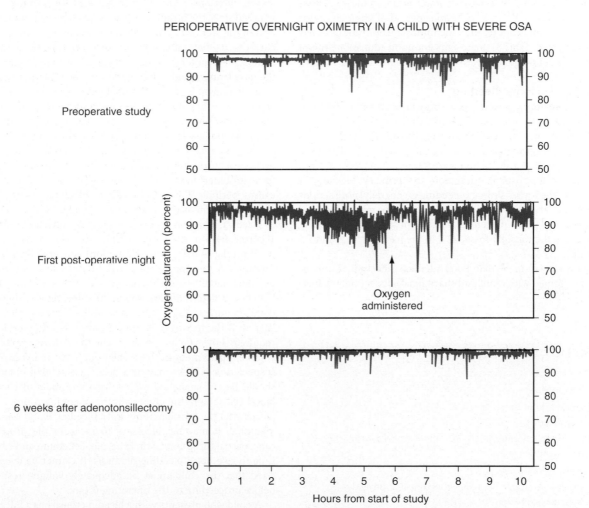

Figure 31-10. Three oximetry trend records from an otherwise healthy child. The x-axis is time ranging from bedtime on the left to arousal the following morning on the right. The *top panel* is the preoperative record showing clusters of desaturation. The *middle panel* is the record from the first night after adenotonsillectomy. With sleep onset, a decrease in saturation is evident that worsens after midnight. Oxygen therapy is administered after midnight. The *bottom panel* is the recording 6 weeks after adenotonsillectomy, which is within normal limits. (From Nixon GM, Kermack AS, McGregor CD, et al: Sleep and breathing on the first night after adenotonsillectomy for obstructive sleep apnea. Pediatr Pulmonol 2005; 39:332-338.)

tonsillitis revealed unexpectedly that 20% had severe obstructive episodes associated with desaturation.[166] Because only a minority of children undergoing adenotonsillectomy undergo diagnostic testing for sleep-disordered breathing, the recently published guidelines on management of OSA have empowered clinical diagnostic criteria such that a child with severe symptoms has moderate to severe OSA until proven otherwise by sleep laboratory testing (Fig. 31-4). Ambulatory programs may now find it cost effective to screen children with a positive clinical history.

In otherwise healthy children, conversion from ambulatory to inpatient status was most frequently prompted by respiratory events in children whose indication for surgery was obstructive breathing.[33] A systematic reduction in postoperative morphine use was associated with a reduced rate of hospital admission from 8% to 2.4%.[45]

Same-day discharge, which abbreviates the postoperative stay in hospital and the minimum period of observation before discharge from hospital, has been the subject of much debate. Because the onset of respiratory complications in these children may be delayed,[54,145,156] a 6- to 8-hour period of observation for respiratory complications after adenotonsillectomy for OSA has been suggested. Table 31-5 presents common admission criteria for children undergoing elective tonsillectomy.

Post-Tonsillectomy Bleeding

Post-tonsillectomy bleeding is a surgical emergency. This can occur either within the first 24 hours (primary) or 5 to 10 days after surgery when the eschar covering the tonsillar bed retracts (secondary). Approximately 75% of postoperative tonsillar hemorrhages occur within 6 hours of surgery. Conversion from ambulatory to hospital admission for primary bleeding is reported to be 1.6%.[33] Primary bleeding is generally more serious than secondary bleeding because it is usually more brisk and profuse. Sixty-seven percent of cases of postoperative bleeding originate in the tonsillar fossa, 27% in the nasopharynx, and 7% in both.[167]

In a review of more than 9000 adenotonsillectomies in children performed with blunt and sharp (cold) dissection, the inci-

Table 31-5. Criteria for Overnight Stay after Tonsillectomy and Adenoidectomy

- Sleep apnea
- Sleep disturbance
- <3 years of age
- Craniofacial abnormalities (e.g., Down syndrome, Treacher Collins syndrome)
- Lives > 1 hour away
- Lives in an unstable home environment that precludes adequate supervision
- Postoperative problems
- Continued vomiting
- Failure to take oral fluids
- Fever

From Zalzal G: Personal communications/Survey of major pediatric hospitals, 2006.

dence of postoperative bleeding was 2.15%, with 76% of the hemorrhages occurring in the first 6 hours postoperatively.[168] An audit of 4800 pediatric tonsillectomies for which hemostasis was secured with electrocautery (hot) techniques reported a primary postoperative hemorrhage rate of 0.9%, with 83% presenting within 4 hours of surgery.[45] The consensus is that the mandatory period of observation for primary hemorrhage depends on the surgical technique: 6 hours and 4 hours for cold and hot dissection, respectively,[45,167,168] although abbreviated periods of observation have been advocated by some.[33]

The management of anesthesia in this situation can be challenging even in the hands of an experienced pediatric anesthesiologist. It often requires dealing with anxious parents, an upset surgeon, and a frightened anemic, hypovolemic child with a stomach full of blood. A thorough review of the anesthetic record of the original surgery will provide pertinent information about any existing medical condition, use of medications such as aspirin, difficulty with airway management, and a rough estimate of intraoperative blood loss and fluid replacement as well as the duration of known bleeding and the volume of blood vomited since the bleeding began. A quick history and examination of the child will provide vital information about the child's current volume status. History of dizziness and presence of orthostatic hypotension may suggest a loss of more than 20% of the circulating blood volume and the need for aggressive fluid resuscitation and crossmatch of blood before induction.[169] Even when severe hypotension is not present, the child with the bleeding tonsil is hypovolemic and has a decrease in cardiac output secondary to ongoing blood loss. If blood loss is severe, and/or fluid resuscitation is not vigorous, lactic acidosis and an eventual state of shock will develop. The compensatory response to acute blood loss is an outpouring of catecholamines. This causes peripheral vasoconstriction, which delays the clinical onset of hypotension in the awake child. When anesthesia-induced vasodilation occurs, profound hypotension is observed. Vigorous fluid resuscitation with crystalloids (repeated boluses of 20 mL/kg of balanced salt solution) and/or colloids is therefore the key to improve the cardiac output and achieve hemodynamic stability before induction of anesthesia. Hemoglobin or hematocrit determination should be interpreted in light of the child's volume status and the type of fluid resuscitation administered. If the hemoglobin concentration is low, blood may be required; however, blood is rarely the primary solution for volume replacement in these children. If severe hypovolemia is suspected or if there may be a delay in obtaining blood, blood should be crossmatched for two or more units of packed red blood cells before the child is in the operating room. If a child bleeds after the tonsillectomy, and a bleeding blood vessel is not identified, it may be necessary to measure the prothrombin time, partial thromboplastin time, platelet count, and a bleeding time to rule out a bleeding diathesis. It cannot be overemphasized that the child must be adequately volume resuscitated before proceeding to the operating room.

A child who presents with a bleeding tonsil has a full stomach (filled with swallowed blood) and may still be hypovolemic. A child who is spitting bright red blood may quickly exsanguinate, but the bleeding may be temporarily controlled by compression of the carotid artery ipsilateral to the bleeding source. The anesthesiologist may have difficulty visualizing the larynx because of the bleeding tonsillar bed and clots in the pharynx. A styletted ETT, two sets of well-illuminated laryngoscopes, and two large-bore rigid Yankauer-type suction catheters must be available before induction of anesthesia (see also Table 39-4 and Chapter 4). On arrival in the operating room and application of routine monitors, the child should be preoxygenated while positioned in the left lateral position and head down to drain blood out of the mouth (Fig. 31-11). The child is then turned supine, and a rapid-sequence induction is carried out with cricoid pressure (Sellick's maneuver) applied by an assistant to minimize the risk of aspirating blood into the lungs.[170] There is no evidence that a rapid-sequence induction with cricoid pressure decreases the risk of aspiration in children with full stomachs, although this practice is commonplace. It should also be recognized that aspiration of blood into the lungs is not synonymous with acid particulate aspiration unless the volume of blood aspirated compromises pulmonary oxygenation. The use of a full induction dose of thiopental or propofol in a hypovolemic child could result in significant hypotension. A reduced dose of these induction agents (e.g., thiopental, 2-3 mg/kg, or propofol, 1-2 mg/kg), or ketamine (1-2 mg/kg) or etomidate (0.2 mg/kg) for induction followed by atropine (0.02 mg/kg) combined with succinylcholine (1.5-2 mg/kg) or rocuronium (1.2 mg/kg) for tracheal intubation will allow rapid control of the airway without producing hypotension.

When possible, a cuffed ETT (one-half size smaller than usual for age or weight) should be used to minimize the chance of blood aspiration around the tube. The use of a stylet is recommended in spite of a previous history of easy intubation. The blood pressure after induction will often reflect the volume status of the child.

Titration of a volatile anesthetic such as sevoflurane or desflurane with nitrous oxide and oxygen[80] supplemented with an opioid such as fentanyl, 1 to 2 μg/kg, will facilitate rapid recovery at the end of surgery.[171] Often these surgeries are not excessively painful because surgery is limited to the area of bleeding. Controlling the bleeding vessel in the tonsillar bed can be accomplished rapidly by the surgeon if the blood pressure is maintained in the normal range. Suctioning the stomach with a large-bore catheter under direct vision after the procedure does not guarantee an empty stomach because much of the blood may be clotted and the clots are often too large to be suctioned. The use of prophylactic antiemetic therapy (e.g., ondansetron 0.1 mg/kg) is indicated.

The most important postoperative consideration is to extubate these children when they are fully awake and able to control their airway reflexes. Extubating the trachea while the child is in the lateral position may be the safest practice to minimize the risk of aspiration. If there is a medical indication to substitute high-dose rocuronium (1.2 mg/kg) for succinylcholine, then a prolonged period of relaxation may be anticipated. Sugammadex may allow early reversal of residual deep neuromuscular blockade with high-dose rocuronium, although at the time of this writing, sugammadex is not approved for use in children. Postoperatively, a repeat determination of the hemoglobin level may be indicated.

Peritonsillar Abscess

Peritonsillar abscess (quinsy tonsil) tends to occur in older children or young adults. It is the most common deep neck space infection treated by otolaryngologists. Infection originates in the tonsil and spreads to the peritonsillar space between the tonsillar capsule and the superior constrictor muscle and usually into the soft palate in the region of the superior pole of the tonsil. Commonly cultured organisms include aerobes such as *Streptococcus pyogenes*, *S. milleri*, *S. viridans*, beta-hemolytic streptococci, *Haemophilus influenzae*, as well as anaerobes such as *Fusobacterium* and *Prevotella* species.[172]

Clinically, these children present with fever, pharyngeal swelling, sore throat, difficulty in swallowing, and often trismus. Trismus is caused by compression of nerves by the tense peritonsillar mass, spasm of the pterygoid muscles, and inflammation of the muscles of the face and neck. Dehydration can ensue because of fever and the persistent difficulty with swallowing.

Preoperative evaluation includes careful assessment of the airway with special emphasis on the degree of trismus. A blood specimen should be sent for total as well as differential white blood cell count to ascertain the response to the infection and for blood cultures for appropriate antibiotic therapy. Computed tomography of the tonsillar area will identify airway deviation and the extent of spread of the abscess (Fig. 31-12).

Treatment should begin with intravenous line placement, fluid hydration, and appropriate antibiotic coverage while awaiting the results of the cultures. The majority of organisms, including anaerobes, are penicillin sensitive. Consequently, penicillin is the antibiotic of choice.[172] The three different procedures currently used to drain a peritonsillar abscess are needle aspiration, incision and drainage, and abscess tonsillectomy.[173] Most children undergo general anesthesia for treatment of peritonsillar abscess by incision and drainage, although in some centers, moderate to deep sedation has been successfully used.[174] If the abscess is small and well confined, immediate tonsillectomy is performed.

The anesthetic management of these children can be challenging. Rupture of the abscess and possible aspiration of purulent material during laryngoscopy and intubation should be avoided during induction of anesthesia. Although the airway may seem compromised, the peritonsillar abscess is most often in a fixed location in the lateral pharynx and does not interfere with mask ventilation. Visualization of the vocal cords is usually

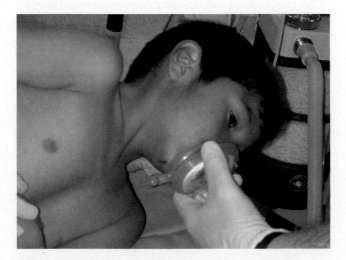

Figure 31-11. Preoxygenation in the lateral position before induction of anesthesia to control post-tonsillectomy bleeding.

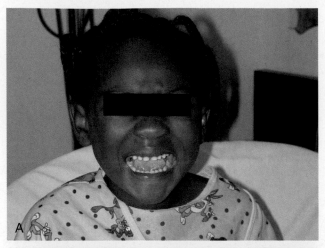

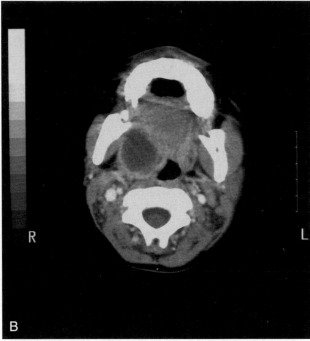

Figure 31-12. A, Peritonsillar abscess with trismus. **B,** Axial enhanced CT scan through the oropharynx showing a 3-cm ring-shaped, enhancing, low-density mass replacing the left tonsil, typical of a tonsillar abscess.

not impaired because the pathology is supraglottic and well above the laryngeal inlet, although a right-sided abscess may interfere with the usual sweeping of the tongue to the left during laryngoscopy. Laryngoscopy must be carefully approached to avoid excessive manipulation of the larynx and surrounding structures. Occasionally, the pharyngeal swelling and the distortion of normal anatomy along with excessive secretions may create difficulty for laryngoscopy and intubation. The operating room should be prepared as for any difficult airway case with different sizes of ETTs, stylets, two sets of well-illuminated laryngoscopes, and a tonsil tip suction catheter attached to a powerful suction device. The surgeon must be present in the operating room during induction of anesthesia should airway obstruction occur. Equipment for cricothyrotomy or tracheotomy must be readily available.

These children are often older and do not require preoperative sedation. If trismus is present, an inhalational induction should be performed using sevoflurane and oxygen while the anesthesiologist assesses mobility of the temporomandibular joint under anesthesia. An oropharyngeal airway is best avoided lest the abscess be traumatized. Usually, apparent trismus resolves once an adequate depth of anesthesia has been achieved. When this is confirmed, or if there was minimal trismus to begin with, then a short-acting muscle relaxant (or propofol) is given to facilitate tracheal intubation. Alternatively, if there is minimal trismus and the preoperative airway assessment indicates minimal distortion, a rapid-sequence intravenous induction after adequate preoxygenation may be the best way to avoid trauma to the pharyngeal structures while struggling with a mask induction, needing to insert an oropharyngeal airway, and possibly causing the abscess to rupture.[1]

To avoid aspiration of purulent material during intubation and drainage, a cuffed ETT is recommended and the child is placed in Trendelenburg position. At the end of surgery, the child should be extubated awake, preferably in the lateral position.[1]

Anesthesia for Endoscopy

Anesthesia for rigid bronchoscopy in young children presents a significant challenge. Not only does the child have a compromised airway, but we also must share that compromised airway with the surgeon. The importance of constant communication between the endoscopist and the anesthesiologist cannot be overstated. In general, the goals of anesthesia for endoscopy are analgesia, an unconscious child, and a quiet surgical field.[175] Coughing, bucking, or straining during instrumentation with a rigid bronchoscope may cause difficulty for the surgeon and damage the child's airway. At the conclusion of the procedure, children should be returned to consciousness quickly with airway reflexes intact to protect the recently instrumented airway. General principles for the anesthetic management will be outlined first. Disease-specific requirements will be discussed under appropriate subheadings.

For most children, a pulse oximeter, blood pressure cuff, electrocardiogram, and precordial stethoscope are applied before induction. Continuous monitoring of ventilation by capnography is not always possible during bronchoscopy. Clinical observation of the chest wall movement and the use of a precordial stethoscope are useful. In many cases, intermittent capnography is possible when the bronchoscope is withdrawn by the surgeon. Although greater than normal CO_2 tensions are inevitable with intermittent ventilation, they are generally well tolerated in the presence of sevoflurane. If halothane is used, ventricular arrhythmias may occur and should be treated by hyperventilation and deepening halothane anesthesia or substituting isoflurane for halothane (see Chapter 6).[176] Hypoxia, on the other hand, is not well tolerated, and the procedure should be stopped while the child is reoxygenated.

In most instances, endoscopists prefer that the child breathes spontaneously throughout the procedure. Inhalation induction by mask is accomplished with oxygen and a volatile agent, usually sevoflurane. Nitrous oxide can be used initially, if tolerated, to speed the induction and then discontinued before the examination. Alternatively, in those children in whom intravenous access was established before anesthesia, an intravenous induction may be achieved with a sleep-dose of propofol, followed by mask ventilation with a volatile agent.

After sufficient depth of anesthesia has been obtained, intravenous access is established and the depth of anesthesia is increased. An antisialagogue (atropine or glycopyrrolate) may be administered intravenously to decrease secretions that may impair the view through the bronchoscope. Topicalization of the vocal cords and airway decreases the incidence of coughing or bucking during instrumentation and allows the child to tolerate a lighter level of anesthesia. Lidocaine, either 2% or 4%, is the most frequently utilized topical anesthetic. It may be applied to the vocal cords either by atomizer or sprayed with a 3-mL Luer-Lok syringe fitted with a 24-gauge intravenous catheter (without the needle). With constant pressure applied on the plunger, a fine stream of lidocaine is directed to the supraglottic structures and through the vocal cords to the tracheal mucosa. The dose of lidocaine should be limited to 3 to 4 mg/kg divided between the laryngeal and tracheal surfaces because rapid absorption via the mucosa occurs. It is important to confirm whether the surgeon intends to observe for movement of the vocal cords or evaluate tracheal or bronchial dynamics so that the anesthetic may be planned accordingly (i.e., spontaneous respirations preserved during light levels of anesthesia versus no respiratory efforts and the use of short-acting muscle relaxants).

Diagnostic Laryngoscopy and Bronchoscopy

Although diagnostic laryngoscopy and bronchoscopy procedures are usually of brief duration, the anesthetic management can be challenging in small infants with an already compromised airway. Stridor, or noisy breathing due to obstructed airflow, is a common indication for a diagnostic laryngoscopy and bronchoscopy in infants and children. Inspiratory stridor results from upper airway obstruction, expiratory stridor results from lower airway obstruction, and biphasic stridor is present with mid-tracheal lesions (see Chapters 11 and 12). Subglottic stenosis may follow prolonged tracheal intubation in a former preterm infant.

The evaluation of a child with stridor begins with taking a thorough history. The age at symptom onset helps suggest a cause; for instance, laryngotracheomalacia and vocal cord paralysis are usually present at or shortly after birth, whereas cysts or mass lesions develop later in life (Table 31-6). Information indicating positions that make the stridor better or worse should be obtained, because placing a child in a position that allows gravity to aid in reducing obstruction can be of benefit during induction.

Physical examination reveals the general condition of a child or infant as well as the degree of the airway compromise. Laboratory examination may include a chest radiograph and barium swallow, which can aid in identifying lesions that may be compressing the trachea. Computed tomography, magnetic resonance imaging, and tomograms may be helpful in isolated instances but are not routinely indicated.

Laryngomalacia is the most common cause of stridor in infants and is most often due to a long epiglottis that prolapses posteriorly and prominent arytenoid cartilages with redundant aryepiglottic folds that prolapse into the glottic opening during inspiration.[177] The definitive diagnosis is obtained by direct laryngoscopy and by rigid or flexible bronchoscopy.

Preliminary examination is usually carried out in the surgeon's office. A small flexible fiberoptic bronchoscope is inserted through the nares into the oropharynx. Nasal insertion provides an excellent view of the movement of the vocal cords and pharyngeal structures. Topicalization of the nasopharynx with lidocaine facilitates passage of the nasal pharyngoscope or bronchoscope. Alternatively, the examination can be accomplished in the operating room in a lightly anesthetized child during spontaneous respiration. Children must be spontaneously breathing so that the vocal cords move freely. After movement of the vocal cords is observed and recorded, the anesthetic level can be increased as appropriate, a rigid bronchoscope (or just the rod-lens-telescope in small infants) is inserted through the vocal cords, and the subglottic area, the lower trachea, and bronchi are evaluated.

The use of premedication in these children should be individualized. Small infants may be brought into the operating room unpremedicated; older children may experience respiratory depression and worsening of airway obstruction if heavy premedication is administered.

Usually an inhalational induction with sevoflurane is performed. Nitrous oxide can be used initially if tolerated to speed the induction and then discontinued before the examination. Because sevoflurane is fairly insoluble and is eliminated quickly, and because ventilation may be intermittently interrupted in these children, supplementation with intravenous agents

Table 31-6. Causes of Stridor

Supraglottic Airway
Choanal atresia
Cyst
Mass
Large tonsils
Large adenoids
Craniofacial abnormalities
Foreign body

Larynx
Laryngomalacia
Vocal cord paralysis
Subglottic stenosis
Hemangiomas
Cysts
Laryngocele
Infection (tonsillitis, peritonsillar abscess)
Foreign body

Subglottic Airway
Tracheomalacia
Vascular ring
Foreign body
Infection (croup, epiglottitis)
Hemangiomas

such as propofol (1 mg/kg boluses or a 50- to 100-μg/kg/min infusion) can help establish an appropriate level of anesthesia without producing excessive respiratory depression. If an inhaled technique is used by insufflation, scavenging may be attempted by inserting a suction device in the mouth.

A propofol-based total intravenous anesthesia (TIVA) technique has the advantage that it can be given continuously during the procedure, resulting in a more stable level of anesthesia than can be achieved with inhalational agents and intermittent ventilation. Propofol can be supplemented with small (0.5 mg/kg) doses of ketamine to enhance analgesia. Opioids can also be used but will frequently induce apnea.

The key to a stress-free bronchoscopy is properly placed topical anesthesia. Although topicalization of the laryngeal structures helps the child tolerate the procedure, it may interfere with assessment of normal vocal cord movement. For that reason, topicalization is often performed after initial evaluation of the upper airway and just before insertion of the broncho-scope for evaluation of the distal airway structures.

After completion of pharyngoscopy/laryngoscopy, the surgeon generally proceeds to rigid bronchoscopy. The size of a rigid bronchoscope refers to the internal diameter. Because the external diameter may be significantly greater than that of an ETT of similar size, care must be taken to select a bronchoscope of proper external diameter to avoid damage to the laryngeal structures (Table 31-7). The rigid bronchoscope can be used for ventilation through the side port attached to the anesthesia circuit with a flexible extension. It is often most useful to para-lyze the child with a fixed lesion, which diminishes the risk of vocal cord injury secondary to movement. For nonfixed lesions, such as aspirated foreign body, and for assessment for broncho-malacia or tracheomalacia, it is preferred to proceed with spon-taneous ventilation, deep level of anesthesia, and good topical anesthesia of the vocal cords and carina. Adequate oxygenation should be maintained in these infants throughout the proce-dure. Because ventilation may be intermittent and at times sub-optimal, it is recommended that 100% oxygen be used as the carrier gas during the bronchoscopic examination. During ven-tilation of the infant with the telescope in place, high resistance may be encountered as a result of partial occlusion of the lumen. This is especially likely when the 2.5-, 3.0-, and 3.5-mm internal diameter scopes are used. Large fresh gas flow rates, large tidal volumes with high inflation pressures, and large inspired volatile anesthetic concentrations (or TIVA) are often necessary to com-pensate for leaks around the ventilating bronchoscope and the high resistance encountered when the viewing telescope is in place. Hand ventilation at greater than normal rates is most effective in achieving adequate ventilation. Sufficient time for exhalation must be provided for passive recoil of the chest. In small infants, there may be room for only the rod-lens-tele-scopic light source, which does not have a ventilation channel. In these cases, insufflation of oxygen via a small tube placed in the hypopharynx via the nose or mouth will delay the onset of desaturation in a spontaneously breathing child. If (when) desat-uration occurs, the surgeon must stop and allow the child to be oxygenated before continuing with the examination.

At the conclusion of bronchoscopy, the surgeon may wish to size the larynx and determine the degree of airway narrowing. A noncuffed ETT is inserted beyond the narrowest portion of the obstructed airway, and the airway is assessed by applying

Table 31-7. External Diameter of Standard Endotracheal Tube Versus Rigid Bronchoscope

Internal Diameter (mm)	External Diameter (mm)	
	Endotracheal Tube*	Rigid Bronchoscope†
2.0	2.9	
2.5	3.6	4.2
3.0	4.3	5.0
3.5	4.9	5.7
3.7 (bronchoscope)		6.3
4.0	5.6	6.7
5.0	6.9	7.8
6.0	8.2	8.2

*Mallinckrodt Medical, Inc., St. Louis, MO.
†Karl Storz Endoscopy-America, Inc., Culver City, CA.

positive pressure between 10 and 25 cm H_2O to the airway and listening with a stethoscope for an air leak around the ETT at the level of the suprasternal notch. The outer diameter of the appropriate ETT is compared with the inner diameter of the child's larynx and trachea, and the percentage of obstruction is calculated. Grade I obstruction involves up to 50% of the airway, grade II is from 51% to 70%, and grade III is greater than 70% (Fig. 31-13).[178]

An alternative method of ventilation during bronchoscopy is the Sanders jet ventilation technique. The principle of jet venti-lation involves intermittent bursts of oxygen delivered under a pressure of 50 psi from a hand-regulated pressure-reducing valve to deliver a maximum pressure of 20-30 mm Hg to the lungs, through a 16-gauge catheter attached to a rigid broncho-scope.[179] Current jet ventilators include adjustable pressure control that permits attenuation of the peak pressure, a desirable feature if this device is to be used in a child. Intermittent flow is accomplished by depressing the lever of an on-off valve. A jet of oxygen is released at the tip of the 16-gauge catheter, creating a Venturi effect that entrains room air into the bronchoscope. This jet of oxygen and room air mixture allows inflation of the lungs to occur. Exhalation is passive and depends on the recoil of the chest wall. Although, in experienced hands, the technique is usually effective for both oxygenation and ventilation, a number of potential problems exist. Because of the high infla-tion pressure, pneumothorax or pneumomediastinum can occur.[180] Blood or infectious or particulate matter in the airway may be forced distally by high-pressure bursts. There is also the possibility of hypoxemia in some children, because the high-pressure oxygen entrains room air, diluting the percent of oxygen.

Dexamethasone in a dose of 0.5 mg/kg IV (maximum dose, 10-20 mg) is frequently administered during the procedure to decrease postoperative laryngeal swelling and the possibility of croup. At the conclusion of rigid bronchoscopy, an ETT can be placed in the trachea to control the airway during recovery from anesthesia or if ventilation is adequate, and the anesthetic depth is not excessive, the child can be allowed to emerge breathing 100% oxygen by a face mask.

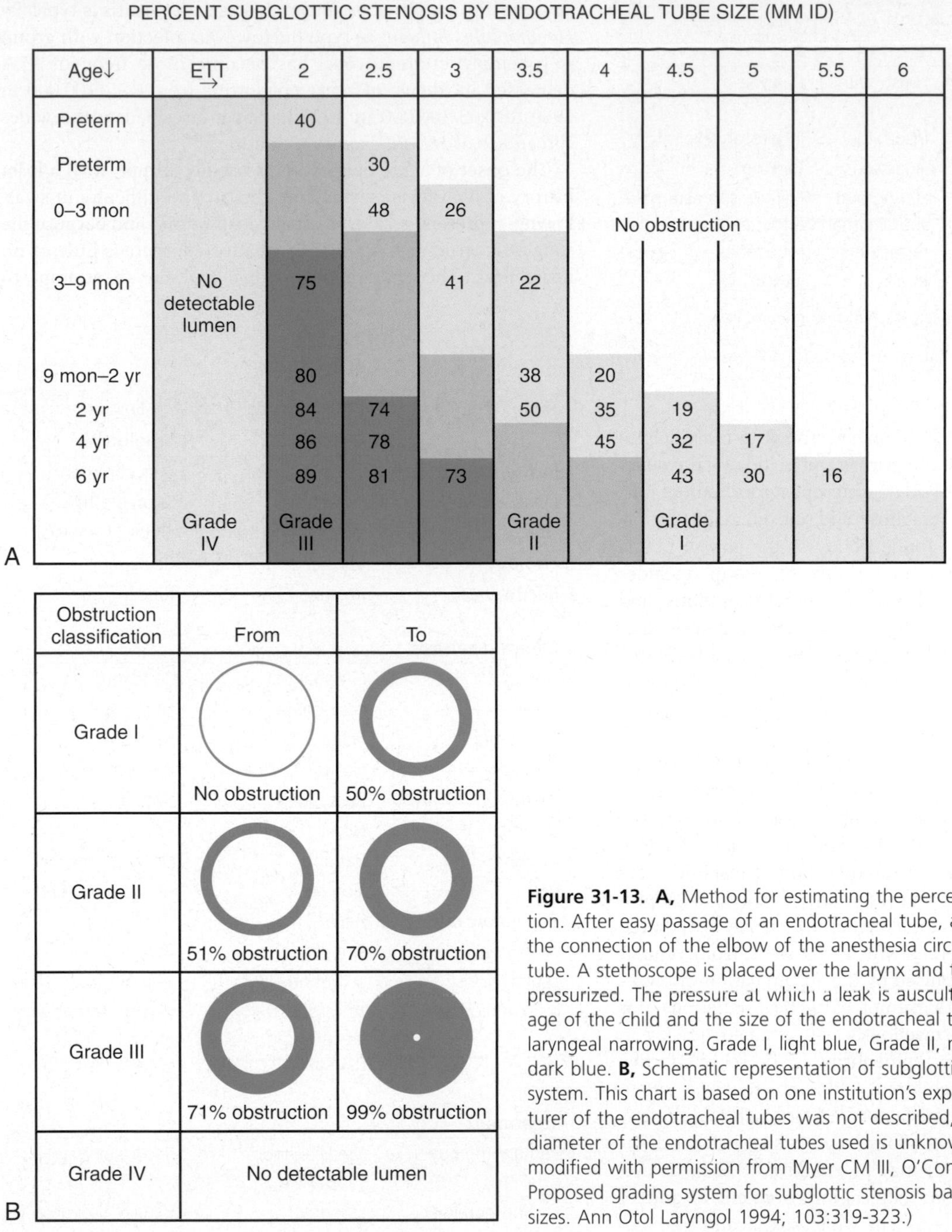

PERCENT SUBGLOTTIC STENOSIS BY ENDOTRACHEAL TUBE SIZE (MM ID)

Age↓	ETT→	2	2.5	3	3.5	4	4.5	5	5.5	6
Preterm		40								
Preterm			30							
0–3 mon			48	26		No obstruction				
3–9 mon	No detectable lumen	75		41	22					
9 mon–2 yr		80			38	20				
2 yr		84	74		50	35	19			
4 yr		86	78			45	32	17		
6 yr		89	81	73			43	30	16	
	Grade IV	Grade III			Grade II		Grade I			

A

Obstruction classification	From	To
Grade I	No obstruction	50% obstruction
Grade II	51% obstruction	70% obstruction
Grade III	71% obstruction	99% obstruction
Grade IV	No detectable lumen	

B

Figure 31-13. A, Method for estimating the percentage of airway obstruction. After easy passage of an endotracheal tube, a manometer is placed at the connection of the elbow of the anesthesia circuit and the endotracheal tube. A stethoscope is placed over the larynx and the circuit is slowly pressurized. The pressure at which a leak is auscultated is matched with the age of the child and the size of the endotracheal tube to assess the degree of laryngeal narrowing. Grade I, light blue, Grade II, medium blue, and Grade III, dark blue. **B,** Schematic representation of subglottic stenosis classification system. This chart is based on one institution's experience and the manufacturer of the endotracheal tubes was not described, thus the actual external diameter of the endotracheal tubes used is unknown. (Reproduced and modified with permission from Myer CM III, O'Connor DM, Cotton RT: Proposed grading system for subglottic stenosis based on endotracheal tube sizes. Ann Otol Laryngol 1994; 103:319-323.)

Croup

Croup is a symptom-complex of inspiratory stridor; suprasternal, intercostal, and substernal retractions; barking cough; and hoarseness. It results from swelling of the mucosa in the subglottic area of the larynx.[1] There are two common entities that account for most cases of infectious croup: spasmodic croup and laryngotracheobronchitis. Spasmodic croup has been diagnosed in about 3% of children with stridor.[181] These children are otherwise healthy and afebrile, presenting with nocturnal episodes of spasmodic cough, which is described as barking and high pitched. The disease is self-limiting. Besides viruses, allergic and psychological factors are blamed for this acute phenomenon. It differs from acute laryngotracheobronchitis in that it is considered an allergic reaction to viral antigens rather than a true viral infection.[182] Besides lack of fever, spasmodic croup is usually remarkable for lack of severe laryngeal inflammation, and supportive therapy on an outpatient basis is all that is recommended.

Viral laryngotracheobronchitis is by far the most common form of infectious croup today. The disease has a gradual onset, usually following an upper respiratory tract infection in a young child. Low-grade fever is common. Children who have more than two episodes of croup requiring hospitalization should be evaluated for subglottic narrowing.[177]

Table 31-8. Clinical Croup Score

	0	1	2
Inspiratory Breath Sounds	Normal	Harsh with rhonchi	Delayed
Stridor	None	Inspiratory	Inspiratory/expiratory
Cough	None	Hoarse cry	Barking
Retractions	None	Flaring and suprasternal retractions	Flaring, suprasternal and intercostal retractions
Cyanosis	None	In air	In 40% O_2

Adapted from Downes JJ, Raphaely RC: Pediatric intensive care. Anesthesiology 1975; 43:238.

Clinical scoring systems based on objective criteria are helpful in following the progress of the disease and in judging the effectiveness of therapy (Table 31-8).[183] Anteroposterior radiographs of the neck will confirm the diagnosis and rule out acute epiglottitis or the possibility of a foreign body in the airway (Table 31-9).[184] The characteristic radiograph of croup includes blurring of the tracheal air shadow on lateral neck films, and symmetric narrowing of the subglottic air shadow, described as a "church steeple" sign on anteroposterior films (Fig. 31-14, see website; see also Fig. 37-5A, B). The lateral neck radiographs show normal supraglottic structures and normal epiglottic shadow.

The majority of cases of croup resolve quickly with simple conservative measures such as breathing humidified air or oxygen. Fewer than 10% of cases require hospitalization because of significant respiratory difficulty, and still fewer children require an artificial airway.[177] Humidification of inspired gases is usually effective in improving respiratory distress, and it prevents drying of secretions. Supplemental oxygen may be required to prevent or treat hypoxemia, which may result from ventilation/perfusion mismatch caused by the accumulation of secretions. Hydration prevents thickening of tracheal secretions; this must be accomplished intravenously and attained quickly in hospitalized cases. Racemic epinephrine is the most effective drug therapy in these children, although the use of L-epinephrine has also been satisfactory.[185] Corticosteroid therapy in viral croup is controversial. Some reports suggest that dexamethasone (0.5-1 mg/kg IV) may be effective.[186] There is evidence that there is significant clinical improvement 12 and 24 hours after corticosteroid treatment, which significantly reduces the incidence of endotracheal intubation.[186] Antibiotics are generally not indicated in the treatment of uncomplicated viral croup. This topic is reviewed in more detail in Chapter 37.

Acute Epiglottitis

Although rare today in children, acute epiglottitis can be fatal because it can produce seemingly unprovoked sudden and complete airway obstruction. This clinical and pathologic entity should more correctly be called supraglottitis because the arytenoids and aryepiglottic folds, as well as the epiglottis, are usually affected. All structures become swollen and stiffened by inflammatory edema (see Figs. 37-3A, B and 37-4).[1] Although the main focus of infection is in the supraglottic structures, the disease produces a generalized toxemia. Epiglottitis is most common between the ages of 3 and 5 years, but it can occur at any age. The causative organism in acute epiglottitis is typically *Haemophilus influenzae* type B. However, infection with group A β-hemolytic streptococci has become more frequent.[187] A decreased incidence of acute epiglottitis from 3.47/100,000 in 1980 to 0.63/100,000 in 1990 has been ascribed to the widespread use of *H. influenzae* vaccination.[188]

The onset of acute epiglottitis is usually abrupt, with a brief history of high fever, severe sore throat, and difficulty in swallowing. If present, stridor is usually inspiratory; and because the subglottic structures are usually unaffected, there is little or no hoarseness. The child appears toxic and, in an attempt to

Table 31-9. Differential Diagnosis of Croup and Epiglottitis

	Croup*	Epiglottitis
Incidence	More common	Less common
Obstruction	Subglottic	Supraglottic
Age	Younger (<3 years)	Older (3-6 years)
Etiology	Viral	Bacterial
Recurrence	Possible (5%)	Rare
Clinical Features		
Onset	Gradual (days)	Sudden (hours)
Fever	Low grade	High
Dysphagia	None	Marked
Drooling	None	Present
Posture	Recumbent	Sitting
Toxemia	None	Present
Cough	Barking	Usually none
Voice	Hoarse	Clear to muffled
Respiratory rate	Rapid	Normal/slow
Larynx palpation	Not tender	Tender
Leukocytosis	+ (Lymphocytic)	+++ (Polyps)
Neck radiographs	Anteroposterior: steeple sign	Lateral: thumb-like mass
Clinical course	Longer	Shorter
Treatment		
Primary therapy	Medical and supportive	Secure airway first
O_2 and humidity	Essential	Usually desirable
Hydration	Oral or IV	Intravenous
Racemic epinephrine	Usually effective	No value
Corticosteroids	Controversial	Not indicated
Antibiotics	Not indicated	Effective
Airway support	Occasionally needed (<3%)	Always indicated (100%)
Preferred airway	Nasotracheal Tracheostomy (rarely)	Nasotracheal
Extubation	4-7 days	1-3 days

*Foreign bodies in the airway should also be considered.
From Hannallah R: Epiglottitis. In Stehling L (ed): Common Problems in Pediatric Anesthesia, 2nd ed. St. Louis, Mosby-Year Book, 1992.

Otorhinolaryngologic Procedures

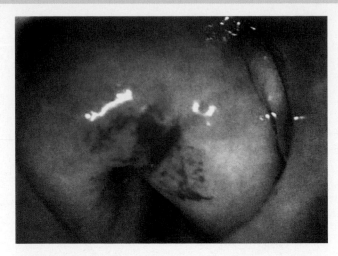

Figure 31-17. A swollen epiglottis seen on direct laryngoscopy. (See also Fig. 37-4.)

improve airflow past the swollen epiglottis, insists on sitting up and leaning forward in the sniffing position (Figs. 31-15 and 31-16 [see website] and Fig. 31-17). The mouth is open, with the tongue protruding. The child frequently drools because of difficulty and pain on swallowing.[1] In addition to high fever, other signs of generalized toxemia may include tachycardia, a flushed face, and prostration. The respiratory pattern is usually slow and quiet to allow more comfortable breathing.

Because of the risk of inducing laryngeal spasm and/or total airway obstruction, examination of the pharynx and larynx should be attempted only in an area with adequate equipment and staff prepared to intervene should upper airway obstruction develop, ideally, the operating room.

The safest, most conservative approach to the management of acute epiglottitis is to establish an artificial airway as soon as the diagnosis is established and, then, with the airway secured, to proceed with appropriate antibiotic and supportive therapy. The child should remain sitting upright at all times and never be forced to lie on his or her back.[184] The management of this problem is described in greater detail in Chapter 37.

Obstructive Laryngeal Papillomatosis

Recurrent respiratory papillomatosis, also known as juvenile laryngeal papillomatosis, is the most commonly found tumor in the larynx and upper airway in children. Recurrent respiratory papillomatosis is caused by the human papillomavirus. The incidence is only 1 in 400 births in spite of evidence of active or latent viral infection in 10% to 25% of pregnant women.[189] The papillomas are usually found in the larynx on the vocal cord margins, epiglottis, pharynx, or trachea (Fig. 31-18). If left untreated, symptoms of aphonia, respiratory distress, hoarseness, stridor, right ventricular hypertrophy, and cor pulmonale may occur.

The current treatment is primarily surgical removal of the papillomatous tissue using the CO_2 laser under microscopic visualization. Alternatively, papillomas can be surgically debulked using an ultrasonic microdébrider or cup forceps before laser treatment. Nonsurgical treatment using interferon alfa-n1 has been beneficial in some children.[190] The main goal of all these treatments is to eliminate the bulk of the lesion without

producing scarring and permanent damage to the underlying mucosa.

Because of the recurrent nature of this condition, most children will return frequently for treatment. Many may require monthly scheduled visits to the operating room to prevent recurring obstruction. If some of these scheduled sessions are missed, or if the progress of the disease is accelerated, the child will present with an acute exacerbation of obstructive symptoms requiring emergent endoscopic resection. In all cases, it is important to obtain a careful history including inquiry about changes in voice or increased difficulty breathing during daily activities that may indicate progressive airway obstruction.

Because of frequent hospitalizations, these children become psychologically sensitized to the perioperative experience. Premedication is usually avoided if the degree of airway obstruction is significant and there are concerns about compromising spontaneous ventilation. In selected cases, the parents (or a child life surrogate) may accompany the child to the operating room for induction to provide emotional support because these children are usually upset.

The perioperative care can be very challenging and often depends on the degree of obstruction to airflow and the type and location of the papilloma. Pedunculated papillomas can produce complete ball-valve obstruction in certain positions. It is therefore prudent to avoid paralyzing these children and to allow them to maintain spontaneous respirations until the airway is examined and the anesthesiologist is certain that assisted or controlled ventilation is possible. These children must be approached the same as any child with anticipated severe airway obstruction (e.g., acute epiglottitis). The surgeon must be present in the operating room, with equipment to deal with total airway obstruction, including rigid bronchoscopes and a tracheostomy/cricothyrotomy set, immediately available. The problem of sharing the already compromised airway with the surgeon is worsened by the need to use a laser beam to excise these lesions. A laser (an acronym for *light amplified by stimulated emission of radiation*) consists of a tube with reflective mirrors at either end with an amplifying medium between

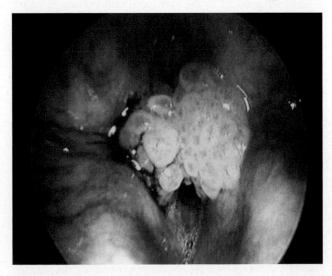

Figure 31-18. Large pedunculated papillomas obstructing the laryngeal inlet.

them to generate electron activity in the form of light. The CO_2 laser is the most widely used in medical practice, having particular application in the treatment of laryngeal or vocal cord papillomas, laryngeal webs, and resection of subglottic tissue and hemangiomas. A laser is useful for endoscopic procedures because the beam may be directed down open-tube endoscopes and is invisible, thereby affording the surgeon an unobstructed view of the lesion during resection. Laser energy is absorbed by tissue water, rapidly increasing its temperature, denaturing protein, and causing vaporization of the target tissue. The thermal energy of the laser beam cauterizes capillaries as it vaporizes tissues; therefore, bleeding is minimal and very little postoperative edema occurs.

These properties give the laser a high degree of specificity; however, they also supply the route by which a misdirected laser beam may cause injury to a child or to unprotected operating room personnel.[191] Laser radiation increases the temperature of absorbent material; therefore, flammable objects, such as surgical drapes, must be kept away from the path of the laser beam. Unprotected surfaces, such as skin, can be burned and must be shielded. Wet towels should be applied to cover the skin of the face and neck when the laser is being used to avoid burns from deflected beams.

The anesthetic management of these children will depend on the approach the surgeon will use to remove the lesions. The basic choice is between intubation and nonintubation techniques. For the latter approach, the use of intermittent apnea versus jet ventilation must be considered.[180] The choice of ETT used during laser surgery can affect the safety of the technique. All standard polyvinylchloride ETTs are flammable and can be ignited and vaporized by a laser beam. Red rubber ETTs do not vaporize but instead deflect the laser beam when wrapped with metallic tape; however, the metallic tape can only be applied up to the cuff and not around it, so the area below the vocal cords may still be vulnerable. Non-latex ETTs have been manufactured specifically for use during laser surgery. Some have a double cuff to ensure protection of the airway in the event that one cuff is damaged by the laser beam. Others have a special matte finish that is effective in deflecting the laser beam throughout its entire length. Nonreflective flexible metal ETTs and specifically wrapped ETTs are also specifically manufactured for use during laser surgery (Fig. 31-19). The outer diameters of these special tubes are considerably greater than the polyvinylchloride counterpart, especially in the small sizes. Thus, they may not be appropriate for very small infants or for children with a severely narrowed airway. Table 31-10 presents a variety of such specialized tubes with a comparison with standard ETTs. Although these ETTs offer some advantage, they are considerably more expensive than metallic tape-wrapped red rubber ETTs. A syringe of normal saline should be immediately available to douse ignited tissues.

In some institutions (after the airway is secured), an intermittent apneic technique using paralysis, TIVA, and topical lidocaine is the usual approach. An antisialagogue such as glycopyrrolate is given at the beginning, along with dexamethasone (0.5 mg/kg; maximum dose 20 mg) to reduce mucosal swelling resulting from repeated intubations. A careful inhalational induction is started using oxygen and sevoflurane with the child initiating each breath and slowly enabling the anesthesiologist to assist until the required depth of anesthesia for laryngoscopy is achieved. Intravenous access is established, and

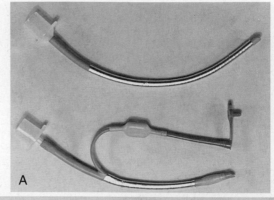

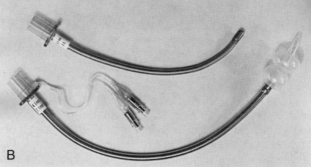

Figure 31-19. Cuffed and uncuffed red rubber endotracheal tubes may be wrapped with reflective metallic tape for use during laser airway surgery. Note that this metallic tape is not approved by the Food and Drug Administration for this application. **A,** Cuffed and uncuffed commercially available foil wrapped laser tubes are available (Laser-ShieldR, II Medtronic Xomed, Jacksonville, FL). **B,** An example of several commercially available stainless steel laser endotracheal tubes (V. Mueller Stainless Co.). Note that the external diameters of these devices are greater than those of standard endotracheal tubes.

the larynx is anesthetized with topical lidocaine (3-4 mg/kg); the airway is then evaluated and tracheal intubation is performed. The ETT chosen is usually several sizes smaller than what is normally appropriate for the child's age because most have some degree of laryngeal scarring from repeated resections and there is the need to avoid obscuring the surgeon's view and access to the lesions with the ETT.

Although the goal is to achieve the desired depth of anesthesia to secure the airway with the child still spontaneously breathing, frequently partial obstruction is encountered before an adequate depth of anesthesia for laryngoscopy is achieved. In these cases, thrusting the jaw forward and applying positive pressure in the anesthetic circuit will maintain an open airway in most situations. If complete obstruction is encountered, then a single intravenous bolus of propofol (2-3 mg/kg) or a short-acting muscle relaxant may be necessary for immediate laryngoscopy and intubation or to allow the surgeon to perform rigid bronchoscopy.

Once the correct position of the ETT is confirmed, a neuromuscular blocking agent (e.g., rocuronium) can be administered and the TIVA technique with propofol (200-300 μg/kg/min) and fentanyl (2-3 μg/kg) or remifentanil infusion (0.1-0.25 μg/kg/min or more, as needed) is started. Muscle relaxation is desirable to produce an immobile surgical field, and its adequacy is best assessed by using a neuromuscular blockade monitor.

Table 31-10. External Diameter of Standard Plastic Versus Endotracheal Tubes Used for Laser Surgery

ID (mm)	OD (mm)						
	Standard ETT (uncuffed)*	Standard ETT (cuffed)*	Laser-Shield (cuffed)†	Laser-flex (uncuffed)*	Laser-flex (cuffed)*	Lasertubus (double cuffed)‡	Red Rubber (cuffed without copper wrap)
3.0	4.2	4.2		5.2			4.7
3.5	4.9	4.9		5.7			5.3
4.0	5.5	5.5	6.6	6.1		6.0	6.0
4.5	6.2	6.2	7.3		7.0		6.7
5.0	6.8	6.8	8.0		7.5	7.3	7.3
5.5	7.5	7.5	8.6		7.9		8.0
6.0	8.2	8.2	9.0		8.5	8.7	8.7

*Mallinckrodt, Inc
†Medtronic, Inc.
‡Lasertubus Rüsch, Inc.

An apneic anesthetic technique without an ETT offers the best unobstructed view of the larynx and avoids the presence of flammable material (e.g., the ETT) in the path of the laser beam. The child is positioned for suspension laryngoscopy with eyes protected with moist eye pads, and the otomicroscope and CO_2 laser equipment are aligned. The ETT is then removed and surgical resection is carried out during repeated periods of apnea. The need for re-intubation is guided by the adequacy of oxygenation as reflected by the pulse oximeter. Re-intubation can be readily performed by the surgeon by introducing the tracheal tube through the suspension laryngoscope under direct vision using the metal suction as a stylet. After each re-intubation the extent of CO_2 retention is assessed by monitoring the end-tidal CO_2 and hyperventilation with 100% oxygen is continued until the tube is removed and surgery is resumed.[1]

A modification of the apneic technique that does not require endotracheal intubation but does provide for oxygenation during laser surgery utilizes a jet ventilator. The operating laryngoscope may be fitted with a catheter through which air is entrained and the lungs are intermittently ventilated by the jet. The advantage of this technique is twofold. The surgical field is extremely quiet because large excursions of the diaphragm are eliminated and ventilation is uninterrupted. Transtracheal jet ventilation carries a greater risk of pneumothorax than the transglottic approach.[180] In morbidly obese children and those with severe disease of the small airways, effective ventilation may be difficult to accomplish with this technique and an alternate approach should be used.[192] Another concern is that, theoretically, jet ventilation may distribute papilloma virus throughout the tracheobronchial tree.

When surgery is completed, the ETT is reinserted and secured until the child is completely awakened. Postoperative measures to prevent laryngeal edema, such as racemic epinephrine inhalation and/or the use of dexamethasone, are usually required.

Aspirated Foreign Bodies

Foreign body aspiration is most common in toddlers 1 to 3 years of age. The majority (95%) of foreign bodies lodge in the right main-stem bronchus.[193] A history of choking while eating or playing, persistent cough, or wheezing that does not respond to medical treatment may be the only manifestations. If the foreign body completely obstructs a bronchus, or creates a ball-valve phenomenon, distal hyperinflation from air trapping may occur; a hyperinflated lung during the expiratory phase may be the only sign seen on chest radiography (Fig. 31-20, see website; see also Figs. 37-6 to 37-8). The more distal the object is lodged in the airway, the more atelectatic changes are noted.

Foreign bodies lodge in the trachea (less than 5% of airway foreign bodies) if they are too large to pass the carina.[194] The signs of a tracheal foreign body may include a brassy cough with or without abnormal voice, bidirectional stridor, or complete airway obstruction in the case of laryngeal foreign bodies. Any sharp object or any object that causes acute upper airway obstruction with cyanosis and an inability to maintain ventilation requires emergent removal. Unroasted peanuts (with unsaturated double bonds in the oils) should be removed promptly because the oil can cause an inflammatory response and subsequent pneumonitis.[195] In contrast, roasted peanuts (with saturated double bonds in the oils) may be present in the lungs for longer periods without inducing as severe an inflammatory response. In addition, peanuts tend to swell, fragment, and crumble over time, making removal "en bloc" extremely difficult. The child who presents with a history of cyanosis after aspiration of a nut very likely has aspirated material bilaterally (as in the case of a broken nut or multiple nuts) and should be examined accordingly.

The anesthetic management of these children depends on the level, degree, and duration of obstruction. A child who aspirates a foreign body while eating, or soon thereafter, presents with the additional risk of a full stomach. Waiting for the stomach to empty may not be appropriate or even effective in the acute situation. Intravenous metoclopramide (0.15 mg/kg) may be used to hasten stomach emptying but will not guarantee that the stomach empties.[196] If time permits, the administration of an anticholinergic agent may be useful to reduce secretions. In the debate of how to anesthetize a child with a full stomach and a compromised airway from the aspirated foreign body, the airway concern takes precedence over the full stomach and an inhalational induction is recommended.

One of the major controversies in the anesthetic management of foreign body aspiration is whether to control ventilation or allow spontaneous respirations during bronchoscopy. Some endoscopists prefer a spontaneously breathing child to prevent movement of the foreign body as it is being retrieved out of the airway. Sevoflurane is preferred over halothane for inhalational induction in these children because it does not cause coughing and maintains hemodynamic stability.[197] Anesthesia is usually maintained with 100% oxygen and halothane or sevoflurane or a propofol-based TIVA technique.[1] Halothane has some advantage over sevoflurane during maintenance because it is more soluble and more slowly eliminated. This allows more time to manipulate the airway without the child becoming too lightly anesthetized and reacting to the procedure. Alternatively, a propofol TIVA technique allows a steady level of anesthesia that is independent of ventilation and does not expose the operating room personnel to waste anesthetic agents that inevitably egress from the airway around the bronchoscope. Often these children have very irritable airways because of the presence of the foreign body. The use of topical lidocaine (3-4 mg/kg) divided between the laryngeal structures and tracheal mucosa is essential to suppress airway reflexes and prevent coughing and bronchospasm (see Chapter 37 for further management suggestions).

Tracheostomy

Tracheostomy in infants and children is usually performed electively as a planned procedure after the airway is already established with an ETT before the child arrives in the operating room. Indications for a planned tracheostomy include lesions such as congenital or acquired vocal cord paralysis, central hypoventilation syndrome (Ondine's curse), craniofacial abnormalities (e.g., Pierre Robin malformation), persistent laryngotracheomalacia, and congenital or acquired subglottic stenosis (see Fig. 33-13A). Usually these children have had a period of watchful waiting, which later results in the need for tracheostomy due to persistent hypoxemia, hypercarbia, or intermittent obstruction that cannot be eliminated with the natural airway. Still other children have acute deterioration of the airway and require tracheostomy on an emergent basis.

In either case, the surgeon will frequently want to perform a thorough examination of the airway (i.e., diagnostic laryngoscopy and bronchoscopy) before proceeding with the tracheostomy. This requires that the tracheal tube be removed, the airway examined with a rigid bronchoscope, and then the child re-intubated for the procedure. After the diagnostic laryngoscopy and bronchoscopy and re-intubation, the child is positioned supine, with the head maximally extended over a shoulder roll and taped to the end of the bed. It is a good practice to have a fresh anesthesia circuit, or an extension, to hand to the surgeon to connect to the freshly inserted tracheostomy cannula.

Anesthesia is maintained with spontaneous respirations of inhalational agents so that if there is airway compromise at any point the child may still be able to maintain oxygenation. One hundred percent oxygen should be administered throughout the procedure because the airway may be lost at any time. Intravenous opioids or local anesthetic infiltration, or both, should be utilized to manage postoperative pain. A thrashing, crying child who is in pain will compromise the integrity of the newly established surgical airway.

Children who cannot be intubated may undergo an "awake" tracheostomy with sedation and local anesthesia. Ketamine, although an attractive alternative, does produce secretions that may further compromise an already marginal airway. The use of an antisialagogue may help control secretions. Children who can be anesthetized with an inhalational agent administered by mask but who cannot be intubated due to severe subglottic ste-

nosis or inability to visualize the vocal cords by direct laryngoscopy may have the airway maintained with spontaneous ventilation and a face mask or an LMA until a surgical airway is obtained.

Once the trachea has been entered, a portion of the delivered tidal volume is lost through the incision and ventilation may become inadequate. This is less of a problem if spontaneous respirations are maintained at this point. It is prudent to leave the ETT within the lumen of the trachea but withdrawn just proximal to the tracheal incision so that it can be readily advanced should difficulty be encountered with passing the tracheotomy tube. Once the tracheotomy tube is in place, the ETT is removed, the sterile distal end of the anesthesia circuit is attached to the tracheotomy tube (and the proximal end to the anesthesia machine), and the wound is closed. In the event of the tracheostomy tube becoming dislodged or removed, the tracheal incision will close and attempts at reinsertion may result in bleeding, the creation of a false passage, or trauma to the tracheal wall. The tracheal lumen is identified by internal traction sutures, which are placed by the surgeon at the end of the surgical procedure (Fig. 31-21, see website). With the surgeon pulling up on the external ends of these sutures, the tracheal incision is identified and the tracheotomy is opened so that an artificial airway can be inserted. The child should not leave the operating room without the potentially lifesaving sutures in place and their laterality (right vs. left) properly identified. Flexible fiberoptic bronchoscopy through the new tracheostomy tube can be performed to confirm appropriate location of the tip of the tracheostomy tube above the carina.

Laryngotracheal Reconstruction

Glottic and subglottic stenosis, although rare, can be life threatening and is difficult to manage from the surgical and anesthesiologic points of view. Congenital laryngeal atresia and congenital laryngeal webs can be incompatible with life unless an emergent tracheostomy is performed at birth. Occasionally this can be done before placental separation as an operation on placental support or ex-utero intrapartum treatment (EXIT) procedure (see Chapter 38). Treatment depends on the severity of laryngeal obstruction. Only a few are severe enough to require immediate intubation or tracheostomy (see Fig. 36-2). Some can be discovered as an incidental finding while trying to intubate a neonate for an unrelated surgical procedure.[198] Most can be broken down by passing a bronchoscope or incised with a surgical knife or scissors. Thin anterior webs can be managed by microendoscopic incision with a microsurgical knife or CO_2 laser, staging the procedure for each side separately to avoid recurrence. The anesthetic management is similar to that for children undergoing laser excision of laryngeal papillomatosis.

Acquired subglottic stenosis is usually the result of prolonged endotracheal intubation for respiratory support of prematurely born infants. In older children, it is often the result of laryngeal trauma. Symptoms usually relate to airway, voice, and feeding and often occur 2 to 4 weeks after the laryngeal insult. Progressive respiratory difficulty with biphasic stridor, dyspnea, air hunger, and retractions are typical. These children usually have a tendency toward prolonged courses of upper respiratory tract infections. Soft tissue radiographs of the neck and computed tomography will help assess the exact site and length of the stenotic segment. Because both gastroesophageal and gastrolaryngopharyngeal reflux disease are thought to play a role in the development and exacerbation of subglottic stenosis, these conditions must be excluded, usually by a 24-hour esophageal pH probe placement. However, direct endoscopic visualization of the larynx is ultimately required to fully evaluate the stenosis. Rigid and flexible endoscopy of the airway and esophagus is performed in the operating room. Because of the small diameter of the airway, the rigid rod-lens-telescope and/or a flexible bronchoscope are used to visualize the larynx and trachea beyond the obstruction. The trachea is then intubated, and the degree of air leak around the tube helps establish the degree of stenosis (see Fig. 31-13; see also Fig. 36-3A).

The surgical management of these infants must be individualized according to the degree of obstruction and the general condition of the child.[199] Most cases of moderate or severe subglottic stenosis require a tracheostomy at or below the third tracheal ring to establish a safe airway. The presence of a tracheostomy also helps to facilitate the airway management during subsequent procedures. For less severe cases, endoscopic dilation or CO_2 laser endoscopic scar excision may be sufficient.

The more severe cases of laryngeal stenosis require external reconstruction. Of the many available options, an anterior cricoid split operation and laryngotracheal reconstruction are more frequently used.

The cricoid split operation is performed with the use of general endotracheal anesthesia. The largest possible tracheal tube is inserted through the nose. An incision is made through the cricoid, and the cartilage springs open. The ETT will be readily visible in the lumen. Frequently, the incision will be extended to include the upper two tracheal rings and even the lower third of the thyroid cartilage (Fig. 31-22). Stay sutures are placed on each side of the incised cricoid, and the skin is loosely approximated. The ETT is left in place for about 7 days to act as a splint while the mucosal swelling subsides and the split cricoid heals. Endoscopy is not usually required, but corticosteroids are administered before extubation.

Open reconstructive surgical techniques are done at the youngest age possible to help the development of speech and language skills. They basically combine the use of laryngeal and cricoid splits, cartilage grafts, and stenting.

For laryngotracheal reconstruction procedures, the infant is positioned with a roll under the shoulders and the head is extended. The tracheostomy cannula is replaced with an ETT that is introduced through the stoma to allow easy and secure access to the airway. A sterile, shortened, preformed oral RAE tube is ideal to allow secure fixation. The distal end is cut to an appropriate length to avoid bronchial intubation and then sutured to the skin of the neck. A costal cartilage graft is harvested and fashioned to fit the intended site of transplantation (anterior or posterior splits). Repair of laryngotracheal stenosis in almost all cases, except anterior subglottic stenosis, requires brief stenting to keep the graft in place and lend support to the reconstructed area. Stents will counteract scar contracture and provide a scaffold for epithelium to cover the lumen of the airway. Many types of stents have been used. T-tubes are popular in adults but are associated with more complications and blockage in children. The lower end of the stent is sutured in place during surgery. The stent is eventually removed endoscopically after cutting the sutures and retrieving the tube.

Single-stage laryngotracheal reconstruction is sometimes used in children without significant obstruction. A full-length nasotracheal tube is used to support the graft for 3 to 7 days depending on the type of graft. The advantages of immediate decannulation and possible avoidance of a tracheostomy altogether make this approach appealing in appropriate candidates (Fig. 31-23).

The anesthetic challenges in these cases are many. The general condition of the child may not be perfect. Residual stigmata of prematurity are often present. The airway will be shared with the surgeon, and the tracheal tube that is placed in the stoma will need to be intermittently removed for surgical access and stent placement. A quiet surgical field is essential. The possibility of a pneumothorax during the cartilage graft harvesting should be kept in mind. The need to ensure that the stent, or the tracheal tube in case of a single-stage laryngotracheal reconstruction, is not dislodged in the intensive care unit cannot be

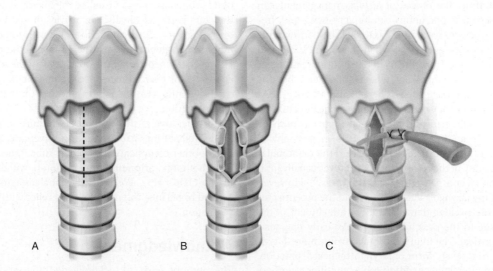

Figure 31-22. Anterior cricoid split. After a midline laryngeal incision through cartilage and mucosa (**A**), the cricoid cartilage is decompressed and the endotracheal tube is ghosted in (**B**). The skin is loosely closed with a drain (**C**). (From Zalzal GH, Cotton RT: Glottic and subglottic stenosis. In Cummings CE [ed]: Otolaryngology Head & Neck Surgery, 4th ed. St. Louis, Elsevier Mosby, 2005.)

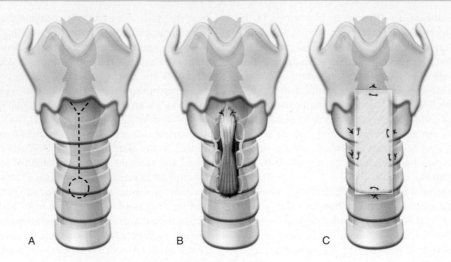

Figure 31-23. (**A**) Laryngotracheal resection with anterior cartilage graft. After a midline incision into the thyroid cartilage (**B**), the intraluminal scar and lining mucosa are incised along the length of the stenotic segment (**C**). Costal cartilage is shaped into a modified boat and placed in position with the lining of the perichondrium facing internally. (From Zalzal GH, Cotton RT: Glottic and subglottic stenosis. In Cummings CE [ed]: Otolaryngology Head & Neck Surgery, 4th ed. St. Louis, Elsevier Mosby, 2005.)

overstated. Accidental extubation cannot be allowed. A combination of sedation techniques and/or pharmacologic relaxation is necessary. The choice is often dictated by the individual policy in each intensive care unit.

Airway Trauma

Nasal fractures are frequently seen in older children and adolescents. They may result from a direct hit (fight) or an accident.[200] Because the nasal mucosa is very vascular, a lot of blood is usually swallowed. A stomach full of blood is to be assumed for the first 24 to 48 hours after the injury. A rapid-sequence tracheal intubation is safest during that period. However, closed reduction of a nasal fracture is often delayed for a few days to allow swelling to subside. At that time, the choice of airway management can include an LMA. These operations can be very brief, and, frequently, the surgeon will leave in a nasal pack and an external splint. The child must be awake enough at the end of surgery to be cooperative and understand the need for mouth breathing. A combative, semi-awake adolescent who is unable to breathe through the nose can hurt himself or herself and others.

Closed or open injuries to the larynx and trachea in children can result from bicycle accidents, falls, direct trauma from sharp objects, and, rarely, a "clothesline" injury. The more cephalad cervical position of the pediatric larynx behind the mandibular arch and the pliability of the cricothyroid structures usually limit the extent of injury and prevent severe fractures.[200] However, the small size of the laryngotracheal airway and the potential for massive soft tissue swelling due to the loose attachment of the submucosal tissue to the perichondrium make early diagnosis and treatment critical. The injury can range from minor laryngeal hematoma to a severe form of laryngotracheal separation. This extreme and often fatal condition can occur after a clothesline mechanism of injury and is often associated with bilateral vocal cord paralysis due to recurrent laryngeal nerve damage.[201]

Hoarseness, cough, dyspnea, hemoptysis, and voice changes suggest laryngeal damage. Clinical subcutaneous emphysema, pneumothorax, and pneumomediastinum signify definite disruption of the laryngotracheal complex. Computed tomography is the most appropriate imaging modality to identify the extent of laryngeal injury.[202]

Positive-pressure ventilation by mask, excessive coughing, or struggling can worsen the subcutaneous emphysema and cause further deterioration of the airway. Administration of nitrous oxide, application of cricoid pressure, multiple vigorous attempts at laryngoscopy and intubation, and passage of blind nasotracheal tubes or nasogastric tubes should be avoided to prevent further trauma by creating a false passage through a mucosal tear. A good approach to this type of injury is to use the fiberoptic bronchoscope to visualize the airway before intubation if the child is stable. Ideally, the airway should be secured in the operating room after induction of general anesthesia with an inhalational agent and with the child breathing spontaneously. However, tracheostomy below the level of the injury under local anesthesia or over a bronchoscope may be necessary if there is extensive injury to the mouth and larynx that requires major reconstruction.

Postoperatively, these children require management in a monitored setting, usually the intensive care unit. The resolution of other complications, such as subcutaneous emphysema, pneumothorax, or pneumomediastinum, will dictate the length of the child's stay. Postoperative analgesia must be carefully titrated to balance the need for pain relief with the adequacy of ventilation.

Acknowledgment

The authors wish to acknowledge the prior contributions to this chapter by Lynne R. Ferrari, MD, and Susan A. Vassallo, MD.

Annotated References

Brown KA, Laferrière A, Lakheeram I, Moss IR: Recurrent hypoxemia in children is associated with increased analgesic sensitivity to opiates. Anesthesiology 2006; 105:665-669

This study makes a clear case that younger children with obstructive sleep apnea syndrome are at increased risk from opioid-induced respiratory depression; equal analgesia can be achieved with one half the usual opioid dose.

Nixon GM, Kermack AS, Davis GM, et al: Planning adenotonsillectomy in children with obstructive sleep apnea: the role of overnight oximetry. Pediatrics 2004; 113:e19-e25

When a full sleep study in a sleep pathology laboratory is not possible, overnight oximetry can be a more practical approach.

Nixon GM, Kermack AS, McGregor CD, et al: Sleep and breathing on the first night after adenotonsillectomy for obstructive sleep apnea. Pediatr Pulmonol 2005; 39:332-338

At-risk children become more hypoxemic on the first night after tonsillectomy than they were preoperatively. This study makes a compelling case for in-hospital monitoring postoperatively.

Practice Guidelines for the Perioperative Management of Patients with Obstructive Sleep Apnea: A report by the American Society of Anesthesiologists Task Force on perioperative management of patients with obstructive sleep apnea. Anesthesiology 2006; 104:1081-1093

A recent practice guideline by a panel of experts discussing different levels of evidence for said guidelines.

Verghese ST, Hannallah RS: Otolaryngological emergencies. Anesthesiol Clin North Am 2001; 19:237-256

A comprehensive review of pediatric airway emergencies is presented.

References

Please see www.expertconsult.com

Ophthalmology

R. Grey Weaver, Jr., and Joseph R. Tobin

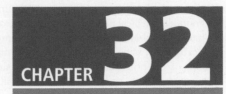

CHAPTER 32

THE INFANT OR CHILD presenting for elective ophthalmic surgery requires careful preanesthetic assessment. In addition to the manifesting ophthalmologic issues, the infant or child may have associated or unassociated systemic disease states. In this chapter we review some of the more important issues that should be addressed preoperatively, as well as some of the difficulties that may be anticipated in the perioperative period after ophthalmologic procedures.

Many ophthalmologic diagnoses can only be confirmed by the ophthalmologist with a cooperative infant or child. Thus, an examination under anesthesia (EUA) is often essential for accurate diagnosis and evaluation of many processes, including trauma, tumors, infiltrative diseases, coloboma, glaucoma and vascular diseases of the retina, Coats disease, and incontinentia pigmenti. Inpatient preterm infants often require serial EUAs to monitor the development and progress of retinopathy of prematurity (ROP) and the response of the disease to surgical therapy. These examinations may be performed in the neonatal intensive care unit or operating room and may require sedation or general anesthesia.[1] Other inpatient trauma victims may require serial EUAs to monitor the development of glaucoma or retinal injury. Serial EUAs are also necessary to monitor progress during outpatient retinoblastoma radiation treatments. The anesthesiologist is therefore a valuable colleague essential to the provision of pediatric ophthalmologic diagnostic and therapeutic techniques.

Certain ophthalmologic procedures require an absolutely immobile child for maximal safety from the surgeon's perspective. These include any surgeries in which the globe is opened, such as cataract removal, vitrectomy, laser or cryotherapy for retinopathy, retinal detachment repair, and anterior chamber paracentesis. Other procedures may only require a child to be cooperative for a nonpainful examination, but because the target organs (orbits) are close to the airway, a strategy must be devised to ensure safe management of the airway.

The child in need of ophthalmologic surgery will almost always require general anesthesia or deep sedation rather than exclusive use of local or regional anesthesia. Many infants and children cannot or will not cooperate for anything beyond a brief eye examination. Although the ophthalmologist may be able to tolerate small movements by the child during an EUA, unnecessary head or eye globe movement during an ophthalmologic procedure should be prevented. Retrobulbar block is sometimes performed for postoperative analgesia in children before emergence from general anesthesia.[2] All complications associated with a retrobulbar block identified in adults may also occur in children.[3,4]

The Preoperative Evaluation

The perioperative environment should be welcoming to the child and their family.[5,6] All team members should be comfortable with anesthesia considerations for infants and children for ophthalmologic procedures.[6] Anticipation and prevention of postoperative nausea and vomiting (PONV) as well as anesthetic emergence and postoperative analgesia are essential.

When scheduled for an elective ophthalmologic procedure, the complete medical history and physical examination, including past surgical/anesthetic history, a current and recently used medication list, known allergies, family history, and review of systems, is essential.[7] Because many ophthalmologic diagnoses are common with systemic conditions, all the implications of the systemic illness are of possible concern for the anesthesiologist.

The physical examination should evaluate whether the ophthalmologic condition will present any need to alter airway management or the ability to obtain an appropriate mask fit. The airway should be carefully assessed for issues arising from other systemic conditions. Cardiorespiratory and neurologic systems assessments are also important in formulating the anesthetic plan.

Common Ophthalmologic Diagnoses Presenting for Surgery

The more common diagnoses and surgical procedures are listed in Table 32-1. Diagnoses may exist in isolation or be one aspect of a more complex group of diagnoses. Many diagnoses will involve systemic illnesses, and the anesthesiologist should be familiar with the implications of the presence of ophthalmologic disease in the evaluation of the child and planning the perioperative experience.

Some procedures and examinations can be performed without insertion of an artificial airway; however, communication with the ophthalmologist for their needs is essential in the planning of the anesthesia. Other procedures may be performed very quickly and require only induction of anesthesia (often by mask in children) and then the face mask is removed from the nasal bridge to allow the ophthalmologist full access to both orbits, eyelids and nasolacrimal ducts. With experience and the newer, soft, inflatable cushion face masks, a close fit can still be obtained to reduce environmental contamination with anesthetic gases and maintain a suitable plane of anesthesia. The EUA may be brief or intermediate in length and, as information is generated, surgical correction may be contemplated during the same anesthetic. Therefore, communication and flexibility become caveats of anesthetic planning. An anesthetic may start with a plan for a brief EUA with mask inhalation anesthesia without a planned intravenous catheter placement. However, if surgical corrective therapy becomes necessary, airway control

Table 32-1. Common Ophthalmologic Procedures in Children

Examination under anesthesia
Strabismus repair
Retinopathy of prematurity—laser or cryotherapy
Ptosis repair
Cataract excision ± intraocular lens placement
Corneal transplant
Evaluation of penetrating eye injuries
Dacryocystorhinotomy and dacryocystocele repair
Enucleation
Retro-orbital cellulitis decompression
Vitrectomy

Table 32-2. Ophthalmologic Conditions Associated with Systemic Syndromes and Illnesses

Syndrome and Illness	Conditions
Fetal alcohol syndrome	Strabismus, optic nerve hypoplasia
Galactosemia	Neonatal cataracts
Mucopolysaccharidoses	Corneal involvement—may require transplant
Retinitis pigmentosa	Heart block
Sturge-Weber syndrome	Glaucoma
Prematurity	Retinopathy of prematurity, strabismus
Fabry disease	Whorled corneal opacities
Tay-Sachs disease	Cherry-red macular spot
Osteogenesis imperfecta	Blue sclerae
Craniofacial syndromes (Crouzon, Apert, Pfeiffer, etc.)	Proptosis, strabismus, glaucoma

may require placement of a laryngeal mask airway (LMA) or an endotracheal tube. Intravenous access may then be needed to administer medications, including those to prevent or treat the oculocardiac reflex (OCR).[8]

For procedures of brief or intermediate duration, the use of an LMA allows excellent access to all periorbital structures and provides good airway control in most circumstances. The LMA also has the advantage of decreasing environmental contamination with anesthetic vapors compared with mask anesthesia. It is relatively easy to insert and secure while avoiding the need for the anesthesiologist to manually maintain a patent airway when a face mask is used. When compared with the endotracheal tube, the LMA does not increase heart rate, blood pressure, and intraocular pressure (IOP) to the same degree.[9]

Some of the more common ophthalmologic presentations with associated systemic illnesses or syndromes are listed in Table 32-2. Some systemic conditions have significant cardiorespiratory or central nervous system implications for perioperative management, and these should be fully evaluated before anesthesia (see Chapter 4). Because many procedures are performed on preterm infants or former preterm infants, prematurity and its complications may have some of the most clinically important implications for anesthetic management.

Association of Ophthalmologic Conditions and Systemic Disorders

Prematurity

The preterm infant may present for many surgical considerations early in life. ROP, congenital cataracts, and glaucoma may require surgery even when the infant weighs less than 1000 g. The preterm infant may have significant systemic illness(es) that will require attention and consideration by the anesthesiologist. Common complications of prematurity include acute and chronic pulmonary disease,[10] respiratory failure and pulmonary hypertension, congenital heart disease (unrepaired or with a limited palliative repair), and intraventricular hemorrhage,[11] with or without obstructive hydrocephalus.

Acutely ill preterm infants and those younger than 1 year of age are at greater risk than older children and adults when elective or urgent surgery is required.[12] Careful attention to airway management, assisted ventilation, and titration of oxygen therapy with specified goals are essential to success.[13] If the preterm infant is already intubated and receiving assisted ventilation, then the anesthesiologist should confirm adequate airway position, transport the infant safely (if coming to the operating room), and minimize exposure to high concentrations of oxygen. Although institutional goals are not uniform regarding supplemental oxygen therapy,[14] communication with the neonatal team is quite helpful in assessing the child's previous oxygen requirement and current targeted goals (e.g., hemoglobin-oxygen saturation levels of 90%-95%). *Because most anesthetics impair hypoxic pulmonary vasoconstriction, a greater fraction of inspired oxygen concentration may be necessary to maintain targeted hemoglobin saturation.*

Hypercarbia and hypoxia may increase choroidal blood volume and increase IOP. Therefore, Pco_2 and Po_2 should be controlled. Infants may be at greater risk for the OCR than older children and adults, and intravenous access should be obtained before the surgical procedure or any examination that will require extraocular muscle traction or pressure on the globe.

Extremely low birth weight infants require many weeks to grow and develop to a weight of approximately 1800 g to maintain normothermia without special environmental control. These infants will commonly have a history of short or intermediate-length assisted ventilation but may currently be without supplemental oxygen support before an EUA or planned operative procedure for ROP.[15] Many of these infants will have received earlier ophthalmologic examinations while ventilated in the neonatal intensive care unit.[16] When surgical therapy (laser or cryosurgical stabilization) of ROP becomes necessary, these infants will require anesthesia to provide optimal conditions (Fig. 32-1). Perioperative apnea may preclude tracheal

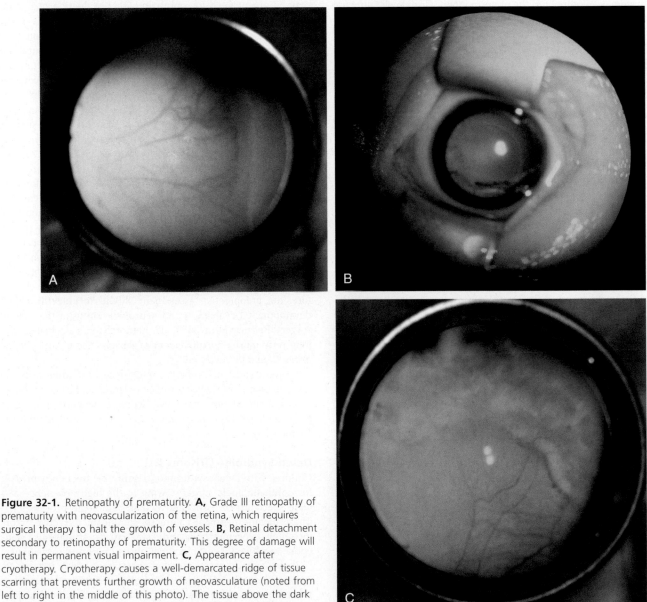

Figure 32-1. Retinopathy of prematurity. **A,** Grade III retinopathy of prematurity with neovascularization of the retina, which requires surgical therapy to halt the growth of vessels. **B,** Retinal detachment secondary to retinopathy of prematurity. This degree of damage will result in permanent visual impairment. **C,** Appearance after cryotherapy. Cryotherapy causes a well-demarcated ridge of tissue scarring that prevents further growth of neovasculature (noted from left to right in the middle of this photo). The tissue above the dark line is scarred and prevents neovascular growth from continuing.

extubation or require close postoperative monitoring after anesthesia.

Perioperative apnea in the preterm infant is widely described.[17,18] Whether still hospitalized or presenting for elective surgery as an outpatient, the preoperative assessment should determine the pattern and frequency of apnea before the planned surgical procedure and anesthetic. If the child has been discharged, the current use of respiratory stimulants (caffeine or theophylline) and oxygen should be determined. Is the apnea monitor still used or has it been discontinued? Hard guidelines have not been developed, but infants still on supplemental oxygen, less than 60 weeks after conception, or monitored for apnea/bradycardia should have continuous cardiorespiratory and oxygen saturation monitoring postoperatively (see Chapter 4). The risk for apnea after anesthesia decreases with advancing gestational age at birth and with advancing postnatal-postconceptual age. The risk of apnea is independent of opioid use and is thought to be multifactorial from the presence of general and neuraxial anesthetics and the immature central nervous system development of the preterm infant. Flexible planning for possible postoperative ventilatory assistance is essential, and families should be informed of this possibility preoperatively.

The airway of the preterm infant who is younger than 52 to 60 weeks' postconceptual age is usually intubated for ophthalmologic surgery (except for a very brief EUA) owing to the immature respiratory drive, unpredictably variable respiratory response to anesthetic agents, and the possible lag to recovery of respiratory drive after completion of the procedure and discontinuation of anesthetic agents. If the infant does not appear to have a stable respiratory drive and strength after anesthesia, then postoperative assisted ventilation should be provided and weaned as they recover. Planning for this contingency is vital. *Ophthalmologic procedures may be brief and with low risk for blood loss; however, general anesthesia and its risks mandate a perioperative environment where postoperative support is available as an inpatient.* Intensive care resources for assisted ventilation in preterm and ex-preterm infants should be available.

Although chronic lung disease secondary to prematurity is prevalent, its intensity has been significantly reduced with the routine utilization of surfactant and advances in ventilator management strategies. Long-lasting respiratory effects from prematurity may include reactive airway disease, subglottic stenosis from prolonged intubation, and alveolar/interstitial disease with an oxygen requirement lasting from weeks to years.[10] Because many anesthetics impair hypoxic pulmonary vasoconstriction, an increased oxygen requirement in the perioperative period should be anticipated. Endotracheal intubation, a light level of anesthesia, or topical use of β-adrenergic antagonists may exacerbate reactive airway disease, requiring further treatment to reduce air trapping and hypercarbia.

Together with airway and alveolar diseases, the anesthesiologist should determine whether pulmonary hypertension or right ventricular dysfunction is or was present.[19] Some infants may be receiving continuing oxygen therapy as treatment for pulmonary hypertension and to reduce intermittent episodes of hypoxemia due to crying or sleeping. If pulmonary hypertension has been previously diagnosed, then an updated or recent evaluation should be reviewed. Because pulmonary hypertension is exacerbated by hypoxia and hypercarbia, endotracheal intubation should be considered to ensure control of ventilation and oxygenation. At the emergence of anesthesia, pulmonary hypertension may be exacerbated when hypercapnia occurs, thereby causing physiologic or anatomic shunting with systemic hemoglobin-oxygen desaturation. Immediate and continued evaluation of the airway is critical to be sure there is not an independent respiratory contribution to systemic hypoxia.

Congenital cardiac disease may be present in the preterm neonate, infant, or child presenting for ophthalmologic procedures. The patent ductus arteriosus may not close spontaneously or with inducement by cyclooxygenase inhibitors in the preterm or full-term infant. This may lead to persistent congestive failure, reduced pulmonary compliance, and complications of fluid management. Congenital cardiac anomalies will require assessment before elective surgery. The varied complex congenital cardiac lesions have a wide spectrum of interactions with multiple anesthetic agents.[20] Many cardiac conditions will require surgery or palliation (e.g., systemic to pulmonary shunts) before elective ophthalmologic procedures. Correction of congenital heart disease is limited by the difficulty of utilizing cardiopulmonary bypass in infants weighing less than 2 kg. There may be urgent need for ophthalmologic evaluation (e.g., congenital tumor, cataract, or glaucoma) before the repair of the congenital cardiac condition. Preoperative consultation with the infant's pediatric cardiologist will provide useful updated information on anticipated perioperative ventricular function and dysrhythmias associated with certain lesions and whether medical management has been optimized before anesthesia.

Intraventricular hemorrhage is a major etiology of morbidity and mortality in the preterm infant.[11] In those who survive, obstructed hydrocephalus may occur and require cerebrospinal fluid diversion procedures to decompress the obstructed ventricular system with associated increased intracranial pressure. Many of these infants require ophthalmologic surgery for strabismus repair secondary to their neurologic insult. If a ventriculoperitoneal shunt is in place, its proper function should be determined by direct evaluation. The anesthesiologist should take specific note whether there is inappropriate macrocephaly or a bulging or tense fontanelle. Obstructed hydrocephalus may occur after the infant's discharge from hospital even though a ventriculperitoneal shunt was previously not required. Therefore, the preoperative assessment should include the child's developmental evaluation and neurologic status at the time of surgery. Because intraventricular hemorrhage is associated with long-term morbidity, the history of seizures and of antiepileptic drugs should be reviewed.

Preterm and small infants rapidly lose heat when anesthetized; prevention of hypothermia is essential in the perioperative environment. Hypothermia will decrease metabolism of most drugs and depresses respiratory drive in preterm infants (see Chapter 25).

Down Syndrome (Trisomy 21)

Children with Down syndrome (trisomy 21) frequently present for ophthalmologic surgery owing to the high prevalence of a wide spectrum of associated ocular pathologic processes.[21-23] These include neonatal cataracts, significant refractive errors including hypermetropia and astigmatism, strabismus, glaucoma, keratoconus, nasolacrimal obstruction, and nystagmus.

It is currently recommended that infants with trisomy 21 receive an ophthalmologic evaluation in the neonatal period. If this requires an EUA, then the anesthesiologist should be prepared for the medical implications associated with trisomy 21, which are extensive.[24,25] Nearly half of these infants are born with congenital heart disease, including septal defects, a complete or partial atrioventricular canal, tetralogy of Fallot, transposition of the great arteries, and valvular insufficiency or stenosis. Any child with a left-to-right shunt may develop pulmonary hypertension, and children with trisomy 21 develop irreversible pulmonary hypertension at an earlier age. A full knowledge and understanding of the cardiac defect(s) present is essential to planning the anesthetic (see Chapters 14, 16, and 21).

Airway abnormalities such as brachycephaly, narrowed nasopharyngeal passages, macroglossia, pharyngeal hypotonia, and subglottic stenosis are frequently observed in children with trisomy 21. These may contribute to the development of chronic intermittent hypoxia, further exacerbating pulmonary hypertension; these children should be anticipated to have exacerbations of airway obstruction and hypoxia after general anesthesia.[26]

Children with trisomy 21 will demonstrate a wide spectrum of developmental delay. Cervical spine instability is noted, and both occiput-C_1 and C_1-C_2 instability have been described.[27,28] Subluxation of the cervical spine has been reported, making it essential that the anesthesiologist use great caution with head position and during laryngoscopy. These infants and children may also have ligamentous laxity of cervical spine and other ligaments. No consensus exists for appropriate radiologic work-up of children who are asymptomatic for cervical disease, although most have been evaluated before school age (~5 years). Positioning the child for ophthalmologic surgery should include attention to neither overextend nor forcibly rotate the neck.

Children with trisomy 21 may be born with congenital hypothyroidism, or it may develop at any time during their life span. They may develop junctional bradycardia during sevoflurane anesthesia.[29] It is not known whether this is associated with or secondary to occult hypothyroidism. If the child is found to have goiter on examination or has symptoms consistent with hypothyroidism (prolonged jaundice, hypothermia, constipation, dry skin, or relative bradycardia), then thyroid function studies should be obtained before anesthesia for an elective procedure.

Alport Syndrome (Progressive Hereditary Nephritis)

Alport syndrome is one of the disorders in the group of familial oculorenal syndromes. This classification includes Lowe (oculocerebral) syndrome and familial renal-retinal dystrophy. Alport syndrome involves sensorineural hearing loss, progressive renal disease, and multiple ophthalmologic presentations, including cataracts, retinal detachment, and keratoconus.[30,31] The major anesthetic implications pertain to the development of myopathy and renal failure. If myopathy is present, it appears prudent to avoid succinylcholine, with the possible risk of a hyperkalemic response. Renal insufficiency may alter the choice of pharmacologic agents to very-short-acting agents or agents that are not renally excreted.

Marfan Syndrome/Ehler-Danlos Syndrome/Homocystinuria

These disorders are considered together only from the perspective of general body phenotype. The metabolic and molecular causes of these syndromes are well described. They share problems with connective tissue development, possible joint laxity, and cardiovascular implications.

Marfan syndrome is caused by a defect in the gene fibrillin-1 with both elastic and nonelastic connective tissues affected. These children have an increased risk of retinal detachment, lens dislocation, glaucoma, and cataract formation (Fig. 32-2, see website).[32] They may have significant pulmonary (scoliosis) and cardiovascular problems.[33] These may include aortic, mitral, or pulmonic valve insufficiency. Preoperative cardiovascular evaluation is indicated to determine the progression of cardiovascular abnormalities that inevitably occur. Blood pressure control is essential to prevent aortic dissection.

Homocystinuria has at least three forms and different inborn errors. There is an enzymatic deficiency of metabolism of sulfur-containing amino acids. The intermediate metabolite (homocystine) builds up. These children suffer from cataracts, retinal degeneration, optic atrophy, glaucoma, and lens dislocation. The cardiovascular pathology includes coronary artery disease at a young age. Thromboembolic phenomena occur more frequently because they appear to have hypercoagulable tendencies.[34] Nitrous oxide should be avoided because it may further augment accumulation of homocystine by its effect on the metabolic pathways.

Ehlers-Danlos syndrome has thus far been differentiated into at least 10 types. Not all types express significant ocular pathology. From the anesthesiologist's consideration, positioning is important to avoid trauma to the skin. These children tend to develop hemorrhages with minor trauma and delayed wound healing. Cardiac lesions may be present, and preoperative screening should be performed. Hypertension should be avoided to reduce the risk of an aneurysm rupture. Local anesthesia may not last as long in some types of these disorders, and the anesthesiologist and ophthalmologist should have flexible plans in dealing with these children for retrobulbar block or general anesthesia.[35]

Mucopolysaccharidoses

The mucopolysaccharidoses are a group of disorders with enzyme defects that result in incomplete degradation of glycosaminoglycans. These children have a variable degree of mental retardation, macroglossia, airway obstruction, cervical spine instability, and systemic involvement with deposition of mucopolysaccharide material. This leads to cardiac and respiratory dysfunction, airway obstruction, and corneal opacities and glaucoma.

The systemic complications of these disorders are sufficiently severe that even well-planned anesthetic management for ophthalmologic procedures may still result in mortality.[36] Airway management can be extremely difficult with poor mask fit, dynamic airway obstruction and narrowed passages, floppy epiglottis, and difficult visualization of the larynx.[37] Infiltrative material may also be deposited in the laryngeal inlet and pretracheal tissues. Endotracheal intubation may require fiberoptic assistance, and the anesthesiologist should have multiple plans for airway management (see Chapter 12). Cardiac evaluation should be considered before an elective procedure to evaluate ventricular function and the presence of infiltrative disease. Intravenous access may be difficult owing to subcutaneous deposition of mucopolysaccharides.

Craniofacial Syndromes

Craniofacial syndromes may have craniosynostosis or only mid and lower facial structure involvement.[38] Apert and Crouzon syndromes are disorders of craniofacial development that differ only in the presence of syndactyly in the former (Fig. 32-3, see website). They share the potential for multiple ocular pathologic processes and potential difficult mask airway management.[39] Other mutations of the fibroblast growth factor receptor-2 gene cause Antley-Bixler and Pfeiffer syndrome. These children may develop chronic airway obstruction, and some will have complete tracheal rings. Tracheal narrowing should be anticipated, and use of a smaller than standard endotracheal tube size should be anticipated. Children with asymmetry of facial and mandibular bone growth may present with limited opening of the mouth. Children with Goldenhar (hemifacial microsomia), Treacher-Collins syndrome, and Pierre Robin sequence can be expected to present a challenge with airway management (see Chapters 12 and 33).[40] Children with craniosynostosis have an increased risk of congenital heart disease, and a cardiac evaluation should be performed before their first anesthetic.[41] Neurologic morbidity and seizure disorders occur more frequently in this group of disorders.

Phakomatoses

The phakomatoses are neurocutaneous syndromes with multiple ocular pathologic processes. These syndromes include neurofibromatosis,[42,43] encephalotrigeminal angiomatosis (Sturge-Weber syndrome),[44] tuberous sclerosis,[45,46] incontinentia pigmenti, and ataxia-telangiectasia. There is variable central nervous system involvement with each of these diseases. Developmental delay, seizures, and significant neurologic morbidity may be present. Anticonvulsant drugs should be continued in the perioperative period, and electrolyte and hepatic function studies and plasma levels of antiepileptic agents should be evaluated preoperatively.

Ophthalmologic Physiology

Two major considerations of ophthalmologic physiology are of great interest to the anesthesiologist. The first is the dynamics of aqueous humor production and transport with ramifications on IOP. The second is the OCR that may occur during any surgical procedure around the orbit. Anesthetic agents are known to have an effect on IOP. Critically, during a penetrating eye injury, any increase of IOP may be associated with extravasation of elements of the globe and irretrievable loss of vision.

Intraocular Pressure

Intraocular pressure is the pressure exerted by the internal components of the globe on the covering (sclera and conjunctiva). The normal IOP is 12 to 15 mm Hg. An IOP greater than 20 mm Hg is considered abnormal. Aqueous humor is a clear fluid produced by the ciliary body that is released into the anterior chamber of the globe. It traverses the anterior chamber and bathes the iris. It drains through the canal of Schlemm into the pores of Fontana and then the episcleral veins (Fig. 32-4). The posterior chamber, which is larger than the anterior chamber, is composed of a gelatinous mix known as vitreous humor. The sclera and globe that encase the intraocular constituents are relatively noncompliant, protected by the bony orbit. However, intraorbital masses may impinge on the globe and increase the relative IOP or alter the flow of aqueous humor, resulting in increased IOP. Any obstruction to the drainage of aqueous humor will cause build up of fluid within the anterior chamber

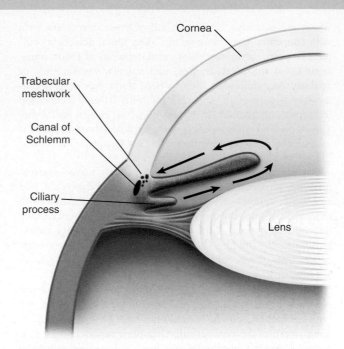

Figure 32-4. Intraocular pressure. Aqueous humor is synthesized in the ciliary process; it then circulates around the iris, past the lens, and into the anterior chamber. After flowing through the trabecular meshwork, aqueous humor enters the canal of Schlemm, which drains into the episcleral venous system. Pathologic conditions that increase venous pressure, obstruct the canal of Schlemm, or increase aqueous humor production may cause an increase in intraocular pressure.

and increase IOP.[47] Increased central venous pressure (such as Trendelenburg position, coughing, Valsalva maneuver, straining, increased intrathoracic pressure) attenuates the drainage of humor from the eye. Arterial pressure does not directly effect changes in IOP. However, as arterial blood pressure increases beyond the normal range, approximately 30% of the increase in systolic blood pressure is reflected in the IOP.

Aqueous humor formation is described in the following equation:

$$IOP = K[(OP_{aq} - OP_{pl}) + P_c]$$

where K is the coefficient of outflow, OP_{aq} is the osmotic pressure of aqueous humor, OP_{pl} is the osmotic pressure of plasma, and P_c indicates capillary pressure. These variables allow the therapeutic intervention of increasing the plasma osmolality acutely with mannitol to lower IOP. This increases the gradient of osmolality and draws water out of the aqueous humor, thereby reducing IOP.

With the relatively noncompliant globe, any pharmacologic or metabolic process that increases choroidal blood volume (hypercapnia, coughing, increased central venous pressure) will lead to choroidal congestion and increased IOP. Although well tolerated in the healthy eye, this congestion may lead to extrusion of contents if the globe is ruptured. The anesthesiologist should carefully control the child's physiology during the induction and maintenance of anesthesia to minimize effects on IOP, regardless if there is a preoperative concern of increased IOP.

Congenital or trauma-induced glaucoma will require therapy to reduce the IOP. If the IOP remains increased, then blood flow in the retina will be impaired, possibly leading to loss of vision. Unfortunately, there are many causes of glaucoma in childhood. Anesthesiologists should utilize their knowledge of physiology and pharmacology to reduce the impact of perioperative care contributing to a process that threatens the child's sight. This includes preventing hypercarbia and hypoxia, avoiding agents known or suspected to increase IOP (succinylcholine and ketamine), and reducing a child's apprehension, crying, and increases in central venous pressure.

The effect of succinylcholine on IOP is well documented.[48,49] Succinylcholine increases IOP 6 to 10 mm Hg, an effect that begins within 1 minute after administration and continues up to 10 minutes, at which time IOP returns to normal. This effect has been attributed to four possible mechanisms:

- Cycloplegia induced by succinylcholine, which obstructs the outflow of aqueous humor
- Tonic contraction of extraocular muscles
- Increased choroidal blood volume
- Relaxation of orbital muscles, which now adds to the external pressure imposed on the globe

Specific muscles appear to develop a sustained tonic tension after succinylcholine that may cause extrusion of intraocular contents if the globe is ruptured.[50] Extrusion of intraocular contents in response to increased IOP depends on the diameter of the orifice: the smaller the laceration (<2 mm), the less the likelihood of extrusion of intraocular contents compared with a larger laceration (>4 mm). Precurarization with a nondepolarizing agent (one-tenth the usual intubating dose) and paralysis with succinylcholine is still advocated by some anesthesiologists to minimize the risk of aspiration in dealing with an open globe injury. Alternatively, rocuronium (1.2 mg/kg IV) can provide optimal intubating conditions in 30 seconds and provides appropriate intubating conditions for the child with the open globe injury while minimizing the risk for aspiration or succinylcholine-associated increases in IOP.

Most general anesthetics decrease IOP,[51] although two are frequently associated with increases in IOP. These are succinylcholine and ketamine.[52,53] Ketamine has been shown to both increase and reduce IOP in children.[53,54] When intravenous access is unavailable or the cardiovascular status of the patient warrants ketamine, the child's overall safety takes precedence over the possible ramifications of ketamine on IOP.

Measurement of IOP is performed by applanation tonometry on the external surface of the globe. Tonometry is often performed along with the EUA during general anesthesia in infants. This prevents an overestimation of IOP in struggling uncooperative infants or children. Borderline measurements must take into account the possible effects of the anesthetic agents temporarily reducing the IOP.

The Oculocardiac Reflex

First described in 1908, the OCR has been recognized as a consequence of ophthalmologic surgery and other conditions.[47] Traction on the extraocular muscles and levator (eyelid elevator) or external pressure applied to the globe may initiate an afferent signal via the trigeminal nerve that evokes an abrupt parasympathetic output of the vagus nerve, resulting in multiple types of dysrhythmias (Fig. 32-5A). These dysrhythmias include sinus or junctional bradycardia, atrioventricular block, ventricular ectopy, or asystole (Fig. 32-5B). Retrobulbar block with local anesthetic may precipitate the trigeminovagal (oculocardiac)

reflex owing to external pressure sensed on the globe, and the local anesthetic may not completely prevent the OCR response to further surgical stimulation or manipulation. For this reason, an anticholinergic medication—atropine (20 µg/kg) or glycopyrrolate (10-20 µg/kg)—is routinely given intravenously at induction of anesthesia or early thereafter. Although these medications do not preclude the occurrence of bradycardia, both decrease its intensity and duration. Because anticholinergics cause pupillary dilatation, they do not present a problem for the ophthalmologist, but these may slightly increase the IOP.

If significant bradycardia occurs, the anesthesia team should have the surgeon release the extraocular muscle or stimulation on the surgical field. An additional intravenous dose of atropine, 5 to 10 µg/kg, will usually interrupt the reflex and correct the situation, but it may recur. Intravenous epinephrine is rarely necessary but should always be available (1-10 µg/kg). The anesthesiologist should ensure adequate oxygenation and ventilation because hypercarbia or hypoxia may compound or intensify the reflex activity.

Other strategies to attenuate the OCR include topically applied lidocaine[55] or intravenous ketamine.[56] In a four-armed study, a ketamine-based anesthetic (10-12 mg/kg/hr) was associated with a decreased incidence of OCR compared with other anesthetic regimens of propofol/alfentanil, sevoflurane/nitrous oxide, and halothane/nitrous oxide.[57] The prevalence of the OCR during sevoflurane and desflurane was similar.[58]

Ophthalmologic Pharmacotherapeutics and Systemic Implications

Topical ophthalmologic medications are usually placed directly on the cornea or in the inferior cul-de-sac. Most of these agents need many minutes to 1 hour for maximal effectiveness. Medications delivered topically to the eye are absorbed through the conjunctiva and nasal mucosa to the systemic circulation. When systemically absorbed, their pharmacologic mechanisms of action predict the systemic consequences; thus, some medications are diluted for use in children to reduce possible systemic toxicity. Anticholinergics, sympathomimetics, and antihistamines can cause pupillary dilation and decrease the movement of aqueous humor, leading to increased IOP. Table 32-3 includes the more commonly used topical agents in pediatric ophthalmology.

Topical mydriatic agents are used to induce pupillary dilatation. The most common agent used is phenylephrine (α_1-adrenergic agonist). Phenylephrine (2.5% solution) is easily absorbed, and in small infants it may cause significant hypertension. Should the hypertension be severe, reflex bradycardia may also occur.

Topical cycloplegic agents dilate the pupil, but in addition these drugs also eliminate lens accommodation by paralyzing the ciliary muscle. This aids in retinal evaluation with the indirect ophthalmoscope and scleral depression and in evaluating refractive errors for which the child is using accommodation for compensation. These agents are muscarinic cholinergic antagonists (also called antimuscarinic agents). Cyclopentolate hydrochloride (0.5%) can cause central nervous system toxicity with disorientation, seizures, and blurred vision. Atropine (0.5%-2.0%) and scopolamine (0.25%) are used for cycloplegia and pupil dilation. Tropicamide (0.5 and 1.0%) is less commonly

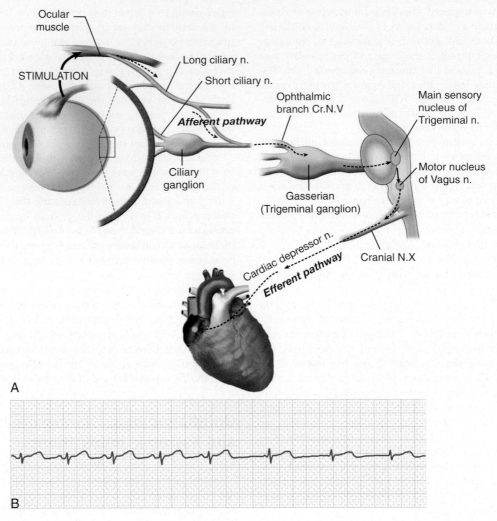

Figure 32-5. Oculocardiac reflex. Traction on the extraocular muscles elicits the oculocardiac reflex. **A,** The afferent limb consists of the long and short ciliary nerves, which synapse in the ciliary ganglion (*dotted arrow*). The ophthalmic division of the trigeminal nerve (cranial nerve V [Cr. N.V]) carries the impulse to the gasserian ganglion; the arc continues to the sensory nucleus of cranial nerve V in the brainstem. Fibers in the reticular formation synapse with the nucleus of the vagus nerve (cranial nerve X [Cranial N.X]). Efferent fibers from the vagus nerve terminate in the heart (*dashed arrow*). The neurotransmitter from the vagus nerve to the sinoatrial node is acetylcholine, and the reflex is blocked by antimuscarinic pharmacologic agents (atropine and glycopyrrolate). **B,** Electrocardiogram showing conversion from normal sinus rhythm to a nodal rhythm.

used in children. When systemically absorbed, these agents may result in antimuscarinic anticholinergic toxicity, including tachycardia, dry mouth, pupillary dilatation, flushing of the skin, heat intolerance/fever, and disorientation (Fig. 32-6, see website).

β-Adrenergic blockers (e.g., timolol, betaxolol) are used to reduce IOP in the treatment of glaucoma. Systemic absorption causes symptoms of sympathetic nervous system blockade. β-Adrenergic antagonists induce bradycardia and cardiovascular collapse and may precipitate bronchospasm. If β-adrenergic intoxication is suspected, then direct-acting cardiovascular stimulants (epinephrine) should be used to antagonize the β-adrenergic blockade rather than ephedrine with its indirect mechanism of action.

Topical local anesthetics are not frequently used in children except for the very cooperative child for tonometry or removal of sutures. Proparacaine and tetracaine are available for topical use, and lidocaine and bupivacaine are used for retrobulbar blocks. Absorption of the esters (proparacaine and tetracaine) has little potential for systemic toxicity owing to the extensive metabolism by cholinesterases. Ophthalmic amide agents, however, do have the potential for systemic toxicity (cardiac dysrhythmias and seizures) but are not frequently used in children. Cocaine is rarely used in pediatric ophthalmology because it has been noted to cause corneal injury. As an excellent vasoconstrictor, it is still utilized to reduce nasal bleeding during nasal and nasolacrimal duct surgery.

Nonsteroidal anti-inflammatory agents are used for certain inflammatory conditions of the eye, but perioperative use in a child is uncommon. The nonsteroidal anti-inflammatory drugs (NSAIDs) are of concern for the ophthalmologist because they may be associated with increased perioperative bleeding locally. Systemically administered NSAIDs (ketorolac, ibuprofen) have anticoagulant profiles and may contribute to surgical bleeding.

Table 32-3. Commonly Used Ophthalmologic Agents

Drugs	Indication	Side Effect Profile
Cholinergic Agonists		
Carbachol	Induce miosis	Corneal edema, retinal detachment
Pilocarpine	Glaucoma	Corneal edema, retinal detachment
Cholinesterase Inhibitors		
Physostigmine	Glaucoma	Retinal detachment, miosis
Echothiophate	Glaucoma	Retinal detachment, miosis
Muscarinic Antagonists		
Atropine Scopolamine Homatropine Cyclopentolate Tropicamide	Similar for all agents in the class: cycloplegic retinoscopy	Similar for all agents in the class: photosensitivity, blurred vision, increased heart rate, dry mouth
Sympathomimetic Agents		
Dipivefrin	Glaucoma	Side effect profiles similar for all agents in the class: photosensitivity, hypersensitivity
Epinephrine	Glaucoma	
Phenylephrine	Mydriasis	
Apraclonidine	Glaucoma	
Brimonidine	Glaucoma	
Cocaine	Local anesthetic	Anisocoria, corneal injury
Hydroxyamphetamine	Glaucoma	Anisocoria
Naphazoline	Decongestant	
Tetrahydrozoline	Decongestant	
α- and β-Adrenergic Antagonists		
Dapiprazole (α)	Reverse mydriasis	Conjunctival hyperemia
Betaxolol (β_1-selective)	Glaucoma	Bradycardia, hypotension
Carteolol (β)	Glaucoma	↓ heart rate, blood pressure, bronchospasm
Levobunolol (β)	Glaucoma	↓ heart rate, blood pressure, bronchospasm
Metipranolol (β)	Glaucoma	↓ heart rate, blood pressure, bronchospasm
Timolol (β)	Glaucoma	↓ heart rate, blood pressure, bronchospasm

Modified from Brunton LL, Lazo, JS, Parker KL (eds): Goodman and Gilman's The Pharmacological Basis of Therapeutics, 11th ed. New York, McGraw-Hill, 2006.

However, five NSAIDs are approved for ocular use: diclofenac, bromfenac, flurbiprofen, ketorolac, and nepafenac. Diclofenac, bromfenac, and nepafenac are used as postoperative anti-inflammatory agents. Ketorolac has been used to treat macular edema after cataract extraction.

Echothiophate (Phospholine Iodide) is a cholinesterase inhibitor used to induce miosis in the treatment of glaucoma. When absorbed systemically, it impairs plasma cholinesterase, thus reducing the metabolism of drugs, including succinylcholine and mivacurium. Decreased metabolism of acetylcholine may result in increased relative cholinergic tone, inducing bradycardia and bronchiolar muscle activity, resulting in bronchospasm. Toxicity from echothiophate may be antagonized by administration of pralidoxime (2-PAM), 25 mg/kg intravenously. Otherwise, its action to reduce effective systemic cholinesterases lasts 4 to 6 weeks.

Pilocarpine is a direct-acting cholinergic agonist and is used to treat glaucoma. Through multiple actions, it improves the flow of aqueous humor. If absorbed, it may acutely cause bradycardia.

Many vitreal substitutes are used in ophthalmologic procedures. These include nonexpansile and expansile gases (i.e., sulfur hexafluoride), perfluorocarbon liquids, and silicone oils. The anesthesia team should be informed when the ophthalmologist plans intraocular use of one of these substances. If a gas pocket will be anticipated, then nitrous oxide should be discontinued or not used at all. When a perforated globe is closed, any residual environmental air pocket could also be expanded by nitrous oxide. Increased ocular pressure and reduced retinal blood flow may result.

Another novel agent being studied in retinal angiogenic diseases is bevacizumab (Avastin).[59] In the doses prescribed, this would not be expected to be of any anesthetic concern but visual outcome of any infant will certainly be monitored for all perioperative care provided.

Emergent, Urgent, and Elective Procedures

One of the greatest controversies in pediatric anesthesia is the best method for induction of anesthesia in a child with an open globe injury and a full stomach.[50] The issue of aspiration while securing the airway versus the possible extravasation of intraocular contents from an increase in IOP is a difficult "risk-balance" assessment. The debate is likely to continue because the risks are real and the incidence of either phenomenon is rare, difficult to study, and probably underreported.

One study has shown that, in adults, aspiration is a relatively rare event with low mortality; there has been no reported mortality in children.[60] Despite the report from more than 60,000 children in the database, the absolute risk of aspiration in children at induction is unknown. Although it is the more rapid-acting muscle relaxant, the use of succinylcholine for rapid-sequence induction in the presence of a perforated globe has been challenged because of its known propensity to increase the IOP. The development of faster-acting nondepolarizing agents such as rocuronium has provided the anesthesiologist alternatives to succinylcholine. High-dose rocuronium provides excellent intubating conditions[61] with the added advantage that rocuronium reduces IOP by its neuromuscular junction blocking effect on extraocular muscles. However, if the child is not adequately induced and fully paralyzed during instrumentation of the airway, then any episodes of coughing, retching, or increased systolic blood pressure may increase IOP. Lidocaine, 1 to 2 mg/kg intravenously, attenuates the hemodynamic responses to laryngoscopy and endotracheal intubation, but this is not a consistent experience.[62,63] Pretreatment with opioids have been proposed to achieve a similar effect (sufentanil [0.05-0.15 µg/kg], morphine [0.03 mg/kg], and remifentanil [0.1 µg/kg]), although they are not consistently recommended. Although reported to blunt the IOP response to intubation, opioids may also induce vomiting, thus increasing IOP.

Intravenous access is essential for a rapid induction of anesthesia. In most instances, children with ruptured globes present with intravenous access because it is critical to begin parenteral antibiotics as soon as possible (i.e., within 6 hours of the rupture) to prevent endophthalmitis, which, if untreated, may result in complete loss of vision in that eye. In some instances, however, intravenous access is not always present. When intravenous access has failed, options to induce anesthesia include:

- Placement of a central line
- Intramuscular ketamine (and succinylcholine or rocuronium)
- Mask induction with sevoflurane/halothane
- Placement of an intraosseous needle
- Rectal methohexital

None of these alternatives is easy. Placement of a central line may be very challenging in a nonsedated or noncooperative child. Absorption of agents given intramuscularly can be quite variable. Although succinylcholine will dependably induce paralysis in a few minutes, the child may cry from pain, develop hypertension, vomit, or experience direct succinylcholine-induced increases in IOP. The latency to action (possibly 2 to 8 minutes) and gradually paralyzed airway reflexes in a child with a full stomach are significant risks.

An argument for placement of an intraosseous needle for induction can be made when intravenous access has not already been established. Even with local anesthetic, the placement of an intraosseous needle would be poorly tolerated by a conscious child. Mask induction with sevoflurane may facilitate induction of anesthesia; but if only a light plane of anesthesia is reached, then coughing and vomiting may occur. The overpressure technique should be used to achieve a rapid and deep plane of anesthesia. Then intravenous access should be attempted. If this is not successful, an intramuscular dose of muscle relaxant is administered.[64-66] In this circumstance the IOP may go up and aspiration is possible. Rectal methohexital (30 mg/kg) is only used in infants; and if the child evacuates part of the dose, then the induction is incomplete.[67] Also there is no rectal absorption of a neuromuscular relaxant so either intramuscular or intravenous administration becomes necessary.

A moderate approach to the child who needs emergent or urgent ophthalmologic surgery is to secure intravenous access as quickly and painlessly as possible. An attempt is made to preoxygenate the child without causing distress. If a tight mask fit is not easily achieved, then forcing the tight fit to the child's face is not desirable owing to the likelihood of increasing IOP as the child resists. Intravenous induction with propofol or thiopental and rocuronium is performed. Either by monitoring 60 to 90 seconds by a watch or clock or train-of-four monitoring, endotracheal intubation is performed as expeditiously as possible and the gastric contents are evacuated as soon as feasible. *The ophthalmologist should be intimately involved in the induction. He or she can physically protect the injured eye with a metal or plastic shield to prevent further injury and assist the anesthesiologist by holding the endotracheal tube and suction apparatus immediately within reach of the field of view of the airway.*

Other urgent procedures might include treatment of retinopathy or decompression of orbital cellulitis. These procedures may be urgent but still allow a number of hours of NPO status. Concern for aspiration may not be as great. Nonetheless, the surgeon will wish to proceed as expeditiously as can be allowed. Options for induction and maintenance may or may not include succinylcholine.

Most ophthalmologic procedures are performed on a scheduled basis, allowing routine preoperative evaluation and planning. This includes establishing all relevant medical information about the child, NPO status, and possible intravenous catheter placement if desired.

Induction and Maintenance of Anesthesia

Intravenous or inhalational induction of anesthesia may be performed in infants and children for most elective ophthalmologic procedures. Most infants will not require a premedicant for anxiolysis, and the use of premedication after the first year of life is usually discussed between the anesthesiologist and the parents and/or child. Separation anxiety or struggling during induction will not usually affect most ophthalmologic diagnoses except for a penetrating eye injury that may become worse if the child struggles.

Intravenous propofol, sodium thiopental, etomidate, or ketamine produce a smooth induction and the anesthesiologist can then support and secure the airway as planned. Inhalation induction with oxygen, nitrous oxide, and either sevoflurane or halothane also produces smooth induction states. Should laryngospasm develop during induction, an intravenous or intramuscular neuromuscular relaxant should rapidly be administered to break the laryngospasm. For planned endotracheal intubation, an intravenous nondepolarizing muscle relaxant is preferred because succinylcholine may raise IOP. Intramuscular administration of succinylcholine or rocuronium[64-66,68-70] may also resolve laryngospasm if an intravenous catheter has not been placed.

Alternate induction methods include intramuscular administration of ketamine (4-10 mg/kg) and, in infants, rectal methohexital (25-30 mg/kg). Ketamine may increase IOP but has been successfully reported in ophthalmologic procedures in children.[56] Rectal methohexital will have a dependable latency to induction of general anesthesia of 7 to 8 minutes, but its elimination may be quite variable and its respiratory depressant effects may linger. Rectal methohexital is infrequently used at the present time.

Endotracheal intubation is our preference for most pediatric ophthalmologic procedures, except for rapid examination under anesthesia or nasolacrimal duct probing. With the secured endotracheal tube, the child and operating table may be safely turned 90 or 180 degrees for optimal positioning for the surgeon. The weight of surgical drapes will be less of an impediment to maintaining ventilation with positive-pressure ventilation than allowing the child to spontaneously ventilate with an LMA or unsecured airway.

An immobile child may be essential to the optimal surgical outcome. If the surgeon requires immobility, the endotracheal tube placement is essential so that neuromuscular relaxants can be safely administered and continued for a possibly undetermined length of time for completion of the procedure. We utilize cuffed and uncuffed endotracheal tubes. If an uncuffed tube does not provide sufficient control of ventilation, we do not hesitate to change to a larger-diameter uncuffed tube or replace the first tube with a cuffed tube to ensure proper ventilation. The endotracheal tube is secured so that the sterile field may be maintained for the procedure. Access to the endotracheal tube and anesthesia circuit by the anesthesia care team without trespass of the surgical field is imperative. It is important to recognize that extensions to the anesthetic circuit have no bearing on the dead space of the circuit, whereas extensions beyond the Y in the circuit (i.e., adjacent to the tracheal tube) will add dead space to the circuit and may compromise ventilation.

Maintenance of anesthesia can be accomplished with many techniques. Inhalation sevoflurane, isoflurane, or desflurane may provide excellent conditions for maintenance of anesthesia[58] and rapid emergence. Emergence from halothane anesthesia is generally slower. We reinforce the need for communication with the ophthalmologist regarding the necessity of an absolutely immobile field. When neuromuscular blockade is necessary, we routinely utilize nondepolarizing neuromuscular relaxants and train-of-four monitoring to ensure the adequacy of surgical conditions. Carefully titrated doses of opioids are used as an anesthetic adjunct if postoperative pain is anticipated.

Strabismus surgery is associated with the greatest incidence of PONV after any surgery in children (45% to 85%).[71] Numerous investigations have identified factors associated with the anesthetic and surgery that affect this incidence. Evidence has shown that the type of ventilation does not attenuate the incidence of PONV.[72] Fluid replacement has a significant effect on the risks of PONV (see later). Avoiding opioids during strabismus surgery may also be effective.[73,74] Nonopioid analgesics such as acetaminophen,[75] diclofenac,[76] and ketorolac[73,74] may be used. If opioids are needed, short-acting medications are preferred: remifentanil, alfentanil, or fentanyl. There is some evidence to suggest that the more extraocular muscles that require surgery[77] and specific muscles that require more traction (inferior oblique) may increase the incidence of PONV, although these data have not been firmly established.

A host of medications can significantly affect the risks of PONV. Preoperative benzodiazepines,[78] avoidance of nitrous oxide,[79] superhydration with balanced salt solutions, propofol,[79,80] clonidine,[81] 5-HT$_3$ receptor antagonists,[82-86] dimenhydrinate,[87,88] metoclopramide,[86,89] dexamethasone,[90-94] and delaying oral fluid ingestions after surgery[95] all attenuate the incidence of PONV. In the cases of clonidine and 5-HT$_3$ receptor blockers, there is a dose-response relationship with PONV,[81,82] although this is not true with dexamethasone.[90] Older antiemetics such as droperidol that have been very effective in attenuating the incidence of PONV[75,96-99] have fallen into disfavor because of their sedative side effects and concerns associated with prolonged QT interval,[100] although the latter has not been a common problem in children.[101]

Anesthesiologists have adopted a multimodal approach to PONV in the case of strabismus surgery. Premedication with oral midazolam, choice of anesthesia, superhydration with intravenous fluid, and the combination of 5-HT$_3$ receptor antagonists and dexamethasone is a commonly used regimen. There is no evidence in children undergoing strabismus surgery that dosing 5-HT$_3$ receptor antagonists at the end of surgery provides better protection against PONV than earlier in the surgery.[102] There is a dichotomy of practice with respect to maintenance of anesthesia. Some avoid nitrous oxide, maintaining anesthesia by propofol infusion and including the just-mentioned supplementary medications. Others use nitrous oxide and an inhalational anesthetic for maintenance but also include the remainder of the preoperative and intraoperative supplementary medications.

Intravenous fluid replacement has been shown to reduce PONV.[103] Children who present for elective surgery drink clear fluids up to 2 hours before surgery, reducing the fasting period. However, it is important to identify those children who have fasted for a prolonged period, to administer sufficient parenteral fluids to replenish their volume status. We recommend calculating the infant or child's fluid deficit and plan to administer 50% to 100% of the calculated deficit to reduce the incidence of PONV. Others have administered large volumes (30 mL/kg) of balanced salt solution and reported that the incidence of PONV is reduced compared with smaller volumes (10 mL/kg).[104] When the surgical procedure is not likely to involve an increased IOP, we routinely replace nearly 100% of the calculated deficit. We have not observed children to experience urinary retention or hypertension from this strategy. However, if the duration of surgery exceeds 3 hours, then we catheterize the bladder to reduce the risk of urinary retention and overdistention of the bladder.

At the completion of surgery, neuromuscular relaxation is antagonized, maintenance agents are discontinued, and the child is allowed to awaken. Deep extubation is preferred by some to reduce coughing and increases in IOP at the time of extubation.[105] Others prefer extubating the trachea when the child is fully awake with intact airway reflexes, although coughing and increases in IOP may occur. For most procedures in children, a short interval of increased IOP will not damage a surgical correction (e.g., strabismus, ptosis, or ROP treatment). Appropriate postoperative analgesics may include local anesthetics, acet-

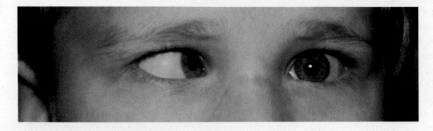

Figure 32-7. Strabismus repair is a common pediatric ophthalmologic procedure. This child demonstrates significant right esotropia that requires surgical correction.

aminophen, and opioids. Nonsteroidal agents are generally not given to these children for concern of perioperative bleeding at the surgical site owing to their mild anticoagulant profile, but ketorolac has been reported as useful.[73] Lorazepam may also have some utility.[78] Postoperatively, withholding oral fluids until the child expresses a desire to drink reduces the incidence of PONV.[95]

Specific Ophthalmologic Procedures

Strabismus repair is common in children.[85] Corrective surgery realigns the divergent visual axes of the eyes by detaching and reattaching extraocular muscles to the globes (Fig. 32-7). The procedures may be brief if only one or two muscles are involved. In infants, inhalation or intravenous induction is performed and neuromuscular blockade is provided with nondepolarizing neuromuscular relaxants. Strabismus may be an isolated finding in a child or a manifestation of other systemic diseases or syndromes.[106] The anesthesiologist should carefully review the birth history, history of prematurity, central nervous system disorders, syndrome identification, possible coexistent myopathy, and cardiovascular and respiratory history. He or she should also anticipate the OCR and pretreat with atropine or glycopyrrolate. PONV is common and may be reduced by multiple strategies (Table 32-4).

We avoid succinylcholine for routine use in children in general; and in this circumstance if succinylcholine is utilized, the surgeon should be informed because it may alter the forced duction testing and thus affect the planned repair.[107] After induction of anesthesia and tracheal intubation, the operating room table is rotated to permit complete access to the orbits. It is common to use a preformed tube that lies flat against the mandible.[108] The endotracheal tube is positioned away from the surgical field. Ventilation may be spontaneous or controlled if the surgery is extraocular. If, however, the surgery is intraocular or medical conditions dictate, controlled ventilation may be preferred. Some anesthesiologists are willing to perform strabismus repair using an LMA with spontaneous ventilation.[109] Although regional block is performed in some adults, strabismus surgery in children is routinely performed with general anesthesia.

Anterior Chamber Paracentesis

An anterior chamber paracentesis may be performed in children for evaluation of uveitis, infection,[110] leukemia[111] or for removal of fluid to decrease IOP. Because the field needs to be sterilized and the needle will enter a small target area of the anterior chamber, the child should be placed under general anesthesia to make the field immobile for the surgeon.

Dacryocystorhinostomy

Infants may be born with nasolacrimal duct stenosis (congenital dacryostenosis) (Figs. 32-8 and 32-9 [see Fig. 32-9 on website]). If conservative measures do not demonstrate improvement, the ophthalmologist may need to dilate the duct or pierce a residual membrane with a solid probe.[112,113] These infants are induced with general anesthesia; and when the level of anesthesia is sufficient, the ophthalmologist can perform the procedure in a few

Table 32-4. Antiemetic Strategies Proposed for Prophylaxis and Treatment of Postoperative Nausea and Vomiting

Strategy	Drug and Dose
Butyrophenone (dopamine antagonist)	Droperidol (10-70 µg/kg)
Serotonin-5HT₃ antagonists	Ondansetron (0.1 mg/kg)
	Granisetron (10-40 µg/kg)
	Dolasetron (0.35 mg/kg)
Propofol-based total intravenous anesthesia	Propofol (100-175 µg/kg/min)
Local anesthetic	Lidocaine local-topical and systemic (1-1.5 mg/kg)
Opioid-sparing analgesics/anesthetics	Retrobulbar block with bupivacaine
Other pharmacology	Dexamethasone (10-500 µg/kg): maximum, 8 mg
	Dimenhydrinate (0.5-1 mg/kg)
	Metoclopramide (0.15-0.25 mg/kg)
	Benzodiazepines (lorazepam, midazolam (10-100 µg/kg)
	Avoid N₂O.
	Avoid opioids; use (ketorolac [Toradol], 0.5 mg/kg PO, IV, IM; acetaminophen, 30-40 mg/kg PR; diclofenac, 1 mg/kg PR) or use short-acting opioids (remifentanil, alfentanil, fentanyl).
Nonpharmacologic adjuvants	Intravenous hydration
	Gastric decompression

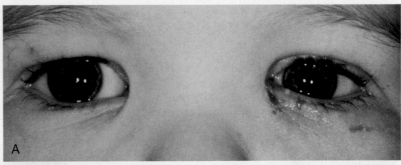

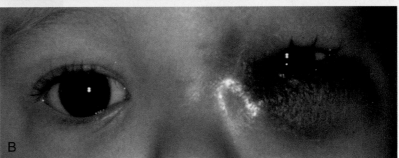

Figure 32-8. Nasolacrimal duct obstruction. Infraorbital inflammation is present to differing degrees from mild obstruction with minor infection and mucoid material accumulation (**A**) to severe obstruction with periorbital or preseptal cellulitis (**B**), and both may require dacryocystorhinostomy procedures.

minutes. The ophthalmologist perforates the membrane with a metal probe. To confirm the duct has been perforated, the ophthalmologist can touch the probe in the duct with a second probe inserted into the nostril. Alternately, the ophthalmologist can inject fluorescein into the nasolacrimal duct and detect the fluorescein in the nasal airway by inserting a pipe cleaner and observing fluorescein on the pipe cleaner. In both instances, fluorescein and/or blood may accumulate in the nasopharynx and reach the larynx. To prevent these secretions from triggering laryngospasm it is prudent to tilt the operating table into Trendelenburg position and place a small roll under the shoulders to pool the fluids in the nasopharyngeal region. These secretions should be suctioned out of the oropharynx and nasopharynx before emergence. Anesthesia may be maintained by mask inhalation or with intravenous agents. The airway and respirations are carefully monitored (visually and by capnography). The infant is awakened, and postoperative analgesia may be offered with acetaminophen and/or opioids as necessary.

Alternatively, an endonasal endoscopic approach may be used for complicated or recurrent dacryorhinocystotomy.[114,115] This makes the procedure significantly longer and will require airway control to facilitate the surgeon's approach and to protect the child from aspirating blood during the procedure.

Ptosis Repair

Ptosis (blepharoptosis) is drooping of the eyelid. This can be congenital or acquired and may be associated with amblyopia or astigmatism. If eyelid closure is complete in infancy, occlusion amblyopia will occur. This may require urgent attention. Otherwise, surgery for ptosis is often performed in later childhood years. The surgical approaches require a quiet surgical field, and the surgeon makes great effort to produce a symmetrical repair.

Cataracts

Cataracts are opacifications of the lens of the eye (Fig. 32-10). Cataracts in children may be congenital, post-traumatic, or metabolic in origin.[116] Congenital cataracts require surgery very early in life to permit photostimulation of the retina.[117] Although the surgery can be performed as an outpatient, the relatively young infant may require monitoring for postoperative anesthetic-induced respiratory depression or apnea. Cataracts are noted in some systemic diseases, and intraocular lens implants are often offered to improve long-term visual prognosis.[118] The child should be examined carefully for dysmorphology, with close attention to issues of airway management and the cardiorespiratory system.

Enucleation

Enucleation of the eye may be necessary when a child has an intraocular tumor (e.g., retinoblastoma) (Fig. 32-11),[119] a ruptured globe or ocular trauma,[120] recurrent/chronic infections, or a blind painful eye. *Leukocoria* is the term used for "white pupil." The differential diagnosis is extensive and includes many intraocular tumors. Other disorders causing leukocoria include Coat's disease, cataract, coloboma, and *Toxocara canis*.

When necessary, the entire globe must be removed. The entire eyeball is removed and all bleeding points are coagulated. The OCR may occur during this procedure and may be attenuated by local infiltration with local anesthetic. PONV is also frequently described.

Vitrectomy

Vitrectomy may be necessary for retinal injury or detachment induced in circumstances of nonaccidental trauma or ROP.[121] Any infant or child presenting acutely with a closed-head injury from suspected abuse should have an ophthalmologic consultation to completely evaluate all orbital structures.[122] These delicate tissues may demonstrate pathology that requires long-term follow-up or urgent medical/surgical therapy. Glaucoma may occur with hyphema or from lens subluxation/dislocation with tearing of the support tissue. Early diagnosis is paramount if surgical intervention is to have the greatest benefit.

Retinopathy of Prematurity

As described earlier, preterm infants may present with multiple ocular pathologic conditions but none are more frequent than ROP. ROP has been extensively studied,[15] and multiple collaborative trials have reported their results and recommendations for medical and surgical intervention.[123-127] The etiology is still unknown, but oxygen-related theories have been described for more than 40 years. Owing to this concern, oxygen range targeting has become more common,[128-130] to reduce the oxidative stress[131] on the infant in general and reduce the effect of oxygen on the neovascularization occurring in the eye.

Laser and cryotherapy are common treatments for this condition.[123,124] With the delicacy and exacting accuracy required in

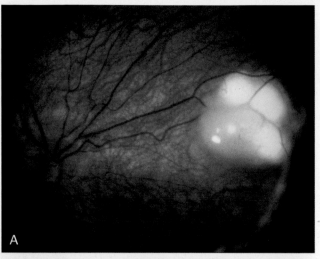

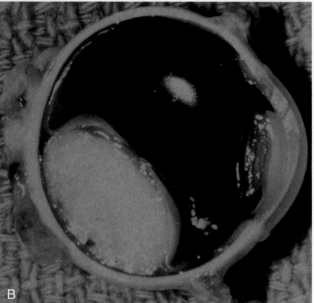

Figure 32-11. Retinoblastoma is one of many intraocular tumors that may require enucleation. **A,** Retinoblastoma seen by direct ophthalmoscopy. **B,** Pathologic specimen of a retinoblastoma in the globe after enucleation.

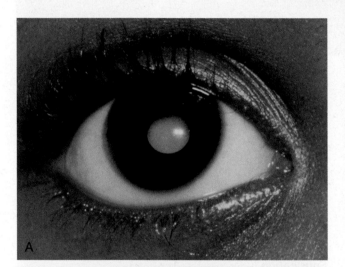

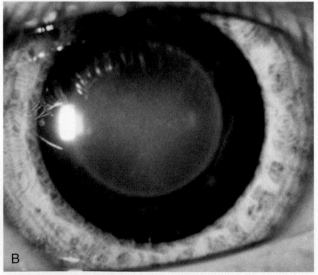

Figure 32-10. Cataracts. **A,** The right red reflex is absent in this child with a cataract that requires removal. **B,** This close-up photograph is of a nuclear cataract, associated with many inborn errors in childhood. Cataracts that are not central or spherical may be caused by trauma or abuse.

laser procedures, we routinely intubate the trachea and utilize neuromuscular relaxants. This facilitates the immobile field necessary for the surgeon and has been demonstrated to provide better perioperative physiologic stability for the infant.[132] The complications of prematurity determine whether extubation is possible, and many infants will require postoperative ventilation, if only for a brief period or overnight. Attention should be made to keep the operative environment warm to reduce thermal stress on the infant.

Acknowledgment

We wish to acknowledge the prior contributions to this chapter of Susan A. Vassallo, MD, and Lynne R. Ferrari, MD.

Annotated References

Askie LM, Henderson-Smart DJ, Irwig L, Simpson JM: Oxygen-saturation targets and outcomes in extremely preterm infants. N Engl J Med 2003; 349:959-967

Advances in neonatology continue to reduce morbidity and mortality in these fragile children. Oxygen-saturation targeting is becoming mainstream. This has implications for the management and oxygen support strategies for infants coming to the operating room for ocular and other surgical procedures. Because volatile anesthetics are known to impair hypoxic pulmonary vasoconstriction, a supplemental oxygen requirement should be anticipated but oxygen-saturation targets should be considered for optimal care.

Borland LM, Colligan J, Brandom BW: Frequency of anesthesia-related complications in children with Down syndrome under general anesthesia for noncardiac procedures. Paediatr Anaesth 2004; 14:733-738

Down syndrome children have multiple systemic conditions of importance to the anesthesiologist. These are not exclusively of interest due to congenital heart disease. Anesthesia-related complications occur more frequently in children with Down syndrome than other children presenting for noncardiac surgery, and prevention of complications is essential with thorough evaluation and planning.

Cunningham AJ, Barry P: Intraocular pressure—physiology and implications for anaesthetic management. Can Anaesth Soc J 1986; 33:195-208

This review elegantly details the physiology of intraocular pressure and conditions that may increase IOP. Structural, physiologic, and pharmacologic considerations are reviewed in detail.

Donahue SP: Clinical practice. Pediatric strabismus. N Engl J Med 2007; 356:1040-1047

Strabismus is a very common presenting condition for surgical therapy in children. Significant improvements in the detection and treatment of strabismus are reviewed. Surgical approach and recent advances are presented.

Stephen E, Dickson J, Kindley AD, et al: Surveillance of vision and ocular disorders in children with Down syndrome. Dev Med Child Neurol 2007; 49:513-515

Children with Down syndrome demonstrate many different ocular disorders. With the multiple systemic issues of concern for the anesthesiologist referenced in the chapter, this reference provides an insight to the ocular diseases that may present for surgical therapy.

References

Please see www.expertconsult.com

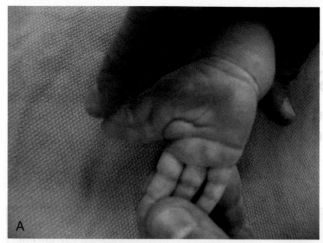

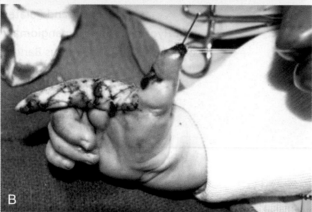

Figure 33-2. Syndactyly of the first and second digit of an infant: dorsal aspect (**A**) and volar aspect (**B**).

perinatal period that lead to the diagnosis, others may go undetected until they present for anesthesia (no familial inheritance pattern has been identified). In these infants, a preoperative electrocardiogram and a cardiology consult are recommended. Surgery is usually performed between 6 and 18 months of age.[11] Unless full-thickness skin grafting is required, regional anesthesia provides excellent intraoperative and postoperative analgesia (see Chapters 42 and 43 for specific limb blocks).

Trauma

A considerable proportion of plastic surgical procedures in children occur for trauma and emergency surgery. Procedures include treatment of simple lacerations, animal bites, tendon and nerve repair, reimplantation of digits and limbs, and treatment of burns (see Chapter 34). The cooperative and fasted child with minor trauma can often undergo minor surgical procedures using local anesthesia, commonly administered by the plastic surgeon in the emergency department. This can be supplemented with inhalation of a 50:50 mixture of nitrous oxide and oxygen (Entonox)[12] or intravenous administration of small doses of a benzodiazepine and opioid (e.g., midazolam, 50 μg/kg, and fentanyl, 0.5 μg/kg) according to locally established sedation protocols (see Chapters 46 and 48).

Surgery for extensive injuries to digits and limbs usually requires general anesthesia because children do not tolerate prolonged tourniquet application. The severity and urgency of the injury dictate the timing of the surgery. The general principles of care for the child with trauma should be followed (see Chapter 39), with particular attention directed to elucidating the presence of other, more life-threatening injuries. For urgent surgery in the presence of a full stomach, precautions against aspiration of gastric contents should be considered. For postoperative pain control, a combination of regional anesthesia and/or systemic analgesia is usually adequate. Continuous brachial plexus or other nerve blocks may improve tissue perfusion[13] and facilitate cooperation during postoperative physiotherapy for procedures such as digital reimplantation. The surgeon must always be cognizant of the risk of continuous nerve blocks in masking the signs associated with compartment syndrome, and frequent and meticulous attention must be paid to perfusion of the extremity.

Specific Plastic Surgical Procedures

Craniosynostosis

Craniosynostosis, a congenital anomaly in which one or more cranial sutures closes prematurely, occurs in approximately 1 in 2,000 births, affecting males more frequently than females. Embryologically, the cranial vault starts to ossify at the eighth week after conception. Fusion of the parietal and frontal bones is usually completed by the seventh month. Postnatally, the anterolateral fontanelle closes by 3 months, the posterior fontanelle by 3 to 6 months, the anterior fontanelle by 9 to 18 months, and the posterolateral fontanelle by 2 years. Premature osseous obliteration of a suture might result from the absence of osteoinhibitory signals from the suture. Craniosynostosis may be categorized as simple, involving one suture, or complex, associated with a variety of syndromes and metabolic diseases (Table 33-1).

Table 33-1. Classification of Craniosynostosis

Nonsyndromic (primary) 95%
Syndromic (more than 150 described)
Crouzon's
Apert's
Pfeiffer
Saethre-Chotzen
Muenke's
Crouzonodermoskeletal
Shprintzen-Goldberg
Loeys-Dietz
Jackson-Weiss
Beare-Stevenson
Cole-Carpenter
Kleeblattschädel
Fibroblast growth factor receptor (FGFR) mutations 1 and 2
Metabolic and Other Causes
Rickets
Bone metabolic disorders (hypophosphatasia)
Achondroplasia
Prematurity

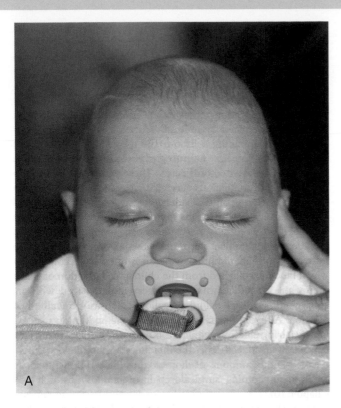

Figure 33-4. A, An infant with classic craniosynostosis. The shape of the child's head may not reflect the severity of the defect. The defect is best appreciated by 3D MRI reconstruction.

In the child with craniosynostosis, the head may assume various shapes depending on the sutures involved (Fig. 33-4 [see website for Fig. 33-4B-D]). The most common sutures involved in order of frequency are sagittal suture, then coronal, then metopic. The coronal suture is more commonly associated with syndrome-based craniosynostoses.

Although most craniosynostoses are isolated, they are associated with more than 150 syndromes (see Table 33-1). Apert's syndrome occurs in approximately 1:100,000 live births, usually owing to sporadic mutations, although autosomal dominant inheritance patterns can occur from affected parents. This syndrome phenotypically manifests as cloverleaf skull (craniosynostosis), hypertelorism, proptosis, midface hypoplasia, and syndactyly (upper or lower extremity). Whether children with Apert's syndrome develop normal IQs is unclear. In a study of 60 children with Apert's syndrome, the authors determined that 32% developed IQs greater than 70.[14] Cranial surgery before 1 year of age was associated with an IQ greater than 70 in more than 50% of children, whereas surgery at beyond 1 year of age was associated with an IQ greater than 70 in only 7%. Two other factors predicted improved IQ results: absence of a defect in the septum pellucidum and noninstitutional residence (i.e., family home residence). Crouzon's syndrome is phenotypically similar to Apert's syndrome but lacks digital involvement. Fifty percent of the cases of Crouzon's syndrome are sporadic mutations, with 40% being familial. Pfeiffer syndrome occurs in approximately 1:25,000 live births. Most cases are familial with an autosomal dominant inheritance pattern, although many remain sporadic. The phenotype of Pfeiffer syndrome is very similar to that of Apert's syndrome with several differences: broad thumb, large

first toe, and polydactyly. Children with Pfeiffer syndrome all develop normal intelligence. A relatively new, but rare syndrome, Shprintzen-Goldberg syndrome, phenotypically resembles Marfan syndrome (with the associated secondary organ involvement) and craniosynostosis.

Indications for cranial vault reconstruction include hydrocephalus, raised intracranial pressure (ICP), and psychosocial reasons. If uncorrected, the deformed cranium may cause severe neurologic sequelae, including visual loss and developmental delay (see Chapter 23).[15-27] Because rapid brain growth during infancy determines skull shape, surgical correction is undertaken within the first months of life to achieve the best cosmetic results. Cranial vault reconstruction may involve the anterior or posterior aspect of the skull or both (total cranial vault reconstruction). Alternatively, surgical correction may employ an extended strip craniectomy in which the cranial vault is split in multiple segments, allowing the skull to grow with the brain (Fig. 33-5 [see website for Fig. 33-5B, C]). This technique is utilized in children younger than 6 months of age and is perceived to be less invasive than total cranial vault reconstruction; however, children are required to wear a protective helmet after surgery.[28,29] Postoperative pain is generally not severe and is managed effectively with a combination of acetaminophen, NSAIDs, and/or intravenous opioids.

Airway Management

Airway management during craniosynostosis surgery can be challenging; meticulous preoperative planning and evaluation of the airway is essential. The face may be difficult to fit with a face mask, nasal passages may be obstructed, and the trachea may be difficult to intubate. External fixator devices on the face may compound the difficulties with the airway (Fig. 33-6, see website).

It is essential that all equipment for management of the difficult airway be present in the operating room before induction of anesthesia (see Table 12-9). Techniques used to gain control of the difficult airway include the use of a flexible fiberoptic bronchoscope, light wand,[30] Glidescope, retrograde intubation, LMA,[31] and others (see Chapter 12). With the "two person intubation technique," the first anesthesiologist applies external

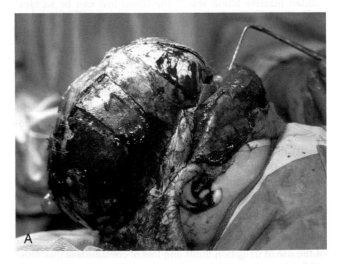

Figure 33-5. A, Child immediately before surgical closure after total cranial vault reshaping using strip craniectomy for sagittal craniosynostosis.

surgery and the transfusion of large volumes of relatively cold intravenous fluids. Effective measures to prevent hypothermia include warming the operating room, insulating the child, and the use of forced air warmers and warming devices for blood and intravenous fluids (see Chapter 25).

Orbital Hypertelorism

The term *orbital hypertelorism* describes abnormally separated orbits. This deformity may occur in isolation or in association with a number of congenital abnormalities, such as facial clefts and Apert's syndrome (Fig. 33-7). Surgical repair involves mobilization and repositioning of the orbit through either a subcranial approach, which leaves the roof of the orbit intact, or an intracranial approach via a frontal craniectomy. This procedure is performed in children older than age 5 years who may have already undergone extensive surgical reconstruction. Surgical manipulation of the globe may elicit the oculocardiac reflex, resulting in bradyarrhythmias or asystole. These arrhythmias are prevented by administering a prophylactic anticholinergic such as intravenous atropine (20 μg/kg) or glycopyrrolate (10 μg/kg). The presence of a difficult airway influences the anesthetic technique, but in most instances an inhalational induction is used. After establishing intravenous access, the airway should be secured using a preformed orotracheal tube. Blood loss from multiple osteotomies may be significant; and, as in the case of craniosynostosis surgery, methods to reduce the use of homologous blood should be considered. Intraoperative management follows the principles outlined for craniosynostosis surgery. At the conclusion of surgery, the trachea is extubated and the child is monitored overnight in a high-dependency setting with the capability of managing acute airway obstruction.

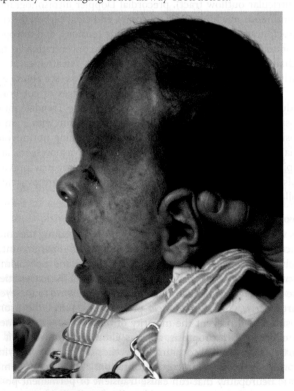

Figure 33-7. Child with Apert's syndrome. Notable features include proptosis, cloverleaf skull, maxillary hypoplasia, and syndactyly (the last feature is present in Apert's syndrome but not in Crouzon's syndrome).

Midface Procedures

Midface advancement to improve facial appearance is commonly required for children with maxillary hypoplasia, such as those with Crouzon's syndrome, Apert's syndrome (which is phenotypically Crouzon's syndrome with syndactyly) (Fig. 33-7), and Pfeiffer syndrome (which phenotypically resembles Apert's syndrome with polydactyly (Fig. 33-8, see website).[77-79] This procedure is typically carried out in preschool children, although complications such as proptosis, corneal ulceration, ocular dislocations, and airway obstruction may necessitate earlier intervention.[79-82] A LeFort II procedure is a similar approach to a LeFort III but the osteotomy is oriented vertically through the infraorbital rim. Thus, the nasal pyramid and the maxilla move forward as a single unit. Le Fort III osteotomy and monobloc procedures (Fig. 33-9) have the potential for significant complications, including massive blood loss, airway difficulties, cerebrospinal fluid leak, and infection.[75,83-85]

Anesthetic concerns are similar to those for orbital hypertelorism and craniosynostosis. Children with Apert's and Crouzon's syndromes often present with incomplete or complete nasal obstruction that results from choanal atresia and/or midface hypoplasia. As a consequence, mask anesthesia can be very difficult even with an oral airway. However, laryngoscopy and tracheal intubation in these children is usually uncomplicated. The diameter of the tracheal tube requires careful consideration because these children may require prolonged postoperative ventilation until postoperative facial and laryngeal edema has resolved. The decision to intubate the trachea via the oral or nasal route must be discussed with the surgeon before induction of anesthesia. A nasotracheal tube can be used throughout the procedure, or the surgeon may request an intraoperative change from the oral to the nasal tracheal position after completing the midfacial osteotomies.[86] To perform the latter maneuver, the anesthesiologist wears a sterile surgical gown and gloves and uses sterile equipment, including laryngoscope, Magill forceps, and tube exchange catheter (see Fig. 12-24). Visualizing the glottis in the midst of the surgery may be difficult because of the presence of airway edema and blood in the hypopharynx. A tube exchange catheter is passed through a naris and into the trachea alongside the orotracheal tube. The nasal tube is then passed over the exchange catheter, and its tip is positioned at the glottic opening. The oral tube is then removed, and the nasal tube is advanced (rotating the bevel 90 degrees clockwise or counterclockwise as needed to pass the arytenoids) and visualized passing through the glottic aperture. Once the tube position is confirmed, the catheter is removed and the nasal tube is sutured securely to the nasal septum. Given the proximity of the tracheal tube to the surgical site, damage to the tracheal tube can occur during surgery.[87,88] Vigilance is required at all times to detect an accidental disconnect or damage to the tracheal tube. The anesthesiologist must be prepared to rapidly respond to an unexpected interruption in ventilation and replace the tracheal tube. A nasogastric tube is placed after surgery to prevent gastric distention and reduce the likelihood of postoperative nausea and vomiting. A wire cutter must be available at the bedside at all times if intermaxillary fixation is used to stabilize the facial bones and mandible. In the intensive care unit, the presence of an audible leak around the tracheal tube is an important criterion to determine the presence of laryngeal or periglottic edema and, therefore, readiness for tracheal extubation.[87]

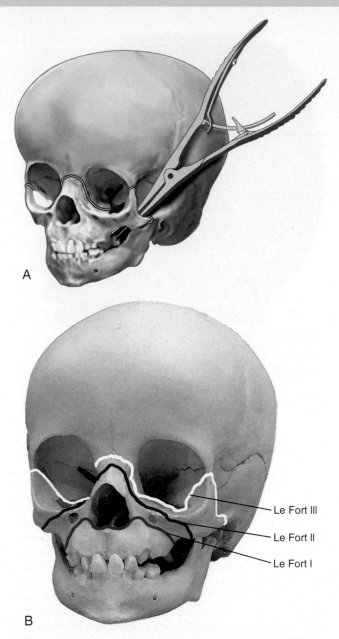

A

B

Figure 33-9. Le Fort III (**A**) and monobloc procedures (**B**) for correction of midface hypoplasia. The osteotomies in the Le Fort III procedure pass through the nasofrontal junction, across the medial orbital wall and floor into the inferior orbital fissure. A cut through the frontozygomatic suture, pterygomaxillary junction, and zygomatic arch allows separation of the midface. The monobloc procedures are similar, but the nasofrontal junction and frontozygomatic suture are not mobilized. This technique allows simultaneous correction of supraorbital and midface deformities at the expense of an increased incidence of postoperative complications.

Le Fort III

Le Fort II

Le Fort I

Orthognathic Surgery

Malocclusion secondary to maxillary or mandibular hypoplasia (such as occurs in hemifacial microsomia and Treacher Collins syndrome), tumors, trauma, as well as temporomandibular joint dysfunction are generally accepted indications for orthognathic surgery. LeFort I procedures for maxillary hypoplasia involve a transverse incision through the maxilla to advance the upper teeth into normal occlusion with the mandible. Children who

are candidates for this surgery are typically adolescents because these procedures are performed once maxillary and mandibular growth is complete. Because this age group usually exhibits increased perioperative anxiety, preoperative assurance and education and premedication with oral midazolam (0.5-0.75 mg/kg, up to 20 mg) are often necessary.

Airway management is a major concern, particularly in those with a hypoplastic mandible or temporomandibular dysfunction.[89] A high index of suspicion of atlantoaxial instability is required if rheumatoid arthritis is the underlying disease process. The anticipated difficult airway can be managed using fiberoptic intubation, with sedation and/or topical local anesthesia or an inhalation induction, as discussed earlier. Nasotracheal intubation using a preformed tracheal tube is the preferred method of intubation. Careful stabilization and fixation of the tube such as trans-septal suturing to prevent unintended extubation is often employed. Excessive pressure on the ala nasi must be avoided by padding the forehead and stabilizing the tube to avoid cranial traction on the tube. If intermaxillary fixation is employed postoperatively, wire cutters must be immediately available and the child must be monitored in an intensive care setting. LeFort I advancements require very close communication between the surgery and anesthesia teams because the nasotracheal tube has been known to become dislodged once the maxilla is fully mobilized.

To reduce intraoperative blood loss, controlled hypotension is commonly employed using any of a range of pharmacologic agents, including inhalational anesthetic agents, β blockers, sodium nitroprusside, and remifentanil. The literature is extensive on the salutary effect of induced hypotension in reducing intraoperative blood loss and improving the quality of the surgical field during orthognathic surgery.[90-99] Invasive blood pressure monitoring is indicated to monitor blood pressure continuously during controlled hypotension and to facilitate intraoperative evaluation of blood gases and hematocrit. In some cases, a mild degree of hypotension is all that is required to provide optimal surgical conditions (systolic blood pressure 85 to 90 mm Hg). Dexamethasone (0.2 mg/kg) may reduce postoperative airway edema.[100] After the return of protective airway reflexes, the trachea is extubated and the child is monitored overnight in a high-dependency setting with the facilities to establish an airway should acute airway obstruction develop.

Hemifacial Microsomia and Treacher Collins Syndrome

Hemifacial microsomias, also known as otomandibular dysostosis (Fig. 33-10), result from a malformation of the first and second branchial arches. These disorders are classified according to the OMENS classification (orbital distortion, mandibular hypoplasia, ear anomaly, nerve involvement, and soft tissue deficiency).[89,101-104] Airway difficulty increases with the complexity of the defect from unilateral to bilateral involvement. The disorder may include mandibular hypoplasia, temporomandibular joint dysostosis, cleft palate, and auricular, ophthalmologic, and facial nerve defects. Goldenhar's syndrome (Fig. 33-11 [see website for Fig. 33-11B, C]) is the most common form of this disorder. Vertebral anomalies are present in 40% and congenital heart defects occur in 35% of children with this syndrome. Airway management in children is complicated because of midfacial hypoplasia, asymmetry of mouth opening, and mandibular retrognathia. Overall, tracheal intubation is easy in 70% and very difficult in 9% of children with unilateral hemifacial micro-

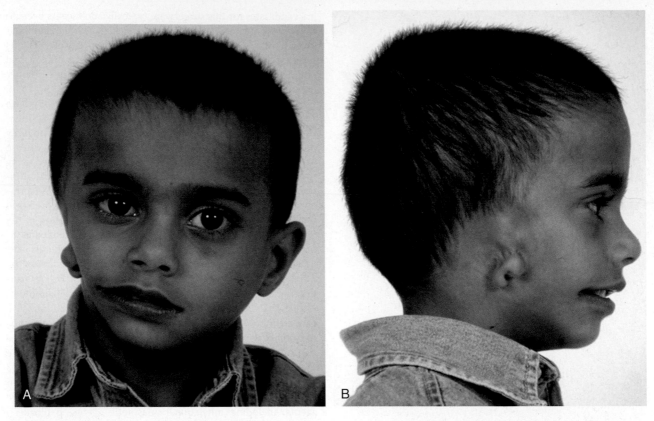

Figure 33-10. Frontal (**A**) and lateral (**B**) views of unilateral hemifacial microsomia. In the lateral view, microstomia and mandibular and ocular deformities are evident. These children may present with either unilateral or bilateral hemifacial microsomia with a hypoplastic mandible and maxilla, together with ear deformities.

somia.[101] In contrast, the incidence of easy, difficult, and very difficult intubation is evenly distributed at 30% to 35% in children with bilateral mandibular hypoplasia.[101] The airway anomalies associated with this syndrome predispose to obstructive sleep apnea.

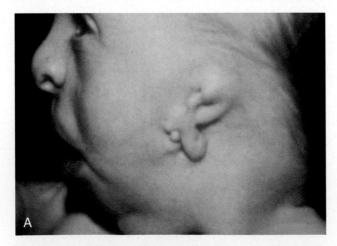

Figure 33-11. A, Goldenhar's syndrome in an infant. This is one of the most common forms of hemifacial microsomia. With unilateral hemifacial microsomia, the airway is usually managed and instrumented without difficulty, but with bilateral mandibular hypoplasia, the airway may be very difficult to manage in one third of afflicted children.

The craniofacial abnormalities of mandibular hypoplasia, macrostomia, and cleft palate in Treacher Collins syndrome (Fig. 33-12, see website) make airway management challenging. The airways in these children become increasingly difficult with age.[89,101] Other clinical features of the syndrome include hypoplastic zygomatic arches, ophthalmic features (including sloping palpebral fissures, coloboma of the eyes, and notched lower eyelids) and microtia, choanal atresia, cardiovascular defects, and renal anomalies. Maintenance of spontaneous respiration until successful tracheal intubation is confirmed is essential. The use of an LMA can be helpful to maintain the airway or if a guide is needed to perform fiberoptic bronchoscopy. The surgical procedure determines whether preformed oral or nasal tracheal tubes are to be used.

Cleft Lip and Palate

Cleft lip and palate are among the more common congenital malformations, occurring with an estimated incidence of approximately 1:700 births worldwide.[89] More common in males than in females, this malformation likely results from both environmental and genetic causes. These disorders are associated with more than 300 syndromes, of which the more common are presented in Table 33-2. Cleft lip and palate occur as a defect of palatal growth in the first trimester. Cleft lip can reliably be diagnosed by ultrasound at 18 to 20 weeks after conception, whereas palatal cleft is diagnosed by examination after delivery. Primary cleft lip repair is undertaken at approximately 3 months of age, and primary cleft palate repair is done at around 6

Table 33-2. Syndromes Commonly Associated with Cleft Lip and Palate

Pierre Robin sequence

Down syndrome

Klippel-Feil syndrome

Treacher Collins syndrome

Velocardiofacial syndrome

Fetal alcohol syndrome

Nager syndrome

Goldenhar's syndrome

months. Surgery for lip and/or nose revision usually takes place in early childhood, and palatal revision and alveolar bone grafts occur at approximately 10 years of age. Rhinoplasty and maxillary osteotomy to complete the repair may take place at 17 to 20 years of age.

Pharyngoplasty may be required for velopharyngeal incompetence secondary to anatomic or neurologic dysfunction to allow normal speech development and to prevent nasal regurgitation during eating.

Anesthetic Considerations

Surgical correction of cleft lip defect is usually performed at 3 months of age to allow sufficient time for maturation and associated abnormalities to become apparent. Preoperative assessment may reveal abnormalities such as mandibular hypoplasia in Pierre Robin sequence (Fig. 33-13 [see website for Fig. 33-13B-D]) and restricted neck movement in Klippel-Feil syndrome (Fig. 33-14, see website).[89] *Pierre Robin sequence* is defined as micrognathia, glossoptosis (caudally displaced insertion of the tongue), and respiratory distress in the first 24 to 48 hours of life. A retrospective study of infants and children who had undergone cleft lip and palate surgery reported that the incidence of difficult intubation was greater in children presenting

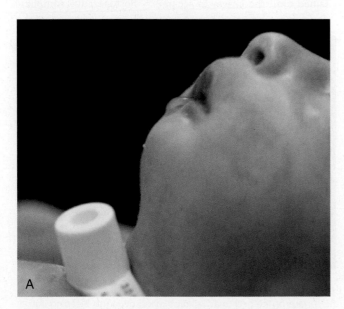

Figure 33-13. A, This child with Pierre Robin sequence required a tracheostomy because of respiratory distress in the first 24 hours postnatally. The retrognathia is often associated with glossoptosis, which makes visualization of the glottic aperture more difficult.

for bilateral cleft lip and cleft palate repair when compared with unilateral lip defects.[105] However, this study included infants and children with micrognathia, which itself could be a cause of difficult intubation because it reduces the hyomental space and displaces the tongue backward. The incidence of difficult laryngoscopy was 50% in those with micrognathia but only 3.8% in those without. Intubation difficulty decreased as age increased, with the greatest difficulty being present in infants younger than 6 months old, which may reflect mandibular growth with increasing age. In our experience, tracheal intubation is not abnormally difficult to achieve in the majority of infants and children with cleft lip or palate.

Induction of anesthesia via face mask is usually uncomplicated in infants with cleft lip and palate. Laryngoscopy should be performed using a straight blade inserted via the right commissure of the mouth into the right pharyngeal gutter so as to displace the tongue to the left (paraglossal approach), taking care to prevent the blade from entering the cleft. If the mandible is hypoplastic, posterior laryngeal pressure may be required to visualize the larynx. In some centers, the tongue is sutured to either the mandible or lower lip to preclude airway obstruction in infants with Pierre Robin sequence in the postnatal period. In such instances, the tongue cannot be displaced to the left to expose the larynx. To facilitate laryngoscopy in such cases, the tongue is released from the lower lip using ketamine sedation; if direct laryngoscopy fails to expose the larynx, a rigid bronchoscope is then inserted after anesthesia is induced by inhalation while the tongue is released.

A variety of tracheal tubes can be used to secure the airway for cleft lip and palate surgery, although the ideal tracheal tube is perhaps the oral RAE tube, which can be fixed centrally to the chin to facilitate optimal surgical access. Reinforced tracheal tubes are a suitable alternative but in either case, care must be taken to fix the tube at the correct length. Throat packs usually impinge on the surgical field and are not normally required for cleft palate repair. The lungs are ventilated for the duration of the procedure, usually 1 to 2 hours. Inhalational or intravenous anesthetics combined with a short-acting opioid such as fentanyl (1-2 μg/kg) can be used for maintenance of anesthesia. Bilateral infraorbital nerve blocks may be used to provide postoperative analgesia for cleft lip repairs; such blocks will reduce the need for opioids and antiemetics and improve the ability to feed.[106]

During cleft palate surgery, the pharyngeal space is reduced dramatically (Fig. 33-15C [see website for Fig. 33-15A, B]). Because the child is at risk for acute upper airway obstruction due to upper airway narrowing, edema, and residual anesthetic effects,[107-112] the trachea is extubated after complete return of upper airway reflexes. Upper respiratory tract infections are common in this age group; antibiotic treatment may reduce the incidence of postoperative respiratory complications.[113]

Blood, edema, and unfamiliar suture lines in the oropharynx can preclude easy laryngoscopy and tracheal intubation should emergency re-intubation be needed after surgery. A nasopharyngeal airway can be inserted by the surgeon before extubation to permit suctioning the airway without damaging the palatal repair and to provide a patent airway. Arm restraints to prevent suture disruption are used in many centers. Observation for signs of upper airway obstruction is required in the recovery period for 48 hours.[107] As soon as the child is awake, feeding with clear fluids is allowed.

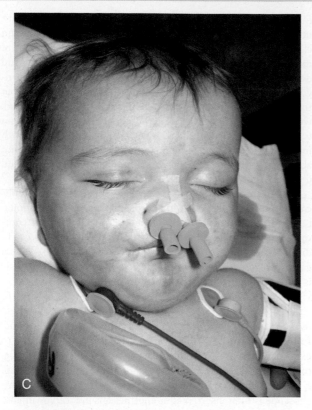

Figure 33-15. C, Nasal airways are often placed at the end of cleft palate or pharyngoplasty surgery to ensure that a patent airway is maintained.

Postoperative pain is managed with opioids in combination with acetaminophen. Sphenopalatine and infraorbital nerve blocks placed by the surgeon at the end of the procedure using a long-acting local anesthetic are particularly useful for management of pain after cleft lip and palate repair.[106] Opioid infusion or nurse-controlled analgesia are effective for the first day after

surgery. The future of cleft lip and palate repair may lie in in-utero techniques, which promise to provide superior wound healing without scarring.[1]

Children who are scheduled for elective pharyngoplasty are usually of school age, having undergone cleft palate repair at an earlier age. The primary objective of this procedure is to restore velopharyngeal competence for speech development, which can be achieved by a pharyngeal flap, sphincter pharyngoplasty, or palatal lengthening (Furlow double-opposing Z-plasty palatoplasty). The anesthetic goals and management are similar to those discussed for cleft palate repair earlier in this section. A careful review of previous anesthetic records may forewarn of a difficult airway.

Cystic Hygromas and Hemangiomas

Cystic hygroma is a rare congenital malformation of the lymphatic system occurring with an incidence of 1 in 16,000 births, most frequently involving the axilla and neck (Fig. 33-16A, B [see website for Fig. 33-16B]). The pathology consists of multiple loculated cysts that contain lymph fluid or blood (see Fig. 33-16C). In most cases, cystic hygromas are present at birth, although 80% to 90% are diagnosed within the first 2 years of life. The natural history is spontaneous resolution, although most require repeated aspirations, sclerotherapy, or surgical excision to debulk the mass (see Fig. 33-16D, on website).[114-116] Cystic hygroma can be associated with other chromosomal abnormalities such as Noonan's and Turner's syndromes, in which case the anesthetic management is guided by the underlying syndrome. Some children will require an urgent tracheostomy in the first hours of life to relieve airway obstruction (see Chapter 38). During the preoperative assessment, the airway should be examined for involvement of supraglottic and infraglottic structures. Acute airway obstruction can occur during induction if cystic lesions are present in the upper airway. Fiberoptic intubation may be required if the larynx is distorted by the lesions, in which case spontaneous ventilation should be maintained until the airway is secured.[117] Postoperative complica-

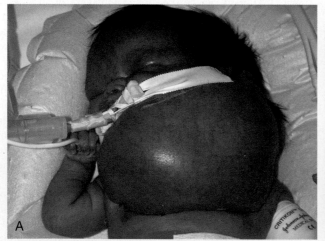

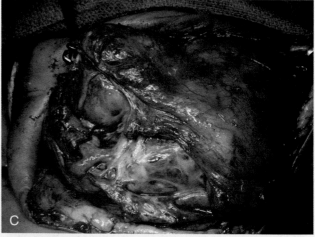

Figure 33-16. A, Cystic hygroma. Note that the bulk of the tumor is extraoral and extralaryngeal, although extension into the tongue and supraglottic region may complicate direct laryngoscopy. The tumor on the surface of the neck may rapidly expand owing to bleeding into the cysts or accumulation of fluid in the lymphatics. Such large tumors may put the overlying skin under great tension. They may also be situated such that they preclude tracheostomy. **C,** Gross pathology in cystic hygromas consists of a combination of multiloculated cysts that may contain a combination of lymph fluid and/or blood. Debulking may result in substantial blood loss. Sequential debulking of the hygroma may be required as the residual cysts expand with fluid and blood and re-expand the hygroma.

tions of surgical excision include laryngeal edema, airway obstruction, pneumonia, facial palsy, and infection.[114,115,118]

Hemangiomas are the most common benign tumors in infancy, affecting up to 10% of infants.[119] The majority of hemangiomas are uncomplicated and require no treatment. The natural course begins with a proliferation phase that starts within the first few months of life, followed by an involution phase of variable length. It is estimated that involution occurs at a rate of 10% per year. Hemangiomas can affect all organs, and intervention is required when the lesion affects the function of vital organs such as the eyes, airway, or liver.[120] Hemangiomas that occur in the subglottic region must be considered in the differential diagnosis of a noninfectious cause of croup in infants younger than 3 months of age. Hemangiomas that are present around the eyes and on the face (Fig. 33-17) are often associated with airway hemangiomas.[121,122] Rarely, large hemangiomas can result in high-output heart failure.

Treatment options for hemangiomas include active nonintervention, systemic corticosteroid treatment, corticosteroid injection, surgical excision, and laser ablation. Surgical treatment is reserved for superficial hemangiomas in locations that are surgically accessible.[120] Laser treatment for superficial lesions is commonly performed as a day case procedure,[123] and routine anesthetic precautions should be taken.

Arteriovenous malformations are present at birth but can go unrecognized for years, especially when they are intracranial. Large arteriovenous malformations may cause high-output cardiac failure, necessitating therapeutic intervention. Treat-

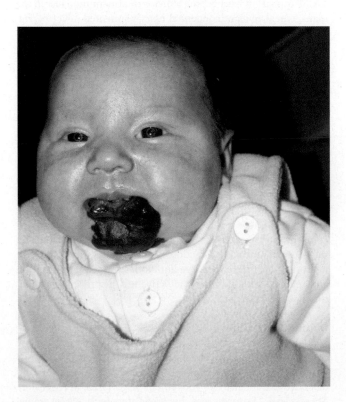

Figure 33-17. Facial hemangioma in the cheek of a child. The hemangioma involves the skin overlying the mandible centrally from the lower lip to the tip of the mandible. Hemangiomas vary widely in size but can enlarge precipitously as a result of bleeding into the tumor.

ment options may include chemotherapy, corticosteroid therapy, embolization, and surgical excision. Children who undergo excision of the hemangiomas often require blood products during surgery, but platelets should be transfused with care because an accumulation within the malformation may increase its size.[124] Nonsteroidal anti-inflammatory drugs should be avoided because of their effects on platelet function.

Congenital Intraoral Fibrous Bands

Congenital intraoral fibrous bands (e.g., pterygium syndrome and syngnathia) can make securing the airway almost impossible to achieve even with advanced pediatric fiberoptic skills (Fig. 33-18, see website). Depending on the severity of the bands, these children may present formidable anesthetic challenges. Intravenous ketamine anesthesia in the spontaneously breathing neonate may allow division of the adhesions in the first few days of life.[125]

Intraoral Tumors

Intraoral tumors are rare in children (Fig. 33-19, see website) but, if massive, may present great challenges in securing the airway. Those that present the greatest difficulties preclude visualizing the larynx (Fig. 33-20, see website) and present an increased risk for intraoperative bleeding. Preoperative radiographic studies should delineate the extent of tumor involvement in the upper airway: that is, is the supraglottic region clear and is the nasopharynx clear for passage of a bronchoscope? If the tumors are sufficiently large that laryngoscopy is not possible, fiberoptic nasal intubation must be considered. If the tumor is resectable, then tracheostomy should be a back-up plan. The risk of bleeding depends on the vascularity of the tumor and the involvement of the tongue. If the vascular supply of the tumor can be isolated, then bleeding should be easily controlled. If, however, the tumor cannot be separated from the tongue, then bleeding can be controlled only by clamping the tongue before resecting the tumor. This should prevent excessive blood loss and permit a hemostatic closure of the resection surface.

Brachial Plexus Surgery

Brachial plexus injury occurs in 0.5 to 4.6 per 1,000 live births as a result of birth trauma.[126] Erb's palsy affects the nerve roots C5, C6, and C7, whereas Klumpke's palsy affects C8 and T1. Complete plexus palsies are the most devastating injuries, resulting in a flail and insensate arm.[127] Although most cases of brachial plexus injury resolve spontaneously, surgical intervention is indicated if the motor function does not improve after 3 months of age.[128,129] For surgery to be successful, the nerve root cannot be completely avulsed from the spinal cord. Therefore, detailed imaging is required to characterize the nature of the injury: avulsion of the nerve root from the spinal cord, disruption of the nerve within the nerve sheath, and disruption of the nerve and the nerve sheath. Because irreversible loss of the neuromotor end plate may occur, surgery is often undertaken before 12 months of age.[126,128-132] Microsurgical repair is currently the treatment of choice and includes resection of neuromas with interpositional nerve grafting.[133] Donor nerves include motor branches of C4, intercostal nerves, inferior branches of the 11th cranial nerve, pectoral nerves, and sural nerves.[134]

Infants who undergo brachial plexus reconstruction are generally completely healthy except for the nerve injury. These cases may be challenging in that the only extremity for intravenous access and monitoring (blood pressure and pulse oximetry) is the contralateral upper extremity. Both lower extremities are usually prepped and draped for harvesting the sural nerves or other donor nerves for the repair. Because these infants are usually 9 to 12 months of age, they are chubby, making intravenous access more difficult. This surgery often takes up to 12 hours, so the considerations for prolonged anesthesia must be implemented. Care must be taken to protect pressure points during positioning. Muscle relaxants are avoided to facilitate intraoperative electrophysiologic testing.[135] An indwelling urinary catheter is essential to decompress the bladder. Analgesic requirement is minimal except during brief periods of surgical stimulation. Remifentanil provides excellent intraoperative analgesia and permits rapid adjustment of the depth of anesthesia. Maintenance of normothermia and prevention of fluid overload are important during this prolonged surgery. Blood loss is minimal, and maintenance fluids usually suffice.[126] Postoperative analgesia requirements are minimal, and acetaminophen and NSAIDs usually provide adequate pain relief. Shoulder spica casts can be applied to avoid sudden neck movements postoperatively if the lower branches of the accessory nerve are used for reconstruction.[136]

Hairy Pigmented Nevi

Congenital melanocytic nevi characteristically vary in size, shape, surface texture, and hairiness. They are frequently excised because they may be disfiguring and have the potential to become malignant. Serial surgical excision is common, but skin grafting and tissue expanders are also used (Fig. 33-21A, see website).[137] The position and size determine the frequency of excision and anesthetic technique. If the face, head, or neck is involved, airway management should be discussed with the surgeon to allow optimal surgical access (Fig. 33-21B).

In general, these children are healthy. In the cooperative and motivated child, local subcutaneous infusion of a very dilute local anesthetic (e.g., ropivacaine 0.08% to 0.3%) mixed with epinephrine 1:1,000,000 can be used to provide painless tumescent anesthesia.[138] The local anesthetic is infused through a 30-gauge needle at an initial rate of 120 mL/hr. Blanching of skin identifies the area that is anesthetized. This method has been

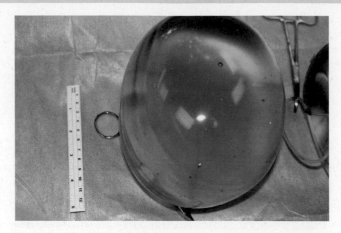

Figure 33-22. Tissue expander that is approximately 18 cm long. These expanders are inserted in a partially deflated state and then expanded by sequentially injecting saline over a period of weeks.

used successfully in children 7 years of age and older.[139] To avoid toxicity, local anesthetic volume and dosing guidelines should be followed (see Chapter 42). The addition of longer-acting local anesthetics to the infiltrate will enhance postoperative analgesia. Repeated reconstructive procedures are often required, and attention should be paid to the need for appropriate premedication where necessary (see Chapter 4)

Tissue Expanders

Tissue expansion has become a major treatment modality in the management of giant congenital hairy pigmented nevi (see Fig. 33-21A on website), hemangiomas, meningomyelocele, abdominal wall defects, and secondary reconstruction of extensive burn scars.[140-148] Tissue expanders effectively allow removal of the affected area and preserve sensation in a durable flap with minimal donor site morbidity.[137] Tissue expanders consist of a silicone shell that stretches to accommodate serial injections of saline when placed subcutaneously or, in the case of the scalp, under the galea, through an incision made in normal tissue adjacent to the lesion or defect (Fig. 33-22).[144,149] Tissue expansion requires at least two surgical procedures, one to insert the expander and a second to remove it, when expansion is complete; some children may require serial insertions.[144] Reconstruction of areas of the head and neck constitute a particular challenge because expansion without oral, visual, or airway compromise is required.[150] Complications of tissue expansion include skin erosion, infection, leakage, migration, and flap necrosis.[147,151-154] Perioperative antibiotics are given at insertion and removal, although their effectiveness in preventing infection has not been established.[137,142,147,152,153]

Möbius Syndrome

Möbius sequence is a rare neurologic disorder characterized by congenital palsy of the facial (VII) and abducens (VI) cranial nerves, resulting in unilateral or bilateral facial weakness and defective extraocular eye movement (Fig. 33-23, see website). These classic features may be associated with other cranial nerves palsies, ophthalmic abnormalities, developmental delay, and various craniofacial, limb, and musculoskeletal malformations, resulting in a variable pattern of clinical expression.[155-159] Involvement of cranial nerves IX and X is associated with pha-

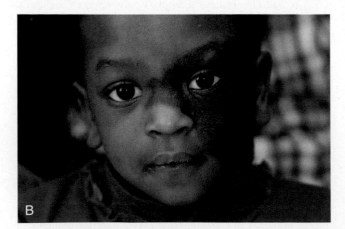

Figure 33-21. B, Here a heavily pigmented nevus covers the lateral aspect of the face from the eyebrow, over the bridge of the nose, and down to the skin covering the mandible. These large and disfiguring pigmented nevi must be resected in staged events.

ryngeal dysfunction, dysphagia, feeding difficulties, retention of oral secretions, and recurrent aspiration pneumonia. Associated micrognathia, microstomia, limited mouth opening, and other orofacial abnormalities may make tracheal intubation difficult.[160] Other associations include gastroesophageal reflux, hypotonia of skeletal muscles, congenital cardiac abnormalities, spinal abnormalities, and peripheral neuropathies. Central alveolar hypoventilation has been described in association with Möbius sequence and may be secondary to hypoplasia of midbrain respiratory centers.[161] Central alveolar hypoventilation, compounded by upper airway hypotonia and the effects of sedatives, opioids, and anesthetic agents, can predispose to postoperative respiratory compromise. The absence of facial expression secondary to paresis of the facial nerve can make it difficult to assess and evaluate postoperative pain.[162] The anesthetic plan for the child with Möbius sequence must be tailored to the individual based on the clinical expression of the syndrome.

The most common surgical procedure performed in children with Möbius sequence is a segmental gracilis muscle transplantation, in which a segment of gracilis muscle is transplanted to the face and revascularized to the facial artery and vein.[163] Motor innervation of the gracilis requires a functioning cranial nerve such as the masseter branch of the trigeminal nerve. The aim of this facial reanimation is to facilitate facial expression and provide lower lip support to reduce drooling and improve speech.[163] Anesthetic considerations for this procedure include those for prolonged surgery, avoidance of neuromuscular block to facilitate intraoperative nerve stimulation, and avoidance of hypocapnia, hypothermia, and hypotension to ensure graft perfusion. The latter considerations are also applicable to the postoperative period. Other surgical procedures commonly performed in children with Möbius sequence include strabismus surgery and orthopedic procedures to improve limb function.

Acknowledgments

The authors thank R. Zuker, MD, FRCS, Professor of Surgery, Division of Plastic Surgery; C. Forrest, MD, FRCS, Associate Professor of Surgery, Head of the Division of Plastic Surgery, The Hospital for Sick Children, University of Toronto, Toronto, Ontario; and J. Girotto MD, Assistant Professor of Pediatrics, Neurosurgery and Plastic Reconstructive Surgery, Director of the Cleft and Craniofacial Center, Golisano Children's Hospital at Strong Memorial Hospital, University of Rochester, Rochester, NY, for providing photographs to illustrate this chapter.

Annotated References

Antony AK, Sloan GM: Airway obstruction following palatoplasty: analysis of 247 consecutive operations. Cleft Palate Craniofac J 2002; 39:145-148

Two hundred and forty-seven children underwent palatoplasty, yielding a 6% incidence of perioperative airway obstruction. The airway obstruction occurred as late as 48 hours postoperatively. Twelve of the 14 children with severe airway compromise required continued tracheal intubation, re-intubation, and tracheostomy. Thirteen of these 14 children (93%) had coexisting craniofacial abnormalities, with 7 having Pierre Robin sequence.

Faberowski LW, Black S, Mickle JP: Incidence of venous air embolism during craniectomy for craniosynostosis repair. Anesthesiology 2000; 92:20-23

This case series of 23 children undergoing craniosynostosis reported an 83% incidence of venous air embolism using precordial Doppler monitoring. Although cardiovascular collapse did not occur, 32% developed hypotension. Detection and early intervention are important strategies to prevent cardiovascular collapse associated with this type of surgery.

Hans P, Collin V, Bonhomme V, et al: Evaluation of acute normovolemic hemodilution for surgical repair of craniosynostosis. J Neurosurg Anesthesiol 2000; 12:33-36

This randomized study of 34 children who required craniosynostosis repair showed no benefit of acute normovolemic hemodilution compared with routine care in terms of blood transfusion. However, this study was not powered a priori. The small volume of surgical blood loss and the limited number of children raise the possibility of a type II statistical error.

Nargozian C: The airway in patients with craniofacial abnormalities. Paediatr Anaesth 2004; 14:53-59

This review summarizes the salient features and airway implications of the major craniofacial disorders that afflict children, including Pierre Robin sequence, Treacher Collins syndrome, Goldenhar's syndrome, and Klippel-Feil syndrome. The anatomic pathology is very well described and the clinical implications of the pathology are thoroughly discussed.

References

Please see www.expertconsult.com

Burn Injuries

Erik S. Shank, Robert L. Sheridan, Charles J. Coté, and
J. A. Jeevendra Martyn

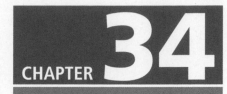

EVERY YEAR IN THE United States about 1.25 million people are treated for burns. Of these burned patients, 500,000 are hospitalized, with an 11% mortality rate.[1,2] Children account for at least 25% of these patients. These patients are well managed only when their care providers thoroughly understand the pathophysiologic and pharmacologic abnormalities associated with burn injury.[3] These abnormalities include metabolic derangements, neurohumoral responses, massive fluid shifts, sepsis, and the systemic effects of massive tissue destruction. In this chapter we address the pathophysiology, the initial evaluation and resuscitation, the anesthetic management, and the pain management of children with burn injury. Some of the principles presented are derived from experiences with adult patients and applied to children, whereas others are the result of more than 30 years of experience in caring for children with burn injuries.

Each year, in the United States approximately 15,000 children are hospitalized with burn injuries.[1] The incidence of fatalities has declined over the past decades, owing mostly to the advent of dedicated hospital burn centers,[4] improved surgical techniques, and safer anesthetic management. However, almost 1,100 children still die each year from fire and burn injuries.

Pathophysiology

Thermal injury to the skin disrupts the vital surface barrier we depend on for thermal regulation, bacterial defenses, and fluid and electrolyte balance. It is essential to appreciate, however, that even minor, localized burn injuries may be associated with diffuse and dramatic systemic responses. These alterations may affect all the systems of the body.[5] Several mediators released from the burned areas activate the inflammatory response and cause local and distant edema. Complement, arachidonic acid metabolites, and oxygen radicals are involved in this response.[6] Cytokines seem to be the main mediators of the systemic effects.[5] Endotoxins are frequently detected in the immediate postburn period, usually correlate with the burn size, and are predictive of the development of multiple organ failure and the subsequent demise of the patient.[6] The clinical symptoms and pathologic changes are relatively more severe in children, and, unfortunately, the gravity of the injury is often underestimated because of their greater ratio of body surface area to weight (Fig. 34-1).

Soon after the injury, massive fluid shifts occur from the vascular compartment into the burned tissue, resulting in sequestration of fluid, even in nonburned areas, causing significant hemoconcentration.[3] Despite the massive fluid loss, systemic blood pressure may be maintained as a result of the outpouring of catecholamines and antidiuretic hormone.[7] In the first 4 days after a burn of moderate size or larger (~40%), an amount of albumin equal to approximately twice the total body plasma content is lost through the wound. In addition to the direct effects of the burn (thrombosis, increased capillary

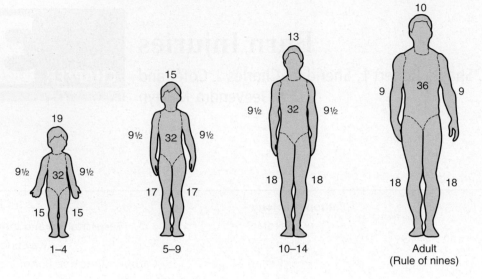

1—4   5—9   10—14   Adult (Rule of nines)

Figure 34-1. The different proportions of body surface area are illustrated for calculation of percentage of burn according to a patient's age. Note the large proportion of body surface area that the head and face account for in an infant. (From Carvajal HF, Goldman AS: Burns. In Vaughan VC III, McKay RJ, Nelson WE [eds]: Nelson's Textbook of Pediatrics. Philadelphia, WB Saunders, 1975, p 281.)

permeability), changes in vascular integrity occur in areas remote from the injury, resulting in tissue edema.[8] In the pulmonary capillary network, these changes may be life-threatening; severe pulmonary edema and vascular congestion may result.

Cardiac

Immediately after injury, cardiac output is strikingly reduced.[9,10] This decrease is often related to the rapid reduction in circulating blood volume or to the severe compressive effects of circumferential burns on the abdomen and chest, impairing venous return.[11] Despite adequate cardiac filling pressures, cardiac output often remains compromised. This finding suggests other contributing factors, such as direct myocardial depression from the burn injury. Some investigators have described circulating myocardial depressant factors such as interleukins, tumor necrosis factors, or oxygen free radicals existing in subjects with extensive third-degree burns.[12-15] At our institution, acutely burned children frequently require inotropic support during the acute period of depressed cardiac function.

Three to 5 days after a burn injury, children develop a hypermetabolic state. This may result in a twofold to threefold increase in cardiac output, which persists for weeks to months, depending on the extent of the injury and the length of time needed for wound closure. During this hypermetabolic period, the child may be hypertensive due to an increased cardiac output. It is important to rule out the most common cause of the hypertension in this period—inadequate pain control. However, a number of other circulating mediators such as increased catecholamines, atrial natriuretic factor, renin, endothelin-1, and others that can cause intermittent or persistent hypertension have been found in burn victims.[16-19] It is also possible to have a depressed cardiac output during this hypermetabolic state if gram-negative sepsis or hypovolemia is present. Closure of the burn wound usually decreases metabolic demand, resulting in a concomitant reduction in cardiac output.[20,21]

Pulmonary

Pulmonary function may be adversely affected from the upper airway to terminal alveoli. The upper airway is an excellent heat exchanger; just as it warms cold air, it cools hot air. The cooling of hot inspired air may result in heat destruction of laryngeal tissues; the air in a closed space (e.g., house or automobile fire) may reach 538° C (1000° F) 2 feet above floor level. Inspiration of superheated air damages the upper airway; airway obstruction occurs as a result of massive edema formation involving all airway structures above the carina (see later). The proximal bronchi may suffer heat destruction of the ciliated epithelium and mucosa. The distal bronchi and alveoli may be damaged by inhalation of toxic fumes, such as nitrogen dioxide and sulfur dioxide, which combine with water in the tracheobronchial tree to form nitric and sulfuric acids. Upper airway damage is therefore usually related to a heat injury, whereas lower airway injury is usually related to chemical or toxic effects. Acid gases such as hydrochloric acid, sulfuric acid, and phosgene penetrate deeply, thereby damaging the alveolar membranes and surfactants.[22] Wool and cotton combustion result in aldehyde formation, which may cause pulmonary edema in concentrations as low as 10 ppm.[23] Combustion of synthetic materials (insulation, wall paneling) releases hydrogen cyanide. Although it is apparently rare,[24] cyanide poisoning can lead to histotoxic hypoxia and death[25] and may mimic carbon monoxide (CO) poisoning. Inhalation of hydrogen cyanide is an often-unrecognized cause of immediate death.

The overall effect of a pulmonary inhalation injury is necrotizing bronchitis, bronchial swelling, alveolar destruction, exudation of protein, loss of surfactant, loss of the protective bronchial lining, and bronchospasm, all of which contribute to the development of bronchopneumonia (Figs. 34-2 and 34-3). Inhalation of particulate matter (smoke, soot) and lower airway edema also result in mechanical airway obstruction. Edema of the bronchi, combined with loss of integrity of the pulmonary capillary endothelium, results in decreased pulmonary compliance. Chest wall compliance may also be diminished by circum-

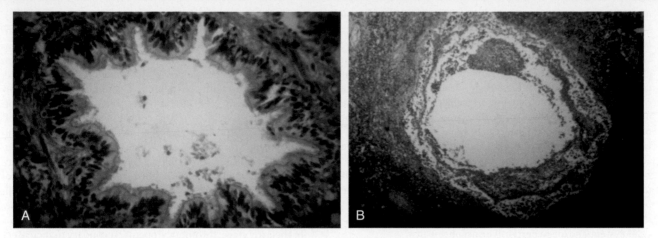

Figure 34-2. A, Cross section of a normal bronchiole. Note the ciliated epithelial layer. **B,** Compare with a cross section of a distal bronchiole from a child who died of an inhalation injury. Note the marked thickening of the bronchial wall, the massive inflammatory cell infiltrate, the sloughing of the mucosa, and the total destruction of the ciliated columnar epithelium.

ferential chest burns, which have a tourniquet-like effect.[11] All of these injuries lead to clinically important ventilation/perfusion abnormalities and right-to-left intrapulmonary shunting, with resultant hypoxemia and hypercarbia. Carbon monoxide inhalation can further compromise both hemoglobin's oxygen-carrying capacity and its ability to deliver oxygen to tissues. Carbon monoxide also impairs oxygen utilization at the cellular level (cellular respiration). Severe smoke inhalation alone may be seen without any externally visible injuries.[26] Extrapulmonary factors such as changes in cardiac output can also contribute to hypoxemia. Measurement of blood gases alone may not indicate these factors. Rational therapy of reduced arterial oxygen saturation requires evaluation of both extrapulmonary and intrapulmonary factors contributing to arterial desaturation.[8,27] Measurements that discriminate extrapulmonary and intrapulmonary factors include cardiac output, mixed venous oxygen content or saturation, and shunt fraction.[9] In general, the prognosis of cutaneous burn is compounded by the simultaneous occurrence of a pulmonary burn. It is estimated that the presence of an inhalational injury doubles the mortality rate from cutaneous burns.[22]

Renal

Renal function may be adversely affected soon after injury as a result of myoglobinuria and hemoglobinuria.[28] The former is most common after electrical injury, whereas the latter is encountered after severe cutaneous burns of about 40% or greater. Hypovolemia, hypotension, and hypoxemia may further aggravate renal dysfunction, resulting in acute tubular necrosis. Increased production of catecholamines, angiotensin, and vasopressin lead to systemic vasoconstriction, compounding the renal insufficiency.[29] Release of vasoactive peptides such as endothelin-1 may cause acute vasoconstriction, which may also have adverse effects on renal function.[30,31] Fluid retention generally occurs during the first 3 to 5 days after injury, and diuresis begins after this. Thus, there may be impairment of renal function soon after injury, which may also delay drug excretion. Three to 7 days after the burn injury, glomerular filtration rate

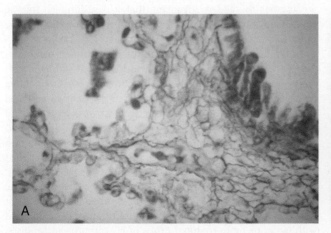
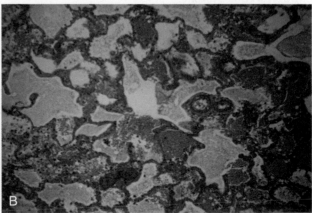

Figure 34-3. A, Normal alveoli. **B,** Inhalation alveolar injury is generally related to noxious fumes such as nitrogen dioxide and sulfur dioxide that are carried far down the tracheobronchial tree, combine with exhaled water, and form nitric acid and sulfuric acid, resulting in pulmonary congestion, alveolar injury, and hyaline membrane formation.

increases pari passu with cardiac output and increased metabolic rate.[32] The serum half-life of many antibiotics as well as other medications excreted through glomerular filtration may be altered as a result of changes (increased or decreased) in glomerular filtration rate.[33-36] Patients suffering a burn that covers more than 40% of their body surface area demonstrate renal tubular dysfunction, mainly an inability to concentrate the urine.[7] Even during hyperosmolar states, antidiuresis is not observed, suggesting an inadequate renal response to antidiuretic hormone and aldosterone. Thus, it is possible to observe adequate urine output even in the presence of hypovolemia.[37] Episodic or persistent hypertension is frequent in children; it may in part be mediated by increased renin and catecholamine production.[38,39] If hypertension is persistent, then treatment should be instituted to avoid excessive stress on the cardiovascular system and/or hypertensive encephalopathy.

Hepatic

The liver may be damaged by hypoxemia and/or hypoperfusion during the early post-burn phase as a result of hypovolemia or hypotension and by inhaled or absorbed chemical toxins.[40,41] Reperfusion injury may harm the liver when adequate circulation is reestablished. Hepatic dysfunction may later result from drug toxicity, sepsis, or blood transfusions. Studies in adults have found increased hepatic blood flow, increased protein synthesis and breakdown, and increased hepatic gluconeogenesis during the hypermetabolic phase of burn injury. With the onset of sepsis, hepatic glucose output and alanine uptake may decrease sharply but hepatic blood flow and oxygen utilization can remain increased.[40,42] Fatty infiltration of the liver has also been reported. Sustained increases in hepatic blood flow deliver more drug to the liver; this effect, combined with drug-induced enzyme induction, may result in a reduced drug half-life.[43] Although all studies of animals suggest a depressed clearance of drugs after burn injury, clinical studies of the capacity of the liver to metabolize drugs are conflicting, even for the same class of drugs.[44-49] The magnitude of the burn, the time after injury, and the effects of co-administered drugs, alone or in combination, as well as alterations in protein binding and volume of distribution, may have a role in these conflicting reports.

Central Nervous System

The central nervous system (CNS) may be adversely affected by inhalation of neurotoxic chemicals or by hypoxic encephalopathy; other contributing factors include sepsis, hyponatremia, and hypovolemia.[50] CNS dysfunction includes hallucinations, personality changes, delirium, seizures, abnormal neurologic symptoms, and coma.[51] These effects may be due to the burn injury itself or to the administration of drugs necessary for sedation, anxiolysis, and analgesia.[52] Such effects usually clear after several weeks. Abnormalities of CNS neurotransmitters have been postulated to mediate the anorexia associated with extensive burn injury.[53] The possibility of cerebral edema and increased intracranial pressure must also be considered during the initial phases of burn injury. Under such circumstances, the usual measures for treating increased intracranial pressure would be instituted (see Chapter 23). Data suggest that rapid overcorrection of hyponatremia may also be associated with cerebral injury.[54]

Hematologic

Blood viscosity may increase as a result of hemoconcentration secondary to fluid shifts and because of alterations in plasma protein content.[55] The hematopoietic system is also adversely affected; an ongoing microangiopathic hemolytic anemia secondary to the burn injury is common.[56] An inhibitor of erythroid stem cells has also been found in the sera of burn patients; it may, in part, contribute to the anemia of burn injury. Another study has demonstrated a normal erythropoietin response to anemia in patients with burn injury.[57] The half-life of red blood cells is diminished in burn patients, and multiple blood draws may also contribute to the development of anemia.[58,59] The possible role of artificial erythropoietin for the care of burned patients has yet to be defined.[60,61]

In the early stage, thrombocytopenia, secondary to increased platelet aggregation and trapping of platelets in the lungs, is followed by an increase in platelet count 10 to 14 days after burn injury. This elevation persists for several months.[59] An increase in fibrin split products (disseminated intravascular coagulopathy), which lasts for 3 to 5 days, may occur.[62] Factors V, VII, and VIII and fibrinogen are also increased severalfold over baseline for the first 3 months after severe injury uncomplicated by sepsis.[62,63] We have observed a number of children with increased platelet counts (>1 million/mm^3) who experienced a marked reduction in platelet count with the onset of sepsis. The sudden onset of thrombocytopenia calls for an evaluation for sepsis. Likewise, there can be massive variations in fibrinogen values (up to 2 g/dL), although there does not appear to be an increased incidence of thrombotic events.

Gastrointestinal

Gastrointestinal function is diminished immediately after thermal injury secondary to the development of gastric and intestinal ileus.[64] Because of the danger of pulmonary aspiration of gastric contents during this time, the stomach should be adequately vented and appropriate gastric acid prophylaxis instituted. At 48 to 72 hours after a burn, when generalized edema is diminishing, gastrointestinal function is usually restored. Enteral feeding should be established at this time to provide calories, to blunt the hypermetabolic response, and to attenuate gluconeogenesis and stress ulceration.[55,65] Early enteral feeding has the added advantage that it can diminish muscle catabolism and even reduce bacterial translocation through the intestinal mucosa.[88]

In children who do not tolerate enteral feeding, parenteral nutrition must be initiated.[65,67] Stress ulcers (Curling ulcers) are associated with any burn injury and may be life-threatening; however, the incidence has decreased in critically ill patients, perhaps in part as a result of better pharmacologic control of gastric acidity.[68] Prospective studies of pediatric and adult burn victims and patients in intensive care indicate that cimetidine in the usual doses may not adequately protect seriously ill patients from increases in gastric acidity.[33,34] This increased requirement is related to pharmacokinetic or pharmacodynamic alterations.[33] Therefore, frequent feedings when tolerated, the liberal use of antacids, combined with larger or more frequent doses of H$_2$-receptor antagonists, may be required to help prevent the development of stress ulceration.[33,55,64]

Endocrine

The endocrinologic response to acute thermal injury is complex, involving most organ systems. Stimuli that trigger endocrine responses include the thermal injury itself and subsequent fluid shifts, as well as stress responses seen with any critical illness.[69] These may include depressed levels of certain hormones (e.g., triiodothyronine, dehydroepiandrosterone, and testosterone) as well as increased levels of many others (antidiuretic hormone, catecholamines, renin, angiotensin II, and cortisol).[70] Glucose control may be poor, owing to the increased levels of cortisol and insulin resistance.[71] Tight control of hyperglycemia may decrease the incidence of urinary tract infection and improve survival of critically ill burn patients, although further investigation is necessary.[72] Avoidance of hyperglycemia may attenuate cerebral injury due to hypoperfusion states (see Chapters 23 and 39).

Skin

Extensive skin destruction results in the inability to regulate body heat, to conserve fluids and electrolytes, and to protect against bacterial invasion. Permeability of burned tissues is markedly increased and proportional to the number of layers of tissue damaged.[73] Because children have a much greater ratio of body surface area to weight compared with adults, they are even more likely to become hypothermic (see Fig. 34-1). Thus, it is important to keep these children covered as much as possible; to increase the environmental temperature; and to use radiant warmers, plastic wrap around extremities, reflective insulated blankets, artificial "noses" (in-line moisture and heat exchangers), and hot-air heating blankets. Late complications affecting the skin include progressive scar formation, which results in movement-restricting contractures.[11,74] Topical antibiotic and antibacterial therapy is necessary to prevent burn wound sepsis.[75,76]

Metabolic

Many metabolic alterations follow extensive burn injury. Increased utilization of glucose, fat, and protein results in greater oxygen demand and increased carbon dioxide (CO_2) production.[2,40,55,67,77-83] Mediators that have been implicated in these metabolic changes include interleukin-1, tumor necrosis factor, catecholamines, prostanoids, and other stress hormones.[2,84] Centrally mediated or sepsis-induced hyperthermia also increases oxygen consumption and CO_2 production. Some of these abnormalities may persist even after complete closure of the burn wounds, when metabolic demand is already reduced.[21,85] Intravenous alimentation, particularly with increased glucose concentrations, may also increase CO_2 production and therefore increase ventilatory requirements.[67] Increase in oxygen demand and CO_2 production must be compensated for during controlled mechanical ventilation.

Calcium Homeostasis

Many acutely burned patients demonstrate an abnormally low ionized calcium levels. Marked abnormalities in the indices of calcium metabolism in both acute and recovery phases may persist for as long as 7 weeks after injury (Fig. 34-4).[86] Hypophosphatemia and hypermagnesemia revert toward normal during the latter phase of recovery from the acute injury. The usual reciprocal relationship between calcium and inorganic phosphate is not evident in patients with major burn injury. Therefore, supplemental calcium therapy is extremely important, particularly during extensive surgical procedures in which ionized hypocalcemia may have adverse cardiovascular effects. In general, frequent small boluses would be safer and more effective than intermittent large boluses (see also Figs. 10-8 and 10-9).[87] Doses of 2.5 mg/kg calcium chloride or 7.5 mg/kg calcium gluconate ionize at equivalent rates and produce equivalent increases in calcium concentration.

Psychiatric

It is imperative to recognize not only the physical assault to the pediatric burn victim but also the psychological trauma associated with the severely burned child. Thirty percent of acutely burned children present with acute stress disorders. Risk factors for acute stress disorders include size of burn, degree of pain, pulse rate, and parental issues.[88] Treatment with fluoxetine or imipramine may help ameliorate these stress disorders.[89-91] There is an increased incidence of attention-deficit disorders in pediatric burn victims, likely owing to the impulsivity.[92,93] Finally, the normal psychosocial support network may be impaired in the families of the burn victim, even before the burn injury.[94,95]

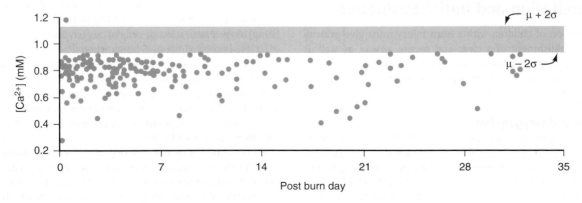

Figure 34-4. Ionized calcium values from burned children and adults are plotted for the first 35 days after burn injury. Note that the majority of values are abnormally low. (From Szyfelbein SK, Drop LJ, Martyn JA: Persistent ionized hypocalcemia during resuscitation and recovery phases of body burns. Crit Care Med 1981; 9:454-458.)

circumferential burns of the chest, abdomen, and extremities must be performed urgently because impaired hemodynamics and respiratory mechanics can cause irreversible damage within hours after the burn injury. Escharotomy often may be accomplished without the need for general anesthesia because a full-thickness burn usually destroys skin innervation.

Electrical Burns

Electrical burns occur with household voltage (electric cords/sockets) and non-household high-voltage current (power line/lightning). Children often disconnect extension cords by stabilizing one end in their mouths and pulling the other end with a hand, resulting in circumoral and lingual burns. High-voltage injuries are often associated with loss of limbs and other injuries that are not immediately obvious.[217-220] The extent of the injury is unpredictable. The surface injury is often small, but the extent of underlying tissue damage and necrosis is massive. Such an injury is a combination of electrical and thermal damage.[220,221] Victims often have concurrent injuries such as fractures of vertebrae or long bones, ruptured organs, myocardial injury, or numerous contusions. Even children with low-voltage injuries may have abnormalities of cardiac conduction.[218] Children with electrical burns may be admitted comatose or seizing. Muscle tissue surrounding bone is usually more affected than superficial muscles because electrical current tends to travel along neurovascular bundles. Early fasciotomy is needed to preserve the blood flow to extremities (Fig. 34-10). It necessitates general anesthesia during the first day of injury at the time when fluid shifts, hyperkalemia, and myoglobinuria are maximal. Massive myonecrosis and hemolysis may result in hyperkalemia, as well as myoglobinuria and hemoglobinuria. In the presence of hemoglobinuria or myoglobinuria, an increased urine flow (>1 mL/kg/hr) should be ensured by the administration of increased fluids and mannitol.[222,223] Alkalization of urine may prevent the precipitation of these proteins in the renal tubules. Follow-up of patients with electrical injuries often reveals unpredictable sequelae, which may manifest months to years later; these injuries may occur in organs or areas that do not appear abnormal during the acute course of illness. These late complications most frequently include neurologic dysfunction, ocular damage, damage to the gastrointestinal tract, circumoral strictures, changes in the electrocardiogram, and delayed hemorrhage from large vessels.[221,223]

Guidelines to Anesthetic Management

Anesthetic management of children with severe thermal injury begins with the initial resuscitation and continues for many years through reconstructive surgery. Knowledge and understanding of the pathophysiology of burn injury enable anesthesiologists to plan appropriate anesthetic management and to recognize and treat complications arising as a result of burn injury or its therapy (Table 34-2).[2,224]

Children who require surgery for burn wound excision and grafting must be properly prepared physiologically and psychologically, and specific equipment must be available in the operating room.

Psychological support must be provided by parents, nurses, physicians, and trained psychologists. It is important for anesthesiologists to understand that the families of children who have sustained a severe burn injury feel a great deal of psychological stress and guilt. This stress may be transferred to anger at the physicians, nurses, and other members of the burn care team. The parents are angry that their child has sustained a devastating injury and occasionally vent this anger and frustration. It is therefore vital that the entire burn care team understand this familial response, that they spend as much time as possible listening to parents' concerns, and that they emphasize all that is being done to ensure the very best for their child. Specific nurses and physicians should be designated to communicate with the family to avoid misunderstandings and confusion about issues of patient care. The anesthesia care team, while explaining the risks of anesthesia, must emphasize the extensive monitoring and the central role that anesthesiologists have in assuring the well-being of their child. Special emphasis must be placed on methods for minimizing physical and psychological pain during transport to the operating room, in the operating room, and postoperatively.

Nutrition: Since keeping children with severe burn injuries NPO for eight or more hours prior to sedation for a dressing change or anesthesia for a surgical procedure would severely compromise caloric intake, we advocate the use of continuous oro-jejunal or naso-jejunal alimentation. Generally children can receive calories up until approximately four hours prior to sedation/induction without fear of significant gastric residual volumes and then feeding can be resumed almost immediately following the procedure.

Adequate sedation and pain control are necessary before moving children to the operating room; this move is painful, both physically and emotionally. Intravenous opioids, such as fentanyl, which has minimal histamine release, are particularly helpful; intravenous midazolam is also helpful for its sedative and amnestic properties. Drug doses should not be based on standard doses used in children without thermal injury. Burned children develop tolerance to most narcotics and sedatives, thus requiring higher doses over time to achieve a satisfactory clinical response.[225,226] The dose of sedative or narcotic should be titrated to effect while the child is carefully observed and monitored. Children with burn injuries rapidly develop tolerance; it is not unusual for children with burns over more than 25% of

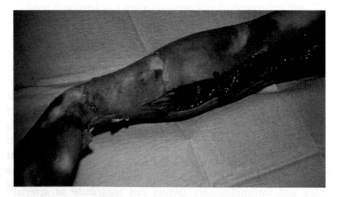

Figure 34-10. Electrical injuries tend to follow neurovascular structures and have an entry as well as an exit wound. The skin might appear normal but the underlying structures may have had extensive injury. These children require a fasciotomy rather than just a simple escharotomy to preserve blood flow to the deep structures. Generally, this is required on the first day of injury for best results in tissue preservation.

Table 34-2. Systemic Effects of Burn Injury

System	Early Effects	Late Effects
Cardiovascular	↓ CO due to decreased circulating blood volume, myocardial depressant factor	↑ CO due to sepsis ↑ CO two to three times > baseline for months (hypermetabolism) Hypertension
Pulmonary	Upper airway obstruction due to edema	
	Lower airway obstruction due to edema, bronchospasm, particulate matter	
	↓ FRC	Bronchopneumonia
	↓ Pulmonary compliance	Tracheal stenosis
	↓ Chest wall compliance	↓ Chest wall compliance
Renal	↓ GFR	↑ GFR secondary to ↑ CO
	Secondary to ↓ circulating blood volume	
	Myoglobinuria	Tubular dysfunction
	Hemoglobinuria	
	Tubular dysfunction	
Hepatic	↓ Function due to ↓ circulating blood volume, hypoxia, hepatotoxins	Hepatitis
		↑ Function due to hypermetabolism, enzyme induction, ↑ CO
		↓ Function due to sepsis, drug interactions
Hematopoietic	↓ Platelets	↑ Platelets
	↑ Fibrin split products, consumptive coagulopathy, anemia	↑ Clotting factors
Neurologic	Encephalopathy	Encephalopathy
	Seizures	Seizures
	↑ ICP	ICU psychosis
Skin	↑ Heat, fluid, electrolyte loss	Contractures, scar formation
Metabolic	↓ Ionized calcium	↑ Oxygen consumption
		↑ Carbon dioxide production
		↓ Ionized calcium
Pharmacokinetics	Altered volume of distribution	Tolerance to narcotics, sedatives
	Altered protein binding	Enzyme induction, altered receptors
	Altered pharmacokinetics	Drug interaction
	Altered pharmacodynamics	

↓ Decrease in; ↑, increase in; AIDS, acquired immunodeficiency syndrome; CO, cardiac output; FRC, functional residual capacity; GFR, glomerular filtration rate; ICP, intracranial pressure; ICU, intensive care unit.

the body surface to require 1 mg/kg/hr of both morphine and midazolam to provide adequate analgesia and sedation.

Correction of intravascular volume before induction of anesthesia may require fluid boluses during and after sedation and before transport. Establishing adequate intravenous access preoperatively may be especially difficult in children with large burns. We utilize both topical anesthetic creams as well as needle-free subcutaneous local anesthetics to help make this process painless and stress free.

It is critically important to *minimize heat loss* and maintain euthermia. This is difficult because of the massive evaporative heat loss that occurs through open wounds. Operating room temperatures during extensive excisions are commonly maintained near 37°C.[84] Attention must be paid to minimize heat loss both during transport and in the operating room. Multiple blankets or thermal reflective covers are helpful. Special equipment is used to maintain body temperature, including a warming blanket, radiant warmer, blood warmer, and heat/moisture exchangers and forced hot air warmers. Simply wrapping the extremities in sterile plastic bags and covering the head

with plastic or thermal insulation material markedly reduces heat and fluid losses (see Fig. 34-8). Although a hot operating room is uncomfortable for staff, maintaining the child's temperature may be helpful in maintaining normal blood clotting. Each calorie that does not have to be spent to maintain body temperature is one more that can be used in the healing process.

Adequate monitoring for major blood loss and fluid shifts includes arterial and central venous cannulas, a urinary catheter, an electrocardiogram, a pulse oximeter, a capnograph, and an esophageal stethoscope. A secure intravenous route for volume infusion is essential. If the potential for rapid blood loss exists, multilumen catheters may not be adequate because of their high-flow resistance. Rapid infusion devices may be particularly helpful (see Chapter 53).[227-229] The femoral vein is an alternate cannulation site, in addition to the internal jugular and subclavian veins (see Chapter 49).

Specific anesthetic equipment is used, including various sterilized laryngoscope blades, endotracheal tubes, airways, and blood pressure cuffs.

cheal tube type and size. As mentioned previously, cuffed endotracheal tubes should usually be used and a record maintained of the size of endotracheal tube, volume of air inflated into the cuff, and pressure at which leakage occurs around the endotracheal tube for each anesthetic procedure. It is common to note the use of smaller diameter endotracheal tubes as weeks go by, heralding the development of a subglottic lesion (stenosis, granuloma, polyps), which should be investigated with bronchoscopy. When nitrous oxide is used, the intraoperative cuff pressure should be checked to avoid excessive pressure on the tracheal mucosa. We generally inflate the cuff to the minimum pressure that allows controlled ventilation.

Airway Control

The pediatric burn patient may present an especially difficult airway challenge to the anesthesiologist. This may be due to external airway factors such as temporomandibular joint limitation, macroglossia from thermal injury, and neck contractures. It may also be due to direct thermal/inhalational injuries to the glottis and respiratory tree. A detailed history and physical examination focusing on airway injury is vital. History details such as victim of fire in a closed space (e.g., house or automobile fire [very commonly associated with inhalational injuries]), vocal changes, stridor, and hoarseness may be important predictors of difficulty in establishing an airway.

Fiberoptic intubation is a very useful method of securing the airway. We utilize this technique frequently after induction when we are confident we can maintain a mask airway as well for "awake" but sedated children who are breathing spontaneously. Recently, we have utilized dexmedetomidine as our sole sedative while performing fiberoptic intubations on spontaneously breathing children. Dexmedetomidine, an α_2 agonist, supplies a relatively stable hemodynamic environment, without respiratory depression, making it an ideal sedative when loss of respiratory drive could be catastrophic.

Fiberoptic intubation is aided in these children often with manual distraction of the tongue (especially if macroglossia is present) and a jaw lift (Fig. 34-15). Sometimes fiberoptic intubation is easier facilitated if the bronchoscope is guided through a laryngeal mask airway that has already been seated and used to ventilate the lungs. This can be especially advantageous if there is a lot of perioral edema from inhalational burn injury.

Besides direct laryngoscopy, fiberoptic intubations and laryngeal mask airway–assisted intubations other techniques have been described, including retrograde wires and light-wand intubations. These techniques may be difficult to use in a child with a severely burned neck and contractures. In children with severe neck or oral contractures, the contracture may be released by the surgeon during ketamine sedation and spontaneous ventilation to facilitate access to the airway. The airway may then be instrumented either directly or indirectly (see Chapter 12).

Hyperalimentation

Hyperalimentation fluids are frequently administered to burned children.[65,264] These fluids should be continued intraoperatively; however, we generally reduce the rate of infusion to one half to two thirds of the initial infusion rate because metabolic rate is usually decreased as a result of anesthetic drugs as well as reduced body temperature. These fluids should be administered with a constant-infusion pump to avoid accidental overinfusion or underinfusion. If the hyperalimentation fluids must be terminated (e.g., to permit blood transfusion), then monitoring of blood glucose levels is recommended. Dangerous rebound hypoglycemia may occur if infusion of these solutions is abruptly interrupted and no compensation is made with other glucose-containing solutions. It should be noted that most blood products, particularly whole blood and FFP, provide a significant glucose load. Compatibility of hyperalimentation solutions with drugs, blood, and other infusions must be addressed.

Awakening

In the immediate postoperative period, oxygen consumption increases even in the absence of shivering.[265] If oxygen debt develops (metabolic acidosis), appropriate measures must be taken to correct it. Special consideration must also be given to the likelihood of severe pain. Analgesic drugs should be administered in increasingly liberal doses because of increased drug tolerance. Adequacy of air exchange and patency of the airway, however, must be given first priority. It is important to assess the leak pressure at the end of the surgical procedure. The airway patency of the burn child is highly dynamic, and the child whose airway had minimal edema at the beginning of a procedure, may have a very edematous airway at the end and be a poor candidate for extubation.

Pain Management

The treatment of burn child with pain, both perioperatively and in the intensive care unit, remains a major challenge for anesthesiologists and intensivists. Nearly every maneuver involving care of the burn child is associated with pain. This includes dressing changes, excision and grafting, physical therapy, weighing, and line placements. Our experience is that the pain is proportional to the size of the thermal injury.

Part of the challenge in managing burn pain is due to the overlay of physiologic and psychosocial responses to thermal injury. Besides physical stimulation of nociceptors and other direct pain mechanisms, there is also the very real anticipation, anxiety, and fear associated with these procedures. Evidence suggests that skillful communication and explanations of why certain treatments are necessary, despite the pain caused, decreases analgesic requirements.[225,266-268]

Opioid administration for pain control has been an evolving science for the child with a burn. Twenty years ago there was a significant fear that treatment of pain with opioids would create "addictions." However, no studies of children have documented addiction, and studies of adults reveal a very low addiction rate.[269-273] This has led to a liberalization of opioid dosing at our institution. It is not unusual to find burn children receiving more than 1 mg/kg/hr of morphine intravenously while recovering from burn injuries in our intensive care unit. Once the thermal wounds are closed, opioid requirements rapidly decrease (Fig. 34-16).

Although the fear of post-burn care addiction to opioids has not been realized, there are other reasons why this class of drugs may be detrimental to the child with a burn. Recent evidence from rats suggests that thermal injury itself may lead to a hyperalgesic state with both a reduced efficacy of morphine (presumably from downregulation of spinal mu receptors) and increases in N-methyl-D-aspartic acid (NMDA) receptors. The increases in NMDA receptors induced by burns provides the rationale for use of ketamine to treat pain. Opioids may also increase sensi-

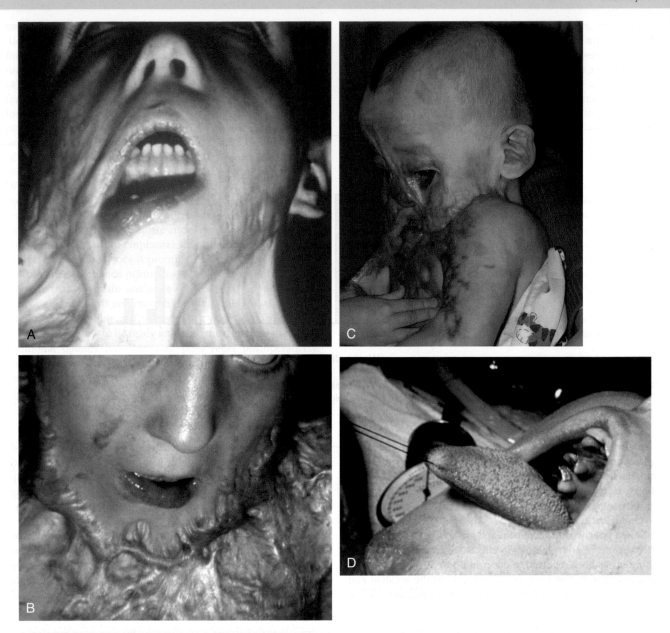

Figure 34-15. A, Child with inadequately treated facial burn; note that skin contracture has resulted in complete distortion of the face with inability to close the right eye. **B,** Child with another example of an inadequately treated neck burn; note that her chin is fused with the sternum, resulting in very difficult airway management. **C,** An acute burn injury with an even more extreme example of inability to access the airway. To manage this child safely for the initial neck release, ECMO was utilized. This child is also unable to close her eyes. **D,** Some children with severe neck burns may only have their airway visualized by pulling back on the tongue (zero silk suture or grasping forceps may be utilized) so as to pull the tongue and larynx cephalad.

tivity to pain from an apoptosis of spinal inhibitory interneurons.[274,275] Opioids in mice may also lead to post-burn immunosuppression.[276]

The fact that opioids may have significant detriments in pain management has led to searches for alternative agents. Among these are potentially dexmedetomidine,[277-283] gabapentin,[284] and, until their recent withdrawal from the market, cyclooxygenase-2 inhibitors.[285-287]

Dexmedetomidine is a parenterally administered α_2 agonist with good sedative and anxiolytic properties. In adults, it has been demonstrated to decrease opioid requirements postopera-

tively.[278-282,288] In children with burns, it has been successfully for sedation.[277] Of note is the observation that larger dexmedetomidine doses may be required than for adult patients or nonburned children.[277] Dexmedetomidine, in and of itself, does not appear to be a remarkable analgesic for children with burns. At our institution, we are beginning studies to evaluate its ability to decrease opioid requirements.

Dressing changes sometimes present one of the greatest analgesic challenges. This is because they are very painful, cause a rapid rise above baseline pain, and are also associated by the child with anticipation of impending pain. A number of methods

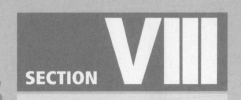

The Extremely Premature Infant (Micropremie)

James P. Spaeth and C. Dean Kurth

THE PRETERM INFANT IS defined by birth before 37 weeks of gestation. Preterm infants can be classified as low birth weight infants (<2500 g), very low birth weight infants (<1500 g), and extremely low birth weight infants (<1000 g). Morbidity and mortality in this population has decreased over the past 25 years, especially in those of extremely low birth weight in which the mortality is now less than 50%, compared with 80% in 1980.[1,2] This decrease in mortality is the result of many factors, including the use of surfactant shortly after birth, antenatal glucocorticoid administration, specialization of neonatal care units, and changes in mechanical ventilator therapy. However, many of these surviving infants develop coexisting diseases that require care by an anesthesiologist. For the purpose of this chapter, we will focus on the very low and extremely low birth weight infant, or "micropremie," and discuss developmental physiology and its impact on anesthetic care; neonatal emergencies are discussed in Chapter 36.

Physiology of Prematurity Related to Anesthesia

Respiratory System

The small airways predispose the micropremie to obstruction and difficulty with ventilation. Resistance to airflow is inversely proportional to the fifth power for large airways and to the fourth power of the radius for small airways (see also Fig. 12-7). As a result, insertion of an endotracheal tube increases resistance and work of breathing far greater for the micropremie (2.5 or 3 mm inside diameter [ID]) than for an infant (4 mm ID), child (5 mm ID), or adult (7 mm ID) (Fig. 35-1). Similarly, partial occlusion of the endotracheal tube by secretions, blood, or kinking increases work of breathing to a much greater extent in the micropremie. Partial occlusion of the natural airway from loss of muscle tone during anesthesia and sedation also increases work of breathing more in the micropremie. Consequently, general anesthesia often requires placement of an endotracheal tube to ensure airway patency and assisted ventilation to overcome the increased work of breathing.

Diseases that narrow the airway such as subglottic stenosis, tracheal stenosis, and tracheobronchomalacia occur commonly in the micropremie, and the associated reduction in airway diameter increase both resistance to airflow and work of breathing. Subglottic stenosis necessitates the placement of a smaller endotracheal tube than would otherwise be placed, further increasing airflow resistance. Tracheal stenosis often occurs near the carina and, although not necessitating a smaller endotracheal tube, it increases airway resistance from the stenosis distal to the endotracheal tube. With tracheobronchomalacia,

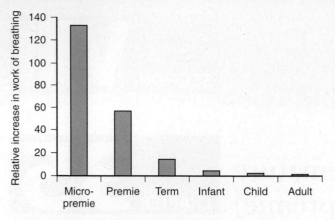

Figure 35-1. Change in work of breathing after placement of an appropriate endotracheal tube in extremely low birth weight infants (<1000 g), premature infants (1500 g), full-term infants, children, and adults (see text for details). (Redrawn with permission from Spaeth JP, O'Hara IB, Kurth CD: Anesthesia for the micropremie. Semin Perinatol 1998; 22:390-401.)

the intrathoracic airways collapse during exhalation, again increasing resistance and work of breathing (see also Fig. 12-10). Positive end-expiratory pressure (PEEP) or continuous positive airway pressure (CPAP) helps stent open the airway. Mechanical ventilation, rather than spontaneous ventilation during anesthesia, prevents fatigue from increased work of breathing and maintains ventilation and oxygenation. During anesthesia, reduced ventilatory rates *and shorter inspiratory to expiratory (I:E) ratios* prevent air trapping and hyperinflation of lung segments.

The structure and function of the immature lung predisposes to hypoxia. The alveoli are primarily composed of thick-walled saccular spaces that decrease lung compliance. Production of surfactant begins at between 23 to 24 weeks of gestation, although surfactant concentrations often remain inadequate until 36 weeks of gestation. Because surfactant content is decreased, lung volumes and compliance are decreased. Low lung volumes and poor compliance increase intrapulmonary shunt and ventilation/perfusion ($\dot{V}/\dot{Q}$) mismatch and increase the risk of hypoxia. Decreased lung volumes and $\dot{V}/\dot{Q}$ mismatch may also occur as a consequence of anesthesia. The effects of immature structure, disease, and anesthesia on lung function all increase the risk of hypoxia during surgery and anesthesia. Mechanical ventilation with continuous PEEP (~5 cm H_2O) during anesthesia maintains lung volume to prevent $\dot{V}/\dot{Q}$ mismatch and hypoxia.

Micropremie lungs are particularly susceptible to oxygen toxicity, barotrauma, and the development of bronchopulmonary dysplasia (BPD).[3] A severity index for BPD based on the need for supplemental oxygen and/or positive-pressure ventilation or nasal CPAP has been developed and shown to identify a spectrum of risk for adverse pulmonary and neurodevelopmental outcomes in prematurely born infants (Table 35-1).[4] Although this severity index has not been studied in the context of anesthetic risk, experience suggests that such infants requiring supplemental oxygen, positive pressure, or medications for reactive airways are at greater risk for perioperative pulmonary complications. Anesthetic goals include minimizing inspired oxygen concentration and peak inspiratory pressures while maintaining oxygenation and ventilation. High peak inspiratory pressures increase the risk of pneumothoraces and interstitial emphysema.

Respiratory Control

Micropremies possess a biphasic ventilatory response to hypoxia. Initially, ventilation increases during hypoxia, but after several minutes, ventilation decreases and apnea may ensue.[5] The ventilatory response to carbon dioxide is decreased in the micropremie, and hypoxia further blunts this response.[6] Anesthetic drugs depress the ventilatory responses to both hypoxia and hypercapnia. Hypoxia and hypercapnia occur commonly as a result of apnea and hypoventilation during emergence and recovery from anesthesia. Thus, the combination of anesthetic effects and an immature respiratory control system increase the risk of hypoxia, hypercapnia, and apnea in the postoperative period.

Apneic episodes occur commonly in the micropremie but decrease with advancing postconceptual age.[7] These apneic episodes usually involve both a failure to breathe (central apnea) and a failure to maintain a patent airway (obstructive apnea). Central apnea results from decreased respiratory center output. Although it may be precipitated by abrupt changes in oxygenation, pulmonary mechanics, brain hemorrhage, hypothermia, or airway stimulation, apnea usually occurs without a precipitating event (i.e., idiopathic). Preterm infants with apnea do not increase ventilation in response to hypercapnia, compared with those without apnea, thereby delaying resumption of breathing and prolonging the apneic episode.[8] During obstructive apnea, the airway becomes obstructed in the hypopharynx and larynx as a result of pharyngeal muscle incoordination. Anesthetic drugs may further decrease pharyngeal muscle tone, precipitating airway obstruction during recovery from anesthesia. The combination of anesthetic effects and immature respiratory control place the micropremie at risk for central and obstructive apnea for a prolonged period of time during recovery from anesthesia.

Not surprisingly, apnea occurs commonly after anesthesia and surgery in preterm infants.[9,10] Like apnea of prematurity, postoperative apnea may be central, obstructive, or mixed in origin.[11] The term *postoperative apnea* usually means prolonged apnea (>15 seconds) or brief apnea accompanied by bradycardia

Table 35-1. Severity-Based Diagnostic Criteria for Bronchopulmonary Dysplasia (BPD)

Gestational age	<32 weeks
Time point of assessment	36 weeks post menstrual age or discharge home, whichever comes first
	Therapy with oxygen >21% for at least 28 days *plus:*
Mild BPD	Breathing room air
Moderate BPD	Need for <30% oxygen
Severe BPD	Need for ≥30% oxygen and/or positive-pressure ventilation or nasal continuous airway pressure

From Ehrenkranz RA, Walsh MC, Vohr BR, et al: Validation of the National Institutes of Health consensus definition of bronchopulmonary dysplasia. Pediatrics 2005; 116:1353-1360.

(heart rate = 80 beats per minute). Postoperative apnea typically occurs as a cluster of episodes over several minutes, with minutes of normal breathing in between the clusters. Bradycardia may occur with apnea, usually beginning at the onset of apnea and not in response to hypoxia. Arterial desaturation usually follows the apnea, although many apneic episodes may not have any associated desaturation.[11] Arterial desaturation is worse with obstructive apnea than with central apnea.[11]

The incidence of postoperative apnea depends on postconceptional and gestational age, hematocrit, and the type of surgical procedure (Fig. 35-2; see also Figs. 4-13 and 4-14).[9-12] The most significant risk factor is postconceptual age; the lower the postconceptual age, the greater the risk, with the incidence of postoperative apnea in the micropremie greater than 50%.[9,10] Postoperative apnea can occur in the micropremie even without a history of apnea during prematurity.[9] Anemia (hematocrit <30%) and younger gestation increase the risk of apnea for a given postconceptual age.[10,12]

Postoperative apnea usually begins within an hour of emergence from anesthesia.[9] In the micropremie, it can continue to occur up to 48 hours postoperatively, despite the elimination of anesthetic agents (see Fig. 35-2). In fact, postoperative apnea can occur after surgery with desflurane- or sevoflurane-based anesthetics or even after surgery for which a regional anesthetic was performed and no general anesthetic drugs were used.[13] Postoperative apnea is more common after major procedures, such as a laparotomy, compared with peripheral surgical procedures, such as inguinal hernia repair. These observations indicate that the neurohormonal response to surgery and postoperative pain may play an important role in the origins of postoperative apnea. Management of postoperative apnea includes close observation with a cardiorespiratory monitor and pulse oximeter, administration of intravenous caffeine,[14] and prevention of anemia or hypovolemia. Nasal CPAP or tracheal intubation and mechanical ventilation may be required for several days postoperatively if these measures fail.

Cardiovascular System

The micropremie remains at greater risk of cardiovascular collapse during anesthesia and surgery than the full-term infant for

Table 35-2. Circulating Blood Volume in Micropremature Infants, Premature Infants, Full-Term Neonates, Infants, and Children

	Blood Volume (mL/kg)	Weight (kg)	Total Blood Volume (mL)	25 mL Blood Loss Percentage Total Blood Volume (%)
Micropremie	110	1	110	23
Premie	100	1.75	175	14
Full-term neonate	90	3	270	9
Infant	80	10	800	3
Child	70	20	1400	2

several reasons. The fetal heart differs from the infant heart in that it has more connective tissue, less organized contractile elements, and increased dependence on extracellular calcium concentration. In addition, the less compliant fetal heart has a flatter Frank-Starling curve and is less sensitive to catecholamines because of near-maximal baseline β-adrenergic stimulation (see Chapter 16).[15,16] Consequently, cardiac output depends more on heart rate in the micropremie than in the term neonate. The high resting heart rate in the micropremie also does not permit cardiac output to increase to the same extent as an infant or child. The micropremie has a small absolute blood volume (Table 35-2). Therefore, relatively little blood loss during surgery can cause hypovolemia, hypotension, and shock. Because autoregulation is not well developed in the micropremie, heart rate may not increase with hypovolemia, and blood flow and oxygen delivery to the brain and heart may decrease with relatively little blood loss.[17] Anesthesia blunts baroreflexes in the micropremie, further limiting the ability to compensate for hypovolemia.[18] The combination of limited ventricular stroke volume reserve, high heart rate, low blood volume, and little autoregulation predispose the micropremie to cardiovascular collapse during major surgery.

Failure of the ductus arteriosus to close in the micropremie further increases this risk. A patent ductus arteriosus (PDA) promotes pulmonary hypertension and congestive heart failure. Changes in systemic or pulmonary vascular resistance alter the direction of flow through the PDA. Increased pulmonary vascular resistance predisposes to right-to-left shunting that worsens with hypoxia, hypercarbia, acidosis, and hypothermia. Fluid restriction and diuretic therapy, often used to treat congestive heart failure from left-to-right shunting through a PDA, further increase the risk of hypotension during surgery. In contrast to full-term neonates, the success of inhaled nitric oxide in the micropremie with hypoxic respiratory failure and pulmonary hypertension remains unclear.[19,20]

Neurologic Development

Although mortality in extremely preterm infants has improved over the years, many survivors experience cognitive impairment and long-term disability.[21,22] Regions of the central nervous system develop at different times during gestation; consequently, the impact of premature birth on the central nervous system (CNS) depends on gestational age at birth and the severity of cardiovascular, respiratory, and other postnatal stressors. The

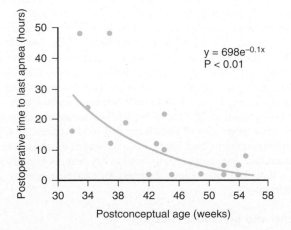

$y = 698e^{-0.1x}$
$P < 0.01$

Figure 35-2. Time from the end of anesthesia to the last episode of postoperative apnea in prematurely born infants. Postconceptual age is gestational age plus postnatal age. (Redrawn with permission from Kurth CD, Spitzer AR, Broennle AM, et al: Postoperative apnea in preterm infants. Anesthesiology 1987; 66:483-488.)

area of the brain most susceptible to injury in the micropremie is the periventricular white matter.[22] The white matter consists of preoligodendrocytes, astrocytes, and neuronal axons. Late in the second trimester (24-27 weeks' gestation), preoligodendrocytes and astrocytes multiply tremendously and most cortical and subcortical structures begin to develop.[22] During this period, the periventricular white matter is particularly susceptible to neurologic injury. The periventricular white matter is perfused by arteries penetrating from the cortical surface and by lenticulostriate arteries from the circle of Willis. As a result, the periventricular white matter is a "watershed region" and susceptible to poor perfusion and hypoxic-ischemic injury during conditions of hypotension, low cardiac output, hypoxemia, and hypocarbia.

Neural pathways allowing for perception of pain develop during the first, second, and third trimesters (see Chapter 38).[23] During the first trimester, peripheral sensory receptors and spinal reflex arcs develop that lead to the presence of a "withdrawal reflex" to non-noxious stimuli. Neurons allowing for nociception appear in the dorsal root ganglia at 19 weeks of gestation, and afferent neurons from the thalamus reach the cortical subplate and cortical plate between 20 and 24 weeks of gestation. It is not until early in the third trimester (29 weeks) that pathways between the thalamus and somatosensory cortex function. Significant controversy exists regarding the exact gestational age at which perception and memory of pain occur. Nevertheless, our approach in the micropremie is to administer anesthesia during surgery and provide pain management postoperatively.

Long-Term Neurologic Complications of Prematurity

Long-term neurologic and developmental disabilities remain common in the micropremie and include cerebral palsy, cognitive deficits, behavioral abnormalities, as well as hearing and visual impairment. In one cohort of extremely low birth weight infants, only 25% were classified as normally developed at age 5, whereas 20% exhibited major disabilities.[21] Brain magnetic resonance imaging (MRI) identifies a spectrum of abnormalities. The most common abnormality is diffuse high signal intensity on T2-weighted imaging in the periventricular cerebral white matter. Diffusion-weighted imaging shows increased apparent diffusion coefficient values (ADC), indicative of increased water content and delayed white matter maturation, suggesting ischemia-reperfusion injury in periventricular white matter, which has activated microglia and damaged preoligodendrocytes.[22,24] Damage to preoligodendrocytes impairs myelination of cerebral white matter axons and accounts for many of the fine motor, speech, and cognitive deficits. On MRI, tissue volumes in the basal ganglia, corpus callosum, amygdala, and hippocampus are reduced and correlate with lower full-scale, verbal, and performance IQ scores.[25] Collectively, these MRI findings indicate that different regions of the brain vary in their susceptibility to injury during development and that such injuries lead to specific long-term disturbances in neurocognitive function.

Intraventricular Hemorrhage

Intraventricular hemorrhage (IVH) occurs in as many as one third of micropremie infants. The severity of IVH, as defined by head ultrasound, is graded as follows:

- Grade 1: hemorrhage limited to the germinal matrix
- Grade 2: hemorrhage extending into the ventricular system
- Grade 3: hemorrhage into the ventricular system and with ventricular dilatation
- Grade 4: hemorrhage extending into brain parenchyma.

Although micropremie infants with grade 3 or 4 IVH are more likely to exhibit severe long-term neurocognitive sequelae, even infants with grade 1 and 2 IVH display poorer neurodevelopmental outcomes compared with those without IVH.[26] Early onset of IVH appears during the first day of life. Risk factors include fetal distress, vaginal delivery, low APGAR scores, metabolic acidosis, hypercapnia, and the need for mechanical ventilation.[27,28] Late onset of IVH appears days to weeks after birth. Risk factors include respiratory distress syndrome, seizures, pneumothoraces, hypoxemia, acidosis, severe hypocarbia, and the use of vasopressor infusions.[27] Rapid fluctuations in cerebral blood flow, cerebral blood volume, and cerebral venous pressure appear to play a role in the development of IVH.[29] Factors that may decrease the incidence and severity of IVH include administration of sedation with opioids, antenatal glucocorticoids, or indomethacin.

Retinopathy of Prematurity

Retinopathy of prematurity (ROP) occurs in approximately 50% of extremely low birth weight infants, with the incidence being inversely proportional to birth weight and gestational age (see Chapter 32).[30] Although the pathogenesis of ROP is not completely understood, variations in arterial oxygenation (hypoxia or hyperoxia) and exposure to bright light appear to play a role.[31] One theory holds that the combination of hyperoxic vasoconstriction of retinal vessels, induction of vascular endothelial growth factor, and free oxygen radicals damage the spindle cells in the retina.[32] During anesthesia, we use the lowest inspired oxygen concentration that provides oxygen saturations between 92% and 96% and strive to avoid significant fluctuations in oxygen saturations.

Temperature Regulation

The micropremie is susceptible to hypothermia. Heat transfer occurs by convection, conduction, radiation, and evaporation (see Chapter 25). Evaporative heat loss and insensible fluid loss are increased in the micropremie because the epidermis has less keratin.[33] Conductive and convective heat loss are also increased because there is little fat for insulation and a large surface area to mass ratio. Thermal regulation is not well developed in the micropremie. Nonshivering thermogenesis, which depends on brown fat stores, is decreased in the micropremie, and regulation of skin blood flow is less efficient.[34] During anesthesia, measures taken to minimize convective heat loss include transporting the child in a thermoneutral incubator and warming the operating room to 78° to 80° F before the neonate arrives in the operating room. Use of a warming pad on the operating table reduces conductive heat loss; use of overhead heat lamps reduces radiant heat loss; and keeping the skin dry reduces evaporative heat loss. The most effective means for warming is a hot air mattress.

Renal and Metabolic Function

In the micropremie, kidney function is decreased as a result of fewer nephrons and smaller glomerular size.[35] Glomeruli continue to form postnatally until approximately 40 days.[36] During this period, low cardiac output, hypotension, and nephrotoxic drugs may inhibit glomerular growth and development. Baseline plasma creatinine levels are higher with increasing prematurity and remain elevated until 3 weeks of age.[37] In addition, the normal increase in creatine clearance seen in term infants occurs more slowly in the micropremie.

Very preterm infants easily become hyponatremic because of reduced proximal tubular reabsorption of sodium and water and reduced receptors for hormones that influence tubular sodium transport. As many as one third of extremely low birth weight infants develop hyponatremia.[38] Frequent assessment of sodium and free water requirements is important during critical illness. Elevation of the plasma potassium concentration occurs in preterm infants during the first few days of life and results from a shift in potassium from the intracellular to extracellular space.[39] These elevations are greater with decreasing gestational age and birth weight.[40] Low cardiac output and urine output may further increase serum potassium concentrations and predispose to cardiac arrhythmias.[41]

Glucose Regulation

The micropremie is at risk for hypoglycemia as well as hyperglycemia. Decreased glycogen and body fat predispose to fasting hypoglycemia, whereas decreased insulin production with infusion of dextrose predisposes to hyperglycemia.[42,43] Glucose production is poorly regulated within a large range of glucose and insulin concentrations. The micropremie is also relatively insulin resistant and requires a higher insulin infusion rate to reach normoglycemia.[44] The use of total parenteral nutrition and glucocorticoids places them at high risk for hyperglycemia.

Glucose and the Brain

Multiple animal models and clinical studies implicate hyperglycemia as detrimental to the adult brain during global and focal ischemia.[45] In contrast, hyperglycemia in neonates appears to protect the brain from ischemic damage.[46-48] Studies in both neonatal rat and pig hypoxia-ischemia models observed less brain damage with higher glucose levels. Many mechanisms exist for this strikingly different outcome between neonates and adults.[49] Relatively mild hypoglycemia is known to cause brain damage in preterm infants.[50] Micropremies with critical illness are especially prone to hypoglycemia because they contain limited stores of glucose and consume glucose anaerobically. Thus, the administration of dextrose-containing fluids (carefully controlled with an infusion pump so as to minimize wide fluctuations in glucose values) and close monitoring of blood glucose levels is vital during anesthesia. Mild or moderate hyperglycemia during surgery is best managed by reducing the rate of infusion of dextrose-containing solutions and not administering insulin, with its attendant risk of hypoglycemia.

Hepatic and Hematologic Function

Immature hepatic function leads to a reduction in many hepatic proteins important for drug metabolism. In addition, reduced albumin synthesis decreases albumin levels compared with term neonates, thus enhancing the "free" concentration of anesthetic drugs such as thiopental that are highly bound to albumin (see Chapter 6). The micropremie is at particular risk for spontaneous liver hemorrhage.[51,52] This occurs most commonly during laparotomy for necrotizing enterocolitis (NEC), is associated with large intravenous fluid resuscitation, and is difficult to control surgically. Recombinant factor VIIa has been used to stop liver hemorrhage when administration of other blood products has been unsuccessful.[53]

The ideal hematocrit level for the micropremie remains controversial. In the micropremie with low oxygen saturations or cardiac output, tissue oxygen delivery will be maximized by maintenance of the hematocrit between 44% to 48%. A study comparing infants between 500 and 1300 g, randomly assigned to either a liberal or restrictive transfusion group, found that the restrictive transfusion group had a higher incidence of intraparenchymal brain hemorrhage, periventricular leukomalacia, and episodes of apnea.[54] The risks of blood transfusion in the micropremie must be weighed against the benefits of improved oxygen delivery and fewer medical complications.

Thrombocytopenia ($<150,000/mm^3$) occurs in as many as 70% of micropremature infants.[55] Although the etiology of thrombocytopenia is often not known, pathophysiologic processes such as sepsis, disseminated intravascular coagulation, and NEC are common causes. Preoperative evaluation should include a recent platelet count and the availability of platelets for major procedures.

Anesthetic Agents and the Micropremie

Anesthesia provides insensibility to pain during surgical procedures. Although anesthesia may be provided by regional or general techniques, general anesthesia is the most commonly used technique in the micropremie. During the past 25 years, general anesthesia has been delivered using both inhaled and intravenous drugs in very premature infants for a variety of surgical procedures.

Anesthetics and the Immature Brain

Research in immature animal models indicates that anesthetic agents possess neuroprotective as well as neurotoxic properties. The inhaled agents conferred neurologic protection against hypoxic-ischemic injury in neonatal pigs and rats.[56-58] The agent must be administered before and during the ischemic event at a concentration of 1 MAC. Thus, for surgery in which there is a risk of brain ischemia, use of an inhaled agent affords some advantages over intravenous agents. Cardiac surgery, ventricular shunt insertion, and vein of Galen embolization represent examples of procedures that are performed in preterm infants that carry a risk of brain ischemia.

Of particular concern are the reports in immature rats showing that prolonged exposure to isoflurane, ketamine, or midazolam precipitates apoptosis in many regions of the brain.[59,60] Exposure for at least 2 hours at 1 MAC of isoflurane was required to produce apoptosis. The cocktail of isoflurane, midazolam, and nitrous oxide produced more neuronal degeneration than isoflurane or midazolam alone.[59] Nitrous oxide by itself was not neurotoxic. As adults, the rats that had been exposed to nitrous oxide as neonates displayed less ability to learn tasks than those that had not been exposed. The neurotoxicity was brain region specific and highly dependent on developmental age. In rats, postnatal age 7 day was more sensitive to neurotoxicity than postnatal age 4 day, whereas postnatal age 14 days did not exhibit toxicity.[61] The postnatal 10-day rats exhibited neurodegenerative changes that were less severe than the postnatal age 7-day rats. Based on the life cycle of the rat compared with the human, the 4-day, 7-day, 10-day, and 14-day postnatal age rat corresponds to 28-week gestation, 32-week gestation, 40-week gestation, and 55-week postconceptual age human. Thus, the potential for neurotoxicity from inhaled anesthetics, midazolam, and ketamine may be greater in preterm infants than full-term infants, although there is no evidence that similar neurotoxicity occurs in humans at any age exposed to any anesthetics.

The mechanism for the neurotoxicity appears to be attributed to the neurotransmitters glutamate and γ-aminobutyric acid, which act as trophic factors in the developing brain.[62] In the immature brain these trophic factors promote synaptic growth and plasticity and are obligate for neuronal survival. The inhaled anesthetics, ketamine, and midazolam exert their anesthetic effects by altering synaptic transmission through blockade of glutamate and γ-aminobutyric acid receptors. In the immature brain, this blockade also precipitates neuronal cell death by apoptosis.[63] A confounding factor is that neurodegeneration and apoptosis is a normal developmental phenomenon in the maturing fetal brain and not all immature animal brains display neurotoxicity to isoflurane and midazolam. In piglets and rabbits, neuronal death was not observed after prolonged exposure.[64] In mice, neuronal degeneration was observed only in postnatal day 7 animals and not other ages and was mild and limited to one brain region.[65] Furthermore, the adult mice that had been exposed to isoflurane as neonates learned equally well in a battery of tests as the adult mice that had not been exposed as neonates.[66] Moreover, immature animals that undergo painful procedures without anesthesia experience neuronal degeneration.[67,68] Preterm infants who receive anesthesia and sedation for painful procedures experience less morbidity and mortality than those who do not.[69,70] Taken together, the neurodegeneration precipitated by inhaled anesthetics, ketamine, and benzodiazepines depends on the species, developmental age, the brain region, and the duration of exposure. Based on the animal models, the micropremie exposed to several hours of high concentrations of inhaled agents with nitrous oxide and midazolam is potentially at risk, as is the micropremie exposed to surgery with insufficient anesthesia. Thus, our approach at the present time for emergency surgery is to use low concentrations of inhaled agent with opioids and regional anesthesia whenever possible.

Inhaled Agents

Minimum alveolar concentration (MAC) defines the anesthetic depth for inhaled agents at which 50% of patients respond to painful stimulus with movement; this measure allows comparison of the effects of inhaled anesthetics at equipotent doses. Ledez and Lerman found that MAC in the micropremie is considerably less than in full-term infants (Fig. 35-3), and that isoflurane administered at equipotent dose (1 MAC) resulted in similar reductions in systolic arterial pressure (20% to 30%).[71] For many years, halothane was recognized to cause significant hypotension and cardiovascular instability in young infants.[72] Halothane (1 MAC) decreases arterial pressure by 33% to 54%, mainly by decreasing ventricular ejection fraction and cardiac output.[73] Because of this cardiovascular depression, we rarely use halothane to anesthetize preterm infants. In contrast to halothane, the decrease in arterial blood pressure seen with isoflurane occurs primarily through a reduction in systemic vascular resistance and not cardiac output.

Sevoflurane and desflurane, newer inhaled anesthetic agents, afford a rapid induction and emergence from general anesthesia.

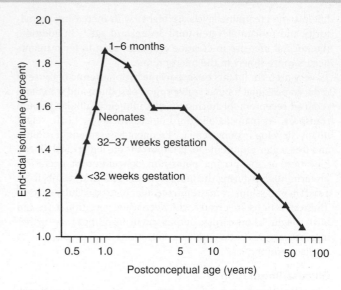

Figure 35-3. The minimal alveolar concentration (MAC) for isoflurane in preterm infants, full-term infants, children, and adults. (Note data are plotted in postconceptual years.) (Reprinted with permission from LeDez KM, Lerman J: The minimum alveolar concentration [MAC] of isoflurane in preterm neonates. Anesthesiology 1987; 67:301-307.)

Sevoflurane has replaced halothane as the agent of choice for inhalational induction. Desflurane is contraindicated for induction of anesthesia but is widely used for maintenance of anesthesia administered through an endotracheal tube. Desflurane and sevoflurane behave similarly to isoflurane in terms of cardiovascular profile. However, desflurane possesses more airway irritability than isoflurane or sevoflurane and is not recommended for infants with severe BPD. Nitrous oxide is not routinely used in the micropremie. First, nitrous oxide must be delivered in inspired concentrations ranging from 50% to 75% to reduce the MAC of other agents; therefore, its role in micropremies, a group often requiring supplemental oxygen, is limited. Second, because of its blood gas solubility, nitrous oxide rapidly enters air-filled cavities; therefore, it is not recommended for use in infants with bowel obstruction, NEC, pulmonary interstitial emphysema, or pneumothoraces.[74] Many micropremies present for surgery with these conditions.

Intravenous Agents

Intravenous agents include opioids, benzodiazepines, barbiturates, propofol, ketamine, and dexmedetomidine. Fentanyl, a synthetic opioid, possesses analgesic and sedative properties. However, it does not reliably produce unconsciousness or amnesia and, by itself, is not considered an anesthetic in children or adults. Nevertheless, the use of fentanyl as an anesthetic has been justified in preterm infants because they were deemed to be inherently amnestic by virtue of their age, even though the age at which "consciousness" and memory occurs is unknown. Preterm infants (<1500 g) who received intravenous fentanyl (30 to 50 μg/kg) and pancuronium for ligation of a PDA exhibit remarkable hemodynamic stability with only a 5% decrease in blood pressure.[75] In addition, hypertension and tachycardia does not occur with skin incision, suggesting that analgesic levels necessary for surgery are produced with this dose of fentanyl.

Collins and colleagues evaluated the pharmacokinetics of fentanyl in preterm infants.[76] After fentanyl administration

(30 µg/kg), plasma concentrations remained constant for up to 120 minutes, indicating a slow clearance of the drug. Indeed, Koren and coworkers found that the elimination half-life of fentanyl ranged from 6 to 32 hours, significantly longer than the 2- to 3-hour half-life observed in children and adults.[77] These studies demonstrate that the half-life, clearance, and volume of distribution of fentanyl are increased compared with the same factors in adults.[78] Thus, for a given dose of fentanyl, higher plasma fentanyl concentrations and a slower clearance of the drug will occur in the micropremie, which serves to prolong analgesia as well as prolong respiratory depression, increase the risk of postoperative apnea, and slow recovery of consciousness. In the micropremie, mechanical ventilation may be required for several days after large doses of fentanyl.

Similarly, the elimination half-life of morphine is markedly prolonged in preterm infants compared with children and adults.[79] The elimination half-life of morphine ranges from 6 to 16 hours in the micropremie compared with 2 to 4 hours in the adult. We prefer fentanyl over high-dose morphine (2 to 3 mg/kg) for anesthesia because it has fewer hemodynamic side effects.

Remifentanil, a relatively new synthetic short-acting opioid, is rapidly inactivated by esterases in the blood and tissues and because of its short half-life is administered by continuous infusion. The half-life of remifentanil in adults is 3 to 4 minutes, independent of the length of infusion, and not significantly different in infants or children.[80] A multicenter study comparing halothane and remifentanil for maintenance of anesthesia in infants undergoing pyloromyotomy showed that infants receiving remifentanil exhibited intraoperative hemodynamic stability without an increase in postoperative apnea or respiratory depression.[81] Remifentanil has not been studied in extremely premature infants.

Ketamine, a phencyclidine derivative, affords several advantages compared with inhaled and other intravenous agents. It provides analgesia, amnesia, and unconsciousness yet minimally depresses cardiovascular function (Fig. 35-4).[82,83] Ketamine is also a potent bronchodilator, a property that may be of particular benefit to the micropremie. However, ketamine anesthesia depresses ventilation and airway reflexes, which predisposes to airway obstruction, apnea, and gastric aspiration. Thus, we recommend the use of an endotracheal tube when ketamine is used for surgical procedures in the micropremie. In the setting of brief painful procedures, we find intravenous ketamine can be used as an anesthetic without an endotracheal tube.

Other intravenous agents include thiopental, propofol, and benzodiazepines. These agents induce loss of consciousness but possess less analgesia than ketamine. Unfortunately, little information exists on the pharmacokinetics or pharmacodynamics of these drugs in preterm infants. Thiopental is a short-acting barbiturate primarily used for the induction of anesthesia. The micropremie requires less thiopental for induction than infants (2-3 mg/kg vs. 5-6 mg/kg) a relationship similar to the MAC of isoflurane.[84] In the micropremie, we only use thiopental for neurosurgical procedures involving increased intracranial pressure. The disadvantage of thiopental is that it depresses cardiac output and causes venodilation and may precipitate cardiovascular collapse in the setting of hypovolemia; it also has a very long half-life in preterm and term infants.

Like thiopental, propofol is primarily used to induce anesthesia. In our experience, the micropremie can be anesthetized

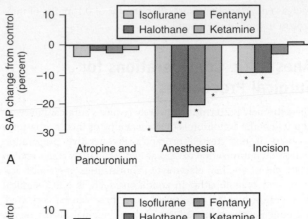

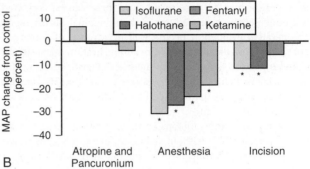

Figure 35-4. A, Changes in systolic arterial pressure (SAP) in preterm infants after anesthesia with either isoflurane, halothane, fentanyl, or ketamine and after surgical incision. **B,** Changes in mean arterial pressure (MAP) in premature infants after anesthesia with either isoflurane, halothane, fentanyl, or ketamine and after surgical incision. (Reprinted with permission from Friesen RH, Henry DB: Cardiovascular changes in preterm neonates receiving isoflurane, halothane, fentanyl, and ketamine. Anesthesiology 1986; 64:238-242.)

with a propofol infusion (50 to 200 µg/kg/min) supplemented with fentanyl as needed for analgesia. The selection of infusion pumps that allow for delivery of small volumes accurately is vital. Recovery from propofol anesthesia is slower in micropremies compared with term infants because they have less fat and muscle tissue to redistribute the drug. Infusions of propofol are used for sedation in many adult intensive care units. In pediatric intensive care units, propofol infusions have been implicated in unexpected deaths.[85] Until the safety of long-term administration of propofol has been examined in preterm infants, other alternatives for prolonged sedation in this population should be seriously considered.

Benzodiazepines such as midazolam and diazepam have been used in the neonatal intensive care unit (NICU) for sedation. As with thiopental and propofol, these drugs do not provide analgesia and are not recommended as the sole anesthetic for surgery. However, the combination of a benzodiazepine and opioid provides complete anesthesia for surgery. Benzodiazepines are eliminated by the liver and thus can last several hours in the micropremie with decreased liver function. Midazolam can cause systemic hypotension, depress ventilation, and impair airway reflexes in preterm infants. The hypotension caused by midazolam is greater in the presence of fentanyl; thus, both drugs must be titrated in small doses when administered concomitantly.[86] Van Straaten and colleagues noted an 8% to 23%

decrease in arterial pressure after a bolus of 0.1 mg/kg of mid-azolam in premature infants.[87]

Anesthetic Considerations for Surgical Procedures

The extremely preterm infant rarely requires surgical intervention unless the condition is life threatening or incurs long-term disability if not treated promptly. Preoperative preparation focuses on optimization of cardiac and respiratory status and on treatment of anemia, electrolyte abnormalities, metabolic acidosis, and coagulopathy. In conditions such as NEC, surgical intervention may be necessary before these can be corrected. For nonemergency procedures such as inguinal hernia repair, preoperative evaluation occurs well in advance of surgery to optimize the medical status before administration of anesthesia. Communication between the anesthesiologist, surgeon, and neonatologist before and after surgery is vital for safe care. For almost all surgeries, packed red blood cells should be available in the operating room.

In the past, some surgeons chose to perform surgery at the bedside in the NICU without an anesthesiologist because it was deemed unsafe to transport the infant, there was lack of an operating room or anesthesiologist to perform the surgery in a timely manner, or it was believed that the micropremie did not need anesthesia. The neonatologist often administered sedation or muscle relaxants during surgery. We believe that this care model does not provide the highest level of patient care; there is ample evidence that the micropremie requires anesthesia for surgery. As far as operating at the bedside is concerned, there is reduced access to the child, suboptimal lighting, reduced sterility, and an inability to control room temperature, which predispose to poor outcomes. In our institution we have addressed the issue of transporting an unstable infant several floors to the operating room by building a surgical suite in the NICU, thus minimizing the period of transport and providing optimal surgical conditions.

Exploratory Laparotomy for Necrotizing Enterocolitis

Necrotizing enterocolitis, a life-threatening condition mainly afflicting preterm infants, occurs in about 5% of extremely low birth weight infants (see Chapter 36).[88] Although NEC may be treated medically, the micropremie with NEC is more likely to require surgery that carries a mortality ranging from 10% to 50%.[89-91] The pathogenesis of NEC is incompletely understood; intestinal mucosal ischemia is thought to play a key role. Other key factors include inflammation of bowel mucosa, alterations in normal intestinal flora by antibiotic therapy, gastric alkalinity, and low systemic cardiac output.[92-94] Early signs of NEC include feeding intolerance, increased work of breathing, lethargy, and temperature instability; later signs include hypotension, abdominal distention, apnea, thrombocytopenia, coagulopathy, and multisystem organ failure. Classic radiographic findings include gas in the intestinal wall (pneumatosis intestinalis) and biliary tract and free air within the abdomen. Indications for surgical exploration include the presence of perforation or continued clinical deterioration despite medical management (Fig. 35-5).

Surgical management of the micropremie with NEC involves either initial primary peritoneal drainage or a laparotomy with resection of necrotic bowel. Primary peritoneal drainage requires

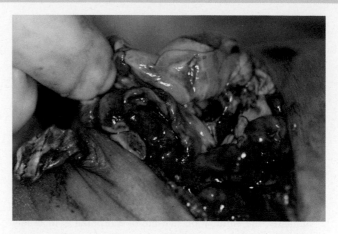

Figure 35-5. Early necrotizing enterocolitis with bowel perforation. Note that the perforation was diagnosed early and that there is soiling of the peritoneum but there does not appear to be any dead bowel. This type of perforation is generally associated with a positive outcome.

a small surgical incision and fewer anesthetic requirements and can be performed at the bedside. Some infants who undergo initial peritoneal drainage will subsequently require laparotomy if their condition worsens. Peritoneal drainage has generally been favored in the smaller and more unstable preterm infants for logistical reasons; thus, the ability to compare the two management strategies has been difficult because of multiple confounding variables.[88,95] A prospective randomized, multicenter trial comparing laparotomy and peritoneal drainage in infants weighing less than 1500 g with perforated NEC found no difference in survival, development of short-gut syndrome, or length of hospital stay between the two approaches.[96]

NEC is a surgical emergency, and preoperative preparation in a timely fashion is vital. NEC predisposes to hypovolemia, cardiovascular and respiratory failure, capillary leak syndrome, disseminated intravascular coagulation, and hypoglycemia. It is important to prepare for all these sequelae. We have albumin, fresh frozen plasma, platelets, and packed red blood cells available; calcium gluconate, dopamine and epinephrine are prepared for treatment of hypotension and low cardiac output. Because pulmonary function may deteriorate, we ensure the availability of sophisticated ventilators for increased mechanical ventilatory support. In our institution we often have the ventilator used in the NICU brought to the operating room in case severe respiratory failure ensues. Coagulopathy and thrombocytopenia increases bleeding and necessitates blood product administration during surgery. Before bringing the micropremie to the operating room, we note the current medications, size and location of intravenous catheters, and dextrose infusion rate and obtain a current plasma glucose concentration.

Vascular access remains critical for this surgery. At least two venous cannulas and an arterial catheter should be considered for optimal care. A central venous catheter facilitates the delivery of infusions such as dopamine or epinephrine. In our institution, many preterm infants have peripherally inserted central catheters, allowing for delivery of vasopressors. These catheters are not well suited for rapid delivery of anesthetic drugs or blood or for measurement of central venous pressure. An arterial catheter provides continuous blood pressure monitoring and the ability to sample blood gases, electrolytes, complete blood cell count (CBC), platelet count, and prothrombin time/partial thromboplastin times (PT/PTT). Blood pressure cuffs often fail to measure arterial pressure during this surgery. A Foley catheter allows for the assessment of urine flow. A nasogastric tube should be present. Time spent by the anesthesia and surgical team to place these lines must be weighed against the need for urgent laparotomy.

General endotracheal anesthesia with neuromuscular blockade remains the anesthetic technique for NEC surgery. NEC increases the risk for aspiration. Tracheal intubation may be achieved by "awake intubation" or rapid sequence anesthetic induction. We prefer an awake intubation in the micropremie because effective cricoid pressure is difficult to apply for rapid sequence induction and arterial desateration occurs rapidly during apnea. After the administration of intravenous atropine, awake intubation is performed using an oxyscope, a laryngoscope with an oxygen port to allow for oxygen delivery during direct laryngoscopy (see Fig. 12-35). In infants whose tracheas are already intubated, anesthesia is effected with ketamine, fentanyl, or an inhaled agent in combination with a nondepolarizing muscle relaxant.

The anesthetic regimen that we prefer includes (1) intravenous fentanyl (5-10 µg/kg), an inhaled anesthetic such as isoflurane, sevoflurane, or desflurane, and muscle relaxant (balanced technique); (2) intravenous fentanyl (20 to 50 µg/kg), intravenous midazolam (0.1 mg/kg), and muscle relaxant (high-dose opioid technique); or (3) ketamine (4 mg/kg/hr) and muscle relaxant. We select the high-dose opioid or ketamine technique for hemodynamically unstable infants. Pancuronium is an ideal muscle relaxant when combined with high doses of fentanyl because of its anticholinergic properties but should be avoided in infants with renal dysfunction. If hypotension persists despite a trial of 10 to 20 mL/kg of intravenous fluid, we begin an infusion of dopamine (5 to 20 µg/kg/min). Hypocalcemia after administration of blood products may contribute to hypotension and requires replacement with either calcium chloride or calcium gluconate (see Chapter 10). When severe shock persists despite intravenous fluid resuscitation, calcium, and dopamine, rescue treatment with "stress dose" glucocorticoids may be beneficial. Treatment with hydrocortisone and dexamethasone has been effective in improving arterial pressure in low birth weight infants with refractory hypotension.[97,98]

Intraoperative fluids consist of maintenance fluids (4 mL/kg/hr), third space loss (at least 10 mL/kg/hr), and replacement of blood loss. Third space losses include evaporation and vascular leak and are replaced with an isotonic salt solution. Blood losses are replaced with packed red blood cells and fresh frozen plasma to maintain the hemoglobin greater than 10 g/dL and the PT/PTT within normal range. Platelets are administered to keep the platelet count greater than 100,000/mm^3. It is common for the micropremie to receive 100 mL/kg of fluid during exploratory laparotomy for NEC. Continuous measurement of arterial pressure and serial measurement of urine output, blood gases, CBC, platelet counts, and PT/PTT aid in the fluid replacement process. Arterial blood gas analysis helps guide ventilation and inspired oxygen concentration. Warming of the operating suite to 80° F, a forced air warmer underneath the infant, and warmed fluids help maintain normothermia during surgery. In preterm infants with NEC, postoperative mechanical ventilation remains the rule. Postoperative analgesia can be provided with a continuous infusion of fentanyl (1-3 µg/kg/hr) or intermittent doses of morphine (0.1 mg/kg every 4 to 6 hours). The time it takes for the micropremie to emerge from anesthesia depends on the anesthetic technique (balanced vs. high-dose opioid vs. ketamine) and the need for postoperative analgesics. After a high-dose opioid technique, the micropremie may take 12 to 24 hours to emerge, as compared with several hours for a balanced or a ketamine technique.

Ligation of Patent Ductus Arteriosus

Failure of the ductus arteriosus to close after birth is common in the micropremie.[99] Indomethacin therapy is less likely to close the PDA in micropremies compared with preterm infants and is more likely to produce complications, including thrombocytopenia, renal failure, hyponatremia, and intestinal perforation.[100] In the micropremie, the PDA incurs significant left-to-right shunting of blood, causing severe pulmonary overcirculation, congestive heart failure, and respiratory failure. In fact, the diameter of the PDA may be greater than the aorta. In the micropremie with respiratory distress syndrome or persistent pulmonary hypertension, right-to-left shunting across the PDA may occur producing cyanosis. Significant controversy remains regarding the timing of surgical intervention and the merits of medical versus surgical therapy. When surgery is performed by experienced teams, the incidence of major complications is small.[101] However, substantial late morbidity and mortality have been reported from long-term complications of prematurity.[102]

During preoperative preparation, arterial pressure, heart rate, arterial blood gases, ventilator settings, and inspired oxygen concentration should be noted. The PDA is ligated through a left thoracotomy and requires retraction of the left lung, which decreases lung compliance, ventilation, and oxygenation. Preoperative difficulty with ventilation and oxygenation forecasts trouble in the operating room. Because the aorta and pulmonary artery lie in proximity to the PDA, severe bleeding may occur abruptly and unexpectedly during the procedure. Packed red blood cells should be immediately available for transfusion. Intraoperative monitoring includes a blood pressure cuff (right arm), continuous end-tidal carbon dioxide monitoring, and a pulse oximeter placed on digits on the right arm and a lower extremity. This will help the surgeon to be certain that the vessel about to be ligated (clipped) is in fact the ductus and not the aorta; it should be noted that with a left-sided arch that the pulse oximeter may need to be applied to the left hand instead of the right to ensure monitoring of a preductal blood vessel. Invasive monitoring of arterial pressure and blood gases is helpful in the micropremie with significant heart failure and/or lung disease, although we do not consider it a requirement for surgery. An intravenous catheter through which blood can be rapidly administered should be available.

The anesthetic technique of choice for PDA ligation remains fentanyl (20 to 50 µg/kg) and pancuronium (0.2 mg/kg). Although this technique usually does not cause hypotension or bradycardia, reduction in arterial pressure after anesthetic induction does occur because of loss of sympathetic tone, especially in the setting of hypovolemia from diuretic therapy. Thus, we commonly administer albumin (10 mL/kg) before induction. During mechanical ventilation, mild hypoventilation and reduction of the inspired oxygen concentration help to reduce pulmonary overcirculation from the PDA. However, during surgical retraction of the lung it is usually necessary to increase ventilator

Annotated References

Anand KJS, Soriano SG: Anesthetic agents and the immature brain: are these toxic or therapeutic. Anesthesiology 2004; 101:527-530

This article written in response to studies in neonatal rats implicates commonly used anesthetic agents as neurotoxic to the developing brain. The authors discuss methodologic problems with these studies and the consequences of withholding anesthesia to infants undergoing painful procedures.

Baum VC, Palmisano BW: The immature heart and anesthesia. Anesthesiology 1997; 87:1529-1548

This article examines developmental aspects of cardiac function and, in particular, how anesthetic agents affect the immature heart.

Coté CJ, Zaslavsky A, Downes JJ, et al: Postoperative apnea in former preterm infants after inguinal herniorrhaphy. Anesthesiology 1995; 82:809-822

This is a combined analysis of eight papers that studied postoperative apnea after general anesthesia for inguinal herniorrhaphy.

Friesen RH, Henry DB: Cardiovascular changes in preterm neonates receiving isoflurane, halothane, fentanyl, and ketamine. Anesthesiology 1986; 64:238-242

This is one of the few studies comparing the cardiovascular effects of different anesthetic agents on the preterm infant.

Jevtovic-Tedorovic V, Hartman RE, Izumi Y, et al: Early exposure to common anesthetic agents causes widespread neurodegeneration in the developing rat brain and persistent learning deficits. J Neurosci 2003; 23:876-882

This publication generated national media attention and questioned the safety of common anesthetic agents used in neonates and premature infants.

Mikkola K, Ritari N, Tommiska V, et al: Neurodevelopmental outcome at 5 years of age of a national cohort of extremely low birth weight infants who were born in 1996-1997. Pediatrics 2005; 116: 1391-1400

This study assesses neurodevelopmental outcome at 5 years of age in a cohort of extremely-low-birth-weight infants. The authors found that only 25% of these children were classified as developmentally normal.

References

Please see www.expertconsult.com

Neonatal Emergencies

Jesse D. Roberts Jr., Thomas M. Romanelli, and I. David Todres

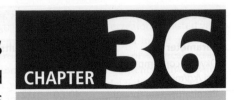

CHAPTER 36

Neonatal Physiology Related to Anesthesia	Preparation for Surgery
Cardiopulmonary	The Operating Room
Temperature Regulation	The Family
Renal and Metabolic Function	**Emergency Surgery**
Gastrointestinal and Hepatic Function	Respiratory Problems
Neurologic Development	Gastrointestinal Problems

ADVANCES IN PERINATAL CARE have greatly reduced the morbidity and mortality of critically ill neonates. Anesthesiologists have contributed to the improvement in neonatal outcome by integrating knowledge of developmental biology and pharmacology and applying these principles in the care of critically ill neonates undergoing surgical procedures. The goals of this chapter are to describe developmental processes in neonates and how they affect the anesthetic management of neonatal emergencies.

Neonatal Physiology Related to Anesthesia

Cardiopulmonary

Oxygen Consumption

The cardiopulmonary system of the neonate is driven by the need to deliver sufficient oxygen to maintain a high metabolic rate. The oxygen consumption of an average neonate is 5 to 8 mL/kg/min, whereas that of an adult is 2 to 3 mL/kg/min (Table 36-1). Primarily, it is this high rate of oxygen consumption that leads to the rapid decrease in blood oxygen levels in the neonate during periods of hypoventilation. Although ventilatory gas exchange volume in adults is nearly 10-fold greater than in neonates, the tidal volume relative to body weight for both is approximately equal (6 mL/kg). In the neonate, increasing the respiratory rate facilitates CO_2 elimination; alveolar ventilation in the perinatal period is approximately 130 mL/kg/min, compared with 60 mL/kg/min in adulthood. In a neonate, the thoracic gas volume on a weight basis is similar to that in an adult.

Pulmonary Gas Exchange

In the neonate, apnea decreases gas exchange in the lung and is associated with hypoxemia and bradycardia. Conceptually, apnea is differentiated in terms of its etiology: (1) *central apnea*, due to immaturity or depression of the respiratory drive; (2) *obstructive apnea*, due to an infant's inability to maintain a patent airway; and (3) *mixed apnea*, a combination of both central and obstructive apnea.[1]

Apnea of central origin may be secondary to the poor organization and integration of afferent input from proprioceptive receptors, which are located in the diaphragm and intercostal muscles, and from medullary and peripheral chemoreceptors. Preterm infants are at greater risk of central apnea because of the responsiveness of chemoreceptors to hypercarbia and hypoxia that develops with advancing conceptual age. Decreased input from chemoreceptors despite periods of mild hypercarbia and hypoxia can cause apnea in preterm infants. Susceptibility to central apnea is exacerbated by metabolic disturbances such as hypothermia, hypoglycemia, and hypocalcemia. For these reasons, central apnea may be exacerbated by anemia and sepsis in neonates. Blood transfusions of preterm infants with a hematocrit less than 27% may reduce the incidence of apnea[2,3]; however, data suggest a poor correlation between anemia and the incidence of apnea/bradycardia spells.[4] Central apnea due to immaturity of the respiratory drive center is often treated with xanthine derivatives, such as caffeine and theophylline (Table 36-2).[5-8] Of particular importance to the anesthesiologist is that central apnea in neonates can be exacerbated by opioids. In these cases, the neonates require careful continuous monitoring of blood oxygen saturation and heart rate in the postoperative period. In some cases, apnea in neonates exposed to opioids may be alleviated by treatment with naloxone.

Apnea of an obstructive or mixed origin is responsible for the majority of apneic episodes in preterm infants.[9-11] Obstructive apnea may be due to incomplete maturation and poor coordination of upper airway musculature. These forms of apnea often respond to changes in head position, insertion of an oral or nasal airway, or placing the infant in a prone position. Application of continuous positive airway pressure may also reduce obstructive apnea.[12]

Recurrent postoperative apnea has been described in neonates with a history of prematurity, apnea, or chronic lung disease.[13] Postoperative apnea is a common morbidity associated with anesthesia in infants who were born prematurely.[14]

pulmonary vascular resistance (e.g., hypoxia, hypercarbia, or acidosis) may result in a return to the fetal-type circulatory pattern with shunting of deoxygenated blood from the right-to-left side of the heart via the PFO or PDA. This right-to-left shunting explains in part why some infants remain hypoxemic despite ventilation with 100% oxygen after severe desaturation.

The ductus arteriosus may remain patent in neonates, especially in prematurely born ones.[72] Bounding peripheral pulses, a harsh systolic ejection murmur at the left sternal border, and widened pulse-pressure difference suggest the presence of a PDA. The presence of a PDA and of right-to-left shunting of blood may contribute to ventilation/perfusion mismatch as deoxygenated blood is shunted from the pulmonary arteries to the systemic circulation through the PDA and differential upper and lower extremity oxygen saturations. Later, as the pulmonary vascular resistance decreases, left-to-right shunting of blood from the systemic to pulmonary circulation across the PDA may cause flow-mediated endothelial cell injury and abnormal pulmonary artery remodeling and hypertension. Infants with a PDA often require increased ventilatory support.

A PDA in the neonate may be treated with indomethacin. Later, if the PDA is not responsive to medical treatments, coil occlusion or surgical ligation may be used.[73-75] Treatment with indomethacin is associated with renal or platelet dysfunction. Although experience suggests that infants who have received large volumes of intravascular fluid have an increased incidence of PDA,[76] the mechanism behind this is unknown and the relationship may not be causal. In fact, if the PDA is associated with ventricular dysfunction and poor organ perfusion, it is *imperative* to provide adequate intravascular volume and to improve cardiac output rather than have the infant be exposed to hypotension mediated by left-to-right shunting across the PDA and hypovolemia. Occasionally, systemic perfusion may be improved in infants with PDA with dopamine infusions and judicious fluid administration.

In neonates, increased pulmonary vascular resistance causes intracardiac shunting of desaturated blood through the PFO and PDA and thereby causes severe systemic hypoxemia. Although the etiology of *persistent pulmonary hypertension of the newborn* (PPHN) is incompletely understood, it is associated with increased muscularization of pulmonary arterial vessels[77] and sepsis and aspiration syndromes.[78] PPHN is suspected in severely hypoxic neonates who do not have a significant increase in postductal oxygen saturation when they breathe 100% oxygen. A difference in preductal and postductal oxygen saturations supports the diagnosis because it reflects the extrapulmonary right-to-left shunting of deoxygenated blood via the PDA. PPHN is diagnosed when pulmonary hypertension and no other structural heart lesions are observed by cardiac ultrasonography.

Treatment of PPHN is directed at decreasing pulmonary vascular resistance and the extrapulmonary shunting of deoxygenated blood. In cases of pneumonia and aspiration syndromes, in which airway disease can lead to atelectasis and intrapulmonary shunt, positive end-expiratory pressure and exogenous surfactant are sometimes used to recruit alveoli. To treat the pulmonary vasoconstriction that is pathognomonic of PPHN, hyperoxia and alkalosis therapies are utilized. Although oxygen is a potent vasodilator, maximum dilatation of the pulmonary vasculature is achieved by relatively low levels of oxygen. For this reason, increasing the F_{IO_2} often does not improve gas exchange in PPHN. Through means that are incompletely understood, alkalosis causes pulmonary vasodilatation. In many infants with PPHN, alkalosis induced by hyperventilation and/or the infusion of base decreases pulmonary vascular resistance and increases systemic oxygen levels. Generally, the vasodilatation induced by alkalosis occurs when the arterial pH is 7.55 or greater. Intravenous vasodilator drugs cause inconsistent vasodilatation in infants with pulmonary hypertension.[79] Unfortunately, because these agents dilate the systemic as well as the pulmonary vasculature, they often cause severe systemic hypotension.

Inhaled NO selectively decreases pulmonary vascular resistance and increases systemic oxygen levels in infants with PPHN.[80-82] NO is a gas that is synthesized by NO synthase in endothelial cells from L-arginine and oxygen diffuses into subjacent smooth muscle cells where it stimulates soluble guanylate cyclase to increase cyclic guanosine monophosphate (cGMP) levels. It is probably through cGMP's stimulation of cGMP-dependent protein kinase I that NO causes vascular relaxation (Fig. 36-1). Recently, it was discovered that inhaling low levels of NO causes selective pulmonary vasodilatation, decreased right-to-left shunting of blood, and increased systemic oxygen levels in neonatal animals and infants with pulmonary hypertension.[83-85] Acutely breathing up to 80 ppm, by volume, of NO rapidly and selectively decreases pulmonary vascular resistance and increases systemic oxygen levels by decreasing extrapulmonary shunting of deoxygenated blood. Although methemoglobin is produced during the metabolism of NO, no important increases in methemoglobin were observed in infants breathing low levels of NO gas. Recent large multicenter studies suggest that breathing as little as 20 ppm NO decreases the requirement for extracorporeal membrane oxygenation (ECMO). Although ECMO is lifesaving for several severely hypoxemic neonates,[86-88] it is expensive, invasive, sometimes causes important complications, and not available at most hospitals. For these reasons, inhaled NO is used in most intensive care nurseries to treat the severe hypoxemia associated with PPHN.

Studies also suggest that chronic NO inhalation protects the neonatal lung from injury.[46] In cell cultures, NO has been

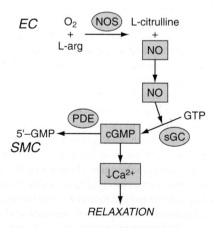

Figure 36-1. Nitric oxide (NO) produced by nitric oxide synthase (NOS) in endothelial cells (EC) diffuses into subjacent smooth muscle cells (SMC), interacts with soluble guanylate cyclase (sGC), and increases the concentration of cyclic guanosine monophosphate (cGMP) to cause vascular relaxation. The effect of NO is decreased by metabolism of cGMP by specific phosphodiesterases (PDE).

observed to decrease pulmonary smooth muscle cell proliferation and increase programmed cell death (apoptosis). Inhaled NO has been observed to decrease pulmonary artery neomuscularization in animals with lungs injured by breathing gases with low levels of oxygen. Although inhaled NO may decrease lung artery remodeling by preventing hypoxic pulmonary vasoconstriction, studies suggest that it prevents abnormal pulmonary artery remodeling in injured lungs without hypertension.[89] Although the protective mechanism of inhaled NO is not known, it has been observed to decrease smooth muscle cell proliferation in vitro,[90] possibly by altering the expression of transcriptional regulators and the progression of the cell cycle.[91-93] New experiments are underway to test whether chronically inhaled NO prevents lung disease, such as BPD, in neonates exposed to increased levels of oxygen and ventilator support.[94-96] It is likely that studies that identify the protective mechanisms of NO/cGMP signaling will guide the development of novel therapies to prevent pulmonary disease in the injured lung.

Temperature Regulation

The neonatal body habitus favors heat loss. The large surface area of the head relative to that of the body of neonates increases heat dissipation. A head cover may significantly reduce temperature loss.[97,98] Neonates do not shiver or sweat effectively to maintain body temperature and rely primarily on brown fat metabolism to maintain body heat. Brown fat cells begin to differentiate at 26 to 30 weeks' gestation and hence are not available in extremely preterm infants to provide fat for metabolism and heat generation.[99] Warming the operating room to 85°F (30°C), using radiant warming units and underbody, forced-air heating pads, and adding humidity to the inspired gases in the ventilator circuits help maintain the neonate's temperature in the neutral thermal range.[100-102] Warming intravenous and irrigation fluids before use may also be beneficial (see Chapter 25).

Renal and Metabolic Function

Renal Function

The placenta acts as an excretory organ of a fetus. A neonate's kidneys are not fully developed until late in gestation, and development is closely related to conceptual age.[103,104] At full-term birth, the glomerular filtration rate is only 15% to 30% of normal adult levels. The glomerular filtration rate reaches adult values at approximately 1 year of age (see Chapter 26 and Fig. 6-7). The kidneys' tubular function, and hence sodium-retaining ability, does not develop until about the 32nd week of gestation.[104,105] The immaturity of the kidney at birth also affects the metabolism of many drugs in the neonate. The renal excretion of medications such as penicillin, gentamicin, and some neuromuscular blocking agents such as pancuronium may be prolonged, resulting in increased duration of action or the development of excessive blood concentrations. This effect is particularly important when administering medications to an extremely preterm infant (see Chapter 6).

The total body water of neonates is greater than in infants, children, or adults. In the preterm infant 75% to 85% of body weight is water; in general, the lower the postconceptional age of the neonate, the greater the percentage of water (see Figs. 6-4 and 6-5). In a term infant, 70% of body weight is water.[106] By 6 to 12 months of age, 50% to 60% of body weight is water. Dif-

ferences between the total body water, renal maturity, and serum protein concentrations in a neonate affect the volume of distribution of most medications. Because of the increase in the volume of distribution of some drugs in the neonate, the initial doses of some medications may be greater on a weight basis than for adults in order to achieve the desired blood concentration. In contrast, because of immaturity of renal function, the interval between dosages of some drugs may be increased (see Chapter 6).

Fluid Management

The basic principles of fluid maintenance in neonates are similar to those in older children and adults. The highly variable body fluid composition, degree of renal maturity,[107] neuroendocrine control of intravascular fluid status, and insensible fluid loss with age[108] make precise estimates of fluid requirements in neonates very difficult (see Chapter 8). Urine volume and concentration may be difficult to determine intraoperatively and may not always correlate with volume status. Moreover, blood pressure and heart rate may not correlate with intravascular volume status in preterm infants and anesthetics may mask subtle cardiovascular responses that occur with changes in intravascular volume. Increased insensible fluid loss, which often occurs in the operating room environment, requires judicious titration of intravenous fluids. Congenital abnormalities (e.g., gastroschisis and omphalocele) may markedly increase insensible fluid loss through exposure of large mucosal surfaces. The use of humidified gas mixtures reduces insensible fluid loss through the respiratory tract.

Methods of Intravenous Access and Monitoring

Infants who are dehydrated after a prolonged period of fasting or vomiting or because of increased insensible fluid losses may require special procedures for intravenous access. With severe hypovolemia, scalp and peripheral veins may be difficult to cannulate. Many of the superficial veins may be thrombosed from prior use. Fiberoptic light sources may help visualize deeper veins and peripheral arteries. Femoral and axillary veins may be accessed percutaneously or via a surgical approach to use in the delivery of fluids and medications.[109-112] Knowledge of the femoral artery and vein anatomy decreases the incidence of accidental injury of the femoral head joint and possible septic arthritis.[113] The external or internal jugular veins can also provide alternative sites for venous access.

In neonates, fluids and many medications may be infused through the umbilical vessels. The tip of umbilical arterial lines should be placed either in a "low" position, at the level of the bifurcation of the femoral arteries (L3-L4), or in a "high" position, in the descending aorta above the diaphragm (T6-T9). The catheter tip of the umbilical artery catheter should not be left in the descending aorta in the area of the renal or mesenteric arteries (L1-L2) because renal or mesenteric artery thrombosis might result (see Fig. 48-7). Aortic thrombosis occurs in approximately 1% of umbilical artery catheterizations, although thrombi can be detected with radiologic techniques in 20% to 95% of infants.[114-116] Infants with renal artery thrombosis may present with hypertension, oliguria, hematuria, and elevated blood creatinine levels. The tip of an umbilical venous catheter should rest in the inferior vena cava above the level of the ductus venosus and hepatic veins so that solutions are not directly infused into the liver parenchyma. The delivery of hypertonic solutions into the liver might result in liver damage and portal cirrhosis. Aspiration of arterial oxygenated blood suggests that the venous catheter has entered the left atrium through the foramen ovale. Catheters in the left atrium should be pulled back to the level described earlier.

Some drugs may be effectively delivered through the endotracheal tube. Rapid uptake and minimal effects on gas exchange or the pulmonary parenchyma occur with epinephrine, atropine, and lidocaine. The dose of some drugs administered through the endotracheal tube (e.g., epinephrine) is increased in comparison with that delivered through the intravenous route. It is important to keep in mind that administration of solutions via the endotracheal tube can cause adverse effects. For example, complications associated with the endotracheal administration of exogenous surfactant include occasional transient hypoxia and bradycardia and are likely due to the relatively large volume of fluid (4-6 mL/kg) associated with the proper dose of surfactant.

Intraosseous cannulation of the tibia with a special intraosseous infusion needle or a styletted spinal needle provides a rapid route for emergency fluid and drug administration and can be lifesaving (see Fig. 49-6).

Glucose Homeostasis

Although the placenta allows the delivery of glucose from the maternal circulation to the fetus, the development of significant glycogen stores does not occur until late in gestation. A number of conditions may lead to hypoglycemia in a neonate. Preterm and small-for-gestational-age (SGA) infants have very high glucose requirements; they require glucose infusion rates of 8 to 10 mg/kg/min. In full-term infants, a glucose infusion rate of 5 to 8 mg/kg/min is required to prevent hypoglycemia. Full-term infants who have been excessively fasted, SGA infants, and infants of diabetic mothers are particularly prone to develop hypoglycemia. Although hypoglycemia may result in respiratory distress, apnea, cyanosis, seizures, tremors, high-pitched cry, irritability, limpness, lethargy, eye rolling, poor feeding, temperature instability, and sweating, the signs and symptoms in infants are often blunted and nonspecific.[117,118] In infants younger than than 24 hours old, a plasma glucose concentration of less than 40 mg/dL is a cause for concern and should be treated (see Chapter 2).[119] After 24 hours of life, plasma glucose values less than 45 mg/dL should be considered abnormally low. Although hypertonic glucose administration has been used to treat hypoglycemia in neonates, studies reveal that administration of hypertonic solutions increases the incidence of intraventricular hemorrhage in preterm infants.[120] For this reason, it is prudent to avoid bolus administration of hypertonic glucose to treat hypoglycemia to prevent sudden changes in blood tonicity and hyperglycemia. A bolus of 3 to 4 mL/kg of $D_{10}W$ (0.1 to 0.2 g/kg of glucose) and an increase in the basal glucose infusion may increase the steady-state glucose level. It is extremely important to reassess the blood glucose concentration after these treatments to determine the effectiveness of the therapy.

Infants undergoing surgical procedures often require less glucose supplementation.[121] This reduced need may be attributed to hormonal responses that decrease glucose uptake as a result of catecholamine release in excess of insulin activity, as well as a decrease in metabolic demand owing to the effects of the anesthetic agents.[122-124] Nevertheless, it is important to administer glucose-containing solutions using a constant-infusion device to avoid large fluctuations in blood glucose values and to monitor blood glucose values in critically ill newborns. All other fluids replaced (third-space losses, blood loss, deficits) should be glucose free to avoid hyperglycemia.[121] Because infants treated with high levels of glucose via total parenteral nutrition (TPN) may develop severe hypoglycemia if the infusion level is abruptly changed, it is important to continue these infusions (possibly at a slightly reduced rate) during surgery and to check the serum glucose levels.

Calcium Homeostasis

Calcium exists in the serum in three fractions: (1) protein bound, (2) chelated to bicarbonate, phosphate, and citrate, and (3) free or ionized calcium (Ca^{2+}). The ionized fraction is the physiologically active component. The serum calcium concentration is mainly regulated by the action of parathyroid hormone (PTH) and vitamin D metabolites. PTH acts directly in the bone and kidneys and indirectly through calciferol in the gut.[125]

Hypocalcemia has been observed in nearly 40% of critically ill neonates.[126] Causes of hypocalcemia include (1) PTH insufficiency and peripheral resistance to PTH, (2) inadequate calcium supplementation, and (3) altered calcium metabolism caused by transfusion with citrated blood products (see Chapter 10), bicarbonate administration, or diuretics (furosemide). Hypocalcemia may be asymptomatic or accompanied by nonspecific symptoms (e.g., seizures and tremors). Thus, the diagnosis rests on the determination of total and ionized calcium levels. In critically ill children, total calcium concentrations do not accurately reflect the ionized calcium concentrations; therefore, the diagnosis of hypocalcemia in these infants should be determined by direct measurement of ionized calcium with an ion-specific electrode.[127] Neonatal hypocalcemia may be defined as a serum ionized calcium less than 1 mmol/L in full-term infants and less than 0.75 mmol/L in preterm infants. Persistent hypocalcemia necessitates determination of magnesium, phosphorus, PTH, and vitamin D levels.

Treatment of hypocalcemia is not effective in the presence of hypomagnesemia. In this situation, administration of supplemental magnesium and calcium as well as treatment of the underlying cause of hypocalcemia are necessary.[126] Symptomatic hypocalcemia is treated with 100 mg/kg calcium gluconate (10%) by slow intravenous infusion (5 minutes) through a patent intravenous line. Thereafter, maintenance calcium is administered at 100 to 200 mg/kg/day elemental calcium and the clinical response and serum ionized calcium levels are carefully monitored.

Gastrointestinal and Hepatic Function

The fetal gut is not functionally developed until late in gestation. In full-term neonates, the maturation of esophageal function occurs soon after birth. However, in comparison with adults, gastric emptying in neonates is prolonged and lower esophageal sphincters are incompetent and reflux of stomach contents is common. Early feeding of hypertonic formulas in preterm infants increases intestinal energy demands and is associated with bowel ischemia and necrotizing enterocolitis.[128] On the other hand, the use of hypocaloric or trophic feeds in preterm infants is associated with subsequent feeding intolerance, indirect hyperbilirubinemia, cholestatic jaundice, and metabolic bone disease.[129,130]

After birth, increased levels of unbound serum bilirubin carry the risk of kernicterus, particularly in infants who are preterm, hypoxemic, and acidotic and have low serum protein levels.[131] Highly protein bound agents such as furosemide, sulfonamides, and benzyl alcohol (found as a preservative in many drugs such as diazepam) may displace bilirubin and increase the possibility of kernicterus (see Chapter 6).[132] Hepatic metabolism is immature in neonates and particularly in preterm infants. Drug metabolism may be prolonged as a result of both immaturity of enzymatic processes and a relatively low hepatic perfusion (less drug delivered to the liver). Any factor that further compromises hepatic blood flow (e.g., increased intra-abdominal pressure) may have profound adverse effects on hepatic drug metabolism.[133] Therefore, careful titration of all hepatically metabolized drugs (e.g., opioids, barbiturates, benzodiazepines, muscle relaxants) is required to optimize therapeutic effects and prevent toxicity.

Neurologic Development

The central nervous system is incompletely developed at birth. However, early in gestation, the pain pathways are integrated with the somatic, neuroendocrine, and autonomic systems. The hormonal responses to pain and stress may be exaggerated in neonates,[122,123] although the clinical importance of this has not been defined. The potential lack of autoregulation of cerebral blood flow and an infant's fragile cerebral blood vessels may be important factors in the development of intraventricular hemorrhage.[134,135] Although an association has been noted between the incidence of intraventricular hemorrhage and fluctuations in blood pressure,[136,137] it is difficult to confirm any causal relationship. This association may be a concern during "awake" or nonanesthetized laryngoscopy and intubation of neonates; however, one study reported no significant change in blood pressure or heart rate in neonates even after awake intubation.[138] In addition, another study questions the lack of autoregulation of cerebral blood flow in preterm infants. Using near-infrared spectroscopy, investigators found that preterm infants could maintain adequate cerebral perfusion at a mean arterial blood pressure in the range of 23 to 39 mm Hg.[139]

In neonates, the spinal cord extends to a lower segment of the spine than in older children and adults. The volume of cerebrospinal fluid and the spinal surface area are proportionally larger in neonates, whereas the amount of myelination is less than in older children and adults (see Fig. 42-4).[140,141] These factors may account in part for the increased amount of local anesthetics (mg/kg) required for a successful spinal anesthetic in infants (see Fig. 42-6).

Hyperoxia has been associated with retinopathy of prematurity (ROP).[142,143] Although two case reports of ROP associated with anesthesia in preterm infants implicated hyperoxia as a primary etiologic factor, the etiology of ROP appears to be multifactorial.[144-153] ROP has been reported in full-term infants, in preterm infants never exposed to greater than ambient oxygen, unilaterally, and even in infants with congenital cyanotic heart disease.[142] The association between arterial oxygen tension and ROP is unclear. ROP begins as retinal vascular narrowing and obliteration followed by increased vascularity (neovascularization), hemorrhage, and, in the most severe cases, retinal detachment and blindness. Factors other than hyperoxia are likely to be important in the development of ROP (see Chapters 6 and 32 and Fig. 32-1 A-C).[154]

Preparation for Surgery

The Operating Room

Conditions that require emergency surgery in neonates are often accompanied by medical problems and, as a consequence, management and monitoring considerations can be complex. Routine standard monitoring equipment includes an electrocardiograph, precordial or esophageal stethoscope, blood pressure monitor, temperature probe, pulse oximeter, and a CO_2 analyzer. Rapid decreases in arterial oxygen content in neonates after brief periods of ventilatory compromise, coupled with the possible risk of ROP due to hyperoxia, dictate the need for continuous oxygen saturation monitoring. A pulse oximeter probe placed in a preductal position (right hand) can be compared with one placed in a postductal position (foot or left hand) to determine the severity of extrapulmonary shunting of deoxygenated blood via the PDA. Pulse oximetry may prove to be particularly useful for infants in whom the risk of intra-arterial monitoring cannot be justified.[155] This device can diagnose hypoxemia but not hyperoxia; however, maintaining the oxygen saturation at 93% to 95% (preductal) places most infants on the steep portion of the oxygen-hemoglobin dissociation curve and avoids severe hyperoxia.[156]

Expired CO_2 can be measured using capnography. However, dilution of the exhaled gases with those of the dead space of the endotracheal tube or by the fresh gas may underestimate the CO_2 levels in the exhaled gases. If desired, a more accurate estimate of expired CO_2 levels may be obtained by using special endotracheal tubes that have a sample port located at its tip or by using a needle introduced through the side wall of the endotracheal tube 2 to 3 cm distal to the tube's 15-mm connector (see Chapter 53).[157,158] Using a circle system may allow reasonably accurate measurement of expired CO_2 values. However, regardless of the circuit configuration, the value obtained by the capnograph may not accurately reflect $Paco_2$ in the presence of congenital heart disease or significant intrapulmonary shunting.[159]

In neonates, changes in blood pressure, heart rate, and the intensity of heart sounds are excellent indicators of cardiac function, intravascular volume status, and depth of anesthesia. Under most circumstances, a urinary catheter permits adequate determination of urine output and aids in the monitoring of fluid balance during prolonged operations. In cases in which major blood or fluid losses are expected, or the physiology is complicated by the presence of cardiac disease, central venous catheters or rarely pulmonary artery catheters are warranted. Any neonate with significant underlying cardiovascular instability should have an intra-arterial catheter placed for continuous monitoring of blood pressure and to provide the means to obtain arterial blood samples for determination of blood pH and gas levels and serum glucose and electrolyte levels. Many neonates arrive in the operating room from the intensive care unit with an umbilical artery line in place. Because of the risk for renal artery thrombosis with these lines, it is important to verify the location of the tip of the umbilical artery catheter. Infrahepatic umbilical venous lines may not be reliable under operative conditions because they may become wedged in the liver. In this position, infusion of hypertonic solutions may lead to parenchymal necrosis and, ultimately, fibrosis.[160,161]

Non-rebreathing (open) circuits are simple and effective for delivering anesthetic agents to infants weighing less than 10 kg.

The system must have provisions for a humidifier to warm and hydrate the cold, dry anesthetic gases. There is, however, a trend away from the use of non-rebreathing circuits in order to save money and reduce air pollution.[30-33] With the increasing need for cost savings there appears to be no significant disadvantage to using circle systems, which allow the use of low fresh gas flows. This substitution should be made only if the provider has a clear understanding of the marked increase in compression volume/compliance volume losses compared with non-rebreathing circuits (see Chapter 53).[30-33] The anesthesia machine should also provide compressed air in addition to oxygen and nitrous oxide (N_2O). The use of air allows regulation of inspired oxygen levels in cases in which nitrous oxide is contraindicated and high levels of O_2 are not desired. Table 36-3 lists basic equipment for conducting emergency anesthesia in neonates.

The Family

Close interaction between the parents and the anesthesia, medical, surgical, and nursing staff promotes effective communication of medical concerns and continued emotional support for parents. The birth of a preterm infant or illness in a full-term infant does not allow time for emotional preparation for or acceptance of the situation by the family because of the suddenness of the event. With the institution of aggressive medical and surgical interventions, parents sometimes feel excluded from the care of their infant and develop feelings of isolation and lack of control. The development of rapport between the parents of critically ill infants and hospital staff is essential to ensure adequate psychological support during this intense anxiety-provoking event.

Emergency Surgery

Respiratory Problems

Lesions of the respiratory system can be categorized into those that involve the large airways or the small airways and lung parenchyma.

Abnormalities of the Airway

Choanal Atresia/Stenosis

Not all neonates are able to change to oral breathing when nasal obstruction occurs.[28,29] Choanal atresia can manifest as cyanosis at rest that resolves with crying or placement of an oral airway. Choanal atresia and stenosis result from the failure of the bone or membranous portion of the nasopharynx to undergo regression during development. The incidence is approximately 1:8000 births. Unilateral lesions are seldom symptomatic and may escape early detection. Although bilateral lesions may be asymptomatic, occasionally they may lead to respiratory distress.[162] Choanal atresia/stenosis are generally not associated with other craniofacial anomalies. Choanal atresia may be found as part of a constellation of congenital anomalies, the CHARGE association: **C**oloboma, **H**eart disease (tetralogy of Fallot, PDA, double-outlet right ventricle with atrioventricular canal, ventricular septal defect, atrial septal defect, right-sided aortic arch), **A**tresia choanae, **R**etarded growth (including other central nervous system anomalies), **G**enital anomalies (hypogonadism), and **E**ar anomalies.[163,164] These infants may develop airway obstruction during anesthetic induction. Early placement of an oral airway, facilitated by preinduction topical application of viscous lidocaine to the tongue, aids in airway management.

Table 36-3. Suggested Equipment for Emergency Neonatal Anesthesia

Airway Equipment

Suction catheters

Oral airways

Face masks

Breathing circuit

Miller 0, 1, blades and handles

Uncuffed endotracheal tubes 2.5, 3.0, 3.5, 4.0

Stylet

Environment

Room temperature (80°-85°F)

Underbody warm air delivery device

Warming blanket

Circuit humidifier

Intravenous fluid warmer

Agents

Gases
  Air/oxygen/nitrous oxide
  Volatile anesthetics

Intravenous anesthetics
  Propofol
  Thiopental
  Ketamine

Muscle relaxants
  Succinylcholine
  Cisatracurium
  Vecuronium
  Rocuronium
  Pancuronium

Narcotics
  Remifentinal
  Fentanyl
  Morphine

Local anesthetics
  Lidocaine (1%)
  Tetracaine (1.0%)
  Bupivacaine (0.25%)

Emergency drugs:
  Atropine
  Epinephrine (1:10,000)
  Dopamine
  Calcium
  Bicarbonate
  Isoproterenol

Intravenous Fluids

Lactated Ringer's

$D_{10}W$

Normal saline

5% albumin

Functional choanal obstruction may result from traumatic nasal suctioning. Obstructive symptoms are often ameliorated by treatment with cool mist therapy or vasoconstrictors such as phenylephrine. The upper airway may also be stented open by nasal placement of a shortened endotracheal tube. Such treatment, however, is only temporary; prolonged use of a nasal airway may increase edema and obstruction.

Laryngeal and Upper Tracheal Obstruction

Obstruction at the level of the larynx or upper trachea may be due to laryngeal and tracheal webs or subglottic lesions. Subglottic lesions may be due to congenital stenosis, hemangioma, web, or vascular ring. Anesthetic management of obstructive lesions in older children and adults usually includes an inhalation anesthetic induction while maintaining spontaneous respirations. This method may be difficult in neonates for the following reasons: (1) the combined effects of inhalation anesthetic agents and immature ventilatory drive regulation may predispose to hypoventilation; (2) hypoventilation leads to increased alveolar CO_2, which displaces alveolar oxygen; and (3) anesthetic agents decrease intercostal muscle function, resulting in decreased functional residual capacity (FRC).[165,166] The hypoventilation and reduced FRC combined with increased oxygen consumption predispose infants to desaturation during anesthetic induction while the infant maintains spontaneous ventilation.

Webs. Laryngeal or tracheal webs generally produce incomplete fibrous membranes, leading to obstruction of the airway with acute respiratory distress or stridor occurring shortly after birth (Fig. 36-2).[167] Complete airway obstruction occasionally results in an emergency in the delivery room. An endotracheal tube may stent open an incomplete lesion. If intubation is not possible, an intravenous catheter passed through the cricothyroid membrane may allow oxygenation and be lifesaving (see Figs. 12-27 and 12-28).[168] A tracheostomy is then established.

Congenital Subglottic Stenosis. The severity of the symptoms resulting from congenital subglottic stenosis is dependent on the degree of airway occlusion (Fig. 36-3A). Treatment depends on the location and length of stenosis. For severe narrowing, a tracheostomy is placed and a series of dilatations is attempted.[169] Tracheal dilatations may cause airway disruption,

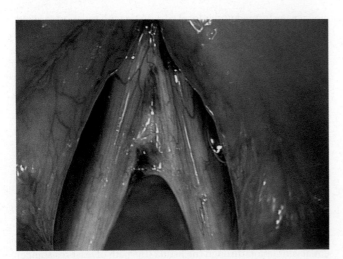

Figure 36-2. Laryngeal web in a neonate. (Courtesy of Dr. Christopher Hartnick.)

pneumomediastinum, and pneumothorax. Anesthesia induction is performed with an inhalation technique with a facemask and appropriate ventilatory assistance. If a tracheostomy is considered, a small-diameter endotracheal tube may be placed to facilitate ventilation until a tracheostomy is performed. If an endotracheal tube is inserted, it should be of smaller diameter so that it passes beyond the level of obstruction. As resistance increases inversely with the airway radius to the fifth power, ventilatory assistance is required to overcome this significant increase in the work of breathing. The greater time constants due to the increased airway resistance then require a prolonged expiratory time to avoid gas trapping.

Subglottic Hemangioma. Subglottic hemangioma may produce respiratory distress during the first few weeks of life as it rapidly increases in size (see Fig. 36-3B and C). The presence of other hemangiomas on an infant's body, especially on the face, is a clue that a subglottic hemangioma may be the source of the respiratory distress.[170] These infants often present with symptoms of upper airway obstruction, which may be life threatening when additional exacerbating factors such as upper respiratory tract infections or other causes of inspissated mucus result in further airway compromise.[171] Any infant who is younger than 3 months of age and presents with symptoms of "croup" must be considered to have causes other than infection as a source of the airway obstruction. If endotracheal intubation is required, it should be carried out as gently as possible because bleeding may occur secondary to trauma from the intubation procedure.

Esophageal Atresia and Tracheoesophageal Fistula. Esophageal atresia and tracheoesophageal fistula (TEF) are often associated with other congenital abnormalities, in particular the VATER association (**V**ertebral abnormalities, imperforate **A**nus, **T**racheo-**E**sophageal fistula, **R**adial aplasia, and **R**enal abnormalities),[172] or the more recently described VACTERL association that includes **C**ongenital heart disease and **L**imb abnormalities in addition to those mentioned with VATER association.[173] The specific cause of these associations is not known. In 90% of cases, esophageal atresia is associated with TEF. Esophageal atresia may be an isolated occurrence.

Affected neonates usually present with excessive oral secretions, regurgitation of feedings, and occasionally respiratory distress exacerbated by feedings; recurrent pneumonia is associated with an H-type TEF and is usually diagnosed later in life. The diagnosis is confirmed by the inability to pass a moderately rigid orogastric tube into the stomach or the demonstration of a blind esophageal pouch by air contrast or radiopaque dye and radiographic studies. The presence of bowel gas suggests a TEF; on occasion, the abdominal distention may be severe enough to cause atelectasis and impede ventilation. In the most common form of TEF, the esophagus ends in a blind proximal pouch with the distal end of the esophagus connected to the trachea (usually posteriorly) just above the carina. In the less common form of isolated TEF without esophageal atresia, radiologic studies may be inconclusive (Fig. 36-4 [see website for Fig. 36-4C]).

Neonates with TEF should be nursed preoperatively prone or in a lateral position on an incline of 30 degrees head up to decrease the risk of pulmonary aspiration. A sump suction catheter placed in the upper esophageal pouch preoperatively and connected to constant suction decreases the accumulation of saliva and reduces the potential for aspiration. Infants with

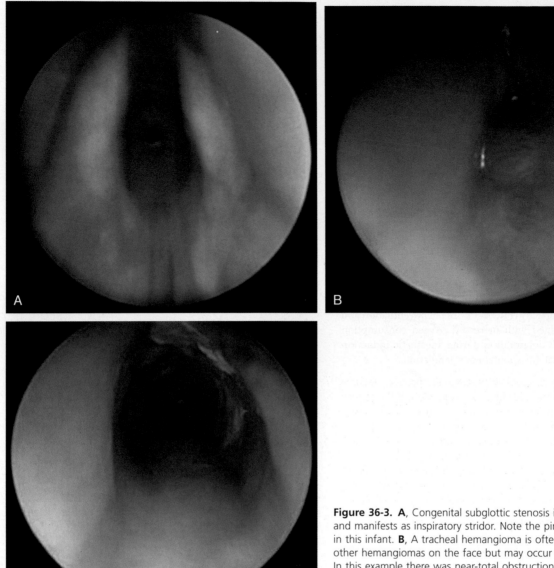

Figure 36-3. A, Congenital subglottic stenosis is usually concentric and manifests as inspiratory stridor. Note the pinhole-sized opening in this infant. **B**, A tracheal hemangioma is often associated with other hemangiomas on the face but may occur as an isolated lesion. In this example there was near-total obstruction of the airway. **C**, Note the patency of the airway after resection. (Courtesy of Dr. Christopher Hartnick.)

esophageal atresia and TEF may have a staged repair of their lesions. A gastrostomy tube, to vent the stomach, and central line, for parenteral nutrition, may be placed under sedation with local anesthesia or general anesthesia. The procedures will permit the infant to receive long-term nutrition so that growth may occur and an esophageal anastomosis can be performed when the infant is older and the distance between the esophageal pouch and stomach decreases.

To establish an airway for general anesthesia, infants with TEF may undergo intubation while they are awake with topical anesthesia of the airway or, if they are medically stable, with intravenous sedation. To properly position the endotracheal tube, an intentional right main-stem endobronchial intubation is initially performed; subsequently, the endotracheal tube is slowly withdrawn while auscultating the left thorax until breath sounds are heard. At this position, the tip of the endotracheal tube is just above the carina and usually below the fistula. When the endotracheal tube is secured in this location, less gastric insufflation is likely through the fistula. A gastrostomy is occa-

sionally performed under local anesthesia with sedation to avoid gastric rupture if the fistula is large and positive-pressure ventilation is required. With a gastric vent in place, an infant may undergo an inhalation induction even if positive-pressure ventilation is necessary. The endotracheal tube is still secured in a position with the tip distal to the fistula. *The endotracheal tube should be carefully secured; if the endotracheal tube is withdrawn to the position of the fistula opening, adequate pulmonary ventilation cannot be guaranteed.* A stethoscope placed over the left chest (usually best in the axilla) may be helpful in detecting accidental advancement of the endotracheal tube into the right main-stem bronchus. Arterial access allows monitoring of blood gas values during the procedure in unstable infants. Pulse oximetry is particularly helpful in detecting partial displacement of the endotracheal tube. Preterm infants with poorly compliant lungs occasionally require positive-pressure ventilation. Preferential ventilation through the fistula (the path of least resistance) may result in inadequate pulmonary ventilation because the air leak through the fistula and out the stomach through the

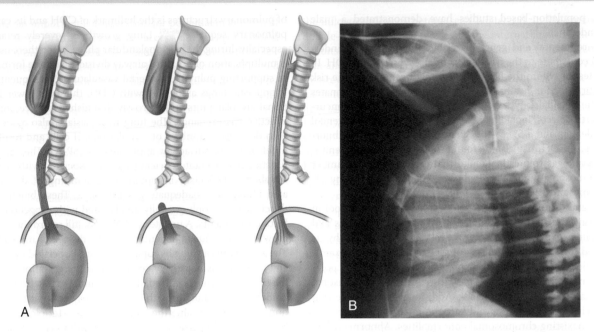

Figure 36-4. A, The three most common forms of esophageal atresia are presented. The most common form (approximately 85%) consists of a dilated proximal esophageal pouch and a fistula between the distal trachea and esophagus (*left*). The second most common form consists of esophageal atresia alone (*middle*). Neonates with tracheoesophageal fistula alone (*right*) often present with pneumonia as the initial manifestation. **B,** The classic presentation is of a newborn with excessive secretions who spits up during the initial feeding; inability to pass a nasogastric tube is pathognomonic. **C,** H-type tracheoesophageal fistula is most often diagnosed with a contrast study (see website). (**A** from Coran AG, Behrendt DM, Weintraub WH, Lee DC: Surgery of the Neonate. Boston, Little, Brown & Co, 1978, P 46; **B** and **C** courtesy of Dr. Daniel P. Doody.)

gastrostomy is excessive. In this instance, a Fogarty catheter passed retrograde through the gastrostomy can be used to occlude the esophagus from below. This approach offers the advantage of avoiding bronchoscopy to pass a Fogarty catheter into the fistula through the trachea in an infant with pulmonary compromise.[174] An epidural catheter threaded from the caudal to the thoracic space may provide a means to give postoperative analgesia in infants who have had TEF repairs (Fig. 36-5, see website).

After correction of the defect, absorptive atelectasis in pulmonary segments may require ventilation with greater inspiratory times to reexpand alveoli. This measure is generally a transient necessity. Early extubation after surgery is desirable because it prevents prolonged pressure of the endotracheal tube on the suture line; however, a high proportion of these infants will require re-intubation due to secretions. Obviously the decision to extubate at the end of the procedure is a joint decision made with the surgeon, balancing the child's cardiopulmonary stability with the desire to remove the endotracheal tube as soon as possible. Conversely, some surgeons prefer to leave the endotracheal tube in place for several days.

Diseases of the Lung Parenchyma

Parenchymal lesions may be congenital or acquired. Lesions may include lung hypoplasia if interruption of parenchymal growth occurs early in gestation. Pulmonary cysts may be clinically insignificant until inflation with N_2O or excessive positive-pressure ventilation leads to gas trapping followed by atelectasis of adjacent areas by compression. Shift of mediastinal contents due to marked cyst distention may compromise cardiovascular function.

The small diameter of a neonate's airway makes double-lumen endotracheal tubes impractical. Nevertheless, selective bronchial intubations may be successful, especially on the right. Fiberoptic bronchoscopes and guide wires aid in the placement of left-sided endotracheal tubes. Bronchial blocking with 5-Fr embolectomy catheters or the intrathoracic use of a clamp by the surgeons may allow selective ventilation of the lung.[175-177]

Avoiding increases in pulmonary artery pressure by preventing hypoxemia, hypercarbia, acidosis, hypothermia, and surgical stress is an essential aspect of managing neonates with compromised pulmonary systems.

Specific Lesions

Congenital Diaphragmatic Hernia

As the diaphragm completes its formation during the 7th to 10th weeks of gestation, anatomic defects that occur will permit the intrusion of abdominal contents into the thoracic cavity, resulting in congenital diaphragmatic hernia (CDH). Although infrequent, this defect in the diaphragm has profound consequences for the further development of the fetus's cardiopulmonary structure, necessitating extensive tertiary care center interventions.

Failure of the diaphragm tissues to fuse appropriately most often appears as the posterolateral Bochdalek-type hernia (90%). Approximately 9% are anterior, Morgagni-type defects. Less than 1% present as bilateral hernias, which are often fatal. The incidence of CDH ranges from 1 : 2000 to 1 : 5000 live births, the variation being attributable to underdiagnosed post-delivery deaths among those neonates severely affected. There tends to be an equal representation between the genders, although some

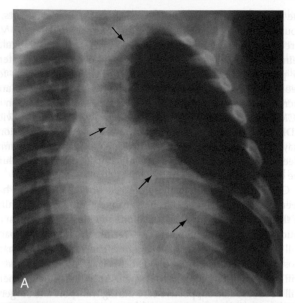

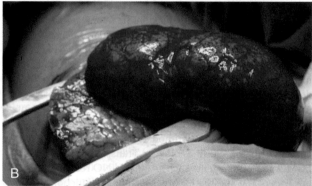

Figure 36-7. A, Radiograph from an infant with congenital lobar emphysema demonstrates hyperinflation of the left lung with herniation across the midline (*arrows*) and mediastinal shift. **B,** Intraoperative photograph shows the emphysematous lobe bulging through the thoracotomy incision.

trapping by a ball-valve effect. Those located in the hilum, in the paratracheal region, or in the lung parenchyma may lead to chronic respiratory illness from infection and abscess formation.[209,210] Congenital cysts are occasionally diagnosed only after rupture of the cyst produces hemorrhage and bronchopulmonary fistula formation.[207,210]

Anesthetic management is directed at minimizing further enlargement of the cyst because a communication may exist with the airway. Awake (sedated) intubation or intubation with an inhalation induction, followed by maintenance of spontaneous ventilation if possible until the thorax is opened, may reduce the potential for sudden enlargement of the cyst. If assisted ventilation is required, low peak inspiratory pressures should be used. Should the cyst be fluid filled or infected, selective bronchial blocking may be helpful in protecting the unaffected lung.[175,176] N_2O and positive-pressure ventilation without adequate expiratory time should be avoided to decrease the potential for cyst enlargement. If these attempts are not successful and cyst enlargement occurs to the point of occluding the airway or causing cardiovascular compromise, then needle aspiration with reduction of cyst size and hence facilitation of oxygenation and

ventilation should be attempted. If this method is unsuccessful, emergency thoracostomy may be lifesaving.

Congenital Lobar Emphysema

Congenital lobar emphysema most commonly affects the left upper lobe but may involve the entire lung (Fig. 36-7).[211,212] Congenital heart disease coexists in approximately 15% of infants.[213] Infants usually present with progressive respiratory failure, unilateral thoracic hyperexpansion, atelectasis of the contralateral lung, and possibly mediastinal shift with cardiovascular compromise.[214] The anesthetic care is focused on minimizing expansion of the emphysema and is similar to that for infants with pulmonary cysts.

Gastrointestinal Problems

The types of emergency surgical conditions that present to an anesthesiologist can be categorized as (1) lesions that are obstructive, (2) those that represent a compromise in intestinal blood supply, and (3) a combination of these two.

Obstructive lesions may be congenital or acquired. Congenital obstruction of the gastrointestinal tract may be suggested by an abnormal increase in maternal weight, polyhydramnios, fetal size greater than normal for gestational age, and fetal abdominal distention detected by ultrasonography. Neonates with acquired lesions may present soon after birth with vomiting, abdominal distention, and late passage of meconium (Fig. 36-8). Associated findings may include aspiration pneumonia, dehydration, hypovolemia, and metabolic abnormalities. These lesions require emergent care only if life-threatening compromise of organ blood flow occurs. Otherwise, a priority is to reestablish euvolemia and a metabolically stable state before surgery.

Infants with obstructive lesions usually undergo general endotracheal anesthesia. Induction of general anesthesia may follow awake intubation if difficulty is anticipated with intubation or if active vomiting occurs; a rapid-sequence induction may be used if no airway anomaly is apparent. A rapid-sequence intubation may proceed in a manner similar to that for children and adults. Desaturation after apnea is more rapid, however,

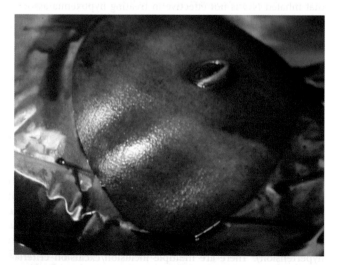

Figure 36-8. Neonate with clear evidence of a bowel obstruction. Note the distended loops of bowel. Because of the high potential for aspiration, this infant will require either an awake intubation or a rapid-sequence induction.

because the oxygen consumption of a neonate is twice that of an adult. If surgery is an emergency and the intravascular volume status of the infant is tenuous, ketamine may be used for induction in place of a short-acting barbiturate or propofol. A stylet within the endotracheal tube may be used to facilitate placement; however, a stylet may cause injury to the airway if improperly used. After intubation, general anesthesia with either an inhalation or opioid technique and neuromuscular blockade, while avoiding N_2O, may be used. Air should be blended with oxygen to decrease the inspired oxygen concentration to safe levels. These infants may have poor renal perfusion; therefore, pancuronium bromide and many antibiotics may have prolonged action. In addition, if hepatic blood flow is compromised, metabolism of opioids and muscle relaxants may be delayed.[133,215]

Infants with lesions that compromise bowel blood flow, leading to ischemia, are extremely ill. These infants may present with a tender and distended abdomen, bloody stools, vomiting, hypotension, metabolic abnormalities, anemia, leukopenia, and thrombocytopenia. Abdominal radiographic examination may reveal distended intestinal loops, decreased bowel gas, and perforation. These infants are not appropriate candidates for regional anesthesia techniques.

Emergency surgery is required and directed at removing necrotic tissue, closing perforations, and reestablishing normal perfusion to the intestine. Blood and blood products should be immediately available, including uncrossmatched blood if crossmatched blood is not available, fresh frozen plasma, and platelets. Before anesthetic induction, adequate venous access should be ensured because these neonates require increased amounts of intraoperative fluids and rapid transfusion of blood products. The umbilical arterial line may be replaced with a peripheral arterial line if it is in a position that may obstruct mesenteric blood flow. The infant's volume status should be optimized by volume administration and dopamine infused to increase blood flow to the gut. If poor peripheral perfusion occurs secondary to a PDA, volume administration should be carefully titrated. In this instance, sympathomimetics may improve cardiac output and organ perfusion.

Specific Lesions

Hypertrophic Pyloric Stenosis

Pyloric stenosis usually manifests within the second to sixth week of life with nonbilious vomiting. This lesion occurs more frequently in males; the incidence is approximately 1:500 live births (Fig. 36-9).[216] Pyloric stenosis represents hypertrophy of the muscularis layer of the pylorus and can often be palpated as an olive-shaped mass between the midline and right upper quadrant. The lesion is most commonly delineated by ultrasonography[217] or rarely with a barium swallow and radiographic examination.

The renal response to vomiting is twofold: (1) serum pH initially is defended by excretion of alkaline urine with sodium and potassium loss; (2) with depletion of these electrolytes, the kidneys secrete acidic urine (paradoxic acidosis), further increasing the metabolic alkalosis. Hypocalcemia may be associated with the hyponatremia. With further fluid loss prerenal azotemia may portend hypovolemic shock and metabolic acidosis. Hemoconcentration may result in polycythemia. This lesion does not mandate an emergency surgical procedure; therefore, intravascular volume and metabolic stabilization and correction

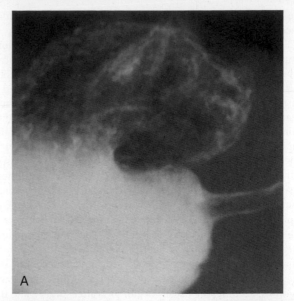

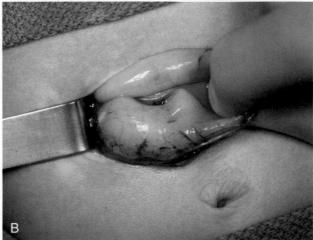

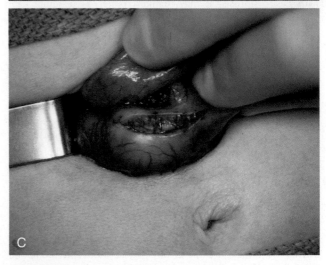

Figure 36-9. A, Barium swallow and abdominal radiograph of an infant with pyloric stenosis demonstrates a high degree of obstruction of the gastric outflow tract with a "wisp" of barium escaping through the pylorus (*arrow*). **B**, The hypertrophied pylorus. **C**, Surgical myotomy relieved the obstruction. (Courtesy of Dr. Daniel P. Doody.)

are a priority. With protracted vomiting, these infants may become hypokalemic, hypochloremic, and alkalotic.[218]

Suctioning an in-situ orogastric or nasogastric tube seldom empties the stomach. A freshly inserted wide-bore orogastric tube almost always removes additional residual gastric contents; this step is especially important for infants who have had a barium contrast radiographic study. One study has shown a nearly complete emptying of the gastric contents if the infant's stomach is suctioned in the right and left lateral as well as the supine positions with a vented catheter (e.g., Salem sump).[219] Therefore, immediately before induction, the stomach is aspirated using a large-bore orogastric tube as described. These infants should not have a gaseous anesthetic induction because vomiting during induction might result in serious pulmonary aspiration. A rapid-sequence induction is preferred. However, if the intubation is anticipated to be difficult, an awake intubation is carried out before the induction of anesthesia. Inhalation or balanced anesthesia may then be used for maintenance. The trachea should be extubated once the infant is fully awake and vigorous. Feedings are usually begun soon after surgery, and the postoperative course is generally uncomplicated. Local infiltration of the incision site with a long-acting local anesthetic generally provides complete analgesia. Some centers place these infants on apnea monitors for the first 12 hours after surgery because several cases of apnea have been reported.[220]

Duodenal and Ileal Obstruction

Congenital duodenal and ileal obstructions (atresia, stenosis, annular pancreas, meconium ileus) are often associated with other anomalies. For example, 20% to 30% of infants with duodenal atresia have trisomy 21 and these infants in turn may have cardiac lesions such as atrial septal defect, ventricular septal defect, or atrioventricular canal. Neonates with intestinal atresia are frequently preterm or may have other associated anomalies such as malrotation of the gut, volvulus, and abdominal wall defects.[221] Meconium ileus occurs in 10% to 15% of neonates with cystic fibrosis. It may manifest either as terminal ileal obstruction by viscid meconium or as bowel atresia. Hyperosmolar enemas are frequently administered to these infants in an effort to clear the viscid meconium plugs; these enemas may result in serious shifts in intravascular volume, leading to hypovolemia requiring aggressive treatment before anesthetic induction.

Duodenal atresia is associated with bilious vomiting beginning within the first 24 to 48 hours after birth. Radiographs of the abdomen demonstrate the pathognomonic double-bubble sign formed by air contrast of the dilated stomach and proximal duodenum; the remaining bowel is devoid of air (Fig. 36-10). With jejunoileal atresia, air-fluid levels are observed throughout the abdomen. With distal ileal obstruction, a barium enema may demonstrate a microcolon. The typical radiographic presentation of meconium ileus is a soap-bubble mass in the right lower abdomen and absence of air-fluid levels. Initial stabilization of infants with these lesions is directed at fluid and metabolic resuscitation. Anesthetic management proceeds after suctioning of contrast agent and other stomach contents. Awake intubation is generally advocated in volume-depleted or actively vomiting infants; rapid-sequence induction may be used in hemodynamically stable neonates with normal airway anatomy. N_2O should be avoided to minimize intestinal distention. Muscle relaxation is generally necessary to facilitate abdominal explora-

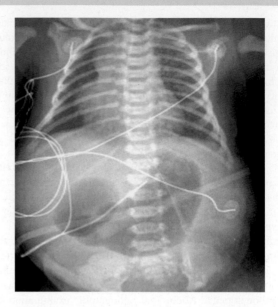

Figure 36-10. Abdominal radiograph of a neonate with congenital duodenal atresia demonstrating a classic double-bubble sign. Note that the remainder of the bowel is devoid of air, indicating complete obstruction.

tion; use of a neuromuscular blocking agent also decreases or avoids the need for large concentrations of potent inhalation agents, which are poorly tolerated by hypovolemic neonates.

Infantile Hernia

Infantile hernia usually manifests within the first 6 months after birth. Although the potential for incarceration through the inguinal canal is present in more than 90% of neonates, it occurs in only 3% to 5% of full-term infants and 30% of preterm infants.[222] With incarceration or strangulation of bowel or gonads, emergency correction is indicated. Incarcerated hernias with or without strangulation should be treated similarly to bowel obstruction. A rapid-sequence or awake intubation should be used at the induction of general anesthesia. An inhalation technique without N_2O or an opioid technique may be used after intubation.

Elective repair of a nonincarcerated hernia can be carried out with either general or regional anesthesia when there is no acute bowel obstruction (e.g., a reduced inguinal hernia).[223-226] An intravenous line should be placed before anesthetic induction if there is any concern about the volume status of an infant. Because blood pressure instability is unusual in infants undergoing spinal anesthesia,[227] placement of an intravenous line in the lower extremity may follow the onset of sensory block. Similarly, blood pressure monitoring may be accomplished by using a blood pressure cuff placed on the lower (anesthetized) extremity. Swaddling and a pacifier often are all that is required for sedation.

Spinal anesthesia may be administered through a 1½-inch, 22-gauge spinal needle. Once the block is placed, the infant should be maintained in a supine position. Leg lifting, especially during placement of the electrocautery grounding pad, should be avoided because it has been associated with a high spinal blockade (see Fig. 42-8 A,B).[228] Apnea or sudden cessation of crying may be the presenting sign of a high spinal blockade in a neonate.

Because hernia repair is a common operation in former preterm infants, this population is at greatest risk for postoperative life-threatening apnea.[14-17,22] Outpatient repair of inguinal hernia in former preterm infants may be contraindicated in those infants 55 weeks' postconceptual age or younger. Because apnea may occur after even regional anesthesia, provision for postoperative monitoring must be instituted for all infants at risk (see Chapter 4).[20]

Imperforate Anus

Imperforate anus is generally recognized at the initial physical examination or by failure to pass meconium within the first 48 hours of life. Neonates with imperforate anus are likely to have associated anomalies of the urogenital sinus as well as those associated with the entire spectrum of the VACTERL syndrome.[173] Some of these infants require a decompressive colostomy before definitive surgery. Before anesthetic induction, it may be prudent to perform echocardiography to rule out associated congenital heart disease. Preductal and postductal oxygen saturation determinations may be of value. If these infants exhibit signs of bowel obstruction, they should undergo anesthesia in a manner similar to that in other infants with obstructive lesions.

Necrotizing Enterocolitis

Necrotizing enterocolitis is not an anomaly but an illness found predominantly in preterm infants.[229] The incidence is 5% to 15% in infants less than 1500 g birth weight, and the mortality rate is 10% to 30%.[230] Morbidity associated with necrotizing enterocolitis includes short bowel syndrome, sepsis, and adhesions associated with bowel obstruction. Associated conditions include birth asphyxia, hypotension, RDS, PDA, recurrent apnea, intestinal ischemia, umbilical vessel cannulation, systemic infections, and early feedings.[114,231-233]

Early signs of necrotizing enterocolitis include temperature instability, poor feeding with gastric residuals or vomiting, malabsorption of feedings (positive stool-reducing substances), lethargy, hyperglycemia, and heme-positive or overtly bloody stools. Affected infants may appear very toxic and have a distended and tender abdomen. Radiographic examination may initially suggest an ileus with edematous bowel and later demonstrate gas in the intestinal wall (pneumatosis intestinalis) and in the biliary tract (Fig. 36-11). When perforation has occurred, free air within the abdominal cavity can be appreciated by radiologic examination of the abdomen.

Infants generally have metabolic and hematologic abnormalities, including hyperglycemia, thrombocytopenia, coagulopathy, and anemia. Hypotension, metabolic acidosis, and prerenal azotemia are other significant findings in severe cases. Initial treatment includes discontinuation of enteral feedings and decompression of the abdomen by means of low-pressure intermittent nasogastric or orogastric suctioning. Wide-spectrum antibiotics are administered, although specific bacteria are not associated with necrotizing enterocolitis. Dopamine infusions may be required to increase the cardiac output and improve intestinal perfusion. Umbilical arterial lines are replaced with a peripheral arterial line so that mesenteric blood flow is not compromised. Indications for surgery can vary from surgeon to surgeon but may include abdominal viscus perforation resulting in free air, persistence of a bowel loop on serial abdominal

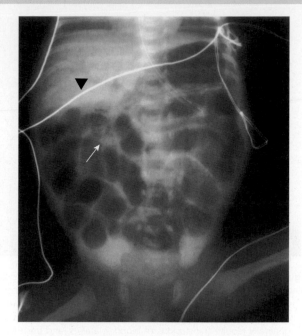

Figure 36-11. Abdominal radiograph in an infant with necrotizing enterocolitis demonstrates generalized bowel distention (ileus), small amount of pneumatosis intestinalis in left upper quadrant (*arrow*), and gas outlining the intrahepatic portal vein (*arrowhead*). (Courtesy of Dr. Sjirk J. Westra.)

radiographs, or persistent metabolic acidosis with hyperkalemia indicating the presence of necrotic tissue.[234]

Adequate preparation before surgery is important. Blood, fresh frozen plasma, and platelets will likely be required. Dopamine infusions may be necessary to improve renal and intestinal perfusion as well as cardiac output. Infants often are already intubated; otherwise, rapid-sequence or awake intubation is indicated. Because they are septic and volume depleted, potent inhalation agents are poorly tolerated and are generally avoided. An opioid and muscle relaxant technique, avoiding N_2O, is preferred. These infants usually have massive volume requirements; it is common for one or more blood volumes of 5% albumin to be required as a result of massive third space losses. In addition, a severe coagulopathy may result in sudden, catastrophic generalized hemorrhage (Fig. 36-12). Platelet transfusion is often needed before surgical incision.

Omphalocele and Gastroschisis

Neonates with omphalocele and gastroschisis have defects in the abdominal wall and may manifest with impaired blood supply to the herniated organs, intestinal obstruction, and major intravascular fluid deficits. The differences between omphalocele and gastroschisis are summarized in Table 36-4.

Omphalocele represents a failure of the gut to migrate from the yolk sac into the abdomen during gestation (Fig. 36-13A).[235,236] It occurs in 1:6000 births.[237] Infants with omphalocele may have associated genetic, cardiac, urologic (exstrophy of the bladder; see Fig. 36-13B), and metabolic abnormalities (Beckwith-Wiedemann syndrome, visceromegaly, hypoglycemia, polycythemia).[238] The herniated viscera are covered with a membranous sac; the bowel is morphologically and usually functionally normal.

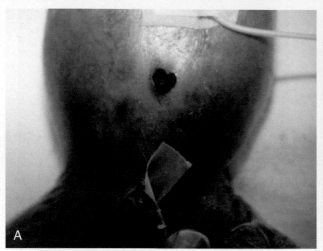
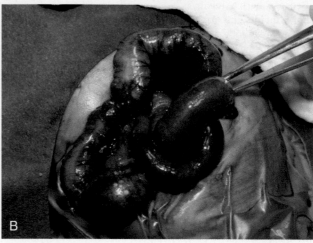

Figure 36-12. A preterm neonate with severe necrotizing enterocolitis and intestinal necrosis. **A,** Abdominal discoloration consistent with dead bowel. **B,** Necrotizing enterocolitis with segment of dead bowel (*top*) and evidence of free stool in the abdomen (*lower right*). These infants often have bowel perforation and hemorrhage from bowel and/or liver. They can have severe hypotension requiring vasopressor support and enormous volume requirements. Moreover, because of hemorrhage and disseminated intravascular coagulopathy, these infants will generally require transfusions of blood, platelets, and fresh frozen plasma. Some practitioners also advocate administration of vitamin K. (Courtesy of Dr. Daniel P. Doody.)

Gastroschisis develops as a result of occlusion of the omphalomesenteric artery during gestation.[236,239] It is usually not associated with other congenital anomalies, and its incidence is 1:15,000 births. The herniated viscera and intestines are exposed to air after delivery, resulting in inflammation, edema, and dilated, foreshortened, and functionally abnormal bowel (see Fig. 36-13C).[240,241]

Management of these lesions from birth until surgery is directed at reduction of fluid loss from exposed visceral surfaces by covering the mucosal surfaces with sterile, saline-soaked dressings. A plastic wrap further decreases evaporative volume losses and the tendency to develop hypothermia. These anomalies represent a wide spectrum of pathology and require individualized assessment of intravascular volume status and fluid replacement. When these infants arrive in the intensive care unit, fluid resuscitation is instituted; neonates with gastroschisis require multiple boluses of 20 mL/kg lactated Ringer's solution and 5% albumin to replace evaporative and third space losses.[242]

Anesthetic management is directed at continued volume resuscitation and measures to prevent hypothermia. Aspiration of stomach contents should be performed. Rapid-sequence induction or awake intubation is carried out. Muscle relaxation facilitates reduction of the eviscerated organs and bowel; however, abdominal closure may be associated with markedly increased intra-abdominal pressure (Fig. 36-14A, see website). The effects of increased intra-abdominal pressure are twofold: (1) decreased organ perfusion and (2) decreased ventilatory reserve. The increase in intra-abdominal pressure may lead to decreased intestinal, renal, and hepatic perfusion and secondarily impaired organ function. This may lead to markedly altered drug metabolism and prolonged drug effect. The bowel may become edematous, and urine output may be reduced as a result of renal congestion. Venous return from the lower body may also be reduced, resulting in lower extremity congestion and cyanosis. Blood pressure and pulse oximetry determinations from a lower extremity may be different from those in the upper extremity. Significantly decreased diaphragmatic function and bilateral lower lobe atelectasis may occur, leading to respiratory failure.[243] Transduction of intragastric or bladder pressures may be a diagnostic adjunct.[244]

If complete reduction is not possible, a staged reduction is then carried out. The intestine is covered with a prosthetic Silon pouch, and the size of the pouch is subsequently reduced in stages either in the operating room or intensive care unit, thus allowing the abdominal cavity gradually to accommodate the increased mass without severely compromising ventilation or organ perfusion (see Fig. 36-14 B to D on the website).[245,246]

Table 36-4. Comparison of Omphalocele and Gastroschisis

	Omphalocele	Gastroschisis
Etiology	Failure of gut migration from yolk sac into abdomen	Occlusion of omphalomesenteric artery
Location	Within umbilical cord	Periumbilical
Associated Lesions	Beckwith-Wiedemann syndrome (macroglossia, gigantism, hypoglycemia, hyperviscosity) Congenital heart disease Exstrophy of bladder	Exposed gut inflammation, edema, dilation and foreshortening

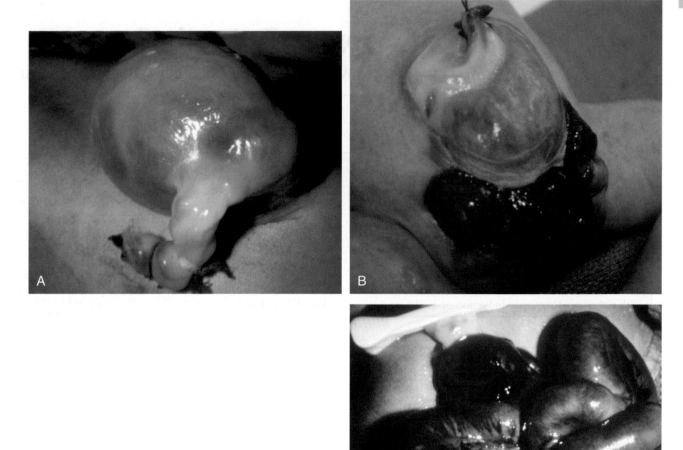

Figure 36-13. A, Omphalocele covered with a membranous sac; the defect arises at the umbilicus. **B**, Omphalocele with associated exstrophy of the bladder. **C**, Gastroschisis; note the absence of a membranous sac. In contrast to omphalocele, the gastroschisis anomaly is periumbilical.

Malrotation and Midgut Volvulus

Malrotation and midgut volvulus result from abnormal migration or incomplete rotation of the intestines from the yolk sac back into the abdomen.[247] Rotation of the intestine around the mesentery may produce the abnormal location of the ileocecal valve in the right upper quadrant and kinking or compression of its vascular supply. If the malrotation occurs during development, atretic segments of bowel are formed. If the kinking or compression occurs after the bowel is normally developed, bowel necrosis results.

These infants present with a tender, distended abdomen and increasing abdominal girth; bloody stools are an ominous sign. These infants may have hypotension, hypovolemia, and electrolyte abnormalities. Because delay in surgery may result in necrosis of the entire small intestine, fluid and electrolyte resuscitation begins preoperatively and continues during surgery. This is a true neonatal emergency and surgery should proceed as reasonably as possible. Blood and blood products should be available in the operating room. Note that the hematocrit may be falsely increased secondary to marked intravascular volume depletion. The indications for intra-arterial monitoring depend on the severity of the infant's illness. Central venous pressure monitoring may improve assessment of intravascular volume status and replacement and postoperative fluid management; however, if there is adequate peripheral venous access, the operation should not be delayed to insert the central venous pressure catheter.

Hirschsprung Disease and Large Bowel Obstruction

Hirschsprung disease is the most common cause of neonatal colon obstruction and consists of the absence of parasympathetic ganglion cells (Auerbach and Meissner plexus) in the large intestine.[248,249] This deficiency creates a nonperistaltic segment of variable length, a tonically contracted anorectal sphincter, and delayed passage of meconium. Functional obstruction occurs at the level of the affected segment. The bowel may occasionally become distended to the point where its blood supply is compromised; perforation may occur, with resultant peritonitis. If the condition is not recognized and is left untreated, enteric bacteria may invade the bowel wall and subsequently enter the bloodstream, producing the toxic megacolon syndrome. Infants thus affected present with a distended, tender abdomen and hypotension and require massive volume replacement as well as vasopressor support (Fig. 36-15).

The majority of these cases are diagnosed early because of bowel distention and failure to pass meconium. Bowel obstruction may be intermittent. Initial management is directed at

limits the time the anesthesiologist has to develop rapport with the child and parents. The anesthesiologist who appears calm and reassuring is of great benefit to both parties, making induction of anesthesia smoother. The importance of offering children and their parents a clear and straightforward explanation of all procedures cannot be overemphasized.

Special Problems

Airway

Respiratory symptoms in children may be related to physical airway obstruction (epiglottitis or foreign body) or pulmonary diseases (asthma, bronchiolitis, or pneumothorax) that result in functional obstruction of the small airways. Once the basic principles of airway management have been followed, then the specific therapy for the underlying cause may be undertaken.

Children arriving in the emergency department with acute upper airway obstruction may exhibit inspiratory stridor, tachypnea, sternal and intercostal retractions, agitation (which may be due to hypoxemia), cyanosis, and tachycardia.[31] It is important to appreciate that they may also manifest few of these symptoms and signs yet their condition may rapidly become life-threatening.

The initial response to these critically ill children should be to administer oxygen, to correct the hypoxemia, and to keep them calm to prevent dynamic collapse of the airway associated with agitation (see Fig. 12-10).[32] If a child does not appear to be tiring, is not cyanotic (not significantly desaturated on pulse oximetry), and has stable vital signs, then radiographic evaluation of the airway may help to clarify the cause of the obstruction.[33] It cannot be overemphasized that it is essential that the child be stable and accompanied by a person who is capable of managing the child's airway should problems arise. In addition, radiographs should be obtained with the child in the upright position to avoid further airway obstruction associated with the supine position.

Blood gas analysis is generally not essential; whether the arterial oxygen tension (PaO_2) is 80 mm Hg or 60 mm Hg does not alter clinical events or the response of the anesthesiologist. It is also difficult to interpret the PaO_2 when the precise amount of inspired oxygen is unknown. Although the arterial carbon dioxide tension ($PaCO_2$) may provide a useful index of ventilatory efforts, obtaining an arterial sample may be so disturbing to a child that severe dynamic airway collapse may precipitate worsening of the respiratory failure (see also Fig. 12-10). Pulse oximetry provides a noninvasive, immediate, and continuous means for assessing oxygenation and is recommended as a continuous monitoring modality in all airway emergencies.

The need for inserting an intravenous line is usually not immediate in cases of moderate airway obstruction. Placing an intravenous line may upset the child and may produce severe dynamic collapse of the airway. The primary focus of attention should be on the major problem, the airway. Placement of the intravenous line may be postponed until after induction of inhalation anesthesia in the operating room.

If there is any doubt as to whether the airway obstruction is imminently life-threatening, the child should be transported directly to the operating room, where a clear airway can be established under controlled anesthesia and monitoring. This would include cases of suspected epiglottitis or foreign body with significant airway obstruction. Preparation for laryngos-copy and bronchoscopy includes establishing a plan with the entire operating team for the sequence of events. The anesthesia team must be familiar with all of the airway-related equipment present and ensure that all connections are appropriate to provide oxygenation and ventilation if necessary. Age and size appropriate equipment and a surgeon with skills to establish a surgical airway should also be present.

The presence of parents during induction of anesthesia may provide a very calming influence on the child, preventing further hypoxemia due to dynamic airway collapse that may occur with crying and agitation. Induction of anesthesia with the child in the sitting position or head-up position may be more comfortable and prevent further obstruction. Halothane has been the mainstay in this situation for many years, but, more recently, sevoflurane has supplanted it because the latter is less likely to induce laryngospasm and hemodynamic instability.[34,35] Anesthesia is induced by inhalational anesthesia using a plastic face mask or by cupping one's hands to form a face mask over the mouth. Once anesthesia is induced, cricoid pressure is applied to decrease the risk of aspiration.[36-39] If the anesthesiologist places his or her fingers gently over the neck and gradually increases the pressure, then effective cricoid pressure can be obtained without distress to the child. With the child anesthetized, an intravenous line is inserted, appropriate fluids and drugs are administered and an airway established. These children may be significantly dehydrated, especially if they are febrile with a prolonged period of inadequate oral intake; rapid rehydration with 10 to 30 mL/kg of lactated Ringer's solution or other balanced salt solution is appropriate. Administration of atropine or glycopyrrolate may be helpful in (1) diminishing secretions, (2) increasing heart rate and thus maintaining cardiac output in the presence of the myocardial depressant effects of the potent inhalation agents, and (3) blocking vagal reflexes associated with laryngoscopy or bronchoscopy.

In children with a compromised or potentially compromised airway, it is important to maintain spontaneous respirations during induction of anesthesia. Administration of a muscle relaxant may result in inability to provide effective ventilation once supporting musculature of the upper airway relaxes. As induction proceeds, incomplete upper airway obstruction may become apparent with the development of stridor and chest wall retractions. This may be immediately remedied by the introduction of continuous positive airway pressure (5 to 15 cm H_2O) by adjusting the "pop-off" valve and maintaining gentle manual pressure on the reservoir bag, while allowing the child to breathe spontaneously.[40] This technique stabilizes the upper airway by opposing the forces that result in dynamic airway collapse (Fig. 37-2). If continuous positive airway pressure does not completely remedy the obstruction, digital pressure should be applied to the coronoid notch at the superior end of the mandible bilaterally and lifting toward the forehead (*jaw thrust*), which will anteriorly translocate the mandible and rotate the temporomandibular joint.[41] A jaw thrust applied at the angle of the mandible is for less effective. As anesthesia is deepened, hypoventilation may occur, in which case the child's respirations must be assisted to prevent hypoxemia and hypercarbia. A child who has been anesthetized with halothane but whose airway has not been instrumented is at risk for developing cardiac dysrhythmias, particularly if hypercarbia and/or catecholamine release occur.[42] The risk of dysrhythmia as well as of myocardial depression during sevoflurane anesthesia is

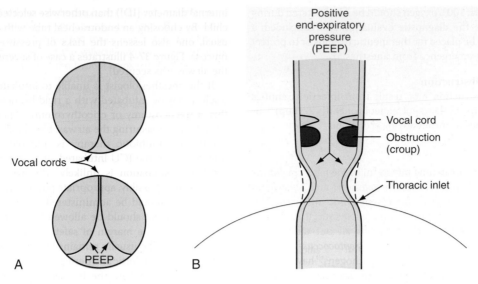

Figure 37-2. When a child has upper airway obstruction caused by laryngospasm (**A**) or mechanical obstruction (**B**), application of approximately 10 cm H_2O of positive end-expiratory pressure (PEEP; *arrows*) during spontaneous breathing often relieves obstruction. PEEP helps to hold the vocal cords apart (**A**) and the airway open (*broken lines* in **B**). (From Coté CJ: Pediatric anesthesia. In Miller RD [ed]: Anesthesia, 6th ed. New York, Churchill Livingstone, 2005, pp 2367-2407.)

attenuated compared with halothane. Some practitioners still prefer to use halothane during stimulating and difficult airway procedures, because more minimal alveolar concentration (MAC) multiples can be delivered with a halothane vaporizer than with a sevoflurane vaporizer (see Table 6-6). However the down side of this approach is that assisted ventilation with high concentrations of halothane may place the child at risk for an anesthetic overdose and cardiac arrest.[43] The end-tidal carbon dioxide monitor tracing (shape of the expired carbon dioxide waveform) may be helpful in guiding the necessary degree of assisted ventilation, continuous positive airway pressure, or both.

With airway obstruction and potential hypoventilation, inhalational induction is slow. The anesthesiologist must recognize this issue, because if laryngoscopy is performed at a light plane of anesthesia, laryngospasm may develop. When the child's eyes are centered and the rectus abdominis muscles are flaccid, the depth of anesthesia should be adequate for laryngoscopy. If sevoflurane does not effect an adequate depth of anesthesia, an intravenous agent (e.g., propofol) may be administered to rapidly deepen the level of anesthesia and provide suitable conditions for laryngoscopy and intubation.[44] During laryngoscopy, the larynx should be examined for the cause of the obstruction. If the supraglottic structures are normal and the cause of obstruction remains unclear, then bronchoscopy may be indicated to examine the airway below the glottis, to rule out a foreign body in the trachea or bronchus. Throughout the procedure, close attention should be paid to the oxygen saturation (pulse oximetry) and the heart rate by means of a precordial stethoscope and/or electrocardiogram. Evidence of compromised oxygenation such as hemoglobin desaturation precedes the onset of bradycardia.[45] The differential diagnosis of a slowing heart rate in a child includes hypoxemia (until proven otherwise), vagal reflexes, or excessive potent anesthetic agent. In any case, this requires urgent attention to stop and reverse the decreasing heart rate. Softening or loss of the heart tones as noted through

a precordial stethoscope indicates severe myocardial depression or hypovolemia. Intravenous atropine (0.02 mg/kg) should be given immediately; and if there is an inadequate response and the heart rate has already slowed to dangerous levels, then epinephrine, 1 to 5 μg/kg, should be administered.

As laryngoscopy proceeds while the child is breathing spontaneously, the child will awaken because of redistribution and elimination of the volatile anesthetic from the brain. If the child is allowed to "lighten" excessively, laryngospasm and other airway events are likely. Some practitioners prefer halothane for maintenance of anesthesia in airway procedures once intravenous access has been established. Volatile anesthetics and oxygen can be delivered through nasal prongs or a tracheal tube placed in the nasopharynx or oropharynx, although this creates serious operating room pollution.[46] Propofol infusion may be used to supplement sevoflurane, or a total intravenous anesthetic (TIVA) technique may be used with propofol and an opioid. If remifentanil is used as a component of TIVA, very low doses (on the order of 0.05 to 0.075 μg/kg/min) must be used to avoid hypopnea or apnea. Negative pressure pulmonary edema may complicate existing hypoxemia.[47-49] The primary pathogenesis of this noncardiogenic pulmonary edema is related to the sudden relief of airway obstruction in the presence of marked negative intrapleural pressures associated with the upper airway obstruction. Negative pressure pulmonary edema usually lasts for a brief period and responds to supportive therapy such as oxygen, morphine, and furosemide.

When bronchoscopy is required, the anesthesiologist and surgeon in consultation should decide whether to intubate the trachea orally initially to stabilize the child or to proceed directly from face mask to bronchoscopy. Oxygenation, ventilation, and visualization of the chest must be adequate at all times to ensure the safe conduct of anesthesia. If a child begins to experience oxyhemoglobin desaturation, the bronchoscope should be withdrawn into the trachea and ventilation of both lungs continued until the oxyhemoglobin saturation has been restored. To

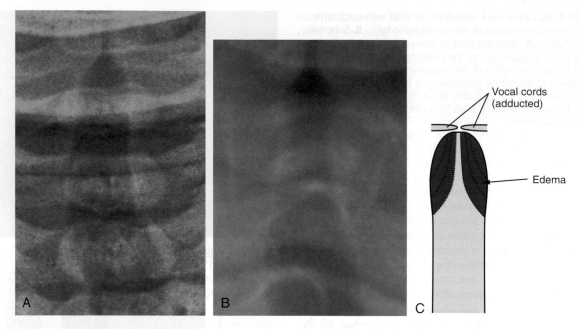

Figure 37-5. A, Radiograph of the normal upper airway (anteroposterior view). Note that the subglottic area is rounded. **B,** Laryngotracheobronchitis (croup) produces swelling (edema and inflammation), which obliterates the normal rounded subglottic area, producing the so-called "sharpened pencil" or "steeple sign." **C,** Schematic representation showing progressive swelling of the subglottic area.

secondary bacterial infections in moderate to severe laryngotracheobronchitis are lacking.[83]

The timing of extubation depends on when an air leak appears around the tracheal tube, and when resolution of the subglottic pathology has occurred. With an adequate air leak (appearing at 10 to 20 cm H_2O peak inflation pressure), awake extubation may be undertaken in the pediatric ICU. Intravenous morphine may be helpful if a child is especially anxious. In cases in which the air leak is minimal (at pressures above 30 cm H_2O), we believe that extubation is more safely carried out in the operating room with the child under general anesthesia. When stabilized, the child is returned to the pediatric ICU. In the pediatric ICU, stridor due to glottic edema after extubation may necessitate treatment with racemic epinephrine inhalation. A single dose of corticosteroid before extubation is thought by some investigators to protect against postextubation edema.[84]

Foreign Body Aspiration
Any child who arrives at the emergency department with a presumptive diagnosis of foreign body aspiration requires immediate assessment. A child who is cyanotic, agitated, tachypneic, and tachycardiac requires urgent care because the cyanosis suggests either a foreign body in the trachea or multiple foreign bodies in both bronchi. A history of choking and cyanosis while eating (particularly peanuts and popcorn) must arouse the strongest suspicion of foreign body aspiration (Fig. 37-6). *A wheezing child may not necessarily be "asthmatic" but may have aspirated a foreign body.*[85,86] Agitation may be misinterpreted as a state of emotional upset when it is due to serious underlying hypoxemia.

If a child is severely distressed because of partial occlusion of the airway, immediate plans should be made to remove the foreign body in the operating room. If the child is stable, then radiographic examination of the airway may be helpful in iden-

tifying and localizing the foreign body. Although most foreign bodies are not radiopaque, the location of the foreign body may be deduced based on evidence of hyperinflation (due to a ball-valve effect) or atelectasis on inspiration/expiration chest radiographs (Fig. 37-7).

Removing the foreign body requires skilled anesthetic and surgical management, as well as careful planning and communication between the two teams. Anesthetic problems include the potential for aspiration and loss of the airway due to a full stomach. In addition, induction of anesthesia by inhalational anesthetics may be prolonged because of abnormalities associated with the airway obstruction. The principles of the anesthetic management for a tracheal foreign body are similar to those for epiglottitis or laryngotracheobronchitis.

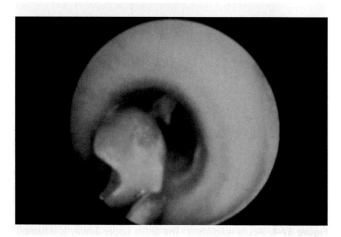

Figure 37-6. A classic peanut in the bronchus. Note the irritation caused by the oil of the peanut.

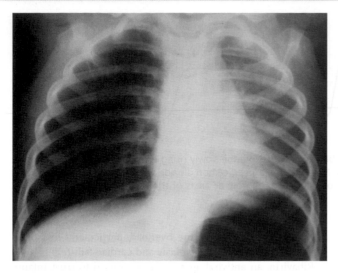

Figure 37-7. Expiratory radiograph of the chest demonstrates marked right-sided hyperinflation due to air trapping by the ball-valve effect of the foreign body. (Courtesy of Sjirk J. Westra, MD, Division of Pediatric Radiology, Massachusetts General Hospital.)

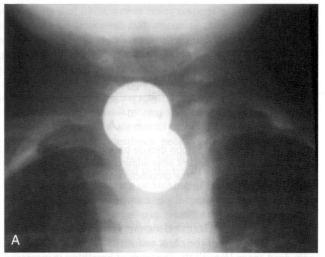

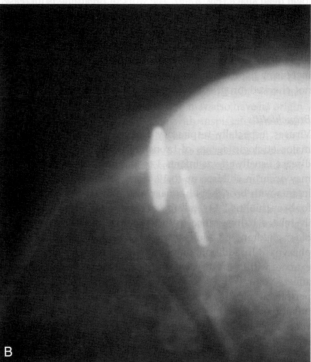

Figure 37-8. Anteroposterior (**A**) and lateral (**B**) neck radiographs of a child who swallowed two coins. Note tracheal compression due to these foreign bodies in the esophagus.

The possibility of forcing the foreign body distally in the airway with assisted ventilation during anesthetic induction has caused much concern. For this reason, spontaneous ventilation is often advocated. Although spontaneous ventilation may be preferable, gentle assisted ventilation may become necessary if oxygenation and ventilation are inadequate. Topical spray of the larynx and vocal cords with 2% to 4% lidocaine (5 mg/kg maximum) before laryngoscopy may reduce the incidence of laryngospasm and coughing.

If a peanut has been aspirated, bronchoscopy should be undertaken without delay; an intense reaction to the peanut oil (if the peanut is not roasted) in the bronchus may lead to complete obstruction and atelectasis together with difficulty extricating the peanut if it has been in the airway for several days. Aspiration of objects such as a watch battery can also result in exposure of the airway mucosa to toxic material. In a child suspected of having foreign body aspiration causing airway obstruction, one must also consider the possibility that a foreign body that is lodged in the esophagus is producing external and posterior compression of the trachea, leading to symptoms of airway obstruction (Fig. 37-8).

As soon as the foreign body has been identified by the bronchoscopist, communication between the surgeon and anesthesiologist is crucial. Most aspirated foreign bodies are too large to be removed through the lumen of the pediatric bronchoscope; therefore, the bronchoscope and object must be removed as a unit. It is particularly important that the child not cough or move during this time, to prevent increasing the possibility of dropping the foreign body in the proximal airway. In addition, the anesthesiologist must be prepared to take control of the airway as soon as the bronchoscopist removes the foreign body from the airway. Frequently, the bronchoscopist will survey the airway again after removal of a foreign body, to remove secretions and assess edema. Residual airway edema is possible after removal of foreign bodies, and the team must carefully assess the child during emergence from anesthesia and in the postoperative period.

Lower Airway Obstruction

Anesthesiologists should be familiar with the conditions of bronchiolitis and status asthmaticus. In terms of pathology, lower airways (terminal bronchioles) are obstructed by edema, bronchiolar cellular infiltrate, mucus plugs, and various degrees of bronchospasm. In young infants with bronchiolitis, bronchospasm is thought to be less significant because of the relative lack of smooth muscle in the terminal bronchioles.[87] Bronchospasm becomes a critical factor in children with asthma (see Chapter 11).

THE ADVENT OF FETAL intervention introduced the concept of surgically correcting a known congenital defect in utero to avoid certain fetal demise. With improvements in prenatal imaging and surgical techniques, fetal interventions have grown to include diagnoses associated with intrauterine demise as well as diseases associated with significant postnatal morbidity. The goal of fetal intervention is to improve the chances of normal fetal development and minimize postnatal morbidity. Advances have changed some procedures from open in-utero interventions, which are associated with significant maternal risk, to percutaneous or fetoscopic techniques, thus improving the maternal risk-to-benefit ratio while diminishing postoperative uterine contractions associated with open procedures.

Fetal surgery differs from any other branch of surgery in that the physician must care for two or possibly three patients at once, all with distinctive and, at times, conflicting requirements. The first is the mother who can tell you of any discomfort, can be monitored directly, and can have drugs administered easily. For the other(s) we have to infer nociceptive capability from indirect sources, monitoring is limited at best, administering drugs is more complicated, and there is the possibility of long-term effects from procedures and drugs administered during early development. The anesthesiologist is required to provide both maternal and fetal anesthesia and analgesia while ensuring both maternal and fetal hemodynamic stability; a plan must be prepared to resuscitate the fetus if problems occur during the intervention.

A Range of Anesthetic Options for Mother and Fetus

Mother

Fetal interventions have been successfully performed with various anesthetic techniques; both maternal and fetal anesthetic requirements must be considered and may, in fact, be quite different. With some endoscopic interventions, the site of surgical intervention is not innervated; thus, the fetus may not sense a noxious stimulus and its anesthetic requirements are presumably minimal. Nevertheless, fetal immobility remains essential to procedural safety and success. Other interventions require needle insertion into the fetus, which elicits a noxious stimulus and perhaps even induces fetal pain. Clearly, open procedures have the capacity to produce significant noxious stimuli. In addition to surgical demands, each mother and fetus exhibits a unique physiologic, pharmacologic, and pathophysiologic profile; the anesthesiologist must weigh the advantages and disadvantages of each anesthetic technique to select the safest anesthetic prescription.

Local Anesthesia

Local anesthesia is almost exclusively used for trocar insertion sites with percutaneous procedures. The most obvious advantage is maternal safety, because the mother receives no intravenous medications. The disadvantages of this technique include increased risk of injury to the nonanesthetized, nonparalyzed fetus, no fetal analgesia, and no uterine relaxation. Those patients on tocolytic therapy or those with polyhydramnios and uterine contractions may be placed at further risk of worsening contractions.

Monitored Anesthesia Care

Intravenous sedation involves the maternal administration of benzodiazepines, opioids, and occasionally low-dose induction agents. The advantages include possible provision of anesthesia and analgesia to the fetus via transplacental transfer of agents, as well as decreased maternal anxiety and pain. Depending on the amount and effect of the drugs administered, this sedation may increase the mother's risk of aspiration due to an unprotected airway. This technique also provides no uterine relaxation.

Regional Neuraxial Blockade

Neuraxial techniques (spinal, epidural, or combined spinal and epidural anesthesia) have been used with fetoscopic techniques and, rarely, without an adjunct general anesthetic, for open techniques. A T4 sensory level blockade is required for most surgical uterine manipulations. This technique has been used with limited success in cases of anterior placentas when externalization of the uterus is mandatory for safe trocar insertion.[1,2] Neuraxial techniques provide no uterine relaxation, nor do they provide any fetal anesthesia or analgesia. Neuraxial anesthesia is associated with an increased maternal risk (failed block, high spinal, total spinal, intravascular injection of local anesthetic).

Regional Neuraxial Blockade with Sedation

The addition of intravenous sedation to regional anesthesia may provide the fetus with anesthesia and analgesia via placental drug transfer. Although intravenous fentanyl, propofol, and benzodiazepines can be administered to patients receiving regional anesthesia, they may place the mother at increased risk of bradyarrhythmias, respiratory depression, and pulmonary aspiration; the need for a T4 sensory block may produce alterations in respiratory mechanics additive to those caused by pregnancy. In addition, the level of sympathetic blockade is often two to six levels higher than the sensory level.[3] Hence, a T4 sensory block may completely block cardiac accelerator fibers (T1 to T4); severe bradyarrhythmias and cardiac arrest have been reported.[4-6] When intravenous agents with vagotonic properties are administered in this clinical setting, the risk of significant bradyarrhythmias may be increased.[7]

General Endotracheal Anesthesia

General anesthesia provides both maternal and fetal anesthesia and dose-dependent uterine relaxation. General anesthesia with halogenated agents provides dose-related uterine relaxation in patients who have received prior tocolytic therapy for preoperative uterine premature contractions.[8-11]

Combined Regional and General Endotracheal Anesthesia

A combined regional and general anesthetic technique is often used for open procedures as well as for those patients with anterior placentas in which externalization of the uterus for safe trochar insertion is anticipated. In addition to providing the advantages of both the regional and the general anesthetic techniques listed previously, this method allows for planned postoperative pain control.[12] The window for trocar insertion is often smaller in this patient cohort, necessitating either externalization of the uterus or extreme lateral decubitus position. Externalization of the uterus requires a larger surgical incision than for standard cesarean sections.

Fetus

Most maternal anesthetic techniques do not provide adequate anesthesia and analgesia for the fetus. There are a number of methods to deliver anesthetic and analgesic medications directly to the fetus. Potential methods include transplacental, direct intramuscular, direct intravascular, and intra-amniotic administration; each is associated with advantages and disadvantages that can have a direct impact on overall outcome.

Transplacental Access

Many fetal interventions (open or endoscopic) employ transplacental drug administration to provide anesthesia and analgesia for both mother and fetus. Many, but not all, drugs cross the placenta via Fick's law of passive diffusion (Fig. 38-1). Lipid solubility, the pH of both maternal and fetal blood, the degree of ionization, protein binding, perfusion, placental area and thickness, and drug concentration are factors that influence transplacental drug diffusion.[13] The most obvious disadvantage with this technique is that the mother must be exposed to every drug that the fetus is intended to receive, often at high concentrations so as to achieve an adequate fetal drug level. In addition, the uptake of drugs may be impaired if there is reduced placental blood flow. This has implications for successful anesthesia and analgesia both in terms of the delivered fetal dose and the time interval that must be allowed from maternal administration to the start of the intervention. All inhaled anesthetics cross the placental barrier, but uptake in the fetus is slower than in the mother.[13] However, because the fetus has a reduced minimal alveolar concentration (MAC) for anesthesia, this takes no longer than maternal anesthesia.[2] Fetal anesthesia is also important to reduce the fetal stress response, which, through catecholamine release, can reduce placental blood flow and exacerbate any asphyxia.[14-17]

Intramuscular Access

Intramuscular injection involves inserting a needle under ultrasound guidance into a fetal extremity or buttocks (Video Clip 38-1, see website). Unlike umbilical cord injection, a noxious stimulus to the fetus is provided at the time of intramuscular injection, thereby stimulating the fetal stress response. Although the bleeding risk from intramuscular injection is less than that with intravascular injections, there is still a risk of bleeding and injury from the needle itself. Furthermore, if the fetus is already stressed, blood will be diverted away from muscle (the site of drug administration) and toward the fetal heart and brain. In this case, it may be impossible to estimate how much drug has been absorbed from the intramuscular site.

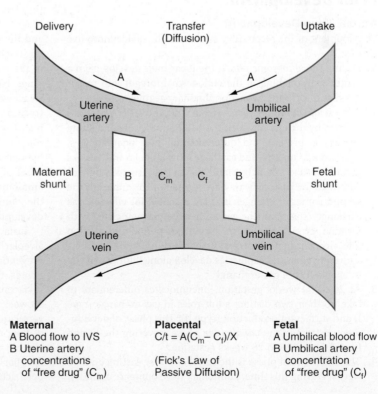

Figure 38-1. Fick's law of passive diffusion. IVS, intervillous space; Cm, maternal uterine artery "free drug" concentration; Cf, fetal umbilical artery "free drug" concentration

Maternal	Placental	Fetal
A Blood flow to IVS	$C/t = A(C_m - C_f)/X$	A Umbilical blood flow
B Uterine artery concentrations of "free drug" (C_m)	(Fick's Law of Passive Diffusion)	B Umbilical artery concentration of "free drug" (C_f)

Intravascular Access

Intravascular fetal drug administration ensures immediate drug levels, and no additional dosing calculations are necessary because placental perfusion does not significantly alter dosing. Intravascular access can be obtained via the umbilical cord (which is not innervated), larger fetal veins (e.g. hepatic vein), or intracardiac, as the specific intervention dictates (Video Clip 38-2, see website). One advantage of administering analgesia via the umbilical vein is the ability to provide analgesia before the surgical insult. Muscle relaxants, analgesics, and vagolytic agents, as well as resuscitation drugs, can be given with assurance of immediate access to the fetal circulation. This method is also useful when alterations in peripheral blood flow occur (i.e., a "central sparing response"), which significantly diminishes the blood distribution to sites of potential intramuscular access.

Fetal intravascular access requires needling in a fetus that is often not sedated from maternally administered agents. The needle may injure the moving fetus, and there is a risk of bleeding from the fetus, umbilical cord, and placenta. Uncontrolled bleeding could impair the surgical view and it places the fetus and mother in jeopardy because an open hysterotomy may be necessary to control bleeding. Needling of the umbilical cord vessels may also produce vascular spasm, potentially compromising fetal perfusion.

Intra-amniotic Access

Intra-amniotic fentanyl, sufentanil, thyroxine, vasopressin, and digoxin have been safely administered in large animal models, with minimal associated maternal drug levels.[18,19] If the safety and efficacy of this method of drug delivery hold true in human trials, intra-amniotic drug administration may become the preferred method for fetal drug delivery.

Fetal Development

Normal Lung Development

Development of the respiratory system can be divided into five phases:

1. During the *embryonic phase*, the lobar buds develop from a ventral outpouching of the endodermal foregut into mesoderm and form the bronchopulmonary segments.
2. The *pseudoglandular phase* (from 7 to 16 weeks gestation) follows, by the end of which the adult number of conducting airways is present and differentiation into pneumocytes, cilia, smooth muscle, and cartilage has begun. From 13 weeks gestation, cilia are active and goblet cells secrete mucus. Although the basic airways have formed by this time, it is the second trimester changes that are essential for effective gas exchange. The acini (the gas exchange units associated with terminal bronchioles) form during this period and develop into alveolar ducts and sacs. Essential thinning of the interstitium begins, and capillaries develop along with the alveoli to enable future gas exchange.
3. At 20 to 22 weeks gestation, pneumocytes differentiate to take up their two distinct adult roles in gas exchange (type I) and surfactant production (type II). This phase of development is termed the *canalicular phase*, covering the period from 16 until 26 to 28 weeks gestation.
4. The last prenatal phase is the *saccular phase*, lasting until 36 weeks. During this time, pulmonary development continues; with further interstitial thinning, the columnar epithelium changes to cuboidal and the gas exchange surface increases in area as mesenchymal ridges form septations within the acini. Surfactant begins to accumulate in lamellar bodies within type II pneumocytes from around 20 weeks gestation.[20-22]
5. During the final *alveolar phase* of lung development, further alveoli form to reach the final adult number of approximately 300 million.

Pathologic Lung Development

In the context of fetal interventions, there are two important causes of respiratory morbidity to consider: insufficient amniotic fluid and prematurity. With either, the timing of the insult in terms of the stage of lung development is critical to estimating the degree of likely morbidity. Deficiency of amniotic fluid may be due to prelabor premature rupture of the amniotic membranes (PPROM), which may be spontaneous or iatrogenically induced either directly through trauma or by introducing infection into the uterus. Small amniotic fluid volume may also be secondary to reduced fetal urine output, from either poor renal function (e.g., with renal agenesis or urinary tract obstruction) or growth restriction secondary to placental insufficiency. Amniotic fluid deficiency contributes to pulmonary hypoplasia. In general, the likelihood is inversely related to gestation at membrane rupture, a long latency to delivery, and the amount of residual amniotic fluid.[23-25] The risk is small if PPROM occurs after 24 weeks gestation,[26] as demonstrated by one series of fetuses with PPROM before 26 weeks reporting pulmonary hypoplasia in only 27% of patients.[27] In contrast, with severe oligohydramnios of more than 2 weeks duration after PPROM arising before 25 weeks gestation, the predicted neonatal mortality is more than 90%.[28]

Studies in sheep show that oligohydramnios causes spinal flexion, which compresses the abdominal contents, displacing the diaphragm upward and thus compressing the developing lungs.[29] This increase in the pressure gradient between the lungs and the amniotic cavity causes a net loss of lung fluid through the trachea, preventing lung expansion.[29] Lung fluid produced in the airways[30] is thought to act as a stent for the developing lungs. Normally, it passes out through the trachea and is either swallowed or passes into the amniotic cavity. Ligation of the trachea causes lung hyperplasia[31] or ipsilateral lung hyperplasia if a main bronchus is ligated.[32] Experimental drainage of amniotic fluid in animals has been shown to result in pulmonary hypoplasia.[33] Later restoration of amniotic fluid prevents the onset of pulmonary hypoplasia.[34] There is evidence to support amnioinfusion in humans to maintain fluid volumes around the fetus after PPROM in an effort to improve lung development.[28,35]

Surfactant is a complex of phospholipids secreted by type II alveolar cells, which reduces lung surface air tension, thereby preventing the lungs from collapsing at low volumes. Glucocorticoids, thyroid hormones, and β-adrenergic agonists stimulate surfactant synthesis. It is first detected in the lungs around 23 weeks gestation, but mature levels necessary for unassisted ventilation are not present until about 34 weeks. The degree of lung maturity can be evaluated by amniocentesis using the lecithin to sphingomyelin (L/S) ratio or, more recently, by the lamellar body count.[36] Acceleration of surfactant synthesis has been achieved using corticosteroids.[37]

Fetal Cardiovascular Development

The differences between the fetal and postnatal circulations are complex (Fig. 38-2). In the fetal circulation, oxygenated blood returns from the placenta via the umbilical veins and ductus venosus (bypassing the liver) into the right atrium. At 20 weeks, 30% of the umbilical venous return (40-60 mL/min/kg) is shunted through the ductus venosus.[38] This flow decreases over the second half of gestation as hepatic blood flow increases so that, by term, only 20% of umbilical venous return (<20 mL/min/kg) is shunted through the ductus venosus.[38] Hypoxia and hemorrhage produce increased resistance in the liver and hence a greater proportion of blood being shunted toward the brain

and heart via the ductus venosus.[39] The proportion of blood that passes through the liver, which is 15% less oxygen saturated, rejoins the ductus venosus blood in the inferior vena cava. However, this deoxygenated blood has lower kinetic energy and so it forms a slower stream in the right atrium, which passes toward the right ventricle.[39] The higher-velocity oxygenated blood from the ductus venosus is preferentially directed through the foramen ovale into the left side of the heart and out via the aortic arch to the developing head and upper body. The integrity of the foramen ovale is thus imperative. Blood returning from the placenta along the umbilical vein is 80% to 85% saturated in oxygen. Despite streaming within the right atrium, some mixing

FETAL CIRCULATION

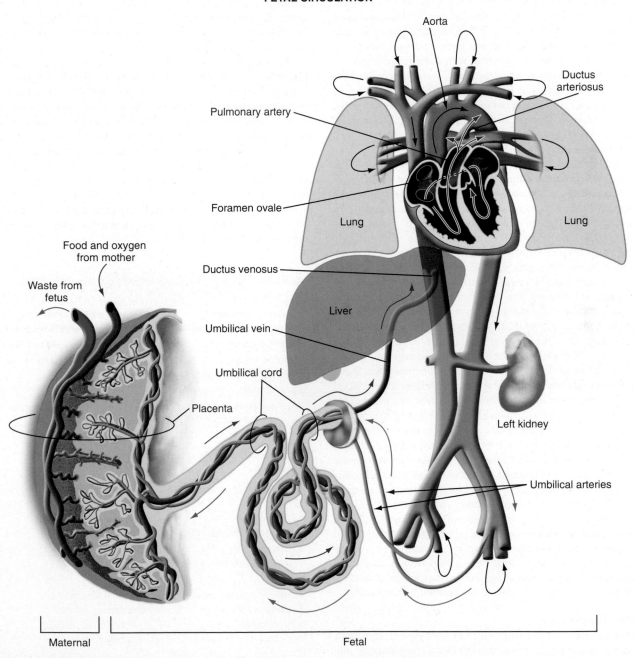

Figure 38-2. Fetal circulation.

does occur, making the blood in the ascending aorta approximately 65% saturated. The blood in the left ventricle, however, is 15% to 20% more saturated in oxygen than the blood in the right ventricle. Most of the deoxygenated blood in the right ventricle bypasses the high-resistance pulmonary vasculature to enter the ductus arteriosus and from there it flows through the descending aorta to supply the lower body or pass via the umbilical arteries for reoxygenation in the placenta. In contrast to extrauterine life, when the two ventricles function in series and thus have equal outputs, before birth they function in parallel. Their outputs, therefore, do not have to be equal and, in fact, are not. In the third trimester, the right side of the heart has a greater flow rate, with Doppler ultrasonography studies showing a 28% greater stroke volume than the left side.

Fetal heart rate is maintained above the intrinsic rate of the sinoatrial node by a combination of vagal and sympathetic inputs as well as circulating catecholamines.[40-42] Fetal heart rate decreases throughout gestation,[43,44] accompanied by an increase in stroke volume as the heart grows. Hypoxic stress in late gestation produces a reflex bradycardia, with a normal heart rate or tachycardia developing a few minutes later. The chemoreflex nature of the bradycardia is demonstrated by its abolition after section of the carotid sinus nerves.[45] The later tachycardia is due to an increase in plasma catecholamines causing β-adrenergic stimulation.[46] Hemorrhage can also produce increases in fetal heart rate, probably via a baroreflex.

Fetal cardiac output is determined largely by heart rate.[47] The combined ventricular output of the left and right ventricles in the human fetus is 450 mL/kg/min.[48] During development, the ability of the fetus to increase stroke volume is limited due to a reduced proportion of functioning contractile tissue and a limited ability to increase heart rate because of a relatively reduced β-receptor density and immature sympathetic drive. Thus, if blood volume is reduced by hemorrhage, the heart cannot compensate by increasing stroke volume, or, conversely, if volume is increased, the walls are less able to distend and cardiac efficiency is reduced (although this second effect is reduced substantially by the huge, relatively compliant placental circulation). Thus, the only way for the fetus to increase cardiac output is to increase heart rate. Despite this homeostatic limitation, the fetus is able to withstand significant hemorrhage. Sheep studies have shown that the fetal lamb can restore arterial blood pressure and heart rate very quickly, without any measurable disturbance in acid-base balance after acute loss of 20% of their blood volume.[49] Even after a 40% reduction in blood volume, the ovine fetal blood pressure recovers to normal within 2 minutes and the heart rate within 35 minutes.[50] Oxygen delivery to the brain and heart is maintained secondary to vascular redistribution ("central sparing effect") and blood volume replacement from the placenta and extravascular space, with 40% of the hemorrhaged loss being corrected within 30 minutes.[50] The development of acidemia indicates that the fetus is not able to compensate; acidosis shifts the oxygen dissociation curve to the right thereby decreasing fetal hemoglobin oxygen saturation. Blood flow during periods of asphyxia increases more than 100% to the brainstem but only 60% to the cerebral hemispheres.[51]

Fetal Oxygenation

The fetus exists in an environment of low oxygen tension, with arterial oxygen partial pressure (Po_2) being approximately one fourth that of the adult. The maximum Po_2 of umbilical venous blood is approximately 30 mm Hg. The affinity of fetal hemoglobin for oxygen is modulated in utero by two principal factors: fetal hemoglobin and 2,3-diphosphoglycerate (2,3-DPG). The hemoglobin oxygen dissociation curve is shifted to the left due to fetal hemoglobin (hemoglobin F), thereby increasing the affinity for oxygen. 2,3-DPG is also present and might be expected to shift the oxyhemoglobin dissociation curve to the right, decreasing the affinity of the fetal hemoglobin for oxygen and favoring oxygen unloading. However, 2,3-DPG only appears to exert approximately 40% of its effect on fetal hemoglobin as it does on adult hemoglobin, thereby preserving a net leftward shift on the oxyhemoglobin dissociation curve. Thus, for any given Po_2, the fetus has a greater affinity for oxygen than the mother. The P50 (the Po_2 at which hemoglobin is 50% desaturated) is approximately 27 mm Hg for the adult and 20 mm Hg for the fetus. The concentration of 2,3-DPG increases with gestation, as does the concentration of hemoglobin A[52]; the greater hemoglobin concentration (18 g/dL) results in a greater total oxygen carrying capacity.

Oxygen supply to fetal tissues depends on a number of factors (Table 38-1). First, the mother must be adequately oxygenated. Second, there must be adequate flow of well-oxygenated blood to the uteroplacental circulation. This blood flow may be reduced from maternal hemorrhage (reduced maternal blood volume) or compression of the inferior vena cava (reduced venous return), which increases uterine venous pressure, thus reducing uterine perfusion. Additionally, aortic compression reduces uterine arterial blood flow.[53] Care must be taken to position the mother in such a way as to prevent aortocaval compression. The surgical incision of hysterotomy itself reduces uteroplacental blood flow by as much as 73% in sheep, whereas fetoscopic procedures with uterine entry have no effect.[54]

Table 38-1. Causes of Impaired Blood Flow and Oxygenation to Fetal Tissues

Causes of Impaired Uteroplacental Blood Flow/Oxygenation	Causes of Impaired Umbilical Blood Flow/Fetal Circulatory Redistribution
Reduced maternal oxygenation/ hemoglobin concentration	Umbilical vessel spasm
Maternal hemorrhage	Reduced fetal cardiac output
Aortocaval compression	Fetal hemorrhage/reduced hemoglobin concentration
Drugs reducing uterine blood flow	Fetal hypothermia
Uterine trauma	Impaired uteroplacental blood flow/oxygenation
Uterine contractions	Umbilical cord kinking
Placental insufficiency (PET, IUGR)	
Polyhydramnios: pressure effect	
Maternal catecholamine production increasing uteroplacental vascular resistance	Fetal catecholamine production increasing fetoplacental vascular resistance

PET, preeclamptic toxemia; IUGR, intrauterine growth retardation.

Even if the uterine circulation is adequate, the fetus still depends on uteroplacental blood flow and umbilical venous blood flow for tissue oxygenation. Care must be taken not to interrupt umbilical vessel blood flow by kinking the cord or by manipulation of the cord, which can cause vasospasm. Umbilical vasoconstriction can also occur as part of a fetal stress reaction due to release of fetal stress hormones. Increases in amniotic fluid volume increase amniotic pressure and impair utero-placental perfusion.[55,56] Placental vascular resistance can be increased, raising fetal cardiac afterload, by the surge in fetal catecholamine production stimulated by surgical stress.[57] Fortunately, animal studies suggest that uteroplacental perfusion has to be reduced by 50% or more before there are adverse effects on arterial fetal blood gas status.[58]

Inhalational anesthetics may cause maternal vasodilatation and, thus, in theory, could cause or exacerbate preexisting fetal hypoxia. Studies of anesthetics in hypoxic ovine fetuses have shown that isoflurane exacerbates preexisting acidosis.[59] It also causes blunting of the usual vascular redistribution response to fetal hypoxia, but, owing to a reduction in cerebral oxygen demand, the balance of cerebral oxygen supply and demand is not affected. β-Adrenergic blockade renders a fetus less able to cope with asphyxia. Compared with controls, these fetuses have a lesser increase in heart rate, cerebral blood flow, and cardiac output and recover more slowly from acidosis.[60]

Central and Peripheral Nervous System Development

By the beginning of the second trimester, the spinal cord is largely formed; development of the brain and spinal cord begins as early as the third postconceptual week. Neural crest cells migrate laterally to form peripheral nerves from about 4 weeks, with the first synapses between them forming a week later.[61] Synapses within the spinal cord develop from about 8 weeks gestation, suggesting the first spinal reflexes may be present at this time. Between 8 and 18 weeks gestation is the time of maximal neuronal development. The first neurons develop in the ventricular zone (an epithelial layer) along with glia, along which the newly formed neurons migrate out in waves to form the neocortex. Synaptogenesis occurs after neural proliferation, first in peripheral structures and then more centrally from around 20 weeks; this process is at least partly dependent on sensory stimulation.[62]

The development of the nociceptive apparatus proceeds in parallel with basic central nervous system development. The first essential requirement for nociception is the presence of sensory receptors, which develop first in the perioral area at around 7 weeks gestation. From here, they develop in the rest of the face and in the palmar surfaces of the hands and soles of the feet from about 11 weeks gestation. By 20 weeks, they are present throughout all of the skin and mucosal surfaces.[63] The nociceptive apparatus are initially involved in local reflex movements at the spinal cord level without higher cortical integration. As these reflex responses become more complex, they, in turn, involve the brainstem, through which other responses, such as increases in heart rate and blood pressure, are mediated. However, such reflexes to noxious stimuli have not been shown to involve the cortex and, thus, are not thought to be available to conscious perception. The nature of fetal consciousness itself is complicated both physiologically and philosophically and a discussion of such is beyond the scope of this chapter. However, there is a working consensus that for consciousness to be present there must be electrical activity in the cerebral cortex.[64] It is suggested that far from being "switched on" at any one moment, consciousness evolves in a gradual process that has been likened to a "dimmer switch," making attribution of fetal consciousness to any particular developmental moment a difficult undertaking.[65]

If we posit cortical integration of ascending stimuli as necessary for conscious interpretation of noxious stimuli, then we must consider the structural and functional development of the thalamus. The thalamus is the structure responsible for relaying afferent signals from the spinal cord to the cerebral cortex. Thus, if cortical functioning is necessary for pain perception, arguably, it cannot be until the thalamocortical connections are formed and functional that the fetus becomes aware of nociceptive stimuli. The thalamus is first identified in primitive form at day 22 or 23 after conception. Its connections grow out in phases, initially only as far as the intermediate zone of the cerebral wall. The neurons then advance further into the cerebral hemispheres, eventually becoming localized into their specific functional fields. The final thalamocortical connections are thought to be in place by about 26 weeks, although estimates differ.[66] In fact, there are thought to be transient cholinergic neurons with functioning synapses connecting the thalamus and cortical plate from about 20 weeks.[67] This time point could be taken as the absolute earliest time in gestation when a fetus could be aware of nociceptive stimuli, or to "feel pain." Certainly, evoked potential studies illustrate cortical sensory impulses from 29 weeks.[68]

Descending inhibition is the process whereby the sensation of pain transmitted in the ascending spinal neurons is dampened via inhibitory descending serotonin neurons of the dorsal horn of the spinal cord.[69] These develop only late in gestation and are still immature at birth. Indeed, in the rat, descending inhibition has been found to not be functionally effective until the 10th postnatal day.[70] This makes it possible that the third trimester fetus, far from being incapable of the sensation of pain, actually perceives pain as being more severe than in the adult.

Cortical Activity

The link between consciousness and electrical activity within the brain can be measured and patterns defined using the electroencephalogram (EEG). Brainstem electrical activity has been shown to be present from 12 weeks. Before 25 weeks, the electrical activity on EEG recordings is discontinuous, with periods of inactivity lasting up to 8 minutes and bursts of activity of only 20 seconds (accounting for only 2% of the total time). From 25 to 29 weeks, the periods of activity increase, such that by 30 weeks, although EEG activity is still not continuous (indeed, in some infants, it does not become continuous during quiet sleep until several weeks after term), two distinct patterns can be recognized as the precursors of adult patterns. At first, these are not necessarily concordant with behavioral state. However, over the next few weeks, the degree of concordance improves.[71] By 34 weeks, electrical activity occurs 80% of the time; from 34 to 37 weeks, sleep/wake cycles become more defined.

It is arguable when electrical activity in the fetal brain first becomes indicative of a state of consciousness, but the lack of cortical electrical activity detected at less than 20 weeks sets the minimum possible limit. As periods of electrical activity gradually increase, again it would seem likely that no sudden event marks the start of consciousness but that as the gaps between periods of electrical activity gradually reduce, consciousness emerges incrementally. The more mature patterns seen from 30 weeks could well be taken as a pragmatic rational cutoff.[72]

Fetal Pain and the Justification for Fetal Anesthesia and Analgesia

Given current knowledge, it is impossible to know exactly when the fetus first becomes aware of pain. One school of thought insists that the entire cytoarchitecture of nociceptive signal transduction and processing is necessary to translate noxious inputs into subjective instantiations of "pain." Others suggest that although the cytoarchitecture present in adults may not be fully developed in the fetus, there are transient structures present during fetal development that may allow such signal transduction and processing on an intermittent basis. At present it is not known if either of these suggestions is correct; instead, we must rely on fetal responses that could serve as indicators of aversion to a stimulus. Observed responses fall under four main categories: motor, endocrine, circulatory redistribution, and cortical activity.

Motor Response

A motor response can first be seen as a whole-body movement away from a stimulus and observed on a sonogram. It is difficult to know if these first movements represent a coordinated and cognitively integrated reaction or simply a reflex response to external stimuli. The perioral area is the first part of the body to respond to touch at approximately 8 weeks, but by 14 weeks most of the body is responsive to touch. As gestation progresses, fetal movements become increasingly complex, with the fetus showing limited responses to stimulation, such as an isolated limb movement, by 26 weeks.[73]

Preterm infants in a neonatal intensive care unit provide a good opportunity to observe facial expressions and behavior in relation to potentially painful procedures. In a study observing ventilated infants from 28 to 32 weeks' gestation, the use of fentanyl analgesia significantly reduced pain-related behaviors such as agitation, inconsolability, and facial expressions consistent with discomfort.[74] Oral sucrose given during heel lancing reduces infant crying time by 31%.[75] Similar findings are observed in infant rats, with the reduction in behavioral distress being reversed by the administration of naltrexone,[76] suggesting that the analgesic effect from sucrose is mediated by endogenous opioids. Unlike the other physiologic responses observed in relation to pain, these behavioral observations provide some indication that the preterm infant is indeed sensate, but whether this is an integrated, cognitively bound experience that might qualify as conscious perception of pain is unclear. Furthermore, the assumption that the prematurely born infant is directly comparable to the fetus, even at the same gestation, is not necessarily correct.

Fetal Endocrine Response to Stress

There is little disagreement about the capacity for a fetal physiochemical stress response from early gestation. Human fetal endocrine responses to stress have been demonstrated from as early as 18 weeks gestation (Fig. 38-3); increases in fetal plasma concentrations of cortisol and β-endorphin have been documented in response to prolonged needling of the intrahepatic vein for intrauterine transfusion.[77] Fetuses receiving the same procedure of transfusion, but via the non-innervated placental cord, failed to show these hormonal responses. Intrahepatic vein needling studies have shown an increase in β-endorphin and norepinephrine during intrahepatic transfusion from 18 weeks gestation, which was noted throughout pregnancy independent

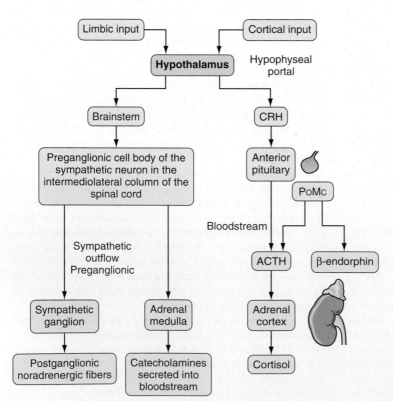

Figure 38-3. Human fetal endocrine responses to stress. ACTH, adenocorticotropic hormone; CRH, corticotropin-releasing hormone; PoMc, pro-opiomelanocortin.

of both gestation and the maternal response.[78] A fetal cortisol response, again independent of the mother's, was observed from 20 weeks gestation.[78] The level of this response increased throughout gestation. Fetal intravenous administration of an opioid ablated the β-endorphin response and partially ablated the cortisol response to the stress of intrahepatic vein needling, suggesting an analgesic effect.[79] A randomized controlled trial of fentanyl analgesia during surgery for patent ductus arteriosus in infants of a mean gestation of 28 weeks found that the increase in β-endorphin in controls was prevented in the treatment group.[80] Treated infants also had reduced levels of lactate and pyruvate and fewer complications during the postnatal period. Administration of low-dose morphine by infusion reduced neurologic sequelae in preterm infants requiring ventilatory support to 4% compared with a rate of 24% in a placebo group in one randomized controlled trial.[81] A reduced cortisol response after fentanyl administration has been observed in preterm ventilated neonates as young as 28 weeks.[77]

Thus, from these studies, one can conclude that the human fetal hypothalamic-pituitary-adrenal axis is functionally mature enough to produce a β-endorphin response by 18 weeks and to produce cortisol and norepinephrine responses from 20 weeks gestation and that these may be modulated by μ-receptor agonism. Although this does not indicate that the fetus is aware of pain at these gestational ages, the mechanisms for physiologic endocrine reactions to noxious stimuli are certainly in place.

Fetal Circulatory Redistribution

Adults respond to extreme cold, hypoxia, or significant hemorrhage by a sympathetically derived redistribution of blood flow to maximize blood flow to the body's more vital organs, the brain, heart, and adrenal glands, at the expense of the peripheral circulation. These changes have also been demonstrated in the fetal animal in response to reduced uterine blood flow,[82] hypoxemia,[83,84] and hemorrhage.[50] Human studies are limited because fetuses can only be observed if they are undergoing clinically indicated procedures. Consequently, many of these fetuses will be abnormal to begin with. However, human fetal intrauterine needling studies that involve perturbation of the fetal trunk have suggested that brain-sparing effects occur in the human fetus from as early as 16 weeks gestation.[85]

The mechanisms responsible for the cardiovascular responses to hypoxia have been characterized in animal models.[86] The carotid chemoreceptors are likely to provide the afferent limb of the reflex because denervating them abolishes the increase in peripheral resistance.[87] Chemical ablation studies suggest that the efferent limb involves α-adrenergic sympathetic fibers.[88] Fetuses in a chronic state of redistribution are still able to maintain control of their circulation, as evidenced by their unimpaired ability to respond with heart rate accelerations and reductions in both cerebral and umbilical vascular waveform pulsatility indices when exposed to vibroacoustic stimulation.[89]

Programming Effects

When considering the effects of noxious stimuli on the developing fetus and the rationale for fetal anesthesia and analgesia, we must consider not just the humanitarian need to alleviate the possible distress of pain sensation but also whether being subjected to surgical stress during early development might cause permanent alterations in physiology. This concept is known as *programming*, defined as "the process whereby a stimulus or

insult at a critical, sensitive period of development has permanent effects on structure, physiology, and metabolism."[90] Studies in rats and nonhuman primates have shown permanent reductions in the numbers of hippocampal and hypothalamic glucocorticoid receptors in the offspring of antenatally stressed animals. This attenuates the negative feedback response, resulting in increased basal and stress-induced cortisol levels in the offspring, which last into adulthood. Behavioral changes, such as poor coping behaviors, have also been observed.

Data in humans are comparatively sparse. Taddio and colleagues demonstrated that boys circumcised in the first 4 to 5 days of the neonatal period had worse behavioral scores and cried longer in response to their vaccination injection at 4 to 6 months of age. This response was partially attenuated with the use of local anesthetic cream at the time of circumcision[91-93]; other investigators have found an increased cortisol response to vaccination at 4 and 6 months in infants stressed at delivery.[94]

Preterm infants in the neonatal intensive care unit may provide insight into this programming phenomenon. At 18 months, extremely low birth weight preterm infants had reduced pain thresholds than infants born at term.[95] One study compared pain responses to heel prick in two groups of infants at 32 weeks: one group born 4 weeks earlier and the other group delivered within the last 4 days. The earlier-born group had dampened behavioral responses to pain, with the number of invasive procedures predictive of pain response.[96] Fitzgerald and colleagues observed hypersensitivity to an innocuous stimulus in an area of local inflammation owing to heel lances. Use of local anesthetic cream reversed this hypersensitivity.[97]

Fetal Monitoring

The goal during any fetal intervention is to optimize fetal well-being by avoiding fetal hypoxia and hypothermia while optimizing stable fetal hemodynamics. It is essential that the physiologic response of the fetus to anesthetic and surgical stresses be understood and addressed to avoid the known detrimental effects of stress on an already compromised fetus. However, access to the fetal patient is limited at best and the technologies for continuous intraoperative and postoperative fetal vital sign monitoring are still in development.

A hysterotomy is not needed for many surgical interventions; thus, the fetal patient remains within the uterus, making access for direct monitoring often impossible. Even for those fetuses that are partially delivered for an invasive procedure, monitoring is obtainable only intermittently and is frequently unreliable because the fetus must remain within a fluid environment during the procedure, making the direct placement of available monitors difficult. Current methods for monitoring fetal well-being include fetal heart rate monitoring (FHR), direct measurement of fetal blood gases, fetal electrocardiography (ECG), fetal pulse oximetry (FPO), fetal echocardiography, and Doppler ultrasonography of fetal cerebral blood flow.

Use of Fetal Heart Rate Monitoring for Fetal Interventions

Currently, FHR monitoring with Doppler ultrasonography is the standard for the intrapartum assessment of fetal well-being. FHR monitoring is also used perioperatively during fetal interventions. The FHR is documented before maternal induction of anesthesia to serve as a baseline for comparison and to reassure the perinatologist, surgeon, and anesthesiologist that the fetus is stable. The FHR may be continuously monitored intraoperatively by fetal echocardiography and with intermittent palpation of the umbilical cord in open cases. It is known that the most commonly used anesthetic induction agents at appropriate doses (thiopental and propofol) rapidly cross the placenta and thus also rapidly reach the fetus.[98,99] The inhalation agents also cross the placenta,[100] but the uptake of the agent occurs more slowly in the fetus than in the mother.[101,102] These anesthetic agents decrease FHR and FHR variability. Although it is reassuring if the FHR is within the normal range for the gestational age, fetal bradycardia is a reliable indicator of fetal distress that needs to be immediately addressed.

Implantable radiotelemeters were developed in an attempt to monitor intra-amniotic fluid pressure as a measure of uterine contractility and also monitor the FHR response to uterine irritability.[103] The entire telemeter with sensory leads was placed subcutaneously in early third trimester sheep and continuously monitored the fetal ECG and temperature.[103,104] A similar device was successfully used for intraoperative monitoring in four human fetuses and then removed at the end of the procedure; in five other human fetuses, the device was placed intraoperatively and then left in the fetus for long-term monitoring, with removal after delivery.[104]

With the advent of minimally invasive fetal endoscopic surgery, new problems in monitoring have surfaced. The fetus is no longer physically accessible to the surgical team, and the trocars used for fetoscopic surgery currently prohibit the placement of radiotelemeters. At present, fetoscopic or cardiac intervention uses the direct visualization of the heart with fetal echocardiography, which gives an accurate estimation of the FHR. Although very beneficial, the continuous use of fetal echocardiography requires the presence of a skilled ultrasonographer in the operative field.

Use of Fetal Blood Sampling During Fetal Interventions

In suspected cases of fetal compromise during an open intervention, fetal blood can be obtained from capillary vessels, a peripheral vein, a central vein, or a puncture of the umbilical vessels. The fetus' small size and friable tissue make vascular access difficult, and puncture of the umbilical vessels can lead to cord spasm, hematoma, and even fetal death and thus should be reserved only for those cases in which no other options are available. Intraosseous access for blood sampling has been possible in fetal sheep, with blood gas values obtained from the medullary cavity nearly identical to fetal venous blood values; the intraosseous route was also useful for the administration of drugs and fluids.[103] During an endoscopic intervention, access to the fetal circulation is possible through puncture of the umbilical vessels. With most fetal cardiac interventions, a needle and/or catheter is placed directly through the fetal myocardium, allowing access for blood samples; only a very small sample should be withdrawn because of the small circulating fetal blood volume.

Fetal Electrocardiography

Several groups have used fetal ECG analysis to determine whether changes in time interval (PR and RR interval) and signal morphology (T to QRS ratio) correlate with fetal or neonatal outcome. Studies in animals and humans have shown that under normal conditions, there is a negative correlation between the PR interval and the FHR: as the FHR slows, the PR interval lengthens, and as the FHR increases, the PR interval shortens. *The opposite relationship occurs in acidemic infants.*[105-111] During periods of fetal compromise, it is hypothesized that the sinoatrial node and the atrioventricular node respond differently.[109] Periods of mild hypoxemia will induce increases in epinephrine levels, which will increase the FHR and shorten the PR interval. However, with periods of prolonged hypoxemia, the oxygen-dependent calcium channels of the sinoatrial node will demonstrate reduced sensitivity to epinephrine, resulting in a decrease in FHR. The fast sodium channels of the atrioventricular node are not affected by the reduction in the oxygen supply, and the increased levels of epinephrine will shorten the PR interval. As a result, the relationship between the PR interval and FHR changes from negative to positive.[109] Measurements of this relationship have been divided into short-term and long-term measures.[109,110] The short-term measure or the conduction index can be intermittently positive over short periods of time without an adverse outcome. However, a prolonged positive conduction index (>20 minutes) has been associated with an increased risk of fetal acidemia.[111]

Use of Fetal Electrocardiography During Fetal Interventions

Attempts at monitoring the fetal ECG during open fetal surgical interventions using either surface or subcutaneously placed electrodes have been frustrating and unreliable. The fetus is naturally bathed in amniotic fluid or isotonic crystalloid solutions that disperse the small electrical ECG signal of the fetal heart, making interpretation difficult. ECG monitoring during endoscopic fetal interventions is not possible because neither the leads nor a radiotelemeter can be placed through the small trocars.

Fetal Pulse Oximetry

Fetal pulse oximetry uses the principle of optical plethysmography and spectrophotometry to measure pulse rate, oxygen saturation, and peripheral perfusion.[112] Pulse oximetry measures the ratio of oxyhemoglobin to the sum of oxyhemoglobin and deoxyhemoglobin in blood. The fetal blood vessels are much smaller and have a smaller pulse pressure than those of the adult, making saturation readings more difficult to accurately detect.[113] In addition, the fetus lives in a relatively oxygen-poor environment with the arterial blood in the maternal circulation at the placenta having a partial pressure of only 20 to 30 mm Hg. Thus, the fetus survives at a much lower normal range of oxygen saturation values (30%-70%) compared with the healthy adult (95%-100%), a difference that, when combined with the presence of 60% to 90% hemoglobin F in the fetus, often yields imprecise measurements in fetal applications using standard technologies.[111,112]

Standard pulse oximeters use the transmission and absorption of light through a vascular bed to a photodetector on the opposite side of the tissue. However, the development of reflectance oximetry allowed measurement of oxygen saturation from light-emitting diodes that are positioned next to each other on the same skin surface and absorption is determined from the light that scatters back to the tissue surface[114,115]; any fetal condition that can decrease vascular pulsations (hypotension, vasoconstriction, shock, strong uterine contractions) can produce inaccurate oximetry readings.[116] Because direct contact of the oximeter must be made with the fetal skin surface, anything that interferes with light transmission or skin adhesion (e.g., fetal or maternal movement, vernix caseosa, caput succedaneum) can influence the quality and accuracy of the oximeter.[117-121] Oximetry readings also vary in relation to the site of sensor application; several studies have found reduced baseline oxygen saturation values with the use of the oxygen sensor on the fetal buttock compared with the fetal head.[122-125]

The development of a 735/890-nm wavelength system (compared with the older 660/890-nm system) has improved the accuracy in fetal arterial oxygen saturation ($FSpo_2$) readings[126]; because the normal range of $FSpo_2$ of 30% to 70% lies in the middle of the oxygen hemoglobin dissociation curve, small changes in pH or oxygen partial pressure (Po_2) will cause large changes in $FSPO_2$.[127] FPO can also identify an acidotic fetus. Increased concentrations of both the hydrogen ion and 2,3-DPG cause a rightward shift of the oxygen dissociation curve (Bohr effect) such that a chronically acidemic or hypoxemic fetus will have a low $FSPO_2$ even though the Po_2 is within normal limits.[127]

Fetal Echocardiography

When technically feasible, fetal echocardiography should be available to assess fetal myocardial contractility and function, heart rate, intravascular volume status, and amniotic fluid volume. We have also used echocardiography to correctly identify proper endotracheal tube placement during an EXIT procedure[128]; a sterile sleeve is placed over the ultrasonographic probe that is then placed over the fetal chest.

Doppler Ultrasonography of Fetal Cerebral Blood Flow

Antepartum Doppler ultrasonography studies of the fetal circulation in cases of intrauterine growth restriction with presumed hypoxia have shown a compensatory redistribution, with an increase in peripheral vascular resistance in the fetal body and placenta and a compensatory reduction in peripheral vascular resistance in the fetal brain, producing a brain-sparing effect.[129] Intrapartum Doppler ultrasonography and FPO have verified the brain-sparing response in the presence of intrapartum arterial hypoxemia ($FSPO_2$ <30% for ≥5 minutes), as reflected by increased mean flow velocity in the fetal middle cerebral artery.[130] Preliminary studies of the middle cerebral artery pulsatility index in minimally invasive procedures such as fetal blood sampling, transfusion, shunt insertion, tissue biopsy, and ovarian cyst aspiration have demonstrated significant cerebral hemodynamic responses (decreases in the middle cerebral artery pulsatility index) in those fetuses that underwent procedures involving transgression of the fetal body. This response was not noted in the fetuses undergoing procedures at the non-innervated placental cord insertion.[131]

Although not yet advocated for routine intrapartum management, it has been suggested that the combination of reduced arterial oxygen saturation and increased cerebral blood flow may indicate an ominous phase during labor. The redistribution of the fetal circulation is not an unlimited protective mechanism[132]; and with persistent cerebral hypoxia, the active vasodilation of the cerebral vessels may fail, leading to disastrous consequences for the fetus.

Physiologic Consequences of Pregnancy

Respiratory and Airway Considerations

There is an increase in metabolic demand of both the mother and the fetus, and this, along with anatomic and hormonal influences, accounts for the changes in maternal pulmonary physiology (Table 38-2). Pregnancy results in progressive increases in oxygen consumption and minute ventilation, along with a decreased residual volume and functional residual capacity (FRC).[133] Parturients are prone to hypoxia because of a tendency for closure of small airways in dependent areas when lung volumes fall below closing capacity. The increased metabolic demands and anatomic changes can make adequate oxygenation and perfusion of the parturient and the fetoplacental unit a constant challenge during maternal general anesthesia. During periods of apnea or hypoventilation, the parturient is prone to rapid development of hypoxia and hypercapnia. Even after adequate preoxygenation, the Pao_2 in an apneic anesthetized parturient decreases by about 8 mm Hg more per minute than in nonpregnant women.[134] Acidosis rapidly develops from hypoxia during difficult airway situations because of a decreased buffering capacity during pregnancy. With increasing gestational age, maternal airway mucosa becomes edematous, abdominal contents shift with increasing uterine size, the diaphragm rises, and the laryngeal structures shift to a more anterior position. These changes increase the frequency of a difficult intubation (failed intubation = approximately 1 in 300 general anesthesia obstetric cases). The decreased pulmonary oxygen stores and increased oxygen consumption make parturients more susceptible than nonpregnant women to the consequences of airway mismanagement.

Not all physiologic changes of pregnancy are deleterious to the performance of an anesthetic. For example, the induction and emergence from anesthesia with inhaled agents occur faster in parturients than in nonpregnant women because the combination of increased alveolar ventilation and decreased FRC speeds the rate at which denitrogenation occurs and at which inspired and alveolar concentrations of inhalational agents reach equilibrium[135]; a faster induction, coupled with a decreased

Table 38-2. Anesthetic Considerations of Respiratory Changes of Pregnancy

Decreased functional residual capacity
  Faster denitrogenation
  Rapidly prone to hypoxia during apnea
  Faster induction and emergence of anesthesia with inhaled agents

Increased oxygen consumption
  Rapidly prone to hypoxia during apnea

Capillary engorgement of the respiratory mucosa
  Predisposes upper airway to trauma, bleeding, and obstruction
  Laryngeal edema increases the frequency of difficult intubation

Decreased $Paco_2$ and no $ETco_2$-$Paco_2$ gradient
  Capnograph reading similar to $Paco_2$
  Hyperventilation may lead to a reduction in uterine blood flow

inhalational anesthetic requirement, make parturients susceptible to relative anesthetic overdose and severe hypotension.[136]

Cardiovascular Considerations

Cardiovascular function is appropriately increased during pregnancy to meet the increased metabolic demands and oxygen requirements of the mother (Table 38-3). Cardiac output increases by as much as 35% to 40% by the end of the first trimester[137] and continues to increase throughout the second trimester until it reaches a level 50% greater than in nonpregnant women. Heart rate increases 15% to 25% above prepregnancy levels and remains stable after the second trimester, but stroke volume progressively increases by 25% to 30% by the end of the second trimester and remains stable until term.[138,139] Aortocaval compression by the gravid uterus can cause a 30% to 50% decrease in cardiac output; lesser decreases occur in the sitting or semirecumbent positions. Maternal position is a major factor contributing to hypotension and fetal well-being.[140]

Maternal blood flow and pressure are directly linked to fetal perfusion via the placenta, and uterine blood flow represents about 10% of maternal cardiac output. The avoidance of aortocaval compression by left or right uterine displacement is imperative to prevent a decrease in the maternal blood pressure. Because large doses of inhalational agent are often necessary for uterine relaxation during fetal intervention, prompt treatment of hypotension is vital. Because uteroplacental blood flow is not autoregulated, a decrease in maternal blood pressure will ultimately cause a decrease in blood flow to the fetus. Intravenous ephedrine (5-10 mg) should be used to treat maternal hypotension unless contraindicated or not effective. In such a situation, phenylephrine should be the vasopressor of choice. Although preliminary animal studies using larger doses of phenylephrine showed fetal asphyxia,[141] more recent studies in parturients given small doses of phenylephrine (40-80 μg) did not demonstrate deleterious effects in the neonate.[142,143] Use of angiotensin II is thought to cause less vasoconstriction in the uterine vessels and to decrease the incidence of fetal acidemia.[144,145] In addition, angiotensin II does not cross the placenta, placing the fetus at no increased risk from potential side effects.[146]

Careful attention to the volume status of the parturient is imperative; aggressive volume hydration, the normal decrease in colloid oncotic pressure that occurs during pregnancy, the decrease in colloid oncotic pressure post partum, and the use of tocolytic agents (magnesium, β agonists) may all predispose the parturient to pulmonary edema.

Table 38-3. Anesthetic Considerations of Cardiovascular Changes of Pregnancy

Aortocaval compression
  Supine position leads to a decline in cardiac output
  May lead to supine hypotensive syndrome
  Mostly prevented by left or right uterine displacement

Decreased colloid oncotic pressure
  Parturient is at higher risk of pulmonary edema

Increased maternal blood volume
  Parturient tolerates more blood loss than nonparturients
  Hypotension and acidosis may develop with significant blood loss

---

Hematologic Considerations

Blood volume increases 35% by the second trimester; the majority of this increase is composed of plasma volume, which increases to 50% to 55% above normal levels and then remains relatively stable to term. The increase in plasma volume above red blood cell volume leads to a decrease in hemoglobin by mid gestation (the "physiologic anemia" of pregnancy).[147] This hemodilution helps maintain the patency of uteroplacental blood flow by reducing blood viscosity and preventing placental thrombosis and infarction.

Central and Peripheral Nervous Systems

Pregnancy-mediated analgesia is affected by changes in spinal opioid antinociceptive pathways and peripheral processes, including the effect of ovarian sex steroids (estrogen and progesterone) and uterine afferent neurotransmission. It is thought that pregnancy-mediated analgesia increases the woman's threshold for pain during the latter stages of pregnancy before labor.[148,149] Pregnant women are more sensitive to the action of many anesthetic agents and require less local and volatile anesthetic than their nonpregnant counterparts for spinal and epidural anesthesia. The MAC of inhalational agents is decreased by approximately 30%; and for this reason the concentration of inhalational agents needs to be carefully titrated.[150]

Pharmacologic Consequences of Pregnancy

Physiologic changes of pregnancy alter the pharmacokinetics and pharmacodynamics of many anesthetic drugs. An increase in total body water and adipose tissue and a decrease in plasma protein levels alter the volume of distribution. An increased renal blood flow and glomerular filtration rate can enhance the elimination of renally excreted drugs; hepatic metabolism of drugs may be inhibited by competition with steroid hormones during pregnancy. Therefore, drug administration must consider the pharmacokinetics within the maternal-placental-fetal unit. Most drugs cross the placenta to some extent, and the proportion transferred increases with gestation. The fetus has decreased levels of plasma protein binding, producing relatively large concentrations of free (unbound-active drug).[151] Despite the fact that oxidation and reduction reactions have been detected in the fetal liver from as early as 16 weeks, enzyme concentrations and reaction rates are minimal, exposing the fetus to more prolonged drug effects than the mother.[152] Early in gestation, the primary mode of drug excretion is via the placenta, but, later, as the fetal kidneys mature, they become the chief route of drug excretion into the amniotic fluid. The latter, however, can act as a reservoir for drugs, from which they can be reabsorbed.[151]

Induction

Pregnancy increases the parturient's sensitivity to induction agents.[153] Propofol has been safely used for induction of anesthesia for cesarean delivery in doses of 2 mg/kg, with minimal effects on the neonate.[154] Ketamine has also been used as the sole induction agent for parturients undergoing elective cesarean section; ketamine (1.5 mg/kg) has not been associated with maternal awareness or neonatal depression at delivery and parturients required fewer analgesics in the first 24 hours after delivery.[155] It is speculated that ketamine's analgesic properties may reduce the sensitization of pain pathways and subsequently confer extended benefit into the postoperative period. Induction agents decrease spontaneous uterine contractions of isolated pregnant rat myometrium but only in concentrations greater than those seen in clinical obstetric practice.[156]

Muscle Relaxants

Although serum cholinesterase activity decreases 30% during pregnancy, recovery from a dose of 1 mg/kg of succinylcholine is not prolonged.[157] Succinylcholine has a very low placental transfer, owing to its low lipid solubility and high degree of ionization.[158] Similarly, mivacurium has been safely used for cesarean section without routine neostigmine antagonism despite a decreased plasma cholinesterase activity.[159] Pregnant women may be more sensitive to the action of nondepolarizing muscle relaxants, with the administration of vecuronium resulting in a more rapid onset and delayed recovery of neuromuscular block when compared with nonpregnant control patients. The prolonged action of vecuronium persists into the postpartum period for at least 4 days[160]; the clinical duration of vecuronium in term and postpartum women is twice that of nonpregnant women.[161] However, in a study comparing cisatracurium 0.2 mg/kg for intubation in immediate postpartum and nonpregnant women, both the mean onset and recovery times in the postpartum period were significantly shorter.[162] Nondepolarizing muscle relaxants have no effect on uterine relaxation.

Volatile Agents

Pregnant women are more sensitive to the anesthetic action of the volatile agents (reduced MAC).[163] This may lead to a deeper level of anesthesia than predicted during fetal surgery and a relative overdose associated with maternal cardiac depression and hypotension. All inhaled anesthetics rapidly cross the placenta, but the uptake of inhaled anesthetics occurs more slowly in the fetus than in the mother.[164,165] At light (1.0 MAC) isoflurane or halothane anesthesia, maternal pulse rate, cardiac output, and acid-base status did not significantly change, nor did fetal pulse rate, acid-base status, or oxygen saturation.[166] During moderately deep (1.5 MAC) isoflurane or halothane anesthesia, maternal arterial pressure and cardiac output decreased. Uterine vasodilation occurred, and uteroplacental perfusion was maintained; fetal oxygenation and base excess were also maintained. However, at greater concentrations of inhaled anesthetic (2.0 MAC), maternal hypotension decreased uteroplacental perfusion despite uterine vasodilation, leading to fetal hypoxia and acidosis. Volatile anesthetic agents produce dose-related uterine relaxation.[167] It usually takes 0.5 MAC of enflurane, isoflurane, or halothane to produce a 20% decrease in contractility and 1.5 MAC to produce a 60% decrease in uterine contractility.[168] Sevoflurane produces a dose-dependent depression of uterine muscle contractility, and uterine activity is virtually abolished at greater than 3.5 MAC.[169] The large concentrations of inhalation agent necessary for uterine relaxation generally require endotracheal intubation and aggressive use of vasopressors.

Fetal Preoperative Evaluation

Prenatal imaging of all fetal anomalies, including anatomic areas of involvement, the relationship to normal structures, and tracheal location, is needed to plan the most appropriate surgical and anesthetic interventions. The accuracy and quality of preoperative fetal ultrasonography and magnetic resonance imaging (MRI) are of the utmost importance because some lesions, especially pulmonary lesions, may spontaneously regress in utero; an inaccurate diagnosis could lead to suboptimal or inappropriate intervention. In addition, extremely valuable information can be obtained that would aid in the decision-making process for a given treatment, namely, the presence of ascites, hydrops, mediastinal shift, degree of lung hypoplasia and lesion involvement, airway involvement and potential tracheal distortion, or compression from intrathoracic masses. Preoperative imaging can also determine other anticipated alterations in anatomy that may acutely alter fetal cardiopulmonary physiology (e.g., mediastinal shift and the known associated potential alterations in fetal preload). Serial radiologic examinations can also monitor the growth of certain masses, the development of hydrops, and the response to treatment medications (e.g., transplacental digoxin). Significant fetal ventricular dysfunction or heart failure should alert the anesthesiologist to the possibility of fetal cardiac arrest during a fetal intervention. Other congenital abnormalities may be detected that may warrant a potential fetal intervention useless.

In addition, a fetal karyotype must be obtained to rule out the presence of any genetic disorders that are associated with significant fetal morbidity or mortality, making further intervention pointless. A fetal karyotype can be performed using amniocentesis or through percutaneous umbilical blood sampling. An estimated fetal weight, obtained by ultrasonography immediately before surgical intervention, allows for preparation of unit doses of fetal medications. Any previous attempts at fetal intervention should be evaluated, including the number of interventions, fetal tolerance of the procedures, transient reversal in fetal symptoms, the presence of fetal cardiac dysfunction, and the reason or reasons for failed intervention. Assuming that fetal hydrops is present, any attempts to treat this condition should also be documented, including the effectiveness of digoxin therapy, total dose administered, method of administration, and response to treatment.

Maternal Evaluation

A complete medical history and physical examination, especially a focused airway evaluation, are of the utmost importance. Details regarding fetal pathophysiology and its effects on secondary maternal morbidity should be addressed. Any patient with significant polyhydramnios and associated preterm contractions is at great risk for preterm labor and rupture of membranes with uterine manipulation. Patients with significant polyhydramnios despite multiple amnioreductions have required greater amounts of intraoperative tocolysis and greater inhalational anesthetic concentrations to obtain uterine relaxation and acceptable surgical conditions.

The presence of fetal hydrops should alert the practitioner to the possibility of maternal mirror syndrome. Mirror syndrome refers to characteristic maternal pathophysiologic changes associated with a variety of fetal disorders, including nonimmune hydrops, molar pregnancies, congenital cystic adenomatoid malformation (CCAM) of the lung, and sacrococcygeal teratoma. Polyhydramnios and placentomegaly are usually present. Although the etiology of this condition is unclear, the end result is a maternal hyperdynamic state with associated hypertension and total body edema.[170] Respiratory insufficiency or pulmonary edema may develop, requiring prompt and aggressive treatment. If preterm uterine contractions develop, treatment options may be limited because tocolytic agents can greatly exacerbate respiratory decompensation. Treatment is aimed at maternal supportive care; even correction of the underlying fetal pathology will not completely resolve the maternal abnormalities. Delivery of the fetus is the only sure method to completely reverse this maternal pathologic process.

The anesthesiologist should specifically investigate for the presence of placentomegaly; increased placental blood flow may alter pharmacologic treatment in both the mother and the fetus because increased metabolism of certain drugs may occur. The presence of placentomegaly may also increase risk for acute intraoperative bleeding, and preparation must be made to rapidly transfuse the mother. Several reports describe inadvertent inclusion of the placental edge during the hysterotomy incision, causing a sudden, massive loss of blood with a completely relaxed uterus[171,172]; immediate surgical control, resuscitation with blood products, and administration of vasopressors that do not increase placental vascular resistance must be administered.

Tocolysis and Tocolytic Agents

The occurrence of contractions and preterm labor is an expectation for the first few postoperative days. Fortunately, in many cases, delivery can be postponed until after 32 weeks, giving the fetus time to heal from the procedure and allowing the lungs to mature. However, for many women, the onset of surgically induced preterm contractions heralds premature labor and delivery that, at best, eliminates the positive results of the procedure, and, at worst, ends in the loss of the pregnancy. Although most fetal surgery patients can now be successfully prevented from delivering immediately after surgery, the current generation of medications used for tocolysis have been ineffective in preventing premature labor and delivery. Preterm labor remains the single most common complication that limits the success of fetal surgery.

Hormonal Receptors in Labor

The adrenergic hormonal system plays a very influential part in the activity of the myometrium; several types of adrenergic receptors are found in the uterus (Fig. 38-4). Stimulation of the α-adrenergic receptor causes an increase in the rate and intensity of uterine contractions, whereas activation of the $β_2$-adrenergic receptors produce myometrial relaxation.[173] In addition, the term uterus is heavily populated with receptors for endogenously released oxytocin responsible for initiating uterine contractions. Prostaglandins also play a significant role in modulating myometrial tone. Generally, prostaglandins are produced in or near the local environment where they exert their effect; both uterotonic and tocolytic prostaglandins have been identified. The balance of intrauterine and maternal uterotonic prostaglandins is believed to play an essential part in the preparation for both term and preterm labor. Prostaglandins, especially prostaglandin E_2, are an essential component of every aspect of natural labor.[174]

Treatment of Acute Preterm Labor

Nonsteroidal Anti-inflammatory Drugs

Nonsteroidal anti-inflammatory drugs (NSAIDs) block the action of cyclooxygenase, preventing the formation of prostaglandins. In-vitro studies of indomethacin have found consistent inhibition or complete arrest of overall myometrial activity.

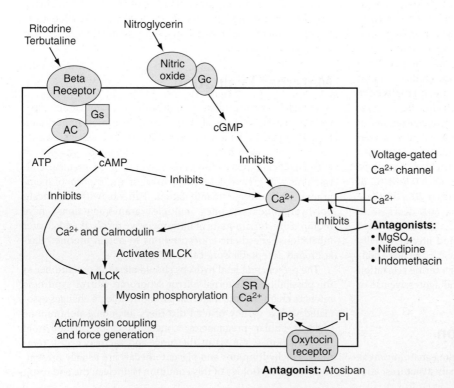

Figure 38-4. Biochemistry of uterine contraction and its inhibition. AC, adenylate cyclase; ATP, adenosine triphosphate; cAMP, cyclic adenosine monophosphate; cGMP, cyclic guanosine monophosphate; IP3, inositol triphosphate; MLCK, myosin light-chain kinase; NTG, nitroglycerin; PI, phosphatidylinositol; SR, sarcoplasmic reticulum.

It is hoped that local delivery of indomethacin through slow-release systems may be developed in the future that may effectively prevent preterm delivery after fetal surgery.

β-Mimetic Agents

Currently, only β_2-selective medications are routinely used for acute preterm labor. Most side effects result from their lack of pure specificity, that is, simultaneous stimulation of β_1- and β_2-adrenergic receptors. Side effects include fetal tachycardia, maternal tremors, palpitations, tachycardia, a decreased or increased blood pressure, lethargy, sleepiness, ketoacidosis, and pulmonary edema. Pulmonary edema occurs in up to 5% of patients, especially when used with other tocolytics (e.g., magnesium).[175] Because the β-mimetic agents are nonspecific receptor agonists, in large concentrations these agents can stimulate α-adrenergic receptors, which promotes uterine contractions, leading to treatment failure.

Magnesium

Magnesium competes with calcium for transmembrane channel entry into cells.[176] Because the myometrium is dependent on stores of calcium for adequate contraction, a decrease in intracellular transport prevents the activation of the actin and myosin complex, resulting in uterine relaxation.

Nitric Oxide Donors

Nitroglycerin is an effective uterine relaxant used in select situations to produce rapid uterine relaxation (e.g., extraction of a retained placenta and uterine inversion). In pregnant sheep, nitroglycerin causes a decrease in mean maternal arterial pressure and increase in heart rate, without compromising uterine blood flow.[177] During fetal surgery, nitroglycerin has been used to relax the myometrium and halt breakthrough contractions. Side effects include maternal hypotension, tachycardia, headache, development of tachyphylaxis, and a high incidence of maternal pulmonary edema.[178]

Calcium-Channel Blockers

Calcium-channel blockers are better tolerated than β-mimetic agents. Nifedipine may be more effective than β_2-adrenergic agonists in postponing delivery in patients treated for preterm labor, especially in those women with intact membranes.[179] Neonates born to women treated with calcium-channel blockers have a reduced frequency of respiratory distress, necrotizing enterocolitis, and intraventricular hemorrhage.[180] The most serious side effect is maternal hypotension; the combination of calcium-channel blockers and magnesium sulfate should generally be avoided.

Oxytocin Receptor Antagonists

The introduction of the oxytocin antagonist atosiban (Tractocile) in Europe for preterm labor produced initial hopes for successful tocolysis. Unfortunately, a double-blind randomized placebo controlled trial did not demonstrate a significant effect on neonatal outcome.[181]

Pain Control

Pain control after fetal surgery is an essential component of tocolytic therapy, because it is believed that adequate pain control prevents the stress-induced hormonal impetus for preterm labor. Surgical stress elicits the release of adrenocorticotropic hormone that increases production of cortisol; cortisol production, in turn, leads to the deleterious changes in the placenta that increase fetal estrogen and prostaglandin production, promoting increased uterine activity. One study[182] found that baboons receiving larger doses of analgesics had smaller concentrations of maternal estrogens, cortisol, and oxytocin than were found in baboons that received a lesser dose. Furthermore, myometrial contractile activity was significantly less in those animals that received more opioids.

Fetal Complications of Tocolytic Therapy

The fetal side effects of tocolytics present a number of problems, albeit usually less so than in the mother. β-Sympathomimetics cause fetal tachycardia.[183] Whereas cyclooxygenase inhibitors have been shown to be more effective than others in delaying labor,[184] the side effects of fetal oliguria and ductus arteriosus constriction have limited their long-term use.[185] However, after short-term use, these side effects are fully reversible within 72 hours from cessation of treatment.[185] Longer-term use of indomethacin has been associated with renal dysfunction and increased rates of necrotizing enterocolitis, intracranial hemorrhage, and patent ductus arteriosus in infants delivered at less than 30 weeks' gestation.[186] Calcium channel blockers such as nifedipine inhibit contractility in smooth muscle cells. No adverse fetal effects have been reported in humans, although, in animals, nifedipine has been shown to cause a reduction in uterine blood flow and fetal metabolic acidosis.[187,188] Magnesium sulfate reduces fetal heart rate variability[189] and depresses fetal right ventricular function.[190] Because this drug rapidly crosses the placenta but is excreted more slowly by the fetal kidneys than by the maternal kidneys, there are concerns about fetal toxicity, resulting in respiratory and central nervous system depression.[191] Atosiban, an oxytocin antagonist, so far has not been found to cause any fetal side effects.[192] Nitric oxide donors such as nitroglycerin appear to have minimal fetal side effects.[193]

Postoperative Pulmonary Edema

Noncardiogenic pulmonary edema is a known complication of tocolysis. Most often, obstetric pulmonary edema is due to increased hydrostatic pressures and resolves rapidly with diuretics, cessation of tocolytics, and fluid restriction. One study observed a prevalence of pulmonary edema of 0.5%, but that rate increased to 23% in fetal surgical patients[178]; 93% of those with pulmonary edema required intensive care and 20% required tracheal intubation. It has been hypothesized that extensive uterine manipulation during surgery may result in release of mediators that increase the permeability of lung vasculature. The class of medications most strongly associated with pulmonary edema is β-mimetic agents. An additional important observation is that patients receiving nitroglycerin for tocolysis have demonstrated more pronounced pulmonary edema (more severe hypoxemia, longer time to resolution, worse chest radiograph, and a greater composite lung injury scores) than those who received other tocolytics.[178]

Congenital Cystic Adenomatoid Malformation: The Open Procedure

Congenital cystic adenomatoid malformation serves as a prime example of a fetal condition requiring open intervention. Fetuses with lung masses presenting before extrauterine viability represent a complex group of congenital disorders. Before the advent of preterm fetal intervention, management of fetal lung masses consisted of limited options, which included (1) delivery with hydrops once fetal viability was determined with regard to lung maturity while acknowledging the potential need for emergent postpartum resuscitation, (2) transplacental digoxin therapy in an effort to treat severe forms of cardiac dysfunction,[194,195] and (3) termination of the pregnancy if the fetus was considered nonviable. Fetuses demonstrating in-utero tumor regressions as documented by serial sonograms are allowed to progress to term gestation. Most infants with smaller lung masses or those with masses demonstrating in-utero regression do well with standard delivery and neonatal resection.[196] However, a subset of fetuses experience significant fetal lung mass growth, ultimately compromising normal lung development. Treatment options for these fetuses have expanded to include cyst aspiration, thoracocentesis, double-J stents for permanent thoracic drainage, and in-utero resection of the lung mass.[196-198] All treatment options aim to reduce the size of the lung mass to allow the remaining fetal lung to develop.

Congenital Cystic Adenomatoid Malformation of the Lung

Congenital cystic adenomatoid malformation (CCAM) of the lung consists of cystic masses of pulmonary tissue and bronchial structures, neither of which participate in gas exchange[199,200] that may represent a form of pulmonary hypoplasia.[201] CCAMs can compress surrounding lung tissue and impede normal lung development, resulting in pulmonary hypoplasia.[202] Of all of the fetal lung masses, CCAM is the lesion most often associated with hydrops fetalis that often indicates a premorbid fetal state. Although the exact mechanisms for the development of hydrops are unclear, it has been suggested to be secondary to either cardiac compression or vena caval obstruction from the intrathoracic mass.[203,204] This condition is associated with a significant imbalance of fetal fluid, resulting in accumulation of fetal fluid causing increases in fetal interstitial and total body water, pericardial and pleural effusions, ascites, anasarca, polyhydramnios, or placental thickening.[205,206]

Fetal lung abnormalities themselves may lead to excessive fluid accumulation because the fetal lung is an important organ for amniotic fluid balance. The average fetal lung fluid production is estimated to be approximately 300 mL/day or about 4 mL/kg/hr[207]; fetal urine output is approximately 700 mL/day, and fetal swallowing is about 700 mL/day. The remaining 300 mL/day is postulated to exit the amnion through the chorioamnionic membrane. CCAMs may impair fetal swallowing via esophageal obstruction and therefore disrupt normal fluid balance; fetal swallowing is the major method by which amniotic fluid water is returned to the fetal vascular compartment. A second possibility is hypersecretion or transudation of fluid from the CCAM itself.

Management

Experts have formulated guidelines for the fetal surgical management of fetuses diagnosed with CCAM lesions; overall prognosis depends on the size of the lung mass and the presence of secondary physiologic derangements.[196] Special consideration is given to fetuses exhibiting signs of hydrops fetalis, especially those who are less than 32 weeks gestation.[208] Although these conclusions were based primarily on the experience with CCAM infants, it might be appropriate to extend this experience to the management of fetuses with other lung lesions. The primary goal of treatment is to reduce lesion size so that the fetal lung has an improved chance of normal development.

Historical Interventions and Outcomes

Adzick and associates reviewed their experience with fetal lung lesions (Fig. 38-5).[196] For the hydropic fetus with a lung mass, management depends on gestational age. For fetuses greater than 32 weeks gestation, delivery should be considered. The lung lesion can then be resected immediately after delivery, although neonatal outcomes are poor. For fetuses less than 32 weeks gestation, fetal thoracotomy and in-utero resection of the mass should be considered. Of the 13 fetuses with lung lesions and hydrops, 8 fetuses underwent in-utero lobectomy, which resulted in resolution of the hydrops, improved in-utero lung growth, and neonatal survival. In this series, six fetuses with large solitary cystic lesions and no evidence of hydrops underwent thoracoamniotic shunting with five survivors. Maternal complications from in-utero fetal lung resection included seroma, wound infection, blood transfusions, mild postoperative pulmonary edema, and one uterine wound dehiscence.

Operating Room Preparation

Like all other types of fetal intervention, ultrasonography should be performed before the induction of anesthesia to assess fetal well-being and to obtain an estimated fetal weight. In addition to the normal preanesthesia preparation checklist, additional maternal airway equipment, resuscitation drugs, and tocolytic agents should be prepared and immediately available. The availability of type-specific packed red blood cells for the mother and O-negative irradiated packed red blood cells, divided into 50-mL aliquots, for the fetus must be confirmed. The operating room temperature should be warmed to at least 80°F to prevent hypothermia of the partially exposed fetus during thoracotomy. Resuscitation drugs for the fetus (atropine 10 to 20 µg/kg, epinephrine 1 µg/kg), as well as a muscle relaxant (e.g., vecuronium 0.2 mg/kg), and fentanyl (10 µg/kg) are prepared under sterile conditions, thus making them available during the procedure.[209] A rapid infusion system with warmed isotonic saline is used to replace amniotic fluid loss during fetal lung resection and ready to administer onto the surgical field via a sterile tubing system. A pulse oximeter with a sterile extension cord should be available for application to the upper extremity of the fetus.

Induction

The preferred method of maternal anesthesia for these cases is general endotracheal anesthesia. Before entering the operating room, an intravenous line is started and sedation is administered as needed. If the mother has not received indomethacin (50 mg rectal suppository) for tocolysis before arrival, it is administered after induction of general anesthesia. Indomethacin is used in conjunction with magnesium in the postoperative period for tocolysis but does not play a significant tocolytic role in the intraoperative period. Once inside the operating room and after placement of standard monitors, a lumbar epidural catheter may be inserted for postoperative pain management. With the exception of a test dose, most practitioners avoid local anesthetic administration through the epidural catheter until the fetal intervention is completed. This is done to avoid possible decreases in maternal mean arterial pressure from an epidural-associated sympathectomy. The mother is then positioned in a uterine displacement position and preoxygenated, and a rapid-sequence induction is performed with an induction agent, suc-

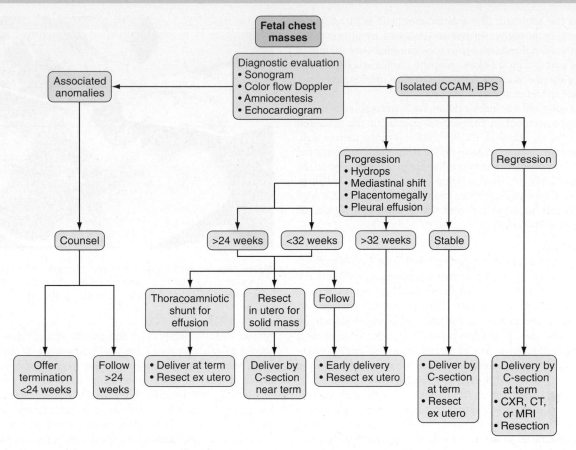

Figure 38-5. Algorithm for the management of fetal chest masses. CCAM, congenital cystic adenomatoid malformation; BPS, bronchopulmonary syndrome; CT, computed tomography (CAT scan); CXR, chest radiography; MRI, magnetic resonance imaging. (Reprinted with permission from Myers LB, Bulich LA [eds]: Anesthesia for Fetal Intervention and Surgery. Philadelphia, BC Decker, 2005.)

cinylcholine, and a rapid-acting opioid. Anesthesia is maintained with 1 MAC of the inhaled anesthetic agent of choice (usually sevoflurane or desflurane should a rapid reinstatement of uterine tone be required) in 100% oxygen while an ultrasonographic examination maps out surface anatomy with respect to the placenta and fetus, as well as reassuring fetal well-being after the anesthetic induction. A second large-bore peripheral intravenous catheter, radial arterial catheter, urinary catheter, and nasogastric tube are then inserted. Because the maternal anesthesia induction is the same as a standard cesarean section, invasive blood pressure monitoring is not necessary until the inhaled anesthetic agent is increased to 2 to 3 MAC. Fetal hemodynamics (heart rate, right ventricular contractility) are monitored intraoperatively by continuous fetal echocardiography.[209]

Maintenance

Before maternal skin incision, the volatile anesthetic is increased to 2 MAC to ensure myometrial relaxation and tocolysis.[209-211] Satisfactory uterine relaxation can be achieved, but these concentrations may decrease maternal arterial pressure, uteroplacental perfusion, and fetal oxygenation and may require pressor support.[209,212] While only small increments in fetal PaO_2 occur with maternal inspired oxygen concentrations of 100%, this small increase may be advantageous. Additionally, the increased inhaled anesthetic requirement dictates the use of only agents that will augment uterine relaxation.[213] Given that nitrous oxide does not affect the uterine tone to any measurable degree and

thus provides no direct benefit when complete uterine relaxation is desired, the use of 100% oxygen is preferred. Maternal eucapnia ($PaCO_2$ of 31-33 mm Hg) is the physiologic goal,[205] because animal and human studies demonstrated that maternal hyperventilation may lead to decreases in fetal PaO_2.[214,215] Some have suggested that maternal hypercarbia can, in fact, increase fetal PO_2.[216] At this time, however, extrapolation of these conclusions to fetal intervention cases should be done with caution.

Once return of neuromuscular function from the short-acting paralytic agent has been determined with the aid of a peripheral nerve stimulator, further doses of nondepolarizing muscle relaxants are titrated as indicated. If preoperative tocolytic agents were administered, combined with the anticipated administration of magnesium sulfate during the abdominal closure, it is recommended to avoid any long-acting nondepolarizing agent so as to ensure the later ability to adequately antagonize neuromuscular blockade.

Meticulous attention to maternal blood pressure is essential to ensure adequate uterine blood flow and uterine perfusion; maternal systolic pressure is maintained at mean awake values with intravenous ephedrine or phenylephrine as needed. Total intravenous fluids are limited unless blood loss is excessive so as to minimize the risk of postoperative maternal pulmonary edema.[217]

Once the uterus has been completely exposed, the surgeons assess uterine tone. Because there is no objective method to assess the degree of uterine relaxation, surgical palpation remains the standard. The volatile anesthetic is increased as necessary, or nitroglycerin boluses (followed by infusion) are administered to diminish uterine tone if needed. Any attempted surgical manipulation before complete uterine relaxation may increase uterine vascular resistance, reduce uterine perfusion, and place the fetus at risk of hypoxia.

After adequate uterine relaxation, the hysterotomy site is prepared by placement of two sutures parallel to the proposed incision site and through the full thickness of the uterine wall. A hemostatic uterine stapling device is inserted; and once the stapler is deployed, the amniotic membranes are secured to the uterine wall, effectively minimizing excessive maternal bleeding. However, if the stapling device misfires or if the placental edge is mistakenly incorporated into the hysterotomy, significant hemorrhage may occur.

Intervention

The fetal hemithorax and upper extremity are delivered through the hysterotomy. Warm fluids are continuously infused into the uterine cavity from a high-volume fluid warmer to replace amniotic fluid losses, provide a thermoneutral environment for the fetus, and prevent umbilical cord kinking or stretching. Limiting the size of the uterine incision helps prevent fetal evaporative fluid loss, uterine hemorrhage, and postoperative uterine contractions. Once the fetal hemithorax and upper extremity have been delivered into the operative field, fentanyl (5 to 20 μg/kg), atropine (20 μg/kg), and a muscle relaxant (usually vecuronium 0.2 mg/kg) are given intramuscularly as a single injection into the exposed shoulder of the fetus.[209] Fentanyl is administered for intraoperative and postoperative fetal analgesia and to suppress the fetal stress response, atropine ablates the expected bradycardic response with fetal surgical manipulation, and a muscle relaxant will ensure an immobile fetus during surgery. Although the fetus receives anesthesia from transplacental transfer of maternal inhaled halogenated anesthetic agents, these additional intramuscular medications augment the fetal anesthetic and ensure fetal analgesia before thoracotomy.

A pulse oximetry probe can be applied to the exposed fetal extremity. Fetal echocardiography provides information about fetal heart rate and ventricular filling, which is particularly useful in those procedures in which blood loss is anticipated (Fig. 38-6). Before fetal thoracotomy, peripheral vascular access can be obtained in the exposed upper extremity and is highly recommended. Fetal lung lesions, especially if composed of multiple tissue types, may have a very irregular vascular supply, and significant fetal hemorrhage is possible. Direct vascular access allows immediate resuscitation and blood administration as needed. Even surgical manipulations alone can lead to hemodynamic instability, requiring urgent resuscitation. This may be secondary to inadvertent mediastinal torsion, resulting in a sudden loss of cardiac preload.

Intraoperative Fetal Resuscitation

Fetal bradycardia (fetal heart rate <100 beats per minute) usually results from hypoperfusion with low cardiac output, umbilical cord kinking, or surgical manipulation, but it may also be a result of increased uterine vascular resistance or unrecognized bleeding from the tumor site. Other expected surgery-related complications include blood loss from the tumor, hypothermia, dehydration, and inadvertent delivery of the fetus. Despite identification and correction of precipitating factors, the fetus may

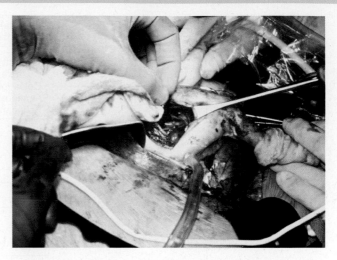

Figure 38-6. In-utero thoracotomy in a 22-week fetus after excision of congenital cystic adenomatoid malformation. (Courtesy of N. Scott Adzick, MD, Children's Hospital of Philadelphia.)

remain severely bradycardic and require resuscitation. Efforts should be made to maximize fetal perfusion and ensure adequate fetal intravascular volume. Maneuvers include confirming maternal FIO2 of 100%, increasing maternal mean arterial pressure to 15% to 25% above awake values, increasing the halogenated agent concentration to ensure minimum uterine vascular resistance, confirming adequate intrauterine volume with warmed replacement Ringer's lactate solution, and identifying the umbilical cord via ultrasonography to verify that twisting or kinking has not occurred. Pharmacologic support may also be needed. In cases with no fetal intravascular access, intramuscular epinephrine (1-2 μg/kg) and atropine (20 μg/kg) can be administered and repeated if necessary. If intravascular access is available, pharmacologic resuscitation should be administered via this route to guarantee immediate effect. In addition, blood transfusions (5-10 mL/kg O-negative irradiated packed cells) can be administered in cases of severe fetal hypovolemia by either an upper extremity intravascular route or by percutaneous access to the umbilical vein with ultrasound guidance.

Closure

Once the lung lesion has been resected and fetal well-being is confirmed, the fetus is returned to the intrauterine environment and the hysterotomy incision is closed. Closure consists of two separate layers, thus minimizing the risk for postoperative amniotic fluid leak and uterine wall dehiscence (Fig. 38-7). It is important to maintain complete uterine relaxation during closure because uterine manipulation can alter blood flow and place the fetus at risk of hypoperfusion. Before the last uterine stitches, intra-amniotic volume is assessed via ultrasonography and any deficit is replaced with warmed Ringer's lactate solution.

Once uterine closure is completed, maternal abdominal wall closure begins. At this time, a magnesium sulfate bolus (6 g) can be administered intravenously over 20 minutes, followed by a 3-g/hr infusion that should be continued into the postoperative period. The epidural catheter can be dosed with local anesthetic (15-20 mL of 0.25% bupivacaine) and an opioid (e.g., fentanyl 1-2 μg/kg) as the inhaled agent is decreased or discontinued. Careful attention to the degree of neuromuscular blockade is

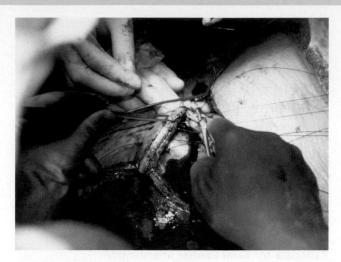

Figure 38-7. Hysterotomy closure. (Courtesy of N. Scott Adzick, MD, Children's Hospital of Philadelphia.)

needed as magnesium sulfate potentiates the action of the muscle relaxants. Extubation occurs as soon as the usual criteria for extubation are met.

Postoperative Management

As soon as the procedure is completed, the mother should be monitored by experienced staff and necessary equipment to immediately address any complications that might occur. Ultrasonography is performed in the immediate postoperative setting and frequently over the subsequent week to monitor fetal hemodynamic stability. Tocodynamometers to assess the degree of uterine activity and irritability are used to guide tocolytic therapy.

Serious postoperative complications include premature labor, pulmonary edema, amniotic fluid leak, wound seroma and infection, and fetal demise.[205,209,218-222] Virtually all patients experience premature uterine contractions in the immediate postoperative period, thereby necessitating a continuous magnesium sulfate infusion. In some instances, additional tocolytic agents may be necessary. Despite maximal tocolytic therapies, continued uterine irritability may result in premature delivery. Amniotic fluid leak can lead to oligohydramnios and significant reductions in amniotic fluid volume that may necessitate replacement. In refractory cases, the mother may return to the operating room for reclosure of the hysterotomy incision.

The etiology of fetal demise after open fetal surgery is usually a secondary consequence of a primary complication (see earlier). As such, every effort is made to minimize and promptly treat potential postoperative complications to ensure a positive fetal intervention and to provide an environment for a successful term gestation. Surgical stress and pain can lead to release of cortisol and inflammatory cytokines in both the mother and the fetus, which, in turn, may lead to premature uterine maturation and contractions.[223] Maternal pain control can be provided by patient-controlled analgesia and epidural or spinal analgesia. One disadvantage to epidural analgesia is that lower systemic opioid concentrations are achieved; therefore, less is transferred to the fetus for postoperative analgesia. The appeal of the greater systemic opioid concentration produced by intravenous analgesia is the possibility of improved fetal analgesia. However, intravenous analgesia does not reliably prevent a maternal stress response. To overcome this disadvantage, the best choice of solution for epidural analgesia may be a reduced concentration of the local anesthetic with a large concentration of a fat-soluble opioid, such as fentanyl. One such reduced epidural solution combines bupivacaine (0.05%) and fentanyl (10 µg/mL)[218]; the large fentanyl concentration allows significant systemic absorption and possible delivery of opioid to the fetus.

Other Diseases Eligible for Open Procedures

Pulmonary Sequestration

Pulmonary sequestration, also known as bronchopulmonary sequestration, accessory lung, or bronchopulmonary foregut malformation, represents 0.5% to 6% of all cases of congenital lung disease (0.15% and 1.7% of live births).[32-34] Pulmonary sequestrations are lesions consisting of nonfunctional lung tissue that do not communicate with the normal tracheobronchial tree and hence do not participate in gas exchange.[33] Pulmonary sequestration may be differentiated from CCAM by investigation of its blood supply. Unlike pulmonary sequestrations, CCAMs derive their blood supply and venous drainage from the pulmonary circulation. A multitude of somatic anomalies have been associated with sequestration, most commonly diaphragmatic hernia. If not treated in utero, these lesions often present as respiratory distress in the neonatal period or as chronic respiratory infections in older children. Although hydrops fetalis occurs with greater frequency in cases of CCAM, hydrops can also develop in the presence of any congenital pulmonary mass lesion. As such, in-utero presentations of pulmonary sequestration are often associated with hydrops fetalis, polyhydramnios, and placentomegaly. Hydrothorax is often associated and may be lymphatic in origin, stemming from the impaired lymph drainage from the sequestration itself.[12,37,38]

Bronchogenic Cysts and Mixed or Hybrid Pulmonary Lesions

Bronchogenic cysts are embryonic abnormalities considered to be a type of bronchopulmonary foregut malformation.[224] These cysts are thought to result from an abnormal budding of the primitive bronchial tree between the fourth and eighth week of gestation, thus representing abnormal lung development at an early stage of ontogeny.[225] In most cases, bronchogenic cysts are asymptomatic in the first months of life. A notable exception is a mediastinal cyst that usually manifests as stridor.

Although in-utero complications are less likely than with the other fetal lung lesions previously described, the propensity of these lesions to cause life-threatening postnatal complications warrants close attention throughout the prenatal period. Common clinical presentations are the result of compression of the tracheobronchial tree, pulmonary artery, or esophagus[226-228]; compression of the bronchus can lead to distal airway obstruction.[229] Postnatal evaluation may reveal bronchial atresia, tracheomalacia, bronchomalacia, or a direct result of distortion or compression of the developing larger airways. Fetal intervention with intermittent or continuous drainage of cysts can prevent the secondary morbidity; definitive fetal surgery with thoracotomy has also been successful.[230]

Sacrococcygeal Teratoma

Sacrococcygeal teratomas (SCTs) are one of the most common congenital tumors in the neonate (1/40,000 live births).[231-233] A variety of tissues from the three primary germ layers are usually found within the tumors; the size can be highly variable.[234,235] Most SCTs are external, usually protruding from the perineal region. The majority of SCTs are a combination of solid and cystic components, with only 15% being entirely cystic.[236,237] SCTs, although usually benign, can cause significant secondary morbidity in selected cases because of the tumor's mass effect and vast blood supply.[238] With smaller tumors, complete surgical resection usually occurs after delivery under elective, controlled conditions. In extreme cases, the tumor can cause fetal congestive heart failure (usually high output failure) and even fetal demise if no treatment is performed.[239] Death is usually secondary to an enlarged tumor mass and associated polyhydramnios, resulting in preterm labor and delivery, with ultimate survival dependent on fetal lung maturity. Massive hemorrhage into the tumor with fetal exsanguination may occur spontaneously in utero or be precipitated by labor and delivery. Dystocia, secondary to tumor bulk or tumor rupture, may occur during vaginal delivery or cesarean section. Prenatal intervention may be necessary, including intrauterine transfusion or fetal surgery for those fetuses that develop significant secondary morbidity (hydrops).

Preoperative Preparation

Preoperative fetal imaging provides information regarding the extent of tumor growth, anatomic location (intrapelvic vs. extrapelvic tumor), and any evidence of cystic components, making the tumor amenable to possible decompression. If there is evidence of hemorrhage into the tumor on MRI or ultrasonography, a preoperative fetal hematocrit is strongly recommended. If open fetal surgery and tumor resection are planned, a transfusion of the anemic fetus before surgery is recommended to allow the fetus to better withstand the anticipated blood loss during tumor resection. Furthermore, the ability to transfuse the fetus during open fetal surgery may not be possible because only the buttocks and tumor of the fetus are usually exposed through the hysterotomy incision (Fig. 38-8). Great care is taken to deliver

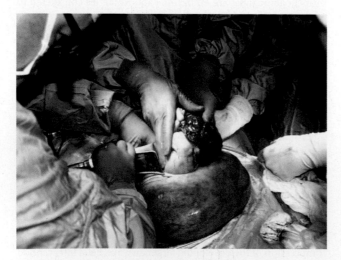

Figure 38-8. Fetal sacrococcygeal teratoma before in-utero resection in a 22-week fetus. (Courtesy of N. Scott Adzick, MD, Children's Hospital of Philadelphia.)

only the fetal part that is absolutely necessary because further delivery could increase the risk of placental separation, uterine contractions, umbilical cord kinking, and inadvertent delivery.

Hypoplastic Left Heart Syndrome: Percutaneous and Fetoscopic Procedures

A variety of congenital heart defects (CHDs) may be considered for fetal intervention. To date, the most studied defects include severe aortic stenosis with evolving hypoplastic left heart syndrome (HLHS) and pulmonary valve atresia with an intact ventricular septum (PAIVS) with evolving hypoplastic right heart syndrome (HRHS).[240-244]

Rationale for Fetal Cardiac Intervention

Most CHDs can be safely repaired in infancy with excellent surgical survival and long-term prognosis. For these defects, there would be no need for in-utero intervention; and for many defects, in-utero intervention would not be technically possible (e.g., arterial switch procedure for transposition of the great arteries). For other defects, surgical correction itself may not be possible and the only option is staged surgical palliation, which is often associated with significant surgical morbidity and mortality.[240,245,246] As such, the risk of performing any fetal intervention must be weighed against the potential benefits of improving the anticipated surgical outcome of the specific cardiac defect performed in the neonatal period. It is the intention of prenatal intervention for certain types of CHD to reverse the pathologic process in an attempt to preserve cardiac structure and function and, thus, it is hoped, prevent serious postnatal disease. A secondary aim of prenatal intervention is to modify the severity of the disease and improve postnatal surgical outcomes.

Defects Amenable to In-Utero Repair

Certain congenital heart defects cause aberrations in blood flow, which are usually secondary to valvular stenosis or regurgitation. Regardless of the etiology, the end result is often an abnormally developed ventricle.[247] Several case reports have characterized the progression of valvular stenosis to ventricular hypoplasia from reduced flow through the chamber during gestation.[248-250] It has been hypothesized that relief of valvular stenosis in utero could reverse the progression toward ventricular hypoplasia. In these cases, there may be a window of opportunity in which ventricular growth can be salvaged. Because most routine prenatal ultrasonographic screening is performed between 16 and 24 weeks gestation, the window of opportunity for prenatal intervention is likely between 20 and 26 weeks gestation.

To date, the defect most amenable to correction is severe aortic stenosis with evolving HLHS.[248-251] Without prenatal intervention, severe aortic stenosis can lead to marked left ventricular dysfunction, diminished flow through the left heart, arrest of left ventricular growth, ventricular fibroelastosis, and, consequently, HLHS. Aortic valve dilation may be performed percutaneously with ultrasound guidance. Optimal fetal positioning, placental location, or maternal habitus may require exposure of the uterus through an abdominal incision to obtain ideal access to the fetal thorax. These procedures have been performed under both maternal regional and general anesthesia, although general anesthesia is often preferred to obtain optimal uterine relaxation and an anesthetized fetus. Preliminary results are promising, but larger prospective investigations are warranted to determine long-term outcomes.[252]

Two right-sided heart defects may be considered for in-utero intervention: (1) pulmonary atresia with intact ventricular septum (PAIVS), also referred to as hypoplastic right heart syndrome (HRHS), and (2) tetralogy of Fallot (TOF) with pulmonary atresia and hypoplastic pulmonary arteries.[253] Unlike the left ventricle, the right ventricular cavity has the capacity to grow postnatally. HRHS is defined as a spectrum from mild disease, in which a biventricular circulation can eventually be achieved through balloon valvuloplasty and surgical palliation at birth, to the most severe form, in which a right ventricle-dependent coronary artery supply develops. There have been no reports of a successful valvuloplasty in which the treated fetus did not also require postnatal surgery.[253]

TOF with pulmonary atresia and hypoplastic pulmonary arteries requires substantial palliative surgery and interventional catheterizations in both infancy and childhood.[254] Prenatally, there is often an identifiable hypoplastic pulmonary valve that may be amenable to balloon dilation. If antegrade flow can be established during gestation, the increased flow could potentially lead to pulmonary artery growth and possibly improve the postnatal options for surgical repair. This in-utero procedure would be technically challenging to perform.

Technical Aspects of Fetal Cardiac Interventions

Open cardiac surgery on the fetus is not presently technically possible.[255-259] In humans, all of the reported procedures to date have been attempted using the transcutaneous or transuterine approach with ultrasound-guided access into the fetal heart.[242-244] Although hysterotomy would provide means for more direct fetal access (e.g., femoral artery, transumbilical or carotid artery access), maternal morbidity would be significantly increased and postoperative premature labor certain, hence requiring additional tocolytic medications in the perioperative period. After valvuloplasty, the fetus requires time for the ventricle to recover. Therefore, any procedure that substantially increases the likelihood of early delivery would likely thus be counterproductive.

Although initial percutaneous techniques for fetal cardiac valvuloplasty were performed with only the mother receiving sedation,[242,243] recent advances in surgical techniques have led to provision of maternal and fetal anesthesia and analgesia.[260] The mother usually receives general anesthesia. After ultrasonographic confirmation of placental location, the maternal abdomen and uterus are punctured with a 22-gauge spinal needle. An intramuscular injection of fentanyl, atropine, and a muscle relaxant is delivered to the fetus. A 19-gauge needle is subsequently directed into the fetal thorax, and access to the fetal heart is obtained. A small coronary balloon-tipped catheter is threaded over a guidewire through the needle and passed through the stenotic valve or closed septum. The catheter balloon is then dilated, and blood flow is confirmed using Doppler ultrasonography (Video Clip 38-3, see website; Fig. 38-9). The technique has been modified in certain cases such that a laparotomy to expose the uterus is performed. Using this technique, better ultrasonography and ideal fetal positioning are possible to achieve optimal access to the fetal thorax.

Anesthetic Management for the Mother

Most cases of fetal cardiac intervention are performed using a percutaneous technique or through a laparotomy incision with direct uterine exposure followed by a transuterine needle approach into the fetal thorax. The surgical approach will vary according to patient habitus, placental position (anterior vs. posterior), and fetal position. For the less invasive percutaneous approach, the choice of a regional anesthetic accompanied by intravenous sedation for the mother may be acceptable. However, it must be remembered that although the placental transfer of sedative drugs administered to the mother may sedate the fetus, an anesthetized or immobile fetus is not guaranteed. Excessive fetal movement makes most cardiac interventions impossible and even dangerous to both the fetus and mother. Some percutaneous approaches are later converted to a laparotomy approach.

Patients who received an epidural anesthetic technique required significantly more intravenous fluids but less intravenous opioid. The administration of large amounts of crystalloid and tocolytics during fetal surgery increases the risk of maternal pulmonary edema.[261,262] Neuraxial techniques (spinal, epidural, and combined spinal-epidural anesthesia) have been used in other percutaneous and fetoscopic procedures; a T4 sensory level blockade is required. It should be noted that neuraxial anesthesia provides no uterine relaxation and no anesthesia or analgesia to the fetus unless supplemented with intravenous maternal analgesics and sedatives (fentanyl, benzodiazepines, propofol). Because of these issues, it is generally recommended, even in anticipated percutaneous procedures, to deliver a general anesthetic to the mother. If there is a high suspicion of a laparotomy being performed, a dose of spinal Duramorph (morphine sulfate) may be delivered to the mother before the anesthetic induction for postoperative pain relief and resultant suppression of myometrial contractility after laparotomy.[248,249]

Anesthetic Management for the Fetus

Anesthesia for percutaneous and fetoscopic interventions, of which fetal cardiac interventions are a significant subset, pose several unique challenges for the anesthesiologist. The combination of immature organ systems and the underlying cardiac anomaly places the fetus at considerable anesthetic risk. Unlike adults and older children, fetal cardiac output depends more on heart rate than on stroke volume. Because fetal myocardial contractility is likely maximally stimulated, the fetus has a limited ability to increase stroke volume. Therefore, it is plausible that fetal patients with congenital heart disease and evidence of failure (i.e., hydrops) will exhibit more pronounced physiologic limitations. Notably, anesthetic-induced decreases in contractility, combined with intracardiac catheter manipulation in a structurally compromised heart, can result in fetal hypotension, bradycardia, and eventual cardiac collapse and death. It is generally accepted that neonates manifest a greater degree of hypotension in response to isoflurane and halothane at equipotent anesthetic concentrations when compared with older children.[263,264] The effects of halothane anesthesia on fetal physiology during fetal surgery have been studied.[265] Pregnant ewes received halothane or nonvolatile, intravenous maintenance anesthetics, and the fetuses were then instrumented for cardiovascular evaluation. In the stressed, acutely instrumented fetal lamb, halothane anesthesia significantly reduced fetal cardiac output and placental blood flow, whereas fetal vascular

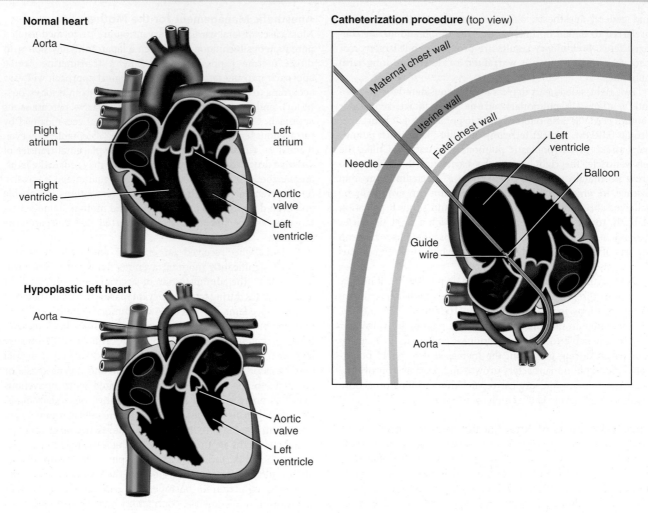

Figure 38-9. Technique for balloon dilation of a stenotic aortic valve in a fetus with hypoplastic left heart syndrome. (Reproduced with permission from Dream Magazine–Children's Hospital Boston 2002; Spring/Summer:20. www.childrenshospital.org)

resistance increased. Placental vascular resistance increased above systemic vascular resistance, which resulted in a shunting of blood away from the placenta and had a harmful effect on fetal respiratory gas exchange. Unfortunately, given the currently available anesthetics, volatile agents are required in such cases to produce uterine relaxation and maintain placental perfusion, thus necessitating fetal exposure and potential fetal risk.

Because direct exposure of the fetus is not warranted during most cardiac interventions, intraoperative monitoring is limited to echocardiography. An ultrasonographer continually monitors the fetal heart during placement of the intracardiac needle and during catheter balloon inflation. A continuous echocardiogram is also useful for measuring fetal heart rate, contractility, and volume status.

Intraoperative Fetal Resuscitation During Percutaneous Interventions

If fetal bradycardia (heart rate <100 beats per minute) or significantly reduced ventricular function develops, resuscitation proceeds immediately. Because direct vascular access to the fetus may not be immediately available, several other treatments can be employed. Intracardiac and intramuscular administration of epinephrine (1-2 µg/kg) may be used to treat severe sustained bradycardia. Other maneuvers improve uterine perfusion and hence fetal oxygenation and include increasing maternal mean arterial pressure to 15% to 25% above awake values with volume loading and ephedrine or phenylephrine and decreasing uterine vascular resistance by ensuring adequate uterine relaxation. Occasionally, pericardial tamponade may cause impaired cardiac function; needle drainage of the effusion may be necessary for fetal survival. If fetal echocardiography indicates a decreased ventricular volume, an intracardiac blood transfusion with O-negative irradiated blood (5-10 mL/kg) may be indicated.

Postoperative Considerations

The fetus is monitored postoperatively with intermittent ultrasonographic examinations. The incidence of premature contractions and labor is less after fetoscopic surgery than after open hysterotomy.[266,267] Fetoscopic intervention also appears to have reduced requirements for tocolysis and a reduced rate of premature delivery.[267] If early delivery should occur, many of these fetuses are considered nonviable owing to their young gestational age (usually <24 weeks gestation) and serious cardiac disease.

Unfortunately, the decrease in incidence and severity of premature contractions is balanced by an increase in the rates of PPROM.[268] Access during fetoscopic surgery requires one or multiple punctures through the amniotic membranes. These sites are not directly closed, leading to high rates of membrane rupture and amniotic fluid leak. Whereas the overall risk of PPROM after amniocentesis is 1% to 2%, the occurrence after single-port fetoscopic cases reaches 5% to 10% and 60% after fetal procedures requiring multiple entry sites.[269,270] Two techniques, such as introducing a plug during removal of the access devices and sealing the membrane rupture with fibrin glue to prevent the rupture of membranes, have been attempted but neither has proven to be ideal.[271,272]

Other Diseases Eligible for Fetoscopic Procedures

Twin-Twin Transfusion Syndrome

Twin-twin transfusion syndrome (TTTS) is a serious complication occurring in 10% to 15% of monozygotic monochorionic twin pregnancies.[273] Although all monochorionic twin pregnancies demonstrate one or more placental vascular anastomoses, TTTS represents a pathologic form of circulatory imbalance between the monochorionic twin fetuses.[274] As a result of this imbalance, a net fetofetal transfusion occurs, from one twin (the donor) to the other (the recipient) (Fig. 38-10). Symptoms develop rapidly and include hypovolemia, oliguria, oligohydramnios, and growth retardation in the donor twin. In turn, the recipient twin develops hypervolemia, polyuria, polyhy-

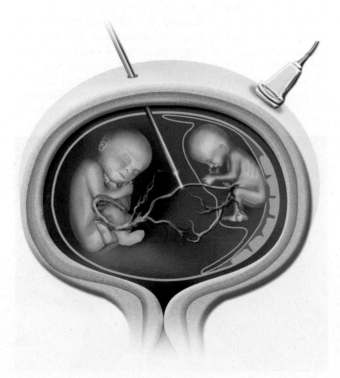

Figure 38-10. Schematic representation of umbilical cord ligation in twin reversed arterial perfusion sequence. (Courtesy of T. M. Crombleholme, MD.)

dramnios, and signs of circulatory volume overload, resulting in congestive heart failure.[273-277] In severe cases, if untreated, TTTS may result in intrauterine fetal death and miscarriage. Even if twins with TTTS survive, there remains a high incidence of secondary neurologic and pulmonary morbidities.

Fetoscopic laser photocoagulation of the communicating vessels associated with TTTS is based on three fundamental assumptions: (1) the syndrome occurs in the presence of vascular communications between fetuses in a monochorionic gestation, (2) obliteration of these vessels can halt the pathophysiologic process, and (3) both deep and superficial communications can be interrupted at the surface of the placenta.[278] Fetoscopic laser surgical occlusion of superficial communicating vessels is associated with a reported survival rate between 55% and 83% and a reduced neurologic complication rate (5%) among survivors.[273,275]

There are few data on the reported anesthetic techniques used for fetoscopic laser ablation. The procedure has been performed with local, general, epidural, and combined general and epidural anesthesia.[279-282] Factors that may influence the anesthetic technique include (1) the planned surgical approach and probability of converting to open fetal surgery; (2) the likelihood of surgical perturbation of innervated fetal tissues; (3) maternal preference; and (4) a history of prior uterine activity. The surgical approach for fetoscopic laser photocoagulation is determined by (1) the location of the placenta (anterior vs. posterior), (2) the position of the fetuses, and (3) the potential window(s) for trocar insertion.[283]

Twin Reversed Arterial Perfusion Sequence

Twin reversed arterial perfusion (TRAP) sequence denotes a common pathophysiology of several different conditions, all of which describe a twin pregnancy in which one twin is normal and the second twin exhibits multisystem malformations, including anencephaly or acardia. The twin with the hemodynamic advantage is denoted as the "pump" twin, perfusing deoxygenated blood in a retrograde direction to the other twin, "the recipient twin." The term *reversed perfusion* is used to describe this scenario because blood enters the acardiac or anencephalic twin through its umbilical artery and exits through the umbilical vein. This eventually places the normal or "pump" twin at a hemodynamic disadvantage because this normal twin provides cardiac output to both itself and the nonviable sibling. This anomaly places the pump twin at risk of cardiac overload and congestive heart failure, often with associated hepatosplenomegaly.

Perinatal complications with TRAP sequence range in severity, with reported death rates for the pump twin ranging from 39% to 59% in untreated pregnancies.[284] Treatment options include observation, medical therapy with digoxin and indomethacin, selective delivery, umbilical cord blockade with a coil, and fetoscopic cord ligation. Although all endoscopic procedures have the primary aim of interrupting umbilical cord blood flow to the nonviable twin, this invasive technique is generally employed after failed medical therapy or after signs of cardiac failure develop in the viable twin.[285,286]

Hydronephrosis and Bladder Outlet Obstruction

Bladder outlet obstruction is most commonly due to posterior urethral valves in males and urethral atresia in females.[287] In severe cases, infants present at birth with respiratory insufficiency secondary to pulmonary hypoplasia and renal failure from renal dysplasia. This severe form of bladder outlet obstruction is heralded by profound oligohydramnios, distended bladder, bilateral hydroureteronephrosis, and dysplastic changes in the kidneys. In some cases, pulmonary hypoplasia can lead to respiratory failure.[288]

Until recently, treatment options were limited to observation and serial prenatal sonograms followed by neonatal surgical intervention. Some groups have attempted to restore amniotic fluid volume to promote lung development and avoid neonatal demise secondary to pulmonary hypoplasia.[289,290] In animal studies, bladder decompression in utero has prevented the progression of renal dysplastic changes and improved pulmonary development.[291] The severity of renal dysplasia depends on both the timing and the severity of obstruction before delivery, which suggests that relief of obstruction between 20 and 30 weeks gestation may reduce the degree of renal dysplasia.[292] These studies have encouraged the development of vesicoamniotic shunts. Although these procedures are associated with a very low maternal morbidity, many fetal risks, including iatrogenic gastroschisis, infection, catheter obstruction or dislodgement, inadequate decompression, and fetal bodily injury, make this technique inappropriate for early-gestation urinary tract decompression as first-line therapy. Fetoscopic techniques to create vesicocutaneous fistulas for decompression and laser ablation of posterior urethral valves have been reported, with promising initial outcomes.[290,293,294] However, these procedures are technically difficult, and the exact role of fetoscopic intervention for correction of bladder outlet obstruction has yet to be determined.

Needle Aspiration and Placement of Shunts

A variety of fetal disorders may benefit from in-utero needle aspiration or shunt placement. These disorders include posterior urethral valves, aqueductal stenosis, fetal hydrothorax, ovarian cyst, and fetal ascites. Various shunts have been attempted to provide long-term decompression, with variable results.[288]

The EXIT Procedure

Ex utero intrapartum treatment, or the EXIT procedure, was initially described as a method for reversal of tracheal occlusion in fetuses with prenatally diagnosed severe congenital diaphragmatic hernia that had undergone in-utero tracheal clip application.[295] Although these infants demonstrated no reduced morbidity compared with those who underwent conventional treatment, this novel technique provided a new therapeutic option for fetuses with a variety of potentially fatal diseases. Improvements in prenatal imaging and widespread use of prenatal ultrasonography have increased the identification of potentially lethal fetal structural malformations, which has had a direct impact on perinatal management and outcomes.

Also referred to as the OOPS procedure (operation on placental support),[296] the EXIT procedure allows for a controlled delivery and intrapartum assessment strategy to treat fetuses with certain life-threatening diseases. By maintaining uteroplacental circulation with only partial delivery of the infant, crucial time is provided to perform procedures critical to infant survival. These procedures include direct laryngoscopy, bronchoscopy, intubation, tracheostomy, tumor decompression and

resection, and extracorporeal membrane oxygenation (ECMO) cannulation before clamping the umbilical cord (Fig. 38-11). In this way, continuous oxygenation is maintained at all times to the threatened infant thereby improving the chances of overall survival. The EXIT procedure is now used for infants in whom prenatal imaging suggests a very low probability of survival with conventional treatment methods. This group includes fetuses with known tracheal obstruction and other life-threatening airway abnormalities, as well as those who will likely require ECMO support (i.e., congenital cardiac disease and diaphragmatic hernia).

Like other types of fetal intervention, the EXIT procedure requires the anesthesiologist to care for two patients at once, often with different and, at times, conflicting requirements. Unlike many other fetal interventions, however, a planned delivery of the infant is the end result of these interventions. This unique difference creates significant increases in maternal morbidity because these procedures require complete uterine relaxation and serious maternal hemorrhage could result.[297] An intimate understanding of the EXIT procedure, the fetal pathophysiology involved, and pregnancy-induced alterations directly affecting anesthesia care is required to minimize maternal and fetal morbidity and mortality.

Historical Perspective

The first published report of an EXIT procedure for fetal airway management in 1989 described a fetus with complete tracheal obstruction secondary to a prenatally diagnosed cervical teratoma.[295] Intubation was attempted while maintaining fetoplacental circulation for 10 minutes, after which time the fetus's condition deteriorated and a nonviable infant was delivered. Although this procedure resulted in a poor outcome, the possibility of successful intervention was introduced.

In a case series,[297] indications for EXIT procedures were (1) reversal of tracheal occlusion in patients with giant fetal neck masses, (2) resection of congenital cystic adenomatoid malformation (CCAM) of the lung, (3) unilateral pulmonary agenesis, (4) congenital high airway obstruction syndrome (CHAOS), (5) ECMO placement, and (6) aid in separation of conjoined twins.

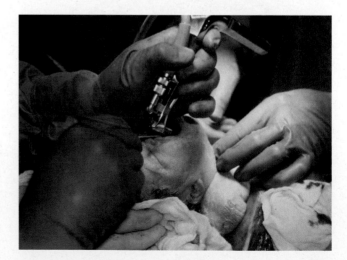

Figure 38-11. Fetal rigid bronchoscopy during ex-utero intrapartum treatment (EXIT) procedure. (Courtesy of N. Scott Adzick, MD, Children's Hospital of Philadelphia.)

Fetal diseases eligible for the EXIT procedure must demonstrate that without intervention, there would be a minimal chance of survival. Perhaps the best argument for perinatal intervention lies in fetal airway management.

Fetal Diseases Eligible for the EXIT Procedure

Cervical Teratoma

Cervical teratomas are rare (1/20,000 to 40,000 live births) and can extend from the mastoid process to the sternal notch inferiorly and to the trapezius muscle posteriorly. They can also invade the oral floor and extend into the anterior mediastinum. Many of the larger teratomas diagnosed prenatally cause maternal polyhydramnios, which is secondary to esophageal compression by the tumor and impaired fetal swallowing. Most of these tumors are benign but are associated with substantial mortality rates caused by airway compression and difficulty in establishing an adequate airway after delivery (Fig. 38-12).[298] Thirty percent of neonates with cervical teratomas die of airway obstruction shortly after delivery[299]; for infants not diagnosed prenatally, mortality rates are even greater.[300,301] In addition, some larger tumors may interfere with normal delivery methods and necessitate emergent alterations in maternal care, which places the mother at increased risk.[298,302]

Until recently, treatment options for infants with cervical teratomas who survived the intrauterine period were limited. The standard of care incorporated scheduled cesarean section followed by various airway maneuvers, including the establishment of a surgical airway. Even with skilled help immediately available, dismal outcomes were common.[298-300] Even if an airway is established, critical time is needed to perform this task, often at the expense of neonatal oxygenation. With the introduction of the EXIT procedure, precious time is provided to locate the trachea and secure a definitive airway before clamping the

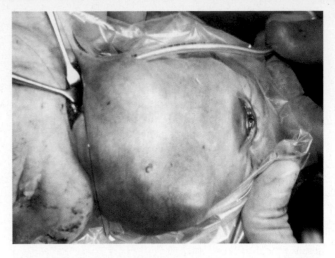

Figure 38-13. Fetus with a cystic hygroma that underwent EXIT to establish a surgical airway before delivery. (Courtesy of N. Scott Adzick, MD, Children's Hospital of Philadelphia.)

umbilical cord, thereby maintaining continuous fetal oxygenation and decreasing morbidity and mortality.

Cystic Hygroma

Cystic hygromas arise from the failure of the jugular lymph sacs to join the lymphatic system early in fetal development, resulting in the development of endothelium-lined cystic spaces that eventually compress normal surrounding structures. This compression may result in fetal hydrops, including skin edema, ascites, and pleural or pericardial effusions (Fig. 38-13).[300,301] In infants with isolated cervical cystic hygroma and no evidence of hydrops, airway compromise at birth or shortly thereafter is the main therapeutic concern. These infants are considered candidates for EXIT procedures.

Congenital High Airway Obstruction Syndrome

Congenital high airway obstruction syndrome (CHAOS) is a clinical syndrome consisting of extremely large echogenic lungs, flattened or inverted diaphragms, a dilated tracheobronchial tree, ascites, and evidence of nonimmune hydrops, including fetal ascites, placentomegaly, and pleural or pericardial effusions.[303-305] Airway obstruction may be due to laryngeal atresia, laryngeal cyst, and tracheal atresia. Diagnosis of prenatal CHAOS is confirmed by ultrasonographic evidence of complete or near-complete upper airway obstruction. Most diagnostic findings result from increased intratracheal pressure and distention of the tracheobronchial tree secondary to the accumulation of fluid in the lungs. Cardiac changes include the appearance of an elongated heart, septal shift, and small, compressed heart chambers.[300]

Management guidelines for fetuses with CHAOS are not definitive. In third trimester fetuses with a diagnosis of CHAOS and no evidence of hydrops, there is most probably incomplete airway obstruction, and management is aimed at establishing an airway before complete delivery. This subset of fetuses would likely benefit from an EXIT procedure.[300,306] Those fetuses with a diagnosis of CHAOS made in the second trimester and those with evidence of complete airway obstruction and/or nonimmune hydrops present a dilemma because insufficient data exist to determine their best treatment options.

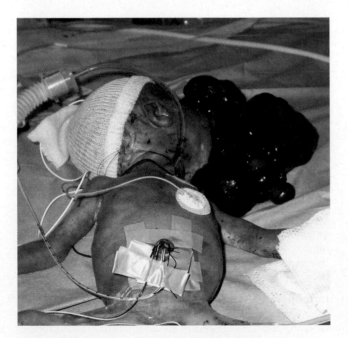

Figure 38-12. Newborn with a massive oropharyngeal cervical teratoma immediately after ex utero intrapartum treatment (EXIT procedure) was performed to secure the airway. Immediate resection of the teratoma followed in an adjacent operating room.

Congenital Goiter

Congenital goiter is associated with fetal hypothyroidism, euthyroidism, or hyperthyroidism. Goiter associated with fetal hypothyroidism is almost always associated with the transplacental passage of a thyroid-stimulating immunoglobulin G antibody from the mother. Such antibodies are present in 90% of women with Graves disease. These antibody levels may not reflect maternal thyroid status, making the fetus of any woman with Graves disease at increased risk for fetal goiter. Less common causes include iodine deficiency, iodine intoxication, congenital metabolic disorders of thyroid hormone synthesis, or hypothalamic-pituitary hypothyroidism. Ultrasonographic findings of fetal hyperthyroidism include cardiac hypertrophy, tachycardia, or nonimmune hydrops fetalis. Fetal hypothyroidism may be associated with fetal cardiomegaly and heart block. Fetal blood sampling is required to determine the fetal thyroid status.[300,307,308]

The possibility of significant airway compression immediately after delivery is similar for all fetuses with goiter. In severe cases, even the presence of experienced personnel in the delivery room may not ensure prompt ability to secure the airway. These infants may benefit from the EXIT procedure, providing the time that may be necessary to identify and secure the compromised fetal airway.

EXIT to ECMO

In addition to airway management, the EXIT procedure may be considered for other instances in which separation from uteroplacental support is expected to cause critical cardiac or pulmonary compromise. Fetuses with congenital heart disease who are expected to need emergent ECMO at birth and fetuses with poor prognosis congenital diaphragmatic hernias may benefit from the "EXIT to ECMO" strategy.[297,309] Neonates undergoing this procedure are partially delivered via the EXIT procedure, and arterial and venous cannulas are inserted while uteroplacental perfusion is maintained. Although CDH remains the most common disease entity considered for potential EXIT to ECMO therapy, this technique has been used for neonates with other disease processes associated with almost certain chance of immediate cardiorespiratory collapse after conventional delivery.

EXIT Procedure Versus Cesarean Section: Anesthetic Perspective

Despite their apparent similarities, the EXIT procedure and cesarean section are vastly different procedures, each having its own potential risks. Both surgical procedures require specific anesthetic techniques, and the ultimate success of both depends on a well-planned and executed anesthetic. Most elective cesarean sections are performed under a regional neuraxial technique (e.g., epidural, spinal, or combined spinal and epidural) with the goal of delivering a healthy infant as safely and expeditiously as possible while maintaining maternal safety. Delivery of a vigorous infant involves minimizing medications that, through placental transfer, may have adverse or depressant effects on the neonate. In those cases in which a general anesthetic is employed, concentration of inhalational agents is kept to a minimum to avoid respiratory depression in the neonate and diminish the risk of uterine atony, minimizing maternal hemorrhage, and facilitating placental separation after delivery. However, even in a routine cesarean section, the hysterotomy incision causes alterations in uterine perfusion such that the infant may be at increased risk for hypoxemia. In addition, after the uterine incision, continual bleeding occurs from the uterine edges of the incision, which can lead to significant maternal blood loss and hypotension, further placing the fetus at risk.

The EXIT procedure, in contrast to a routine cesarean section, requires complete uterine relaxation before hysterotomy by means of large inhaled anesthetic concentrations[301] for several reasons: (1) surgical manipulation often requires delivering the fetal head, shoulders, and neck mass through the hysterotomy incision, which is often not possible with a normal low transverse segment incision used in routine cesarean sections without complete uterine relaxation; (2) the fetus may undergo a surgical procedure and thus will require anesthesia that is delivered via transplacental transfer of inhalation agent; and (3) maintaining fetal oxygenation depends on uterine perfusion and minimal uterine vascular resistance. Complete uterine relaxation places the mother at risk for acute hemorrhage, but with the use of a uterine stapling device that seals the membranes and uterine edges during EXIT procedures, the amount of blood loss is markedly reduced. High-dose anesthetic requirements also place the mother at risk of hypotension from profound vasodilation and myocardial depression, which will, in turn, cause fetal hypoxia from decreased uterine perfusion if it is not aggressively and promptly treated.

Short-term maternal outcomes do not appear to differ between patients receiving EXIT procedures and those undergoing standard cesarean sections. Although the EXIT procedures take approximately twice as long to perform, there appear to be no significant differences in estimated blood loss, length of hospital stay after delivery, incidence of endometritis, superficial wound infections, total infections, thromboembolic events, or maternal deaths.[311]

Maternal Preoperative Evaluation

A detailed maternal history regarding exposure to any prior drugs that may affect the fetus is important. A maternal physical examination, including clinical signs of hypothyroidism or hyperthyroidism and a focused airway examination, should be performed. For fetuses with suspected goiter, maternal blood analysis, including thyroxine levels, thyroid-stimulating hormone levels, and thyroid-stimulating antibodies, is performed. A history of chronic uterine irritability and contractions may indicate a fetus that may be borderline acidotic, thus making this fetus more susceptible to the physiologic and pharmacologic alterations associated with the EXIT procedure. The presence of fetal acidemia, regardless of the cause, may necessitate aggressive resuscitation immediately after delivery and may even require the administration of resuscitation medications, including blood products and bicarbonate, before beginning the fetal intervention.

Intraoperative Considerations

A multidisciplinary team consisting of an obstetrician, pediatric surgeon, ultrasonographer, anesthesiologist, neonatologist, scrub nurses, and technicians provides the expertise in each respective field to aid in the overall success of the procedure. In cases in which immediate surgical intervention is planned (e.g., resection of a neck mass), a prepared adjacent operating room with separate personnel should be available. A meeting of the entire team is held before the start of the case to clearly identify individual roles and to discuss any concerns or questions. This is also a good opportunity to address any clinical changes, either in radiographic findings or in fetal position, or other factors that may alter the surgical plan.

Uterine Relaxation and Perfusion

It is of primary importance to ensure complete uterine relaxation throughout the duration of fetal uteroplacental support to preserve maternal-fetal gas exchange at the placental interface, ensure fetal oxygenation, and avoid life-threatening hypoxemia. Factors affecting uterine blood flow include, but are not limited to, anesthetic induction agents, maternal hyperventilation, maternal hypotension, maternal catecholamine release, and other causes of increased noradrenergic activity and uterine tone. Any increase in uterine vascular resistance will decrease uterine perfusion, as is seen with uterine contractions. Of all factors ensuring the overall success of the EXIT procedure, minimal uterine vascular resistance is the most important because decreases in uterine blood flow will cause fetal hypoxemia, acidosis, and, potentially, fetal demise.

Surgical Procedure

After the hysterotomy site has been created and hemostasis achieved, the fetal head, neck, and shoulders are delivered. Because many of these procedures involve large neck masses, a generous hysterotomy incision is needed to partially deliver the fetus without injury to the mass or fetus. Furthermore, if a uterine contraction occurs at this time, inadvertent expulsion of the fetus could occur, interrupting the fetoplacental unit and thus critically jeopardizing the viability of the fetus. In some cases, a fetal extremity may be delivered to apply a pulse oximetry probe and to obtain intravenous access.[312,313] Although the fetus is anesthetized via placental transfer of maternally administered inhaled anesthetics in most cases, additional analgesia and paralytics are administered (e.g., fentanyl, atropine, muscle relaxant). The additional medications may be given as a single intramuscular dose in an upper extremity or can alternatively be delivered under ultrasound guidance before hysterotomy. An advantage to earlier administration is increased time for fetal absorption via the intramuscular route. If peripheral intravenous access is obtained, additional medications can be given through this route.

Access to the Fetal Airway

Most EXIT procedures are currently performed to access a compromised fetal airway before delivery; successful access depends on meticulous preoperative evaluation and careful preparation. Portions of the trachea can be completely compressed and distorted such that even successful intubation may result in an inability to achieve adequate ventilation. For this reason, most surgeons perform a direct laryngoscopy and rigid bronchoscopy to examine the status of the fetal airway. In one series successful endotracheal intubation by conventional means was reported in 77% of cases.[297] In those cases in which tracheal intubation is impossible, a surgical tracheostomy can be performed as soon as the trachea is identified. The trachea can be located with the aid of preoperative radiographic studies, often identifying the tracheal location relative to fixed external anatomic landmarks. Gentle surgical palpation may also aid in the identification of cartilaginous tracheal rings. In cases in which the former options have failed, ultrasonography with the sterile probe inserted directly into the surgical incision may help to locate the trachea.[314] When tracheal rings are identified, the trachea may be accessed directly with an endotracheal tube by tunneling through the fetal soft tissue or with the aid of a retrograde wire inserted by the Seldinger technique. The trachea, exposed through a neck incision, may be incised via a temporary tracheotomy to allow passage of a feeding tube or wire from the trachea to the mouth or nose. The guidewire is then attached to the endotracheal tube, which is then pulled down into the proper position. After suturing the endotracheal tube securely to the mouth, the tracheotomy can then be closed.

Regardless of the method used to secure the trachea, the anesthesiologist must be prepared to control ventilation in the fetus. In some institutions, an anesthesiologist may be scrubbed at the operative field to assume this responsibility. In other institutions, one of the surgeons or neonatologists assumes this role. Adequate ventilation may be difficult to achieve for several reasons. Certain types of tumors, specifically cervical teratomas, may secrete thick mucus into the trachea, and this must be aggressively removed before ventilation. As soon as the airway is satisfactorily cleared, surfactant should be administered (calfactant, 3 mL/kg) via the endotracheal tube to diminish expected airway resistance. Surfactant is provided for two principal reasons. First, the majority of infants treated for such lesions are delivered at some point before term and their pulmonary development (considered both by gestational age and underlying pathophysiology) cannot be assumed to be normal. Second, the thick mucoid secretions and the aggressive lavage necessary to clear them may interrupt the normal surfactant layering and functionality, suggesting that surfactant therapy may provide a benefit if administered before lung ventilation. These steps should result in increases in fetal oxygen saturation to levels greater than 90%. If this does not occur, the position of the endotracheal tube should be rechecked and the lungs should be auscultated with the aid of a sterile stethoscope. In addition, ultrasound examination for the presence of air bronchograms may be used to confirm tracheal intubation. Ventilation occurs most commonly with the aid of a sterile Jackson-Rees circuit. When adequate ventilation has been established, the fetus can be delivered.

Delivery of the Infant and Maternal Management

Before umbilical cord clamping and delivery, coordination between the surgery and anesthesia teams is crucial to prevent uterine atony and excessive maternal hemorrhage. Because a decrease in the tocolytic agent, whether an inhaled or an intravenous agent, would result in increased uterine vascular resistance and decreased fetal oxygenation, reversal of the tocolysis must not occur before the umbilical cord is clamped. However, at clamping, a near-total reversal of tocolysis is required to limit uterine bleeding. This is best achieved with low-solubility halogenated inhaled anesthetics (e.g., desflurane). As the cord is clamped, the anesthetic agent is immediately discontinued and oxytocin is administered as a bolus followed by a continuous infusion and titrated to uterine response (e.g., 40 units oxytocin in 500 mL NS over 30 minutes, followed by 20 units over 8 hours). Additional uterotonic medications may be necessary and must be immediately available should uncontrolled maternal hemorrhage occur. These medications include methylergonovine, carboprost,

Trauma

Joseph Tepas and Hernando DeSoto

MODERN MEDICAL CARE OF infants and children has become increasingly sophisticated and effective. The common diseases of childhood are better understood and more effectively treated, producing more cures with higher quality of life. Little of this progress, however, has significantly affected what we now define as "the disease of injury." Injuries remain the leading cause of death and disability in the pediatric population of the United States.[1] Injury has also emerged as the most common public health threat to children of the world. This is especially so in areas of civil strife, where the real victims of armed conflict are the orphans of the combatants and the unwitting victims of ordnance left behind. In this modern era of medicine it is unimaginable that our approach to the largest pediatric public health problem in the world, that is, traumatic pediatric injuries, is neither standardized nor driven by protocol.[2,3]

This chapter is a review of modern principles of management of the acute phase of the "disease of injury"; it is intended to augment the standard principles of advanced trauma life support as promulgated by the American College of Surgeons Committee on Trauma, as well as the concepts of advanced pediatric life support defined by the American Academy of Pediatrics and the American College of Emergency Physicians.[4,5] Both the *Advanced Trauma Life Support* and the *Advanced Pediatric Life Support* courses are readily available and serve as excellent references for the basic protocols, policies, and procedures for triage, initial assessment, acute resuscitation, and definitive initial management.

Anesthesiologists are essential participants in the care of injured children. Obviously, emergent, urgent, and elective operative interventions demand full involvement of the anesthesia care team; in many institutions, the anesthesia service also provides critical care management. Thus, from the perspectives of airway control, ventilation, hemodynamic resuscitation, metabolic management, and effective control of pain, anesthesiologists play a critical central role in determining the injured child's survival and quality of life (Fig. 39-1). In Canada and some European countries initial resuscitation of injured patients is performed by specially qualified physicians, particularly anesthesiologists, both at the scene and during initial transport. These physicians are charged with assessing the patient, securing the airway, initiating treatment to assure hemodynamic stability, and coordinating with a base hospital the details of management and transport of the patient to an appropriate trauma center, so-called *stay and play*. Many aspects of this type of system design are now being integrated into existing American trauma systems as part of mass casualty disaster management plans.[6,7] Other countries (e.g., the United States) have a different system more in keeping with the military approach whereby emergency medical technicians are the initial team to make rapid assessments, to make initial efforts at stabilization via radio contact with the emergency medical facility, and to return the patient to a hospital environment as rapidly as possible, so-called *scoop and run*.

Epidemiology

The epidemiology of the "disease of injury" reflects its continued growth as a health risk for the children of the world. Table 39-1 illustrates the recent population incidence of pediatric injury types per 100,000 U.S. population.[1] These trends are similar for previous years and are a distressing reflection of American societal failures in accident prevention. Vehicular trauma is the major threat to children in the United States, and research has begun to identify methods to improve protection of children

Table 39-3. The Pediatric Trauma Score (PTS)

	Score			Total*
	+2	+1	−1	
Size	>20 kg	10-20 kg	<10 kg	
Airway	Normal	Maintainable	Not maintainable	
Systolic Blood Pressure	>90 mm Hg	90-50 mm Hg	<50 mm Hg	
Central Nervous System	Awake	Obtunded/loss of consciousness	Comatose	
Open Wound	None	Minor	Major/penetrating	
Skeletal Trauma	None	Closed fracture	Open/multiple fractures	

*Score is sum of all rows. Maximum score of 12 indicates minor injury; severe injury is defined as <7; a minimum score (−6) is uniformly fatal.

attempts at intubation must not contribute to injury and be pursued only as necessary. Portable end-tidal carbon dioxide monitors and carbon dioxide detectors have reduced the incidence of unrecognized esophageal intubation (Fig. 39-2). For children who are injured in remote settings and for whom prolonged transport is likely, elective intubation may be needed to ensure effective airway control.

In many trauma systems the anesthesiologist is routinely summoned to provide emergency department airway support. Children who have received pre-hospital care commonly present with significant aerophagia and may well be developing edema of the airway structures as a result of manipulation during initial care at the scene of the accident. Those responsible for acute airway management in the trauma center must know what occurred in the field. Specific data regarding the reasons for

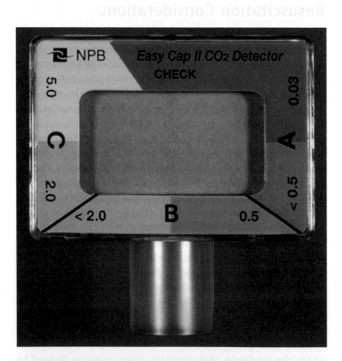

Figure 39-2. The confirmation of appropriate endotracheal intubation is best accomplished by a measurement of exhaled CO_2. When a capnograph is unavailable, portable products such as the Easy Cap II (Mallinckrodt, Inc., Pleasanton, CA 94588), which has a dead space of 25 mL and is generally indicated for patients weighing less than 15 kg, or the PediCap, which has a dead space of 3 mL and is for children who weigh 1 to 15 kg, may be used.

intubation, number of attempts, and possibility of aspiration will directly affect success and efficiency of airway care during resuscitation and initial management when the child arrives in the hospital setting. Regardless of site or mode of endotracheal intubation, proper position, airway patency, and correct endotracheal tube size must be confirmed as soon as the child arrives in the trauma center or emergency department.[30] Table 39-2 lists the appropriate size by specific age category for critical resuscitation equipment that must be immediately available in any pediatric resuscitation facility. In our trauma center emergency department, this equipment is stored in an open-shelf color-coded system that presents the age-appropriate size of each item on sequential shelves, beginning with the smallest on top (Fig. 39-3).

The most effective approach to initial airway management, especially if the child is being appropriately oxygenated by bag-valve-mask ventilation, is to follow a protocol for rapid-sequence intubation because such children invariably have a full stomach.[31-34] "Awake intubation" is generally reserved for infants with severe airway obstruction (blood, vomitus, foreign body, or edema) or infants and children with sufficiently depressed consciousness that no medications are needed. Protocols for acute airway management should include (1) administration of analgesic and sedative medications (e.g., fentanyl and midazolam); (2) administration of a vagolytic (so as to avoid succinylcholine- or reflex-induced bradycardia); (3) lidocaine (1-2 mg/kg) to reduce hemodynamic responses to intubation and either propofol (2-3 mg/kg), thiopental (4-6 mg/kg), ketamine (2-3 mg/kg), or etomidate (0.2-0.3 mg/kg); and (4) succinylcholine (2 mg/kg) or high-dose rocuronium (1.2 mg/kg), if there is a contraindication to the use of succinylcholine. The selection of drugs will depend on the individual patient circumstances (e.g., head injury, hypovolemia, contraindication to succinylcholine) and condition on arrival in the emergency department. Table 39-4 lists the possible choices of agents and dosing, with advantages and disadvantages. In situations in which there is hemodynamic instability and the possibility of a head injury, etomidate is our preferred induction agent.[35] Figure 39-4 presents an algorithm for management of children with traumatic brain injury, and Figure 39-5 presents an algorithm for management of children with multiple trauma but without a brain injury. In a child with a normal airway, the goals of any drug regimen in the emergency setting are to produce amnesia, analgesia, and unconsciousness and to facilitate intubation with the use of neuromuscular blockade. The process of airway management should not exacerbate hemodynamic responses,

ing cl
acces
occur
in the
ponac
fluid
this p
ing vc
Ideall
and li
space.

Int
both i
access
pediat
placer
media
These
femor:
failed
istratic
they a
crystal
ucts.[57]
or trau
effecti
matic-
been c
difficul
manuf:
A new
like a b

Stra…
the S…

The adv
acles i
an incr
comorb
natal pr
for acu
attentio
disorde
psychos
ment. F
"gradua
margina
of sever
conside
care.

Bette
and, in
ongoing
redefine
acute r
trauma
nally wa
ing volu
to tissue

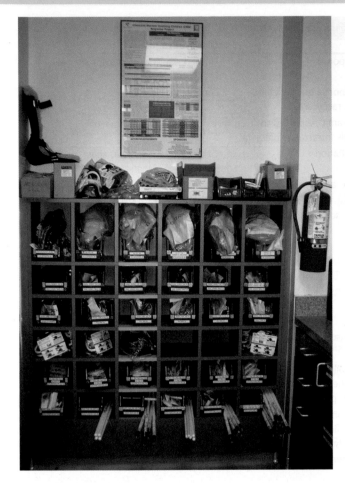

Figure 39-3. This shelving system, devised by Robert Luten, MD, in 1984, remains the most effective and efficient way to store age- and weight-based resuscitation equipment and to ensure that all compartments are always stocked.

especially in children with head injury and possible increased intracranial pressure. Regardless of the venue of endotracheal intubation, it is essential that a device to measure the presence of expired carbon dioxide be used to confirm proper placement within the trachea (see Fig. 39-2). This may take the form of simple devices that change color (e.g., Easy Cap II [Mallinckrodt, Inc., Pleasanton, CA]), or with a hand-held portable device that measures expired carbon dioxide and pulse oximetry (e.g., Oridion, Inc., Needham, MA).

Injury to the cervical spine is less common in children than in adult trauma patients because the child's spine is more elastic and mobile; the incompletely calcified vertebrae in the child's spine are less likely to fracture with minor trauma. Nevertheless, the risk of spine injury in the pediatric patient is increased whenever the child is subjected to inertial force from falls or the chaotic rotary forces associated with motor vehicle crashes.[10,36] Any child with a suspected neck injury should have cervical spine precautions implemented (i.e., collar device immobilization). In-line stabilization should always be maintained when airway manipulation is attempted (Figs. 39-6 and 39-7). It is difficult to rule out spinal cord injury in children by standard radiography alone because up to 50% of spinal cord injuries may exist without radiographic findings (SCIWORA, spinal cord

injury without radiologic abnormality).[37,38] Often the radiograph does not include a view below C6, the odontoid process is not seen, and/or pseudosubluxation of C2-C3 or C3-C4 may occur and be missed. As computed tomography (CT) technology has advanced to more rapid and precise imaging, many centers have replaced standard radiographic examinations with routine CT for evaluation of the cervical spine for injury. When we compared the diagnostic yield of plain film screening to CT in our unit, we doubled the rate of fractures identified![39] In light of the complex nature of interpretation of the child's cervical spine and the frequent incidence of potential spinal cord injury, without immediate radiologic evidence of fracture or subluxation, the safest course is to assume there may be a potential cervical spine injury in any symptomatic or unevaluable child.

In the operating room, the induction of anesthesia is individualized depending on the child's injuries, condition at the time of presentation, whether the airway has already been secured, and anticipated airway difficulty. For trauma patients for whom we anticipate an operative procedure of at least 1 hour, we normally use high-dose rocuronium (1.2 mg/kg) instead of succinylcholine when hyperkalemia is a risk.

Alternate approaches should be considered in children in whom a difficult intubation is anticipated.[40,41] In a nonemergent situation, the fiberoptic bronchoscope (FOB) is very helpful, especially in children with limited mouth opening, limited neck movement (common in the trauma victim with a head collar), or associated congenital syndrome that makes direct laryngoscopy difficult or impossible.[42,43] In emergency situations, blind placement of a supraglottic device such as a laryngeal mask airway (LMA) is most commonly used. The LMA does not protect the airway from aspiration but it may be used as a conduit to facilitate either a blind or fiberoptic intubation of the trachea.[44] The development of an LMA with a modified cuff and drainage tube designed specifically for emergency airway management may make this process even safer because evacuation of the stomach is possible.[45,46] The development of the "Fast-Track" LMA provides an additional supraglottic device that is useful when direct visualization of the laryngeal inlet is not possible. However, this is only of benefit in larger children because a pediatric version is not yet available. Another useful device in the pediatric trauma victim is the lightwand[47] or light-assisted device. This is a rigid stylet with a light at its tip; the lightwand (Anesthesia Medical Specialties, Beaumont, CA) utilizes the technique of transtracheal illumination for blind intubation of the trachea in older children. Advantages in the trauma patient include its ease of learning and its usefulness of not having to align the airway planes in a child with a potential cervical spine injury. Also, blood and secretions are not an impediment to success as with use of the FOB (see Chapter 12 for more detailed discussion).

Ventilation

One of the most common areas of miscommunication between the team providing initial assessment and that which continues definitive management concerns ventilatory care. The successful acquisition of a reliable airway frequently leads to overaggressive ventilation that rapidly induces pathologic hypocapnia. Conversely, use of an inadequately sized endotracheal tube, the presence of blood and secretions, coexisting pulmonary injury, or pneumothorax may alter the mechanics of ventilation so that "routine" initial ventilator settings are inadequate, thus ventilat-

that hyperventilation, even during "rescue" from acute intracranial hypertension, preferentially decreases blood flow to the penumbra of injured neurons surrounding the area of acute brain injury, thereby actually worsening flow to the area most in need of perfusion.[100,101]

Besides control of airway, ventilation, and adequacy of oxygenation, management of brain injury must also address excessive elaboration of excitatory neurotransmitters that are a common characteristic of neuronal damage. One multi-institutional study has demonstrated that seizure prophylaxis in the pediatric trauma patient was associated with decreased mortality.[102] Whether this is a cause-and-effect relationship or a confounding variable has not been defined. Although this observation has not been validated in follow-up multi-institutional studies, routine administration of anti-seizure medications such as phenytoin or phenobarbital seems reasonable.[103] The basic pathophysiology underscores the fact that optimizing neuronal recovery demands minimizing ongoing sources of "secondary injury." The practical application of this process for most modern trauma systems and trauma centers is the immediate administration of opioids and benzodiazepines titrated to an appropriate level of analgesia and sedation that supports convalescence without causing overactivation of the excitatory neurotransmitters.[15] This "calming" of the brain can induce deep sedation and potential for hypoventilation; however, because these children are routinely intubated and mechanically ventilated, this latter problem is usually not a concern.

Intraoperatively, opioids (e.g., fentanyl, sufentanil, or remifentanil) are frequently administered as intermittent bolus doses or continuous infusions to supplement volatile anesthetics. Postoperatively, such infusions may be continued along with other measures to reduce intracerebral pressure. Because the use of these drugs may have important hemodynamic implications in the management of the child with head trauma, judicious use of opioid infusions must be accompanied by careful monitoring of hemodynamic parameters because avoidance of further brain injury is dependent on maintaining an adequate cerebral perfusion pressure in the presence of increased intracranial pressure. Use of propofol, combined with mannitol and hyperventilation, in adult patients with closed-head injury has been reported to provide significant reduction of intracranial pressure without affecting mean arterial pressure.[104] Despite sporadic reports of successful use of propofol in management of intracranial hypertension associated with pediatric traumatic brain injury, a number of reports suggest that administration of propofol by continuous infusion is associated with a syndrome of lethal metabolic acidosis.[105-109] Because these risks do not outweigh benefits of alternative therapies, continuous infusion of propofol for either sedation or management of refractory intracranial hypertension in severe pediatric traumatic brain injury is not recommended.[110]

When intracranial hypertension and cerebral perfusion pressure do not respond to mannitol, diuretic therapy, sedation, analgesia, and administration of pentobarbital, we supplement this with bolus administration of hypertonic saline. Our preferred concentration is 23.4%, infused through a central venous catheter in a dose of 0.75 times the child's weight in kilograms administered over 30 minutes. Hypertonic saline has been demonstrated to be more efficacious than mannitol and it exerts an anti-inflammatory effect.[111] It can be used whenever serum sodium concentration is less than 150 mEq/L and serum

osmolality is less than 300 mOsm/L. When this therapy fails, and maximum "pentobarbital coma" has been achieved, rescue craniectomy is considered. Our results, and those of others, have been encouraging and suggest that success is related to early and aggressive intervention.[112]

One source of continued potential morbidity in multidisciplinary management of the brain-injured child is inadequate communication of clinical data among specialists involved in the child's care. For the past 15 years we have used a standardized daily assessment system based on the concept that the injured child is a "hot potato" (*a spud is a slang term for a potato*). The "potato note" is based on the mnemonic "PASS A SPUD." The PASS reflects the core of neurologic critical care management and specifically addresses the need for *P*aralytics, *A*nalgesics, *S*edation, and *S*eizure prophylaxis as discussed earlier. The "A" represents *A*ntibiotics and sits as a separate issue to focus attention on the fact that overuse of antibiotics is an invitation to nosocomial sepsis. The second tier of management, "SPUD," reflects the need for *S*teroids if so indicated for spinal cord injury or as an associated adjunct for therapy of certain pulmonary disorders. The "P" represents both *P*entobarbital and *P*ressors (vasopressors) to emphasize that use of pentobarbital therapy should stimulate consideration of the other to offset the hypotension caused by pentobarbital therapy and thus maintain an adequate cerebral perfusion pressure. "U" stands for *U*lcer prophylaxis, which, in our unit, is treated with sucralfate rather than histamine blockers or proton pump inhibitors. We prefer to supplement the efficacy of the mucus barrier with a physical protectant rather than alter gastric pH and parietal cell function with histamine antagonists or proton pump inhibitors. The balance between bleeding risk (stress ulcer) and nosocomial infection is not well defined for the pediatric trauma patient. Because the former is more common and the latter is relatively rare, the potential benefits of sucralfate on mucosal perfusion and its cytoprotective properties render it a better choice for use in injured children who require mechanical ventilation.[113-115] Finally, the "D" reflects use of *D*iuretics, which are frequently administered in the acute phase of resuscitation for suspected intracranial hypertension and which require careful monitoring of serum osmolality and electrolyte balance. Daily notes follow this system, thereby enabling all members of the care team to track the status of each of these components and review any plans for change. Table 39-7 lists the drug doses and infusion rates for these components and our current management regimen.

The basic premise of traumatic brain injury critical care is tiered management intended to optimize neuronal recovery and minimize secondary injury, especially from uncontrolled cerebral edema. We consider the clinical management just described as first-tier therapy.

Electrolyte Management

Regardless of whether lactated Ringer's or normal saline is used for initial fluid resuscitation, maintaining serum electrolytes within limits of normal is critical for rapid restoration of homeostasis. Severely injured infants and children are frequently not significantly hypovolemic as a result of their trauma. When these children are administered "resuscitative" fluids, they may quickly become volume overloaded and begin a diuresis that is frequently also a natriuresis.[70-72] Because the stress of injury produces a catecholamine-driven elaboration of aldosterone

Table 39-7. Current Traumatic Brain Injury Protocol at University of Florida Health Science Center, Jacksonville

Paralytics	Vecuronium 0.1 mg/kg/hour
Analgesic	Morphine 0.05-0.1 mg/kg/hour
Sedation	Midazolam 0.05-0.1 mg/kg/hour
Seizure Treatment/ Prevention	Phenytoin (15-20 mg/kg loading dose given slowly followed by 5-6 mg/kg/day in four divided doses)
	Phenobarbital (loading dose 20 mg/kg given slowly followed by 10-20 mg/kg/day in four divided doses)
	Blood concentrations of both are measured after 24 hours to assess therapeutic blood values.
Antibiotics	Careful selection as indicated
Corticosteroids	Spinal cord injury protocol (corticosteroids may be indicated as adjunct treatment of spinal cord injury)
Pressors/Pentobarbital	Dopamine 3-20 µg/kg/min
	Pentobarbital 0.5-5.0 mg/kg/hour (must maintain mean cerebral perfusion pressure >50 and ideally <80 mm Hg)
Ulcer Prophylaxis	Sucralfate (not an H_2 blocker such as ranitidine)
Diuretics	Mannitol 0.25-1.0 g/kg

and antidiuretic hormone, there is an obligatory retention of free water, which will result in a transient hyponatremia. Use of normal saline will blunt this phenomenon and limit free water available to shift into the extravascular space. Because young children have an increased ratio of body surface area to body volume, unaccounted evaporative free water loss can lead to hypernatremia, especially if the child is febrile. If the brain injury includes dysfunction of the posterior pituitary, diabetes insipidus may rapidly drive serum sodium levels in excess of 160 mEq/L. It is essential, therefore, that serum sodium and chloride concentrations be closely monitored along with urine specific gravity and output. Our management targets are serum sodium concentrations between 138 and 148 mEq/L and serum chloride levels between 95 and 105 mEq/L. Under most circumstances excess sodium is excreted in the urine. To maintain these guideline concentrations, we frequently use a combination of sodium chloride and sodium acetate to deliver a maintenance sodium concentration of 140 mEq/L and a chloride concentration of 70 mEq/L. When the child's central nervous system status has stabilized, we gradually introduce enteric nutrition and drop exogenous sodium chloride supplement to standard maintenance. Because urgent surgical intervention may be required during the early phases of acute central nervous system injury, intraoperative management of fluid compartments must be based on ongoing assessment of these changing factors. This translates to ensuring that central circulation is adequate as indicated by monitoring of filling pressures. It is also based on adequacy of oxygen transport and extraction as determined by an $S\bar{v}o_2$ between 65% and 75%.[116] Effective blood component therapy must consider rheology, coagulation status, and balance between oncotic and hydrostatic pressures.

Glycemia Control

The stress response associated with multisystem trauma stimulates hyperglycemia, which represents a combination of immediate mobilization of glycogen stores and catecholamine-induced proteolysis in peripheral skeletal muscle. The resultant hyperglycemia is commonly associated with "insulin resistance," which results from a combination of factors that undermine functionality of insulin receptors, thereby diminishing glucose uptake and enhancing even further the "stress response" stimulation of proteolysis. Studies in adult patients who have sustained uncontrolled hyperglycemia demonstrate a statistically significant increase in mortality and in infectious morbidity.[117] A somewhat similar investigation by Cochran and colleagues demonstrated a statistically significant relationship between initial hyperglycemia and adverse outcome.[118] While these investigators were primarily focused on the predictive value of a single, initial glucose assay, their data strongly reinforce the concept that effective control of blood glucose values will enhance the potential for improved outcomes.[119] Thus, it is critical that glucose homeostasis be maintained as aggressively and precisely as possible. The "optimal range" is between 80 and 120 mg/dL. Use of insulin is critical to maintain glucose values within the desired range and so that exogenous insulin may also exert a trophic effect on cellular function; such tight glucose control demands constant and ongoing monitoring.[120-122] From a practical perspective, this translates to frequent and careful glucose monitoring in the operating room and intensive care unit.

Nutritional Management

Over the past 2 decades the role of the gastrointestinal system as a major source of sepsis and secondary organ system dysfunction has become better understood and has emerged as a major consideration in understanding initial management and prophylaxis of necrotizing enterocolitis in the high-risk neonate.[123-125] From the perspective of the acutely injured child, there are two major components of clinical management. First is avoidance of hypoperfusion, which may undermine integrity of the mucosal barrier, thereby stimulating the enterocyte and underlying submucosal macrophages to inordinate proliferation of proinflammatory cytokines.[126-128] Because this process may also involve activation of specific receptors that decrease caspase-driven apoptosis, these activated polymorphonuclear neutrophils and macrophages continue to elaborate proinflammatory cytokines and various activated free radicals that stimulate the systemic inflammatory response. The second component is the early use of the gut for nutritional support, possibly with special formulations intended to accelerate neuronal recovery.[129,130] Both of these goals are best accomplished by initiation of enteric feeding as soon as physiologically and clinically appropriate. Even in

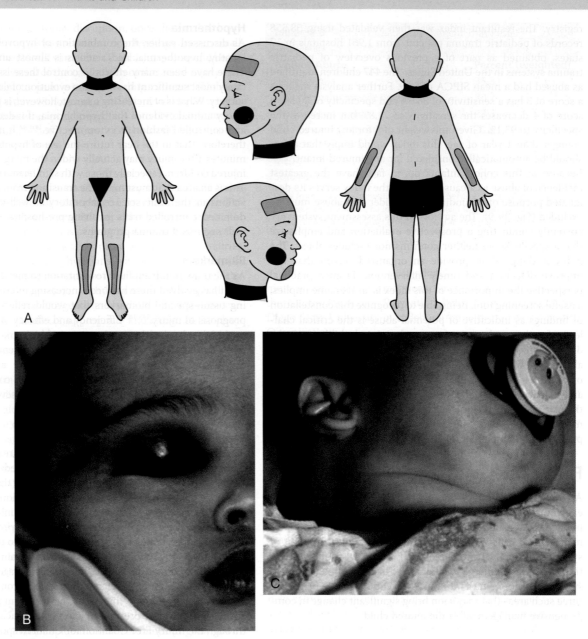

Figure 39-10. This series of pictures is intended to illustrate common examples of child abuse. In the operating room we have a perfect opportunity to examine children from head to toe as we prepare them for their surgical procedure. It is during this time that we can become powerful child protection advocates. **A,** Typical areas where children might present with bruises due to daily living activities. The blue areas indicate normal areas where one would expect to see bruising. The black areas are unusual areas of bruises. Any bruise in the black areas must be suspect for possible child abuse. Cutaneous manifestations of child abuse are varied. **B,** A child with obvious facial trauma.

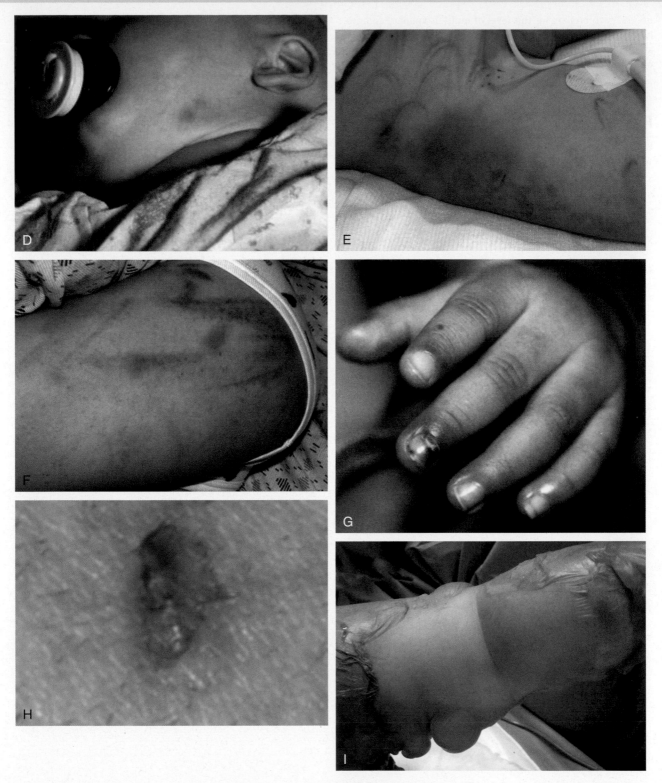

Figure 39-10, cont'd C and **D,** An infant with bilateral facial bruises on either side of the neck. **E,** A whipping injury from an electrical cord. **F,** A whipping injury from a belt plus additional bruises. **G,** Unusual finger injuries in an infant. **H,** A cigarette burn. **I,** An immersion burn; note sparing of the popliteal fossa typical of such a child abuse injury. (Photographs courtesy of a number of child advocates from several institutions who asked to remain anonymous.)

necessary to prepare for this level of multidisciplinary comprehensive care is well worth the return in diminished mortality and, more importantly, in a quality of life for survivors that any of us would wish for our children.

Acknowledgment

We wish to thank Alexsandra J. Mazurek, MD, and Steven C. Hall, MD, for their prior contributions to this chapter.

References

Please see www.expertconsult.com

Cardiopulmonary Resuscitation

Marilyn C. Morris, I. David Todres, and Charles L. Schleien

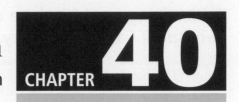

THE PEDIATRIC ANESTHESIOLOGIST MUST be prepared to resuscitate a child who suffers a cardiac arrest in the course of a routine elective anesthetic, during a high-risk surgery, or outside the operating room, where anesthesiologists often function as a vital part of the "code team." The goal of this chapter is to provide pediatric anesthesiologists with an in-depth understanding of cardiopulmonary-cerebral resuscitation physiology and recommended resuscitative techniques.

Historical Background

Neonates were successfully resuscitated with mouth-to-mouth resuscitation in the early part of the 19th century, but this technique was abandoned because of the fear of contracting a contagious disease. In 1814, a description in poetical form of the Rules of the Humane Society for recovering drowned persons included the following description of mouth-to-mouth resuscitation[1]:

*Let one the mouth, and either nostril close
While through the other the bellows gently blows.
Thus the pure air with steady force convey,
To put the flaccid lungs again in play.
Should bellows not be found, or found too late,
Let some kind soul with willing mouth inflate;*

*Then downward, though but lightly, press the chest.
And let the inflated air be upward prest.*

External cardiac massage was successfully conducted more than 100 years ago in two children (ages 8 and 13 years) after circulatory arrest precipitated by chloroform anesthesia.[2] In 1904, Crile described the effectiveness of external cardiac compressions in maintaining the circulation of dogs.[3]

After reports by Elam and coworkers,[4] Gordon and colleagues,[5] and Safar[6] demonstrating the effectiveness of mouth-to-mouth resuscitation, in 1958 the National Academy of Sciences National Research Council recommended mouth-to-mouth resuscitation with maximum backward tilt of the head as the preferred technique for all individuals requiring emergency artificial ventilation. External cardiac compression as a resuscitation technique was revived in 1960, when Kouwenhoven and coworkers[7] demonstrated the effectiveness of external cardiac compressions combined with artificial respirations. Before this study, internal cardiac compression was the accepted technique, with its effectiveness demonstrated by experience in cardiac bypass surgery. In 1947, Beck and associates[8] successfully internally defibrillated the human heart; and in 1956, Zoll and colleagues[9] performed the first successful external defibrillation of a human heart.

Epidemiology and Outcome of In-hospital Cardiopulmonary Arrest

A 2006 review of cardiac arrest events submitted to the National Registry of Cardiopulmonary Circulation included 880 pediatric events, excluding events in a delivery room or neonatal intensive care unit (ICU). The majority of children who suffered a cardiac arrest (46%) were admitted for medical management of a noncardiac condition. Fifty-eight percent had preexisting respiratory insufficiency, 36% had preexisting hypotension and hypoperfusion, 31% had preexisting congestive heart failure, and 29% had preexisting pneumonia, septicemia, or other infections. The median age was 5.6 years.[10] Sixty-five percent of the inpatient cardiac arrests reported took place in an ICU, 13% in an emergency department, 14% in a general inpatient area, and 3% in an operating room or postanesthesia care unit. Twenty-seven percent of the children survived to hospital discharge, 58% of these with a good neurologic outcome. The mean duration of cardiopulmonary resuscitation (CPR) for the children who survived to hospital discharge was 27.3 minutes (median, 15 minutes).[10] Other large series of in-hospital pediatric cardiac arrest report survival ranging from 14% to 44%,[11-13] with the 44% survival representing cardiac arrests that took place in a pediatric cardiac ICU.

Diagnosis of Cardiac Arrest

For the child who suffers a cardiac arrest in the operating room, electronic monitoring will generally alert the anesthesiologist of an actual or impending cardiac arrest. The electrocardiogram (ECG) will indicate nonperfusing rhythms such as ventricular fibrillation and asystole, end-tidal carbon dioxide (ETco$_2$) will decrease precipitously when lack of cardiac output results in decreased delivery of CO$_2$ to the lungs, and a pulse oximeter will lose its regular waveform in the absence of pulsatile blood flow. Granting the importance of these monitors, the diagnosis of cardiopulmonary arrest still rests on the absence of a major pulse (carotid, femoral, brachial) by palpation in the presence of unconsciousness and apnea.

Attention must be paid in the early minutes of resuscitation to determine the cause of the arrest. Many children will not be successfully resuscitated without correction of the underlying problem. A focused physical examination should be conducted and a brief history elicited if it is not already known. If not present, a cardiorespiratory monitor should be placed and the ECG examined. In an intraoperative arrest, the surgeon may be able to provide clues to diagnosis, whether based on blood loss, compression of vessels, decreasing venous return to the heart, or manipulation of anatomic structures (e.g., manipulation of the vagus nerve resulting in severe bradycardia or asystole). Equipment malfunction must always be considered as a potential cause of arrest. Early in the course of an attempted resuscitation, a blood gas analysis should be performed and key electrolytes measured (ideally as point-of-care testing).

Mechanics of CPR

Management proceeds along the well-known ABC algorithm (Airway, Breathing, Circulation) with the exception that the child with ventricular fibrillation or pulseless ventricular tachycardia should receive electrical defibrillation without delay. Airway access in children with ventricular fibrillation or pulseless ventricular tachycardia should be done secondarily. CPR should be conducted up until the earliest moment when the shock can be delivered.

Airway

The child's airway generally can be managed effectively before tracheal intubation with bag-valve-mask (BVM) ventilation with proper head positioning and jaw thrust. While tracheal intubation ensures optimal control of the airway for effective ventilation, multiple attempts at intubation by the inexperienced operator may seriously compromise the child's ability to recover. In the child without an artificial airway, the use of BVM devices may result in a significant risk of gastric inflation, followed by pulmonary aspiration of gastric contents. Abdominal distention (gastric and bowel) can significantly compromise oxygenation; therefore, the stomach should be vented when excessive gastric inflation occurs. In one study, there was a 28% incidence of pulmonary aspiration in a series of failed resuscitations.[14] For this reason, excessive inflation pressures should be avoided. However, effective bilateral ventilation is best judged by visualizing bilateral chest excursions and listening to the quality of breath sounds rather than setting a preset maximal inflation pressure.

Endotracheal intubation should be attempted as soon as appropriate personnel and equipment are available. The ETco$_2$ is a valuable method of confirming the correct intratracheal position of the endotracheal tube. A disposable colorimetric ETco$_2$ is useful in verifying endotracheal tube placement in children when in-line capnography is not available. However, it is important to appreciate that ETco$_2$ measurements are only meaningful when there is effective pulmonary circulation, such that a lack of color change may reflect either improper tube positioning or lack of effective chest compressions.

Breathing

In the inpatient environment, equipment necessary to ventilate a child emergently should be readily available. Because the equipment provided for emergency ventilatory support may differ depending on the location within a hospital, an anesthesiologist needs to be familiar with all of the types of equipment used in the hospital in which he or she practices. Anesthesiologists are skilled providers of ventilatory support, but in the context of a cardiac arrest one must return to the basics and remember that *if there is no chest movement, there is no ventilation*. If no chest movement occurs during BVM ventilation despite an apparently good seal between the mask and the child's face, upper airway obstruction, whether anatomic or due to a foreign body, as well as bilateral tension pneumothorax must be considered.

Overventilation is common during CPR, resulting in greater mean intrathoracic pressure which decreases venous return and reduces cardiac output.[15] In cardiopulmonary arrest, a less than normal minute ventilation may be appropriate, because cardiac output and delivery of CO$_2$ to the lungs are low. If there is no artificial airway in place, two breaths should be given after each 15 chest compressions. Once an artificial airway is in place, ventilations should be given at a rate of 8 to 10 per minute *without* pausing during chest compressions (Table 40-1).

Table 40-1. Ventilation and Chest Compressions During Pediatric CPR (All Ages)

	Respirations	Chest Compressions	Notes
Bag-mask ventilation	2 respirations after each 15 chest compressions (if one rescuer only, 2 respirations after each 30 compressions)	100 per minute	Aspirate (vent) the stomach if gastric inflation interferes with ventilation.
Endotracheal intubation	8 to 10 per minute	100 per minute	Do not pause compressions during ventilation.

Circulation

During cardiac arrest, chest compressions provide the sole perfusion to a child's vital organs; therefore, great attention should be paid to performing this task optimally. Key elements to providing quality chest compressions include (1) ensuring adequate rate (100 compressions per minute), (2) ensuring adequate chest wall depression (one third to one half of the anteroposterior chest diameter), (3) releasing completely between compressions to allow full chest wall recoil, (4) minimizing interruptions in chest compressions, and (5) ensuring that the child is on a sufficiently hard surface to allow effective chest compressions.[16] In short, "push hard and push fast," release completely, and don't interrupt compressions unnecessarily.

If a child is small enough (usually 6 months of age or younger) that the person providing chest compressions can comfortably encircle the chest with his or her hands, then chest compressions should be performed using the circumferential technique, with thumbs depressing the sternum and the fingers supporting the infant's back and circumferentially squeezing the thorax (Fig. 40-1). In larger infants, the sternum can be compressed using two fingers; and in the child, either one or two hands can

be used, depending on the size of the child and of the rescuer.[16] Whichever method is used, focused attention must remain on delivering effective compressions with *minimal interruptions*. In all cases other than circumferential CPR, a backboard must be used. Properly delivered chest compressions are tiring to the provider, and providers should rotate as frequently as necessary such that compressions are not compromised by muscle fatigue on the part of the provider.

Mechanisms of Blood Flow

External chest compressions provide cardiac output through two mechanisms: the cardiac pump mechanism and the thoracic pump mechanism. By the cardiac pump mechanism of blood flow, blood is squeezed from the heart by compression of the heart between the sternum and the vertebral column, exiting the heart only anterograde because of closure of the atrioventricular valves. Between compressions, ventricular pressure decreases below atrial pressure, allowing the atrioventricular valves to open and the ventricles to fill. This sequence of events resembles the normal cardiac cycle. While the cardiac pump is likely not the dominant blood flow mechanism during most closed-chest CPR, specific clinical situations have been identified in which the cardiac pump mechanism is more prominent. For example, a smaller, more compliant chest may allow for more direct cardiac compression (Fig. 40-2). Increasing the

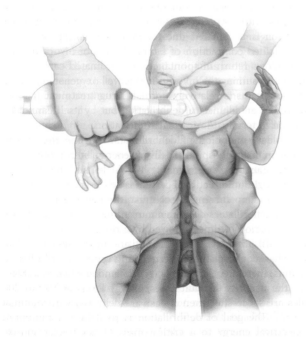

Figure 40-1. Chest-encircling method for cardiac compressions in a neonate: thumbs are placed one finger's breadth below the nipple line. (Modified from Todres ID, Rogers MC: Methods of external cardiac massage in the newborn infant. J Pediatr 1975; 86:781-782.)

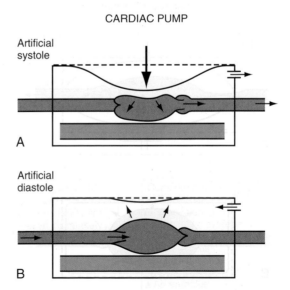

Figure 40-2. A, The cardiac pump mechanism by which the heart is directly squeezed between the sternum and vertebral column, representing artificial systole. **B,** Artificial diastole occurs with relaxation of the compressions. (From Babbs CF: New versus old theories of blood flow during CPR. Crit Care Med 1980; 8:191-195, © by Williams & Wilkins.)

resumed. Approximately 2 minutes of CPR should be delivered before a second attempt at defibrillation (4 joules/kg).[16]

If ventricular fibrillation/pulseless ventricular tachycardia persists beyond the second attempt at defibrillation, standard dose epinephrine should be administered (with subsequent doses every 3 to 5 minutes during persistent cardiac arrest). After 2 minutes of chest compressions, defibrillation should be attempted again, followed by administration of amiodarone or lidocaine with subsequent defibrillation attempts. It is not necessary to increase the energy dose on each successive shock during defibrillation. However, successful defibrillation without known adverse effects at greater current in excess of 4 joules/kg has been reported.[16]

Open-Chest Defibrillation

If the chest is already open, ventricular fibrillation should be treated with open-chest defibrillation, using internal paddles applied directly to the heart. These should have a diameter of 6 cm for adults, 4 cm for children, and 2 cm for infants. Handles should be insulated. Saline-soaked pads or gauzes should be placed between the paddles and the heart. One electrode is placed behind the left ventricle and the other over the right ventricle on the anterior surface of the heart. The dosage used should begin at 5 joules in infants and 20 joules in adults.

Automated External Defibrillation

Use of automated external defibrillators (AEDs) is now standard therapy in out-of-hospital resuscitation of adults.[29] AEDs are now deemed appropriate for use in children older than 1 year of age. If available, use of pediatric attenuator pads or a pediatric mode on the AED should be used in children 1 to 8 years of age, but if they are unavailable (and a standard defibrillator is similarly unavailable) an unmodified AED should be used.

Transcutaneous Cardiac Pacing

In the absence of in-situ pacing wires or an indwelling transvenous or esophageal pacing catheter, transcutaneous cardiac pacing (TCP) is the preferred method for temporary electrical cardiac pacing in children with asystole or severe bradycardia. TCP is indicated for children whose primary problem is impulse formation or conduction, with preserved myocardial function. It is most effective in those with sinus bradycardia or high-grade atrioventricular block with slow ventricular response but adequate stroke volume. TCP is not indicated for children in prolonged arrest, because in this situation it usually results in electrical but not mechanical cardiac capture and its use may delay or interfere with other resuscitative efforts.

To set up pacing, one electrode is placed anteriorly at the left sternal border and the other posteriorly just below the left scapula. Smaller electrodes are available for infants and children, but adult-sized electrodes can be used in children weighing more than 15 kg. ECG leads should be connected to the pacemaker, the demand or asynchronous mode selected, and an age-appropriate heart rate used. The stimulus output should be set at zero when the pacemaker is turned on and then increased gradually until electrical capture is seen on the monitor. After electrical capture is achieved, one must ascertain whether an effective arterial pulse is generated. If not, other resuscitative efforts should be employed.

The most serious complication of TCP is the induction of a ventricular arrhythmia. Fortunately, this is rare and may be prevented by pacing only in the demand mode. Mild transient erythema beneath the electrodes is common. Skeletal muscle contraction can be minimized by using large electrodes, a 40-msec pulse duration, and the smallest stimulus required for capture. If defibrillation or cardioversion is necessary, one must allow a distance of 2 to 3 cm between the electrode and paddles to prevent arcing of the current.

Vascular Access and Monitoring During CPR

Vascular Access and Fluid Administration

One of the key aspects of successful CPR is the early establishment of a route for the administration of fluids and medications. If an intravenous line cannot be established rapidly, the intraosseous or endotracheal route should be used (see Chapter 49).

Intravenous Access

Many children who suffer an in-hospital cardiac arrest will already have established vascular access. For children with impending cardiac arrest and no vascular access, a brief attempt should be made to start a peripheral intravenous line. If access is not achieved quickly, then an intraosseous needle should be placed. For young children in cardiac arrest without vascular access, an intraosseous needle should be placed immediately, to avoid any delay that could come with repeated attempts at establishing intravenous access.

Intraosseous Access

All medications and fluids used during CPR, including whole blood, can be given by the intraosseous route. An intraosseous needle may also be used to obtain initial blood samples, although acid-base analysis will be inaccurate after administration of sodium bicarbonate via the intraosseous needle. The use of intraosseous lines should be considered a temporary measure during emergencies when other vascular sites are not available. The placement of an intraosseous needle in the older child or adult, although possible, is difficult owing to the thick bony cortex; however, a 50% success rate has been reported in adults and children older than 10 years of age.[30]

The technique of placing an intraosseous line is straightforward. A specialized intraosseous needle or, if not available, a standard 16- or 18-gauge needle, a spinal needle with stylet, or bone marrow needle is inserted into the anterior surface of the tibia 1 to 2 cm below and 1 cm medial to the tibial tuberosity. The needle is directed at a 90-degree angle to the anteromedial surface of the tibia, just distal to the tuberosity (see Fig. 49-6). When the needle passes through the cortex into the marrow there is loss of resistance. The infusion is successful if the needle is in the marrow cavity, as evidenced by the needle standing upright without support. It loses the upright position if it has slipped into the subcutaneous tissue. Free flow of the drug or fluid infusion without significant subcutaneous infiltration should also be demonstrated. The technique has a low complication rate,[31] although possible complications include osteomyelitis, fat and bone marrow embolism, and compartment syndrome. For this reason, the intraosseous needle should be replaced by a definitive intravenous line as soon as practical.

Endotracheal Medication Administration

In the absence of other vascular access, medications including lidocaine, atropine, naloxone, and epinephrine can be given through the endotracheal tube. The use of ionized medications such as sodium bicarbonate or calcium chloride is not recommended by this route. The peak level of epinephrine or lidocaine administered via the endotracheal route may be lower compared with the intraosseous route. The peak drug concentration of epinephrine was only 10% as high after endotracheal administration compared with intravenous administration in anesthetized dogs. The recommended dose of endotracheal epinephrine is 10 times the intravenous or intraosseous dose: 0.1 mg/kg for bradycardia or pulseless arrest.

The volume and the diluent in which the medications are administered through an endotracheal tube may be important. When large volumes of fluid are used, pulmonary surfactant may be altered or destroyed, resulting in atelectasis. The total volume of fluid delivered into the trachea with each drug administered should not exceed 10 mL in the adult or 5 mL in the infant.[32] However, dilution of drug is important so as to achieve drug application to a wide area of mucosal surface beyond the tip of the endotracheal tube. Absorption into the systemic circulation may further be enhanced by deep intrapulmonary administration. This distal placement of drug can be performed by passing a catheter deep into the bronchial tree. The risk associated with the endotracheal route of drug administration is the formation of an intrapulmonary depot of drug, which may prolong the drugs' effect. This could theoretically result in post-resuscitation hypertension and tachycardia or the recurrence of fibrillation after normal circulation is restored.

Monitoring During CPR

A basic clinical examination is vital during cardiac arrest. The chest is carefully observed for adequacy of bilateral chest expansion with artificial ventilation and for equal and normal breath sounds. In addition, one should constantly reevaluate the depth of compression and the position of the rescuer's hands in performing chest compressions by palpation of a major artery. Palpation is essential in establishing pulselessness and in assessing the adequacy of blood flow during chest compressions. Palpating the peripheral pulses may be inaccurate, especially during intense vasoconstriction associated with the use of epinephrine.

The use of an indwelling arterial catheter, when available, is a valuable monitor in assessing the arterial blood pressure. Specific attention should be paid to diastolic blood pressure as it relates directly to adequacy of coronary perfusion during CPR. In addition, an arterial line allows for frequent blood sampling, particularly for measurement of arterial pH and blood gases. Pulse oximetry can be used during CPR to determine the oxygen saturation and may be of value in assessing the adequacy of cardiac output, as reflected in the plethysmograph. The ECG can suggest metabolic imbalances and diagnose electrical disturbances.

The $ETCO_2$ monitor can provide important information during a resuscitation attempt. Because the generation of exhaled CO_2 depends on pulmonary blood flow, it can provide a useful indicator of the adequacy of cardiac output generated by chest compressions. As the cardiac output increases, the $ETCO_2$ increases and the difference between end-tidal and arterial CO_2 becomes smaller.[33] In animal models, $ETCO_2$ during CPR correlates with coronary perfusion pressure and with return of spontaneous circulation.[34,35] In adults with cardiac arrest, an $ETCO_2$ of greater than 10 mm Hg is associated with return of spontaneous circulation and with hospital survival.[36,37]

When the $ETCO_2$ monitor reads less than 10 mm Hg, efforts should be taken to enhance the quality of chest compressions (push hard, push fast, release completely, optimize hand position). A low $ETCO_2$ may occur transiently in the presence of adequate chest compressions after administration of epine-phrine owing to an increase in intrapulmonary shunting.

Temperature should be monitored during and after CPR. The resuscitation of the child with hypothermia as the cause of cardiac arrest must be continued until the child's core temperature has increased above 35°C (95°F). Use of a glass bulb thermometer allows measurement of temperature to very low levels. Repeated measurements of core body temperature should be made at several sites (rectal, bladder, esophageal, axillary, and tympanic membrane) if possible to avoid misleading temperature readings from a single site, which might be affected by alterations in regional blood flow during CPR. Hyperthermia should be aggressively treated in the peri-arrest period, because post-arrest fever is associated with worse outcomes in children,[38] with animal models strongly suggesting causation.[39] Accumulating data indicate a benefit to induced hypothermia after resuscitation from cardiac arrest in adults[40,41] and after perinatal hypoxic/ischemic injury.[42] Clinicians may choose to control a child's temperature in the range of 33°-35°C (91.4°-95°F) for 12 to 48 hours after resuscitation with slow subsequent rewarming.

Medications Used During CPR

α- and β-Adrenergic Agonists

In 1963, only 3 years after the original description of closed-chest CPR, Redding and Pearson showed that early administration of epinephrine in a canine model of cardiac arrest improved the success rate of CPR.[43] They also demonstrated that the increase in aortic diastolic pressure with the administration of α-adrenergic agonists was responsible for the improved success of resuscitation. They theorized that vasopressors such as epinephrine were of value because the drug increased peripheral vascular tone and, hence, coronary perfusion pressure.

The relative importance of α- and β-adrenergic agonist actions during resuscitation has been widely investigated. In a canine model of cardiac arrest, only 27% of dogs that received a pure β-adrenergic receptor agonist along with an α-adrenergic antagonist were resuscitated successfully, compared with 100% of dogs that received a pure α-adrenergic agonist and a β-adrenergic antagonist. Other investigators have demonstrated that the α-adrenergic effects of epinephrine resulted in intense vasoconstriction of the resistance vessels of all organs of the body, except those supplying the heart and brain.[44] Because of the widespread vasoconstriction in nonvital organs, adequate perfusion pressure and thus blood flow to the heart and brain can be achieved despite the fact that cardiac output is very small during CPR.[44-46]

The increase in aortic diastolic pressure associated with epinephrine administration during CPR is critical for maintaining coronary blood flow and enhancing the success of resuscitation. Even though the contractile state of the myocardium is increased by the use of β-adrenergic agonists in the spontaneously beating heart, β-adrenergic agonists may actually decrease myocardial blood flow by increasing intramyocardial wall pressure and vascular resistance during CPR.[47] By its inotropic and chronotropic effects, β-adrenergic stimulation increases myocardial oxygen demand, which, when superimposed on low coronary blood flow, increases the risk of ischemic injury.

Any medication that causes systemic arterial vasoconstriction can be used to increase aortic diastolic pressure and resuscitate the heart. For example, pure α-adrenergic agonists can be used in place of epinephrine during CPR. Phenylephrine and methoxamine, two α-adrenergic agonists, have been used in animal models of CPR with success equal to that of epinephrine. Their use results in a higher oxygen supply to demand ratio in the ischemic heart and at least a theoretical advantage over the combined α- and β-adrenergic agonist effects of epinephrine. These agonists, as well as other classes of vasopressors such as vasopressin, have been used successfully for resuscitation.

The merits of using a pure α-adrenergic agonist during CPR have been questioned by some investigators. While the inotropic and chronotropic effects of β-adrenergic agonists may have deleterious hemodynamic effects during CPR for ventricular fibrillation, increases in both heart rate and contractility will increase cardiac output when spontaneous coordinated ventricular contractions are achieved.

Epinephrine

Epinephrine (adrenaline) is an endogenous catecholamine with potent α- and β-adrenergic stimulating properties. The α-adrenergic action increases systemic and pulmonary vascular resistance, increasing both systolic and diastolic blood pressure. The rise in diastolic blood pressure directly increases coronary perfusion pressure, thereby increasing coronary blood flow and increasing the likelihood of return of spontaneous circulation.[48,49] The β-adrenergic effect increases myocardial contractility and heart rate and relaxes smooth muscle in the skeletal muscle vascular bed and bronchi. Epinephrine also increases the vigor and intensity of ventricular fibrillation, increasing the likelihood of successful defibrillation.[50]

Larger than necessary doses of epinephrine may be deleterious. Epinephrine may worsen myocardial ischemic injury secondary to increased oxygen demand and may result in postresuscitative tachyarrhythmias, hypertension, and pulmonary edema. Epinephrine causes hypoxemia and an increase in alveolar dead space ventilation by redistributing pulmonary blood flow.[33,51] Prolonged peripheral vasoconstriction by excessive doses of epinephrine may delay or impair reperfusion of systemic organs, particularly the kidneys and gastrointestinal tract.

Routine use of large dose epinephrine in in-hospital pediatric cardiac arrest should be *avoided*. A randomized controlled trial in 2003 compared high-dose to standard-dose epinephrine for children with in-hospital cardiac arrest refractory to initial standard-dose epinephrine. This study demonstrated reduced survival at 24 hours and a trend toward decreased survival to hospital discharge in the children receiving large doses of epinephrine.[52] Despite this report, large doses of epinephrine may be considered in special cases, particularly when diastolic blood pressure remains low despite excellent chest compression and several standard doses of epinephrine.

Vasopressin

Vasopressin is a long-acting endogenous hormone that causes vasoconstriction (V1 receptor) and reabsorption of

water in the renal tubule (V2 receptor). In experimental models of cardiac arrest, vasopressin increases blood flow to the heart and brain and improves long-term survival compared with epinephrine.[53,54] In a randomized trial comparing the efficacy of epinephrine to vasopressin in shock-resistant out-of-hospital ventricular fibrillation in adults, vasopressin produced a greater rate of return of spontaneous circulation.[55] In a study of adult in-hospital cardiac arrest, vasopressin produced a rate of survival to hospital discharge similar to epinephrine.[56]

In a pediatric porcine model of prolonged ventricular fibrillation, the use of vasopressin and epinephrine in combination resulted in greater left ventricular blood flow than either vasopressor alone and both vasopressin alone and vasopressin plus epinephrine resulted in superior cerebral blood flow than epinephrine alone.[57] By contrast, in a pediatric porcine model of *asphyxial* cardiac arrest, return of spontaneous circulation was more likely in piglets treated with epinephrine than in those treated with vasopressin.[58] A case series of four children who received vasopressin during six prolonged cardiac arrest events suggests that the use of bolus vasopressin may result in return of spontaneous circulation when standard medications have failed.[59] Because of a paucity of pediatric data, vasopressin is considered Class Indeterminate by the American Heart Association for use during pediatric cardiac arrest[16] although Class IIB for adults (40 U to replace the second or third dose of epinephrine, dose not repeated).

Atropine

Atropine, a parasympatholytic agent, blocks cholinergic stimulation of the muscarinic receptors of the heart, increasing the sinus rate and shortening atrioventricular node conduction time. Atropine may activate latent ectopic pacemakers. Atropine has little effect on systemic vascular resistance, myocardial perfusion pressure, or contractility.[60]

Atropine is indicated for the treatment of asystole, pulseless electrical activity, bradycardia associated with hypotension, second- and third-degree heart block, and slow idioventricular rhythms. Atropine is particularly effective in clinical conditions associated with excessive parasympathetic tone. *However, epinephrine is the medication of choice for children with asystole or bradycardia associated with severe hypotension.*

The recommended pediatric dose of atropine is 0.02 mg/kg, with a minimum dose of 0.1 mg and a maximum dose of 2.0 mg. Smaller doses than 0.1 mg even in small infants may result paradoxically in bradycardia due to a central stimulatory effect on the medullary vagal nuclei by a dose that is too low to provide anticholinergic effects on the heart.[61] Atropine may be given by any route, including intravenous, intraosseous, endotracheal, intramuscular, and subcutaneous. Its onset of action occurs within 30 seconds, and its peak effect occurs between 1 and 2 minutes after an intravenous dose. The recommended adult dose is 0.5 mg every 5 minutes until the desired heart rate is obtained, up to a maximum of 2.0 mg.

Sodium Bicarbonate

The routine use of sodium bicarbonate during CPR remains controversial, and it remains American Heart Association Class Indeterminate. Acidosis itself may depress myocardial function, prolong diastolic depolarization, depress spontaneous cardiac activity, decrease the electrical threshold for ventricular fibrillation, and reduce the cardiac response to catecholamines.[62-64] Acidosis also vasodilates systemic vessels and attenuates the vasoconstrictive response of peripheral vessels to catecholamines,[65] which is the opposite of the desired vascular effect during CPR. In children with a reactive pulmonary vascular bed, acidosis causes pulmonary hypertension. Therefore, correction of even mild acidosis may be helpful in resuscitating children with increased pulmonary vascular resistance. Additionally, the presence of severe acidosis may increase the threshold for myocardial stimulation in a child with an artificial cardiac pacemaker.[66] Other situations in which administration of bicarbonate is indicated include tricyclic antidepressant overdose, hyperkalemia, hypermagnesemia, or sodium channel blocker poisoning.

Potentially deleterious effects of bicarbonate administration include metabolic alkalosis, hypercapnia, hypernatremia, and hyperosmolality. All of these side effects are associated with a large mortality rate. Alkalosis causes a leftward shift of the oxyhemoglobin dissociation curve and thus impairs release of oxygen from hemoglobin to tissues at a time when oxygen delivery may already be reduced.[67] Alkalosis can also result in hypokalemia by enhancing potassium influx into cells and in ionic hypocalcemia by increasing protein binding of ionized calcium. The marked hypercapnic acidosis that occurs during CPR on the venous side of the circulation, including the coronary sinus, may be worsened by the administration of bicarbonate.[68] Myocardial acidosis during cardiac arrest is associated with decreased myocardial contractility.[64] Hypernatremia and hyperosmolality may decrease tissue perfusion by increasing interstitial edema in microvascular beds.

Paradoxical intracellular acidosis after bicarbonate administration is possible due to the rapid entry of CO_2 into cells with a slow egress of hydrogen ions out of cells; however, in neonatal rabbits recovering from hypoxic acidosis, bicarbonate administration increased both arterial pH and intracellular brain pH as measured by nuclear magnetic resonance spectroscopy.[69,70] Likewise, intracellular brain adenosine triphosphate concentration did not change during severe intracellular acidosis in the brain produced by extreme hypercapnia in rats.[70] The rats who maintained adenosine triphosphate concentration, even in the presence of severe brain acidosis, had no functional or histologic differences from normal control animals. In a separate animal study, investigators demonstrated that bicarbonate administration slowed the rate of decrease of both arterial and cerebral pH during prolonged CPR, indicating that the blood-brain pH gradient is maintained during CPR.[71] Given the potentially deleterious effects of bicarbonate administration, its routine use should be limited to cases in which there is a specific indication, as discussed earlier.

Calcium

Calcium administration during CPR should be restricted to cases with a specific indication for calcium (e.g., hypocalcemia, hyperkalemia, hypermagnesemia, and calcium channel blocker overdose). These restrictions are based on the possibility that exogenously administered calcium may worsen ischemia-reperfusion injury. Intracellular calcium overload occurs during cerebral ischemia by the influx of calcium through voltage-dependent and agonist-dependent (e.g., N-methyl-D-aspartate [NMDA]) calcium channels. Calcium plays an important role in the process of cell death in many organs, possibly by activation of intracellular enzymes such as nitric oxide synthase, phospholipase A and C, and others.[72]

The calcium ion is essential in myocardial excitation-contraction coupling, in increasing ventricular contractility, and in enhancing ventricular automaticity during asystole. Ionized hypocalcemia is associated with decreased ventricular performance and the peripheral blunting of the hemodynamic response to catecholamines.[73,74] Severe ionized hypocalcemia has been documented in adults suffering from out-of-hospital cardiac arrest[75,76] and in animals during prolonged CPR.[77] Thus, children at risk for ionized hypocalcemia should be identified and treated as expeditiously as possible. Both total and ionized hypocalcemia may occur in children with either chronic or acute disease. Ionized hypocalcemia also occurs after massive or rapid transfusion of blood products because citrate and other preservatives in stored blood products bind calcium. Because of this effect, ionized hypocalcemia is a known cause of cardiac arrest in the operating room and should be treated immediately with calcium chloride or calcium gluconate. The magnitude of hypocalcemia in this setting depends on the rate of blood administration, the total dose, and the hepatic and renal function of the child. Administration of fresh frozen plasma at a rate greater than 1 mL/kg/min causes a significant decrease in ionized calcium concentration in anesthetized children.[78]

The pediatric dose of calcium chloride for resuscitation is 20 mg/kg with a maximum dose of 0.5 to 1 g. Calcium gluconate is as effective as calcium chloride in increasing the ionized calcium concentration during CPR.[79,80] Calcium gluconate is given at a dose of three times that of calcium chloride (mg/kg) (i.e., 20 mg/kg calcium chloride is equivalent to 60 mg/kg calcium gluconate), with a maximum dose of 2 g in pediatric patients. Calcium should be given slowly through a large-bore, free-flowing intravenous line, preferably a central venous line. When administered too rapidly, calcium may cause bradycardia, heart block, or ventricular standstill. Severe tissue necrosis occurs when calcium infiltrates into subcutaneous tissue.

Glucose

The administration of glucose during CPR should be restricted to children with documented hypoglycemia because of the possible detrimental effects of hyperglycemia on the brain during or after ischemia. The mechanism by which hyperglycemia exacerbates ischemic neurologic injury may be due to an increased production of lactic acid in the brain by anaerobic metabolism. During ischemia under normoglycemic conditions, brain lactate concentration reaches a plateau. In a hyperglycemic milieu, however, brain lactate concentration continues to increase for the duration of the ischemic period.[81]

Clinical studies have shown a direct correlation between the initial postcardiac arrest serum glucose concentration and poor neurologic outcome,[82-84] although the greater glucose concentration may be a marker rather than a cause of more severe brain injury.[85] However, given the likelihood of additional ischemic and hypoxic events in the post-resuscitation period, it seems prudent to maintain serum glucose concentration in the normal range. Additional studies need to be carried out to determine if the benefit from tight control of serum glucose concentration after cardiac arrest or the use of insulin outweighs the risk of iatrogenic hypoglycemia.

Some groups of children, including preterm infants and debilitated children with small endogenous glycogen stores, are more prone to developing hypoglycemia during and after a physiologic stress such as surgery.[86] Bedside monitoring of serum glucose concentration is critical during and after a cardiac arrest and allows for intervention before the critical point of small substrate delivery has been reached. The dose of glucose generally needed to correct hypoglycemia is 0.5 g/kg given as 5 mL/kg of 10% dextrose in infants or 1 mL/kg of 50% dextrose in an older child. The osmolarity of 50% dextrose is approximately 2700 mOsm/L and has been associated with intraventricular hemorrhage in neonates and infants: therefore, the more dilute concentration is recommended in infants.

Amiodarone

Amiodarone has now supplanted lidocaine as the first drug of choice for medical management of shock-resistant ventricular tachycardia and fibrillation. The role of amiodarone was established for cardiac arrest after a series of studies demonstrated efficacy and superiority over lidocaine in the management of refractory tachyarrhythmias in adults. Compared with lidocaine, amiodarone results in an increased rate of survival to hospital admission in patients with shock-resistant out-of-hospital ventricular fibrillation.[87]

Early reports on the use of oral amiodarone in children were favorable.[88-90] Recent data on amiodarone use in children are limited to case reports and descriptive case series. Nevertheless, it is now used widely for serious pediatric arrhythmias in the nonresuscitation environment and appears to be effective and have an acceptable short-term safety profile. This growing pediatric experience among experts and inference from adult studies led to its inclusion in the 2000 American Heart Association Pediatric Advanced Life Support guidelines.[91]

The pharmacology of amiodarone is complex and may explain the wide range of its usefulness. It is primarily classified as a Vaughn-Williams class III agent that blocks the adenosine triphosphate–sensitive outward potassium channels causing prolongation of the action potential and refractory period; however, this effect requires intracellular accumulation. On intravenous loading, the antiarrhythmic effects are primarily due to noncompetitive α- and β-adrenergic receptor blockade, calcium-channel blockade, and effects on inward sodium current causing a decrease in anterograde conduction across the atrioventricular node and an increase in the effective atrioventricular refractory period. The α-adrenergic blockade leads to vasodilation, which may increase coronary blood flow. It is poorly absorbed orally, requiring intravenous loading in urgent situations. The full antiarrhythmic impact requires a loading period of up to 1 to 3 weeks to achieve intracellular levels and full potassium channel–blocking effects.

Hypotension is commonly reported with intravenous administration of amiodarone and may limit the rate at which the drug can be given. The overall hemodynamic impact of intravenous administration will depend on the balance of its effect on rate control, myocardial performance, and vasodilation. Dosage recommendations for children are based on limited clinical studies and from extrapolation of adult data. For life-threatening arrhythmias, the recommended intravenous dose is 5 mg/kg. This dose can be repeated if necessary to control the arrhythmia. Intravenous loading doses are followed by a continuous infusion of 10 to 20 mg/kg/day if there is a risk of arrhythmia recurrence. The ideal rate of bolus administration is unclear; in adults, once

diluted, it is given as an IV push. As recommended by the manufacturer of the drug, it is best administered over 10 minutes so as to avoid the potential for profound vasodilation. We recommend slow IV push (2-3 minutes) until the arrhythmia is controlled and then a slower bolus (up to 10 minutes) for the remainder of the dose. An alternative dosing regimen for children is 1 mg/kg IV push every 5 minutes up to 5 mg/kg. The use of the small aliquot bolus technique may be particularly appropriate for infants younger than 12 months of age.

Amiodarone-induced torsades de pointes has been described in case reports.[92] The use of amiodarone should be avoided in combination with other drugs that prolong the QT interval, as well as in the setting of hypomagnesemia and other electrolyte abnormalities that predispose to torsades de pointes. Severe bradycardia and heart block have also been described, especially in the postoperative period, and ventricular pacing wires are recommended in this setting. Both amiodarone and inhalation anesthetic agents prolong the QT interval; however, there are no specific data to evaluate the use of amiodarone for ventricular dysrhythmias in children receiving inhalation anesthetics. It would seem prudent to be especially vigilant for this side effect in this circumstance.

Noncardiac side effects are often seen, especially with chronic dosing.[93] The most serious of these has been the development of interstitial pneumonitis seen most often in patients with pre-existing lung disease.[94] The incidence in children is unknown. Rarely, an acute adult respiratory distress syndrome–like illness has been reported in both infants and adults at the initiation of treatment.[80,95] The lung disease may remit with early discontinuation of the drug. Hypothyroidism, hepatotoxicity, photosensitivity, and corneal opacities may occur with chronic use.

Lidocaine

Lidocaine is a class IB antiarrhythmic that decreases automaticity of pacemaker tissue that prevents or terminates ventricular arrhythmias due to accelerated ectopic foci. Lidocaine abolishes reentrant ventricular arrhythmias by decreasing the action potential duration and the conduction time of Purkinje fibers and increases the effective refractory period of Purkinje fibers, reducing the nonuniformity of contraction. Lidocaine has no effect on atrioventricular nodal conduction time, so it is ineffective in the treatment of atrial or atrioventricular junctional arrhythmias. In healthy adults, no change in heart rate or blood pressure occurs with lidocaine administration. In patients with cardiac disease there may be a slight decrease in ventricular function when a lidocaine bolus is administered intravenously.

In children with normal cardiac and hepatic function, an initial intravenous bolus of 1 mg/kg of lidocaine is given, followed by a constant intravenous infusion at a rate of 20-50 μg/kg/min. If the arrhythmia recurs, a second intravenous bolus at the same dose can be given.[96] In children with severe diminution of cardiac output, a bolus of no greater than 0.75 mg/kg, followed by an infusion at the rate of 10 to 20 μg/kg/min, is administered. In children with hepatic disease, dosages should be decreased by 50%. Children with renal insufficiency have normal lidocaine pharmacokinetics; however, toxic metabolites may accumulate in children receiving infusions over a long period of time. In children with hypoproteinemia, the dose of lidocaine should also be lowered, due to the increase in free fraction of drug.

Toxic effects of lidocaine occur when the serum concentration exceeds 7 to 8 μg/mL and include seizures, psychosis, drowsiness, paresthesias, disorientation, agitation, tinnitus, muscle spasms, and respiratory arrest. The treatment of choice for lidocaine-induced seizures is a benzodiazepine (midazolam or lorazepam) or a barbiturate (phenobarbital), which also increases the hepatic metabolism of lidocaine.[96] Conversion of second-degree heart block to complete heart block has been described,[97] as has severe sinus bradycardia.

Special Cardiac Arrest Situations

Perioperative Cardiac Arrest

The incidence, causes, and risk factors associated with perioperative cardiac arrest have been evaluated by the Pediatric Perioperative Cardiac Arrest registry.[98] In this analysis (1994-1996), cardiac arrest or death in the perioperative period occurred at a rate of 2.8 per 10,000 anesthetic procedures. Twenty-one percent of cardiac arrests occurred during induction, with 67% during maintenance. Death occurred in 43% of these cases within 24 hours after cardiac arrest and in another 4% in the following 3 weeks. Twenty-five percent of the total number of arrests occurred in infants younger than 1 month of age; their mortality rate was greater than in all other age groups, although their American Society of Anesthesiologists (ASA) classification was also greater. It is noteworthy that only 8% of cases were respiratory in origin, the majority of which were related to airway obstruction. Among the cardiovascular causes, hemorrhage was responsible for the largest number of cardiac arrests. Relative overdose of inhalation anesthetic accounted for 6% of the cardiac arrest events in the series; all of these children were successfully resuscitated.

Cardiac arrest in the operating room should have the greatest potential for a successful outcome, because it is a witnessed arrest with virtually instantaneous availability of skilled personnel, monitoring equipment, resuscitative equipment, and drugs. Whenever a cardiac arrest occurs in the operating room, the circumstances causing the arrest should be rapidly determined. The circumstances of the arrest may provide a clue as to the cause, such as hyperkalemia after succinylcholine or rapid blood transfusion, hypocalcemia during a rapid infusion of fresh frozen plasma or large blood transfusion, or a sudden fall in $ETco_2$ indicating air, blood clot, or tumor embolism. A bradyarrhythmia always must be assumed to be first due to hypoxemia, second due to anesthetic overdose (real or relative), and third possibly related to a vagal reflex due to a surgical or airway manipulation. Administering 100% oxygen and ensuring adequate ventilation is always the first maneuver regardless of the cause of the bradycardia. In reflex-induced bradycardia, atropine may be the first drug of choice but in extreme cases of bradycardia, whatever the mechanism, epinephrine should be used. Hypotension and a low cardiac output state must be rapidly corrected by appropriate administration of vasopressors, intravenous fluids, and adequate chest compressions to circulate drugs to have the needed clinical effect. Once there is need for chest compressions, then the standard American Heart Association recommendations for CPR generally apply and this includes the frequent administration of epinephrine. Figure 40-5 presents an algorithm for the differential diagnosis and treatment of more common causes of acute operating room–associated cardiac dysfunction.

Hyperkalemia

A child with a hyperkalemic cardiac arrest may be identified by history, by the progression of ECG changes leading up to the arrest, or by initial laboratory results. A high index of suspicion must be maintained for hyperkalemia as a cause of cardiac arrest because it requires specific therapy. Along with the usual resuscitation algorithms, immediate therapy to antagonize the effects of an increased serum potassium level is necessary. Calcium gluconate or calcium chloride will antagonize the effects of hyperkalemia at the myocardial cell membrane, increasing the threshold for fibrillation. Sodium bicarbonate and hyperventilation will increase the serum pH and shift potassium from the extracellular to the intracellular compartment; insulin (with concomitant dextrose) will also cause potassium to shift intracellularly (0.1 unit/kg of insulin with 0.5 g/kg of dextrose; 2 mL/kg of dextrose 25%). The serum potassium level must be monitored frequently during this treatment, preferably by point-of-care testing modalities. Because these therapies shift potassium intracellularly, therapy to remove potassium from the body (furosemide, hemodialysis) may also be indicated.

Anaphylaxis

Anaphylaxis is an unusual, but usually reversible, cause of cardiac arrest. Manifestations of anaphylaxis include skin reaction (usually flushing, pallor, or urticaria), airway edema and possible obstruction, bronchospasm, and cardiovascular collapse. Anaphylaxis may be particularly severe in situations of decreased endogenous catecholamines, such as in a child taking β blockers or in children receiving spinal or epidural anesthesia.

Resuscitation of the child with anaphylaxis rests on reversing airway obstruction and restoring intravascular volume and vascular tone. In the child with cardiac arrest, standard dose epinephrine should be administered intravenously. In the child with impending cardiac arrest, 0.01 mL/kg of subcutaneous epinephrine (1:1000 concentration) may be preferred. Children with anaphylactic shock have profound intravascular depletion requiring rapidly administered, large volume fluid resuscitation. In addition to the usual resuscitation medications, treatment should include an antihistamine and corticosteroid, such as diphenhydramine (Benadryl), 1 mg/kg, and methylprednisolone (Solu-Medrol), 2 mg/kg. Inhaled bronchodilators such as albuterol may help reverse bronchospasm. If severe airway obstruction occurs, endotracheal intubation or even cricothyroidotomy may become difficult or impossible. Therefore, the airway should be secured early on by a skilled practitioner.

Supraventricular Tachycardia

Supraventricular tachycardia (SVT), a common arrhythmia in infants and children, may be associated with severe circulatory compromise or even cardiac arrest. Therapy for this arrhythmia should be based on the child's hemodynamic status. SVT associated with inadequate circulation should be immediately treated with synchronized cardioversion beginning at a dose of 0.5 J/kg. If intravenous access is available, adenosine can be administered as cardioversion is being prepared; however, cardioversion should not be delayed while intravenous access is being obtained.

Adenosine is the medical treatment of choice for SVT. The underlying mechanism in children is usually a reentry circuit involving the atrioventricular node. Adenosine causes a temporary block in the atrioventricular node and interrupts this reentry circuit. The initial dose is 0.1 mg/kg given as a rapid intravenous bolus. Central venous administration is preferable because the drug is rapidly metabolized by red blood cell adenosine deaminase and therefore has a half-life of only 10 seconds. When the drug is given peripherally, the intravenous line should be immediately and rapidly flushed with 10 mL of saline. If there is no interruption in the reentry circuit, successive doses of 0.2 and 0.4 mg/kg should be given. In neonates, a smaller initial dose of 0.05 mg/kg is given and increased by 0.05 mg/kg/dose until termination of the arrhythmia up to a maximum dose of 0.25 mg/kg.[99] When SVT appears without any circulatory compromise, conversion of the arrhythmia may first be attempted with a vagal maneuver such as ice to the face. If this is ineffective, then adenosine should be utilized.

Other medications to treat SVT have a greater incidence of side effects. Digoxin is often ineffective and causes frequent arrhythmias. Verapamil should be avoided in infants because of its association with congestive heart failure and cardiac arrest due to its negative inotropic effects.[100] Flecainide is effective in treating SVT but has many cardiac and noncardiac side effects[101]; its role for hemodynamically unstable SVT still needs to be established. Other therapies include β-adrenergic blockers, edrophonium, and α agonists. If SVT persists despite medical therapy and the child progresses to circulatory instability, electrical cardioversion should proceed immediately.

Pulseless Electrical Activity

Pulseless electrical activity (PEA) is defined as organized ECG activity, excluding ventricular tachycardia and fibrillation, without clinical evidence of a palpable pulse or myocardial contractions. It may occur spontaneously after cardiac arrest or as an intervening rhythm associated with treatment for cardiac arrest. The etiology of PEA is divided into primary (cardiac) and secondary (noncardiac) causes. Primary PEA, associated with cardiac arrest, is due to depletion of myocardial energy stores and, as such, responds poorly to therapy. Drugs used to treat primary PEA include epinephrine, atropine, calcium, and sodium bicarbonate.

The causes of secondary PEA are often remembered using the 4 H's and 4 T's mnemonic: *Hypovolemia, Hypoxia, Hypothermia,* and *Hypo-* or *Hyper-electrolytemia, Tension pneumothorax,* pericardial *Tamponade, Thromboembolism,* and *Toxins* (anesthetic overdose). In secondary PEA, intervention is directed at the underlying disorder and usually results in a successful resuscitation. When the cause of PEA is unknown and the child does not respond to medications, one should consider giving a fluid bolus and inserting needles into the pleural space to rule out pneumothorax and into the pericardial space to rule out cardiac tamponade.

Adjunctive CPR Techniques

Open-Chest CPR

The use of open-chest cardiac massage, although generally replaced by closed-chest CPR, still has an active role in the operating room and ICU especially during and after thoracic surgery. Compared with closed-chest CPR, open-chest CPR generates greater cardiac output and vital organ blood flow. During open-chest CPR there is less elevation of intrathoracic, right atrial, and intracranial pressure, resulting in greater coronary and cerebral perfusion pressure and greater myocardial and cerebral blood flow.[102-104]

Typically in the operating room and the ICU, open-chest CPR is preferable to closed-chest CPR in the child who has had a recent sternotomy. Open-chest CPR is also indicated for selected children when closed-chest CPR has failed, although exactly which children should receive this method of resuscitation under this condition is controversial. When initiated early after failure of closed-chest CPR, open-chest CPR may improve outcome.[105-107] When performed after 15 minutes of closed-chest CPR, open-chest CPR significantly improves coronary perfusion pressure and the rate of successful resuscitation.[49]

Extracorporeal Membrane Oxygenation

In institutions with the ability to rapidly mobilize an extracorporeal circuit, extracorporeal CPR should be considered for refractory pediatric cardiac arrest when the condition leading to arrest is reversible and when the period of no flow (cardiac arrest without CPR) was brief. Survival with a good neurologic outcome is possible after more than 50 minutes of CPR in selected children who were resuscitated via extracorporeal CPR.[108,109] Cardiopulmonary bypass requires major technical support and sophistication but can be rapidly implemented in hospitals set up to do so. Extracorporeal CPR should be reserved for children who have effective CPR initiated immediately after cardiac arrest.

Active Compression-Decompression

Active compression-decompression CPR utilizes a negative-pressure "pull" on the thorax during the release phase of chest compression using a hand-held suction device. This technique has been shown to improve vascular pressures and minute ventilation during CPR in animals and humans.[110-114] The hemodynamic benefit of this technique is attributed to enhancement of venous return by the negative intrathoracic pressure generated during the decompression phase. Thus, when this technique was used with a device adding impedance to inspiration, vascular pressures and flow increased further.[115] Its effectiveness in adults shows promise, with increased survival and a trend toward neurologic improvement in pre-hospital victims.[116-118] However, two recent, larger trials did not demonstrate improved survival in in-hospital or pre-hospital victims of cardiac arrest, nor did any subgroup demonstrate benefit from active compression-decompression CPR.[119-121] The complication rate, including fatal rib and sternal fractures, may be greater with this technique.[122]

Interposed Abdominal Compression

Interposed abdominal compression CPR (IAC-CPR) represents the delivery of an abdominal compression during the relaxation phase of chest compression. IAC-CPR may augment conventional CPR in several ways. First, IAC-CPR may return venous blood to the chest during chest relaxation.[123,124] Second, IAC-CPR increases intrathoracic pressure and augments the duty cycle of chest compression.[125] Third, IAC-CPR may compress the aorta and return blood retrograde to the carotid or coronary arteries.[124]

In animal experiments, cardiac output and cerebral and coronary blood flow were improved when IAC-CPR was compared with conventional CPR[123,125,126] but not in an infant model.[127] Human studies also demonstrated an increase in aortic pressure and coronary perfusion pressure during IAC-CPR compared with conventional CPR.[22,128,129] Clinically, IAC-CPR requires additional manpower and equipment and remains experimental until additional outcome studies prove its superiority over conventional techniques of CPR. The risk of injury to intra-abdominal organs during IAC-CPR has not been evaluated.

Annotated References

American Heart Association: 2005 American Heart Association guidelines for cardiopulmonary resuscitation and emergency cardiovascular care. Circulation 2005; 112(suppl 1) IV-1-IV203

This publication provides comprehensive guidelines for pediatric and adult advanced life support, with comprehensive references.

Nadkarni VM, Larkin GL, Peberdy MA, et al: First documented rhythm and clinical outcome from in-hospital cardiac arrest among children and adults. JAMA 2006; 295:50-57

In this multicenter registry of in-hospital cardiac arrest, the first documented pulseless arrest rhythm was typically asystole or pulseless electrical activity in both children and adults. Because of improved survival after asystole and pulseless electrical activity, children had better outcomes than adults despite fewer cardiac arrests due to ventricular fibrillation or pulseless ventricular tachycardia.

Perondi M, Reis A, Paiva E, et al: A comparison of high-dose and standard-dose epinephrine in children with cardiac arrest. N Engl J Med 2004; 350:1722-1730

This blinded, randomized controlled trial compared high-dose to standard-dose epinephrine as rescue therapy in children with in-hospital cardiac arrest. No benefit of high-dose epinephrine was detected. The data suggest that high-dose therapy may be more deleterious than standard-dose therapy.

References

Please see www.expertconsult.com

Malignant Hyperthermia

Jerome Parness, Jerrold Lerman, and Robert C. Stough

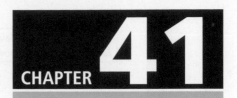

CHAPTER 41

MALIGNANT HYPERTHERMIA (MH) is a pharmacogenetic disease of skeletal muscle that in the presence of triggering anesthetics may precipitate a potentially fatal sequence of metabolic responses. The primary triggers for MH—inhalational anesthetics and succinylcholine—induce an uncontrollable release of intramyoplasmic calcium (Ca^{2+}) that results in sustained muscle contractures, which, in turn, produce a hypermetabolic response. The hypermetabolic syndrome is manifest by hyperpnea, hypercarbia, tachycardia, and a mixed metabolic and respiratory acidosis. Clinically, it is usually accompanied by some form of muscle rigidity, either isolated muscle rigidity (as in the temporomandibular joint, e.g., masseter muscle tetany ["jaws of steel"]) or total-body muscle rigidity (sustained contraction of major peripheral muscle groups). The mortality from MH has markedly decreased from more than 80% in the 1960s to less than 5% in recent years (Fig. 41-1).[1,2] This decrease in mortality is attributable to several factors: (1) better identification of MH-susceptible individuals; (2) the routine use of capnography and pulse oximetry, thus facilitating early identification of the signs and symptoms of an acute MH reaction[3,4]; (3) a better understanding of the pathogenesis of MH; and (4) the widespread availability of dantrolene, which, in the majority of cases, rapidly aborts the reaction (see later).

MH was first described by Denborough and Lovell in 1960, reporting on a 21-year-old man with compound fractures of his right tibia, who, with great trepidation, underwent a general anesthetic with halothane.[5] After 10 minutes of anesthesia, he became hemodynamically unstable with hypotension, tachycardia, and mottled skin that was "hot" to the touch. Interestingly, the soda lime canister was also noted to be hot and was changed because it appeared to be exhausted. The anesthetic was discontinued, the patient was packed in ice, and he recovered without sequelae. Postprocedural examination did not reveal any known medical abnormalities. A careful family history, however, disclosed that 10 relatives in his family had previously died after ether anesthesia, thus suggesting an autosomal dominant pattern of inheritance. This patient required a subsequent operation and was administered a spinal anesthetic without incident, thus demonstrating the effectiveness of nontriggering anesthetics.[6] Subsequent reports from around the world established this disorder as a familial entity that was potentially fatal.[7,8] The term *malignant hyperpyrexia* (later changed to *malignant hyperthermia*) was coined in 1967 in Toronto, Canada, at the first international meeting of this disorder.

The incidence of MH in the population based on occurrences of MH reactions has been variously reported as ranging from 1:50,000 to 1:100,000 in adults and from 1:3,000 to 1:15,000 in children.[9,10] In a subsequent survey of suspected MH reactions in adults in Denmark, the incidence of suspected MH was 1:16,000 anesthetics overall, an incidence that increased to 1:4,200 when an inhaled anesthetic and succinylcholine were combined.[11] A survey of anesthetics in a pediatric hospital in the United States during the halothane era revealed an incidence of MH in children of 1:20,000 to 1:40,000, almost half of that reported previously.[12] The incidence of fulminant MH (defined by a rapid increase in temperature accompanied by life-

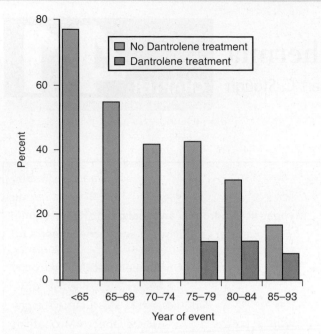

Figure 41-1. The trend in fatality rate in malignant hyperthermia is shown over time. The *blue bars* represent data from 361 patients, and the *magenta bars* represent data from 142 patients. Note the marked improvement in mortality with dantrolene treatment. (Modified from Strazis KP, Fox AW: Malignant hyperthermia: a review of published cases. Anesth Analg 1993; 77:297-304.)

threatening metabolic changes, arrhythmias, and increased serum creatine kinase [CK]) is reported to be 1:250,000 cases of general anesthesia in Denmark.[11] A similar incidence of fulminant MH, 1:200,000, was reported from the United Kingdom.[13] An important and new observation in the survey from Denmark was a 1:12,000 incidence of masseter muscle spasm in patients who received succinylcholine, whether in combination with inhaled or intravenous anesthetics.[11] Clinically, the demographic data suggested that the incidence or suspicion of MH was greater in children compared with that in adults; the incidence was even greater in children in whom succinylcholine was used, and this use was common. The data suggested that the incidence of MH reactions in the past 1 to 2 decades has markedly decreased for two reasons: (1) many families with a genetic predisposition to MH have been identified and bring it to the attention of their surgical and anesthetic care providers preoperatively, and (2) the routine use of succinylcholine has decreased dramatically as a result of concerns regarding rare complications, such as hyperkalemic cardiac arrest. The latter has resulted in a black box warning admonishing against the routine use of succinylcholine in children, particularly male children younger than the age of 8 years who might have unrecognized muscular dystrophy or other myopathy.[14,15] What is still certain is that all inhalational anesthetics and succinylcholine remain potent triggers of MH reactions in susceptible patients.[16-20] No other drugs in use today for intravenous or regional anesthesia are triggering agents. A comprehensive list of triggering agents and nontriggering drugs is available on the website of the Malignant Hyperthermia Association of the United States (MHAUS).* Morbidity and mortality from MH has decreased as a result of the introduction of intravenous dantrolene as

first-line pharmacotherapy and greater awareness of MH and vigilance on the part of practitioners.[21]

Clinical Presentation

The most common presentation of MH is as a hypermetabolic response to one of the inhalational anesthetics or succinylcholine (Table 41-1). The earliest clinical sign of an MH reaction is an increase in end-tidal CO_2 that is difficult to control with mechanical ventilation or that cannot be compensated for by a rapidly increasing minute ventilation in the spontaneously breathing patient.[2,22] Other nonspecific signs include autonomic activation (tachycardia and hypertension). Severe masseter muscle spasm after the use of succinylcholine is considered highly suspicious for MH susceptibility; in-vitro live muscle biopsy testing reveals that 28% to 50% of these patients are MH susceptible (Table 41-2).[23-25] Severe masseter muscle spasm (also known as *masseter tetany*) refers to the inability to insert a laryngoscope blade between the teeth in the mouth, the so-called jaws of steel (Fig. 41-2). Generalized muscle rigidity develops as a result of the excessive accumulation of myoplasmic Ca^{2+} concentrations in MH-susceptible skeletal muscle, causing the muscles to contract continuously. This occurs even in the face of neuromuscular blockade with a nondepolarizing muscle relaxant. Hyperthermia, often a late sign, results from the greatly increased aerobic and anaerobic metabolic activity of triggered skeletal muscle. The overlying skin soon becomes hot to the touch; and, often, but not always, large muscle groups such as calf or thigh muscles can be felt to be tight or knotted. This is accompanied by exaggerated CO_2 production (usually the first indication of an MH event) and accumulation of lactate

Table 41-1. Clinical and Laboratory Findings Associated with Malignant Hyperthermia

Clinical Findings	Laboratory Findings
Tachycardia, tachypnea and hypertension	Increased $Paco_2$
Hypercarbia ($ETco_2$)	Acidosis (mixed respiratory/ metabolic)
Greatly increased minute ventilation	Relative hypoxia, increased alveolar to arterial partial pressure gradient for oxygen
Generalized muscle rigidity (unresponsive to nondepolarizing muscle relaxants)	Hyperkalemia
Skin mottling	Elevated plasma lactate
Hyperthermia (late sign)	Abnormal coagulation studies (late sign)
Cardiac arrhythmias (hyperkalemia induced: PVC, VT, VF)	Myoglobinuria Myoglobinemia
Cola-colored urine (late sign)	Increased CPK (generally late sign)
Disseminated intravascular coagulation (late)	

PVC, premature ventricular contraction; VT, Ventricular tachycardia; VF, ventricular fibrillation.

*http://www.mhaus.org.

Table 41-2. Limited Excursion of the Mandible: Differential Diagnosis

- Temporomandibular joint dysfunction: congenital, inflammatory/infectious, trauma, neoplasm, collagen vascular disease (rheumatoid arthritis)
- Muscle disease: malignant hyperthermia, Duchenne or Becker muscular dystrophy, myotonia congenita
- Integumentary disease: inflammatory/infectious, neoplasm, radiation, collagen vascular disease (scleroderma)
- Neurologic injury
- Abnormal response to succinylcholine (Nietlich or Cynthiana [C5] pseudocholinesterase variant) (for details see Chapter 6)
- Ineffective succinylcholine

Table 41-3. Arterial Blood Gas Data from a Child in Early Malignant Hyperthermia

Time	08:52	08:59	09:05	09:27
pH	7.34	7.03	7.29	7.39
PCO_2	46.3	109.4	47.9	42.7
PO_2	236	159	589	635
B.E.	−1	−2	−3	1
HCO_3^-	25.1	29	23.1	25.6

Note the pure respiratory acidosis in this patient from Figure 41-3 and the rapid decrease in $PaCO_2$ after dantrolene administration between 08:59 and 09:05.
BE, base excess.

fueled by markedly increased glycogenolysis and glycolysis.[26,27] This runaway metabolic process is reflected in arterial blood gases as a mixed metabolic and respiratory acidosis. If an acute MH reaction is diagnosed early in its evolution, before the body becomes unable to maintain the aerobic metabolic rate, the arterial blood gas analysis demonstrates a nearly pure respiratory acidosis, which can make the diagnosis of MH difficult (Table 41-3). A (mixed) venous or peripheral venous blood gas analysis is most helpful in establishing the presence of hypermetabolism because it is more likely to demonstrate an increase in CO_2 levels, significant oxygen desaturation consistent with increased oxygen consumption (PVO_2 < 40 mm Hg despite the child receiving supplemental oxygen as part of his or her anesthetic management where the expected PVO_2 would be >60 mm Hg), and increased lactate production.

Untreated MH progresses to uncontrolled temperature elevation increasing as rapidly as 1°C every 10 minutes in fulminant cases. In one case a patient's temperature is documented to have reached 43.8°C (110.8°F) within 18 minutes![28] The runaway metabolic process in MH results in severe hypoxia, exaggerated hypercarbia, skin mottling, exuberant metabolic acidosis, rhabdomyolysis, and hyperkalemia. Unstable hemodynamics and ventricular arrhythmias inevitably follow. Patients may die of intractable ventricular arrhythmias, pulmonary edema, disseminated intravascular coagulation, cerebral hypoxia/edema, and/or renal failure due to myoglobin deposition in the renal tubules. In the early years of treating acute MH reactions, before dantrolene was identified as the specific antidote, symptomatic treatment was the mainstay of therapy. This included treatment of acidosis and hyperkalemia with bicarbonate and insulin-glucose, respectively; active cooling of the patient with iced saline gastric lavage; infusion of cold intravenous saline; and infusions of procainamide, the last shown later to be ineffective. These interventions helped to reduce mortality to about 50%.

The presenting signs of MH under general anesthesia are variable (Table 41-1). The syndrome may be fulminant or indolent, not all the features of a classic MH reaction may be immediately evident, and it may occur intraoperatively or postoperatively. The latest recorded presentation of MH, for example, is 11 hours postoperatively.[29] The likelihood that an MH-susceptible patient will develop MH in the presence of inhalational anesthetics is exasperatingly unpredictable, and susceptible individuals can have a number of uneventful general anesthetics before an MH event is triggered.[2] Indeed, the majority of patients lack a family or personal history of MH. Therefore, a negative history should not be considered as evidence that a child is not MH susceptible. Furthermore, other disease states may be confused with MH (Table 41-4) and must be distinguished from them for correct therapy to be instituted.

Given both the variability of the clinical presentation of MH and the dearth of pathognomonic signs of this syndrome, establishing the diagnosis of MH can be exceedingly difficult. In response to the need for some objective measure of the likelihood of a clinical episode being MH, a retrospective, multifactor clinical grading scale was developed by an international panel of experts.[30] This grading scale was devised to clarify a cutoff for a positive caffeine-halothane contracture test (see later). It was not intended to be a clinical guide in the operating room. Despite the recommendations in the paper not to use this scale to guide treatment and to be more conservative, we include their tables to educate the reader and help to identify a true MH reaction (Tables 41-5 and 41-6). Although this clinical grading scale is somewhat cumbersome, and has not been prospectively validated in clinical settings for use by nonexperts, we maintain that it remains a useful guide for the clinician who faces a possible MH reaction.

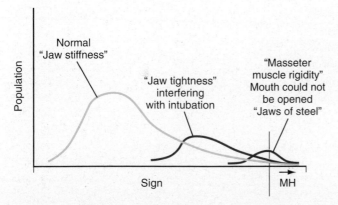

Figure 41-2. The spectrum of masseter muscle responses to succinylcholine varies from a slight jaw stiffness that does not interfere with endotracheal intubation to the extreme "jaws of steel," which is masseter muscle tetany not allowing the mouth to be opened. It is likely the latter response that is highly associated with malignant hyperthermia (MH). Even with the inability to open the mouth, the child's lungs should still be able to be ventilated by bag and mask, because all other muscles are relaxed. (From Kaplan RF: Malignant Hyperthermia, Annual Refresher Course Lectures. Washington, DC, American Society of Anesthesiologists, 1993.)

Table 41-4. Differential Diagnosis of Malignant Hyperthermia

Diagnosis	Distinguishing Traits
Hyperthyroidism	Symptoms and physical findings often present; blood gas abnormalities rise gradually; creatine phosphokinase value does not increase substantively.
Sepsis	Usually normal blood gases early, metabolic acidosis late; creatine phosphokinase remains normal.
Pheochromocytoma	Similar to MH except marked blood pressure swings
Metastatic carcinoid	Flushing, diarrhea, hypotension
Cocaine intoxication	Fever, rigidity, rhabdomyolysis similar to NMS
Heat stroke	Similar to MH except that the patient is outside the operating room
Masseter spasm (MMR)	May progress to MH; total body spasm more likely than isolated MMR
Neuroleptic malignant syndrome (NMS)	Similar to MH; usually associated with the use of antipsychotics
Serotonergic toxicity	Similar to MH and NMS; associated with the administration of mood-elevating drugs (e.g., SSRIs)
Nonmalignant hyperthermia syndrome	Reported only once; severe hyperthermia seemingly associated with fentanyl

SSRIs, selective serotonin reuptake inhibitors.

Patient Preparation

The best treatment begins with prevention and preparation, that is, obtaining an accurate family history of suspicious or unusual reactions to a general anesthetic in blood relatives. For children, it is important to ask the parent(s) whether anyone in the family has had untoward anesthetic events, including death, and/or neuromuscular disease. For male children in particular, it is important to inquire about muscle diseases such as muscular dystrophy. These questions assume a classic nuclear family, but with increasing levels of adoption, artificial insemination, surrogate motherhood, and egg donors, such probing may not elicit clear family histories. The anesthesiologist must be sensitive but decisive in determining the true genetic relationship between

Table 41-5. Clinical Indicators for Use in Determining the Malignant Hyperthermia Raw Score

Process	Indicator	Points
Rigidity	Generalized muscular rigidity	15
	Masseter spasm	15
Muscle breakdown	Creatine kinase >20,000 IU after succinylcholine	15
	Creatine kinase >10,000 IU with no succinylcholine	15
	Cola-colored urine in perioperative period	10
	Myoglobin in urine >60 µg/L	5
	Myoglobin in serum >170 µg/L	5
	Blood/plasma/serum K^+ > 6 mEq/L, no renal illness	3
Respiratory acidosis	PET_{CO_2} > 55 mm Hg with controlled ventilation	15
	Arterial Pa_{CO_2} > 60 mm Hg, controlled ventilation	15
	PET_{CO_2} > 60 mm Hg with spontaneous ventilation	15
	Arterial Pa_{CO_2} > 65 mm Hg, spontaneous ventilation	15
	Inappropriate hypercarbia, anesthesiologist's call	15
	Inappropriate tachypnea	10
Temperature increase	Inappropriately rapid increase	15
	Inappropriately increased temperature >38.8°C (101.8°F)	10
Cardiac involvement	Inappropriate sinus tachycardia	3
	Ventricular tachycardia or fibrillation	3
Family history	Positive family history in first-degree relative	15
	Positive family history, more distant relative	5
Others	Arterial base excess more negative than −8 mEq/L	10
	Arterial pH < 7.25	10
	Rapid reversal of MH signs after intravenous administration of dantrolene	5
	Positive MH family history with another indicator from the patient's anesthetic experience other than increased creatine kinase	10
	Elevated creatine kinase and a family history of MH	10

From Larach MG, Localio AR, Allen GC, et al: A clinical grading scale to predict malignant hyperthermia susceptibility. Anesthesiology 1994; 80:771-779.

Table 41-6. Scoring Rules for the Malignant Hyperthermia Clinical Grading Scale: Interpreting Raw Score, MH Rank, and Qualitative Likelihood

Raw Score Range	MH Rank	Description of Likelihood
0	1	Almost never
3-9	2	Unlikely
10-19	3	Somewhat less than likely
20-34	4	Somewhat greater than likely
35-49	5	Very likely
≥50	6	Almost certain

From Schulte-Sasse U, Hess W, Eberlein HJ: Postoperative malignant hyperthermia and dantrolene therapy. Can Anaesth Soc J 1983; 30:635-640.

the guardians and the child. One author (JP) was associated with a case in which an adopted child died secondary to succinylcholine-induced hyperkalemic cardiac arrest, even though the parent denied that anyone in the family had anesthetic problems or muscle disease during the preoperative assessment. Only during the immediate post-event period did the parent reveal that the child had been adopted and had an uncle diagnosed with muscular dystrophy.

If the anesthesiologist is informed that the child has a blood relative who has had an MH episode or has a myopathy with high concordance to MH, then, in the absence of a definitive diagnosis, the most prudent course of action is to plan for a nontriggering anesthetic—either total intravenous or regional anesthesia or a combination of both. In the rare circumstance in which such prudence cannot be followed, extreme vigilance and preparation to treat MH are of the utmost importance.

When a child with known susceptibility to MH is scheduled for general anesthesia, the workstation must be prepared to preclude the accidental delivery of triggering agents. First, succinylcholine should not be readily available for administration. Second, all vaporizers should be either physically disengaged from the anesthesia machine (which is the preferable plan), because they can contribute trace concentrations of inhalational anesthetics even in the "off" state, or, if they cannot be removed, tape placed across the on/off dials so that one does not accidentally switch them on.[31] The CO_2 absorbent should be replaced and a new anesthetic circuit installed. These measures are designed to produce the lowest trace anesthetic gas concentrations possible because the lower MH-triggering limits of inhalational anesthetic gases are not known (but believed to be approximately 10 ppm). Third, the anesthetic machine should be flushed with 10 L/min of oxygen for a period of time that depends on the manufacturer and age of the anesthetic machine; some machines may benefit from replacing various internal components (see later).

Newer anesthesia workstations are more complex in construction than older machines and contain internal working parts that are plastic (which might serve as a reservoir for trace anesthetics) rather than metal. Hence, no one guideline for flushing an anesthetic machine free of inhalational anesthetic can be applied to all machines. When older Datex-Ohmeda (Datex-Ohmeda, Madison, WI) machines are flushed with 10 L/min oxygen/air for 6 to 10 minutes, the detected concentration of inhalational anesthetic in the breathing circuit is approximately 10 ppm.[32-35] Not only should a fresh gas flow in excess of

10 L/min be used, but the ventilator bellows also should be flushed and then left in the "on" mode during the period of flushing.[34] Preliminary data demonstrate that if the anesthetic breathing circuit is left on the Drager Primus (Dräger Medical, Telford, PA), and oxygen flush flows maintained at 10 L/min, then the time to reach a concentration of inhalational anesthetic of 10 ppm increases.[35] To wash the inhalational anesthetic from the newer anesthetic workstations such as the Drager Primus in a timely manner, one must replace the ventilator diaphragm and integrated breathing system with autoclaved components and flush the workstation for 10 minutes at a fresh gas flow of 10 L/min without a breathing circuit on the machine.[36] Leaving a breathing circuit in situ while the anesthesia machine is flushed dramatically increases the time to wash out the inhalational anesthetic.[31,32,37,38] Flushing the Drager Primus with high flow oxygen (10 L/min) for more than 10 minutes without the circuit in place and with the vaporizer removed should reduce volatile anesthetic concentrations to the 10- to 20-ppm range, a range that has not been associated with MH triggering in susceptible patients. Similar studies with the Siemens KION (Siemens Medical Solutions, Malvern, PA) anesthesia machine have demonstrated that with the CO_2 absorber out of the circuit, a fresh gas flow of 10 L/min reduces the concentration of halothane or isoflurane down to 10 ppm in 25 minutes.[34] These data support the notion that the previously held guidelines to wash out inhalational anesthetics in older anesthetic machines do not hold true for newer machines. We submit that it should be incumbent on each manufacturer to examine the washout times of inhalational anesthetics from their machines and to develop guidelines for use of each of their machines with MH-susceptible patients.

Monitoring

Body temperature should be measured in all children who undergo general anesthesia, except for the briefest procedures. One of us (JL) recommends monitoring the axillary temperature site (opposite the extremity with the intravenous line) rather than a core site for early detection of an MH reaction because the axillary region is surrounded by large muscle bulk in the pectoral shoulder girdle. Furthermore, capnography and pulse oximetry are required of all children during general anesthesia, irrespective of the duration of the procedure.*

Diagnosis

Because the first systemic effect of MH is increased metabolism (increased oxygen consumption and CO_2 production), the cardiovascular and respiratory systems respond to this increased oxygen demand by increasing cardiac output, heart rate, and respiratory rate. Therefore, the first clinically evident signs and symptoms of this syndrome in a spontaneously breathing patient are tachycardia and tachypnea (see Table 41-1). However, an increased $ETCO_2$ value generally precedes these signs and symptoms and is usually evident in the child either breathing spontaneously or on controlled ventilation. On the other hand, in the case we present here (Fig. 41-3), the heart increased dramatically at least 10 minutes before a significant increase in $ETCO_2$ was detected; tachycardia may be a more common pre-

*See http://www.asahq.org/publicationsAndServices/standards/02.pdf.

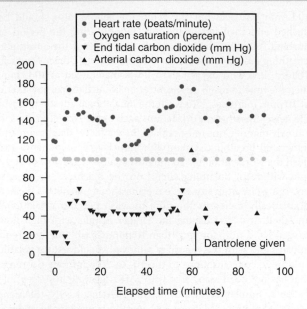

Figure 41-3. Response of physiologic parameters to dantrolene during an apparent intraoperative episode of malignant hyperthermia. Note the rapid fall in both arterial and end-tidal carbon dioxide after dantrolene administration. (Courtesy of Steven C. Hall, MD.)

sentation than previously thought. Sudden unexpected cardiac arrest, especially during induction of anesthesia, is not a common presentation of an MH episode and generally suggests a cause other than MH, such as acute rhabdomyolysis and resultant hyperkalemia after succinylcholine.

A child's response to surgery during "light" anesthesia often includes tachycardia. However, a dramatic and unexpected increase in heart rate from 120 to 180 beats per minute in a healthy child of 7 years (or an increase from 70 to 120 beats per minute in an adult) strongly suggests the presence of a pathologic process and a differential diagnosis beyond light anesthesia should be seriously considered. It is reasonable to deepen anesthesia to address the light anesthesia, but it is also essential to immediately rule in or out other causes, including mechanical factors (e.g., endobronchial intubation, hypoventilation, or circuit problems that can lead to rebreathing), endocrinopathy (thyroid storm, pheochromocytoma), hypovolemia, sepsis, medication-related (excess anticholinergic), drug overdose (cocaine), and primary cardiac disease (supraventricular tachycardia, atrial fibrillation, and others). A rapid increase in the inspired concentration of desflurane or isoflurane may also cause tachycardia. If none of these factors appears to be causative, and a brief trial of deeper anesthesia fails to slow the heart rate, then simultaneous venous and arterial blood should be sampled to determine whether a hypermetabolic state is present or developing (see earlier). In this respect, an $ETCO_2$ (end-tidal) carbon dioxide monitor is particularly valuable. During hypermetabolic states such as thyrotoxicosis or infection, as well as airway obstruction, a rapidly increasing $ETCO_2$ can be easily corrected with mild to moderate hyperventilation. In contrast, during MH reactions, it is very difficult to reduce the $ETCO_2$ to the normal range, even with vigorous mechanical hyperventilation. Indeed, sometimes the CO_2 production is so great that the in-circuit CO_2 absorbent becomes rapidly exhausted in an exo-

thermic reaction, and the absorbent container becomes hot to touch.

Differential Diagnosis

A moderate but gradual temperature increase may occur in children excessively draped, those with air mattress warming devices, and those covered with plastic occlusive wrap. However, the sudden onset of a high fever must be more thoroughly investigated and may be due to sepsis, neurologic injury, thyroid storm, metastatic carcinoid, cystinosis, pheochromocytoma, or nonmalignant hyperthermia of unknown origin, the last reported only once (see Table 41-4).[39-42]

Treatment

If one suspects that a child is experiencing an MH episode during an anesthetic, the inhalational anesthetic should be immediately discontinued, 100% oxygen should be administered at a high fresh gas flow, minute ventilation should be increased to control the $Pa/ETCO_2$, the surgeon should be informed of your suspicion, and help should be sought. Surgery must either be aborted, or if that is not possible, then completed in the most expeditious manner possible. The call for help should bring the MH cart containing dantrolene, the specific pharmacotherapy for MH, to the operating room (Table 41-7). Additional personnel will be needed to help to dissolve dantrolene if the child is adult size.

Native dantrolene is quite insoluble in water, so several strategies have been developed to speed its solubility. The current formulation is packaged as a lyophilized yellow powder in 20-mg vials that contain 3 g of mannitol and enough base to maintain the pH at 9.5. The lyophilized preparation, mannitol, and the alkaline pH all speed the dissolution of dantrolene in water. Sixty milliliters of sterile water should be added to each vial to dissolve the dantrolene, with a resultant dantrolene concentration of 0.33 mg/mL. Warming the sterile water will speed the dissolution.[43] Most of the dantrolene in a vial will dissolve within 60 seconds of adding the water. As soon as the vial is shaken, the solution turns clear orange and dantrolene should be withdrawn and administered, although sometimes one to two additional minutes are required to dissolve the last few crystals. Given the highly alkaline pH of the dantrolene solution, dantrolene should be rapidly infused into a large vein. Extravasation of dantrolene or prolonged infusions may cause thrombophlebitis or thrombosis of both large and small veins.[44] Indeed, one of us (JL) cared for a child in whom a continuous and prolonged dantrolene infusion caused complete thrombosis of the veins of the ipsilateral arm. Alternately, short-term infusions may be more effective than intermittent bolus administration to maintain adequate serum dantrolene concentrations to prevent recrudescence of the syndrome after the success of initial therapy, and may be superior to bolus dosing every 6 hours according to a study in adults.[45] A new formulation of dantrolene that rapidly dissolves is currently under Federal review.

For a 70-kg child, a minimum of nine vials of dantrolene for an initial bolus of 2.5 mg/kg should be immediately available; if 10 mg/kg were needed to ultimately control the MH reaction in this individual, 36 vials of dantrolene would be needed. The response to dantrolene should be evident within minutes (with a marked reduction in expired carbon dioxide tension, heart rate and respiratory rate; see Fig. 41-3); all physiologic parameters

Table 41-7. Contents of Pediatric Malignant Hyperthermia Emergency Cart

	Fluids		
2000 mL D₅ 0.2 NaCl 500-mL IV bottles			
3000 mL 0.9 NaCl 500-mL IV bottles			
1 Regular insulin 100 Units/mL 10-ml vial			
4 Ice packs			

Drugs Number	Drug	Dose	Vessel
10	Dantrolene IV	20 mg (dilute with 60 mL sterile water)	
10	100 mL sterile injectable water *for Dantrolene use only* (red label)		
10	18-gauge and 20-gauge needles		
4	Sodium bicarbonate	1 mEq/mL	50-mL vial
1	Sodium bicarbonate	1 mEq/mL	50-mL syringe
1	50% dextrose	500 mg/mL	50-mL vial
10	Sterile injection NaCl		10-mL vial
4	Mannitol 25%	12.5 g/50 mL	50-mL vial
10	Furosemide (Lasix)	10 mg/mL	4-mL ampule
10	20-and 22-gauge IV catheters		
8	Syringes: TB, 6 mL, 12 mL, 20 mL, and 60 mL		

To rapidly mix dantrolene, use 18-gauge needles on 60-mL syringes to rapidly transfer sterile water to dantrolene vials. Have a colleague vigorously shake the vial while diluting the next dantrolene vial to ensure adequate dissolution and reduce the time of preparation. Final concentration is 0.33 mg/mL. Administer 2.5 mg/kg. *Note:* for larger patients, several individuals may be needed to vigorously shake the multiple dantrolene vials.

IV, intravenous; TB, tuberculin.

should rapidly normalize over 45 minutes. The clinical endpoints include (1) complete cessation of tachycardia and tachypnea, (2) a resolution of the muscle rigidity, (3) restoration of urinary output, (4) return of normal consciousness, (5) self correction of blood gas abnormalities, and (6) resolution of electrolyte disturbances. If these do not occur or are incomplete, then further doses of dantrolene should be repeated until the signs of MH have abated.[46] An initial bolus dose of 2.5 mg/kg has been shown to control most MH reactions provided the dantrolene was administered soon after the onset of the reaction (see Fig. 41-3).[46] There is no known upper limit to the amount of dantrolene that can be given acutely. Most acute MH reactions are completely controlled with 10 mg/kg of intravenous dantrolene, although in some instances 20 mg/kg has been required.

Although dantrolene is effective in terminating acute MH reactions, this effect may wane as the blood concentration of dantrolene decreases, permitting a recrudescence to occur. The prevalence of recrudescence has recently been reported at a surprisingly high rate, about 20%, and was associated with a number of predictors, including muscular body type and a greater time interval between induction of anesthesia and the development of the initial reaction.[47] Importantly, the first episode of recrudescence may occur any time after the initial reaction was successfully treated, up to and as late as 36 hours later.[48] The possibility of recrudescence must always be considered when an MH reaction has occurred. In the event that a child had been discharged from the hospital before recrudescence begins, it is essential that the parents have instructions on how to proceed should signs and symptoms of an MH reaction or recrudescence occur. Currently, MHAUS recommends that 1 mg/kg of dantrolene be administered intravenously every 6

hours for 24 to 48 hours after an MH reaction to prevent recrudescence. However, at the present time, this recommendation remains empirical because there are no data to support the effectiveness of any dose of prophylactic dantrolene to prevent a recrudescence. We recommend continued vigilance, frequent physical examinations for muscle tightness, and repeated laboratory tests (blood gases) and monitoring of vital signs for evidence of a recrudescence of MH. If a recrudescence occurs, then intravenous dantrolene should be administered until the reaction abates once again.

The pharmacokinetics of intravenous dantrolene have been studied in MH-susceptible children ages 2 to 7 years.[49] A loading dose of 2.5 mg/kg produces predictable blood concentrations (3 μg/mL) similar to those reported in adults (Fig. 41-4).[49] Based on their data, half the dose of dantrolene that was required to stop the initial MH reaction may be administered every 6 hours (as a bolus) to maintain a therapeutic blood concentration of dantrolene in children and possibly prevent a recrudescence.

Acute administration of dantrolene causes skeletal muscle weakness that could lead to respiratory embarrassment. Not surprisingly, neostigmine and nondepolarizing skeletal muscle blockers are ineffective in reversing the effects of dantrolene, because the site of action of dantrolene is intracellular. It may therefore be advisable to maintain control of the airway until there is no further evidence of a continued MH event. Indeed, orally administered dantrolene, which was recommended preoperatively for 2 to 3 days in MH-susceptible children 2 decades ago, caused skeletal muscle weakness, dysarthria, sialorrhea, and diplopia to such a degree that many children eschewed the premedication. There is no evidence that this recommendation prevented MH events, particularly when a nontriggering anesthetic technique is utilized.

ingly, no overt myopathies have been reported in these affected individuals.

Normal Skeletal Muscle

Excitation-Contraction Coupling: a Basic Review of Muscle Physiology

The neurochemical signal that triggers excitation-contraction coupling begins with the release of acetylcholine from the motor nerve terminal at the skeletal muscle nicotinic synapse, resulting in depolarization of the surface membrane, the sarcolemma. Sarcolemmal membrane depolarization is transmitted into the interior of the muscle cell by specialized invaginations of the surface membrane known as transverse tubules (TT), which occur at regular intervals along the muscle cell (Fig. 41-6). The TT membrane is studded with the skeletal muscle isoform of the voltage-dependent Ca^{2+} channel known as the dihydropyridine receptor (DHPR). In skeletal muscle, this channel does not transmit Ca^{2+} in response to sarcolemmal depolarization. Rather, this channel functions as a sarcolemmal voltage sensor. In response to depolarization, intrachannel charge movement across the TT membrane results in conformational change of the DHPR. The TT is surrounded by specialized portions of the cellular organelle that are responsible for maintaining the cellu-

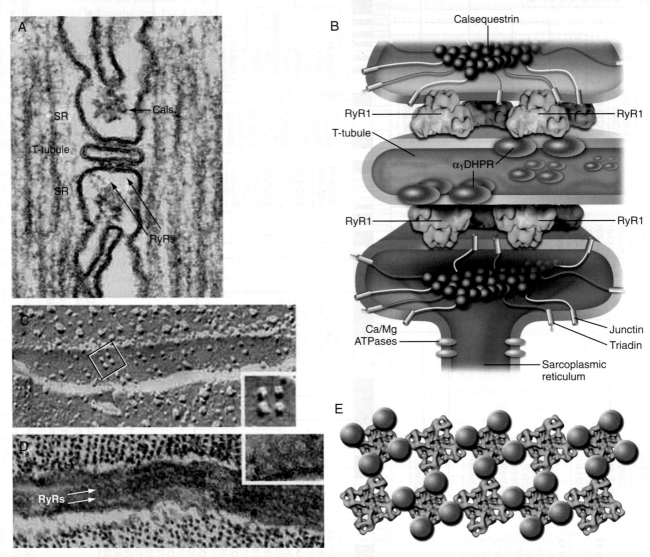

Figure 41-6. Structure of calcium release units in adult skeletal muscle fibers. In adult skeletal muscle, junctions are mostly triads: two sarcoplasmic reticulum (SR) elements coupled to a central transverse tubule (T-tubule). **A,** A triad from the toadfish swimbladder muscle in thin-section electron microscopy: the cytoplasmic domains of the SR Ca^{2+} release channel (RyR1), or feet, and calsequestrin (Cals.), the SR Ca^{2+} storage protein, are well visible. **B,** A tridimensional reconstruction of a skeletal muscle triad showing the ultrastructural localization of RyRs, DHPRs, calsequestrin, triadin, junctin, and Ca^{2+}/Mg^{2+}-ATPases. Note the localization of DHPRs in the T-tubule membrane: DHPRs are intramembrane proteins that are not visible in thin-section electron microscopy but can be visualized by freeze fracture replicas of T tubules (see **C**). **C,** DHPRs in skeletal muscle form tetrads, group of four receptors (see *inset*), that are linked to subunit of alternate RyRs (see **B** and **E**). **D,** In sections parallel to the junctional plane, feet arrays (RyRs) are clearly visible (toadfish swimbladder muscle): feet touch each other close to the corner of the molecule (see *inset*). **E,** Model that summarizes finding of panels **C** and **D**: RyRs form two (rarely three) rows and DHPRs form tetrads that are associated with alternate RyRs (RyRs in *green;* DHPRs in *orange;* T-tubule in *green*). (**A** courtesy of Clara Franzini-Armstrong; **B,** courtesy of T. Wagenknecht; reproduced with permission from Protasi F: Structural interaction between RYRs and DHPRs in calcium release units of cardiac and skeletal muscle cells. Front Biosci 2002; 7:d650-658.)

lar Ca^{2+} store, the SR. The face of the SR junctional membrane apposing the TT contains a packed, regular array of RyR1 in close apposition to the DHPR. Physically, the DHPR and RyR1 overlie each other in a unique arrangement of four DHPR (tetrad) per RyR1, with every other RyR1 lacking a tetrad (see Fig. 41-6).[110] Physical interaction of the DHPR with RyR1 after depolarization causes RyR1 to open, and SR-stored Ca^{2+} is released into the myoplasm. There, the troponin-C subunit of the troponin complex is bound to tropomyosin, which, in the resting state, inhibits myosin interaction with actin, thus maintaining a relaxed muscle. Ca^{2+} binding to troponin-C causes a conformational change in troponin, thereby allowing the complex to move away from tropomyosin, which now rotates along the actin filament so as to allow myosin head interaction with this fibrous protein. Fiber shortening and muscle contraction then occur in a myosin-ATPase–driven ratcheting reaction. The muscle relaxes when the SR membrane–bound Ca^{2+}-ATPase transports free myoplasmic Ca^{2+} back into the SR against its concentration gradient in an energy-dependent reaction, thereby driving myoplasmic Ca^{2+} concentrations down to resting levels. Troponin I, with its bound Ca^{2+} now removed, moves back to block the myosin interaction with actin, thereby preventing muscle contraction and inducing its relaxation. While detailed description of the complexity of this process is beyond the scope of this chapter, interested readers are referred to the many wonderful reviews of excitation-contraction coupling that abound in the literature, a few of which are referenced here.[111,112]

Pathophysiology of Malignant Hyperthermia

The advancement in our knowledge of the pathophysiology of MH has been reviewed in great depth, and the reader is referred to these articles for more detail.[113-116] At the cellular level, MH is characterized by an inhalation anesthetic–induced, uncontrolled rise in intramyoplasmic Ca^{2+} levels[117,118] which precedes the metabolic and clinical signs of this syndrome[119] (Fig. 41-7). This increase in intramyoplasmic Ca^{2+} has been demonstrated by direct measurement of intracellular Ca^{2+} in MH-triggered swine,[117] as well as in Ca^{2+} release sensitivity of isolated SR from MH-susceptible pigs.[85,86,120,121] There is also a significant loss in the ability of Mg^{2+}, the natural, inhibitory divalent cation that competes with Ca^{2+} for binding sites on RyR1, to inhibit Ca^{2+} release in MH skeletal muscle.[122-124] Furthermore, RyR1 isolated from MH-susceptible pigs demonstrate greater open probabilities, greater sensitivity to Ca^{2+} activation, less sensitivity to Ca^{2+} inactivation, as well as reduced inhibition by Mg^{2+}. As a result, these affected RyR1 channels spend more time in the open state and less time in the closed state, when compared with normal channels.[125-129] This presumably underlies both the sensitivity of MHS RyR1 channels to volatile anesthetics and to the increase in intramyoplasmic Ca^{2+} seen in MH-triggered skeletal muscle, although this mechanism is not formally proven. Similar single channel studies of the Ca^{2+} responsiveness of human MH susceptible RyR1 yielded more equivocal results,[130] presumably owing to the genetic heterogeneity of the human MH-susceptible population. Even within a single individual, heterozygosity for an MH mutation would permit a given RyR1 channel that is supposed to be made up of four identical subunits to contain any combination of zero to four MHS subunits in combination with wild type, normal RyR1 subunits. Hence, when examining single channels from a population of channels isolated from a single heterozygous MHS patient, one would expect a wider range of channel responses than in the homozygous, inbred, porcine population.

Recently, several laboratories have reported the creation of knock-in mice containing one of two known *RYR1* MH mutations: Tyr522Ser and the Arg163Cys.[61,62] In contradistinction to the pig model, and like their MH-susceptible human counterparts, the knock-in MH mice are heterozygous. Their homozygous litter mates die in utero on day 17. These heterozygous mice become rigid, hyperthermic, and hypermetabolic and die after exposure to inhalational anesthetics or heat stress, and respond therapeutically to dantrolene. They display exaggerated responses to the RyR1 agonists caffeine and 4-chloro-m-cresol, as well as to potassium depolarization. As with MH-susceptible humans and pigs, their muscle is less sensitive to inhibitory Mg^{2+} and possesses higher resting Ca^{2+} concentrations than wild-type animals. These experimental animals, therefore, display a physiologic MH phenotype remarkably similar, if not identical, to the human syndrome and should prove extraordinarily useful in working out the details of MH pathophysiology.

Interestingly, the development of MH seems to require some form of neural input to muscle, because complete epidural anesthesia in the porcine MH model completely inhibits the development of MH.[131] On the other hand, complete inhibition of neural input into skeletal muscle in this model by the use of competitive, nondepolarizing, nicotinic cholinergic receptor antagonists such as *d*-tubocurarine, pancuronium, and vecuronium before a halothane challenge does not inhibit the development of MH.[132,133] Together, these results suggest that a neurologically significant contribution to MH arises from the central nervous system, either via sympathetic outflow and/or via the neuroendocrine axis, rather than direct skeletal muscle stimulation. Such a theory is consistent with the "awake" or stress-related episodes of MH described earlier.

Dantrolene: Molecular Mechanism

Dantrolene (Fig. 41-8) is a hydantoin derivative originally synthesized as part of an effort to examine the muscle relaxant properties of a series of substituted furan derivatives.[134] Believing they might have a neuromuscular blocking drug, scientists began to work out the mechanism of action but found that it acted like no other known skeletal muscle relaxant at the time: it affected the intrinsic properties of skeletal muscle without affecting the central nervous system, neuromuscular transmission, the electrical properties of the sarcolemma or the T-tubule, the electromyogram, or the "train of four." In short, its action was intracellular (Fig. 41-9).[135] Indirect evidence pointed to dantrolene affecting the Ca^{2+} fluxes that were intrinsic to skeletal muscle contraction.[136-138] Direct observations[139,140] demonstrated that dantrolene suppressed the rate and amount of Ca^{2+} released from SR without completely abolishing it. Subsequently, it was demonstrated that dantrolene inhibited halothane-induced Ca^{2+} release from the isolated SR of MH-susceptible pigs,[120,141,142] while the drug had no effect on calcium reuptake back into SR.[143,144]

Once SR Ca^{2+} release was identified as the likely target of dantrolene activity, a number of unsuccessful attempts were made at identifying a dantrolene binding partner in SR, mainly because of the difficulties of doing detailed pharmacologic receptor analyses with a drug as hydrophobic as dantrolene.[145,146]

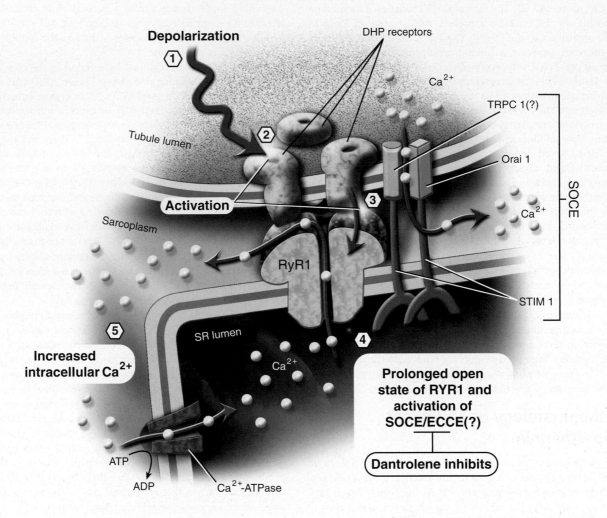

Figure 41-7. Schematic of the known pathophysiology of malignant hyperthermia (MH). Exposure of an individual who has a genetic susceptibility (ryanodine receptor [*RYR1*] or dihydropyridine receptor [*DHP*] mutation) to an anesthetic triggering agent may result in MH. Normally, muscle cell depolarization (1) is sensed by the DHP receptor (2), which signals RyR1 opening by a direct physical connection (3). The conventional view of the genesis of malignant hyperthermia is that RyR1 opening is easier and more sustained in the presence of volatile anesthetics (4), allowing for a sustained rise of Ca^{2+} in the myoplasm (5) that surpasses the sarcoplasmic reticulum Ca^{2+} reuptake activity of the Ca^{2+}/Mg^{2+}-ATPase. This results in unrelenting muscle contraction and uncontrolled anaerobic and aerobic metabolism, which translate into the clinical manifestations of respiratory and metabolic acidosis, muscle rigidity, and hyperthermia. If the process continues unabated, adenosine triphosphate (ATP) depletion eventually causes widespread muscle fiber hypoxia with resultant cell death and rhabdomyolysis. Rhabdomyolysis manifests clinically as hyperkalemia and myoglobinuria and an increase in serum creatine kinase. Dantrolene sodium has been shown to bind to RyR1, presumably causing it to favor the closed state and stemming the uninhibited flow of calcium into the myoplasm. The recently described contributions of Store Operated Ca^{2+} Entry (SOCE) to myoplasmic Ca^{2+} fluxes and its inhibition by dantrolene suggest that MH may have a significant component from SOCE and/or ECCE (excitation-coupled Ca^{2+} entry), and it is the RyR1-dependent activation of SOCE and/or ECCE that dantrolene may inhibit (see text and Addendum). (Modified from Litman RS, Rosenberg H: Malignant hyperthermia: update on susceptibility testing. JAMA 2005; 293:2918-2924.)

It was not until 1995 that an assay for radioactively labeled dantrolene helped elucidate specific binding sites in porcine skeletal muscle SR.[147] Dantrolene inhibits RyR1-dependent cellular Ca^{2+} fluxes in skeletal muscle, albeit incompletely, yet does not seem to affect RyR1 channel activity or its ability to transport Ca^{2+}.[148] The question then becomes with what does dantrolene interact and how does this interaction relate to reduced Ca^{2+} fluxes in skeletal muscle and MH?

Recent evidence demonstrates that there is a second physiologic process called Store Operated Ca^{2+} Entry (SOCE) that contributes to the increase in intracellular Ca^{2+} as a result of

RyR1 opening in skeletal muscle.[149-151] SOCE is a process by which the SR store of Ca^{2+} is replenished from the extracellular milieu after significant loss of Ca^{2+} from SR.[152] Surprising results from experiments with azumolene, a more water-soluble congener of dantrolene, have demonstrated that the drug inhibits skeletal muscle RyR1-dependent SOCE, not SR Ca^{2+} release![153] These results raise profound questions. Are the induced Ca^{2+} fluxes during excitation-contraction coupling, experimental manipulation, and MH that result in a rise in intracellular Ca^{2+} all due to RyR1-dependent-Ca^{2+} release, RyR1-dependent-Ca^{2+} entry, or both? Our elucidation of the pathophysiology of MH

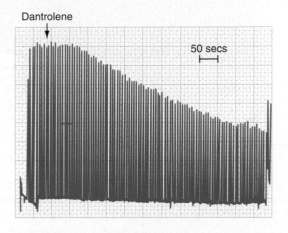

EMHG measures the response to graded increases in halothane concentration to 2% and incremental increases in caffeine concentration, also in different fascicles. The diagnosis of MH susceptibility in the IVCT requires a positive response to both challenges, whereas a positive response to one of the challenging agent results in "equivocal" diagnostic categorization (malignant hyperthermia equivocal [MHE]).[160-162]

Even though the EMHG protocol may prevent excess false-positive and false-negative results relative to the NAMHG protocol, overall results are comparable to NAMHG.[163] The EMHG reports that the sensitivity and specificity of its protocol are 99% and 94%, respectively,[161] whereas the NAMHG reports that its sensitivity and specificity are 97% and 78%, respectively.[164] Because the North American protocol is less specific and tends to overdiagnose MH susceptibility, this allows for a very small likelihood of missing an MH-susceptible individual. The fact that there are some false-positive findings in the contracture testing demonstrates that other myopathic conditions that are

Figure 41-8. Dantrolene and congeners. Both dantrolene and azumolene are equipotent drugs, but azumolene is far more water soluble. Only dantrolene is approved by the U.S. Food and Drug Administration for treatment of malignant hyperthermia. Amino-dantrolene is a poorly active congener, demonstrating how small changes in drug structure can result in large changes in activity. (Redrawn with permission from Parness J, Palnitkar SS: Identification of dantrolene binding sites in porcine skeletal muscle sarcoplasmic reticulum. J Biol Chem 1995; 270:18465-18472.)

and the mechanism of action of dantrolene is bringing fundamental changes to our understanding of muscle physiology and pathophysiology. As our understanding continues to evolve, the future for advances in therapy and testing capabilities hold great promise (see Addendum).

Laboratory Diagnosis

Contracture Testing

The standard for testing susceptibility to MH in the human population is an in-vitro contracture test in which live human muscle fibers from the vastus lateralis are tested in a physiologic bath. With one end of the muscle tissue attached to a strain gauge, the degree of tension developed at baseline and on electrical stimulation is measured as a function of the concentrations of halothane or caffeine. The test is based on the observation that fresh muscle isolated from MH-susceptible patients behaved abnormally when subjected to halothane or caffeine in vitro (Fig. 41-10).[154-157] Two variations of this test have been developed and adopted, one by the North American Malignant Hyperthermia Group (NAMHG), known as the caffeine-halothane contracture test (CHCT), the other by the European Malignant Hyperthermia Group (EMHG), known as the in-vitro contracture test (IVCT). The NAMHG measures the response in separate muscle fascicles to either a bolus of 3% halothane or incremental increases in caffeine concentration[158,159] and requires a positive response to one of the challenges for a diagnosis of MH susceptibility. Those not responding are considered normal. The

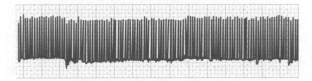

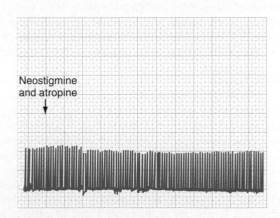

Figure 41-9. Intraoperative electromyogram of a child given intravenous dantrolene 2.4 mg/kg. The twitch tension decreased about 75% after dantrolene but was not reversed by administration of neostigmine, demonstrating the lack of involvement of the neuromuscular junction in the action of dantrolene.

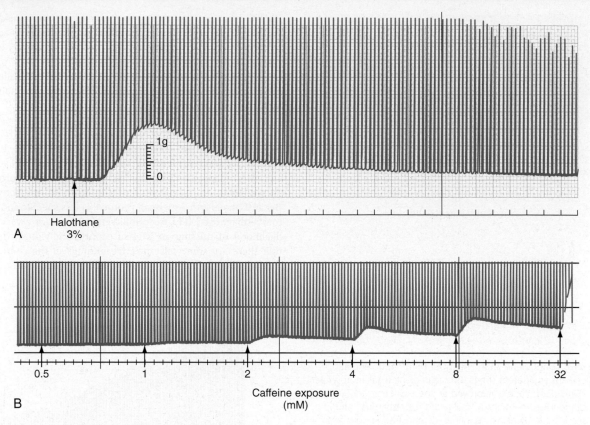

Figure 41-10. Caffeine-halothane contracture test. **A,** Abnormal (positive) response to 3% halothane. Each small box represents 0.1 g tension. The contracture response in this case is 1.6 g. A normal response to 3% halothane is a contracture up to 0.7 g. After exposure to halothane, 32 mm caffeine is added to the bath to determine maximal response. **B,** Abnormal (positive) response to caffeine. Caffeine exposure is to 0.5, 1.0, 2.0, 4.0, 8.0, and 32 mm for 4 min. A contracture of greater than 0.3 g to 2 mm caffeine or less indicates susceptibility. (Redrawn with permission from Rosenberg H, Antognini JF, Muldoon S: Testing for malignant hyperthermia. Anesthesiology 2002; 96:232-237.)[229]

not necessarily concordant with MH have muscle tissue that is also capable of giving an abnormal response to halothane and caffeine exposure. Discordance between the results of an IVCT and the presence of MH mutations in *RYR1* can occur in MH families in that 3.1% to 19.4% of family members who do not carry an MH mutation respond positively to IVCT challenge.[161,165] This presumably indicates that there are other factors (a second MHS mutation in *RYR1*, a separate MHS locus, or a sensitivity to caffeine and halothane that does not reflect MH susceptibility) in these individuals that will give a positive IVCT but it does not necessarily mean that they are MH susceptible

Genetic Testing

Limited examination of the *RYR1* gene is available for the purpose of diagnosing MH susceptibility at two CLIA-approved laboratories in North America (see earlier). Any physician can write a prescription for "the ryanodine receptor gene test for MH susceptibility" or fill out the requisition form and send blood through the mail to one of these two laboratories. Because the understanding of the genetics of MH and even the clinical phenomena produced by this condition are not completely described, it is strongly recommended that all patients who undergo such testing contact the North American MH Registry and report their medical history to this confidential research registry.*

*www.mhreg.org; telephone number: 888-274-7899.

It is recommended that individuals who have the diagnosis of MH confirmed by CHCT, or the finding of a known MH causative mutation (see www.ehmg.org for a listing of these), wear *Medic Alert* bracelets obtainable from www.mhaus.org that indicate "Inhalation Anesthetics and Succinylcholine are potentially lethal."

Myopathic Syndromes and Malignant Hyperthermia

Central Core Disease and King-Denborough Syndrome

An incriminatory association between various myopathies and malignant hyperthermia susceptibility, now known to be far more restricted than originally thought, was described in the 1970s and 1980s, with much debate over the biochemical and pathophysiologic character of the clinical episodes that resulted from exposure to MH-triggering agents.[166] Did the clinical episodes represent true MH, did the episodes relate to the instability of myopathic muscle membrane with attendant destruction of muscle cells and release of intracellular proteins, and was there sometimes a hyperthermic reaction to these exposures? Although both types of episodes might result in increased CK, hyperkalemia, myoglobinemia, and myoglobin-uria, one results from exaggerated ramping of cellular energy and heat production and the other results from a mechanism(s) of cellular destruction that does not involve cellular metabolism as a primary cause. Of the true congenital myopathies, central core disease (CCD) and the related multi-minicore disease (MmD), as well as the myopathy of King-Denborough syndrome, are the only myopathies known today to have a definite relationship with true MH.

CCD is a congenital myopathy in which type 1 skeletal muscle fibers contain characteristic amorphous central areas (cores) that lack mitochondria and oxidative enzyme activity running the length of the fiber.[74] The syndrome can be transmitted in both autosomal dominant or recessive modes of inheritance,[167] has a variable clinical presentation that commonly includes muscle atrophy, lower limb muscle weakness, and floppy infant syndrome, and is often accompanied by hip displacement and scoliosis. Skeletal muscle from MmD patients show multifocal cores on oxidative staining, typically present in only a few sarcomeres along the long axis of the fiber, and affect both type 1 and type 2 fibers. MmD may evolve into CCD over time, both clinically and histologically. MmD patients present with a variety of clinical symptoms: a severe form of autosomal recessive inheritance with severe axial muscle weakness leading to life-threatening respiratory insufficiency and scoliosis; a moderate form characterized by generalized muscle weakness particularly in the pelvic girdle and hands and accompanied by amyotrophy and hyperlaxity of joints; and two classic forms, one with the addition of ophthalmoplegia, the other affected during the fetal period and accompanied by arthrogryposis.[168-170]

King-Denborough syndrome (KDS) is an extremely rare congenital entity characterized by dysmorphic facies that includes ptosis, downslanting palpebral fissures, hypertelorism, epicanthic folds, low-set ears, malar hyperplasia, micrognathia, high-arched palate, clinodactyly, palmar simian line, pectus excavatum, winging of the scapulae, lumbar lordosis and mild thoracic scoliosis, mildly delayed motor development with mild proximal muscle weakness, and diffuse joint hyperextensibility.[171] Both CCD and KDS have high concordance with MH.[74,172-175] Case reports have demonstrated MH occurring in KDS,[172] and a CHCT (MH-positive) has been successfully performed on a 3-year-old child with KDS.[176] Finally, CCD mutations are all linked to RyR1; MmD mutations are linked either to *RYR1* or the gene for selenoprotein N of unknown function.[74,177]

Duchenne Muscular Dystrophy

This congenital muscular dystrophy is found in the class of dystrophinopathies. It is X linked, and female carriers most often have mild clinical manifestations, if any. From a clinical standpoint, these children present many significant concerns for the anesthesiologist. One form of Duchenne muscular dystrophy (DMD) exhibits X-linked cardiomyopathy without any associated striated muscle dystrophinopathy. These children are at risk for a dilated cardiomyopathy (usually starting in adolescence) that can result in acute cardiac failure during especially long and stressful anesthetics. Another form of DMD is the classic presentation of "calf pseudohypertrophy," as well as resting increase in of CK. These children often demonstrate rhabdomyolysis with hyperkalemic cardiac arrest when exposed to succinylcholine.[15,178] There have been reports of rhabdomyolysis and hyperkalemic cardiac arrest after exposure to inhalational anesthetic agents alone, even in the immediate postoperative period.[179-183] Early studies of responses of muscle biopsy contracture tests of DMD and Becker muscular dystrophy (BMD, see later) demonstrated positive contracture tests in some children, indicating suscepti-

bility to MH in a subset of these children.[166,184] On the other hand, contracture testing did not reveal MH susceptibility in the dystrophin deficient *mdx* mouse model,[185] and one study did not find positive contractures in muscle from a 2-year-old child with Becker-Duchenne muscular dystrophy.[186] Quite likely the syndrome of muscle cell breakdown that sometimes results when these children are treated with inhalational anesthetics is due to rhabdomyolysis, rather than true MH, and loss of Ca^{2+} homeostasis does seem to play a role in the pathogenesis of DMD and other dystrophinopathies.[187,188] The best practice approach arguably would be to avoid inhalational anesthetics because they would be expected to produce some myocardial depression and may predispose to skeletal muscle membrane instability (i.e., rhabdomyolysis) with resultant MH-like effects. Succinylcholine is to be eschewed to avoid hyperkalemic cardiac arrest.

Becker Muscular Dystrophy

Related to, but distinct from DMD, is Becker muscular dystrophy (BMD). In this dystrophinopathy, as opposed to DMD, these children have a less malignant course even with the common calf pseudohypertrophy, likely because they retain the presence of a semifunctional, truncated dystrophin or reduced levels of full-length dystrophin.[189] Serious neuromuscular effects are generally seen only rather late in the disease. Nevertheless, succinylcholine has been associated with massive rhabdomyolysis and fatal hyperkalemia (see DMD, earlier). Again, inhalational anesthetics that would be expected to produce myocardial depression should be avoided, especially in children with significant cardiomyopathy, noting, however, that such cardiomyopathy may be subclinical, particularly in younger children. No true evidence of association of this milder form of dystrophinopathy with MH has been forthcoming. Inhalational anesthetics and succinylcholine are likely to have effects in these children similar to those seen with DMD. Prudent practice would suggest using a nontriggering anesthetic technique in these individuals. Even with that caveat, it would also be prudent in these dystrophic syndromes to check CK and potassium levels before, immediately after, and for 6 to 24 hours postoperatively.

Emery-Dreifuss Muscular Dystrophy

Emery-Dreifuss muscular dystrophy (EDMD) is a congenital muscular dystrophy that is either X linked or autosomal dominant, the genes for both of which code for nuclear envelope proteins called lamins.[190] Indeed, there are now known to be more than 180 mutations in the lamin genes *LMNA*, *LMNB1*, and *LMNB2*, which are associated with a series of diseases, collectively known as laminopathies, that include premature aging syndromes, myopathies, neuropathies, lipodystrophies, and dermopathies.[191] Because these are nuclear lamina proteins, the pathogenesis of this form of muscular dystrophy, as well as the other diseases just mentioned, continues to baffle scientists. EDMD lies between DMD and BMD in clinical presentation in that it is associated with less rapidly progressive muscle disease and fewer early contractures than with DMD but a greater incidence of cardiac defects. These cardiac defects are predominantly conduction defects, rather than the dilated cardiomyopathy one sees in BMD. Furthermore, the level of CK is less than that found in DMD disease. There have been no cases of MH, inhalational anesthetic-induced rhabdomyolysis, or succinylcholine-induced hyperkalemia reported with EDMD. As with the two aforementioned myopathies, a conservative practice in the past has been to avoid inhalational anesthetics and certainly succinylcholine because of the potentially fatal increase in serum potassium concentration,[192] although it is not at all clear that this is necessary. Indeed, the greatest anesthetic difficulties in these children may be cardiac in origin.

Miscellaneous Myopathies

Despite linguistic association, there is little evidence in the literature to substantiate any claims to MH susceptibility in other myopathies, such as the limb-girdle muscular dystrophies, the myotonic dystrophies, distal myopathies, or the mitochondrial myopathies. Given the potential for dysfunctional muscular responses in some of the myopathies with sarcolemmal protein dysfunction to succinylcholine or inhalational anesthetics, it might be prudent to avoid succinylcholine, and possibly inhalational anesthetics, as well. On the other hand, children with myotonic dystrophy have received succinylcholine without incident.[193] The paucity of literature on negative outcomes due to inhalational anesthetics or succinylcholine in these children makes such recommendations simply a conservative approach, rather than a guideline. There is no evidence that intravenous anesthetics achieve better outcomes than inhalational anesthetics.[194-197] Indeed, a recent review of anesthetic techniques and myotonic dystrophy reported that inhalational anesthetics have been used without ill effect on muscle.[198] Great controversy continues to rage with regard to the use of inhalational agents in children with muscular dystrophy despite the occasional case report of cardiac arrest secondary to rhabdomyolysis in the perioperative period in these children.[199] There is much yet to be learned.

Heat Stroke and Malignant Hyperthermia

Heat stroke and MH share a common pathophysiologic endpoint—rampant hyperthermia that can lead to death—and can be mistaken for one another.[200] Denborough presented the possible association between MH and heat stroke in 1982 and later demonstrated that MH-susceptible piglets could be triggered into an MH crisis by overheating alone.[59,60] Not surprisingly, there have been sporadic reports in the literature claiming a similar association in adult humans.[63,65,201] Indeed, a patient is reported to have developed MH on rewarming after hypothermic cardiopulmonary bypass.[71] Even the recently developed mouse knock-in models of MH are susceptible to heat-induced triggering of MH.[61,62]

If the vast majority of cases of exertional heat stroke were manifestations of MH susceptibility, then dantrolene should be of significant therapeutic benefit in heat stroke, but this has not proven to be the case.[202] It is likely that there are subsets of patients with MH susceptibility who may be susceptible to exertional heat stroke, but they remain an infinitesimally small proportion of patients who get heat stroke. It is clear that patients who demonstrate such a propensity should be alerted to the hazards of overheating from whatever the cause (sports, military action, extremely hot climates). Because genotype-phenotype correlations between MH susceptibility and susceptibility to heat stroke are as yet unavailable, predicting such susceptibility is beyond our capabilities.

Given our present state of knowledge, if signs and symptoms of heat stress, muscle cramping, or stiffness occur during exposure to environmental heat or vigorous exercise, MH-

susceptible individuals should rest, remain well hydrated, and refrain from similar activity in the future. If heat stroke occurs in an MH-susceptible individual, dantrolene may be life saving and urgent treatment is indicated. Confirmation of the diagnosis of MH susceptibility usually precludes active duty service in the military given the high likelihood of experiencing severe physical stress and the potential for heat stroke. Furthermore, a confirmed diagnosis of MH susceptibility has sometimes compromised the availability of health insurance. Knowledge of the presence of increased risk of adverse metabolic reactions to anesthesia can prevent severe morbidity and mortality by simply avoiding agents and situations that trigger the syndrome.

Emerging Malignant Hyperthermia Mimics

Malignant Hyperthermia-like Syndrome in Pediatric Diabetes Mellitus

Diabetes mellitus is a fairly common chronic disease of childhood that has two well-characterized life-threatening presentations: diabetic ketoacidosis (DKA) and hyperglycemic hyperosmotic nonketotic syndrome (HHNS).[203-206] The former, associated with type 1 diabetes, usually presents as nausea, vomiting, dehydration, and weakness, with shock and coma being fairly uncommon (1%-2%) in the absence of cerebral edema. Fever is rarely a symptom and usually spurs a search for an underlying infection. HHNS is usually associated with type 2 diabetes and commonly presents as the classic symptoms of increasing polyuria, polydipsia, and lethargy that develop over a few days. Mortality is estimated to be between 12% and 46%, somewhat more dramatic than that seen in DKA (2%-10%), presumably because the vast majority of cases of HHNS occur in adults with multiple other medical problems. Indeed, the greatest rates of mortality with HHNS occur in adults older than 75 years of age or those with osmolarities greater than 350 mOsm/L. Surprisingly, the incidence of HHNS in the U.S. pediatric population has been rapidly rising and seems to be associated with the increase in childhood obesity. Despite this, HHNS is rare in children and the presence of fever, as in DKA, usually prompts the search for underlying infection.

Recently, a new syndrome of a malignant hyperthermia-like syndrome (MHLS) on the background of pediatric diabetes mellitus was described in six adolescent males, 14 to 18 years of age, that were culled from cases in three tertiary care facilities in the United States.[207] The features of the syndrome included HHNS with coma, fever, rhabdomyolysis, and severe cardiovascular instability. All six were adolescents, five were obese, five had *acanthosis nigricans*, four were African-American, and four died. Subsequent to this report, two more cases were described: one died 14 hours after admission due to too rapid a correction of serum osmolarity and resultant cerebral edema and cardiovascular collapse, and a second was treated with dantrolene and completely recovered despite developing compartment syndrome in her left upper extremity due to rhabdomyolysis.[208] The survivor was tested for metabolic abnormalities, and a deficiency in short-chain acyl-CoA dehydrogenase was found. The authors recommend that anyone presenting with symptoms of both HHNS and MHLS should be treated with dantrolene as soon as the syndrome is recognized, as well as the fluid and insulin therapy necessary for an appropriate rate of correction of serum osmolarity. A search of the literature reveals a similar case described 10 years earlier as fulminant MH associated with

DKA in a patient who survived with the addition of dantrolene to his treatment regimen.[209]

Although it is difficult to ascertain the efficacy of dantrolene in abrogating the deleterious effects on skeletal muscle and in saving critically ill patients with MHLS during HHNS with such a small number of patients treated, it seems prudent to initiate immediate treatment with dantrolene in these cases until such time as data can inform us as to the true efficacy of this drug in MHLS.

Disorders of Fatty Acid Metabolism

In recent years, a growing number of reports have documented cases of rhabdomyolysis in patients with disorders of fatty acid metabolism, in some ways mimicking "awake" MH. There have been case reports of rhabdomyolysis and cardiac arrest in patients with carnitine palmitoyltransferase II deficiency.[210-212] Various forms of acyl-CoA dehydrogenase deficiencies (very long-chain, long-chain, medium-chain, and short-chain) give rise to different types of myopathy that can have severe clinical consequences, including severe hypoglycemia and rhabdomyolysis with attendant multiorgan dysfunction, which in some deficiencies are brought about by stress—particularly heat and severe exercise.[213,214] These diseases can manifest as early onset in childhood or as late onset in adolescence or young adulthood and can be a particular problem for these individuals in the military or who participate in intense sports.[214] Indeed, patients with the very long chain acyl-CoA dehydrogenase deficiency can present with acute hypercapnic respiratory failure.[215] Dantrolene has been used successfully to treat one case of recurrent rhabdomyolysis in a patient with very long chain acyl-CoA dehydrogenase deficiency,[216] and it, therefore, may be useful in the treatment of acute intraoperative rhabdomyolysis in these patients. Currently there is no literature to help us in deciding this matter.

Children may present for surgery without a diagnosis of an inborn error of fatty acid metabolism, and intraoperative rhabdomyolysis, mimicking aspects of fulminant MH, may be the first presentation for the anesthesiologist. Preoperative increases in serum CK and uric acid, presumably due to subclinical rhabdomyolysis, may be a hint that there is an inborn error of metabolism or myopathy,[217] but such tests are not part of the usual preoperative panel of blood tests in normal anesthetic practice. Perioperative stress as a result of fasting, fear, disease state, and so on, can induce metabolic decompensation and hypoglycemia, so use of an intravenous glucose-electrolyte solution is imperative in known affected children.[218] Because of the few case reports of these patients experiencing rhabdomyolysis when anesthetized with inhalational anesthetics, there has been a general reluctance to use inhalational anesthetics in these patients when their disease entity is diagnosed preoperatively.[218,219] It is likely, however, that the number of patients with inborn errors of fatty acid metabolism who undergo surgery is far greater than the paucity of reports of adverse outcomes during inhalational anesthetics. There is likely to be a wide variation in sensitivity of these patients to various kinds of stress, and the vast majority will likely do well with any well-managed anesthetic. Because it is impossible, at present, to predict which affected children fall into the "safe" category, prudence would dictate that one avoid the inhalational anesthetics in these children, if at all possible.

The avoidance of inhalational anesthetics, however, is not without its own theoretical difficulties and leaves the anesthesiologist with two major anesthetic choices: total intravenous anesthesia (TIVA) or regional anesthesia. In the pediatric population, peripheral surgery often allows for the use of intravenous sedation and regional anesthesia, as in the successfully treated case described by Steiner and colleagues.[217] Not all surgery is peripheral, and not all peripheral surgery can be managed using regional anesthesia. TIVA is commonly used in pediatric anesthetic practice, and the most commonly used drug infusion today is propofol.[220] Propofol infusion syndrome, a rare, usually lethal complication of prolonged infusions is diagnosed by the presence of bradycardia in association with lipemic plasma, enlarged fatty liver, severe metabolic acidosis, and rhabdomyolysis and/or myoglobinuria.[221] In this syndrome, a large increase in particular fatty acids (malonylcarnitine and C5-acylcarnitine) that points to impaired entry of long-chain fatty acids into mitochondria and to resultant failure of mitochondrial respiration at complex II has been identified.[222] Others suggest that propofol infusion syndrome may be uncovering medium-chain acyl-CoA dehydrogenase deficiencies.[221] The suggestion that propofol can impair fatty acid uptake and subsequent oxidation makes one wonder whether the acute administration of propofol to someone whose fatty acid metabolism is already impaired can precipitate a metabolic crisis. Indeed, Uezono and colleagues have queried whether the acquired lipid load of a propofol infusion in the absence of adequate carbohydrate intake in these children can uncover carnitine deficiency and in that sense is a model for propofol infusion syndrome.[223] Moreover, propofol itself has been shown to inhibit mitochondrial respiration, also mimicking the effects of fatty acid oxidation deficiencies.[221] In these children, the use of propofol is clearly associated with an undefined risk of inducing metabolic crisis. If their metabolic abnormalities are subclinical, there is no easy, inexpensive preoperative screening method that will establish a diagnosis for a rare metabolic abnormality. Even if the child is diagnosed with one of the subsets of fatty acid oxidation deficiencies there is no way to preoperatively predict which children will be sensitive to propofol and if they are sensitive how sensitive they will be. In these instances, careful discussion of the anesthetic issues with parents, children, and surgeons is mandatory.

Neuroleptic Malignant Syndrome

Neuroleptic malignant syndrome (NMS) is a rare, potentially lethal reaction to neuroleptics (0.1%-2.5% of patients) characterized clinically by fever, muscle rigidity, altered consciousness, and autonomic instability, with laboratory findings that include increased CK, leukocytosis, raised liver enzymes, and reduced serum iron or potassium concentrations.[224] The similarity to MH is obvious, and the distinction between the two is often difficult to make, except by medication history, with neuroleptics in NMS and inhalational anesthetics and/or succinylcholine in MH. The development of NMS is associated with children who are taking neuroleptics that block all dopamine D_2 receptors (high-potency neuroleptics [e.g., haloperidol], atypical neuroleptics [e.g., thiothixene], low-potency D_2-receptor antagonists [e.g., metoclopramide and tricyclic antidepressants]) and with withdrawal of anti-parkinsonian medications. It is suggested, but not proven, that the syndrome results from a deficiency of central dopamine. Indeed, many other mechanisms of pathophysiologic origin have been proposed to explain the many clinical findings that cannot be explained by lack of dopamine. Successful therapy for NMS requires early recognition, cessation of offending medications, and intensive medical and nursing care geared toward hydration and restoring electrolyte balance.[224] Specific pharmacologic therapy with dopamine agonists such as bromocriptine or with dantrolene have been advocated, the latter with much controversy. Despite the fact that textbooks of psychiatry list dantrolene as first-line pharmacologic treatment of NMS, there are no good data that it has a therapeutic effect in NMS, except for the occasional case report declaring that dantrolene is effective.[224-226]

Children with psychiatric diagnoses requiring treatment with neuroleptics make up a significant percentage of pediatric psychiatric patients, and NMS in this population is well described. NMS in the pediatric population continues to be a problem, even with the newest of drugs. The perioperative period for the pediatric patient on neuroleptics is one fraught with potential diagnostic dilemmas: is this MH or NMS? Indeed, there is a recent report of postoperative NMS in a child with severe cerebral palsy and seizure disorder who was not taking any neuroleptics and who was successfully treated three times with dantrolene.[227] Was this NMS or a mild form of MH? The answer is unclear.

Summary

There are many clinical scenarios in pediatric anesthesia with the potential to mimic MH and to challenge both our diagnostic acumen and our ability to deliver safe anesthetic care. Not all metabolic syndromes that reveal themselves under inhalational anesthesia are MH, and not all metabolic syndromes that respond to dantrolene are MH. The examples given here impress the need once again for expert advice during a case of suspected MH, and the reader is once again urged to make use of the Malignant Hyperthermia Hotline when the need arises.

Acknowledgment

The editors wish to thank John F. Ryan, MD for his prior contribution to this chapter.

Addendum

Recently, new evidence of a dantrolene-sensitive, excitation-coupled Ca^{2+} entry mechanism of skeletal muscle (ECCE) that is more easily activated in MH skeletal muscle has been published.[1-4] ECCE is different from SOCE in that it does not require depletion of the SR Ca^{2+} store, and is activated simply by high frequency electrical stimulation of the skeletal muscle membrane. ECCE, along with SOCE, present new physiological targets of investigation in to the pathophysiology of MH that involve Ca^{2+} entry, rather than Ca^{2+} release (see Fig. 41-7).

Addendum References

1. Cherednichenko G, Hurne AM, Fessenden JD, et al: Conformational activation of Ca^{2+} entry by depolarization of skeletal myotubes. Proc Natl Acad Sci U S A. 2004; 101:15793-15798.
2. Hurne AM, O'Brien JJ, Wingrove D, et al: Ryanodine receptor type 1 (RyR1) mutations C4958S and C4961S reveal excitation-coupled calcium entry (ECCE) is independent of sarcoplasmic reticulum store depletion. J Biol Chem 2005; 280:36994-37004.
3. Yang T, Allen PD, Pessah IN, Lopez JR: Enhanced excitation-coupled calcium entry in myotubes is associated with expression of RyR1 malignant hyperthermia mutations. J Biol Chem 2007; 282:37471-37478.
4. Cherednichenko G, Ward CW, Feng W, et al: Enhanced excitation-coupled calcium entry in myotubes expressing malignant hyperthermia mutation R163C is attenuated by dantrolene. Mol Pharmacol 2008; 73:1203-1212.

Annotated References

Brandom BW: Genetics of malignant hyperthermia. Sci World J 2006; 6:1722-1730
Excellent review of our state of knowledge of the genetics of MH and testing, the reporting of MH cases, and the populations involved.

Kolb ME, Horne ML, Martz R: Dantrolene in human malignant hyperthermia. Anesthesiology 1982; 56:254-262
The classic report of dantrolene efficacy in treating MH.

Krause T, Gerbershagen MU, Fiege M, et al: Dantrolene—a review of its pharmacology, therapeutic use and new developments. Anaesthesia 2004; 59:364-373
Very good review of different aspects of dantrolene pharmacology.

Larach MG, Localio AR, Allen GC, et al: A clinical grading scale to predict malignant hyperthermia susceptibility. Anesthesiology 1994; 80:771-779
Retrospective clinical grading scale for likelihood of an MH episode.

Lerman J, McLeod ME, Strong HA: Pharmacokinetics of intravenous dantrolene in children. Anesthesiology 1989; 70:625-629
The first and only treatment of this subject.

Litman RS, Rosenberg H: Malignant hyperthermia: update on susceptibility testing. JAMA 2005; 15:2918-2924
Excellent, simple review of clinical pathophysiology and testing strategies.

Robinson R, Carpenter D, Shaw MA, et al: Mutations in *RyR1* in malignant hyperthermia and central core disease. Hum Mutat 2006; 27:977-989
Comprehensive clinical and genetic review of MH and CCD. The most up-to-date annotation of all published RyR1 mutations, comparing data from the United States and the United Kingdom, showing that "hot spots" of mutation in RyR1 may be population specific. All the data together show that there are many mutations outside hot spot regions. Which mutations are concordant for both MH and CCD and which are not discussed.

Rossi AE, Dirksen RT: Sarcoplasmic reticulum: the dynamic calcium governor of muscle. Muscle Nerve 2006; 33:715-731
Wonderful review of our state of knowledge of the molecular pathophysiology of MH and CCD from experts.

Treves S, Anderson AA, Ducreux S, et al: Ryanodine receptor 1 mutations, dysregulation of calcium homeostasis and neuromuscular disorders. Neuromuscul Disord 2005; 15:577-587
Another excellent review and a different perspective of the pathophysiology of MH and CCD from the laboratory that has enabled the establishment of white blood cell lines from MH patients.

References

Please see www.expertconsult.com

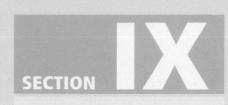

Regional Anesthesia

David M. Polaner, Santhanam Suresh, and Charles J. Coté   CHAPTER 42

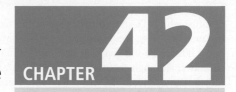

THE USE OF REGIONAL anesthesia techniques in children has increased dramatically in the past two decades.[1,2] Regional anesthesia is most commonly used in conjunction with general anesthesia in children, although in certain circumstances regional anesthesia may be the sole technique. In addition to central neuraxis blocks, peripheral nerve blocks are now employed with increasing frequency, and the introduction of high-resolution portable ultrasound imaging has opened up new vistas for the pediatric anesthesiologist. Ultrasound-guided visualization of anatomic structures permits both greater precision of needle or catheter placement and confirmation that the drug has been deposited at the site of choice (see Chapter 43). Supplementing a general anesthetic with a nerve block can result in a pain-free awakening and postoperative analgesia without the potentially deleterious side effects associated with parenteral opioids (see Chapter 44).[3] This benefit may be of particular importance to neonates and former preterm infants and in children with cystic fibrosis and other conditions.[4] There is also evidence that suggests that regional anesthesia may improve pulmonary function in children who have undergone thoracic or upper abdominal surgery.[5-7] Lastly, the greatly increased number of "same day surgery" cases in recent years has made the advantages of regional anesthesia such as the rapid awakening, enhanced postoperative analgesia with no sedation or altered sensorium, and lack of opioid-induced nausea or vomiting even more apparent. The safe and effective use of these techniques in children,

however, requires an understanding of both the developmental anatomy of the region in which the block is placed and the developmental pharmacology of local anesthetics.

Pharmacology and Pharmacokinetics of Local Anesthetics

There are two classes of clinically useful local anesthetics, the amino-amides (amides) and the amino-esters (esters) (Table 42-1). The amides are degraded in the liver by cytochrome P450 enzymes, whereas the esters are hydrolyzed primarily by plasma cholinesterases.[8-12] These degradation pathways are important because they account for some of the differences in distribution and metabolism of local anesthetics in children, particularly when neonates are compared with adults.

Amides

Amide local anesthetics commonly used in pediatric anesthesia include lidocaine, bupivacaine, and ropivacaine. The choice of agent most often depends on the desired speed of onset and duration of action of the block, but in small infants and children issues related to potential toxicity are also important. Compared with an adult, the neonatal liver has limited enzymatic activity to metabolize and biotransform drugs (see Chapter 6). The ability to oxidize and to reduce drugs, in particular, is

Table 42-1. Commonly Used Local Anesthetics

Esters	Amides
Procaine	Lidocaine
Tetracaine	Mepivacaine
2-Chloroprocaine	Bupivacaine
	Levobupivacaine
	Ropivacaine
	Etidocaine

diminished.[11-17] Despite differences in the oxidative activity of the neonatal liver, the rates of plasma decay of single doses of both lidocaine and bupivacaine are similar in adults and neonates, although there are conflicting data. Neonates do not metabolize mepivacaine, with most of it excreted unchanged in the urine.[18-24] Conjugation reactions are severely limited at birth and do not reach adult levels until approximately 3 months of age.[13-16,20]

Older children also differ from adults with respect to the pharmacokinetics of local anesthetics. Children achieve peak plasma concentrations of amide local anesthetics more rapidly than adults after intercostal nerve blocks but at similar times (approximately 30 minutes with lidocaine and bupivacaine) after caudal epidural administration.[25-27] Ilioinguinal nerve blocks in children weighing less than 15 kg produce plasma concentrations of bupivacaine in the toxic range if more than 1.25 mg/kg is administered.[28] The steady-state volume of distribution (Vdss) for amides in children is greater than in adults, whereas their clearances (Cl) are similar.[27,29,30] Because the elimination half-life ($t_{1/2}$) is related to the volume of distribution and clearance,

$$t_{1/2} = (0.693 \cdot VDss)/Cl,$$

a larger steady-state volume of distribution directly prolongs the elimination half-life. This prolongation of the half-life, however, is probably of little clinical importance for single-dose administration but may have profound consequences for continuous administration; that is, the drug may accumulate over several days, with an insidious onset of toxicity. The risk of drug accumulation with repeated doses as well as continuous infusions appears to be significantly increased in infants and children.[31,32]

Bupivacaine

Bupivacaine remains the most commonly used amide local anesthetic agent for regional blockade in infants and children. After a single administration, analgesia may be expected for up to 4 hours, although its duration of action is somewhat less in small infants. The concentration used depends on the site of injection, the desired density of blockade, consideration of the toxic threshold of the drug, and the dosage limitations imposed by the concomitant administration of other local anesthetics, such as local infiltration by the surgeon or intravenous or topical laryngotracheal administration of lidocaine. The most commonly used concentration for peripheral nerve blocks is 0.25%, with reduced concentrations of 0.0625% to 0.1% used for continuous epidural administration. The 0.5% concentration is less commonly used in children, although it may be employed for peripheral nerve blocks where subsequent doses and drug accumulation are not of concern.

Bupivacaine is highly bound to plasma proteins, particularly to α_1-acid glycoprotein. It is a racemic mixture of the *levo* and *dextro* enantiomers; the *l*-isoform is the bioactive one with regard to clinical effect, and the *d*-isoform contributes more to toxicity. The major advantage of levobupivacaine, the *l*-enantiomer of bupivacaine, over the racemic preparation is the reduced cardiac and central nervous system (CNS) toxicities. Levobupivacaine retains similar efficacy and duration of blockade as the racemic formulation; retention of efficacy has been demonstrated in both an bovine model and in adult volunteers.[33,34] The use of this local anesthetic appears to reduce the toxic threshold by up to 30%. Although levobupivacaine is used widely outside North America, recently it has become difficult to obtain in the United States.[35]

Several new experimental preparations of bupivacaine have the prospect to offer dramatically prolonged analgesia with a reduced potential for toxicity. Bioerodible encapsulated microspheres of bupivacaine administered for peripheral neural blockade[36] release local anesthetic over many hours to several days depending on the formulation of the microsphere, thus producing very prolonged analgesia.[37] The addition of dexamethasone to the microspheres prolonged the effect of the blockade up to 13-fold, and plasma bupivacaine concentrations in animal studies were far below the toxic threshhold.[38] No adverse local reactions were noted. Several different preparations have been developed and studied, including synthetic bioerodible microspheres, protein/lipid/sugar spheres, and liposheres.[39-41] If these formulations become available for the clinician, they may be particularly useful for children who cannot have an indwelling catheter for a regional anesthetic but still require prolonged neural blockade for analgesia. Potential applications include intercostal blockade for children with rib fractures, postoperative analgesia for ambulatory surgery, and children in whom an indwelling epidural catheter poses an excessive risk of infection.[42]

Ropivacaine

Ropivacaine is an amide local anesthetic. Like levobupivacaine, it is an *l*-enantiomer that has reduced risks of cardiac and neurologic toxicities compared with bupivacaine.[43] The lethal dose in 50% of animals (LD_{50}) appears to be greater than that of bupivacaine. Rats of different maturity exhibited a threefold greater tolerance to equipotent doses of ropivacaine than to bupivacaine when administered for a femoral nerve block.[44] Ropivacaine is also reputed to have a lesser degree of motor blockade for equianalgesic potency, but data are conflicting in this regard. Some studies report a greater sparing of motor function compared with bupivacaine, whereas others have found no difference in motor and sensory blockade. Ropivacaine has been reported to produce denser blockade of the Aδ and C fibers than bupivacaine when low concentrations are used, lending mechanistic credence to the idea of differential blockade.[45] Much of the infant animal data, however, do not support the existence of a greater sensorimotor differential block than that after bupivacaine. The few clinical studies in infants and children currently available do not report a detectable motor-sensory differential, in contrast to the data in adults.[44,46] Several clinical studies in infants and children report a prolonged duration of analgesia with ropivacaine, despite using a solution of reduced potency.[46-48] Although there are still only limited data available in children, the decreased potential for toxicity makes ropivacaine an attractive agent in this age group. Most reports in the literature have used an 0.2% solution (2 mg/mL). The volume of drug injected was similar to that of bupivacaine and depended on the type of block and size of the child. We use concentrations of 0.1% for infusions with opioid for continuous postoperative analgesia.

Esters

The pharmacokinetics of the ester local anesthetics are also affected by the quantitative and qualitative difference in plasma proteins. Plasma pseudocholinesterase activity in infants is decreased compared with adults[49]; thus, the plasma half-life of the ester local anesthetics may be prolonged. Despite a prolonged elimination half-life in infants, 2,3-chloroprocaine has been recommended for neonatal regional techniques, including epidural blockade.[50,51] Limited data suggest that 2,3-chloroprocaine may be safe in this setting and that potentially toxic accumulation does not occur after several hours of use with a 1.5% concentration.

Another enzymatic system with decreased activity in neonates is methemoglobin reductase, which is responsible for maintaining hemoglobin in a reduced valence state where it is capable of binding and transporting oxygen. Hepatic metabolism of prilocaine yields o-toluidine, which can produce methemoglobinemia, thereby rendering red blood cells less capable of carrying oxygen.[52] The decreased activity of methemoglobin reductase and the increased susceptibility of fetal hemoglobin to oxidization make prilocaine an unsuitable local anesthetic for use in neonates. Although prilocaine is no longer available for use in the United States as an injected local anesthetic, it is one of the components of EMLA cream (Eutectic Mixture of Local Anesthetics), a commonly employed transdermal local anesthetic. The total dose and surface area for EMLA application is therefore limited in neonates because methemoglobinemia has been reported in this age group.[53] Other local anesthetics, particularly topical agents such as benzocaine, are potentially dangerous in infants because of the risk of methemoglobinemia by this same mechanism.[54] EMLA should only be applied to normal intact skin in appropriate doses[55] (<10 kg applied to a maximum of approximately 100 cm² surface area; 10-20 kg applied to a maximum of approximately 600 cm² surface area; >20 kg applied to a maximum of approximately 2000 cm² surface area). The duration of action is 1 to 2 hours after the cream is removed. Adverse reactions include skin blanching, erythema, itching, rash, and methemoglobinemia. EMLA should be used with caution and with strict attention to the amount of cream and surface area of application in children younger than 1 month of age. Infants receiving drugs that may induce methemoglobinemia, such as phenytoin, phenobarbital, and sulfonamides may be at increased risk, and caution is warranted. It is contraindicated in children with congenital or idiopathic methemoglobinemia. Ametop, a topical preparation of amethocaine, has a more rapid onset of analgesia and increased depth of penetration through the skin and produces minimal vasoconstriction of the skin as compared with EMLA.[56] Iontophoresis of lidocaine can also produce excellent transdermal skin analgesia with much faster onset of action (10 minutes) and greater depth of skin penetration than EMLA.[56]

Toxicity of Local Anesthetics

With the exception of uncommon effects such as producing methemoglobinemia, the major toxic effects of local anesthetics are on the cardiovascular system and the CNS. Local anesthetics readily cross the blood-brain barrier to cause alterations in CNS function. A consistent sequence of symptoms can be observed as plasma local anesthetic concentrations progressively increase, although this may not be readily apparent in infants and small children. Because of the lower threshold for cardiac toxicity with bupivacaine, cardiac and CNS toxicity may occur virtually simultaneously in infants and children or cardiac toxicity may even precede CNS toxicity. During the intraoperative use of bupivacaine, the risk of cardiac toxicity may be increased by the concomitant use of volatile anesthetics and the CNS effects of the general anesthetic may obscure the signs of CNS toxicity until devastating cardiovascular effects are apparent.[57]

In adults, the earliest symptom of local anesthetic toxicity is circumoral paresthesia, which is due to the high tissue concentrations of local anesthetic rather than CNS effects. The development of circumoral paresthesias is followed by the prodromal CNS symptoms of lightheadedness and dizziness, which progress to both visual and auditory disturbances, such as difficulty in focusing and tinnitus. Objective signs of CNS toxicity during this time are shivering, slurred speech, and muscle twitching. As the plasma concentration of local anesthetic continues to increase, CNS excitation occurs, resulting in generalized seizures. Further increases in the local anesthetic concentration depresses the CNS, with respiratory depression leading to a respiratory arrest. In adults, cardiovascular toxicity usually follows CNS toxicity. In this case, the systemic blood pressure decreases because the peripheral vasculature dilates and because of direct myocardial depression, leading to a progressive bradycardia. These effects culminate in a cardiac arrest. In large doses, bupivacaine produces ventricular dysrhythmias, including ventricular tachycardia, and ST segment changes suggestive of myocardial ischemia, especially when epinephrine-containing solutions are used. Bupivacaine has a particularly strong affinity for the fast sodium channels as well as the calcium and slow potassium channels in the myocardium. These effects explain why it is frequently so difficult to resuscitate children from a toxic dose of bupivacaine.[58-60] Stereoselectivity of the sodium channel in the open state, however, has not been demonstrated. There is also evidence that the slow or flicker potassium channels may play a significant role in bupivacaine toxicity.[61]

With an intravascular injection of bupivacaine with epinephrine, characteristic changes on the electrocardiogram (ECG) may be seen without any observable symptoms of CNS toxicity. Figure 42-1 shows an ECG tracing obtained during an intravenous injection of bupivacaine with and without epinephrine. Even a small intravenous dose of 1 to 2 µg/kg of epinephrine in a 1:200,000 solution with 0.25% bupivacaine will produce peaked T waves with ST segment elevation on the ECG, particularly in the lateral chest leads.[62-64] As opposed to the serious risk of ischemia and dysrhythmias with larger unintended doses of bupivacaine with epinephrine, the use of small test doses produces only brief transient changes in the ECG and may therefore be useful in the detection of an intravascular catheter or needle placement. Tachycardia is not a reliable indicator of an intravascular injection of bupivacaine, occurring in only 73% of intravascular injections during general anesthesia. These data suggest that careful observation of the ECG during test-dose administration may be a sensitive indicator of unintended intravascular injection of bupivacaine in the child anesthetized with a volatile agent. All leads appear to be equally sensitive for detecting these changes.[65] The ECG changes after the epinephrine-containing test dose appear to be the result of the

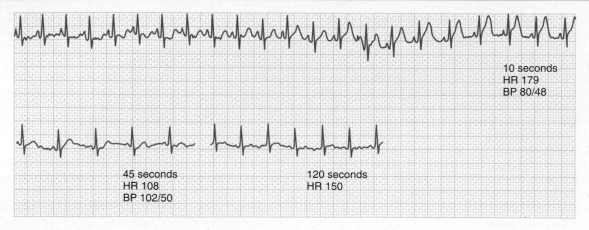

Figure 42-1. ECG changes associated with the intravenous injection of bupivacaine and epinephrine 1:200,000. Note the marked increase in the height of the T wave. (Reproduced with permission from Freid EB, Bailey AG, Valley RD: Electrocardiographic and hemodynamic changes associated with unintentional intravascular injection of bupivacaine with epinephrine in children. Anesthesiology 1993; 79:394-398.)

combination of the two drugs and not what would occur with either drug alone (see further).

Plasma protein binding is the most important pharmacologic factor that determines the toxicity of local anesthetics, particularly for amides, because it is the free (unbound) fraction of the drug that produces toxicity. Reduced plasma protein concentrations cause more drug to remain in the unbound active form with greater potential for toxicity (see Chapter 6). Concentrations of both albumin and α_1-acid glycoprotein are less in neonates, producing clinically crucial differences in the free fraction of amide local anesthetics among neonates, older children, and adults.[66] The significantly greater concentrations of free lidocaine and bupivacaine in infants and neonates are attributed primarily to the decreased level of α_1-acid glycoprotein, which is the primary binding protein of these drugs.[31,67-70] Current data suggest that the plasma concentration of free drug may be 30% greater in infants younger than 6 months of age and even greater in preterm infants than in adolescents.[70a] α_1-Acid glycoprotein is an acute phase reactant; the levels of this protein have been shown to increase after surgery. Concentrations of α_1-acid glycoprotein in infants were less in those undergoing elective rather than emergency surgery.[71] It is not known whether these increased α_1-acid glycoprotein concentrations are sufficient to afford any protective effect on the risk of toxicity from bupivacaine accumulation in the perioperative period.

Plasma concentrations of lidocaine that depress the cardiovascular and respiratory systems in neonates are about half those that cause similar toxicity in adults.[72] In contrast, 2-day-old guinea pigs were less susceptible to the toxic effects of bupivacaine than 2-week or 2-month-old pigs, even though the blood concentrations achieved in the 2-day olds were greater.[57] Data regarding toxicity in infant versus adolescent versus adult rats for both bupivacaine and ropivacaine are similar.[44] Young dogs, however, have a decreased threshold to both seizure and cardiac toxicity caused by excessive doses of bupivacaine.[73] Because species differences are important in toxicity studies, it is difficult to predict which study better represents the human neonate.[74] No data exist in humans regarding age-dependent differences in the toxic threshold of bupivacaine at a given blood concentration. Seizures and cardiovascular collapse have been reported in human infants at the usual adult blood concentrations of bupivacaine. Whereas data from some animal studies suggest that the greater volume of distribution of amides in younger children may protect against bupivacaine toxicity, retrospective analyses of large databases of infants who have received epidural infusions indicate that these findings may not be applicable to the human infant, particularly during continuous infusions or with repeated dosing. Current data on the pharmacokinetic and pharmacodynamic differences associated with early infancy suggest that caution should be exercised when using local anesthetics in infants. Several reports document that infants and children may develop evidence of systemic toxicity, including dysrhythmias, seizures, and cardiovascular compromise from the accumulation of epidural infusions of bupivacaine.[31,75-78] Meticulous attention must be paid to the total dose, rate of administration, site of injection, and the use of vasoconstrictors to diminish the rate of uptake of the local anesthetic. This is particularly important when a continuous regional anesthetic technique is used postoperatively or during prolonged surgery when repeated doses of local anesthetic are administered.

We recommend that both the bolus and infusion doses of bupivacaine and lidocaine be reduced by 30% for infants younger than 6 months of age to decrease the risk for toxicity. This would result in a maximal bupivacaine rate of not more than 0.3 mg/kg/hr.[32] Whereas these recommendations are particularly applicable to the use of continuous bupivacaine infusions for postoperative analgesia, the same caveats apply to large single injections, repeated injections, and continuous infusions of local anesthetics during long surgical procedures.

The d-stereoisomer of local anesthetics may also be a primary factor in the risk for both cardiac and CNS toxicity.[60] As described earlier, both ropivacaine and levobupivacaine are l-enantiomers and have decreased toxicity compared with bupivacaine, a racemic mixture, in adults and experimental animals.[61] This may be at least partly due to the reduced affinity of cardiac and CNS tissues for the l-enantiomer.[43] The introduction of levobupivacaine and ropivacaine into the clinical armamentarium may prove beneficial in decreasing local anesthetic toxicity.

Prevention of Toxicity

There are few data that correlate the anesthetic block, blood concentration of local anesthetic, and dose in infants and children. Most dosing guidelines have been extrapolated from studies in adults. Table 42-2 lists the maximum recommended doses of local anesthetics as well as their approximate durations of action. To avoid overdose and the possibility of toxic effects, it is prudent to remain within these guidelines until studies in children clarify the pharmacokinetics and pharmacodynamics of local anesthetics for specific nerve blocks. As discussed earlier, all of these doses should be reduced by 30% in infants younger than 6 months of age.

Toxic reactions from the administration of local anesthetics are a function of (1) the total dose administered, (2) the site of administration, (3) the rate of uptake, (4) pharmacologic alterations in toxic threshold, (5) the technique of administration, (6) the rate of degradation, metabolism, and excretion of local anesthetic, and (7) the acid-base status of the child.[79-84]

Total Drug Dose

The dose of local anesthetic should be determined according to a child's age, physical status, the area to be anesthetized, and *weight according to lean body mass*. A severely ill child who is in congestive heart failure, for example, has a reduced capacity to metabolize amide local anesthetics because of a reduced cardiac output and hepatic blood flow. Similarly, a markedly obese child must not be given a larger dose simply on the basis of increased weight. If a large volume of local anesthetic is required for a particular procedure, a lower concentration should be used to avoid exceeding maximal safe dosage recommendations. Dosages are calculated based on the lean body weight of the child (e.g., a 20-kg child could receive up to 50 mg of bupivacaine). An easy approximation for bupivacaine is 1 mL/kg of 0.25% bupivacaine, reduced by approximately one third for infants younger than 6 months of age.

Site of Injection

Injection of local anesthetics into very vascular areas leads to greater blood concentrations than the same dose injected into less vascular areas. The order of uptake (i.e., maximum blood concentration) of local anesthetics (in order from greatest to least) with regional blocks in adults is (1) intercostal nerve blocks, (2) caudal blocks, (3) epidural blocks, and (4) brachial plexus and femoral-sciatic nerve blocks.[85] An easy way to remember this is by the mnemonic ICE Block:

I = intercostal
C = caudal
E = epidural
Block = peripheral nerve blocks

Studies are required to determine whether this order holds true for children. Blood concentrations of bupivacaine twice those measured in older children have been reported in children weighing less than 15 kg after ilioinguinal nerve block for herniorrhaphy using only 1.25 mg/kg of 0.5% bupivacaine without epinephrine, which is half the usual recommended maximal dose.[28] However, the fascia iliaca block in older children produced blood concentrations of bupivacaine that were within the acceptable safe range.[86] Local infiltration of the wound in herniorrhaphy has not been associated with increased blood concentrations of local anesthetics,[87] but scalp infiltration during neurosurgery may produce relatively greater blood concentrations.[88] As would be expected, spinal anesthesia results in very small blood levels, even in neonates.[70]

Rate of Uptake

The rate of uptake of a local anesthetic depends on the vascularity of the site of injection. Increased perfusion increases the uptake of local anesthetic, whereas decreased perfusion decreases the uptake.[89] The rate of uptake in children is usually more rapid than in adults. In general, the addition of a vasoconstrictor to the local anesthetic reduces the rate of uptake and prolongs the duration of the block. In adults, the dose of epinephrine is usually limited when used in conjunction with potent anesthetic agents because of the risk of inducing cardiac arrhythmias. If epinephrine is combined with the ester anesthetics, there is no increased risk of arrhythmias. For example, in adults anesthetized with halothane, the maximum recommended dose of epinephrine is 1.0 to 1.5 µg/kg. In children, however, larger doses of epinephrine may be safe.[90-92] We have used as much as 10 µg/kg of epinephrine in children, with a maximum dose of 250 µg, during halothane anesthesia without evidence of ventricular irritability. An epinephrine concentration of 1:100,000 should not be exceeded, and 1:200,000 or less is generally used. A quick reference for converting local anesthetic concentrations and the amount of epinephrine in various dilutions is presented in Tables 42-3 and 42-4. *Epinephrine is contraindicated in blocks in which vasoconstriction of an end-artery could lead to tissue necrosis, such as for digital and penile blocks.*

Alteration in Toxic Threshold

Medications such as diazepam or midazolam, which increase the seizure threshold (i.e., the threshold for CNS toxicity) can

Table 42-2. Maximum Recommended Doses and Duration of Action of Commonly Used Local Anesthetics

Local Anesthetic	Maximum Dose (mg/kg)*	Duration of Action (min)†
Procaine	10	60-90
2-Chloroprocaine	20	30-60
Tetracaine	1.5	180-600
Lidocaine	7	90-200
Mepivacaine	7	120-240
Bupivacaine	2.5	180-600
Ropivacaine	3	120-240

*These are maximum doses of local anesthetics. Doses of amides should be decreased by 30% in infants younger than 6 months of age. When lidocaine is being administered intravascularly (e.g., during intravenous regional anesthesia), the dose should be decreased to 3 to 5 mg/kg; there is no need to administer long-acting local anesthetic agents for intravenous regional anesthesia, and such a practice is potentially dangerous.
†Duration of action is dependent on concentration, total dose, site of administration, and the child's age.

Table 42-3. Epinephrine Dilution and Conversion to µg/mL

Epinephrine Dilution	µg/mL
1:100,000	10
1:200,000	5
1:400,000	2.5
1:800,000	1.25

Table 42-4. Local Anesthetic Concentration and its Conversion to mg/mL

Concentration (percent)	mg/mL
3	30
2.5	25
2	20
1	10
0.5	5
0.25	2.5
0.125	1.25

be valuable adjuncts to regional anesthesia. Premedication with diazepam (0.15 to 0.3 mg/kg) decreases a child's anxiety but also offers some protection from the toxic CNS effects of a local anesthetic overdose.[93] Although diazepam is no longer in common clinical use in children in the perioperative period, evidence in animal models and considerable clinical experience in humans suggests that midazolam is also effective in terminating seizure activity.[94] Animal data, however, suggest that the concomitant use of diazepam and bupivacaine decreases the elimination of bupivacaine from serum and cardiac tissue in mice.[95] This effect is not due to changes in protein binding.[96] It is not known if this is true for all benzodiazepines or if this is also the case in humans. Although premedication with a benzodiazepine prevents manifestations of CNS toxicity, the threshold for cardiovascular toxicity is unchanged.[97] Thus, after premedication with a benzodiazepine, cardiovascular collapse may occur without any warning because the symptoms of CNS toxicity may be blunted. Because most regional anesthetics that are performed in children are placed after induction of general anesthesia (with the exception of some blocks in former preterm infants), this may be a moot point in most circumstances.

Technique of Administration

Whenever regional anesthesia is performed, the operator must be prepared for an adverse reaction and resuscitation supplies, including drugs, suction, and airway equipment, must be immediately available. The needle or catheter must always be inspected for blood as soon as it is positioned, but before injecting the local anesthetic, to determine if the tip is within an artery or vein. It is preferable to observe the needle or catheter for passive blood flow rather than to actively aspirate for blood because the blood vessels such as the epidural venous plexus are thin walled and collapse readily when negative pressure is applied. As a result, the inability to aspirate blood is not absolute proof that the needle or catheter is not in a blood vessel. For this reason, a small volume of local anesthetic with a marker for intravascular injection such as epinephrine in a concentration of 1:200,000, is employed whenever possible. Data from awake adults indicate that this will result in an increase in heart rate within 1 minute of intravascular administration.[98] When the drugs are administered during a general anesthetic, however, the efficacy of the test dose to detect an intravascular injection may be greatly reduced. Heart rate increases in only 73% of children after an intravenous injection of 0.5 μg/kg of epinephrine during halothane anesthesia, suggesting that this marker of an intravascular

injection is not completely reliable.[99] Administration of atropine several minutes before the test dose increased the rate of positive responders to 92%, suggesting that vagal tone and the anesthetic's blunting of the sympathetic reflexes are responsible for the reduced sensitivity of the test dose. Test doses during isoflurane anesthesia appear to have the same limitations.[100] With sevoflurane, positive results were obtained in 100% of children if the threshold for a positive response was an increase in heart rate of 10 beats per minute and a dose in excess of 0.5 μg/kg of epinephrine was used; in 85% positive results were obtained if 0.25 μg/kg of epinephrine was used.[101] In all children, a change in the T wave amplitude was a reliable indicator of intravascular injection with both doses of epinephrine (Fig. 42-1). All children in that study were pretreated with atropine. It is not known if increasing the dose of epinephrine to 1.0 μg/kg or increasing the concentration of epinephrine in the test dose solution to 1:100,000 during general anesthesia would increase the sensitivity of the heart rate response test without atropine. Systolic blood pressure increased by more than 10% within 60 seconds of the test dose injection, suggesting that an increase in blood pressure may be a more sensitive indicator of intravascular injection than heart rate during inhalation anesthesia. ST segment and T wave changes also appear to be sensitive indicators of intravascular injection of local anesthetic. Observation of the ECG yields a highly sensitive indicator of an intravascular injection of bupivacaine with epinephrine. These ECG changes were present in 97% of infants and children who received an intravenous dose of bupivacaine and epinephrine.[63] These investigators did not confirm the efficacy of pretreatment with atropine on the heart rate. Isoproterenol (added to the local anesthetic rather than epinephrine), 0.075 to 0.1 μg/kg, increases the heart rate in 90% to 100% of children during halothane anesthesia.[102,103] It also increases the heart rate in adults during isoflurane and sevoflurane anesthesia, but this has not been extensively studied in children.[104-106] Until more data are available, it would appear most prudent to use an epinephrine-containing test dose before administering the therapeutic dose of local anesthetic for neural blockade.[101] The test dose should be repeated before any subsequent bolus injections through a catheter. If the child is receiving a general inhalation anesthetic, blood pressure and the ST segment configuration, in addition to the heart rate, should be carefully and frequently observed after injection of the test dose.[65] Pretreatment with atropine may increase the rate of detecting an unintended intravascular injection. In addition, the rate of injection may also be a factor in the development of toxicity. If injection is partially or completely intravascular, a slow injection may not exceed the toxic threshold, whereas a rapid injection could. Thus, slow incremental injection of the therapeutic blocking dose of local anesthetic (over several minutes) may further increase the safety of regional blockade. However, repeated injections within a brief period may also result in toxic reactions.

To date there are no published data testing the reliability of positive test dose criteria during total intravenous anesthesia with propofol and remifentanil. Preliminary unpublished data by one of us (D.M.P.) suggest that T wave changes may be an unreliable indicator of intravascular injection and that intravascular injection can be reliably detected by an increase of blood pressure of more than 10% of baseline, particularly diastolic pressure.

Treatment of Toxic Reactions

Treatment of toxic reactions to local anesthetic overdose requires knowledge of the signs and symptoms previously described. Toxicity from large concentrations of bupivacaine, especially cardiac toxicity, is particularly difficult to treat, and it must be recognized that the signs of local anesthetic toxicity, with the exception of the catastrophic cardiovascular events, are all masked by general anesthesia. Indeed, inhaled anesthetics may actually raise the threshold for seizures and thereby delay the detection of toxicity until cardiovascular collapse occurs. Even in the nonanesthetized child, the progression from prodromal signs to cardiovascular collapse may be very rapid and the initial definitive therapy in some cases may need to be directed at reestablishing circulation and normal cardiac rhythm. As always, initial management should consist of establishing and maintaining a patent airway and providing supplemental oxygen. The timely administration of a CNS depressant that alters the seizure threshold may prevent seizures. Midazolam (0.05-0.2 mg/kg IV), thiopental (2-3 mg/kg IV), and propofol (1-3 mg/kg) effectively prevent or terminate seizure activity. If seizure activity is present, the use of succinylcholine or other relaxant may facilitate tracheal intubation but does not prevent seizure activity. It should be remembered, however, that the acute morbidity from seizures is the result of airway complications (hypoxia and aspiration) and that securing the airway takes precedence over the actual control of the electrical activity of the seizure. CNS excitability is exacerbated in the presence of hypercarbia; it is, therefore, important to mildly hyperventilate children who have seizures.

Recent advances in the treatment of bupivacaine toxicity have dramatically altered the sequence of therapeutic interventions that should be initiated in the event of cardiovascular collapse after a large intravascular injection of bupivacaine. Intravenous lipid emulsion has been shown to be very effective for resuscitation of cardiac arrest due to bupivacaine toxicity. In dogs, successful resuscitation after cardiac arrest and 10 minutes of external cardiac massage was demonstrated after lipid administration.[107] Although 100% of the dogs that received an infusion of 20% lipid emulsion were successfully resuscitated, none of the controls that received a saline infusion survived. These animal studies have been corroborated with several anecdotal reports of rescue from cardiac arrest after intravascular injections of all of the amide local anesthetics in common use.[108-111] The mechanism of action of lipid emulsions in bupivacaine toxicity is not entirely understood, but studies in isolated rat heart preparations concluded that lipid treatment promotes the elution of bupivacaine from the myocardium and accelerates the recovery from bupivacaine-induced asystole.[112] This "lipid sink" hypothesis suggests a novel mechanism of action as compared with more conventional anti-dysrhythmic drugs and appears to be more effective as well. The adult literature suggests that 1 mL/kg of 20% lipid emulsion should be administered over 1 minute and repeated every 3 to 5 minutes up to a maximum of 3 mL/kg, followed by a maintenance infusion rate of 0.25 mL/kg/min until the circulation is restored.[113] To date, there is only one published pediatric report with this intervention but success was achieved with a single injection 3 mL/kg over 3 minutes of 20% lipid emulsion.[109] Therefore, the dose of lipids in children remains speculative. There is a growing consensus that 20% lipid emulsions should be immediately available in any location where regional anesthesia is performed to permit rapid treatment of cardiac toxicity. A lipid emulsion of propofol is not recommended as a substitute for Intralipid for resuscitation from bupivacaine toxicity.

Because the initial stage of cardiovascular toxicity consists of peripheral vasodilation, supportive treatment should include intravenous fluid loading (10 to 20 mL/kg of isotonic crystalloid) and, if necessary, titration of a peripheral vasoconstrictor such as phenylephrine (initial rate of 0.1 µg/kg/min) to maintain vascular tone and systemic blood pressure at acceptable limits. As toxicity progresses to cardiovascular collapse, profound decreases in myocardial contractility occur, followed by dysrhythmias. In dogs, echocardiography showed that decreased systolic function always preceded the development of dysrhythmias. In rats, norepinephrine was more effective than epinephrine, dopamine, isoproterenol, or amrinone to treat bupivacaine cardiac toxicity.[114,115] A report in infants suggested that phenytoin (5 mg/kg administered by a slow intravenous infusion) treated bupivacaine cardiac toxicity.[116] Many toxic reactions are self-limited because the local anesthetic redistributes throughout the body and plasma concentrations rapidly decrease. Excretion of local anesthetic is hastened by hydration and alkalization of the urine by intravenous administration of sodium bicarbonate.[117,118] Cardiopulmonary bypass has also been used to successfully resuscitate an adult with bupivacaine-induced cardiac toxicity.[119] All current data, however, strongly suggest that lipid infusion is the most successful therapy for local anesthetic cardiotoxicity, and immediate administration of this agent should be the first line of therapy.

Hypersensitivity to Local Anesthetics

Hypersensitivity reactions to local anesthetics are rare.[120-122] Ester local anesthetics are metabolized to *p*-aminobenzoic acid, which is usually responsible for allergic reactions in this group. However, these agents may cause allergic phenomena in children who are sensitive to sulfonamides, sulfites, or thiazide diuretics.[123,124] Among the amide local anesthetics, only one case of a true allergic reaction has been documented. These drugs may contain the preservative, methylparaben, which may produce allergic reactions in those sensitive to *p*-aminobenzoic acid.[124,125] When in doubt, local anesthetic allergy must be ruled out. Detailed protocols are described elsewhere.[126]

Equipment

Use of Ultrasound

Recently there has been great interest in the use of ultrasound-guided peripheral nerve blocks in children.[127] The availability of high-resolution portable ultrasound machines has become increasingly commonplace and will likely soon become the new standard of care for many peripheral nerve blocks. Although this requires sophisticated expensive equipment, it may have a larger role in pediatric regional blockade because most blocks are performed while the child is anesthetized. Several manufacturers make ultrasound machines that are about the size of a laptop computer and have been designed for ease of use by the anesthesiologist. The cost-effectiveness of acquiring these devices is justified because they serve a dual purpose for placing invasive central lines. Direct visualization of the nerve may facilitate correct placement of the local anesthetic and may also help reduce the total dose of local anesthetic needed for successful blockade. It is imperative to use an ultrasound machine that is capable of scanning superficially because most of the nerves in children are usually less than a few millimeters from the skin. A more in-depth discussion of ultrasound guidance for peripheral nerve blocks can be found in Chapter 43.

Use of a Nerve Stimulator

Because peripheral nerve blocks are commonly performed in sedated or anesthetized infants and children, the use of a peripheral nerve stimulator is a safe and effective method to locate the nerve to be blocked. A nerve stimulator is not a substitute for anatomic knowledge but is a useful adjunct that allows the performance of the block in an unconscious or uncooperative heavily sedated child. It avoids the need to seek sensory paresthesias or to rely on anatomic landmarks alone and may diminish the potential for injury caused by needle impingement of a nerve. The tiny amount of current flowing from the uninsulated needle tip stimulates the nerve and produces a motor response when the needle is in close proximity to the nerve. The nerve stimulator is connected to a child as shown in Figure 42-2. The cathode (negative pole) cable must be attached to the low output terminal of the nerve stimulator. The cathode cable is attached via a sterile alligator clip to the proximal (uninsulated) shaft of a Teflon-insulated needle or to the plug-in lead of a specially designed block needle, and the anode (positive lead) is connected to the child via an ECG electrode, distant to the block site.[128,129] The needle is advanced in the appropriate anatomic direction, and when it is believed to be in the correct position the nerve stimulator is adjusted to approximately 0.5 mA with repetitive single pulse output at 1-second intervals. Local muscle contraction should be minimal at this setting, although direct muscle stimulation can occur and must be distinguished from neural stimulation. The area innervated by the nerves to be blocked is observed for the appropriate muscle contractions. As the uninsulated needle tip approaches the nerve, the muscle contractions will increase in intensity and become less strong as it moves away from the nerve. One should be able to decrease the current to approximately 0.2 mA with continued elicitation of easily perceptible muscle contraction to be sure that the needle tip is correctly positioned. It should be noted that the injection of even a very small volume of local anesthetic will ablate or dramatically attenuate responses produced by the low current of the nerve stimulator, so the needle position should be optimized before injection. The responses to stimulation of the radial, median, ulnar, and musculocutaneous nerves are

shown in Figure 42-3. Despite the introduction of ultrasound guidance for placement of peripheral nerve blocks, it is still common practice among most practitioners to verify the position of the tip of the needle using a nerve stimulator. The limitation with the use of ultrasound guidance is the absence of echogenic needles.

Specific Procedures

Central Neuraxial Blockade

Anatomic and Physiologic Considerations

Several anatomic and physiologic differences between adults and children affect the performance of regional anesthetic techniques. The conus medullaris (the terminus of the spinal cord) in neonates and infants is located at the L3 vertebral level, which is more caudal than in adults. It does not reach the adult level at L1 until approximately 1 year of age (Fig. 42-4) owing to the difference in the rates of growth between the spinal cord and the bony vertebral column. Thus, lumbar puncture for subarachnoid block in neonates and infants should be performed at the L4-L5 or L5-S1 interspace to avoid needle injury to the spinal cord. The vertebral laminae are poorly calcified at this age, so a midline approach is preferable to a paramedian one in which the needle is "walked off" the laminae. Another anatomic difference is noted in the sacrum. In neonates, the sacrum is narrower and flatter than in adults (see Fig. 42-4). The approach to the subarachnoid space from the caudal canal is much more direct in neonates than in adults, making dural puncture more likely, so the needle must not be advanced deeply in neonates.[130] The presence of a deep sacral dimple may be associated with spina bifida occulta, greatly increasing the probability of dural puncture. Thus, a caudal block may be contraindicated in these children.

The distance from the skin to the subarachnoid space, which is very small in neonates (approximately 1.4 cm), increases progressively with age (Fig. 42-5).[131] The ligamentum flavum is much thinner and less dense in infants and children than in adults, which makes the engagement of the epidural needle more difficult to detect and unintended dural puncture during epidural catheter placement a greater risk for the infrequent operator. Cerebrospinal fluid (CSF) volume as a percentage of body weight is greater in infants and young children than in adults (Fig. 42-6), although these studies are limited.[132-136] This

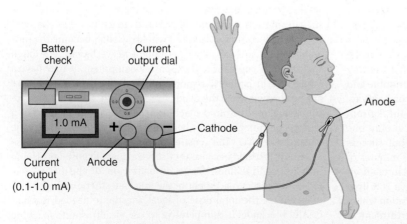

Figure 42-2. A nerve stimulator should be used to locate a nerve in a child who is anesthetized and in the awake, sedated child to avoid the need to seek a sensory paresthesia. In this example, the brachial plexus is sought in the axilla. Note that the appropriate muscle response to nerve stimulation is elicited at 0.5-mA current and should continue to respond with 0.2-mA current.

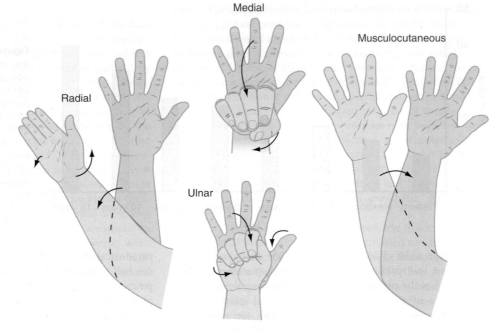

Figure 42-3. Characteristic movements of the fingers, wrist, and elbow in response to nerve stimulation. (Modified with permission from Cousins MJ, Bridenbaugh PO [eds]: Neural Blockade in Clinical Anesthesia and Management of Pain, 2nd ed. Philadelphia, JB Lippincott, 1988, p 406.)

finding may account in part for the comparatively larger doses of local anesthetics required for surgical anesthesia with subarachnoid block in infants and young children. The CSF turnover rate is also considerably greater in infants and children, accounting in part for the much briefer duration of subarachnoid block with any given agent compared with adults. Obviously, these anatomic differences necessitate meticulous

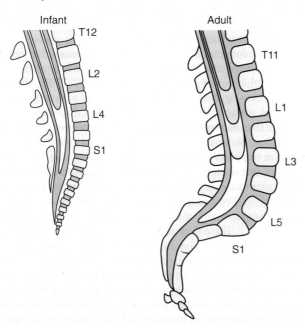

Figure 42-4. Anatomic differences between adults and children that affect the performance of spinal and epidural anesthesia; an infant's sacrum (*left*) is flatter and narrower than an adult's (*right*). Note that the tip of the spinal cord in a neonate ends at L3 and does not achieve the normal adult position (L1-2) until approximately 1 year of age. The relative location of the spinal cord with growth to adulthood is illustrated on the right as different shades of yellow with the darkest being the final adult configuration.

attention to detail to achieve successful and uncomplicated spinal or epidural anesthesia.

In contrast to older children and adults, subarachnoid and epidural blockade in infants and small children is characterized by hemodynamic stability, even when the level of the block reaches the upper thoracic dermatomes.[137,138] Although heart rate variability, as determined by spectral analysis, is lower, the heart rate is preserved, because the parasympathetic activity modulating heart rate appears to be attenuated in infants receiving spinal anesthesia.[139] This attenuated vagal tone allows the heart rate to compensate for any alterations in peripheral vascular tone. This appears to be a greater factor in the preservation of hemodynamic stability than other factors, such as the relatively small venous capacitance in the lower extremities in infants and the relative lack of resting sympathetic peripheral vascular tone.[140] Nonetheless, data suggest that alterations in vascular resistance and blood flow to some vascular beds may occur, at least under certain conditions, in infants. In former preterm infants who received isobaric bupivacaine for subarachnoid block, cerebral blood flow was reduced concomitant with systemic blood pressure changes, although the conditions under which the baseline pressures were measured were not clear.[141] In a study in which changes in regional temperature were used as a surrogate sign of sympathetic activity, extremity but not trunk temperature increased during subarachnoid block, together with small insignificant changes in blood pressure.[142] In our clinical experience, and that of others including the University of Vermont neonatal spinal anesthesia database (more than 1700 cases), clinically significant systemic blood pressure changes do not occur in young infants after a subarachnoid block (R. Williams, personal communication).

Central neuraxial blockade can affect the respiratory mechanics of the chest wall and diaphragm by virtue of the diminution of intercostal muscle activity. This may be particularly relevant in infants and young children, whose chest walls are very compliant due to limited ossification of the ribs.[143] Infants rely to a greater extent on the diaphragm for the maintenance of tidal

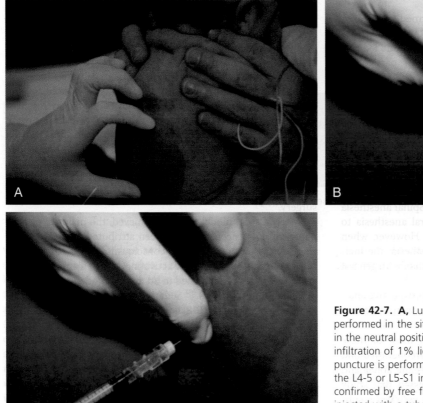

Figure 42-7. A, Lumbar puncture in a neonate or infant is generally performed in the sitting position. Note that the head is maintained in the neutral position to prevent airway obstruction. **B,** After local infiltration of 1% lidocaine with a 25- to 30-gauge needle, lumbar puncture is performed with a 22-gauge 1.5-inch styletted needle at the L4-5 or L5-S1 interspace. Entrance into the subarachnoid space is confirmed by free flow of cerebrospinal fluid. **C,** Local anesthetic is injected with a tuberculin syringe. Care must be taken not to inject rapidly or a high level of blockade might result.

the child's legs should be maintained at the horizontal level to preclude cephalad spread of the local anesthetic and a "total" spinal anesthesia (Fig. 42-8A, B).[189] The grounding pad can be safely placed by lifting the entire infant, while maintaining the body in the horizontal plane, or the pad can be affixed to the anterior thigh if sufficient space and muscle mass are available.

Because spinal anesthesia maintains hemodynamic stability in infants, some pediatric anesthesiologists have advocated

starting the intravenous line after the onset of lower extremity analgesia. Although this may be relatively safe in this setting, if a "total spinal" occurred and the airway had to be instrumented or resuscitation drugs had to be administered, having intravenous access would be important. In addition, should intravenous access prove difficult, valuable operating time would be lost while searching for a suitable vein. We have found that applying the pulse oximeter to a toe of one leg and the blood

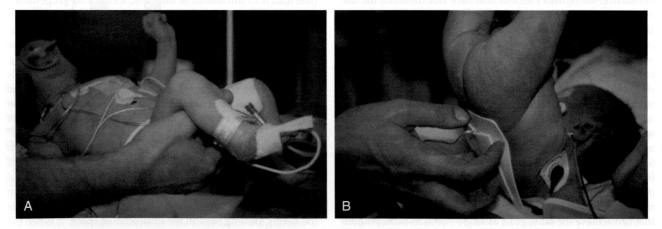

Figure 42-8. A, The proper method of applying an electrocautery pad; the infant's entire body is elevated while maintaining the horizontal position to avoid excessively high spread of subarachnoid blockade. **B,** Improper method of applying an electrocautery pad in a neonate after subarachnoid administration of local anesthetic; the legs should never be elevated.

pressure cuff to the thigh of the other allows the neonate to remain undisturbed during a surgical procedure (e.g., inguinal herniorrhaphy) (Fig. 42-9, see website).

Because the addition of sedatives has been associated with postanesthetic apnea with an incidence at least as great as that of general anesthesia, we try to avoid all sedatives, especially ketamine.[167] Many, if not most, neonates will fall asleep once the block has set, in large part due to the lack of afferent input through the infant's largest sensory organ, the skin. A pacifier dipped in 50% dextrose will also help the infant to remain quiet and still. Gentle restraint is necessary in some cases. It is particularly important for the infant to be still and not bear down when the hernia sac is being dissected to avoid the extrusion of abdominal contents through the open hernia.

Selection of Drug

Neonates and Infants. The proportional dose of local anesthetic required for subarachnoid block in neonates is much greater than that required for adults. When calculated on a per kilogram basis, there is a near 10-fold greater drug requirement in neonates to reach a similar dermatomal distribution as for adults. In addition, the duration of the relatively larger dose lasts only about one third to one half as long as in the adult. As discussed previously, this appears to be at least in part due to the greater volume of CSF per kilogram and to the more rapid turnover of CSF in this age group. The drugs that have commonly been used for spinal anesthesia in neonates and infants include tetracaine, bupivacaine, and lidocaine.[132,190-194] Reported doses of tetracaine range from 0.22 to 1.0 mg/kg, with larger doses used more commonly to achieve an adequate height and duration of blockade. We use hyperbaric tetracaine (0.75-1.0 mg/kg [equal volumes of tetracaine 1.0% and 10% dextrose]) with 0.01 mL/kg of epinephrine (1:100,000). Epinephrine has been shown to prolong the duration of block by more than 30%.[195] We prepare a 1:1,000 epinephrine solution in a tuberculin or glass syringe and expel the contents in the manner of heparinizing a blood gas syringe. This leaves only a residual amount of epinephrine "wash" in the hub of the needle. The tetracaine dose and dextrose, if they are packaged separately, are combined. This dose usually provides adequate analgesia for inguinal hernia repair with a duration of motor block of 90 to 120 minutes and a dermatome height in the mid to upper thoracic region. For surgeries of limited duration that involve a lower extremity, smaller doses (0.5 to 0.6 mg/kg) may be used. Both isobaric and hyperbaric bupivacaine (0.5-1.0 mg/kg of a 0.5% solution) have been used in neonates and infants, with a reported duration similar to that of tetracaine, although the duration of action of the isobaric solution is slightly greater than for the hyperbaric solution.[193,194,196] A dose-ranging study reported that the addition of clonidine (1 µg/kg) prolonged the duration of blockade from a mean of 67 minutes (plain bupivacaine) to 111 minutes.[197] The use of larger doses of clonidine (2 µg/kg), however, caused transient hypotension and apnea, which required treatment with caffeine. Although lidocaine (2 mg/kg) is useful for a block of brief duration, such as for a muscle biopsy of the lower extremity, the duration of useful block is only approximately 30 minutes. In light of concerns regarding lidocaine in the subarachnoid space, we no longer recommend it in infants.[198-200] A summary of doses for commonly used local anesthetics for subarachnoid block in neonates and infants is provided in Table 42-5.

Children. There is little information on the doses of local anesthetics for spinal anesthesia in children, as subarachnoid block is much less commonly used outside the neonatal period. When a regional technique is desirable in children, an epidural or caudal block together with a "light" general anesthetic is preferable. For spinal anesthesia, 0.3 to 0.5 mg/kg of bupivacaine (5 mg/mL concentration) may be used in children 2 months to 12 years of age.[188] Doses of 0.3 to 0.4 mg/kg hyperbaric tetracaine have been used for subarachnoid block in children aged 12 weeks to 2 years and 0.2 to 0.3 mg/kg in children older than 2 years.[201-203] Based on these limited data, the dose requirement for spinal anesthesia decreases with increasing age. Because there are few data available on drug doses and the height of anesthetic block produced in this age group, it is prudent to use these values as an appropriate reference point and to revise the dose as dictated by clinical experience.

Complications

Complications after spinal anesthesia include total spinal anesthesia, post-dural puncture headache, backache, neurologic sequelae, and the risk of lumbar epidermoid tumors if nonstyletted needles are used for subarachnoid puncture.[187-189,204-210]

Total spinal anesthesia has been reported in neonates. It is manifested by apnea with no change in systemic blood pressure.[189] It can occur after a dose of as little as 0.6 mg/kg of tetracaine.[189] Alteration in position, particularly by raising the lower body above the level of the head or thorax, may be the most common factor that predisposes to excessive high levels of blockade. Although the rate of administration of the local anesthetic does not appear to affect the level of spinal anesthesia in adults, no such studies have been carried out in neonates or infants.[211] It is possible that factors such as the use of a relatively large-bore needle (22-gauge) and a tuberculin syringe providing the means for injecting with high pressure, along with the small distance between vertebrae, combine to make the rate of injection an important consideration in neonates and infants by producing unintended barbotage. We have also observed this complication with rapid drug administration. Management consists of assisted or controlled ventilation until the return of spontaneous respiratory function.

The incidence of post-dural puncture headache appears to be infrequent in infants and children, although the incidence in preverbal children is unknown. An early study reported an incidence of spinal headache of approximately 2% using 20- to 22-gauge needles in children 2 to 17 years of age.[203] However, no details were provided about the distribution of headache with respect to age. Other studies reported a 5% incidence of headaches in children ranging from 2 months to nearly 10 years of age, but, again, no age distribution was cited.[187,188] A prospec-

Table 42-5. Local Anesthetics for Spinal Anesthesia in Neonates and Infants

Anesthetic Drug	Usual Dose (mg/kg)	Range (mg/kg)
1% Tetracaine in 5% dextrose	0.75	0.6-1
0.5% Bupivacaine (isobaric)	0.8	0.5-1[191]
0.75% Bupivacaine in 8.25% dextrose	0.6	0.5-1[192]

question of contamination, the catheter should be promptly removed.

It is preferable to place epidural catheters at a lumbar or thoracic interspace. Advantages include exclusion of the insertion site from the diaper area, with less risk of contamination by stool and urine; closer proximity to the desired tip location; and smaller volume of drug required for a more cephalad dermatomal level (if the caudal catheter is not threaded cephalad). Both lumbar and thoracic epidural catheters may be safely placed in anesthetized infants and children by experienced anesthesiologists.[234] Although the risks of neural injury in the unconscious child are theoretically increased, no longitudinal studies have shown this to be the case in practice. They have confirmed the safety of these techniques when performed by experienced pediatric anesthesiologists.[235] Indeed, many of the arguments against regional anesthesia in the unconscious child are of speculative validity, especially when one considers as the alternative a moving and uncooperative child.[234]

The technique for both lumbar and thoracic epidural catheter placement is similar to that in adults, with certain important exceptions (see Chapter 43 for ultrasound techniques). The midline approach is most commonly used, for the same reasons cited earlier regarding subarachnoid block. The ligamentum flavum is considerably thinner and less dense in infants than in older children and adults. This makes recognition of engagement in the ligament more difficult and requires both extra care and slower, more deliberate passage of the needle to avoid subarachnoid puncture. It takes experience to perceive the more subtle differences in "feel" that are characteristic of the tissue planes in small children. The angle of approach to the epidural space is slightly more perpendicular to the plane of the back than in older children and adults, owing to the orientation of the spinous processes in infants and small children. The loss of resistance technique should be used, but only with saline, not air. There are several reports of venous air embolism in infants and children when air was used to test for loss of resistance.[236-238] Another method for identifying the epidural space is to attach an intravenous infusion chamber with a mini-drip or other free-flowing fluid delivery device to the epidural needle; commencement of dripping identifies entry into the epidural space (see Video 42-1).[239-241] We use a short (5 cm) 18-gauge Tuohy needle and a 20- or 21-gauge catheter in infants and children. The shorter length offers much better control than an adult-length (10 cm) needle. These catheters have fewer problems than the 24-gauge needle, and the needle diameter is reasonable for use in small infants. Epidural kits specifically for infants and children are available.

Selection of Drug. The drug dose required for epidural blockade to a given dermatomal level depends on the volume (not concentration) of the local anesthetic and the volume of the epidural space, which may change with age. Numerous studies have discussed the doses of local anesthetic drugs used for caudal anesthesia in children.[213,215-217,219,220,222-228] The volumes of local anesthetic that block from a T4 to a T10 dermatome level span a fivefold range. In our experience, the formula of Takasaki and colleagues[220] has best approximated good clinical results:

Volume (mL) = 0.05 mL/kg/dermatome to be blocked

Thus, in a 10-kg child in whom we wish to produce a T10 dermatome level, we would use a volume of (0.05 mL/kg/dermatome) × (10 kg) × (12 dermatomes) = 6 mL.

Another simple method is to administer 1 mL/kg (up to 20 mL) of 0.125% bupivacaine with 1:200,000 epinephrine; this generally provides a sensory block with minimal motor block up to the T4-T6 level.

Because the level of the block depends on the volume of drug administered, the concentration of the local anesthetic should be based on the desired density of the block (less dense for postoperative analgesia, more dense for intraoperative anesthesia) and on the risk of toxicity.

Continuous Epidural Infusions

Although intermittent doses of local anesthetic are often used to maintain epidural anesthesia during a prolonged surgical procedure, it is also common practice to initiate continuous infusions of local anesthetics during surgery. Continuous infusions maintain the block at a constant level, assuming that the infusion rate is appropriate. This obviates the need for repetitive test dosing. Theoretically, fewer entries into the epidural catheter may reduce the risk of infection and the risk of accidental administration of the wrong drug. Strict attention to the total drug administered per hour (i.e., the drug concentration and infusion rate) is required to preclude potentially toxic drug doses. We recommend that the same dosing guidelines for postoperative infusion rates be followed intraoperatively: *a maximum of 0.4 mg/kg/hr of bupivacaine after the initial block is established, with this dose reduced by 30% for infants younger than 6 months of age.*[32] The concentration of local anesthetic solution that should be used depends on the age of the child, the surgical procedure, and the area that needs to be blocked. When a more dense block is required in a small infant, it may be beneficial to use 2,3-chloroprocaine because it undergoes ester hydrolysis and has a reduced risk of accumulation compared with bupivacaine; a denser block with a more concentrated solution may then be achieved. The newer amides ropivacaine and levobupivacaine may also successfully address these issues and allow the administration of more concentrated agents to produce denser blockade with less potential for adverse effects (see Chapters 43 and 44).

Epidural Opioids

Epidural opioids can be safely used to augment intraoperative anesthesia in children as well as to provide postoperative analgesia. Their use is discussed in detail in Chapter 44. If extubation of the trachea is expected at the end of the surgical procedure, one must take into account both the systemic and the central neuraxial opioid doses to avoid excessive respiratory depression.

Complications

Complications after epidural anesthesia or analgesia include intravascular or intraosseous injection, hematoma, neural injury, and infection. Figure 42-11 illustrates sites of unintended needle placement during the performance of a caudal epidural block. Injection of local anesthetic into an epidural blood vessel or intraosseous injection into the marrow cavity may result in a rapid increase in the blood concentration of the local anesthetic and a toxic reaction. Signs, symptoms, and treatment of such reactions have been discussed previously. It is also possible to pass the needle through the sacrum and perforate bowel or the pelvic organs, particularly in infants in whom ossification of the sacrum is incomplete.

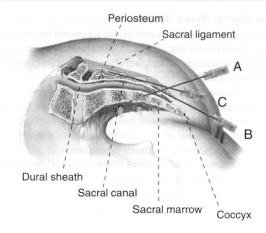

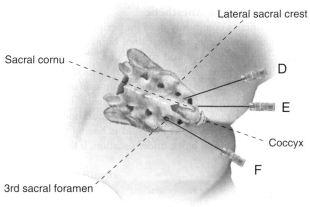

Figure 42-11. Sites of misplacement of local anesthetic for caudal block anesthesia. Note that injection may be made into bone marrow (A), into subperiosteum (B), into posterior sacral ligaments (C), into a false "decoy" hiatus (D), into the anterior sacral wall and possibly out into the pelvis (E), or into a lateral foramen, producing a limited block (F). (Reproduced with permission from Cousins MJ, Bridenbaugh PO [eds]: Neural Blockade in Clinical Anesthesia and Management of Pain, 2nd ed. Philadelphia, JB Lippincott, 1988, p 378.)

Infection is of grave concern when it occurs in either the subarachnoid or the epidural space.[242] A study of 1620 children over a 6-year period found a zero incidence of epidural abscess.[243] Catheters remained in situ for a mean of 2 days (maximum 8 days). The adult literature also suggests that infection is an uncommon complication.[244,245] However, both superficial and deep abscesses may rarely occur, particularly in those patients with immunodeficiency syndromes and cancer who are on long-term infusions.[246] Epidural abscess and meningitis are the most potentially serious complications.[242,247] The development of an epidural abscess is a surgical emergency, because failure to treat it can lead to neurologic injury. The signs and symptoms (Table 42-6) are the same as for epidural hematoma, although fever, increased erythrocyte sedimentation rate, and increased leukocyte count with a leftward shift are also often present. Surgical drainage may be necessary. A large multicenter prospective study of regional anesthesia in children has recently been completed in Great Britain.[248] Over 10,000 children who received continuous epidural blocks were enrolled in the study over 5

years and three serious infections (two epidural abscesses and one case of meningitis) were noted. These infections were all related to insertion site infections. All cultures grew *Staphylococcus aureus.* Twenty-five local infections were reported, mostly *S. aureus,* and 80% were associated with catheters left in place more than 48 hours. Of note is that some localized infections that developed at the catheter insertion site became apparent only days after the removal of the catheter; one of these progressed to an epidural abscess. Whether these infections developed while the catheter was in place, because the bacteria tracked through the open site in the skin after the catheter was removed, or by hematogenous spread is unknown. Infants and toddlers who are in diapers require meticulous management of these catheters and their insertion site. A mild erythema occasionally occurs at the site of catheter insertion when children have indwelling catheters in place for several days, and this must be distinguished from a cellulitis. If there is any question that the site is infected, then the catheter should be removed. Although no serious systemic infection occurred in a prospective study of 210 children with 170 caudal catheters (age 3 ± 1 years) and 40 lumbar epidural catheters (age 11 ± 3 years) that were in place for 3 ± 1 days, 35% were colonized with bacteria.[249] This rate of colonization was similar with both caudal (25%) and lumbar epidural (23%) approaches. These results suggest that colonization is not synonymous with infection. Moreover, the factors that can transform colonization into infection are unknown.

Clinical experience with caudal/epidural catheters has shown that it is common for fluid to leak from the insertion site, especially in the presence of presacral edema. Any child who develops a fever of unknown origin and who also has an indwelling caudal/epidural catheter should have the catheter removed (see Chapter 44).

Epidural hematoma is also a rare complication after epidural blockade. Optimal outcome depends on rapid diagnosis and prompt treatment and decompression. Signs and symptoms are presented in Table 42-6. The presence of clinically important coagulopathy or thrombocytopenia is an unacceptable risk for developing an epidural hematoma and is a contraindication to central neuraxial blockade.

Postoperative, *urinary retention* has been tenuously associated with both epidural and spinal anesthesia. In this regard, it

Table 42-6. Signs and Symptoms of Epidural Hematoma and Abscess

Abscess	Hematoma
Fever	Afebrile
± ↑ WBC	WBC normal
± ↑ Sedimentation rate	Sedimentation rate normal or
± Left WBC shift	slightly elevated
Localized back pain	Localized back pain
Radicular pain	Radicular pain
Paraplegia	Paraplegia
Sensory loss	Sensory loss
Urinary and fecal retention	Urinary and fecal retention
Incontinence	Incontinence
Local tenderness	Local tenderness
Defect on myelography	Defect on myelography
Localized lesion on magnetic resonance imaging	Localized lesion on magnetic resonance imaging

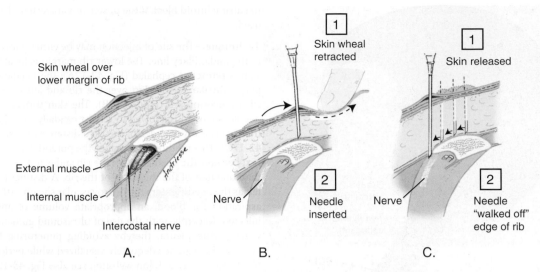

Figure 42-17. Intercostal block. A skin wheal is inserted on the lower rib margin (**A**). The skin wheal is retracted over the body of the rib, and a needle is inserted until contact is made with the rib (**B**). The skin is released, and the needle is carefully "walked" off the edge of the rib margin (**C**).

Technique. The block may be performed either at the beginning of surgery or before the end of general anesthesia. If bupivacaine is used, a minimum of 15 minutes is usually required from the completion of the block until maximal analgesia is obtained. Thus, blocks placed at the beginning of the surgical procedure (our preference) are usually more effective than those performed at the end of surgery. Blocks performed before skin incision may also provide "preemptive analgesia." The duration of postoperative analgesia does not appear to be affected by placement of the block at the beginning of the procedure,

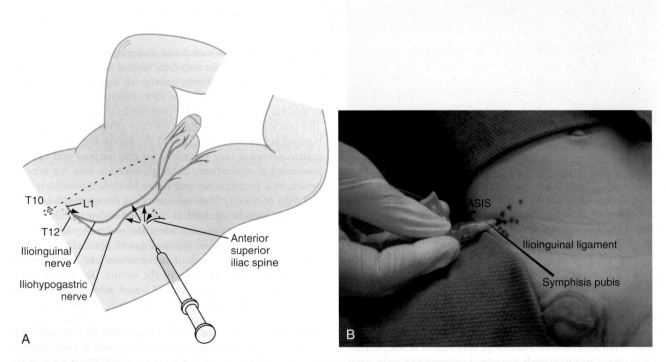

Figure 42-18. Ilioinguinal and iliohypogastric nerve blocks. **A** and **B,** The anterior superior iliac spine (ASIS) is palpated, and a point 1.0 to 1.5 cm cephalad and toward the midline is located (*dashed line*). A 22-gauge needle is passed through the external and internal oblique muscles, and 1.0 to 5.0 mL of local anesthetic is deposited in a fan-like fashion cephalad toward the umbilicus, medially, and caudad toward the groin (*solid arrows*). Just before removal from the skin, another 0.5 to 1.0 mL of local anesthetic is injected subcutaneously to block the iliohypogastric nerve. Blockade of these nerves provide postoperative analgesia for inguinal hernia and orchidopexy procedures.

assuming that the surgical procedure is not of more than 1.5 hours in duration. A short-bevel 27-gauge needle is inserted at a 45-degree angle at a point one fourth of the way toward the midline along a line drawn from the anterior superior iliac spine to the umbilicus (1.0 to 1.5 cm cephalad and toward the midline from the anterior superior iliac spine in a 10- to 15-kg child). As the needle is advanced through the external and internal oblique muscles (Fig. 42-18B), two "pops" are elicited and provide useful guides of proper needle placement. Negative aspiration should be confirmed several times during the incremental injection of local anesthetic. A volume of 0.3 mL/kg of local anesthetic is injected in a fan-like fashion, cephalad toward the umbilicus, caudad toward the groin, and medially. Before removal of the needle from the skin, an additional 0.5 to 1.0 mL of local anesthetic is injected subcutaneously to block the iliohypogastric nerve. Care must be taken to avoid entering the peritoneum, which has been reported after the blind injection approach.[287] For inguinal herniorrhaphy, orchidopexy, or other inguinal procedures, local anesthetic deposited directly into the wound before it is closed has also proved effective for postoperative analgesia.[283] The volume of drug used by this approach, like the volume of drug used for wound infiltration, must be accounted for when calculating the maximal dose of local anesthetic that can be used. As mentioned earlier, an ultrasound-guided technique may be easier and leads to fewer complications while performing the block (see Fig. 42-18C, D [on website]).[286]

Complications. Complications are rare. Care should be taken not to enter the peritoneal cavity. Intravascular injection may be avoided with incremental injection with frequent aspiration.

Penile Block

A penile block is used for anesthesia and postoperative analgesia for circumcision, urethral dilatation, and hypospadias repair. Caudal anesthesia is superior for proximal shaft or penoscrotal hypospadias repair because a penile block provides analgesia only for the distal two thirds of the penis.[224,288,289] The block is easily performed and has a high success rate. Bupivacaine, levobupivacaine, and ropivacaine are the most useful agents because of their prolonged duration of action. *Epinephrine must never be used for this block because the dorsal artery of the penis is an end artery and vasospasm caused by epinephrine could cause necrosis.*

Anatomy. The nerve supply of the penis is from the pudendal nerve and the pelvic plexus (Fig. 42-19A). Along the dorsal artery to the penis are two dorsal nerves that separate at the level of the symphysis pubis; they supply the sensory innervation to the penis.

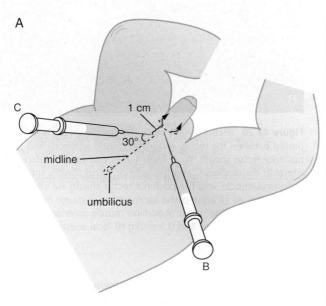

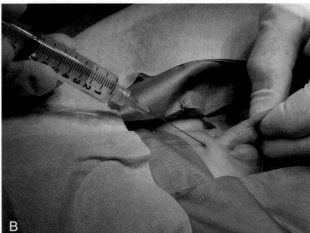

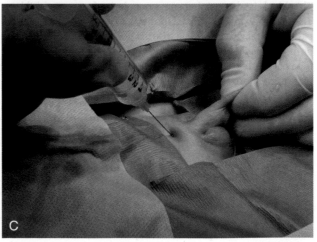

Figure 42-19. Penile block. **A,** Dorsal nerve block: a 27 or 25-gauge needle is inserted in the midline, 1 cm above the symphysis pubis at an angle of 30 degrees from the plane of the abdominal wall and directed caudad. **B,** Ring block: a 25-gauge needle is inserted at the base of the penis at a 45-degree angle, and a ring of local anesthetic is deposited (*curved arrows*). This may be done through a single needle placement by redirecting the needle. This block may be used in children in whom a caudal block is contraindicated. **C,** After piercing the penile fascia (0.5 to 1.0 cm) and negative aspiration for blood, 1.0 to 4.0 mL of local anesthetic without epinephrine is injected.

Technique. Three approaches to perform a paravertebral block in children have been described:

Loss-of-Resistance Technique.[295] The skin is punctured laterally to the spinous process and the needle is advanced in a perpendicular manner until contact is made with the transverse process. A Tuohy needle (19-20 gauge if younger than 1 year, 18 gauge if older than 1 year) is then "walked" below/underneath the transverse process and by means of a loss-of-resistance technique the costotransverse ligament is pierced and the paravertebral space located. Alternatively the needle can be "walked" above/over the top of the transverse process, but by using this approach there is the risk of striking the neck of the rib before entering the paravertebral space. Occasionally this will redirect the needle, making it virtually impossible to obtain access to the paravertebral space. The approach from below the transverse process is clearly advantageous.

Once in the paravertebral space the bolus dose of local anesthetic can be injected after careful aspiration to exclude the presence of blood or air. If a continuous technique is preferred, a catheter can be introduced 1 to 2 cm into the paravertebral space through the Tuohy needle. The insertion of the catheter frequently needs manipulation of the Tuohy needle to be successful, and occasionally one will have to make the injection of the bolus dose to "open up"/"create" a space to allow catheter insertion. One should not insert more than 1 to 2 cm of the catheter into the paravertebral space because further advancement may cause the catheter to migrate into the spinal canal through the intervertebral foramen (causing an epidural distribution of the block) or to go laterally, following the path of the intercostal nerve (giving a dense block of only one dermatome).

An estimate of the distance from the spinous process to the skin puncture site (spinous process/paravertebral space distance) and the distance from the skin to the paravertebral space can be approximated by the following equations[296,297]:

$$\text{Spinous process/paravertebral space distance (mm)}$$
$$= 0.12 \times \text{kg} + 10.2$$

$$\text{Skin/paravertebral space distance (mm)} = 0.53 \times \text{kg} + 21.2$$

The level of the puncture depends on the surgical intervention, but for a thoracotomy the puncture is best performed at T5-6 and for renal surgery at T9-10.

Nerve-Stimulator–Guided Technique.[298] The intervertebral lines corresponding to the specific dermatomes are determined by manual palpation. The site of injection is marked 1 to 2 cm laterally from the midline on the intervertebral line according to the child's weight.[18] A 21-gauge insulated needle of appropriate length, attached to a nerve stimulator (initial stimulating current: 2.5 to 5 mA, 1 Hz), is introduced perpendicularly to the skin in all planes. A contraction of the paraspinal muscles is initially observed, and the needle is advanced until the costotransverse ligament is reached. At this point the contraction of the paraspinal muscles will disappear. After piercing the costotransverse ligament, muscle contractions of the corresponding level are sought and the needle tip is manipulated into a position allowing continued muscular contractions while reducing the stimulating current to 0.4 to 0.6 mA; the desired local anesthetic dose and volume is injected. Manipulation of the needle tip within the paravertebral space is not an "in and out" movement

but is rather an angular manipulation and circumferential rotation around the axis of the needle to reach an optimal position of the needle tip with regard to the nerve within the paravertebral space.

Ultrasound-Aided Approach. With the aid of ultrasound the position of the transverse processes and the depth to the paravertebral space can be determined; ultrasound is very helpful regardless of whether a loss-of-resistance or nerve-stimulator–guided technique is used.

Selection of Drug. After a negative aspiration test and administration of a test dose, 0.5 mL/kg of the local anesthetic (levobupivacaine 0.25% with epinephrine 1:200,000, bupivacaine 0.25% with epinephrine 1:200,000, or lidocaine 1% with epinephrine 1:200,000) is injected in toddlers and older children. This dose will usually spread to cover at least five dermatomes. A typical distribution of the block will be unilateral analgesia of the trunk ranging from T4 to T12 (Fig. 42-21). In neonates and infants, slightly modified dosage regimens are recommended[299-301]; these dosages have been found to be both effective and associated with acceptable plasma concentrations of bupivacaine.[299]

Complications. The use of a percutaneous loss-of-resistance technique in a mixed adult and pediatric population was found to be associated with an overall failure rate of approximately 10% and the complications experienced were hypotension (5%) (only adults), vascular puncture (4%), inadvertent pleural puncture (1%), and pneumothorax (0.5%).[302] The risk for block failure is reduced to less than 5% when a nerve-stimulator–guided technique is used, and this technique also appears to be associated with a reduced risk for complications.[298,303] Use of ultrasound may further improve success while reducing complications.

Upper Extremity Blocks

Brachial Plexus Block

Of the four techniques used to block the brachial plexus (axillary, infraclavicular, supraclavicular, and interscalene), the axillary approach is most commonly used in children.[304] Advantages include ease of insertion, a high rate of success in experienced hands, and low morbidity. The block is also well suited for orthopedic or plastic surgical repairs on the hand or forearm in a child with a full stomach.[305,306] In this situation, deeper levels of sedation, intravascular injection, or drug overdose places the child at risk for aspiration of gastric contents. Because it is unnecessary to elicit a sensory paresthesia, the block can also be performed in an anesthetized child for postoperative pain management. Toxicity is avoided if the dose of bupivacaine is less than 2.5 mg/kg.

Infraclavicular, supraclavicular, and interscalene blocks are not as frequently used as the axillary block in children. The infraclavicular block is our preferred technique for the placement of a continuous catheter in the postoperative period. Unintentional block of the phrenic and recurrent laryngeal nerves is much more common in young children because these nerves are close to the site of injection, especially with an interscalene block. Data suggest that some degree of phrenic nerve blockade is present in all children receiving interscalene blocks.[307,308] Phrenic nerve blockade may cause respiratory failure in very young children whose breathing is almost totally dependent on the diaphragm, whereas block of the recurrent laryngeal nerve may cause increased airway resistance due to vocal cord paralysis. The risk of pneumothorax is greater because the apex of the lung is situated more rostral in infants and small children. Total spinal anesthesia is also more likely with the interscalene approach to axillary plexus blockade.[309]

Anatomy. The brachial plexus arises in the neck from spinal nerves C5, C6, C7, C8, and T1, passes between the clavicle and first rib, and extends into the axilla. At that point, the axillary artery is surrounded by a narrow fascial sheath that contains the median nerve anteriorly, the ulnar nerve posteriorly, and the radial nerve on the posterolateral aspect (Fig. 42-23A). In children, the axillary artery and, at times, the axillary sheath itself may be palpable.

Technique. Several techniques can be used to establish that the needle is within the axillary sheath. The first is by eliciting a sensory paresthesia with the needle, but this has little application in pediatric practice, particularly in young children and in those who are anesthetized. The use of a nerve stimulator allows precise placement of the needle in the neurovascular sheath without either the cooperation of the child or the need for painful sensory paresthesias (see Fig. 42-3). In thin children, the sheath can often be palpated as a cord-like structure inferior to the coracobrachialis muscle, allowing the placement of the needle in the sheath by "feel." A transarterial approach can also be used.[310] With all techniques, it is useful to attach a short piece of extension tubing between the needle and syringe to facilitate precise handling during needle placement, aspiration, and drug injection.

The axillary approach to the brachial plexus is best accomplished by abducting the arm to 90 degrees (see Fig. 42-2). Care

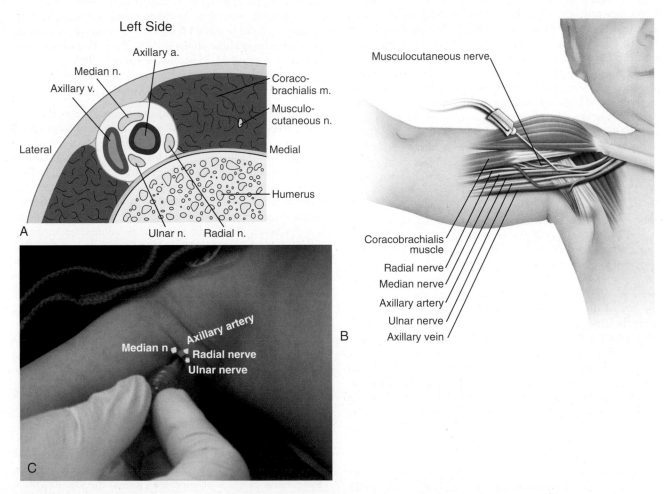

Figure 42-23. A and **B,** The anatomic relationships of the brachial plexus are presented. Note that the fascial sheath envelops the nerves and the axillary artery and vein; the musculocutaneous nerve lies within the body of the coracobrachialis muscle. Local anesthetic injected within the sheath (on either side of the axillary artery) produces a satisfactory block. There may be septation within the sheath in some individuals (not pictured). **C,** The axillary artery is palpated with the arm in abduction in the axilla. A needle is introduced superior to the pulsation to block the median nerve. If a nerve stimulator is used, opposition of the thumb can be elicited as the median nerve is stimulated. The needle is then gently positioned below the artery; the ulnar nerve can be blocked in this position. If a nerve stimulator is used, flexion of the fifth finger is elicited. For blocking the radial nerve that is situated posterior to the artery, it may be necessary to pass the needle posterior to the artery while constantly aspirating to avoid intravascular placement. If the needle does encounter the axillary artery, continue to advance the needle so that the aspirate is negative while the needle is situated posterior to the artery. If a nerve stimulator is used, biceps flexion may be observed. A total volume of 0.1 mL/kg to 0.15 mL/kg in divided doses between all three nerves will provide an adequate blockade of the nerves. If the axillary artery is encountered while accessing the radial nerve, it is imperative to apply pressure after the block is placed to avoid hematoma formation. a, artery; v, vein; n, nerve.

should be taken not to hyperabduct the arm, obscuring the axillary pulse. The artery is palpated in the axilla, and a short beveled needle is advanced toward it (see Fig. 42-23B). When using a nerve stimulator, a distal motor response is elicited in the distribution of the radial, ulnar, or median nerves at a threshold of less than 0.2 mA (see Fig. 42-3). If one is not using a nerve stimulator, the needle is advanced until a distinct pop is felt as the needle pierces the axillary sheath. The axillary sheath may be divided into fascial compartments for each nerve, and these may limit the spread of local anesthetic within the axillary sheath. Although distinct paresthesias to the distribution of all three nerves may be elicited with the nerve stimulator, and divided doses of anesthetic may be administered to each of those locations, in practice it becomes extremely difficult to find the second and third motor paresthesia after the administration of even a very small amount of local anesthetic with the first injection. Alternatively, the transarterial technique, which involves direct puncture of the axillary artery, allows deposition of local anesthetic in two sites within the sheath. The needle is aimed directly toward the axillary pulse. As soon as blood is aspirated, the needle is advanced through the posterior wall of the artery. When blood can no longer be aspirated, half of the dose of local anesthetic is deposited posterior to the artery. The needle is withdrawn through the anterior wall of the artery, and the remainder of the dose is deposited anterior to the artery after reconfirming a negative aspiration for blood. Regardless of technique, the local anesthetic is administered in incremental quantities with intermittent aspiration to confirm that the needle is still outside the blood vessel. Some practitioners advocate applying a tourniquet distal to the site where the block is to be performed. It is sometimes difficult to block the musculocutaneous nerve, which carries sensory fibers to the radial aspect of the forearm, because it exits the brachial plexus proximal in the axillary fossa. Applying a tourniquet may promote proximal spread of local anesthetic and enhance the chances of a successful block of this nerve. Alternatively, the musculocutaneous nerve may be blocked by infiltrating 1 to 3 mL (proportional to the size of the child) of local anesthetic into the body of the coracobrachialis muscle. Regardless of the technique chosen, an additional 1 to 3 mL of local anesthetic is deposited as a subcutaneous cuff to block the intercostobrachial nerve and its communications with the musculocutaneous nerve. These additional quantities of local anesthetic must be accounted for when calculating the total drug dose. An ultrasound may also be used in conjunction with a nerve stimulator to further improve the localization of each nerve bundle (Fig. 42-23C [on website]; also Fig. 43-23D [on website] and Fig. 43-24).[306]

Selection of Drug. Local anesthetics commonly used in our practice include lidocaine and bupivacaine (Table 42-7). As with other regional techniques that involve larger volumes of local anesthetic, the addition of both levobupivacaine and ropivacaine to the armamentarium is likely to prove beneficial in reducing the risk of toxicity from local anesthetics. Because it is desirable to have a prolonged duration of postoperative analgesia, longer-acting agents are usually used in place of lidocaine. To help ensure block of the musculocutaneous nerve, we use large volumes (0.5 mL/kg), diluting the concentration of local anesthetic with normal saline as needed to avoid toxicity. Care must always be taken not to exceed the maximal allowable doses of bupivacaine on a milligram per kilogram basis (2.5 mg/kg).[311]

Adding epinephrine (1 : 200,000) may decrease vascular absorption and the potential for toxicity. Sodium bicarbonate (1 mEq/10 mL of local anesthetic) added to the local anesthetic will speed the onset of blockade by increasing the pH of the solution; this is particularly the case with the premixed anesthetic-epinephrine formulations that have a reduced pH.

Complications. All of the nerves of the brachial plexus occupy a neurovascular bundle and hence are prone to unintended injection into a blood vessel. A hematoma may form at the site of injection; if large enough, the hematoma may compress the neurovascular bundle, rendering the limb ischemic. Hence it is important to know the child's coagulation status before attempting the block. Intravascular injection may be avoided with incremental injection and frequent aspiration. Intraneural injection may be minimized by use of a nerve stimulator.

Infraclavicular Approach. This approach to the brachial plexus is very helpful, particularly in children who may have fractures making it painful to abduct the arm. A vertical approach to the infraclavicular brachial plexus is performed using the coracoid process as a landmark to access the nerve.[312] We routinely use this technique in children who require continuous infusions of local anesthetic solution in the postoperative period.

Technique. With the arm in abduction or adduction, the acromial process is palpated. A line drawn 2 cm below and medial to the coracoid process is usually where the needle is introduced (Fig. 42-24A). At this level, the pleura is not usually affected. A sheathed needle with a nerve stimulator is introduced, and the nerve is stimulated at about 1 mA. Any stimulation other than forearm flexion is taken as a positive stimulation of the brachial plexus. Forearm flexion denotes stimulation of the musculocutaneous nerve. The needle should then be directed medial to provide a blockade of the cords of the brachial plexus (see Fig. 42-24B). An ultrasound-guided technique may also be used (see Fig. 42-24C [on website]; see also Chapter 43 and Figs. 43-19 to 43-22).

Complications. There is the potential for intrapleural injection and pneumothorax, especially if the needle is directed medially. Because of the proximity of the plexus to the subclavian vein and artery, it is imperative that the procedure not be attempted on children who have coagulation abnormalities.

Supraclavicular Approach. This is an easy approach to the brachial plexus in children and can be readily performed particularly with the aid of ultrasound guidance. The risk with performing this procedure without ultrasound guidance is the potential for injection into the vertebral artery. It can be used for most procedures performed on the upper arm and forearm. The cervical pleura is also located close to the supraclavicular plexus; thus, caution should be exercised while performing this block. The entire brachial plexus including the musculocutaneous and the axillary nerves is located medial to the artery. Occasionally, the suprascapular nerve may leave the upper trunk more cranially.

Indications. This block is used for analgesia or anesthesia for upper arm surgery and can be performed with either a single injection or catheter technique.

Technique. The supraclavicular plexus is located above the clavicle and is located superficially approximately at the middle

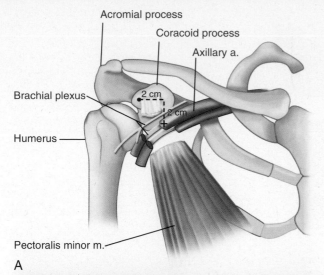

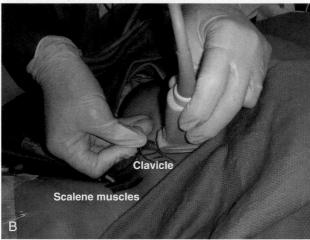

Figure 42-24. A, Anatomic landmarks for the infraclavicular approach to the brachial plexus. Note that the arm is in an abducted position, which may be quite useful for children with fractures (Modified from Wilson JL, Brown DL, Wong GY, et al: Infraclavicular brachial plexus block: parasagittal anatomy important to the coracoid technique. Anesth Analg 1998; 87:870-873.) **B,** The coracoid process is palpated. With the arm abducted, a needle is inserted 2 cm medial and inferior to the coracoid process. A nerve stimulator is used and stimulation is initiated at 1 mA and then decreased to 0.4 mA as the nerve is accessed. Elicitation of hand flexion or extension is used as an indicator of being close to the nerve. After aspiration, 0.2 mL/kg of local anesthetic solution is injected. Use of ultrasound may also improve the success of this block (**C**).

of the sternocleidomastoid. A stimulating needle (1 mA of energy) is passed above the clavicle lateral to the arterial pulsation and close to the inferior margin of the anterior scalene. The plexus is located superficially and can be easily stimulated as soon as the skin is pierced. Any movement of the arm is accepted as an adequate stimualtion to the plexus. The energy is reduced to 0.4 mA and, if continued response to the stimulation is observed, 0.15-0.2 mL/kg of local anesthetic solution is injected in graduated doses after careful aspiration.

The ultrasound-guided technique is now our preferred method for blocking the supraclavicular plexus. We use a linear probe or a hockey stick probe and, using the in-plane technique, pass the needle close to the plexus. If a stimulating needle is used, the needle is advanced until we see movement of the hand. We have been able to decrease the dose of local anesthetic solution to 0.15 to 0.2 mL/kg (Fig. 42-25A-C [see website for C]; see also Fig. 43-18).

Complications. Pleural puncture and intravascular injection can occur from misplacement of the needle.

Interscalene Approach. This approach is not commonly used in children. The main indication for this technique is for children undergoing shoulder surgery; this approach is generally reserved for the older teenager or young adult.

Anatomy. The interscalene groove is formed by the anterior and middle scalene muscles and is located in most children at the lateral border of the sternocleidomastoid muscle (Fig. 42-26A). The upper three nerve roots are superficial, whereas the lower two roots are in a deeper position. In children the lower nerve roots are close to the pleura, which may increase the potential for a pneumothorax. The phrenic nerve is also close to the nerve roots and may often be blocked on the side of the nerve block. Therefore, this block is clearly avoided in children who may have a compromised pulmonary system.

Indications. Shoulder and upper arm surgery and ensuing postoperative analgesia can be provided with this block.

Conventional Techniques. Dalens and associates reported a technique of parascalene brachial plexus blockade for pediatric shoulder surgery using an extended head position and placing the puncture between the lower and middle thirds of the line extending from the center of the clavicle to the C6 transverse process (Chassaignac) (see Fig. 42-25A).[313] The rationale for selecting this puncture site was to avoid the vertebral artery and pleura. With the use of a perpendicular needle orientation, the lower roots (C8 and T1) are not blocked at all or require very large amounts of local anesthetic to be successfully blocked. Ultrasound guidance is greatly advantageous in this situation because it paves the way for safe blockade of both roots (C8 and T1). With the use of a nerve stimulator, diaphragmatic stimulation may be observed as a result of ventromedial needle position (the phrenic nerve runs ventral to the body of the anterior scalene muscle).

Ultrasound-Guided Technique (see Chapter 43). To visualize the anatomic structures of a child's neck, a high-frequency linear ultrasound probe is used. The process is facilitated by slightly turning the child's head to the contralateral side. The probe should be oriented from the medial to the lateral aspect. Medially, the thyroid gland and the major vessels in the neck area (carotid artery and internal jugular vein) are easily identified. Then the probe is moved along the sternocleidomastoid muscle until its lateral border is reached. At the same time, the transducer is moved in a caudal direction such that the posterior scalene gap and the upper anterior roots (C5-C7) of the brachial plexus become visible between the anterior and medial scalene muscles. In very small children, all roots of the brachial plexus (C5-T1) can be simultaneously visualized. The puncture is performed in a tangential direction relative to the neck above the transducer. The C5 nerve root will be encountered superficially, within a few millimeters. As a rule, the needle should be oriented lateral to the C7 root, which will ensure that the neck

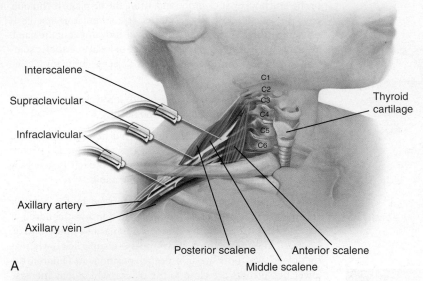

A

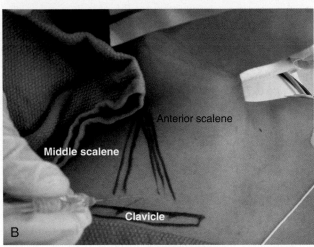

B

Figure 42-25. A right-sided supraclavicular block: landmark technique: The supraclavicular block is used frequently in children for most procedures on the hand and elbow. **A,** The divisions and cords are located around the carotid artery cephalad to the clavicle at the inferior margins of the scalene muscles. **B,** A stimulating needle, using 0.5 mA of energy, is introduced at the inferior border of the anterior scalene muscle. Any movement of the patient's fingers (including flexion or extension) suggests adequate positioning of the needle. After aspiration to avoid intravascular injection, 0.15 mL/kg of local anesthetic solution is injected.

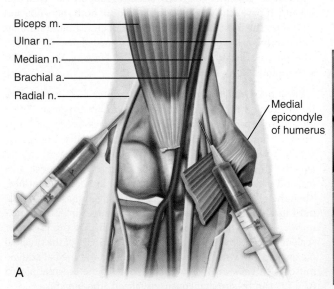

A

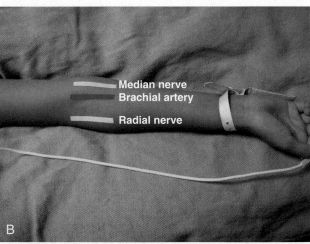

B

Figure 42-26. **A,** Anatomic relationship of the nerves around the elbow. **B,** Radial nerve block: the intercondylar line is marked. After identification of the biceps tendon, a 27-gauge needle is inserted directly toward the bone of the lateral epicondyle toward the lateral margin; 2.0 to 5.0 mL (depending on the patient's weight) of bupivacaine (0.25% with epinephrine 1:200,000) is injected into the area. To block the median nerve, the brachial artery is palpated at the elbow crease. The median nerve is located immediately medial to the brachial artery. A nerve stimulator is used, and flexion of the patient's fingers denotes adequate localization of the nerve.

vessels remain at an adequate distance from the needle insertion site. As soon as the local anesthetic has been injected, it will spread toward the C5 root, which can be visualized in the ultrasound image. Depending on the blockade required, the needle can be advanced to a deeper level for injection after the deep roots (C8 and T1) have been visualized. If the local anesthetic fails to spread adequately in a medial direction, the needle is retracted toward the subcutaneous level and is then repositioned on the medial side of the posterior scalene gap in the area of the C7 root. In the majority of cases, however, the local anesthetic will spread in an adequate manner even when the needle is in a lateral position. The injected volume of local anesthetic should not exceed the amount necessary to fully cover the root surfaces. It is, therefore, inappropriate to recommend a specific volume. In general, however, complete blockade via the scalene route can be expected with local anesthetic volumes of 0.15 to 0.25 mL/kg.

Complications. Pneumothorax, intravascular injection, and temporary phrenic nerve injury are risks of this block.

Intravenous Regional Anesthesia

Intravenous regional anesthesia was first described in 1908 by August Bier and is frequently referred to as the Bier block.[314] This technique has been advocated for upper extremity procedures lasting 30 to 60 minutes in children because of its rapid onset of anesthesia and its ease of performance.[315-317] *Only dilute lidocaine (0.25% or 0.5%) can be used because of the risk of local anesthetic toxicity.* This can be a useful block for upper extremity fracture reduction or suture of a large laceration in children with a full stomach. It is also helpful for chronic painful conditions including complex regional pain syndrome type 1 in children and adolescents.[318] The exsanguination and manipulation of the limb before administering the local anesthetic may prove to be unduly painful for children with a fracture, and many children may not tolerate the discomfort of the tourniquet without significant sedation. Another disadvantage is the possibility of toxic reactions in the event of tourniquet failure. Strict attention to detail—elevation or exsanguination of the extremity to be blocked, proper application of a double pneumatic cuff, careful attention to anesthetic dose, and care not to deflate the tourniquet until 30 minutes after injection of the local anesthetic—is important to avoid serious complications and provide a successful block. This block is unsuitable for children younger than 1 year of age because of the risk of toxic reactions in infants. This technique may also be contraindicated for children in whom the prolonged use of a tourniquet is inadvisable.

Technique. A small-gauge intravenous cannula is inserted in a vein on the dorsum of the hand. Exsanguination of the arm may be accomplished either by wrapping the limb with an Esmarch bandage or by elevation of the limb if wrapping is too painful. The proximal compartment of a double tourniquet is inflated to a pressure of 200 to 250 mm Hg, although some have recommended that it be inflated to 150 mm Hg above the child's systolic blood pressure. If tourniquet pain develops during the course of the procedure, the distal cuff may be inflated, followed by deflation of the proximal cuff. The tourniquet must remain inflated for a minimum of 30 minutes to prevent a rapid intravenous infusion of lidocaine. It is best to deflate the tourniquet incrementally. Because no residual blockade persists after the tourniquet is released, supplementary analgesia must be considered (e.g., intravenous opioids, local infiltration with a long-acting local anesthetic).

Selection of Drug. Only *preservative-free* 0.25 to 0.5% lidocaine without epinephrine (1 mL/kg) should be used for this block because the duration of the block is limited by tourniquet time and because of the potential for cardiac toxicity with longer-acting agents. A very low dose of a nondepolarizing neuromuscular blocking agent, such as rocuronium (0.03 mg/kg), may improve the quality of the motor blockade.

Complications. Unintended deflation of the tourniquet results in release of drug into the intravascular compartment; hence, only a short-acting local anesthetic such as lidocaine should be used. Bupivacaine should never be used for this block because of the risk of cardiotoxicity.

Peripheral Blocks at the Elbow

There is usually no great advantage to blocking the peripheral nerves at the elbow compared with blocking them at the wrist for analgesia/anesthesia of the hand because the forearm is supplied by cutaneous branches that originate in the upper arm. However, on some occasions (e.g., to avoid injections into surgical fields or areas of infection), anesthesia of the hand may be achieved by blocking the appropriate nerves at the elbow because the cutaneous nerve supply to the hand arises at the elbow.

Radial Nerve

Anatomy. The radial nerve supplies the radial side of the dorsum of the hand and the proximal parts of the radial three and a half digits. Block at the elbow is useful for the provision of anesthesia for an arteriovenous fistula. It is also useful to supplement an inadequate brachial plexus block at the axillary level. The radial nerve passes over the anterior aspect of the lateral epicondyle (Fig. 42-26A).

Technique. The intercondylar line is marked. After identification of the biceps tendon, a 27-gauge needle is inserted directly toward the bone of the lateral epicondyle toward the lateral margin; 2.0 to 5.0 mL (depending on the child's weight) of bupivacaine (0.25% with epinephrine 1:200,000) is injected into the area (Fig. 42-26B). Ultrasound guidance can help with determination of exact location of the nerve in the forearm (see Chapter 43 and Fig. 43-27).

Complications. Intravascular injection and intraneural injections are potential complications. The use of a nerve stimulator or ultrasound can reduce unintended intraneural injection. Intravascular injection may be avoided with incremental injection and frequent aspiration.

Median Nerve

Anatomy. This nerve supplies the radial side of the palm and the three and a half digits of the palmar aspect (see Fig. 42-26). It accompanies the brachial artery in its course down the arm. It is initially lateral and then crosses the ventral side of the artery and eventually lies medial to the artery at the bend of the elbow. It is deep to the bicipital fascia and superficial to the brachialis muscle.

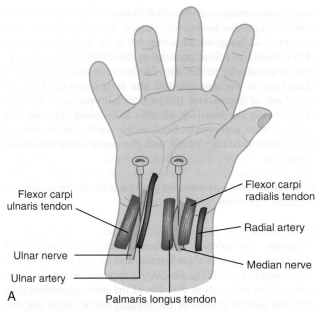

Flexor carpi ulnaris tendon

Flexor carpi radialis tendon

Radial artery

Ulnar nerve

Median nerve

Ulnar artery

A Palmaris longus tendon

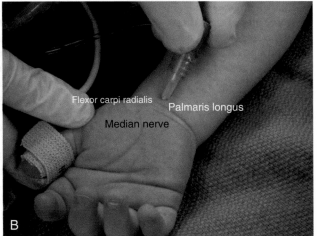

Flexor carpi radialis

Palmaris longus

Median nerve

B

Figure 42-29. Wrist block: median and ulnar nerves. **A,** Median nerve: identify the palmaris tendon by asking the child to flex the wrist against resistance. Distal skin creases are identified. **B,** A 27-gauge needle is inserted at the level of the distal skin crease perpendicular to the skin. The nerve is at a depth of less than 1 cm in teenagers and less than that in younger children. Inject 1.0 to 2.0 mL of bupivacaine (0.25 % with 1:200.000 epinephrine) in the area. If the child is awake, it is better to elicit paresthesias because the needle may be anterior to the neurovascular bundle and can be missed altogether. Ulnar nerve: identify the flexor carpi ulnaris tendon, which lies proximal to the pisiform bone. A 27-gauge needle is inserted just proximal to the pisiform bone and directed radially a distance of approximately 0.5 cm. Two milliliters of bupivacaine (0.25% with epinephrine 1:200,000) is injected. (Modified with permission from Raj P, Pai U: Techniques of nerve blocking. In Raj P [ed]: Handbook of Regional Anesthesia. New York, Churchill Livingstone, 1985, p 185.)

common digital nerves then become the proper digital nerves (digital collaterals) that supply the skin of the palmar surface and the dorsal side of the terminal phalanx of their respective digits. All digital nerves ultimately terminate in two branches: one ramifies in the skin of the fingertips and the other ends in the

pulp under the nail. Smaller digital nerves are derived from the radial and ulnar nerves and supply the back of the fingers. These tend to lie on the dorsolateral aspect of the finger. There are four dorsal digital nerves: (1) ulnar side of the thumb; (2) radial side of the index finger; (3) adjacent sides of index and middle fingers; and (4) communication to the adjacent sides of middle and ring finger.

Technique. There are two techniques for blockade of the digital nerves.

For blockade at the base of the thumb (Fig. 42-30A, B), with the thumb extended, on the palmar surface of the hand, a 27-gauge needle is inserted into the web space between the index finger and thumb. The needle is advanced to the junction of the web space and the palmar skin of the hand a distance of about 1 cm; 0.5 mL of bupivacaine *without epinephrine* is injected. A second needle is inserted into the thenar eminence on the radial aspect of the thumb; 1.0 mL of bupivacaine *without epinephrine* is injected. Caution has to be exercised if the child has collagen vascular disease because this may precipitate acute vascular spasm that may not be relieved.

Blockade of the other fingers is accomplished at the bifurcation between the metacarpal heads (Fig. 42-30B, C). With the fingers extended, a 27-gauge needle is inserted into the web about 3 mm proximal to the junction between the web and the palmar skin; 1.0 to 2.0 mL of bupivacaine *without epinephrine* is injected. This can be performed either from a dorsal approach or a volar approach.

Caution: Vasoconstrictors are avoided when blocking digital nerves because these are end vessels and acute vasospasm due to epinephrine can lead to permanent damage or necrosis of the digits.

Complications. Large volumes of local anesthetic are contraindicated because of the possibility of pressure and vascular compromise. Vasoconstrictors should be avoided because they may cause necrosis of the digit. Intravascular injection may be avoided with incremental injection and frequent aspiration.

Lower Extremity Blocks

The major use of nerve blocks of the lower extremity in children is for managing postoperative pain and as an adjunct to general anesthesia. When considering the sensory and cutaneous innervation of the lower extremity (Fig. 42-31), it is not surprising that few surgical procedures can be accomplished under single nerve blocks. However, combinations of sciatic, femoral, and lateral femoral cutaneous blockade can provide both excellent postoperative analgesia and surgical anesthesia for selected operations; the fascia iliaca block produces anesthesia of multiple nerves with a single injection.

Sciatic Nerve Block

Anatomy. The sciatic nerve arises from the L4 through S3 roots of the sacral plexus, passes through the pelvis, and becomes superficial at the lower margin of the gluteus maximus muscle. It then descends into the lower extremity in the posterior aspect of the thigh, supplying sensory innervation to the posterior thigh as well as to the entire leg and foot below the level of the knee, except for the medial aspect, which is supplied by the femoral nerve (Fig. 42-31A). Although a sciatic nerve block alone is useful for few surgical procedures, it can be combined with a femoral nerve block (Fig. 42-31B) for operations below

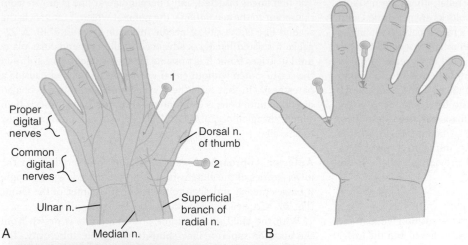

Proper digital nerves

Common digital nerves

Ulnar n.

Median n.

Dorsal n. of thumb

Superficial branch of radial n.

A

B

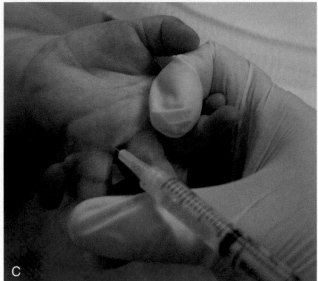

C

FIGURE 42-30. Digital nerve blocks. **A,** Blockade of the thumb: with the thumb extended, on the palmar surface of the hand, a 27-gauge needle is inserted into the web space between the index finger and thumb (**1**). The needle is advanced to the junction of the web space and the palmar skin of the hand a distance of about 1 cm; 0.5 mL of bupivacaine *without epinephrine* is injected. A second needle is inserted into the thenar eminence on the radial aspect of the thumb, and 1.0 mL of bupivacaine *without epinephrine* is injected (**2**). Caution has to be exercised if the patient has collagen vascular disease because this may precipitate acute vascular spasm that may not be relieved. **B,** Blockade of other digits: blockade of the other fingers is accomplished at the bifurcation between the metacarpal heads. With the fingers widely extended, a 27-gauge needle is inserted into the web about 3 mm proximal to the junction between the web and the palmar skin; 1.0 to 2.0 mL of bupivacaine *without epinephrine* is injected. **C,** This can be performed either from a dorsal approach or a volar approach. The web on either side will have to be blocked to provide analgesia for each finger to be anesthetized.

FEMORAL AND OBTURATOR DISTRIBUTION

Lateral femoral cutaneous n.

Anterior femoral cutaneous n.

Obturator n.

Saphenous n.

A   Back   Front   Medial   Lateral

SCIATIC DISTRIBUTION

Posterior cutaneous n.

Lateral femoral cutaneous n.

Tibial n.

Superficial peroneal n.

Deep peroneal n.

Tibial n.

B   Back   Front   Medial   Lateral

Figure 42-31. The sensory innervation of the lower extremity is presented. Note that anesthesia of the lower extremity requires block of the femoral nerve (**A**) (and its branches) as well as the sciatic nerve (**B**).

the knee and for postoperative pain relief. There are multiple approaches to the sciatic nerve.[321] All blocks are performed with the aid of a nerve stimulator to elicit a motor paresthesia in the foot, and, if the block is performed in a lightly sedated trauma victim, the approach that places the child in a greater position of comfort should be chosen. Recently, the use of ultrasound guidance has improved the performance of the nerve block (see Chapter 43). A newer approach to the sciatic nerve using a lateral approach to the popliteal fossa has been described. This offers the additional advantage of being able to provide the block in the supine position. An infragluteal, parabiceps approach is another easy method of providing a sciatic nerve block in children.[322]

Approach of Labat (Posterior Approach)

The child is placed in the lateral decubitus position lying on the nonoperative leg. The leg to be blocked is flexed and the lower leg is extended (Fig. 42-32A). A line is drawn from the posterior superior iliac spine to the greater trochanter of the femur. Another line is drawn from the greater trochanter to the coccyx.

The first line is bisected, and a perpendicular line is drawn from that point to the second line; the point at which it intersects the second line is the site of needle insertion (Fig. 42-32B). A 22-gauge insulated needle is advanced in the perpendicular plane until it strikes bone. It is possible for the needle to pass through the sciatic notch without either encountering bone or causing a paresthesia. In that case, the needle is redirected in a cephalad direction until bone is encountered. A motor paresthesia is then sought using an organized grid-like approach, fanning medially to laterally.

Anterior Approach. As the sciatic nerve emerges from the lower border of the gluteus maximus to extend down the thigh, it passes medial and deep to the lesser trochanter of the femur (Fig. 42-33A; see also Fig. 43-31).

With the child in the supine position, a line is drawn from the anterior superior iliac spine to the pubic tuberosity. The greater trochanter is then located, and another line is drawn parallel to the first line (Fig. 42-33B); at the medial one third of the first line, a perpendicular is dropped to the second line. The

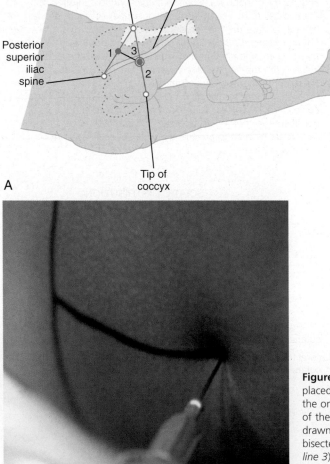

Figure 42-32. A, Sciatic nerve block (approach of Labat). The patient is placed in a lateral position with the lower leg extended and the upper leg, the one to be blocked, flexed; a line is drawn from the greater trochanter of the femur to the posterior superior iliac spine (*line 1*). A second line is drawn from the greater trochanter to the coccyx (*line 2*). Line 1 is bisected, and a perpendicular line is drawn from that point to line 2 (*black line 3*); the point at which the perpendicular broken line intersects line 2 (*circle with dot*) is the point of needle insertion. **B,** A 22-gauge needle is advanced perpendicular to the skin until it strikes bone or, if the child is awake, a paresthesia is elicited. Use of a nerve stimulator will produce either plantarflexion or dorsiflexion of the foot.

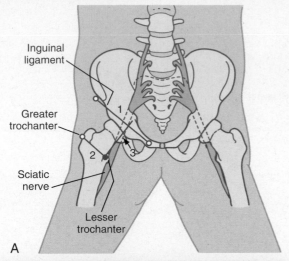

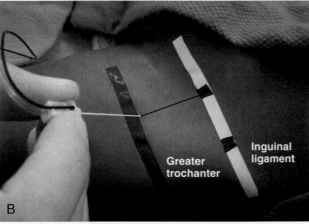

Figure 42-33. A, Sciatic nerve block (anterior approach). With the patient supine, a line is drawn from the anterior iliac spine to the pubic tuberosity (*line 1*). The greater trochanter is located, and another line is drawn parallel to the first (*line 2*). A perpendicular line is dropped from line 1 at a point one third the distance laterally from the pubic tuberosity to the anterior iliac spine (*solid line 3*). **B,** Left sciatic nerve block. A needle is inserted at the intersection of line 2 and the perpendicular line (*in A, solid dot*) until bone is encountered. The needle is redirected off the edge of the femur to the approximate posterior margin of the femur and, after negative aspiration for blood, ease of injection is ascertained. Resistance to injection indicates that the needle is within muscle or fascial bundle; the needle should be advanced until there is minimal resistance to injection or until a paresthesia is elicited.

point of intersection with the line originating at the greater trochanter marks the point of needle entry. The needle is inserted in a perpendicular plane until bone is encountered. It is then partially withdrawn and redirected medially. When the needle is posterior to the medial margin of the femur, ease of injection is determined after negative aspiration for blood. This approach carries a greater risk of unintended puncture of the femoral vessels, and repeated negative aspirations must precede incremental injection. If the needle is in muscle or a fascial bundle, resistance to injection will be felt. In this case, the needle is advanced until minimal resistance to injection is felt. Motor paresthesia is a helpful indicator.

For the previous two techniques, a dose of 0.2 mL/kg of bupivacaine (0.25% with epinephrine 1:200,000) is the dose usually administered for children older than 6 months of age. If the sciatic nerve block is used in conjunction with a femoral nerve block, consideration should be given to diluting the local anesthetic concentration further to limit the injected dose to 2.5 mg/kg of bupivacaine.[323]

Lateral Popliteal Sciatic Nerve Block
This approach to the sciatic nerve can be performed with the child in the supine position.[324] This block provides postoperative analgesia in children undergoing surgery to the foot and knee such as clubfoot repair or triple arthrodesis and in children having knee surgery particularly when combined with a femoral nerve block.[325] It has the advantage of preserving hamstring function and allows early ambulation with crutches.

Anatomy. The popliteal fossa is a diamond-shaped area located behind the knee. It is bordered by the biceps femoris laterally, medially by the tendons of the semitendinosus and semimembranosus muscles, and inferiorly by the heads of the gastrocnemius muscle. The sciatic nerve, after its formation from L4 through S5, innervates all areas of the leg and foot below the knee except the anteromedial cutaneous areas of the leg and foot, which are supplied by the femoral nerve. The sciatic nerve divides into two branches, the larger tibial nerve located medially and the common peroneal nerve located laterally. The nerves are together at the apex of the popliteal fossa where they are in close proximity to each other and are enclosed in a connective tissue sheath for a few centimeters before dividing into the component nerves (Fig. 42-34A).

Technique. After induction of general anesthesia, the lower leg is elevated on a pillow. The biceps femoris tendon is palpated. The tendon is then traced upward for 3 to 5 cm. A 22-gauge insulated needle is inserted anterior to the tendon in a horizontal plane with a cephalad angulation (see Fig. 42-34B). A nerve stimulator is attached to the sheathed needle and with low voltage stimulation (0.2 to 0.5 mV), the foot is observed for plantarflexion or dorsiflexion. On injection of a test dose of 1 mL bupivacaine (0.25% with epinephrine 1:200,000), the twitching is abolished. This confirms the correct placement of the needle (Fig. 42-34C); 5 to 10 mL of additional local anesthetic is then injected. In adult studies, it has been shown that the sciatic nerve block is longer lasting than an ankle block or subcutaneous infiltration and provides excellent postoperative analgesia.[324] Continuous catheter techniques can be used to provide effective analgesia in children in the postoperative period.[326] An ultrasound-guided technique may also be used (see Chapter 43 and Fig. 43-34).

Complications. Intraneural injection must be avoided. Using a low-voltage nerve stimulator ensures the proper placement of the needle. It is rare to see intravascular placement of the needle with this approach. Intravascular injection may be avoided with incremental injection and frequent aspiration.

Parabiceps Infragluteal Approach
This approach is a simple way to access the sciatic nerve.[322] It offers an advantage over the popliteal fossa technique because the posterior cutaneous nerve supplying the posterior portion of the thigh can be blocked with this approach.

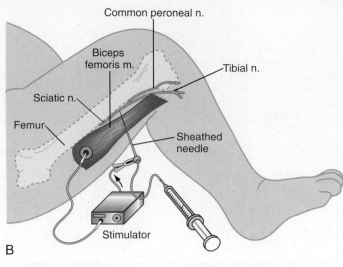

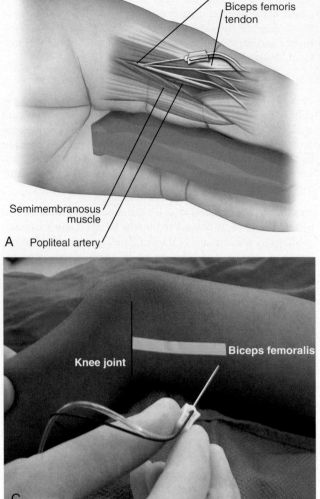

Figure 42-34. Lateral popliteal sciatic nerve block. **A,** Anatomy for lateral popliteal approach to the sciatic nerve. The lower leg is elevated on a pillow and the biceps femoris tendon is palpated. The tendon is traced proximally for 3 to 5 cm. **B,** A 22-gauge insulated needle is inserted anterior to the tendon in a horizontal plane with a cephalad angulation. A nerve stimulator is attached to the needle and with low voltage stimulation (0.2 to 0.5 mV), the foot is observed for plantarflexion or dorsiflexion. With injection of the test dose of 1.0 mL of bupivacaine (0.25% with 1:200,000 epinephrine), the twitching is abolished. This confirms the correct placement of the needle. **C,** Then 5 to 10 mL of additional local anesthetic is injected.

Technique. The child is placed in the supine position or a lateral position to perform this block. The biceps femoris tendon is palpated and traced cephalad to the distal crease of the buttocks (Fig. 42-35A). A stimulating needle is then inserted perpendicular to the femoral shaft, along the biceps femoris tendon (parabiceps) until a twitch is obtained (Fig. 42-35B). Either inversion or eversion of the foot is a reasonable response for localization of the nerve. Next, 0.2 mL/kg of local anesthetic solution is injected into the area. An ultrasound-guided approach may facilitate this block (Fig. 42-35C [on website]; see also Chapter 43 and Figs. 43-31 to 43-33).[327]

Complications. Profound motor block can be seen in most children after a parabiceps subgluteal sciatic nerve block. Caution should be exercised if the child is discharged home because of the motor weakness produced. More recently we have used continuous catheters in hospitalized children having major lower extremity surgical procedures with very good results.[328]

Femoral Nerve Block

A femoral nerve block is particularly useful in children with a fractured femoral shaft so that transport, radiographic, and other manipulations are not painful.[329-331] This block provides analgesia and relieves muscle spasms around the fracture site.

Anatomy. The femoral nerve is located immediately lateral to the femoral artery and deep to both the fascia lata and fascia iliaca (Fig. 42-36A).

Technique. A 22-gauge blunt-bevel needle is advanced lateral to the pulsation of the femoral artery. Two fascial planes can be located by the distinct pop that is felt as the needle traverses these fascial tissues. The nerve is blocked by depositing an appropriate volume (5-10 mL) of local anesthetic lateral to the femoral pulse and deep to the fascia iliaca. The needle is advanced in a perpendicular plane (Fig. 42-36B). It is not necessary to elicit a motor paresthesia provided that the two fascial planes are penetrated. Performance of this block may, on occa-

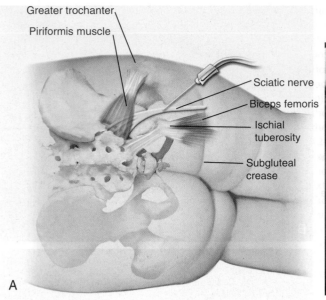

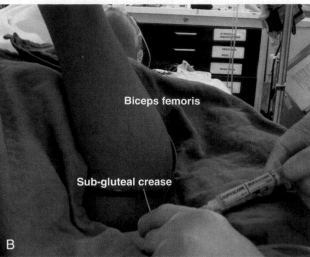

Figure 42-35. A, Artist's rendering of parabiceps infragluteal block. **B,** The gluteal crease is identified (left leg). in the prone or supine position. The biceps femoris muscle is identified (distal portion not illustrated) and followed cephalad to the gluteal crease. A stimulating needle is inserted at the level of the gluteal crease along the medial border of the biceps femoris muscle; with stimulation at 0.5 mA, plantarflexion or extension or inversion or eversion denotes adequate positioning of the needle. After aspiration to rule out intravascular injection, 0.2 mL/kg of local anesthetic solution is injected to provide an adequate blockade of the sciatic nerve.

sion, produce a fascia iliaca block. Repeated aspiration and incremental injection should be used to avoid injection into the femoral artery. With ultrasound guidance, the femoral nerve can be easily visualized and can be blocked (see also Chapter 43 and Fig. 43-29).[327] A catheter can be placed to provide continuous analgesia in the postoperative period.[329]

Complications. It may be preferable to avoid this technique in children who are on anticoagulants or who may have blood dyscrasias owing to the close proximity of the nerve to the femoral artery. Intravascular injection may be avoided with incremental injection and frequent aspiration.

Lateral Femoral Cutaneous Nerve
Anatomy. The lateral femoral cutaneous nerve arises from the L2 and L3 roots of the lumbar plexus. It emerges from the lateral border of the psoas muscle and passes obliquely under the fascia iliaca to enter the thigh 1 to 2 cm medial to the anterior superior iliac crest (Fig. 42-36A). The nerve innervates the lateral aspect of the thigh. One of its anterior branches forms part of the patellar plexus; thus, it must be blocked for regional anesthesia of the knee. Blockade is also indicated for supplementation of femoral and sciatic nerve blocks to provide relief of tourniquet pain. It is also suitable for anesthetizing the lateral aspect of the thigh as a donor site for small skin grafts, fascia iliaca grafts, or muscle biopsy for muscular disorders.[332,333] This block can also be used for diagnostic as well as therapeutic purposes in treating meralgia paresthetica, a condition that leads to chronic pain along the lateral aspect of the thigh.[334,335] In most cases, a fascia iliaca block will block this nerve along with the femoral and obturator nerves, thus obviating

the need for performing an isolated lateral femoral cutaneous block.

Technique. A point approximately 2 cm caudal and 2 cm medial to the anterior superior iliac spine is located (Fig. 42-36C). A blunt needle is then advanced through the skin and then through the fascia lata. A distinct pop is felt at this point. The fascia lata and fascia iliaca compartments are entered as two distinct "pops" can be felt as the needle advances into the fascia iliaca compartment. Two to 10 mL of local anesthetic, depending on the size of the child, is deposited in a fan-like fashion. Recently, we have used an ultrasound-guided technique that allows us to visualize the fascia iliaca compartment as it fills up with the local anesthetic solution on injection.

Complications. It is rare to see any complications associated with a lateral femoral cutaneous nerve block. However, care must be taken to avoid an intraneural placement of the local anesthetic solution. Intravascular injection may be avoided with incremental injection and frequent aspiration.

Fascia Iliaca Block
This block is particularly useful in children to provide unilateral anesthesia or analgesia of the lower extremity. The block has been reported to be less reliable in adults than in children.[336] It produces blockade of the femoral, lateral femoral cutaneous, and obturator nerves with a single injection of local anesthetic.

Anatomy. The compartment is bounded superficially by the fascia iliaca and iliacus muscle, superiorly by the iliac crest, and deeply by the psoas muscle (Fig. 42-36A). It has the advantage

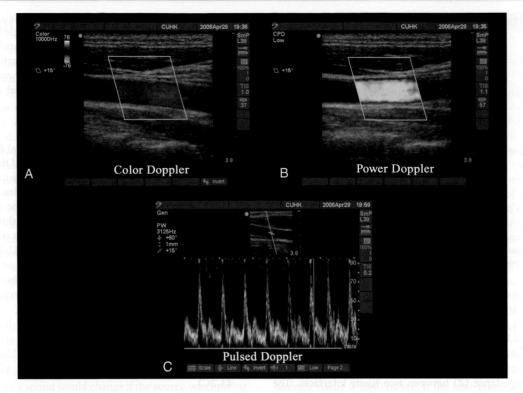

Figure 43-2. Doppler ultrasound. **A,** Color Doppler. **B,** Power Doppler. **C,** Pulsed Doppler.

optimization control. In the "Res" (resolution) setting the highest frequency of the broadband transducer is selected; in the "Pen" (penetration) setting the lowest frequency is selected; and in the "Gen" (general) setting an intermediate frequency is selected.

Gain
The gain control adjusts the amplification of the returning acoustic signals and is used to optimize the US image (Fig. 43-3). Reduced gain produces a dark image (see Fig. 43-3A) and detail is masked. In contrast, too much gain produces a white image and detail is saturated (see Fig. 43-3B). In some US machines there are separate controls for overall gain and gain for the near and far fields. "Auto-gain," whereby the US machine automatically adjusts the gain, is also available in some machines.

Time-Gain Compensation
US energy is progressively attenuated as it travels through tissue. Therefore, signals returning from reflectors at a depth are weaker in strength. By selectively amplifying the echoes from greater depths, using a method called time-gain compensation (TGC), or depth-gain compensation (DGC), equal reflectors at unequal depths are displayed as structures of equal brightness on the monitor. TGC is preset to a large degree, and the operators can make fine adjustments if necessary. The TGC control is presented as a series of sliders arranged in a vertical fashion on the control panel (Fig. 43-4, see website). Each of the sliders adjusts the amplification of the returning US signals at a specific image depth.

Depth
Adjustment in the displayed depth may be necessary depending on the location of the target, the patient's body size, or other anatomic factors. A depth greater than necessary should not be chosen because this reduces the frame rate and resolution of the image.

Focus (Focal Zone)
The focus of the US signal occurs at a point where the beam is at its narrowest width. It is also the region where lateral resolution is the best. The focus point should, therefore, be positioned at the depth where the pertinent anatomic structures are located. In some US machines, the operator can select multiple focal zones, but this markedly reduces the frame rate and thus should not be routinely used.

Freeze and Unfreeze
"Freeze" function allows the operator to lock a static image on the monitor. A number of frames (usually 20 or more) are also simultaneously stored in a memory bank. A trackball or an "arrow" key is then used to scroll back and forth through these frames. The selected still image can then be used for annotation, documentation, storage, review, or teaching. Pressing the freeze button once again will unfreeze the image.

Ultrasound Transducers
The transducer functions both as a transmitter and a receiver of the US signal.[39-41] Three types of transducers are currently used (Fig. 43-5): (1) in a linear-array transducer, the piezoelectric crystals are arranged in a linear fashion and sequentially fired to produce parallel beams of US in sequence, creating a field of view that is rectangular and as wide as the footprint of the transducer (see Fig. 43-5A); (2) a curved linear-array transducer has a curved surface, creating a field of view that is wider than the footprint of the probe (see Fig. 43-5B), but at the cost of reduced lateral resolution in the far field as the scan lines diverge; (3) a phased-array transducer has a small footprint but the US

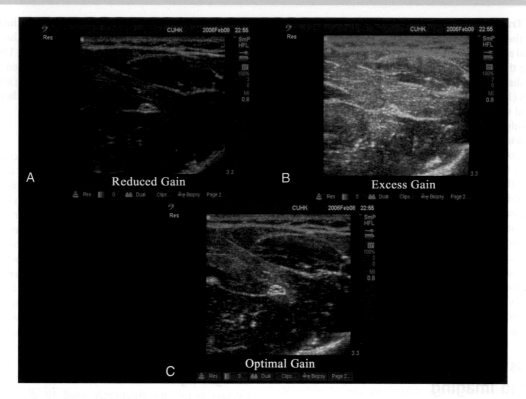

Figure 43-3. Transverse sonogram of the forearm demonstrating reduced gain (**A**), excess gain (**B**), and optimal gain (**C**).

beam is steered electronically to produce a sufficiently wide far field of view. The US beam diverges from virtually the same point in the transducer (see Fig. 43-5C). Phased-array transducers are routinely used for transthoracic echocardiography. The footprints of these transducers are small enough to fit between the ribs and still produce a wide far field of view to

image the heart. US transducers either serve a single frequency or a range of frequencies (broadband). For example, a transducer with the notation HFL38/13-6 indicates that it is a high-frequency broadband (13-6 MHz) linear transducer with a 38-mm footprint. Note that the nomenclature used for transducers varies among manufacturers of US devices.

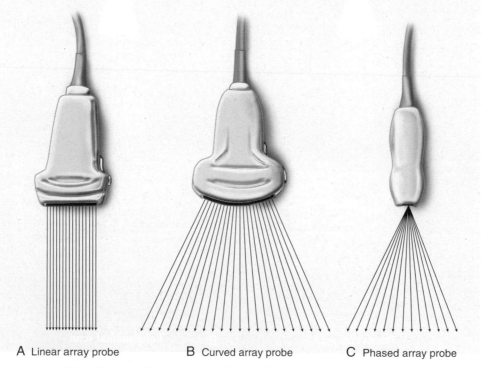

Figure 43-5. Schematic diagram illustrating the different types of ultrasound transducers. Note how the ultrasound beam is emitted from each of these transducers.

Propagation Speed Artifact

These artifacts occur when the media through which the US beam passes does not propagate at 1540 m/sec, resulting in echoes that appear at incorrect depths on the monitor. An example of propagation speed artifact is the "bayonet artifact,"[65] which has been reported during an US-guided axillary brachial plexus block. The shaft of the needle appeared bent when it accidentally traversed the axillary artery. This happens because of the difference in the velocity of sound between whole blood (1580 m/sec) and soft tissue (1540 m/sec).

Acoustic Shadowing

Acoustic shadow is an echo-free area behind surfaces that are highly reflective or attenuating, such as bone (see Fig. 43-12) or metallic implants. The implication for regional anesthesia is that tissues in the area of the shadow cannot be imaged.

Scanning Routine

Being able to consistently produce high-quality images of the area scanned is vital for safety and success during any USGRA procedure. Without optimal images, it is not possible to accurately identify musculoskeletal structures or perform interventions with precision. We have found that following a "scanning routine" or a set of simple steps, which is repeatable, is essential for optimal imaging; the routine that we follow is outlined in Table 43-2. Although the suggested routine may appear complicated at first, with repetition these steps are gradually internalized. Attaching a card with the scanning routine to the US machine facilitates easy recall.

Scout Scan

The aim of the scout scan, or the pre-intervention scan, as the name implies, is to examine the area of interest before the intervention. This has also been referred to as a "mapping scan."[17] During the scout scan steps 8 and 9 described in Table 43-2 are performed, the sonoanatomy of the area is visualized, and the image is optimized. Once an optimal view with the target structure is obtained, and the best possible site for needle insertion is determined, it is advisable to mark the position[44] of the transducer on the patient's skin so that the transducer can be returned to the same position after sterile preparations have been completed. It is common to diagnose anatomic variations during the scout scan. The operator can then decide whether to continue with the block in the same location or to choose an alternative

approach or technique that may be safer. This assessment of anatomic variation is one of the major benefits of using US for regional anesthesia.

General Considerations in Children

Nearly all regional anesthesia techniques that are used in adults can be performed in children (see Chapter 42). Nevertheless published data suggest that central neuraxial blocks are more frequently performed in children than peripheral nerve blocks.[66,67] The reasons for the underusage of peripheral nerve blocks in children may be due to unfamiliarity, lack of experience, or fear of technical and local anesthetic complications. Recent years have seen an increase in interest in the use of USGRA in adults[43,44]; however, it is fair to say that USGRA for children is still in its infancy.

Preparations for an ultrasound-guided nerve block should begin during the preoperative visit by adequately explaining the technique, its benefits and risks, and, more importantly, the possibility of a failed block to the parents. In the event of failure, a contingency plan to quickly convert to general anesthesia or another form of postoperative analgesia must always be in place. In children, most regional anesthetic procedures are performed while the child is anesthetized. However, in a cooperative child or under special circumstances, such as in a child with difficult airway or a child predisposed to malignant hyperthermia, it is possible to perform the block after light sedation. We find that it is easy to explain the procedure to children who are older than 8 years of age. Some of them may even express a wish to stay awake and observe the US images during the block. EMLA (eutectic mixture of local anesthetic) cream applied an hour before the procedure to the skin over the area where the block needle and the intravenous (IV) catheter are to be inserted helps reduce needle-related pain. Parental presence during the nerve block may also be helpful. In older children, allowing the child to listen to favorite music through a personal stereo or watch a video is a are useful distraction technique that makes the whole experience a pleasant one for the child. We have connected a DVD player to our US machine, and this is used to play movies or cartoons through the monitor during the surgical procedure (Fig. 43-16, see website).

Before any USGRA procedure, IV access is established, standard monitoring is applied, and equipment and drugs appropriate for the child are prepared. Aseptic precautions are maintained, and the skin over the needle puncture site is prepared with antiseptic solution in the usual fashion. The US probe is prepared by covering the footprint with a sterile transparent dressing. It is important to avoid trapping any air between the transparent dressing and the footprint. This is done by gently stretching the transparent dressing before applying it on the footprint. The transducer and cable are then covered using a sterile plastic cover. We use the same plastic cover that our surgeons use to cover their laparoscopic camera.

Tips and Tricks for Success

There are certain steps that are common to all US-guided procedures and if they are followed, they may increase success. The lights in the room must be dimmed to avoid any glare or reflection from the US monitor. The operator must assume a comfortable position (Fig. 43-17). For upper extremity blocks, the operator sits at the ipsilateral head end of the child and the US machine is placed directly in front. For lower extremity blocks,

Table 43-2. Scanning Routine

1. Turn on the ultrasound machine.
2. Select a scanning mode.
3. Select an appropriate transducer.
4. Dim the lights in the room.
5. Assume a comfortable position.
6. Apply liberal amount of ultrasound gel.
7. Perform a scout scan.
8. Orient the transducer and image.
9. Select the appropriate ultrasound settings (preset, frequency—for broadband transducers, depth, gain and focus point).
10. Mark the position of the transducer on the patient's skin once an optimal image is obtained before the intervention.

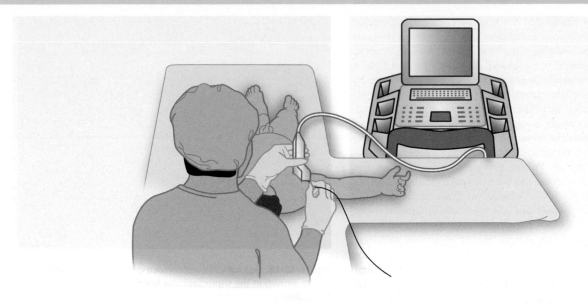

Figure 43-17. Position of the child, anesthesiologist, and ultrasound machine during a USGRA procedure.

such as femoral nerve block, the operator stands on the ipsilateral side of the child and the US machine is placed on the opposite side. For lower extremity or central neuraxial blocks in the lateral position, the operator sits behind the child and the US machine is placed in front with the monitor in the line of view of the operator. Because of the small muscle bulk in young children the nerves are relatively superficial and can most frequently be easily visualized using high-frequency linear transducers. The exact choice of transducer depends on the area scanned, but a high-frequency linear transducer with a small footprint (13-6 MHz, "hockey-stick," 26-mm footprint) is particularly suited in young children. The 15-7 MHz broadband linear-array transducers are used for most blocks in neonates and infants. In older children, a 10-7 MHz broadband linear-array transducer, which allows greater flexibility with the depth of scan, is adequate for most procedures. Low-frequency (5-2 MHz) curved-array transducers are rarely used in children but are useful for imaging deeper structures such as the lumbar plexus and sciatic nerve in older children.

To improve dexterity, hold the transducer with the nondominant hand and perform interventions with the dominant hand. Holding the transducer steady for even short periods of time can be quite testing. We have found that gently resting the hand that is holding the transducer on the child during a procedure helps to keep the transducer steady (see Fig. 43-17). It is important to maintain light contact between the transducer and the skin because excessive pressure in a child will cause the veins to collapse or distort the anatomy of the area of interest. Always apply liberal amounts of US gel to maintain adequate acoustic coupling between the skin and the transducer because even small amounts of air trapped between the two can result in artifacts. We use sterile US gel from single-use sachets for all US-guided peripheral nerve blocks. At any given time during an US-guided intervention one must move either the transducer or the needle. It is impossible to maintain the needle within the plane of imaging if both are moving, a common error by novices. This results in an inability to visualize the needle. If the needle

is not visible in the US image, a good strategy is to keep the needle steady and manipulate the transducer (slide, tilt, or rotate) until the needle becomes visible on the monitor. Thereafter, the transducer should be held steady and the needle should be gently advanced to the target nerve, maintaining it in the imaging plane. When the angle of insertion of the needle is steep (>60 degrees), it is preferable to introduce the needle in the short axis.[45,46] However, if one uses the long-axis approach for all US-guided interventions, as in our case, then inserting the needle a few centimeters away from the edge of the transducer may improve needle visibility by shallowing the angle between the needle and the imaging plane.

One must avoid injecting air into the area of the intervention at all cost because air bubbles in the field of imaging will degrade the US image. We routinely introduce the needle into the subcutaneous tissue and then purge it with saline or the local anesthetic to remove any air from the shaft of the needle, extension, and syringe system before proceeding with the block. An assistant aids with the injection. When the needle tip is close to the target nerve, the assistant gently aspirates to exclude unintended intravascular placement. The assistant must avoid generating excessive negative pressure because small blood vessels are prone to collapse. A short length of extension tubing attached between the needle and the local anesthetic syringe allows the operator to hold the needle steady while the assistant performs the injection.[68] We routinely perform a test injection with 1 to 2 mL of saline or 5% dextrose (when nerve stimulation is also used)[47] and visualize the distribution of the injectate in real time before injecting the local anesthetic. Failure to visualize the injectate in the US image indicates that the needle is not in the plane of imaging or it is intravascular until proven otherwise. No further injection should be made until the needle is repositioned and the distribution of the injectate is confirmed.

Ancillary Equipment

Other than the US machine, equipment required for US-guided nerve block procedures in children is relatively simple. We are

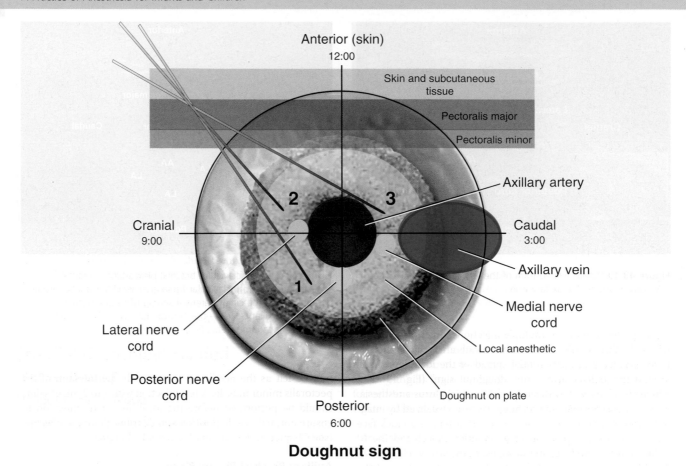

Doughnut sign

Figure 43-22. Infraclavicular brachial plexus block. Schematic diagram showing the positions of the cords of the brachial plexus and the sites at which the local anesthetic is injected: (1) posterior cord, (2) lateral cord, and (3) medial cord.

may also be located very close to the median nerve, and local anesthetic injected close to the median nerve may affect the musculocutaneous nerve. The shape of the musculocutaneous nerve varies along its course, and it may appear oval, round, elliptical, or even triangular.[83]

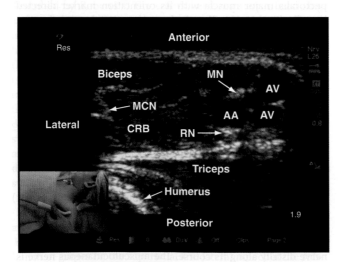

Figure 43-23. Transverse sonogram of the left axilla. AA, axillary artery; AV, axillary vein; CRB, coracobrachialis muscle; MN, median nerve; RN, radial nerve; MCN, musculocutaneous nerve.

We prefer the long axis (in-plane) approach for needle insertion during axillary brachial plexus block in both sedated and anesthetized children. The block needle is inserted from the lateral to the medial side of the arm, keeping it within the plane of the US imaging. A subtle "pop" is often felt when the tip of the needle traverses the perimysium of the biceps muscle and enters the fascial plane containing the neurovascular bundle. Multiple injections are required to block the median, radial, and ulnar nerves. The objective is to produce a circumferential spread of local anesthetic around the artery (i.e., "the doughnut sign"[78] in the US image). To achieve this, local anesthetic is injected close to the anterior (12-o'clock position), posterior (6-o'clock position), and lateral (9-o'clock position) aspects of the axillary artery. The musculocutaneous nerve is then identified and selectively blocked using a few milliliters of local anesthetic.[84] We have found this approach to be technically simple, safe, and effective in producing brachial plexus blockade in children (see Chapter 42 for landmark-guided techniques).

Selective Peripheral Nerve Blocks of the Upper Extremity

Selective blockade of the nerves of the upper extremity is very rarely performed in children. It can be used to rescue incomplete or partial axillary brachial plexus block or provide analgesia or anesthesia over a very specific dermatome. We have also found it to be useful for "US-guided differential nerve blockade"

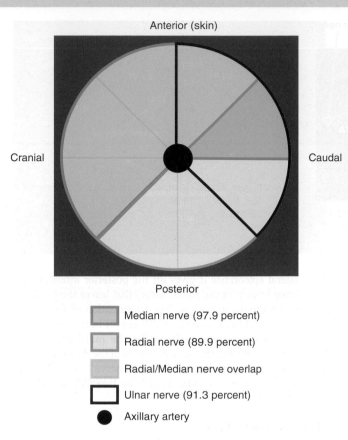

Median nerve (97.9 percent)

Radial nerve (89.9 percent)

Radial/Median nerve overlap

Ulnar nerve (91.3 percent)

Axillary artery

Figure 43-24. Schematic diagram showing the positions of the three main nerves (median, radial, and ulnar) of the brachial plexus in relation to the axillary artery, as identified on transverse ultrasonography, at the axilla.

duration of action of lidocaine compared with bupivacaine or ropivacaine, the child regains protective motor function of the elbow fairly quickly after surgery (2-4 hours) while still enjoying prolonged postoperative analgesia from the distal nerve block. All the major nerves of the upper extremity (median, ulnar, and radial) can be identified[50] using high-frequency linear-array transducers (13-10 MHz) and it is possible to selectively block these nerves at various sites along their course with only a few milliliters (1-2 mL) of local anesthetic. We prefer the in-plane needle insertion technique and use a short-beveled block needle for this purpose.

Median Nerve

The median nerve is closely related to the brachial artery throughout its course in the arm. In the upper part, it is lateral to the artery; in the middle of the arm it crosses the artery from the lateral to medial side and continues on the medial side all the way up to the elbow. In the anticubital fossa, the median nerve lies medial to the brachial artery, behind the bicipital aponeurosis, and in front of the brachialis muscle (Fig. 43-25). In the forearm, the median nerve is deep to the flexor digitorum superficialis and on the surface of the flexor digitorum profundus (see Fig. 43-26) and accompanied by the median artery that is a branch of the anterior interosseous artery. Pulsations of the latter can occasionally be observed on the US image. A few centimeters proximal to the wrist, the median nerve becomes superficial and lies between the tendon of the flexor carpi radialis (laterally) and the flexor digitorum superficialis (medially) and may also be overlapped by the tendon of the palmaris longus. Because the nerve is superficial at this level and it can be difficult to differentiate the nerve from the tendons, we prefer to perform median nerve block at the mid forearm, where it is clearly delineated (see Chapter 42 for landmark-guided techniques).

Ulnar Nerve

In the arm, the ulnar nerve runs on the medial side of the brachial artery up to about the mid-humeral level or the insertion of the coracobrachialis muscle, where it pierces the medial intermuscular septum and enters the posterior compartment of the arm. At the elbow, it passes behind the medial epicondyle to enter the ulnar nerve sulcus. Although the nerve is palpable and superficial at the sulcus, it is often difficult to visualize using US

in adults undergoing ambulatory hand surgery, and the same may also be applicable in children. In this technique an axillary brachial plexus block is performed using a short-acting local anesthetic agent such as lidocaine and combined with a peripheral nerve block (e.g., a median or ulnar nerve block [depending on the dermatomes involved]) in the forearm using a long-acting drug (bupivacaine or ropivacaine). Because of the shorter

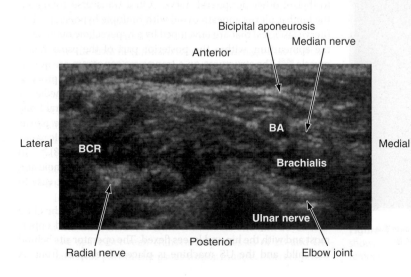

Figure 43-25. Transverse sonogram of the cubital fossa. BA, brachial artery; BCR, brachioradialis.

(in-plane) of the US transducer from the lateral to medial side and directed to the lateral aspect of the femoral nerve. A test injection with saline (1-2 mL) is performed before the local anesthetic is injected to confirm that the needle is deep to the fascia iliaca and to observe the distribution of the injectate in relation to the femoral nerve (see Chapter 42 for landmark-guided techniques).

Subsartorial Saphenous Nerve Block

The saphenous nerve is a branch of the anterior division of the femoral nerve and supplies the skin on the medial aspect of the leg and foot up to the ball of the big toe. In the thigh, the saphenous nerve is located in the subsartorial canal and local anesthetic injected into this intramuscular space produces a saphenous nerve block.[91] The subsartorial canal is also referred to as the "adductor canal" or "Hunter's canal" and is situated on the medial side of the middle one third of the thigh and extends from the apex of the femoral triangle, above, to the tendinous opening in the adductor magnus muscle, below. The canal is triangular in cross section, and its anterior wall is formed by the vastus medialis muscle, the posterior wall or floor is formed by the adductor longus, and the medial wall or roof is formed by a strong fibrous membrane that is overlapped by the sartorius muscle (Fig. 43-30). The subsartorial canal contains the following structures: femoral artery and vein, saphenous nerve, nerve to vastus medialis, and the two divisions of the obturator nerve. The femoral vein lies posterior to the artery in the upper part and lateral to the artery in the lower part of the canal. The saphenous nerve crosses the femoral artery anteriorly from the lateral to the medial side in the canal.

A high-frequency (13-6 MHz) linear-array probe is used to scan the saphenous nerve in the subsartorial canal with the child the supine position. The ipsilateral lower limb is slightly abducted and externally rotated, and the knee is also slightly flexed. For a right-sided block, a right-handed operator stands on the right side of the patient and the US machine is positioned directly in front on the contralateral side. The transducer is positioned in the transverse axis over the middle one third of the thigh. The

triangular subsartorial canal can be identified between the perimysium of the vastus medialis (closely related to the femur), the adductor longus, and the sartorius muscles (see Fig. 43-30). The pulsatile femoral artery lies anterior to the vein in the canal, and the saphenous nerve is seen as a round or oval hyperechoic structure anterior to the artery (12-o'clock position) (see Fig. 43-30). Because the saphenous nerve is a small nerve, it may not always be visible on US imaging in children. However, owing to the close relation of the saphenous nerve to the femoral artery in the subsartorial canal, a perivascular (arterial) injection in the canal will produce saphenous nerve block. The block needle is inserted in the long-axis (in-plane) of the US transducer from the medial to lateral side and is directed to the anterior aspect of the femoral artery. A test injection of saline (1-2 mL) is performed to confirm that the tip of the needle is in the canal, after which the local anesthetic is injected.

Sciatic Nerve Block

The sciatic nerve is the largest mixed nerve in the body and arises from the lumbosacral plexus (L4, L5, S1-3). It innervates the posterior aspect of the thigh and the entire lower limb below the knee except for a small patch of skin on the medial aspect of the leg and ankle, which is innervated by the saphenous nerve. Sciatic nerve block (SNB) is frequently used to provide analgesia for foot (clubfoot) and leg surgery in children. Several different approaches to the sciatic nerve have been described in the literature. Most approaches described to date rely on surface anatomic landmarks (anterior, transgluteal, infragluteal, lateral, posterior subgluteal, proximal thigh, or at the popliteal fossa). Recently, US-guided SNB has also been described.[92] A proximal approach to the sciatic nerve is selected when surgery involves the hip (rare in children) or the block of the posterior cutaneous nerve of the thigh is warranted. Because SNB is most frequently used for foot (clubfoot) surgery in children, a distal approach to the sciatic nerve at the popliteal fossa is usually preferred (see Chapter 42 for landmark-guided techniques).[69,93]

Sciatic Nerve Block at the Subgluteal Space

The sciatic nerve exits the pelvis through the greater sciatic foramen, between the piriformis and the superior gemelli muscles, and enters the subgluteal space below the piriformis muscle. It then descends over the dorsum of the ischium, lying on the dorsal surface of the gemellus superior muscle, tendon of obturator internus, gemellus inferior muscle, and quadratus femoris muscle (in a cranial to caudal relation) before it enters the hollow between the greater trochanter and the ischial tuberosity and then goes on to the posterior compartment of the thigh. The anterior surface of the gluteus maximus covers the upper part of the sciatic nerve; and immediately distal to its lower border (infragluteal position), the sciatic nerve is fairly superficial. In between the greater trochanter and the ischial tuberosity, the sciatic nerve lies in the "subgluteal space," which is a well-defined anatomic space between the anterior surface of the gluteus maximus and the posterior surface of the quadratus femoris muscle (Fig. 43-31).[69] Other structures that are present in the subgluteal space include the posterior cutaneous nerve of the thigh, inferior gluteal vessels and nerve, nerve to the short and long head of the biceps femoris, the comitans artery and vein of the sciatic nerve, and the ascending branch of the medial circumflex artery (see Fig. 43-31). Local anesthetic injected into the subgluteal space blocks not only the sciatic nerve but also the posterior cutaneous nerve of the thigh.[69] The latter is useful

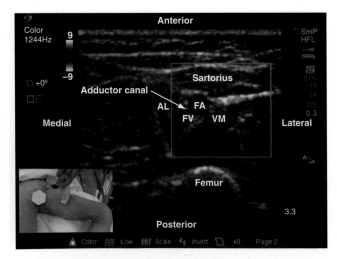

Figure 43-30. Transverse sonogram of the thigh showing the adductor canal. AL, adductor longus; FA, femoral artery; FV, femoral vein; VM, vastus medialis.

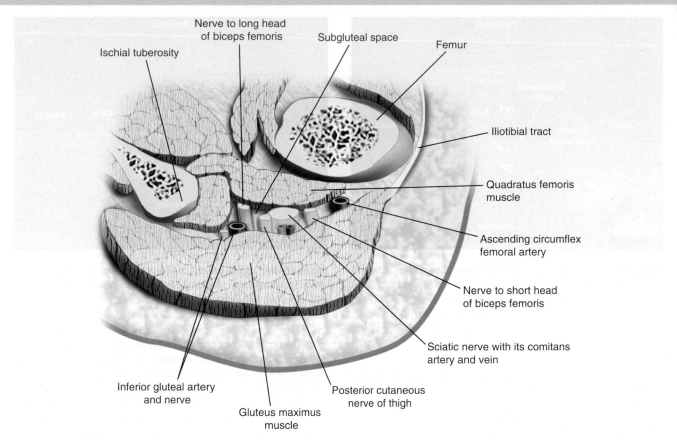

Figure 43-31. Transverse section through the gluteal region at the level of the quadratus femoris muscle showing the subgluteal space and its contents.

when anesthesia over the posterior aspect of the thigh is needed.

US-guided SNB at the subgluteal space is performed with the child in the lateral position. The side to be anesthetized is placed uppermost, and the hip and knees are flexed (Fig. 43-32). The operator sits or stands behind the child, and the US machine is positioned directly in front. In young children, a linear-array transducer (10-5 MHz) is adequate for imaging the sciatic nerve. In older children (>6-8 years), the sciatic nerve can also be imaged using a linear-array transducer (10-5 MHz). However, the increased depth of scan required (due to increased muscle bulk) limits the field of vision because as the depth of scan increases the field of vision becomes narrower when a linear transducer is used. Therefore, a curved-array transducer (8-5 MHz) with a wide field of vision is preferable in older children.

The greater trochanter and the ischial tuberosity are identified, and a line is drawn between these two landmarks. The US transducer is placed parallel to this line with its orientation marker directed toward the greater trochanter to obtain a transverse scan of the sciatic nerve and the subgluteal space. It may be necessary to slide the transducer slightly cephalad or caudad before an optimal image of the sciatic nerve in the subgluteal space can be obtained. On a sonogram, the subgluteal space is seen as a hypoechoic area between the hyperechoic perimysium of the gluteus maximus and quadratus femoris muscle (see Fig. 43-32) extending from the greater trochanter laterally to the ischial tuberosity medially.[69] The subgluteal space

is not so well delineated in young children and is better visualized in older children. The sciatic nerve is seen as an oval or triangular hyperechoic structure within the subgluteal space (see Fig. 43-32). The medial limit of the space is obscured by the attachments of the semimembranosus, semitendinosus, and biceps femoris muscles to the ischial tuberosity. Pulsations of the inferior gluteal artery can often be detected medial to the sciatic nerve on the sonogram.

The block needle is inserted in the long axis (in-plane) of the US beam from the ischial tuberosity side and advanced slowly toward the sciatic nerve. Once the block needle is deemed to be in the subgluteal space, the position is confirmed by injecting 1 to 3 mL of saline through the needle and observing a distention of the subgluteal space (i.e., separation of the perimysium of the gluteus maximus and quadratus femoris muscle) on the US image (Fig. 43-33). However, if the test injection of saline is seen to spread posterior to the perimysium of the gluteus maximus muscle it indicates that the tip of the needle is not in the subgluteal space. The needle should be reoriented and advanced a little farther until the typical distention of the subgluteal space to the saline test injection is seen. Occasionally, a subtle pop is felt when the needle tip traverses the perimysium of the gluteus maximus muscle and enters the subgluteal space. Local anesthetic is then injected in aliquots over 2 to 3 minutes while observing for the distention of the subgluteal space and the spread of local anesthetic in relation to the sciatic nerve. It is also easy to pass a catheter into the subgluteal space when a continuous SNB is planned. Because the catheter is inserted

A linear-array transducer (13-10 MHz) is used for the imaging and the ilioinguinal and iliohypogastric nerves, which are best visualized close to the ASIS. The operator stands on the ipsilateral side to be blocked, and the US machine is positioned directly opposite on the contralateral side. The transducer is positioned close to the ASIS and parallel to a line joining the ASIS and the umbilicus (Fig. 43-37). The ilioinguinal and iliohypogastric nerves are seen as two small, rounded structures lying side by side between the internal oblique and transversus abdominis muscle (see Fig. 43-37). The external oblique is frequently seen only as a hyperechoic aponeurotic layer at the point of needle insertion. Deep to the transversus abdominis muscle the peritoneum and the bowel are also visualized (see Fig. 43-37).

The block needle is inserted in the long axis (in-plane) of the US beam in a medial to lateral direction (Fig. 43-38). We prefer this orientation because it facilitates visualization of the needle (in-plane) and, in the event that the needle is inadvertently inserted too deep, further passage is obstructed by the iliac bone, thus reducing the potential for a major complication such as bowel perforation. When the tip of the needle is close to the two nerves, a test injection is performed with 0.5 to 1.0 mL of normal saline. Correct position of the needle tip is confirmed by observing the widening of the tissue plane between the internal oblique and the transversus abdominis muscle. A calculated dose of a long-acting local anesthetic (0.2 mL/kg) is then injected through the needle, and the spread of the local anesthetic to both the nerves is visualized (see Chapter 42 for landmark-guided techniques).[103]

Spinal Sonography and Central Neuraxial Blocks

Since the early 1980s, spinal ultrasonography has been used as a diagnostic screening tool in neonates and infants suspected of spinal dysraphism and for detecting spinal tumors, vascular malformations, and trauma.[105,106] Today it is considered the first-line screening test for spinal dysraphism with a diagnostic sensitivity comparable to that of MRI. Spinal ultrasonography is possible in neonates and infants because the incomplete ossification of the predominantly cartilaginous posterior spinal ele-

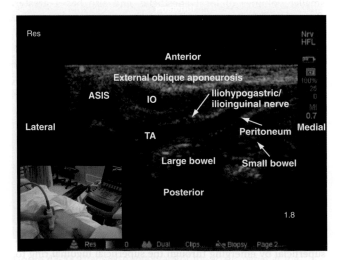

Figure 43-37. Transverse sonogram of the inguinal region showing the ilioinguinal and iliohypogastric nerves and its relation to the abdominal musculature. ASIS, anterior superior iliac spine; IO, internal oblique; TA, transverse abdominis.

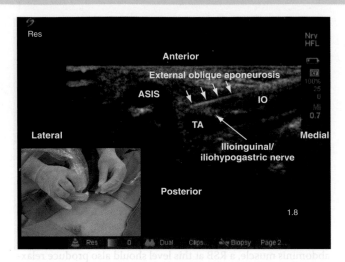

Figure 43-38. Ilioinguinal iliohypogastric nerve block. The in-plane needle insertion technique. ASIS, anterior superior iliac spine; IO, internal oblique; TA, transverse abdominis.

ments creates an acoustic window that allows the transmission of the US beam. The overall visibility of neuraxial structures decreases with age.[107] Neuraxial structures are best visualized in neonates and young infants younger than 3 months of age[107]; progressive ossification of the posterior spinal elements makes detailed sonographic evaluation of the spine difficult beyond 6 months of age[105,106] unless the child has a persistent posterior spinal defect. Some reports have demonstrated that neuraxial structures can still be visualized in older children, although their details are limited.[107,108] The overall visibility of neuraxial structures also decreases as one progresses up the spine, with the best visibility in the sacral level followed by the lumbar and then at the thoracic level.[108]

In diagnostic radiology, spinal US is most frequently performed with the child in the prone position, whereas in an anesthetized child it is generally performed in the lateral position.[107,108] Because the neuraxial structures are relatively superficial in children they are best visualized using high-frequency (10-5 MHz) transducers and they also produce better images than sector transducers.[107] Scans are obtained in both the transverse (axial) and longitudinal (sagittal) axes, and they are performed either through the midline or parallel and lateral (paramedian) to the spinous processes. The paramedian scan is preferable in older children because it avoids the ossified spinous processes that can interfere with US transmission. In neonates and young infants the spinal canal can be scanned with the transducer placed directly over the spinous processes (i.e., a median longitudinal scan). Beyond this age group a paramedian longitudinal scan provides the best overall view of neuraxial structures.[107]

On a longitudinal sonogram, the neonatal spinal cord is seen as a hypoechoic tubular structure with hyperechoic anterior and posterior walls (Fig. 43-39). A thin strip of variable intense echo, "the central echo complex" (see Fig. 43-39), extends longitudinally through the center of the spinal cord and represents the area between the myelinated ventral white commissure and the central portion of the anterior median fissure. This produces the "triplet echoes" that are characteristic of the spinal cord at all levels (see Fig. 43-39). The diameter of the spinal cord varies,

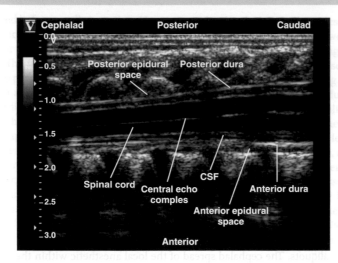

Figure 43-39. Longitudinal paramedian sonogram of the thoracic spine in a neonate.

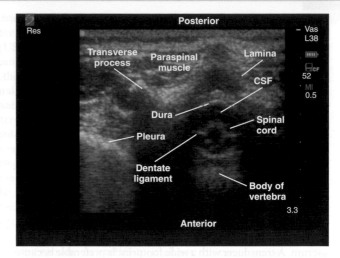

Figure 43-42. Transverse sonogram of the thoracic spine in a neonate.

being largest in the cervical and lumbar regions and smallest at the thoracic region.[109] Anterior and posterior to the spinal cord are two well-defined linear and hyperechoic echoes that represent the arachnoid-dural layer (see Fig. 43-39). The ligamentum flavum, which is relevant for epidural access, is also readily visualized in young children and appears less echogenic than the dura (Fig. 43-40, see website). The dural layers taper distally to close the thecal sac at the S2 level. The epidural space is the hypoechoic area between the dura and the ligamentum flavum (see Figs. 43-39 and 43-40 on website), and arterial pulsations may also be visible on US between these two layers.[107,110] The cerebrospinal fluid (CSF) surrounds the spinal cord as an anechoic layer between the dura and spinal cord (see Fig. 43-40 on website). The vertebral bodies are seen as echogenic structures anterior to the spinal cord. The spinal cord tapers distally to form the conus medullaris (Fig. 43-41) at the level of first and second lumbar vertebral bodies.[107,110] The conus medullaris is continuous with the filum terminale, which extends into the

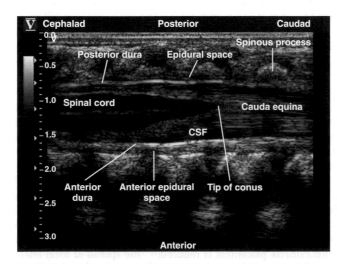

Figure 43-41. Longitudinal paramedian sonogram of the thoracolumbar spine in a neonate showing the termination of the spinal cord.

sacral canal as a hyperechoic structure. It is surrounded by the roots of the cauda equina, which appear as multiple parallel echogenic lines surrounding the filum terminale (see Fig. 43-41). Differentiation of the filum terminale from the roots of the cauda equina can sometimes be difficult. The cauda equina typically lies in the anterior half of the spinal canal when the child is in the prone position, but it moves freely within the CSF with change in position and with crying.[111] Slight anteroposterior movement of the spinal cord, superimposed on the arterial pulsations, is commonly seen during real-time imaging.[110] The spinal cord can also be seen to move in a craniocaudal direction with flexion extension movement of the neck.[105] Rapid fibrillatory movements are also seen in the roots of the cauda equina.[110]

On a transverse (axial) sonogram, the spinal cord is seen as a round or oval hypoechoic structure, with its bright central echo complex (Fig. 43-42). The spinal cord is fixed laterally by the dentate ligament (see Fig. 43-42), which represents the transversely oriented, echogenic arachnoid duplications that are seen in parts of the thoracic spinal canal.[109] Paired (ventral and dorsal) echogenic nerve roots are seen below the L2 level. Farther caudally in the lumbar region, a transverse scan shows the filum terminale surrounded by the nerve roots of the cauda equina (Fig. 43-43, see website). The arachnoid-dura matter complex is hyperechoic and forms the anterior and posterior border of the subarachnoid space with the anechoic CSF and the spinal cord in the thoracic region (see Fig. 43-42) and the cauda equina in the lumbar region (see Fig. 43-43 on website). The vertebral bodies are the hyperechoic structures anterior to the spinal canal. The vertebral arches are also echogenic and cast an acoustic shadow anteriorly (see Figs. 43-42 and 43-43 on website). The paraspinal muscles appear hypoechoic on US (see Chapter 42 for landmark-guided techniques).

Caudal Epidural Anesthesia

Single-shot caudal epidural injection is the most frequently used regional anesthetic technique in children and almost always is used in combination with general anesthesia for surgery involving the lower thoracic, lumbar, and sacral dermatomes.[112] There are several methods of performing a caudal epidural injection.

this scale, the higher rungs of the ladder represent increasing pain. Although moderate to strong correlations have been reported between the VAS, faces pain scales, and the Oucher,[35,41] results regarding the effect of age on VAS ratings are conflicting. An important caveat when using numeric scales in children is to be sure of the denominator that the child is using.

Selection Criteria

Selection of a self-report tool for a child requires careful consideration of the age, and cognitive and developmental level of each child. Figure 44-5 depicts the percentages of children of different ages who are able to self-report their pain and the tools most appropriate for various age ranges. Children who are unable to use a self-report tool may be able to report their pain intensity using simple words such as "small," "medium," and "big." In many cases, it may be necessary to complement self-reported pain scores with behavioral observations, particularly in preschool-aged children. Regardless of the tool selected, assessment of postoperative pain is greatly facilitated by the introduction of the concept of rating pain and of the tool itself during the preoperative preparation of the child.

Observational-Behavioral Measures

Despite several age-appropriate methods for self-report, children may still be unable or unwilling to report their pain, and pain assessment in these children relies on observations of behaviors. Büttner and Finke found five behaviors that were reliable, specific, and sensitive when predicting analgesic requirements. These included facial expression, vocalization/cry, leg posture, body posture, and motor restlessness.[42] Variations in these behaviors have been used in several observational pain tools. Table 44-1 describes the content validity of some of the observational tools that are commonly used in clinical practice. Behavioral measures of pain include behavior checklists that provide a list of pain behaviors that are marked as present or absent and the extent of pain is estimated on the basis of the number of behaviors present at the time of the assessment.[43,44] Behavior rating scales on the other hand incorporate a rating of the intensity or frequency and duration of each behavior.[45] Global rating scales provide a rating of the observer's global impression of the child's pain.

Children's Hospital of Eastern Ontario Pain Scale (CHEOPS)

The CHEOPS is one of the earliest developed behavioral rating scales to systematically assess pain in young children (Table 44-2).[46] This tool incorporates six categories of behavior that are scored individually from 0 to 2 or 1 to 3 and then summed to yield a pain score ranging from 4 to 13. Scores less than

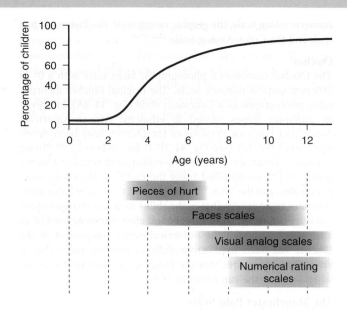

Figure 44-5. Self-report tools most appropriate for different age ranges.

or equal to 6 indicate no pain. Its validity and reliability for brief painful events and for postoperative pain has been well established with good to excellent correlations with faces pain scales and the VAS.[41,47] However, the length and inconsistent scoring system among categories of the CHEOPS makes it somewhat cumbersome and impractical to use in a busy clinical setting.

Face, Legs, Activity, Cry, Consolability Scale (FLACC)

The FLACC scale was developed in an effort to improve on the pragmatic qualities of the existing behavioral pain tools by providing a simple framework for quantifying pain behaviors in children.[45] This tool includes five categories of pain behaviors, including facial expression, leg movement, activity, cry, and consolability (Table 44-3) that were previously found to reliably correlate with pain in young children.[42] The acronym FLACC facilitates recall of these categories, each of which is scored from 0 to 2 to provide a total pain score ranging from 0 to 10. The FLACC tool has been extensively tested and found to have good interrater reliability and excellent validity as demonstrated by changes in pain scores from before to after analgesic administration and excellent correlation with the Objective Pain Scale (OPS), the CHEOPS, the Toddler Preschool Preoperative Pain Scale (TPPPS) and good correlation with self-reported pain scores using faces pain scales.[45,47-49] The FLACC scale has been

Table 44-1. Content Validity of Behavioral Pain Tools: Categories of Behavior in Pain Assessment Tools

FLACC	CHEOPS	OPS	TPPPS	Büttner/Finke
Face	Facial expression		Facial pain expression	Facial expression
Legs	Leg movement	Movement		Leg position
Activity	Torso movement	Agitation	Bodily pain expression	Position of torso
				Motor restlessness
Cry	Cry	Cry	Vocal pain expression	Cry
Consolability	Touching of the wound	Blood pressure		Consolability
	Verbal report of pain	Verbal complaint and body language		

Table 44-2. Children's Hospital Eastern Ontario Pain Scale (CHEOPS)*

Item	Behavioral	Score	Definition
Cry	No cry	1	Child is not crying.
	Moaning	2	Child is moaning or quietly vocalizing silent cry.
	Crying	2	Child is crying, but the cry is gentle or whimpering.
	Scream	3	Child is in a full-lunged cry; sobbing; may be scored with complaint or without complaint.
Facial	Composed	1	Child has neutral facial expression.
	Grimace	2	Score only if definite negative facial expression.
	Smiling	0	Score only if definite positive facial expression.
Child Verbal	None	1	Child is not talking.
	Other complaints	1	Child complains, but not about pain, e.g., "I want to see mommy" or "I am thirsty."
	Pain complaints	2	Child complains about pain.
	Both complaints	2	Child complains about pain and about other things, e.g., "It hurts; I want my mommy."
	Positive	0	Child makes any positive statement or talks about others things without complaint.
Torso	Neutral	1	Body (not limbs) is at rest; torso is inactive.
	Shifting	2	Body is in motion in a shifting or serpentine fashion.
	Tense	2	Body is arched or rigid.
	Shivering	2	Body is shuddering or shaking involuntarily.
	Upright	2	Child is in a vertical or in upright position.
	Restrained	2	Body is restrained.
Touch	Not touching	1	Child is not touching or grabbing at wound.
	Reach	2	Child is reaching for but not touching wound.
	Touch	2	Child is gently touching wound or wound area.
	Grab	2	Child is grabbing vigorously at wound.
	Restrained	2	Child's arms are restrained.
Legs	Neutral	1	Legs may be in any position but are relaxed; includes gentle swimming or separate-like movements.
	Squirm/kicking	2	Definitive uneasy or restless movements in the legs and/or striking out with foot or feet.
	Drawn up/tensed	2	Legs tensed and/or pulled up tightly to body and kept there.
	Standing	2	Standing, crouching, or kneeling.
	Restrained	2	Child's legs are being held down.

*Recommended for children 1-7 years old: A score greater than 6 indicates pain.

translated into several languages, including Chinese, Swedish, French, Italian, Portuguese, Norwegian, and Thai.

Comfort Scale
The Comfort scale (Table 44-4) was developed for use in an intensive care setting and consists of six behavioral and two physiologic measures, each of which has five response categories, thereby allowing detection of subtle changes in the child's distress.[50] Initial evaluation of the Comfort scale found acceptable interrater reliability and good correlations with VAS scores in 37 mechanically ventilated infants.[50] Another study evaluated the reliability and validity of the Comfort scale as a postopera-

Table 44-3. The FLACC Behavioral Pain Scale

	Scoring		
Categories	*0*	*1*	*2*
Face	No particular expression or smile	Occasional grimace or frown, withdrawn, disinterested	Frequent to constant frown, clenched jaw, quivering chin
Legs	Normal position or relaxed	Uneasy, restless, tense	Kicking, or legs drawn up
Activity	Lying quietly, normal position, moves easily	Squirming, shifting back and forth, tense	Arched, rigid, or jerking
Cry	No cry (awake or asleep)	Moans or whimpers, occasional complaint	Crying steadily, screams or sobs, frequent complaints
Consolability	Content, relaxed	Reassured by occasional touching, hugging, or being talked to, distractible	Difficult to console or comfort

Each of the five categories (F) Face; (L) Legs; (A) Activity; (C) Cry; (C) Consolability is scored from 0 to 2, which results in a total score between 0 and 10.
©2002, The Regents of the University of Michigan. All Rights Reserved.

behavior over a 10-minute observation period. The scores of all items are summed to provide a total pain score. A study that evaluated this tool in 25 children with severe cognitive impairment[58] reported good interrater reliability in four of the six behavior categories and good correlations between NCCPC-PV scores and VAS scores. Although this checklist provides a comprehensive pain assessment method for children with cognitive impairment undergoing surgery it may be cumbersome for frequent and repeated pain assessments in the clinical setting.

The Pain Indicator for Communicatively Impaired Children

Stallard and associates interviewed parents/caregivers of 30 communicatively impaired children regarding cues they used to identify pain in their child.[59] Six core pain cues were reported by 90% of the caregivers as signs of definite or severe pain in their child (Table 44-7). Each of these cues is scored on a 4-point Likert scale (not at all, a little, often, all the time) based on the frequency of occurrence of the behavior over the observation period. Caregivers of children with severe cognitive impairment who evaluated this scale at home over a 7-day period reported no significant relationship between crying and the presence of pain. Yet, they found that a "screwed up or distressed looking

face" had the strongest relationship with the presence of pain. In fact, they found that facial expression alone correctly identified 71% of children in pain and 93% of those not in pain, with an overall correct classification rate of 87%. This tool provides a simple method of assessing pain in children with cognitive impairment in the home setting. Further testing of this tool is required in the hospital setting and using shorter observation periods to determine its feasibility of use by clinicians.

Face, Legs, Activity, Cry, Consolability Observational Tool (FLACC)

Initial evaluation of the FLACC tool in children with cognitive impairment found good correlation between scores assigned independently by different observers and by parent global ratings of pain.[60] However, although measures of exact agreement between observers were found to be acceptable for the Face, Cry, and Consolability categories, less agreement was found in the Legs and Activity categories, likely due to coexisting motor impairments such as spasticity. The FLACC tool was therefore revised to incorporate additional descriptors of behaviors most consistently associated with pain in children with cognitive impairment (Table 44-8).[61] Evaluation of the revised FLACC in 52 cognitively impaired children found improved interrater reliability for total FLACC scores as well as for each of the categories. Also, good correlation between FLACC, parent, and child scores supported its criterion validity. Additionally, FLACC scores decreased after opioid administration, supporting the construct validity of the tool. The pragmatic attributes of the revised FLACC (r-FLACC) were compared with those of the Nurses' Assessment of Pain Intensity (NAPI) and the Non-Communicating Children's Pain Checklist-Postoperative Version (NCCPC-PV).[62] Clinicians using these tools to score pain rated the complexity as less and the relative advantage and overall clinical utility of the FLACC and the NAPI to be greater compared with the NCCPC-PV, suggesting that these tools may be more readily adopted into clinical practice.

Table 44-7. Pain Indicator for Communicatively Impaired Children (PICIC)

1. Crying with or without tears
2. Screaming, yelling, groaning, or moaning
3. Screwed up or distressed looking face
4. Body appearing stiff or tense
5. Difficult to comfort or console
6. Flinches or moves away if touched

From Stallard P, Williams L, Velleman R, et al: The development and evaluation of the pain indicator for communicatively impaired children (PICIC). Pain 2002; 98:145-149.

Table 44-8. Revised FLACC for Pain Assessment in the Cognitively Impaired*

	0	1	2
Face	No particular expression or smile	Occasional grimace/frown; withdrawn or disinterested [Appears sad or worried]	Consistent grimace or frown Frequent/constant quivering chin, clenched jaw [Distressed-looking face; expression of fright or panic]
Legs	Normal position or relaxed	Uneasy, restless, tense [Occasional tremors]	Kicking, or legs drawn up [Marked increase in spasticity, constant tremors or jerking]
Activity	Lying quietly, normal position, moves easily	Squirming, shifting back and forth, tense [Mildly agitated (e.g., head back and forth, aggression); Shallow, splinting respirations, intermittent sighs]	Arched, rigid, or jerking [Severe agitation head banging; shivering (not rigors); breath holding, gasping or sharp intake of breath; severe splinting]
Cry	No cry (awake or asleep)	Moans or whimpers, occasional complaint [Occasional verbal outburst or grunt]	Crying steadily, screams or sobs, frequent complaints [Repeated outbursts, constant grunting]
Consolability	Content, relaxed	Reassured by occasional touching, hugging or "talking to", distractible	Difficult to console or comfort [Pushing away caregiver, resisting care or comfort measures]

*Revised descriptors for children with disabilities shown in *brackets*.

Strategies for Pain Management

Pain is a complex phenomenon that occurs due to the transmission of nociceptive stimuli from the peripheral nervous system through the spinal cord to the cerebral cortex. Pain perception is further influenced by emotions, behavior, and previous pain experiences via multiple synapses in the limbic system, frontal cortex, and thalamus. Given the complexity of the pain mechanism, effective treatment of pain requires the use of multimodal therapies that target multiple sites along the pain pathways, as illustrated in Figure 44-6. Analgesics with additive or synergistic effects yet different side effect profiles should be selected so that adequate analgesia can be provided with the least side effects. Thus, pain can be treated at the peripheral level using local anesthetics, peripheral nerve blockade, nonsteroidal anti-inflammatory drugs (NSAIDs), or opioids. At the spinal cord level it can be treated with local anesthetics, opioids, and α_2 agonists, and at the cortical level opioids can be used.[63] Most cases of moderate to severe pain are best treated with a combination of analgesic techniques.

The strategy for postoperative pain management is an integral part of the preanesthetic plan so that informed consent for necessary procedures such as placement of peripheral or regional blocks can be obtained (see Chapters 42 and 43). Additionally, appropriate teaching for techniques such as patient-controlled analgesia (PCA) can begin in the preoperative period. An honest discussion with the child that, although some discomfort is inevitable, every effort will be made to minimize pain after surgery, decreases the anxiety related to the perioperative experience. This, together with the use of nonpharmacologic techniques, may even reduce the need for opioids and other analgesics. Selection of an analgesic regimen requires careful consideration of a number of factors, including scope and requirements of the surgical procedure, age and cognitive abilities of the child, the child's previous pain experience and response to treatment, underlying medical conditions that might alter the response to pain medications, and child and family preferences. In all cases, the goal should be for the child to emerge from anesthesia in reasonable comfort because it is generally easier to maintain analgesia in a pain-free child than to achieve analgesia in a child with severe pain. Figure 44-7 presents a flow chart describing strategies for assessment and management of acute postoperative pain in a child.

Surgical Considerations

The scope and requirements of the surgical procedure as well as specific postoperative issues should be discussed with the surgical team before choosing an analgesic regimen, particularly if a regional technique is planned. For example, the site of placement of an epidural catheter and choice of epidural solution will

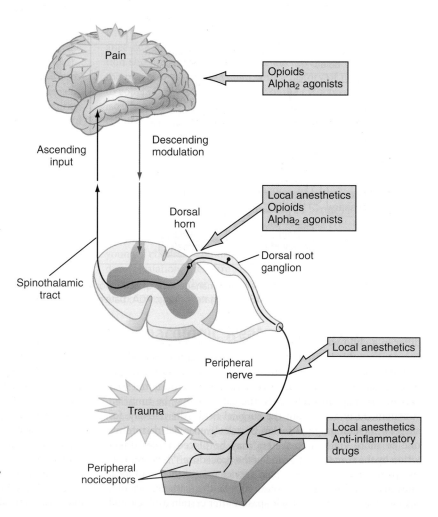

Figure 44-6. Schematic diagram of the pain pathways and multimodal measures to provide pain relief. (From http://old.cvm.msu.edu/courses/VM545/Evans/Pain%20Management%20PDA.htm.)

relatively stable plasma drug concentrations.[156] Although it is used most frequently to facilitate weaning opioid-tolerant children, it has also been recommended for postoperative analgesia and for transitioning children from parenteral to oral opioid therapy.[157-159] Methadone is especially useful for children with cancer or other serious illnesses who require a long-acting oral opioid because it is available in an elixir formulation. Unlike some sustained-release formulations of other opioids, oral methadone is also relatively inexpensive. Note that crushing tablets of most sustained-release formulations of other opioids renders them into immediate release, relatively short-acting medications. Methadone should be thought of as virtually a combination analgesic. It is supplied as a racemic mixture. The l-isomer acts as a μ opioid, whereas the d-isomer acts as an antagonist at the N-methyl-D-aspartate (NMDA) subclass of excitatory amino acid receptors. Action at NMDA receptors may make methadone uniquely useful in the treatment of neuropathic pain. This NMDA-blocking action, and a differential activation of receptor-mediated endocytosis versus protein kinase activation,[160,161] may lead to a relatively slower rate of development of tolerance for methadone compared with some other opioids. Despite these advantages of methadone, it requires careful titration and repeated reassessment to avoid delayed oversedation. This challenge in methadone dosing is due in part to its slow and widely variable clearance but also to the effects of NMDA antagonism on generating incomplete cross tolerance on conversion to methadone from other opioids. In opioid-naive subjects, a single dose of IV morphine is roughly equipotent to a single dose of methadone. Although morphine has active metabolites, the slower clearance of methadone compared with morphine means that, in opioid-naive subjects, daily IV methadone requirements are roughly one third those of morphine. *However, in the setting of marked opioid tolerance, as seen in children with advanced cancer and in the setting of intensive care, the equipotent daily dose of IV methadone may be as small as 1/10 the preceding daily dose of IV morphine.* [105,156,162-164] A convenient calculation tool available on a web site (www.globalrph.com/narcoticonv.htm) has synthesized the information from these and other studies to aid in opioid conversions in both opioid-naive and opioid-tolerant subjects. In our practice, this calculation tool appears quite useful, although it must be noted that it has not received independent assessment for use in children.

Intermittent IV injections with opioids of short or moderate duration administered on an as-needed basis (*pro re nata* or prn) do not achieve a stable blood level and predispose to periods of excessive sedation alternating with periods of inadequate analgesia. Yet this technique remains the most common method of treating postoperative pain in many centers. A partial solution to this problem is prescribing the drug to be administered at closer intervals such as 2 hourly and the use of a "reverse-prn" schedule, in which the medication is offered at the prescribed interval but the child can choose to take it or refuse it. Children should be assessed frequently with the goal of administering the next dose before the recurrence of moderate to severe pain. The use of a long-acting opioid such as methadone has been recommended in an effort to provide more prolonged and even periods of analgesia than could be achieved with shorter-acting opioids, approaching the efficacy of continuous infusions.[165] However, careful titration of dosing and frequent assessment of the child are required owing to methadone's slow and variable clearance. Alternatively, administration of shorter-acting opioids via continuous infusion or a PCA device should be considered.

Continuous IV opioid infusions are an excellent means of providing analgesia to children with moderate to severe pain who are unable to use PCA, such as infants, young children, and those who are cognitively impaired or physically disabled.[166] Once a therapeutic blood level is achieved by administering an initial loading dose, an infusion rate can be selected to maintain that level without excessive fluctuations. Additionally, rescue doses of IV opioids may be required for breakthrough pain. Opioids, however, cause a dose-dependent respiratory depression by shifting the carbon dioxide response curve, reducing its slope, and decreasing the hypoxic ventilatory response. Residual and synergistic effects of sedatives and hypnotics in the early postoperative period further increase the risk of opioid-induced respiratory depression, particularly in preterm and term infants due to age-related differences in elimination and clearance of opioids and other sedating medications (see also Chapter 6). This is of particular concern with the use of continuous opioid infusions because inappropriate dosing or prolonged elimination may lead to drug accumulation, placing children at risk for side effects. Therefore, the rate of the infusion should be carefully selected based on the child's age, comorbidities, and clinical condition. Additionally, children who receive opioid infusions should be monitored and assessed frequently for depth of sedation and respiratory rate. The onset of sedation is an important clinical index of incipient respiratory depression and should alert the nursing staff and physicians to decrease the infusion rate and observe the child more closely. Use of continuous pulse oximetry is widely recommended for continuous opioid infusions in opioid-naive children and other children at increased risk for respiratory depression. Another method of IV opioid delivery is via PCA, which is discussed elsewhere in this chapter.

Intermittent intramuscular (IM) and subcutaneous injections of opioids are obsolete because they are frightening and unpleasant for children and are often perceived as worse than the pain for which they are administered.[167] Additionally, they have the pharmacokinetic disadvantage of unpredictable and erratic uptake if regional blood flow is impaired and they produce pronounced peaks and valleys in blood concentration. The goal of maintaining an even level of analgesia is thus nearly impossible to achieve with these routes of administration. An important exception to this statement involves the use of indwelling subcutaneous catheters for continuous infusions and PCA. Subcutaneous catheters are particularly useful for opioid delivery in palliative care.

Selection of Opioids for Parenteral Use

Morphine is the opioid most commonly used for postoperative analgesia and has been extensively studied in all pediatric age groups. After major abdominal, thoracic, and orthopedic surgery, children who received continuous morphine infusions had reduced pain scores compared with those who received intermittent IM or IV injections.[168-170] However, other investigators were only able to demonstrate reduced pain scores with continuous morphine infusions compared with intermittent IV injections of morphine in children between 1 and 3 years of age and not in infants from birth to 1 year of age.[171,172] Similarly, the data regarding the beneficial effects of opioid analgesia in ameliorating the postoperative response to surgical stress are conflicting. A significant reduction in serum β-endorphin levels has been reported in neonates after the initiation of a continuous infusion of morphine in the postoperative period.[173] In neonates whose lungs were mechanically ventilated, both epinephrine and norepinephrine concentrations decreased significantly after the initiation of morphine or fentanyl infusions.[174] However, β-endorphin levels decreased only in the children who received fentanyl. When the effects of continuous infusions of morphine were compared with those of intermittent IV injections of morphine on the stress response in children between 1 and 3 years of age, reduced glucose concentrations in the continuous infusion group suggested only a modest ablation of the stress response in this age group.[171]

Several studies have described the pharmacokinetics of morphine administered as a continuous infusion and evaluated its effects on respiratory parameters in neonates, infants, and children after various surgical procedures. Lynn and colleagues studied the dose-response characteristics of continuous morphine infusions and established its serum analgesic concentrations in children aged 14 months to 17 years after heart surgery.[175] Infusion rates were adjusted between 10 and 50 μg/kg/hr to minimize discomfort and avoid excessive sedation. Supplemental boluses of 100 μg/kg morphine were given for breakthrough pain. Morphine concentrations reached steady state in 4 hours. Those children who could self-report their pain reported good analgesia when the morphine concentrations were more than 12 ng/mL. Morphine infusions of 10 to 30 μg/kg/hr yielded mean serum concentrations of 10 to 22 ng/mL with rare respiratory depression ($Paco_2 > 50$ mm Hg in 1/44 children). Furthermore, children who were treated with morphine infusions of 10 to 30 μg/kg/hr were noted to breathe spontaneously after extubation of the trachea and those who were weaned from assisted to spontaneous ventilation maintained a normal $Paco_2$. On the other hand, 3 of 5 children who received a greater infusion rate of morphine, 40 to 50 μg/kg/hr, experienced hypercarbia ($Paco_2$ 48-66 mm Hg). A subsequent study by the same investigators evaluated the severity of respiratory depression in infants and children aged 2 to 570 days treated with morphine. They found that 67% to 70% of those with morphine levels greater than 20 ng/mL experienced respiratory depression ($Paco_2 > 55$ mm Hg and/or depressed slope of the CO_2 response curve) compared with 15% to 28% of those with levels less than 20 ng/mL.[176] The investigators suggested a steady-state morphine concentration of 20 ng/mL as a threshold concentration for respiratory depression in this age group.

Previous studies have found that the clearance of morphine is impaired in preterm infants and that it increases with postconceptual age.[177] Additionally, morphine clearance is impaired in full-term infants up to 1 to 2 months of age, at which time it is comparable with that in older children and adults.[80,178] Preterm and full-term neonates, therefore, have a narrower therapeutic window for morphine analgesia compared with older children. Indeed, these groups have been shown to have reduced morphine requirements postoperatively, requiring fewer rescue doses of morphine when receiving either continuous infusions or intermittent bolus doses.[179] Therefore, opioids should be carefully titrated in these infants in a monitored environment with significantly reduced continuous infusion rates. Based on pharmacokinetic modeling and morphine clearance predictions, a target morphine concentration of 10 ng/mL can be achieved with morphine infusions ranging from 5 μg/kg/hr in term neonates to 16 μg/kg/hr in 1- to 3-year-old children (see Chapter 6).[180]

Pharmacodynamic differences between infants and children have been postulated as the mechanism responsible for the greater sensitivity of infants to the respiratory depressant effects of opioids compared with older children. However, this may not be the case. Although rodent data suggest that the brain concentrations of opioids in neonates are greater than those in older children at similar serum concentrations,[181] these findings may not be applicable to humans. Neonatal rats have a relatively immature brain and a far more permeable blood-brain barrier than that in human infants. Consequently, the rodent may not be an appropriate model to depict the human condition.[182] It appears that the "increased sensitivity" is related, at least in part, to pharmacokinetic variables, perhaps in some measure as a result of a neonate's decreased liver blood flow and conjugating ability.

Regardless of the mechanism, respiratory depression remains the most feared side effect of opioids administered by any route. Neonates and infants younger than 6 months of age are at greater risk for opioid-induced respiratory depression because the ventilatory responses to airway obstruction, hypoxemia, and hypercapnia are immature at birth and mature over the first several months of life in preterm as well as full-term infants. Indeed, a previous study reported a 4.5% incidence of failure to wean from the ventilator and a 13.5% incidence of apnea (≥30 seconds that required intervention) or severe respiratory depression in spontaneously breathing neonates who were receiving opioids for postoperative pain.[183] Another report of a 3-year surveillance period for adverse drug reactions described 15 children aged 2 days to 17 years who experienced opioid-induced respiratory depression.[184] Respiratory depression in this study was defined as apnea, hypoxemia, cyanosis, a marked decrease in respiratory rate, or a need for naloxone. Although this study was unable to define the incidence of respiratory depression because the denominator was unknown, it did identify several predisposing factors, including age younger than 1 year (7/15 children), drug errors including prescription and administration errors (6/15), concurrent medical problems (diminished respiratory reserve, hepatic and/or renal impairment), and concurrent sedative drugs. In contrast, no case of respiratory depression was reported in 110 children older than 3 months of age who were receiving opioid infusions postoperatively.[185] Interpretation of this literature is confounded with different monitoring techniques and different definitions of respiratory depression. For instance, in the latter study, a 4.5% incidence of clinically significant hypoxemia was reported but was not included in their definition of respiratory depression. Additionally, children in that study were monitored with hourly documentation of respiratory rate but no pulse oximetry was used after discharge from the PACU, thereby reducing their ability to detect the more subtle episodes of respiratory depression. In summary, the results of these studies suggest that children who receive opioids require careful monitoring for respiratory depression with appropriate age-based reduction of dosage, particularly in neonates and infants younger than 6 months of age.

The most common side effect of opioid therapy is nausea and vomiting. One study reported nausea and vomiting in 34/80, or 42.5%, of children receiving postoperative morphine infusions,

stimulus. Indeed, Crawford and colleagues have reported that children with sickle cell disease self-administered more than double the dose of morphine via PCA, required more nonopioid adjuvant analgesics, reported greater pain scores, and stayed in the hospital for twice the duration compared with non–sickle cell children after laparoscopic cholecystectomy.[218]

In a double-blind, three-period crossover study, the efficacy, side effect profile, and potency of morphine and hydromorphone PCA were compared in 10 pediatric oncology children with mucositis.[200] There were no differences in efficacy or side effects, including nausea, vomiting, pruritus, and sedation, but it was found that children used 27% more hydromorphone than expected when hydromorphone to morphine doses were calculated on the basis of a 7:1 ratio. These investigators suggested that a potency ratio of 5:1 might be more appropriate for this population. Further studies with a larger sample size are required to evaluate whether hydromorphone offers any benefits over morphine via PCA in the chronic and acute pain settings. Fentanyl PCA has been used with success as a first-line and a secondary drug in children with cancer pain as well as acute postoperative pain.[212,219] Most of the side effects including nausea and pruritus were mild and easily managed. However, some reported an overall incidence of apnea and hypoxemia of 3.5% in 212 children receiving PCA of whom 144 had received fentanyl.[212] In children undergoing orthopedic surgery, those receiving morphine PCA experienced improved analgesia with similar side effects compared with those receiving meperidine.[202] Finally, children who received tramadol PCA after heart surgery were extubated earlier and had less sedation, comparable pain scores, and a similar incidence of emesis as those who received morphine PCA.[151] The IV formulation of tramadol is not yet available in the United States, but some studies from Europe and China support its use in the postoperative period.[151,220]

Pump Settings

Most PCA pumps have five settings to adjust:

- A *loading dose* of opioid ranging from 0.025 to 0.1 mg/kg morphine divided into incremental doses is usually given to establish adequate analgesia before therapy is turned over to the child because self-administered doses with this technique are generally small. Further increments of 0.02 mg/kg may be added at 5- to 10-minute intervals if pain persists. A sufficient interval between incremental doses must be allowed so that the morphine achieves its peak effect before the next dose, thereby avoiding an overdose. If PCA is started in the PACU, opioid doses administered during surgery must be considered before prescribing a loading dose. Additionally, it may be desirable to administer the loading dose via the PCA pump so that it is included in the initial 4-hour or hourly limit of the PCA because children who receive IV prn doses of opioids in the PACU followed by initiation of PCA may be at risk for oversedation and respiratory depression due to opioid stacking. Children who have received opioids toward the end of surgery, those who awaken in comfort, or those who receive nerve blocks may not need a loading dose and may start to use the demand doses as needed on awakening.

- A *patient bolus dose*, that is, the dose that will be administered with each child's activation of the pump, must be prescribed. These small boluses are usually in the range of 0.01 to 0.02 mg/kg of morphine in opioid-naive subjects.

- A *lockout interval* of usually 6 to 15 minutes prevents a child from activating the pump until the full effect from the previous bolus is achieved, and it should correspond to the time from IV injection to the peak effect of the drug.

- A *continuous basal infusion* ranging from 0.01 to 0.02 mg/kg/hr of morphine (or more, in opioid-tolerant subjects) may be used in selective cases (see later).

- A *maximum hourly dose or a 4-hour limit* may be chosen to limit the cumulative amount of drug a child can administer. Once this limit is reached, the child cannot activate the pump until the 4-hour limit has passed. Four-hour limits allow for increased flexibility in dosing over longer periods of time and pain intensity. Typically, the maximum hourly dose ranges from 0.05 to 0.1 mg/kg and 4-hour limits from 0.25 to 0.4 mg/kg of morphine in opioid-naive subjects. This amount may be chosen based on the average hourly use of morphine during the past 24 hours or, in children started on PCA immediately after surgery, at the reduced range of the dosage scale.

Figure 44-8 presents sample PCA orders, including choice of drugs, dosing, and suggested monitoring.

Continuous Basal Infusions (CBI)

The use of a CBI of the opioid to supplement child-administered doses remains a subject of controversy. The rationale for the use of CBI is to maintain near-therapeutic plasma opioid levels, particularly during periods of sleep when there may be no self-administered doses, as illustrated in Figure 44-9A. On the other hand, as depicted in Figure 44-9B, a child who receives PCA bolus dosing only with no CBI is likely to awaken with unrelieved pain that may require multiple doses and multiple lockout intervals to again achieve adequate pain relief. Decreased nocturnal awakenings secondary to pain, improved restfulness or sleep patterns, reduced total opioid consumption, fewer side effects, and improved analgesic effectiveness have all been proposed as potential reasons in favor of using CBI. However, the use of CBI commits the child to receiving a fixed dose of opioid regardless of the level of sedation and has the theoretical potential for overriding one of the inherent safety features of PCA, that is, an excessively sedated or somnolent child is unlikely to push the button and therefore receives no additional opioid but, with a fixed infusion, drug may accumulate (Fig. 44-9C) with the potential for hypoventilation.[221] Furthermore, it has also been argued that programming errors with CBI can lead to more serious adverse events because the opioid medication is delivered regardless of the child's level of sedation.[220,222]

Some adult studies have suggested that the use of CBI has limited benefit in terms of efficacy and is associated with a greater incidence of opioid side effects, including respiratory depression.[223-225] Studies in children, however, have yielded conflicting results.[209,210,226-230] The safety and efficacy of morphine PCA with and without CBI and IM morphine as needed were studied.[209] In this study of children aged 7 to 19 years undergoing orthopedic surgery, significantly reduced pain scores were reported in the PCA + CBI group compared with the two other groups and both PCA groups were more likely to experience only mild pain compared with the IM group. There were no differences in morphine consumption or in opioid side effects among the three groups with no incidents of respiratory depression. Notably, child satisfaction was greatest in the PCA + CBI group. Similar pain scores with improved sleeping patterns have

Pediatric Acute Pain Service (APS)	BIRTHDATE
	NAME
Patient Controlled Analgesia (PCA) Initial Orders	Reg. No.

Date: _____ Time: _____

Clerk's Initials: _____ Unit: _____

No other OPIOIDS or SEDATIVES to be administered while on PCA unless Pain Service has ordered them or been notified. Please page Pain Service before discontinuing PCA at pager xxxx. AGE: _____ mo/yr WEIGHT: _____ kg	MODE: ☐ PCA ONLY ☐ PCA & Continuous ☐ Nurse Controlled ☐ Continuous ☐ Other: _____

Select drug to be used	☐ Morphine		☐ Hydromorphone Anesthesia faculty/follow approval needed. Must start at 100 mcg/ml concentration.		☐ Fentanyl _____
Drug Concentration	☐ 1 mg/mL	☐ 100 µg/mL (3000 µg/30 mL use for pts ≤10 kg)	☐ 0.5 mg/mL (use only for pts requiring excessive dosing)	☐ 100 µg/mL (3000 µg/30 mL)	20 µg/mL
PCA Dose	_____mg 0.02–0.03 mg/kg	_____µg 20–30 µg/kg	_____mg 0.002–0.004 mg/kg	_____µg 2–4 µg/kg	_____µg 0.20–0.5 µg
Lockout Interval	_____min 8–15 mins	_____min 8–15 mins	_____min 8–15 mins	_____min 8–15 mins	_____min 8–15 mins
Continuous Infusion Rate	_____mg/hr 0.01–0.02 mg/kg/hr	_____µg/hr 10–20 µg/kg/hr	_____mg/hr 0.002–0.004 mg/kg/hr	_____µg/hr 2–4 µg/kg/hr	_____/hr 0.1–0.5 µg/kg/hr
4 Hour Limit	_____mg 0.25–0.4 mg/kg	_____µg 250–400 µg/kg	_____mg 0.05–0.08 mg/kg	_____µg 50–80 µg/kg	_____µg 7–10 µg/kg
Double Check	Double check pump settings against the order. Document double check on the PCA/Epidural Flowsheet.				

Emergency Measures	**For sedation score >2 or respiratory rate < _____ :**
	   Hold PCA and page Pain Service
	
	For sedation score = 4 or respiratory rate < _____ :
	   Hold PCA, give Naloxone and STAT page Primary Service **FIRST**, then Pain Service
	   Naloxone Dose:
	     Under 10 kg _____ mg IV STAT (0.01 mg/kg/dose, max of 0.1 mg), may repeat q 2 min × 2
	     Over 10 kg 0.1 mg IV STAT, may repeat q 2 min × 2
	
	For O₂ Saturation <_____ : (Consider baseline saturation) Stimulate patient and encourage deep breathing
	   Administer O₂ by face mask or nasal cannula and page the Primary Service and Pain Service				

Antipruritic	☐ Naloxone (Narcan) 0.25 µg/kg/hr. Add 0.25 mg to 100 mL normal saline (0.1 mL/kg/hr = 0.25 µg/kg/hr) to be infused at 0.1 mL/hr × weight (kg) =_____mL/hr or Nalbuphine 0.05 mg/kg =_____mg IV q 4 hrs				
Antiemetic	☐ Ondansetron (Zofran)_____ mg IV q 6 hrs PRN (0.1 mg/kg/dose up to 4 mg) MAX single dose: 4 mg ☐ Per Primary Service ☐ Other: _____				
Other	☐ Other: _____				

1. Monitoring:

   Continuous pulse oximetry while on PCA except while patient is out of bed. Record pulse oximetry readings at same frequency as respiratory rate. Respiratory rate and sedation level:

      Initiation of therapy: q 30 minutes × 1 hr and then q 2 hrs for the first 24 hrs and then q 4 hrs
      Transfer to a new unit: q 30 minutes × 1 hr then either q 2 or 4 hrs (depends upon start of PCA therapy)
      With loading dose and increases in doses, infusions, limits: q 30 minutes × 2 then q 2 or 4 hrs (depends upon start of PCA therapy)
      Regularly scheduled Day/Night changes: q 4 hrs if therapy has been initiated longer than 24 hrs.

   Pain Scores:
      q 2 hrs × 8 hrs, then q 4 hrs. If pain not controlled after 1 hr, page xxxx or xxxx

2. The Acute Pain Service (APS) nurse may change PCA orders by increasing or decreasing pump settings by 20% and stop the continuous infusion.
3. Any order changes in #2 must be documented on a subsequent PCA order form.

Verbal ☐				
Telephone ☐	Print name/title of person giving order	Signature/title of person taking order	Date	Time
	Physician Signature	Dr. #	Date	Time

Figure 44-8. Sample patient-controlled analgesia orders. (Modified from the University of Michigan Hospitals & Health Centers.)

Table 44-13. Causes of PCA Errors

Improper child selection	• Extremes of age: preterm infant, neonate • Significant airway, neurologic or respiratory compromise
Inadequate child education	• Identify PCA button for child • Avoid mixup with nurse call button • Provide education before surgery
Unauthorized activation of PCA device	• Only child or individuals authorized by medical team should push PCA button. • Specific policies and procedures for caregiver-assisted dosing
Inadequate staff training	• Knowledge of programming of PCA pump • Recognition of excessive sedation and/or respiratory depression
Prescription errors	• Inappropriate opioid selection • Incorrect conversion • Dosing error: units μg vs. mg, decimal point
Dispensing errors	• Wrong drug or concentration • Incorrect labeling • Incorrect transcription of prescriptions
Pump programming errors	• Wrong drug, concentration, settings • Failure to double check settings against prescription and with second practitioner
Inadequate monitoring	• Frequency of monitoring • Pulse oximetry, capnography as indicated • Prompt recognition of side effects and timely intervention
Flaws in equipment design	• Default opioid concentrations • Dosing units: mL vs. mg • Activation button resembles nurse call button • No audible signal when child receives PCA dose • Pumps that do not require review of all settings before infusion starts

ensure timely and appropriate clinician response to deteriorating respiratory status of patients on opioid therapy. Recently, a nurse notification system was implemented at one of the authors' institutions where pulse oximetry alarms generated automated nurse call light notification after 15 seconds, a page to the bedside nurse and charge nurse after 1 minute, and an emergency group page after 3 minutes of sustained oxygen desaturation.[232] The impact of implementing such technology on the incidence of PCA-related adverse events requires investigation. It must be emphasized that pulse oximetry can detect hypoventilation only if the child is breathing room air. Oximetry is *not* a measure of ventilation but rather oxygenation. The use of supplemental oxygen has been reported to mask the ability of pulse oximetry to detect respiratory depression by delaying the onset of desaturation.[252,253]

Side stream sampling of end-tidal CO_2 via a nasal cannula or noninvasive capnography detects respiratory depression earlier and more frequently than pulse oximetry or periodic checks of respiratory rate in adults who are receiving opioids via PCA or for procedural sedation/analgesia.[254,255] Although similar data for children receiving PCA therapy are not available, studies in children undergoing procedural sedation in the emergency department and ICU have reported detection of respiratory events using capnography that would have been unrecognized using pulse oximetry, periodic respiratory rate monitoring, and/or clinical examination.[256-259] Additionally, these studies identified instances of respiratory depression that were recognized by abnormal capnography before oxygen desaturation was detected. Thus, capnography may provide the earliest warning of impending respiratory compromise and may alert clinicians to carefully evaluate their children and adjust opioid doses accordingly. Conversely, in real-world practice, capnograph cannulas can be difficult to maintain in proper position in children on a busy postoperative ward, readings can be influenced by mouth breathing, and this technology also has the potential for false-positive and false-negative conclusions. Newer technology incorporates a fully integrated PCA system with modules for continuous monitoring of oxygen saturation and end-tidal CO_2.[260] Some of these pumps also have a feature that shuts off PCA delivery if preset threshold parameters for oxygen saturation and end-tidal CO_2 are reached. Studies evaluating the benefits of such technology in reducing PCA-related adverse events in children are needed. Although electronic monitoring has an important role in patient safety, all available methods are imperfect. Moreover, they generate frequent false alarms that annoy children and families, disturb the restorative sleep of both children and parents, and contribute to desensitization of nurse's vigilance.

Regional Blockade and Analgesia

The use of local anesthetics, both with and without the addition of central neuraxis opioids and other adjuncts, offers many advantages in the postoperative setting. Blockade with long-acting local anesthetics can provide postoperative analgesia for outpatient surgery so that a child can be discharged home in comfort. Reducing or eliminating the need for systemic analgesics diminishes the potential for side effects associated with their use (see Chapters 42 and 43). Regional blockade affords the ability to provide excellent analgesia to children who might otherwise not tolerate larger doses of opioids. This group includes some neonates, especially preterm and former preterm infants, who are at risk for apnea; children with problems of central ventilatory control; children with precarious airways or those who risk obstruction with sedation, (e.g., children with obstructive sleep apnea); and those with respiratory disease.

There are few absolute contraindications to regional blockade. Anatomic anomalies, such as myelodysplasia, sacral dysgenesis, and other abnormalities either disrupting the epidural space or making access to it impossible, may prevent the performance of a caudal or epidural block. A report of epidural analgesia in children with myelodysplasia, however, suggests that catheters may be used safely in these children when placed at a level above the anatomic neural abnormality.[261] In cases involving these types of anatomic anomalies, we encourage consultation with experts in pediatric regional anesthesia, prior review of imaging studies, and consideration of use of fluoroscopic guidance. A needle and block should never be placed through infected tissue or in close proximity to it. Children with burn injuries may be candidates for continuous regional tech-

niques, provided the burned area is distant from the catheter placement site. We do not believe that the benefits of regional analgesia outweigh the potential risks inherent in inserting catheters through burned tissue or close to it. The use of catheters in burned children should be limited to those having burns on less than 30% of body surface area and having no burned areas contiguous with the catheter insertion site. Sepsis presents a similar problem. In general, it is not advisable to place caudal or epidural catheters in children who are septic for fear of seeding the epidural space during a period of bacteremia. Peripheral nerve, plexus, or intrapleural catheters may pose less of a problem in this regard, but there are no data to provide guidance regarding this issue. Coagulopathy and thrombocytopenia are relative contraindications to regional anesthesia, with mild abnormalities in hemostasis not necessarily precluding a regional block. In unusual cases, and with proper consideration of risk-benefit issues, fresh frozen plasma or platelets can be infused at the time of a regional procedure to provide temporary correction of coagulopathy. The considerations regarding regional anesthesia, coagulopathy, and anticoagulation are complex and have been reviewed extensively for adults by consensus groups from the American and European Societies of Regional Anesthesia.[261a] In the absence of additional pediatric data, we recommend clinicians to review these publications (they differ slightly) as provisional guides for pediatric regional anesthesia as well. When a surgical procedure on an extremity has involved a nerve repair or revision, some surgeons may wish to assess motor or sensory function postoperatively. In these cases, consultation with the surgeon should precede a plan for postoperative regional analgesia. If the surgery involves the legs, a caudal or lumbar epidural catheter can be used with opioids or adjunctive drugs such as clonidine rather than local anesthetics. Very dilute concentrations of local anesthetics (e.g., 0.05%-0.075% bupivacaine or ropivacaine) may provide some additive analgesia without significantly impairing motor function.

Opinions differ about whether a block should be placed at the beginning or end of the surgical procedure. However, evidence suggests that placing a block before the onset of surgery offers several advantages.[262] While preemptive or preventive analgesia is a reproducible phenomenon in laboratory studies, results of human studies have been conflicting, and our understanding of how to translate this to clinical practice remains incomplete. Initial studies in adults demonstrated a dramatic decrease in the incidence of phantom limb pain when epidural blockade was administered before amputation, although subsequent studies did not uniformly confirm this initial observation.[263-266] Similarly, children who receive intraoperative neural blockade may experience less postoperative pain than those managed with general anesthesia alone, with the duration of analgesia in some cases lasting beyond the pharmacologic action of the block. On the other hand, a blinded study of caudal anesthesia administered either before or after inguinal surgery failed to show a difference in postoperative analgesia.[267] It is theorized that interruption of nociceptive impulses at the spinal cord level attenuates imprinting of painful stimuli on the sensory cortex or forestalls the development of spinal cord hyperexcitability and "wind up," thereby reducing the neural input and producing prolonged postoperative pain.[265,268-271] It has also become increasingly clear that if preemptive or preventative analgesia is to have a beneficial effect, other conditions must be met: the block must be of sufficient duration in relation to the nociceptive stimulus,

it must extend into the postoperative period, and it must be effective at preventing central transmission of the nociceptive signals.[262] This latter requirement suggests that a multimodal analgesic approach may have the most benefit.[266] The presence of poorly controlled preoperative pain may have already sensitized the CNS, rendering the pain difficult to control via intraoperative or postoperative interventions.[272] Additionally, in an adult double-blind, randomized study, epidural opioids reduced the inflammatory response after surgery as measured by interleukin-2 levels, suggesting that attenuating the stress response to surgery may improve postoperative analgesia.[273]

Further evidence suggests that local anesthetic infiltration of the incision site, especially when performed in conjunction with a regional anesthetic technique, may be an effective means of providing prolonged analgesia after surgery.[274,275] This simple and effective adjunct can be used before or at the end of virtually any surgical procedure. A major limitation of wound infiltration with currently available local anesthetics is that the duration of analgesia is usually only 4 to 6 hours. Because postoperative pain commonly persists for several days, it would be more useful to have local anesthetics that could provide analgesia for 2 to 4 days. One method of providing prolonged analgesia that is currently under investigation involves injection of a suspension of biodegradable polymer microspheres or liposphere containing bupivacaine. Dexamethasone can further prolong the duration of the block. After injection, these microspheres release bupivacaine in a controlled manner to provide blockade of peripheral nerves for periods of 2 to 6 days, depending on dose, formulation, and site of injection.[276-279] An alternative approach to providing prolonged analgesia currently under investigation is the use of modified neurotoxins. Site 1 sodium channel blockers such as tetrodotoxin and saxitoxin have very high affinity for sodium channels in vitro. Tetrodotoxin and saxitoxin are nonneurotoxic, and they do not block sodium channels in the myocardium.[280] Research in animal models showed that combining these toxins with either bupivacaine, epinephrine, or clonidine results in marked prolongation of nerve blockade and reduced systemic toxicity.

Peripheral nerve and plexus blocks tend to have relatively long durations of action as well, commonly providing at least 8 to 12 hours of analgesia and sometimes exceeding 24 hours. Depending on the nature of the surgery, this may permit the child to transition to nonopioid analgesics at the time the block wears off, thereby eliminating or reducing the use of opioids and their potential untoward effects.

Placing a single-injection caudal block before incision does not abbreviate the duration of postoperative analgesia after brief surgical procedures of 1 hour or less. For example, the times from recovery until the first request for analgesics after caudal blocks placed before incision or after surgery for inguinal herniorrhaphy were similar.[281] For more prolonged procedures, the block may be renewed with a second caudal injection before emergence or a catheter placed and redosed at appropriate intervals (usually ~1.5 hours). A volume of one half of the original dose is usually sufficient if less than 2 hours have elapsed. A reduced concentration of local anesthetic is usually effective for postoperative analgesia. If a catheter technique is to be used for postoperative analgesia, it is generally preferable to place the catheter before surgery and maintain the block throughout the procedure. Adjunctive additives such as clonidine have also been shown in some studies to prolong the action of "single shot" central neuraxis and some peripheral blocks (see later). A single-injection block placed before the incision can provide analgesia for prolonged surgery as well as for postoperative pain management. In cases of major surgery on the extremities and shoulders, there is a growing practice trend toward placement of indwelling plexus or peripheral nerve catheters for local anesthetic infusions for several days, both for adults and children, as detailed subsequently in the section on Catheter Techniques.[282,283]

When the duration of pain after surgery is expected to be brief, a single-shot nerve block technique may be chosen. Both peripheral nerve blocks and central neuraxis blocks (caudal or lumbar epidural) may be used. This therapy is particularly indicated for ambulatory surgery. The techniques are discussed in detail in Chapters 42 and 43.

Choice of Local Anesthetics, Additives, and Dosing

Dilute long-acting local anesthetics such as bupivacaine 0.25% or ropivacaine 0.2% are the most commonly used. These anesthetics have the dual advantages of a relatively prolonged duration of action and decreased motor blockade. Epinephrine (1:200,000) is often added to bupivacaine to decrease systemic absorption and increase duration of action but *must be omitted when a digital or penile block is performed because of the risk of inducing ischemia by direct vasoconstriction.* The optimal concentration of bupivacaine that provided maximum sensory blockade without motor blockade for caudal analgesia was determined to be 0.125%,[284] although another study suggests that the optimal concentration of bupivacaine is 0.175% (7 mL of 0.25% combined with 3 mL of saline).[285] More concentrated solutions of bupivacaine (0.25%) may be used for blocks that do not significantly affect motor function, such as for an ilioinguinal-iliohypogastric nerve block after herniorrhaphy. There is no advantage in the use of bupivacaine 0.5% solutions in most settings, and use of several different solution concentrations may increase the risk of erroneous dose calculations and potential overdosage. Our clinical impression is that thoracic epidural analgesia after Nuss bar placement may be enhanced with denser blockade. For these blocks, motor block is of less significance. For thoracic epidural blocks, we use ropivacaine 0.2% with an opioid and clonidine. The maximum allowable dose of bupivacaine is 2.5 mg/kg, and this may be a limiting factor when using the more concentrated solutions in infants and younger children, although less commonly with older children and adolescents.

Ropivacaine, a *l*-enantiomer amide local anesthetic, is widely used in children, particularly in neonates and infants.[286-289] In both pediatric and adult studies, the duration of analgesia after ropivacaine is similar to that after bupivacaine. Although in adults some evidence suggests that there is a selective sensory versus motor blockade, this has not been demonstrated in studies of immature animals or children.[286-288,290-296] Ropivacaine, a *l*-enantiomer, is less cardiotoxic than bupivacaine. In terms of developing terminal apnea, infant rats tolerate 1.5 times the dose of ropivacaine as compared with bupivacaine. The doses for the onset of respiratory distress and the seizure threshold are similarly increased with ropivacaine.[288] These differences are more pronounced in infant rats than in adult rats. Animal data suggest that the toxic thresholds for both CNS and cardiovascular toxicity are increased 20% to 30% with this agent in both adults and infants, although CNS toxicity in terms of

seizures can still occur with ropivacaine if the dose exceeds the toxic threshold. The authors recommend using a *l*-enantiomer such as ropivacaine in preference to bupivacaine in infants younger than 6 months of age because of the potential increased margin of safety.[289,297] Another local anesthetic with a similar decreased toxicity is levobupivacaine (the *l*-isomer of bupivacaine). This drug possesses clinical properties similar to bupivacaine with a moderate reduction in the toxicity risks inherent with bupivacaine.[298-300] Studies in children with this agent are ongoing, but levobupivacaine has become difficult to obtain in the United States.[301]

Other drugs have been added to the local anesthetic in caudal blocks to prolong the duration of the sensory block, an obviously desirable attribute for a single-injection block. Clonidine, in a dose of 0.5 to 2 µg/kg, has been shown to increase the duration of analgesia after bupivacaine in caudal blocks with insignificant hemodynamic effects, mild sedation, and no delay in recovery times.[302-308] Clonidine's appeal as an additive for caudal analgesia is a reflection of the limited nausea, itching, ileus, and urinary retention compared with opioid additives, although it may increase postoperative somnolence or respiratory depression at doses in excess of 1 µg/kg.[309-312] Despite the reported beneficial effects of clonidine in prolonging the duration of analgesia and in increasing the efficacy of caudal analgesia, one investigation found no difference between IV and caudally administered clonidine at equipotent doses.[313] We caution against the use of more than 1 µg/kg for outpatient procedures.

Opioids have been injected in the epidural and intrathecal space for analgesia in children, both with and without local anesthetics. Central neuraxial opioids have been used for more than two decades to produce effective analgesia in children. However, opioids administered into the central neuraxis have the potential to cause delayed respiratory depression and are generally avoided in the outpatient setting to ensure the safety of children after discharge.[314]

Preservative-free ketamine has also been used for caudal analgesia, both alone and in combination with bupivacaine. Doses of 0.5 mg/kg appear to provide adequate analgesia, without untoward behavioral effects such as those reported with IV or oral administration of ketamine.[315] When combined with bupivacaine, the duration of analgesia approached 24 hours.[316-318] *Only preservative-free ketamine should be used because preservatives have been associated with neurotoxicity.*[319,320] In the United States no preservative-free formulation of ketamine is available.[304,321]

When performing a regional block, the total safe dose of local anesthetic should be calculated first and the volume and concentration of the solution should be adjusted if necessary to avoid administering potentially toxic doses. Because most infants and children will have a regional block placed in combination with general anesthesia, surgical concentrations of local anesthetics are not necessary and dilute medications can still provide excellent postoperative analgesia. This is particularly important when performing blocks in infants. For example, a 7-kg infant has a maximal allowable dose of 17.5 mg of bupivacaine; if a 0.25% solution (2.5 mg/mL) were administered, the total volume would be limited to 7 mL. The maximum dose should probably be slightly more restrictive in infants younger than 6 months of age. At this age, the allowable dose should probably be reduced a further 30%; that is, a 4-kg 2-month-old infant would be permitted to receive 2.7 mL (6.6 mg) of the same solution. Children undergoing outpatient surgery may be discharged after a single-injection regional block, but follow-up the next day with the family is necessary to ensure that the block has receded and no complications have developed. This is especially the case after peripheral nerve blocks. Parents must further be cautioned that there may be some degree of motor blockade present and that the blocked limb must be protected from injury. If a lower extremity is blocked, assistance with ambulation is mandatory.

Choice of Block and Techniques

Inguinal herniorrhaphy is frequently performed in children, and the placement of an ilioinguinal-iliohypogastric nerve block provides excellent postoperative analgesia (see Chapter 42). It appears similar in efficacy to a caudal block, with a duration of analgesia of at least 4 hours when bupivacaine with epinephrine is used. For orchiopexy, ilioinguinal nerve block has been found to be as effective as caudal blockade to the T10 level in a randomized and blinded investigation.[322] In our experience, however, postoperative analgesia for procedures that involve considerable manipulation and traction on the spermatic cord and testis may be better managed with caudal blockade. Penile block is effective for both circumcision and distal, simple hypospadias repair; more extensive procedures on the penis, especially repair of penile-scrotal hypospadias, require a caudal, rather than a penile block to produce effective analgesia.[323]

The use of a nerve stimulator, Teflon-coated needles, and ultrasound makes the identification of plexuses and peripheral nerves much easier in an anesthetized child. It is plausible, but unproven, that ultrasound may reduce the risk of injury to nerves and adjacent structures (see Chapters 42 and 43). Note that ultrasound evaluation can be misleading regarding needle positioning if the needle tip is allowed to pass out of the plane of view. Although it remains unknown if ultrasound and more precise needle placement will reduce nerve injury, there is evidence that it reduces the volume of local anesthetic needed to produce an effective block.[324,325] Ultrasound visualization of the local anesthetic surrounding a nerve or plexus provides reliable confirmation that a block will be successful. Nerve blocks of the lower extremity can be used instead of caudal blockade (see Chapter 42). They provide a field of analgesia limited to the operative site, have a prolonged duration of analgesia (usually at least twice that of caudal block), and eliminate some of the potential undesirable effects of central neuraxis blockade, such as urinary retention, widespread motor blockade, and, occasionally, numbness. The fascia iliaca block, which produces analgesia in the distribution of the femoral, obturator, and lateral femoral cutaneous nerves, has been described in children as an excellent alternative for postoperative analgesia of a lower extremity.[326] Blockade of the femoral nerve, the sciatic nerve, and the nerves of the ankle is easily performed in children using similar landmarks to those in adults (see Chapter 42). Regional blockade of the upper extremity may involve an axillary block, supraclavicular or infraclavicular block, or blockade of the individual nerves at the level of the arm or wrist. Intercostal nerve blocks may be used after thoracic or upper abdominal surgery. This block may be considered for procedures of limited scope such as open-lung biopsy or thoracostomy for drainage, but the duration of blockade is limited to several hours. In our view, for most upper abdominal procedures, the duration of single-injection percuta-

neous intercostal blockade is generally too short to warrant the risk of pneumothorax. For open-chest procedures, intercostal blocks by the surgeon pose a low risk and may be indicated, although again their effectiveness is limited by their short duration. Epinephrine is commonly included in the local anesthetic for these blocks to limit the rate of uptake from the site. More extensive surgery can be anticipated to cause postoperative pain of longer duration and may be best managed with a catheter (continuous infusion) technique.

Catheter Techniques

A catheter placed in the epidural space or adjacent to a nerve or plexus affords an anesthesiologist the ability to provide continuous uninterrupted analgesia for prolonged periods after surgery. These catheters are commonly used for about 3 days but may be used for much longer periods in selected situations. If the catheters are tunneled under the skin, the length of time they may be in situ may even exceed 7 days with proper care.[327,328] Catheters can also be placed in intrapleural or extrapleural/retropleural locations to provide analgesia after thoracic surgery. In our experience, intrapleural analgesia reduces but does not eliminate the need for systemic opioids, especially if thoracostomy drains are present. We rarely use this technique because toxic concentrations of local anesthetic have been reported. Continuous extrapleural, intercostal, and paravertebral catheters can be placed either through the operative field or percutaneously. In adult studies, and in a smaller series of pediatric studies, these techniques appear to provide excellent analgesia at rest but with movement they provide only partial opioid sparing. Some clinicians regard these techniques as providing many of the advantages of thoracic epidural analgesia, with the potential for reducing some of the risks and side effects of thoracic epidural analgesia.

Continuous regional blockade is remarkably effective and safe, although as with any technique, monitoring for untoward effects is necessary to prevent complications. New technology for the delivery of drugs to peripheral nerves and plexuses have made it possible for children to receive the benefits of continuous neural blockade after discharge from the hospital or day surgery unit. Catheters may deliver local anesthetics and other medications via controlled infusion devices that use a pressurized elastomer bulb reservoir that controls the infusion rate with a flow limiter (ON-Q pump, I Flow Corporation, Lake Forest, CA) (Fig. 44-10). This device can be used at home after discharge for infusion of medication into a tissue plane to provide a continuous field blockade or a continuous peripheral nerve block. Infusions of local anesthetics in the subcutaneous tissues at the incision site or into the surgical plane using these devices have been employed for prolonged analgesia in both adults and children. Several types of these infusion systems are available, including ones that have a fixed infusion rate, a variable infusion rate, and a continuous infusion with a bolus option. The latter two must be used with caution in smaller children in whom local anesthetic toxicity from excessive dosage may be a risk; we generally use the fixed-rate devices. When continuous peripheral nerve or plexus blocks are used for outpatients there must be a carefully constructed system in place for following these children to avoid complications and achieve early detection of potentially adverse events. Daily follow-up, either by visiting nurses or by phone, is mandatory. We are aware of a small number of anecdotal cases of what may have been excessive

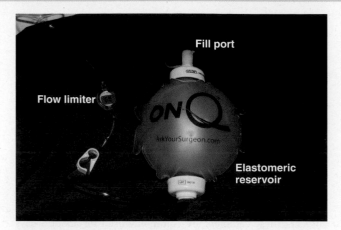

Figure 44-10. ON-Q pump: an elastomeric infusion device for ambulatory continuous regional blockade. The pump bulb is filled with local anesthetic and pressurized. The flow restrictor is readily set to the desired flow rate and the system is disposable.

delivery of local anesthetic from a home local anesthetic infusion pump that resulted in side effects, although no catastrophic events have been reported.

Caudal and Epidural Catheters

For practitioners who are less experienced with lumbar epidural catheterization in young children, the caudal route is recommended for children younger than 6 years. With experience and proper equipment, the lumbar route is feasible at any age but specific expertise is required for infants and toddlers. In infants and children up to about 6 years of age, catheters may be advanced freely from the caudal canal cephalad to lower thoracic levels with excellent success.[329] This is possible in part because young children have a less developed vascular plexus and more compact and globular fat than do older children and adults.[329,330] However, other authors describe less reliability with caudal-to-thoracic advancement of catheters in children larger than 10 kg.[331] This has been attributed to the more mature composition of the contents of the epidural space. With age, the epidural fat appears to lose the spongy gelatinous character noted in infants and the spaces between the fat globules become less distinct.[329,330] Catheters made of nylon or polyamide may be less likely to kink beneath the skin and seem to thread more easily than those made of Teflon or other materials. The catheter should never be advanced if resistance is felt. In addition to problems threading catheters in older children, it has been reported that in neonates weighing less than 3.5 kg one may not be able to pass catheters to higher levels without some risk of the catheter looping back, kinking, or puncturing the dura.[332] In one series of 20 preterm infants, epidurography revealed misplaced catheters in 3 infants. Unpublished data suggest that misplacement of threaded catheters may be more common than is generally recognized. In this series of 724 epidurograms, unexpected misplacement was detected in 11, including 3 intravascular catheters despite negative test doses, 2 intrathecal without cerebrospinal fluid aspiration, 4 that were intraperitoneal, and 1 each in the rectum and psoas compartment. These authors recommended epidurography in all cases, although this

is not the current standard of practice.[333] If specific dermatomal placement of a catheter is sought, one might consider obtaining an imaging study to confirm the dermatomal level of the tip of the catheter. As an alternative to epidurography, Tsui developed the stimulating catheter, which allows real-time monitoring of the location of the tip of the catheter as it is advanced cephalad (using one system available in Canada with the stylette in place) or at least confirmation of tip location on removal of the stylette (using a convenient modification of equipment readily available in the United States) (see Video Clips 44-1, 44-2, and 44-3).[334,335] The technique requires use of saline loss of resistance and avoiding air bubbles in the epidural space or in the catheter-connector-injection system because air impedes electrical conduction. In addition, neuromuscular blockade must be avoided because it abolishes the motor response. Used in conjunction with a nerve stimulator set to very low milliamperage (~6 mA), the muscles supplied by a nerve root twitch as the catheter approaches the segments that supply that dermatome, thereby confirming the catheter tip's location. Specifically, twitches in the feet and ankles occur with catheter tips around L5-S1, hip flexion occurs with catheter tips around T12-S1, abdominal muscle twitches without hip flexion imply thoracic positioning above T12, intercostal muscle twitches imply midthoracic tip positioning. Finger twitches would imply advancement to around T1. This technique can also be used to detect catheter malpositioning. Bilateral twitching at a current less than 0.6 mA generally implies subarachnoid positioning. Unilateral twitches in a narrow motor distribution at a current less than 1 mA may suggest advancement out a root foramen. Unilateral twitches at a current less than 1 mA in a very broad motor distribution may indicate subdural positioning. Absence of twitches as the current is increased to about 15 mA (in the absence of air bubbles or neuromuscular blockade) generally indicates that the epidural catheter is not in the epidural space. Our experience is that the use of one of these confirmatory techniques can help avoid problems with failed or incomplete blocks in the postoperative period.

Choice of drugs for epidural infusions depends on a number of factors, including site of surgery, site of the epidural catheter tip, and child risk factors. Whereas bolus injections spread some distance up and down the epidural space, the spread of infusions is more limited. Local anesthetics, lipophilic opioids, and, to some extent, clonidine all have more restricted cephalad spread during infusions compared with hydrophilic opioids such as hydromorphone or morphine. Experience in adults suggests that the greatest benefits for pain relief with movement occur when local anesthetics are used when epidural catheter tips are positioned at or slightly above the dermatomal levels involved in the surgery. Positioning at levels slightly above the dermatomal levels involved in surgery is more relevant for surgery in lumbosacral dermatomes compared with upper thoracic dermatomes because of the greater distance between root level and dorsal horn level in these two circumstances.[336]

Placement of catheters at thoracic levels requires consideration of risk-benefit tradeoffs. Therefore, if a catheter tip is at the lumbar or caudal level, and the surgery is in thoracic and upper abdominal dermatomes, then continuous infusions containing local anesthetics with or without lipophilic opioids such as fentanyl or sufentanil are likely to be ineffective. Increasing the infusion volume is unlikely to fix this problem because of the limitations posed by maximum allowable systemic local anesthetic concentrations. In this circumstance, there are several alternative choices for upper abdominal or thoracic surgery.

Hydrophilic opioids (e.g., morphine or hydromorphone) can be administered through lumbar or caudal catheters. With these opioids, a wider range of dermatomes can be covered after caudal or lumbar catheter placement and only small increases in dose are required for a surgical site remote from the catheter tip. This same characteristic, unfortunately, also appears to increase the risk for side effects including respiratory depression as a result of rostral spread of morphine in the cerebrospinal fluid to the central respiratory center in the brainstem. Hydromorphone may also offer some advantages because there is less rostral spread when administered by the epidural route and slightly less pruritus than with morphine, although it provides more rostral spread than with fentanyl.[337,338] Lumbar administration spreads sufficiently to provide thoracic analgesia.[339] It should be noted that the potency of hydromorphone relative to morphine in the epidural space is less than when it is administered systemically (2-3:1 epidural vs. 5:1 systemic).[340]

A thoracic epidural catheter can be inserted in a sedated, awake child. With the catheter tip located at a thoracic dermatomal level, local anesthetic-lipophilic opioid infusions (e.g., bupivacaine-fentanyl) may be chosen.

A thoracic catheter can also be placed in an anesthetized child. Some clinicians are hesitant to perform thoracic epidural puncture in anesthetized children because of the inability to use child reports (paresthesia, lancinating pain) as an indicator of improper catheter or needle placement. However, there are few data to suggest that the risk of inserting a thoracic epidural catheter in an anesthetized child by an experienced clinician is actually greater than attempting such placement in an awake child who may not be able to remain still, nor is it clear that a well-sedated child can accurately report what he or she is feeling and differentiate the discomfort of needle passage from more ominous pain. The prospective data from the British National Epidural Audit do not support the contention that there is increased risk with this practice.[341] Although clinical series have reported successful and safe thoracic catheter placement in children,[342,343] this technique should be applied only by experienced practitioners because the tolerances for error are smaller than in adults and older children.[344,345]

It is extremely important to secure the catheter to the skin with a clear occlusive dressing so that the caudal catheter does not become contaminated or dislodged and the catheter site can be inspected daily. In addition, tincture of benzoin or other adhesive solution reduces the incidence of catheter and dressing displacement. For a caudal catheter, the use of an adhesive-edged plastic drape, covering the area from the gluteal crease over the dressing, also helps prevent fecal soiling of the dressing by children who are in diapers. We have not experienced any episodes of contamination of the insertion site or infection using these methods. The use of lumbar catheters removes the insertion site from the diaper area and thereby further reduces the potential for contamination of the catheter and the insertion site.

Management of children with an epidural catheter involves nursing management and monitoring and medical management of drug selection and dosing. It is important to recognize that comprehensive treatment of these children can be successful only if the medical and nursing services coordinate care in all areas. As with PCA or continuous-infusion opioids, the orders should be standardized and written in consultation with the nursing staff so that misinterpretations are less likely to occur (Fig. 44-11). Because the single most sensitive monitor of children receiving epidural opioids is the nurse, rather than a mechanical or electronic device, education of the nursing staff is of paramount importance to ensure safety. Nursing staff can also assess the adequacy of analgesia and thereby help to titrate the drug dose. Catheter insertion sites should be inspected at least once daily, both for the integrity of the dressing and for any evidence of erythema or skin infection (Fig. 44-12). *When continuous infusions are used, the tubing connecting the infusion pump to the catheter should not have any injection ports and it should be clearly labeled as an epidural catheter to preclude unintended epidural administration of drugs intended for IV use.*

A variation of traditional epidural analgesia and PCA is the technique of patient-controlled epidural analgesia (PCEA).[346] With this variation of traditional PCA, children are generally maintained with an infusion of epidural analgesics (frequently opioid alone or an opiate/local anesthetic mixture) and have the capability of self-administering supplemental doses when needed.[347,348] When utilizing this technique, the background infusion is used to provide the majority of the analgesia and the child can add to this when needed. It must be emphasized that the time needed for a bolus dose to effect a change with epidural administration is more prolonged than it is with IV agents. Therefore with PCEA, lockout intervals are greater (often 15-30 minutes) than with PCA.[347,348] The considerations one would employ for choosing this technique include the same child monitoring factors for IV PCA and epidural analgesia.

Selection of Drugs and Doses

Many drugs and combinations have been administered via the epidural space to provide postoperative analgesia.[308] The most common choices involve mixtures of local anesthetics and opioids, such as bupivacaine and fentanyl, although, increasingly, clonidine is being added as well (Table 44-14).

The choice of drug is based on several factors: the age and size of the child, the operation, and the underlying medical conditions that may decrease the margin of safety of one of the agents. Epidural opioids should be used with great caution, or at considerably reduced doses, in children at risk for apnea or hypoventilation (e.g., former preterm infants, children with chronic respiratory failure, or those with obstructive sleep apnea). The risk of accumulation of the amino-amide local anesthetics is particularly problematic in very young or preterm infants, thus toxicity, even with racemic agents such as ropivacaine, is increased.[349,350] Because safe infusion rates of bupivacaine in the neonate frequently provide insufficient analgesia, the amino-ester local anesthetic chloroprocaine may be used in an epidural infusion instead.[351] Because the latter drug undergoes rapid ester hydrolysis with virtually no risk of accumulation, it has been used extensively in infants without reports of CNS or cardiac toxicity.[351]

Local anesthetic and opioid combinations (e.g., 0.1% bupivacaine with fentanyl 2 to 3 μg/mL or hydromorphone 5 μg/mL at infusion rates of 0.1 to 0.2 mL/kg/hr, ranging up to 0.4 mL/kg/hr via lumbar epidural catheters or caudal catheters advanced to a lumbar position provide adequate analgesia in the majority of children undergoing lower abdominal or lower extremity surgery. When a block is not previously established in

Child's weight: _____ kg
Allergies: _____

Continuous regional analgesia via (check appropriate modality)
☐ Caudal epidural   ☐ Lumbar epidural   ☐ Thoracic epidural   ☐ Plexus or peripheral nerve catheter (specify)

_____

The catheter is _____ cm at the skin.   Loss of resistance (for lumbar and thoracic epidurals) was at _____ cm.

Infusion:
(Choose one only) ☐ Bupivacaine   ☐ Ropivacaine   ☐ Chloroprocaine
(Concentration) ☐ 0.075%   ☐ 0.1%   ☐ 0.2%   ☐ 1% (chloroprocaine only)

Additives (caudal and epidural only):
Opioid *(choose one only)* ☐ Fentanyl   ☐ Hydromorphone   ☐ Morphine
Concentration (μg/mL): ☐ 1   ☐ 2   ☐ 3   ☐ 5 (hydromorphone and morphine only)   ☐ 7 (morphine only)
☐ 10 (morphine only)
☐ Clonidine   Concentration (μg/mL): ☐ 0.5   ☐ 1

Infusion rate: Start at _____ mL/hour. Range: _____ to _____ mL/hr. This is a maximum of _____ mg/kg/hr of local anesthetic and _____ μg/kg/hr of opioid.

Dosing guidelines for regional anesthesia/analgesia solution

	Local anesthetics		Opioids			
	Bupivacaine or ropivacaine	Chloroprocaine	Fentanyl	Hydromorphone	Morphine	Clonidine
Concentration	0.05–0.1% (0.5–1 mg/mL) May use up to 0.2% for ropivacaine	1–1.5% (10–15 mg/mL)	1–3 μg/mL	3–7 μg/mL	5–10 μg/mL	0.5–1 μg/mL
Suggested dose	Less than 6 months of age: 0.2–0.3 mg/kg/hr; Maximum dose: 0.3 mg/kg/hr 6 months of age or older: 0.2–0.4 mg/kg/hr Maximum dose: 0.4 mg/kg/hr	0.2–0.8 mL/kg/hr (neonates)*	0.3–1 μg/kg/hr	1–2.5 μg/kg/hr	1–5 μg/kg/hr	0.1–0.5 μg/kg/hr

*Note that the concentration of additives must be proportionally reduced with chloroprocaine if higher infusion rates are administered to avoid overdose.

Treatment of side effects:
Respiratory depression: For RR < _____ BPM, immediately stop epidural infusion and call acute pain service STAT. Administer O_2, ensure clear airway, and assist ventilation if necessary.
☐ Naloxone (Narcan) 1 μg/kg IV = _____ μg, repeat q1 minute as needed

Nausea and vomiting: ☐ Ondansetron 0.1 mg/kg (4 mg max) = _____ mg IV q6hr
☐ Metoclopramide 0.1 mg/kg (10 mg max) = _____ mg IV q6hr

Pruritus: ☐ Nalbuphine 0.05 mg/kg = _____ mg IV q4hr

☐ *For any of above,* begin naloxone infusion at 0.25 μg/kg/hour = _____ μg/hr

Adjunctive medications: ☐ Acetaminophen 10 mg/kg PO q4hr for 24 hours then q4hr prn
Inadequate analgesia: ☐ Morphine 0.05–0.1 mg/kg IV = _____ mg q3–4hr prn pain
☐ Ketorolac 0.5 mg/kg IV = _____ mg q6hr prn pain (up to 15 mg ≤ 50 kg; up to 30 mg > 50 kg)
Muscle spasms: ☐ Diazepam 0.05–0.1 mg/kg IV = _____ mg q6hr prn

Monitoring and equipment: *must choose for patients receiving epidural opioids*
☐ Continuous pulse oximetry and respiratory monitoring
☐ O_2 and bag/mask delivery system, suction at the bedside

Nursing orders:
VS: ☐ q4hr: temp, HR, RR, BP, pain score
☐ Dermatome level for caudal and epidural
☐ Spo2 and sedation score (required if opioids are used). Call acute pain service for RR < _____ bpm.
☐ Record Bromage score q8hr; call acute pain service if 4 or less (choose for children receiving local anesthetics).

Call acute pain service for any questions or problems: inadequate analgesia despite intervention, loose or contaminated dressing, catheter disconnect, sedation score >3, increased somnolence, confusion, agitation, dizziness, tinnitus, hypotension, bradycardia, fever >38.2°C; inflammation, tenderness or swelling at catheter site; Bromage score >0.

Maintain IV access.

For epidural or peripheral nerve block of lower extremity: Ambulate with assistance only with order from primary service and Bromage score of 0. Pad blocked extremities and elevate heels off of bed.

Figure 44-11. Sample epidural orders.

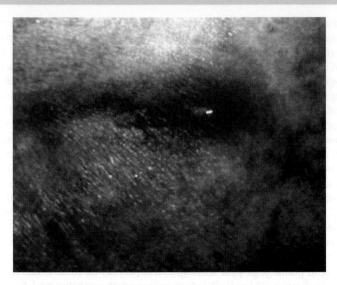

Figure 44-12. Superficial skin infection at the site of an epidural catheter insertion. The catheter was withdrawn, and the problem resolved with local skin care only.

the operating room, it is useful to dose catheters with local anesthetic (without opioids) at a volume of 0.05 mL/kg per spinal segment, not to exceed 5 mg/kg of lidocaine or 2.5 mg/kg of bupivacaine. Bupivacaine infusion rates should not exceed 0.4 mg/kg/hr (e.g, 0.4 mL/kg/hr for 0.1% bupivacaine) for children, because toxicity may result.[352] Similarly, starting epidural fentanyl infusion rates should not exceed 1 μg/kg/hr; the upper limits of epidural fentanyl dosage are determined by clinical effect. Fentanyl alone (0.3 μg/kg/hr) has been shown to provide 90% effective postoperative analgesia after a levobupivacaine

block was established during surgery.[353] If epidural local anesthetic infusions are begun without either opioids or clonidine (e.g., 0.0625% to 0.125% bupivacaine) and inadequate analgesia occurs at infusion rates of 0.3 to 0.4 mL/kg/hr (a maximum dosage of 0.4 mg/kg/hr), further increases in local anesthetic infusion rate or concentration should be avoided. Instead, the placement of the catheter should be confirmed (e.g., with an epidurogram or chloroprocaine/lidocaine test dose). If the catheter is properly located, an epidural opioid or clonidine should be added to the local anesthetic infusion. It is imperative to confirm that an epidural catheter is properly functioning immediately after an infant or child arrives in the PACU or if there is any question of its proper location later. If lidocaine or bupivacaine has been given during or after surgery as an initial bolus followed by a continuous infusion, then use of a repeat bolus dose of either of these amino amides may result in a "staircasing" of plasma concentrations, with a risk for systemic toxicity. Although administration of epidural or systemic opioids may provide analgesia, they may not clarify the site of the epidural catheter. For this reason, confirmation of the catheter location is imperative whenever the clinical picture is not clear. Several means of accomplishing this are described later.

Neonates are at increased risk for potential local anesthetic toxicity because of decreased protein binding (resulting in increased unbound drug) and possibly immature drug metabolism. The manifestations of local anesthetic toxicity in infants and neonates may be more difficult to recognize than in adults. Hence, a conservative maximum infusion dose for bupivacaine of 0.2 mg/kg/hr for no longer than 48 hours in neonates is strongly recommended.[354-356] In general, concentrations of bupivacaine less than 0.05% to 0.1% may not consistently provide adequate analgesia (although they may do so in combination with adjunctive additives such as opioids and clonidine) and

Table 44-14. Commonly Used Medications for Epidural Administration

	Dose Range	Untoward Effects	Comments
Local Anesthetics		Motor block	Reduce dose by 30% in infants younger than 6 months of age
Bupivacaine	0.2-0.4 mg/kg/hour		
Ropivacaine	0.2-0.5 mg/kg/hour		Levo-enantiomer; may have 20%-30% less toxicity than racemic amino amides
Levobupivacaine	0.2-0.5 mg/kg/hour		
Chloroprocaine	1-1.5%; 0.2-0.8 mL/kg/hour (neonates)		
Opioids		Respiratory depression, sedation, pruritus, urinary retention	
Fentanyl	0.3-1 μg/kg/hour		Lipophilic; use when catheter tip is positioned near surgical dermatomes and wide spread is not needed
Hydromorphone	1-2.5 μg/kg/hour		Hydrophilic; use when surgery is more extensive and/or catheter tip is positioned farther from surgical dermatomes
Morphine	1-5 μg/kg/hour	Most rostral spread of opioids	
Adjuncts			
Clonidine	0.1-0.5 μg/kg/hour	Sedation, respiratory depression at higher doses, hypotension (possibly postural) at high doses	Increased risk of apnea with high doses in neonates

respiratory monitors may continue to register breathing efforts when significant airway obstruction exists, as long as the chest wall is still moving, thereby potentially delaying the recognition of respiratory depression. Because electronic monitors that ring only in the child's room can be ignored, it is important that these monitors are configured to either ring at the nurse's station and in the hallways or notify the nurse directly using portable communication devices. Such advanced communication systems are now commercially available and may help to provide early warning of impending complications, although the risk of false alarms, and the complacency caused by their frequent activation, must also be considered. Again, it is emphasized that no monitor can replace vigilance and frequent clinical assessment.

Oversedation, diminished respiratory depth, and slowing of the respiratory rate are treated by decreasing the rate of opioid administration and, if necessary, administering small incremental doses of naloxone. It is only necessary to administer naloxone in small incremental IV doses (0.5 to 1 µg/kg) every few minutes until reversal of the side effects is achieved. Untoward effects can thus be reversed without affecting analgesia. In such a case, however, heightened vigilance must be maintained for several hours, because the duration of action of low-dose naloxone may be outlasted by the duration of the opioid. In such cases, a continuous microinfusion as described earlier (0.25 µg/kg/hr) may need to be instituted. More profound respiratory depression, including inability to arouse the child and apnea, must be treated more aggressively. In this circumstance, the infusion should be discontinued, positive-pressure ventilation with oxygen instituted if respirations are very slow, shallow, or absent, and up to 5 to 10 µg/kg of naloxone administered intravenously. As long as respirations are adequately supported, there is no need to administer very large doses of naloxone. *The new development of respiratory depression in a child receiving what appears to be an appropriate opioid dose should always raise the question of catheter migration into the subarachnoid space. Whenever central neuraxial opioids are administered, facilities must be immediately available at the child's bedside for resuscitation in the unlikely event of an airway emergency.* It is recommended that emergency equipment including a bag-valve device, appropriate sizes of masks and airways, and suction be at the child's bedside or in a "code cart" that is accessible within seconds should the need arise. Naloxone should similarly be immediately available without the need to obtain the drug from the pharmacy. All children receiving continuous regional analgesia should also have an IV line (a heparin lock is adequate in those children not requiring IV fluids).

Pruritus is a common side effect associated with epidural or intrathecal opioid use, occurring in as many as 30% to 70% of children. Antihistamines are ineffective antipruritics in this situation because the mechanism is a central opioid effect not a histamine effect. Thus, opioid antagonists, used in small doses, are most effective. A low dose infusion of naloxone (0.25 µg/kg/hr IV) can be employed with good results. Nalbuphine is used in some centers to antagonize pruritus (25-50 µg/kg q6hr prn), and some studies have found this to be effective. Although we have found this treatment to be effective, others have found it to be no more effective than placebo in reducing pruritus in children.[373]

Nausea and vomiting can also occur in association with opioids and may be more common with morphine than with fentanyl. Children who are fasted during the first 24 hours after surgery do not vomit excessively even when given caudal morphine.[374] As with all other opioid side effects, nausea and vomiting respond to the previously mentioned doses of naloxone. Some antiemetics, such as antihistamines, may cause sedation and should be used with caution. Serotonin receptor antagonists such as ondansetron (0.1-0.15 mg/kg, maximum 4 mg) or dolasetron (0.35 mg/kg, maximum 12.5 mg) have no sedative effects.[375] Metoclopramide in doses of 0.1 to 0.15 mg/kg (100-150 µg/kg) IV every 6 to 8 hours appears to provide adequate relief with minimal sedation. It is sometimes prudent to decrease the infusion rate of the epidural (if the block level permits) or the opioid concentration in the infusate when untoward effects require treatment. If additional analgesia is required, acetaminophen or ketorolac may be administered. Untoward effects of epidural opioids and their treatment are summarized in Table 44-15.

Urinary retention is a relatively common complication of neuraxial opioids. Studies of single-injection caudal blocks have found that this complication does not occur when epidural local anesthetics are used, only when they are combined with opioids.

Catheter-Related Complications

Inadequate analgesia must prompt an examination of the child and a review of the operative procedure and the analgesic technique. The dermatome level should be determined using differentiation between cold and warm sensation in children who are cognitively and developmentally able to cooperate. Presence of a dermatomal level suggests a successful block of inadequate height. No demonstrable blockade suggests a primary malfunction, although low concentrations of local anesthetic may make differentiation of the level difficult in some children. If there were difficulties during catheter placement coupled with a lack of effective analgesia when the child emerges from general anesthesia, the catheter is likely malpositioned. We often use epidurography in this situation to determine whether the catheter is in the epidural space. Misplacement in various locations has been reported, including the subdural space, paravertebral space, tissue planes adjacent to the spine, and even in an epidural blood vessel after a negative test dose.[376,377] The catheter's location can be easily visualized on a plain radiograph (or with fluoroscopy in the operating room) after the injection of a small volume of nonionic contrast. Contrast agent in the epidural space has a characteristic "bubbly" appearance, with the contrast agent centrally located over the spinal column (Fig. 44-13). The existence of a median raphe in the epidural space has been postulated and may be the cause of unilateral multi-dermatome blockade.[378] This has been demonstrated on epidurography when unilateral blockade has occurred (Fig. 44-14). A single unilateral dermatomal band of analgesia or temperature sensation change may indicate that the catheter has passed through a spinal foramen. In some cases, simply withdrawing the catheter 1 or 2 cm may allow proper repositioning within the epidural space. A functional, rather than anatomic, method of confirming epidural placement is the "chloroprocaine test," which has the advantage of both providing rapid analgesia (with a properly located catheter) and confirming the site of placement. A chloroprocaine test is presented in Figure 44-15)

On occasion, a collection of fluid may be found at the skin insertion site and pooling under the dressing. Experience sug-

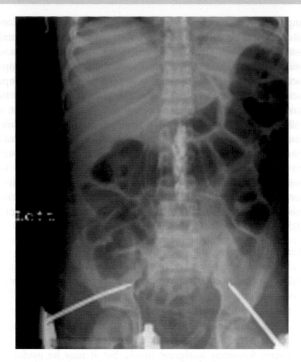

Figure 44-13. An epidurogram shows the appearance of the contrast agent centered in the spinal column and also the bubbly appearance of the contrast agent presumably produced by the epidural fat and plexus.

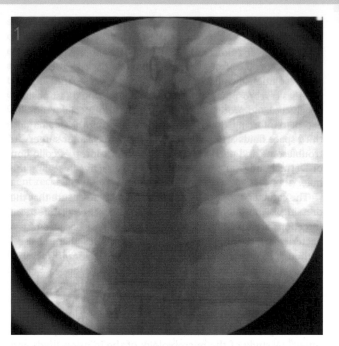

Figure 44-14. Epidurogram taken with fluoroscopy demonstrating unilateral spread of contrast agent. The contrast agent appears to have a very sharp edge precisely in the center of the spinal column, demarcating one side of the epidural space from the other.

PROCEDURE FOR THE CHLOROPROCAINE TEST

An anesthesiologist is present for the procedure with use of standard monitors and supplies for providing respiratory or hemodynamic support.

1. A loading dose of chloroprocaine 3% is divided in 5 equal increments, each given at 1–2 minute intervals (over 5–10 minutes total) according to weight approximately as follows: (doses may be adjusted according to clinical circumstances)

Weight Group	Increment Volume	Total Volume
0–10 kg	0.125 mL/kg	0.6 mL/kg
10–20 kg	0.1 mL/kg	0.5 mL/kg
20–35 kg	2.5 mL (fixed volume)	12.5 mL (fixed volume)
35–60 kg	3 mL (fixed volume)	15 mL (fixed volume)
≥60 kg	3.5 mL (fixed volume)	17.5 mL (fixed volume)

2. Incremental dosing is stopped before giving the full dose if there are clear signs of bilateral lower extremity sensory or motor block, or a very definite reduction in heart rate (e.g., 30 beats per minute) and blood pressure (e.g., 25 mm Hg drop in systolic pressure). In most cases, because you are performing this test because of signs of pain, there is some tachycardia and hypertension relative to baseline values at the start of the test. Transient cessation of crying in an infant or toddler is not a sufficiently specific positive response to warrant interruption of the test.

3. A catheter positioned in the **thoracic** epidural space will generally not show lower extremity sensory or motor block with the chloroprocaine test, but should give a very clear drop in heart rate and blood pressure, as well as a clear and persistent reduction in pain reports or pain behaviors.

4. If the chloroprocaine test is positive (i.e., confirms epidural placement), this implies that a stronger or different epidural solution is needed for steady-state pain relief. Because hydromorphone is sufficiently hydrophilic to spread from lumbar to thoracic spinal levels, **switching the solution from bupivacaine-fetanyl to bupivacaine-hydromorphone will provide good steady-state pain relief in >90% of these cases**. A typical loading dose of hydromorphone of 2 μg/kg (0.002 mg/kg) will provide analgesia within 30 minutes in most cases.

Figure 44-15. Procedure for the chloroprocaine test.

If the chloroprocaine test fails to confirm epidural placement, the catheter is repositioned, removed, or replaced according to clinical circumstances.

- Lockout interval: 8 to 15 minutes
- Four-hour limit of 0.25 to 0.3 mg/kg
- Apnea monitoring, continuous pulse oximetry, and frequent observation
- Add acetaminophen as needed 10-15 mg/kg q4hr (oral) or 35-40 mg/kg initial dose (rectal) followed by 20 mg/kg q6hr (rectal) not to exceed 100 mg/kg/day

CASE 4

An 8-year-old, 18-kg girl with cerebral palsy, severe cognitive impairment, ASA III, presented for femoral osteotomy.

Considerations

- Painful surgery
- Altered/individual pain behaviors: use specific tools for pain assessment such as r-FLACC
- Potential for altered pain perception
- Increased risk of opioid-induced respiratory depression
- May need benzodiazepines for muscle spasms

Alternatives

1. Continuous epidural analgesia
   - Need to cover approximately 10 dermatomes (5 sacral, 5 lumbar); initial bolus, 10 × 0.05 mL/kg/dermatome × 18 kg = 9 mL.
   - Bupivacaine 0.1% with fentanyl, 2 μg/mL, starting at 0.2 mL/kg/hr × 18 kg = 3.6 mL/hr
   - Apnea monitoring, pulse oximetry, and frequent observation
   - Add acetaminophen as needed, 10 to 15 mg/kg q4hr (oral) or 35-40 mg/kg initial dose (rectal) followed by 20 mg/kg q6hr (rectal) not to exceed 100 mg/kg/day (rectal).

2. Femoral nerve, fascia iliaca, or lumbar plexus block
   - There is the need to block the distribution of the femoral nerve and possibly (depending on the location of the incision) the lateral femoral cutaneous and obturator nerves.
   - Single injection block of the peripheral nerves will provide analgesia for 8 to 16 hours; a continuous catheter technique will provide longer duration of analgesia.
   - Blockade of just the upper leg is provided without risks of urinary retention or motor block of the contralateral leg
   - 0.2% ropivacaine or 0.125% to 0.25% bupivacaine; initial dose of 0.3 mL/kg = 5.4 mL, followed by infusion of 0.2 mL/kg/hr = 3.6 mL/hr
   - Add acetaminophen and diazepam as needed.

3. Continuous intravenous morphine infusion
   - Loading dose of up to 0.05 to 0.1 mg/kg × 18 kg = 0.9 to 1.8 mg in incremental doses if needed
   - Infusion starting at 0.02 mg/kg/hr (20 μg/kg/hr) × 18 kg = 0.36 mg/hr
   - Apnea monitoring, continuous pulse oximetry, and frequent observation
   - Add acetaminophen as needed
   - Consider IV/PO diazepam, 0.05 mg/kg, for muscle spasms.

4. Nurse-controlled analgesia with morphine
   - Loading dose 0.05 to 0.1 mg/kg × 18 kg = 0.9 to 1.8 mg administered via PCA pump in PACU
   - Continuous basal infusion of 0.01 to 0.02 mg/kg/hr
   - Bolus dose of 0.02 to 0.03 mg/kg
   - Lockout interval: 8 to 15 minutes
   - Four-hour limit of 0.25 to 0.3 mg/kg
   - Apnea monitoring, continuous pulse oximetry, and frequent observation
   - Add acetaminophen as needed
   - Consider IV/PO diazepam, 0.05 mg/kg, for muscle spasms.

Chronic Pain

Alexandra Szabova and Kenneth Goldschneider

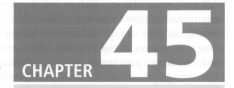

CHAPTER 45

THE PRACTICING PEDIATRIC ANESTHESIOLOGIST will see chronic pain in one of three main venues: a child coming to the operating room for a procedure, after a request for a consultation from a colleague of another specialty, or when making rounds on the acute pain service. The field of chronic pain is broad and extends beyond the realm of practice of most anesthesiologists. Even so, he or she may be asked to provide interventional treatment of postdural puncture headaches, discogenic pain, and complex regional pain syndrome (CRPS). Children with abdominal pain, back pain, and joint pain may be hospitalized for evaluation or treatment (including surgery), and consultation may be requested of the acute pain service. The spectrum of pain diagnoses in children is broad. The nuances of assessment and treatment of each type of pain vary, but some common themes exist. In this chapter we focus on the essential approaches to pain in children and provide some guidelines to assist in helping the patient and colleagues who request your assistance.

Chronic Pain in Children

Chronic pain affects large numbers of children.[1] Back pain has been reported in up to 50% of children by the mid teens,[2] and abdominal pain occurs weekly in up to 17%.[3] Other conditions such as headaches, CRPS, fibromyalgia, limb pain, chest pain, and joint pain are also common. Many of these painful condi-

tions occur in the school-aged child but become much more prevalent after the onset of puberty. Girls are more commonly affected than boys.[1,4,5] Chronic pain can affect the child's sense of well-being, daily function,[6,7] and school attendance. These effects can continue over years if the pain is not adequately treated.[6] Effects on the family can include time away from work for the parents, altered views of the child's health, and increased health care utilization. The complexity of many pediatric pain conditions is greater than can be appropriately treated on an acute pain service or after a brief encounter for consideration of a procedure. The model that has yielded the best results is one in which the multifaceted aspects of pain are addressed in concert.

There are several chronic medical conditions that are strongly associated with pain and blur the boundaries between acute and chronic pain treatment. These conditions include sickle cell disease, cystic fibrosis,[8] epidermolysis bullosa,[9] and cancer. Each disease predisposes children to pain. Headaches, abdominal and chest pain are common in children with cystic fibrosis. Sickle cell disease can cause pain in almost any part of the body, but bone, back, chest, and hip pain are most prominent. Skin and joint pains are prevalent in many forms of epidermolysis bullosa. Cancer and epidermolysis bullosa further complicate pain treatment because the disease causes pain, complications of the disease cause pain, and even the treatment can cause

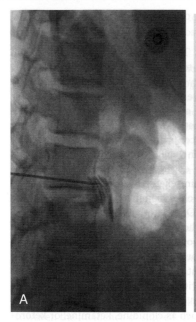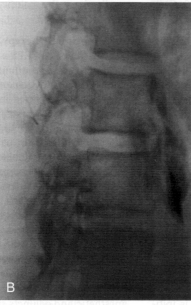

Figure 45-2. Lumbar sympathetic block. **A,** Lateral view. Tuohy needle is in proper position. Note prepsoas spread of contrast agent. **B,** Catheter in situ. Note dye spread and clearing due to injection of local anesthetic through catheter. Catheter is tunneled and can be left in place for a week.

prevalence (1 month to 1 year) of 17.6% to 28%; in different studies, the incidence varied from 16% to 22%. According to one of the reviewed studies, in more than one half of the cases the cause could not be identified and only a minority of children had an underlying disease process (spondylolysis, infection, tumor, disc problem). Radiologic studies correlated poorly with the pain and failed to distinguish between individuals with and without pain. Selected "red flags" for back pain are presented in Table 45-3.

One study attempted to identify biologic risk factors for recurrent nonspecific low back pain in adolescents.[43] This case-controlled study of 28 adolescents with back pain demonstrated that 32% visited physician's office, 46% could not participate in sports and physical activities due to pain, and 32% were absent from school. The main risk factors were decreased hip range of motion, decreased abdominal muscle endurance, and a decrease in lumbar spine flexibility and lateral flexion of the spine. In summary, increased body mass index, moderate (but not competitive) sport activities, sedentary lifestyle, and mechanical causes (heavy book bags) are not associated with increased risk for low back pain. A care pathway for the evaluation and treatment of back pain in children and adolescents is presented in Table 45-7.

Rheumatologic and Musculoskeletal Pain

A special group of children with musculoskeletal pain are those with rheumatologic diseases. The majority of children referred to the rheumatologist's office complain of musculoskeletal pain. Only a portion of these are diagnosed with the true rheumatologic diseases of which juvenile idiopathic arthritis is the most frequent. Besides pain, the diseases often manifest as morning stiffness, fatigue, and sleep problems. The process may progress and cause joint deformities and destruction due to osteoporosis, with resulting growth abnormalities and functional disability. The management is a combination of pharmacologic and non-pharmacologic interventions. The mainstay of therapy is use of NSAIDs, acetaminophen, and, rarely, opioids for severe break-

Table 45-7. Care Pathway for Back Pain

Evaluation

- Medical
- Behavior medicine
- Physical therapy
- Review of records, treatments, history, physical findings
- Consult orthopedics; magnetic resonance imaging/computed tomography, as indicated by history and examination findings

Treatment

- *Medications:*
  Tricyclic antidepressants
  Muscle relaxants (e.g., baclofen, cyclobenzaprine)
  Anticonvulsant (if radicular component)
  Nonsteroidal anti-inflammatory drug of choice
  Cyclooxgenase-2 inhibitor if gastrointestinal/bleeding issues
  If disc disease with radicular pain is documented, up to three epidural steroid injections may be helpful.

- *Behavior medicine:* biofeedback, coping skills, and relaxation techniques

- *Physical therapy:*
  Stretching, postural rehabilitation, general reconditioning, lifting techniques
  Limit bed rest; reactivate
  Transcutaneous electrical nerve stimulation (TENS)
  Exercise program

- *Other:*
  Acupuncture
  Yoga
  Chiropractic (older patients, lumbar only)
  Massage
  Trigger point injections
  Additional modalities for specific indications include back bracing, surgery, bisphosphonate therapy

through pain. The rheumatologist may prescribe agents such as methotrexate, cyclophosphamide, or systemic corticosteroids for severe flareups. Splints, physical therapy, and psychological intervention such as cognitive behavioral therapy are also often used.[44] We have found that some children with Ehlers-Danlos syndrome or other connective tissue disorders suffer from unstable joints that become very painful from repeated dislocations and mechanical stress. These children have commonly required long-term palliation with methadone or similar long-acting opioid. A fair number of young women will present with fatigue, poor sleep, and pain or unusual tenderness in multiple sites. Fibromyalgia is more commonly seen in adolescents than generally expected and can be a significant problem. Therapy includes education, general restorative therapy, with a focus on aerobic reconditioning, and medications. Traditionally, tricyclic antidepressants and cyclobenzaprine have been used, with duloxetine shown to be helpful in adults.[45] As with many chronic pain conditions, cognitive behavioral approaches are valuable components of treatment.[46]

One patient population for whom musculoskeletal pain is a particularly difficult problem is the group of children with cerebral palsy.[47] Spasticity itself can be painful, and certainly the daily stretching exercises are reported to be painful by many patients. Additionally, a subgroup of children with cerebral palsy are nonverbal, making assessment very difficult. The parents or guardians can provide information regarding how their child displays pain and how the pain manifests itself during daily life. If diaper changes seem to hurt, then one should suspect hip or perineal pain. Pain after eating or a history of hard stools may point toward constipation-based abdominal pain. A careful, sometimes staged, examination is required. A thoughtful, empirical approach to therapy and judicious use of radiologic and laboratory evaluations can often lead to diagnosis (Table 45-8).

Pain in Sickle Cell Disease, Trait, and Variants

Sickle cell disease is a hereditary disorder characterized by the presence of abnormal hemoglobin S (with valine substitution for glutamic acid on the β-globulin chain) (see Chapter 9). As a result, a deoxygenated environment causes hemoglobin to turn into an insoluble form and to obstruct the microcirculation. The homozygous form presents as a hemolytic anemia with unique vaso-occlusive features. The heterozygous form is milder and presents as a borderline anemia (sickle cell trait) and rarely with vaso-occlusive features. Hemoglobin SC is another variant, whose clinical presentation is similar to HbSS but whose vaso-occlusive episodes are fewer and usually less intense. About 8% of African Americans carry the gene. From a pain management perspective, the homozygous HbSS genotype manifests as either acute pain attacks (pain crisis, vaso-occlusive episodes, acute chest syndrome) or as underlying chronic pain with acute exacerbations (avascular necrosis, vertebral collapse, joint involvement). Treatment frequently is multidisciplinary with close cooperation between hematologist (transfusions, hydroxyurea, bone marrow transplantation), psychologist (behavioral interventions, relaxation techniques, coping skill development), and pain physician.[48] Most of the episodes can be managed at home with NSAIDs or acetaminophen, supplemented with opioids such as codeine or oxycodone, or tramadol. In severe cases, patients are often hospitalized and treated with intravenous opioids and gradually weaned off as the primary process improves. For episodes of localized, hard-to-control pain, or if

Table 45-8. Care Pathway for Nonverbal Patients

Evaluation

- Medical: often tricky; go slowly
  May need more than one visit to complete the examination
  Try to isolate body part during examination, to avoid generalized effect
  Watch facial/vocal and parent reaction to each examination maneuver
- Behavioral medicine (often not possible)
- Physical therapy (often already engaged in therapy)
- Review of records, treatments, history, physical findings
- Video: the parent may be able to capture pain behaviors for you to view

Treatment

- *Medications:* often on multiple agents at baseline. Coordination with other practitioners is important. Use general principles when choosing medications. Sometimes a long-acting opioid is beneficial for refractory musculoskeletal pain. Watch for worsening of constipation.
- *Physical therapy:* often already engaged. If not, then engage for musculoskeletal pain or help therapist focus efforts of a particular region of the body.
- *Behavioral medicine:* often not possible if patient's cognitive ability is too low. However, sometimes the family can benefit because they carry a large burden when caring for patients with multiple medical problems.
- *Other:*
  Nerve blocks can be used to identify painful areas, if more than one seems active.
  Rarely, a patient needs to be brought to the operating suite for an infusion of remifentanil to identify opioid responsiveness versus potentially centralized or behavioral pain phenomena. The latter may respond to anticonvulsant therapy.
  Intrathecal baclofen (and occasionally morphine)
  Surgical therapy for select conditions

Cautions

- Site of pain is often unclear.
- Don't forget to look in the ears.
- If patient is spastic, strongly consider hip pathology (e.g., subluxation, bursitis, infection).
- Constipation, gallbladder pain, and gastroesophageal reflux are all possible.
- These patients often require more testing than verbal patients.
- Be careful with use of nonsteroidal anti-inflammatory drugs because gastroesophageal reflux can be a problem and reporting abdominal pain as a signal of gastrointestinal side effects may not be possible.

acute chest syndrome develops, epidural analgesia can provide excellent relief.[49] Rarely, children require opioid maintenance with long-acting preparations of morphine sulfate or oxycodone (Table 45-9). The presence of hyperalgesia over the affected area suggests either peripheral or central sensitization, although the role for neuropathic medications is undefined.

related to gabapentin and is reported to have fewer side effects and a significantly faster titration schedule. Currently, it is only approved for postherpetic neuralgia and diabetic neuropathy in adults; experience in children is growing but still limited.

Topiramate

Best studied for the treatment of migraine headaches, topiramate can be applied to the full spectrum of neuropathic pain states.[33] A unique side effect is appetite suppression, and this drug could be chosen in someone with neuropathic pain who is concerned about weight gain when treated with other membrane stabilizers. Topiramate has carbonic anhydrase–inhibiting properties and can result in metabolic acidosis and lead to renal stones in some cases.

Oxcarbazepine

This is the second-generation relative of carbamazepine and has potential for the treatment of neuropathic pain states. Although rare, Stevens-Johnson syndrome can occur with this medication, as with a number of other anticonvulsants. Hyponatremia can also occur, in addition to side effects common to anticonvulsants (sedation, difficulty concentrating, ataxia, mood instability).

Carbamazepine, Valproic Acid, Phenytoin

A summary of effectiveness of these drugs has been presented.[53] Carbamazepine has proven effective in the treatment of trigeminal neuralgia. It was also effective in the treatment of spasticity in multiple sclerosis and spinal cord injury in comparison with tizanidine. Phenytoin has been used in cancer pain, either by itself or in combination with buprenorphine, and provided good pain relief in more than 60% of patients. Despite their effectiveness, the use of these medications is limited owing to potentially serious side effects. For carbamazepine and phenytoin, these include liver and renal toxicity (regular laboratory tests are necessary), aplastic anemia, Steven-Johnson syndrome, and a syndrome of inappropriate secretion of antidiuretic hormone (SIADH)-like picture. Valproate lacks renal side effects but can cause pancreatitis.

Antidepressants

Two major groups of antidepressants are used in the treatment of chronic pain: tricyclic antidepressants (TCAs) (amitriptyline, nortriptyline, desipramine, doxepin, imipramine) and newer selective serotonin reuptake inhibitors (SSRIs) (fluoxetine, paroxetine) and serotonin-norepinephrine reuptake inhibitors (SNRIs) (venlafaxine, duloxetine).[54] The efficacy of TCAs in the treatment of neuropathic pain has been confirmed in meta-analyses.[55,56] The doses required to control chronic pain are usually less than those used in the treatment of depression. The efficacy of antidepressants has been demonstrated in neuropathic as well as non-neuropathic pain, which is a significant difference compared with membrane stabilizers. Examples of chronic non-neuropathic pain in which antidepressants are effective include fibromyalgia and low back pain. When prescribing antidepressants, we recommend vigilance about the potential increase in suicidal ideation and attempts in adolescents and young adults. We inform patients and families in detail, to ensure that they would communicate such ideation with their family and us. We refer patients who appear to be at greater risk for psychiatric comorbidity to a psychologist for evaluation before prescribing this class of medications.

Tricyclic Antidepressants

The major limiting factor in prescribing these medications is their side effects. Onset of side effects can be reduced by slow dose escalation, as with the anticonvulsants. The most frequent side effect is sedation, which is often beneficial in chronic pain patients who have difficulties sleeping. It is important to monitor the child in the mornings, to prevent carryover sedation. In such cases, it is reasonable either to decrease the dose or encourage the child to take the medication earlier in the evening. Because of the anticholinergic effects of TCAs, children will often notice a dry mouth and may experience constipation, urinary retention, or weight gain. TCAs are known to prolong the cardiac QT interval, which can cause a lethal arrhythmia. We take a careful history of cardiac symptoms and conduction abnormalities in the child and family members. It is reasonable to order a baseline electrocardiogram to rule out congenital prolonged QT interval before initiation of therapy. Concomitant use of SSRIs, SNRIs, or tramadol can decrease the seizure threshold in children with a seizure disorder; therefore, their simultaneous use is discouraged. Amitriptyline and nortriptyline are the most commonly used medications of this group. The usual starting dose is 5 to 10 mg orally at night, increased to 20 or 25 mg at night 1 week later. The dose can be escalated up to 1 mg/kg, although this high a dose is rarely required in chronic pain patients. Analgesic effects can be seen in 1 to 3 weeks, as with antidepressants effects. Nortriptyline is a metabolite of amitriptyline, with similar utility for pain but less sedation. The dosing schedule is the same as for amitriptyline. If top-range dosing is required, periodic electrocardiographic monitoring for QTc changes is suggested.

Selective Serotonin (and Norepinephrine) Reuptake Inhibitors

Venlafaxine's starting dose is 37.5 mg/day in adults, which can be increased by 37.5 mg every week up to 300 mg/day. Side effects include headaches, nausea, sweating, sedation, hypertension, and seizures. If the dose is below 150 mg/day, the effects are mostly serotoninergic. If it is above 150 mg/day, the effects are mixed serotoninergic and noradrenergic. Duloxetine has antidepressant effects as well as analgesic effects for both neuropathic pain and fibromyalgia.[45,54] It is usually started at 20 to 60 mg daily to a maximum dose of 120 mg/day. The major side effects are nausea, dry mouth, constipation, dizziness, and insomnia. Use of both medications in younger children is best left to those who prescribe the medications frequently because dosing has not been well established in the pediatric age group.

Muscle Relaxants

Muscle relaxants are frequently used as an adjunct to other medications (mostly NSAIDs) in patients with myofascial pain.

Cyclobenzaprine

Cyclobenzaprine is a centrally acting muscle relaxant. Its major side effects are somnolence, dizziness, and asthenia. The usual starting dose is 5 mg at night time, which can be increased to 10 mg after 5 to 7 days unless the child has difficulties awakening in the morning. The dose can be escalated up to 10 mg three times a day.

Baclofen

Baclofen is one of the most powerful centrally acting muscle relaxants. It interacts with the GABA(b) receptor subtype. It is usually indicated in patients with spasticity such as cerebral palsy or multiple sclerosis. In children 2 to 7 years old, the dose is 10 to 15 mg/day, divided in two to three doses. The dose can be escalated every 3 days by 5 mg to a maximum dose of 40 mg/day. In children older than 8 years of age, the maximum dose is 60 mg/day. Baclofen is one of a few medications approved for intrathecal administration via implanted pumps and is usually administered to children with spasticity (e.g., cerebral palsy, spinal cord injury).

Tramadol

Tramadol is a unique analgesic that cannot be classified in any of the existing groups. It is a very weak mu-receptor opioid agonist. It also blocks monoamine reuptake in the central nervous system (similar to antidepressants). For the latter reason, tramadol is a popular analgesic for neuropathic pain, especially for controlling paresthesias, allodynia, and touch-evoked pain. The likelihood of tolerance and the development of dependence is small, although it has been reported. Despite its weak opioid properties, sudden discontinuation of tramadol can cause withdrawal symptoms. The doses used for chronic pain vary from 25 mg up to 100 mg four times a day (400 mg/day maximum). The dose should be limited in renally impaired children with creatinine clearance less than 30 mL/min up to a maximum 200 mg/day and in those with impaired liver function up to 100 mg/day. Common side effects include nausea/vomiting, sedation, constipation, diarrhea, dizziness, headache, seizures, and hallucinations. Rare side effects include orthostatic hypotension, syncope, and tachyarrhythmia.

Corticosteroids, Local Anesthetics, NMDA Receptor Antagonists, Capsaicin, α_2-Adrenergic Receptor Agonist

There are many drugs utilized in the treatment of chronic pain, with a wide array of mechanisms of action. Oral medications with local anesthetic properties such as mexiletine have been used in the treatment of neuropathic pain in CRPS. The α_2 receptor agonist clonidine finds its application in the same arena. It is used orally or added to local anesthetic solutions in intravenous regional techniques. The major limiting factor in the use of these drugs is their side effect profile, which includes hypotension, sedation, bradycardia, and nausea (especially with mexiletine). There is experience in the adult population, but use of these medications in the pediatric chronic pain population is more limited. α_2-adrenergic agonist blocking properties are also part of the mechanism of action of the muscle relaxant tizanidine. The topical agent capsaicin, originating from hot chili peppers, is also helpful in neuropathic pain, but its application can cause a burning sensation where applied, which is often poorly tolerated. The topical lidocaine patch has been proven effective in the controlling symptoms of postherpetic neuralgia[57] and has also been used for localized myofascial pain, hyperpathia, and allodynia in other neuropathic conditions. Pharmacokinetic studies in adults have found minimal lidocaine blood levels, suggesting a large margin of safety,[58] although similar studies have not been carried out in children. We believe that this is a safe adjunct to symptomatic treatment of chronic pain. NMDA receptor antagonists such as ketamine, amantadine, or dextromethorphan have anecdotal evidence supporting their utility in the treatment of neuropathic pain. It is also thought

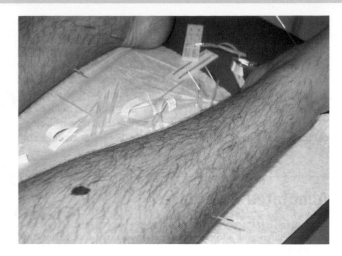

Figure 45-3. Acupuncture needles in situ.

that NMDA receptor antagonists exert an opioid-sparing effect. An important limiting factor of the broader use of ketamine in the treatment of chronic pain symptoms is the potential for psychotropic side effects.

Complementary Therapies

Alternative therapies have held appeal to patients for a long time. Given that "traditional" medical therapies have a high failure rate, patients will continue to search for other possible treatments. There are a variety of treatments, however, that are useful in the treatment of chronic pain. As a consultant, one should consider suggesting some of these therapies in situations where they seem appropriate. TENS and biofeedback have been discussed earlier.

Acupuncture (and its derivative, acupressure) originated in China and is an important part of traditional Chinese medicine (Fig. 45-3). In acupuncture, the body energy or qi (pronounced "chi") circulates in body meridians and collaterals. Meridians and collaterals are pathways that represent body organ systems called the Zang-Fu organs. They resemble Western medicine organs, but they are viewed in a different manner. The meridians and collaterals pertain to organs interiorly and extend over the body exteriorly forming an organic whole between the tissues and organs. In Chinese medicine, pain is caused by obstruction in the circulation of qi in these channels due to multiple causes. Treatment is focused on treating the cause itself, as well as alleviating the symptom—pain. Acupuncture has been utilized in acute and chronic pain conditions such as neck and back pain, dental pain, musculoskeletal and arthritic pain, CRPS, migraine, facial pain, and fibromyalgia. The data from randomized controlled trials is controversial or insufficient to support or deny efficacy of acupuncture.[59] In certain patients, however, acupuncture is effective. Frequently, acupuncture is not covered by insurance companies and requires out-of-pocket coverage by the patient, which excludes many from utilizing this nonpharmacologic modality.

Summary

As a pediatric anesthesiologist you may be called on to assist with the care of a pediatric patient with chronic pain. The basic

2. Monitoring equipment that is MRI safe does not always provide the same monitoring accuracy and consistency as the monitors that are typically used in the operating room.

3. The lighting in the MRI scanner, at best, is often too dim to appropriately assess the child's clinical status.

4. Defibrillators are not MRI safe and have been known to malfunction in the MRI environment.

5. All MRI units that deliver either anesthesia or sedation should have a nonferrous Ambu bag attached to a wall-oxygen source inside the MRI unit.

Difficult Airway Management in the Non–Operating Room (Off-Site) Environment

There are two potential difficult airway scenarios that may occur in non–operating room (off-site) locations: the child with a known difficult airway and the child with an unrecognized difficult airway. In the event that the off-site location is remote to the operating room, it is our preference to secure a pre-identified "potential difficult airway" in the controlled operating room environment. Regardless of an anesthesiologist's comfort level and familiarity with the intended off-site environment, the critical back-up personnel are not always available in those locations. In the radiology suite, fiberoptic intubations are not routine and the radiology nurses are, understandably, unable to assist with facility. It is important to note that a fiberoptic bronchoscope and light source are not MRI compatible. It is easier to perform a fiberoptic intubation, or to have the fiberoptic equipment readily available, in a true operating room. In this environment, both the nursing and anesthesia support staff (technicians, other anesthesiologists, and otolaryngologists) are readily available and prepared to provide assistance. After intubation, the child may be transported to the off-site location for subsequent care.

The alternate scenario, and one that anesthesiologists prefer to avoid, is the unrecognized difficult airway. For this reason, it is important to have alternate airway devices such as LMAs stocked in all anesthesia carts that are designated for off-site locations. In the event that the child cannot be ventilated or intubated, the LMA may be lifesaving.[6,7]

Computed Tomography

Computed tomography (CT) involves ionizing radiation and can provide a good modality for differentiating between high density (calcium, iron, bone, contrast-enhanced vascular and cerebrospinal fluid [CSF] spaces) and low-density (oxygen, nitrogen, carbon in air, fat, CSF, muscle, white matter, gray matter, and water-containing lesions) structures. Because the scan time for current devices is brief, with actual imaging time ranging from 5 to 50 seconds per sequence, most children are able to tolerate CT without sedation or anesthesia. In the uncommon situation that anesthesia is required, it is often for those who have a fragile or unstable respiratory or cardiovascular status, children who are unable to cooperate (cognitively impaired children and those younger than 2 to 3 years of age), or those who require a CT emergently. Emergent indications include head trauma, unstable respiratory status in need of a pulmonary diagnosis, unexplained changes in mental status, or neoplasm work-up in severely debilitated children. Anesthesia management is necessary when there is a potentially unstable airway (peritonsillar abscess, anterior mediastinal mass, craniofacial anomaly, tracheoesophageal fistula, uncontrolled vomiting or gastroesophageal reflux), or the need for breath holding during acquisition of images (three-dimensional dynamic airway studies) (Figs. 46-1 and 46-2).

Children with Down syndrome pose a unique risk for atlantoaxial instability and may require a head or neck CT to evaluate cervical and temporomandibular anatomy, recurrent sinusitis, or choanal atresia. The incidence of atlantoaxial instability varies from 12% to 32%.[8] Many children with Down syndrome require

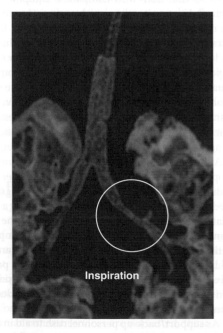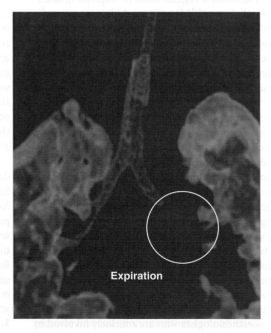

Figure 46-1. Three-dimensional dynamic CT scan demonstrating change in caliber of left main-stem bronchus in an intubated child at end-inspiration (pressure held at 15-18 mm Hg) (*left*) versus end-expiration (*right*).

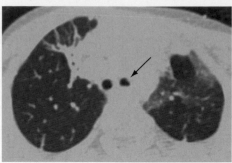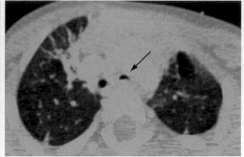

Figure 46-2. Three-dimensional CT scan demonstrating change in caliber of left main-stem bronchus (*arrows*) on inspiration (*left*) versus expiration (*right*).

cervical spine radiographs before entering grade school or participating in the Special Olympics. Usually, the parents know and can relay the results of cervical spine radiographs. These studies alone do NOT indicate to the practitioner whether the child is at risk for dislocation.[9,10] Rather, it is the presence of neurologic signs or symptoms that would herald a spine that is "at risk": abnormal gait, increased clumsiness, fatigue with ambulation, complaints of numbness, tingling in an extremity, weakness of an extremity, or a new preference for sitting games. In infants, these clinical signs may be difficult to assess. In younger patients, developmental milestones (e.g., crawling, sitting up, reaching for objects) should be evaluated. Physical signs may include clonus, hyperreflexia, quadriparesis, neurogenic bladder, hemiparesis, ataxia, and sensory loss. Children with atlantoaxial instability on a radiograph are at less risk for dislocation if they do not exhibit any signs or symptoms of instability. Children who are capable of following commands are asked to perform full neck flexion and extension maneuvers to determine whether pain, sensory, or motor manifestations of cord compression develop.

It is important to recognize that an anesthesiologist should not electively manage any child who displays neurologic signs or symptoms until a neurosurgical or orthopedic consult is obtained. Even those children who are asymptomatic, however, should always be treated with care to avoid unnecessary neck movement. Specifically, during any manipulation of the neck or airway (mask ventilation, intubation), attention is given to avoid excessive flexion, rotation, or neck extension.[11,12] There have been case reports of spinal cord injury secondary to atlantoaxial subluxation after prolonged general anesthetics and extensive, prolonged postoperative stay in an intensive care unit.[13,14]

A challenge for many anesthesiologists is the management of children who require oral contrast for CT. Because children lack abundant retroperitoneal fat, they do not have the natural contrast needed to elucidate abdominal images. For this reason, children may be required to ingest (orally or via nasogastric tube) Gastrografin (Bristol-Myers Squibb, Princeton, NJ) to opacify the stomach and bowel. Oral contrast is useful in the identification of an intra-abdominal abscess, mass, fluid collection, bowel injury, pancreatic injury, or other traumatic injury. The oral contrast comes as 3% Gastrografin and is diluted to a 1.5% to 2.5% strength concentration. 3% Gastrografin is the full-strength concentration; in this undiluted form, Gastrografin is hypertonic (2200 mOsm/L). At this concentration, it can cause pulmonary edema, pneumonitis, osmotic effusions, and death if aspirated. Gastrografin is *never* administered full strength. It

is diluted to 1.5% to 2.5% strength. A review of the pediatric and adult literature confirms that there has never been a documented morbidity, death, or report of clinical aspiration with this dilute form.[15,16]

The volume of oral contrast that is administered orally can be quite large. Neonates typically receive 60 to 90 mL. Infants between 1 month and 1 year of age may receive up to 240 mL. Children between the ages of 1 and 5 years receive between 240 to 360 mL of contrast medium. The risk lies in the need to anesthetize these children within an optimal window after ingestion (usually 30 minutes to 1 hour after receiving the contrast agent) to enhance visualization. By most fasting guidelines (nil per os [NPO]), Gastrografin consumption within 1 to 2 hours of an anesthetic or sedation does not fall within the usual NPO guidelines. Yet, the scan must be completed while the Gastrografin is still in the gastrointestinal tract. Despite the large volume of Gastrografin that may be ingested, we do not believe that there is a significant aspiration risk in this population and do not routinely secure the airway with an endotracheal tube (Fig. 46-3). One study of 337 children found no cases of pulmonary aspiration after sedation. When dilute Gastrografin is used, the risks associated with pulmonary aspiration are small even

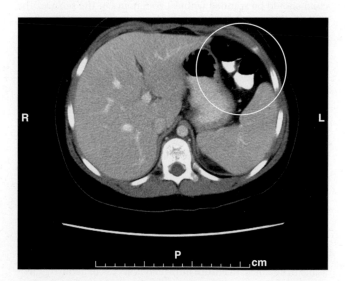

Figure 46-3. Four hours after ingestion of Gastrografin, oral contrast is still present in the stomach and small intestine. Although dilute Gastrografin is still frequently present in the stomach at the time of CT imaging, there are as yet no case reports validating an increase in risk for pulmonary aspiration.

in children who are moderately to deeply sedated.[17] Nonetheless, there is no accepted standard of care for the airway management of these children. Some anesthesiologists will do an intravenous or inhalation induction and maintain the anesthetic with either an LMA or spontaneous ventilation without an airway device. Others perform a rapid-sequence induction and intubation. The lack of consensus among anesthesiologists and the absence of evidence preclude a clear and consistent approach to managing these children. There is no accepted standard of care for these situations.

Nuclear Medicine

Nuclear medicine is one of the oldest functional imaging disciplines. Because of the advances in instrumentation and radiopharmaceuticals, nuclear scanning is becoming an increasingly popular imaging modality. Specifically, these scans are useful for identification of epileptic foci in refractory epilepsy, evaluation of cerebrovascular disease (moyamoya disease), and the evaluation of cognitive and behavior disorders.[18] To complete these scans, the child must remain motionless for at least 1 hour.

The two most common nuclear studies that involve anesthesia are single-photon emission computed tomography (SPECT) and positron emission tomography (PET) scans. SPECT scans use single-photon gamma-emitting radioisotopes and rotating gamma cameras to produce three-dimensional brain images. SPECT scans involve the use of radiolabeled technetium-99m (half-life, 6 hours), which has a high rate of first-pass extraction as well as of intracellular trapping in proportion to regional cerebral blood flow.[19] This scan is useful when seeking to localize seizure foci because seizure foci are associated with alterations in regional cerebral blood flow and metabolism. Injection of the radionuclide during a seizure will tag areas of increased cerebral blood flow and identify the seizure foci. The technetium radionuclide is ideal because it remains intracellular for hours and can be visualized hours after a neurologic event has occurred (e.g., when looking for foci in intractable epilepsy). Ideally, the child should be scanned within 1 to 6 hours of the seizure. The radionuclides are physiologically harmless and nonallergenic. This scan is often requested in preparation for a surgical resection of the identified focus.

PET scans use radionuclide tracers of metabolic activity such as oxygen usage and glucose metabolism. Radionuclide tracers of glucose may be useful when seeking seizure foci or tumor recurrence.[20,21] Unlike SPECT scans, PET scans should be performed during the seizure itself. Because of the short half-life of the glucose tracer (110 minutes), the scan is best completed during the seizure or within 1 hour thereafter. These children must remain motionless during the entire study. Thus, in the event that the child needs a general anesthetic, an anesthesia team must be immediately available. One of the potential concerns for the anesthesia team is the risk of hypovolemia, especially in infants, who remain NPO without intravenous hydration while anticipating the seizure. It is therefore important to work with the neurology and neurosurgery services to plan these scans in advance, to ensure intravenous access to avoid hypovolemia, and to delegate an anesthesia team.

Stereotactic Radiosurgery

Stereotactic radiosurgery (gamma knife) is a major advance in the treatment of selected malignant tumors (ependymoma, glioblastomas), vascular malformations, acoustic neuromas, and pituitary adenomas in children.[22] Radiosurgery is indicated, especially for those children with a tumor located deep in the brain or in an area that could put the child at significant surgical risk (e.g., speech, motor, cerebellum, brainstem areas) or for the recurrent brain tumor that has failed prior treatment. Radiosurgery involves the use of a single large fraction of radiation that is directed at a specific target with minimal radiation exposure to the surrounding normal tissues. Optimal results are achieved with small tumor volumes ($\leq$14 cm^3).[23]

Stereotactic radiosurgery requires the coordination of the departments of radiology, radiation therapy, and anesthesiology. The procedure averages 9 hours but can take up to 15 hours.[24] The stereotactic portion of the procedure begins in the morning in a CT scanner. A stereotactic head frame is screwed into the cranium after induction of general anesthesia and tracheal intubation. Some children tolerate the application of the head frame with local anesthesia alone but then develop anxiety due to the pressure sensation produced by the head frame that can lead to anxiety, nausea, or vomiting. With the head frame in place, it is difficult for the child to turn his or her head to the side in the event of vomiting. In this situation there is a risk of pulmonary aspiration. When the head frame is in place, the key to unlock and remove it should be taped to the frame itself, in the event of a situation necessitating its emergent removal (e.g., vomiting, airway obstruction, or accidental extubation).

Most children are unable to tolerate the head frame and lengthy procedure without general anesthesia. For smaller children, nasal intubation is preferred to provide better stability during transport from the radiology suite to the operating room. After intubation, an oral or nasogastric tube is placed to remove residual gastric contents and an esophageal stethoscope is inserted to monitor breath sounds and temperature. After the head frame is in place and the imaging study is completed, the child is transported (intubated, sedated, and appropriately monitored) to the postanesthesia care unit (PACU). In the PACU the lungs are ventilated and the child is sedated with a propofol infusion to maintain sedation while the radiologists and neurosurgeons review the images and plan the afternoon radiosurgery. The child's care is transferred to the PACU nurse and PACU anesthesiologist in much the same way that intubated children are managed in the ICU setting. The child often remains paralyzed with neuromuscular blockade to minimize the risk of accidental extubation. The recovery room stay can range from 3 to 5 hours, during which time these children require continuous nursing coverage and physiologic monitoring.

After the images are reviewed and the radiosurgery planning is complete, the child is transported to the stereotactic radiosurgery linear accelerator for treatment. In the treatment room there is full anesthesia monitoring and an anesthesia machine. To minimize radiation exposure to health care personnel, only the child remains in the scanner during treatment, observed at a distance with video cameras focused on both the child and monitors. The actual treatment lasts approximately 1 hour.

After the radiosurgery is completed, the child is transferred, with the trachea still intubated, back to the PACU, where the trachea is extubated under controlled conditions. There are inherent risks to this prolonged anesthetic, which requires multiple transports between sites. One study examined 68 radiosurgery procedures in 65 children and reported four potentially serious anesthesia-related events.[24] In those children who received general anesthesia, serious complications included obstruction of the endotracheal tube while in the head frame and lobar collapse requiring prolonged mechanical ventilation.

Radiation Therapy

Radiation therapy for children uses ionizing photons to destroy lymphomas, acute leukemias, Wilms tumor, retinoblastomas, and tumors of the central nervous system. Repeat sessions are typical, requiring motionlessness conditions to precisely target malignant cells. A planning session in a simulator is typically scheduled before the initiation of radiation therapy to map the fields that require irradiation while the child is in a fixed position.

Radiation therapy is typically administered in fractionated doses by dividing the total radiation therapy course among daily or twice-daily sessions. Dividing the total radiation therapy course into discrete daily sessions allows normal tissue repair between sessions while the tumor burden is lessened or destroyed. The rationale for twice-daily fractionation in children is that fractionation to growing bone in rats reduces the growth deficit by 25% to 30%. The hope is that other normal tissues may be similarly spared during growth.[25,26] Twice-daily fractionation is usually reserved for children with leukemia or lymphoma in preparation for a bone marrow transplant.

These children usually have central venous access to obviate repeated venipunctures. Daily anesthetic management typically consists of an intravenous propofol infusion with blow-by oxygen and spontaneous ventilation. Only the child remains in the room during treatment. Most children are receiving adjuvant and simultaneous chemotherapy. As the treatment progresses, nausea, vomiting and respiratory illness stemming from chemotherapy-induced immunocompromise can challenge the anesthesiologist. It is important to recognize that the daily treatments are critical, and any cancellation should be firmly discouraged.

Magnetic Resonance Imaging

Magnetic resonance imaging (MRI) is employed for the evaluation of neoplasms, nonhemorrhagic trauma, vascular lesions, orthopedic lesions (including joint disorders), central nervous system and spinal cord lesions, craniofacial disorders, and other disorders.[27-29] Brain MRI is also indicated for detecting the origin of developmental delay, behavioral disorders, seizures, failure to thrive, apnea, cyanosis, hypotonia, and in the work-up of mitochondrial and metabolic diseases. Magnetic resonance angiography and venography (MRA and MRV) are especially helpful in evaluating vascular flow and can often replace invasive angiography in follow-up evaluations of vascular malformations, interventional therapy, or radiotherapy.[30] MRA and MRV imaging does not require intravascular contrast and thereby avoids the risk of a reaction to a contrast agent. Most MRI systems are superconducting magnets set up in a horizontal configuration within the bore so that the magnetic field is directed lengthwise to the child. The magnet is cooled by liquid nitrogen to a temperature of 4° C. The strength of the magnetic field in these scanners is described in units known as Tesla (T) and range from 0.5 to 3.0 T. One Tesla is the equivalent of 10,000 gauss. The earth's magnetic field is 0.5 gauss. The majority of patient-care magnets are 1.5 T. To put this into perspective, a 1.5-T magnet is the equivalent of 30,000 times the earth's magnetic field. It can take up to 96 hours to generate a

magnetic field, so the magnet should only be quenched in emergency situations.

There are a variety of safety issues with respect to MRI that are important. Significant morbidity with potential mortality can result from ferrous objects unintentionally brought into the scanner room. Projectiles caused by ferromagnetic attraction to the magnetic field are a major hazard in the MRI suite (Fig. 46-4). In the presence of an external magnetic field, a ferromagnetic object can develop its own intrinsic magnetic field. The attractive forces created between the intrinsic and extrinsic magnetic fields can propel the ferromagnetic object toward the MRI scanner. Having a small hand-held magnet outside the MRI scanner is a useful means to test whether objects are ferromagnetic and thus at risk for being pulled into the magnet. This may avoid potential disasters in the MRI scanner. Some objects that have been attracted to the MRI magnet include a metal fan, pulse oximeter, shrapnel, wheelchair, cigarette lighter, stethoscope, pager, hearing aid, vacuum cleaner, calculator, hair pin, oxygen tank, prosthetic limb, pencil, insulin infusion pump, keys, watches, clipboards, and steel-tipped/heeled shoes.[31,32] Mortality can result from projectile disasters, as in the case of a death in 2001 in which a ferrous oxygen tank was inadvertently brought into the MRI scanner after the wall oxygen source failed. The oxygen tank was "pulled" from the hands of the respiratory therapist crushing the skull of the child being scanned (New York Times, July 31, 2001:B1, B5).

Other potential morbidity can result from implanted devices (i.e., cardiac pacemakers, spinal cord stimulators) as a result of inappropriate patient screening or unfamiliarity with a particular implant's MRI compatibility. Recently the U.S. Food and Drug Administration (FDA) has changed the terminology for designating MRI safe objects from MRI-compatible and MRI-incompatible to MRI-safe, MRI-unsafe, and MRI-conditional. This terminology will not be applied retrospectively to objects previously designated as MRI-noncompatible. *MRI-safe* is

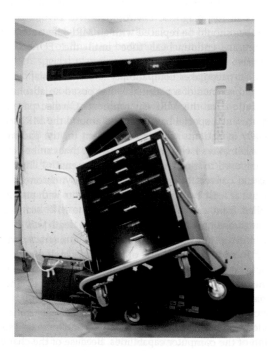

Figure 46-4. Non–MRI-compatible anesthesia cart inadvertently brought into scanner.

outside the scanner, equipped with 30 feet of intravenous infusion tubing. In this circumstance, it is important to determine if the pump is able to infuse accurately through the resistance of the long tubing. An Ambu bag or Mapleson circuit must always be situated in the MRI suite and connected directly to an oxygen source within the scanner. This is critical, especially when the anesthesia machine is far from the child. Regardless of how the anesthetic is delivered, or where the anesthesia machine is situated, the ASA guidelines for monitoring must be followed: pulse oximetry, ECG, expired carbon dioxide, and blood pressure monitoring.

MRI-safe stethoscopes, stylets, laryngoscope, and flashlights should be available. If financial resources are unavailable, intubating in the MRI scanner can be accomplished without investing in laryngoscopes that are "MRI-safe." The only component of the laryngoscope that is usually not MRI-safe is the battery in the handle. Replacing the battery with a lithium battery may be a simple, safe, and less expensive alternative to purchasing a marketed MRI-compatible/safe laryngoscope. As always, before introducing any equipment into the MRI environment, a rudimentary safety check should be performed by first passing a hand-held magnet over the object to confirm that there is no ferrous material within. As a final safety check, an MRI safety expert must carefully introduce the object into the scanner (before bringing in a child) to confirm safety.

Anesthetic management of children in the MRI suite is highly dependent on the availability of support personnel, equipment, the anesthesiologist's personal anesthetic practice, and the child's medical history. Requiring a general anesthetic to complete a noninvasive procedure in children is often a frightening prospect for parents. Parents may not appreciate that although there is no pain or discomfort involved in the procedure, the child may require a general anesthetic to remain motionless for the scan. Some children may not actually require airway control (LMA or endotracheal tube) to tolerate an MRI and may be able to remain motionless with an intravenous sedative. How the anesthetic is delivered will vary from anesthesiologist to anesthesiologist. It is important to recognize that when the small child is down the long bore of the magnet, he or she may be impossible to visualize. If respiratory problems occur, valuable time can be lost while pulling the child out of the bore; because of these considerations, some anesthesiologists may prefer to insert an LMA or secure the airway with an endotracheal tube. Alternatives include spontaneous ventilation with an unprotected airway maintained with a propofol or dexmedetomidine infusion.[85] Nasal prongs that deliver oxygen (2-4 L/min) while aspirating gas for carbon dioxide (capnometry) allow continuous assessment of respirations during spontaneous ventilation.

Most LMAs are MRI compatible. Be aware, however, that the pilot balloon should be taped to the circuit tubing when imaging the head or neck because it will create artifacts on the images (Figs. 46-6 and 46-7). Coating the LMA cuff with lidocaine gel decreases the incidence of sore throat[86] and retching.[87] A retrospective study of 200 patients reveals that sedation and topical anesthesia enable successful LMA insertion in adults.[88] An LMA may provide a suitable alternative for airway management in children with bronchopulmonary dysplasia, cystic fibrosis, severe asthma, and active respiratory issues. A study of children with upper respiratory infections compared the complications after the use of LMAs versus endotracheal tubes. There was a reduced incidence of mild bronchospasm, laryngospasm, breath

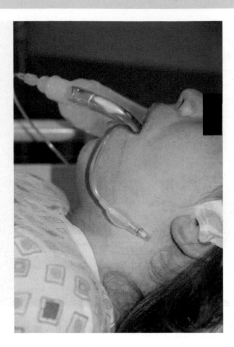

Figure 46-6. Laryngeal mask airway with pilot balloon left adjacent to face.

holding, and "major" oxygen desaturation (less than 90%) in the group that received LMAs as compared with endotracheal tubes.[89] Similarly, the use of LMAs in former preterm infants with bronchopulmonary dysplasia revealed less coughing and wheezing and greater hemodynamic stability in those children receiving LMAs when compared with endotracheal tubes. Children who had LMAs placed (vs. endotracheal tubes) were discharged home earlier after an open-sky vitrectomy for retinopathy of prematurity.[90] LMAs provide for more hemodynamic stability not only during the procedure but also on

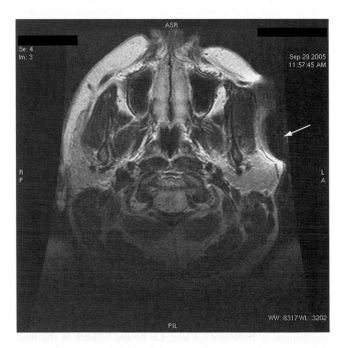

Figure 46-7. MR image of patient in Figure 46-6 demonstrating artifact (*arrow*) created by ferrous material in pilot balloon.

removal of the LMA (as compared with endotracheal extubation).[91] LMAs are very useful in the MRI/CT setting because they allow for spontaneous ventilation, enable the anesthesiologist to follow end-tidal CO_2, and provide a clear airway in a child who may otherwise obstruct under sedation. With the LMA in place, the child can be maintained with minimal anesthetic, allowed to breathe spontaneously, and then rapidly awakened at the conclusion of the scan.

There are various techniques of providing anesthesia within the MRI scanner. Propofol, dexmedetomidine, and inhalation anesthesia have all demonstrated success for diagnostic imaging studies, depending on patient medical history, the comfort level of the anesthesiologist, and the logistics of the environment.[92-97]

Interventional Radiology/Invasive Angiography

Even the simplest procedures such as angiography often require a general anesthetic to ensure motionless conditions in the pediatric population. Many procedures will require intermittent breath holding to acquire better images. When the radiologist encounters vasospasm or wishes to promote arterial vasodilatation, controlled endotracheal intubation is preferred. This will accommodate the radiologist's frequent request to the anesthesiologist to induce hypercarbia to promote vasodilation for enhanced imaging.

Imaging studies of the abdomen and pelvis have unique considerations for the anesthesiologist. Personal experience has demonstrated that nitrous oxide can diffuse into the bowel, causing distention and in some cases can distort or mask the vasculature of interest. It is for this reason that avoidance of nitrous oxide should be considered when angiography involves the abdomen and pelvis; air and oxygen are preferable in these particular circumstances. When angiographic imaging of the abdomen is required, the interventional radiologist may request that the anesthesiologist administer intravenous glucagon, usually in 0.25-mg increments. Glucagon reduces peristalsis and, as a consequence, reduces motion artifact during image acquisition.[98] It is useful for digital subtraction angiography[99] and visceral angiography.[100] Glucagon can have side effects, which include nausea, vomiting, hyperglycemia, depression of clotting factors, and electrolyte disturbances.[101] Children who receive glucagon frequently vomit; thus, it is advisable to administer an antiemetic before awakening them from anesthesia, although the efficacy for this indication is not clearly established.

Cerebral angiography can be challenging. Cerebral angiograms typically require endotracheal intubation to provide hypercarbia and breath holding (when requested by the radiologist). Hypercarbia to end-tidal CO_2 greater than or equal to 50 will promote vasodilation to allow better access and visualization of cerebral vasculature (Fig. 46-8). Orogastric and nasogastric tubes, esophageal stethoscopes, and esophageal temperature probes should not be placed for cerebral angiography because they may cause artifacts on the angiographic images. Cerebral studies may be indicated in the work-up or postoperative follow-up of vascular malformation or tumor resections, stroke, hemorrhagic events, vascular disease, and unexplained mental status changes. Any child requiring a study for the potential or confirmed diagnosis of moyamoya disease should be treated with utmost precaution. These children should have anesthetic techniques that minimize the risk of transient ischemic attacks and stroke during the procedure.[102] Anesthetic care should begin with the pre-induction administration of 10 mL/kg of intravenous fluid to minimize the risk of hypotension (and potential cerebral ischemia) on induction of anesthesia. Hypocarbia should be avoided throughout and mild hypercarbia promoted. In the event of vasospasm or difficult access of small, tortuous vessels, locally administered (through the catheter) nitroglycerin in small doses (25-50 μg) may facilitate visualization and access. The nitroglycerin, although often successful in discretely vasodilating specific areas, will generally not have a clinically important systemic effect on blood pressure; therefore, intra-arterial blood pressure monitoring is usually not required.

The anesthetic management of children with vascular malformations who present for embolization or sclerotherapy procedures can be challenging. Congenital vascular malformations represent aberrant connections between blood vessels that may be composed of lymphatic, arterial, and venous connections. These lesions, although present at birth, are often discrete and not clearly visible. As the child grows, the vascular malformation may expand rapidly, growing with the child. This rapid proliferative phase may occur in response to hormonal changes (pregnancy, puberty), trauma, or other stimuli.[103] Vascular malformations may be classified as high-flow or low-flow lesions, depending on which vessels are involved. High-flow lesions may include arteriovenous fistulas, some large hemangiomas, and arteriovenous malformations. Particularly with large lesions, high-output cardiac failure and congestive heart failure with potential for pulmonary edema should be anticipated and assessed in the physical examination and past medical history

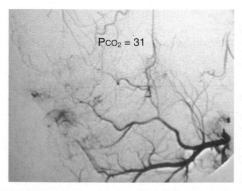
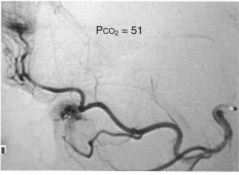

Figure 46-8. Effect of hypercarbia on caliber of cerebral blood vessels.

(Fig. 46-9). Low-flow lesions consist of venous, intramuscular venous, and lymphatic malformations. Surgical resection of symptomatic vascular malformations may be hazardous, as well as unsuccessful: any vascular element not resected may enlarge and cause further problems. It is for this reason that invasive angiography and embolization is becoming a popular alternative to surgical resection.

Not all vascular malformations require intervention. Only those lesions that are symptomatic require intervention. Symptoms that may require intervention include pain, tissue ulceration, disfiguring mass, airway compromise, cardiovascular compromise, impairment of limb function, coagulopathy, claudication, hemorrhage, and progressive nerve degeneration or palsy. Because large vascular lesions require multiple embolizations, parents and children are often reassured and comforted in seeing familiar anesthesiologists. Familiarity with the child, especially those with complex medical issues, is another benefit of having consistent anesthesiologists in the radiology suites. Vascular embolization is often used as a bridge to surgical resection. Successful embolization and sclerotherapy may decrease the size of the malformation, enable a more complete resection, as well as reduce blood flow to the lesion to reduce surgical risks.

When embolizing vascular malformations, radiologists often strive to cut off the feeding vessels with agents that include ethanol, stainless steel coils, absorbable gelatin pledgets and powder, polyvinyl alcohol foam, glues, thread, and ethanol. The choice of agent depends on the clinical situation and the size of the blood vessel. Absolute ethanol (99.9% alcohol) is a powerful sclerosing agent that causes thrombosis even at the level of the capillary bed. It is particularly useful in the embolization of symptomatic vascular malformations. Ethanol causes thrombosis because it injures the vascular endothelium. Ethanol also denatures blood proteins. When permanent occlusion is the goal, polyvinyl alcohol foam and ethanol are often employed because they both occlude at the level of the arterioles and capillaries. Medium- to small-sized arteries may be occluded with coils, which are the surgical equivalent of ligation. In trauma situations, when only temporary (days) occlusion is the goal, absorbable gelatin pledgets or powder is employed.[104]

The embolization and sclerotherapy of vascular malformations usually requires a general anesthetic to ensure motionless conditions, especially during high-risk procedures that involve the injection of a contrast agent and potentially painful sclerosants. These procedures require careful planning and discussion between the interventional radiologist and the anesthesiologist for safe airway management, intraprocedural and postprocedural care, and disposition. The anesthesiologist must have a basic understanding of the procedure and of the risks involved. Some of the risks are inherent to the procedure and the agents used for embolization or sclerotherapy. Other risks may be associated with the type and location of the vascular malformation being treated. Before each procedure, the anesthesiologist and radiologist should discuss the radiologist's specific requirements and concerns and decide on an anesthetic plan. Some procedures, especially embolizations of the head and neck, carry an increased risk of neurologic or cardiovascular complications.[105] It is important for the anesthesiologist to anticipate potential complications and modify the anesthetic technique so that a neurologic assessment may be performed soon after extubation.

The anesthesiologist should be familiar with the mechanism of action and potential risks associated with the various agents and devices used for embolization and sclerotherapy. All sclerosants, when administered into the vascular bed, produce local hemolysis. Large amounts of sclerosant, particularly sodium tetradecyl and ethanol, can cause hemoglobinuria, which can result in renal injury if the child is not adequately hydrated during and after the procedure.[106-108] Most children have a urine catheter placed to follow urine output, enable generous hydration, and monitor any hematuria. The anesthesiologist should generously hydrate the child with intravenous saline. On average, it has been our practice to administer as much as 50-mL/kg intravenous fluids over the course of the procedure. When hemoglobinuria is noted during the procedure, the anesthesiologist should notify the radiologist coincident with increasing the rate of fluid administration (Fig. 46-10). Aggressive and immediate treatment of hematuria is essential so as to minimize the risk of renal damage. Inadequate hydration with subsequent hemolysis has resulted in renal failure with subsequent hemodialysis (personal correspondence). Hemoglobinuria may not occur until the end of the procedure, sometimes after a cumulative large dose of sclerosant has been administered or the tourniquet (if used) has been released. During procedures that involve lower extremity lesions and tourniquets, hemoglobinuria can develop soon after the tourniquet is released. Promoting diuresis with furosemide (0.5-1.0 mg/kg) helps to facilitate the resolution of gross hematuria. Occasionally, hemoglobinuria develops 1 to 2 hours after the procedure, usually while in the PACU. It is important to carefully balance the fluid administered with the urine output. At our institution, in the event of persistent hemoglobinuria, in the recovery room, sodium bicarbonate (75 mEq/L in D5W) is administered at two times maintenance rate to alkalinize the urine and minimize precipitation of hemoglobin in the renal tubules.[109]

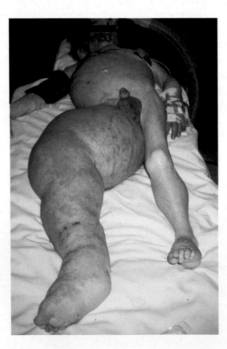

Figure 46-9. Arteriovenous malformation of the leg with high-output cardiac failure.

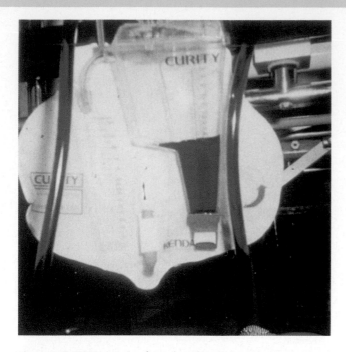

Figure 46-10. Hematuria after ethanol embolization.

Administration of ethanol has the potential for severe complications. The most infrequent but serious risk is cardiovascular collapse, which is generally preceded by hypoxemia and bradycardia. Most reported cases of cardiovascular collapse involved lower extremity malformations.[110] The etiology of the cardiovascular collapse associated with ethanol is unclear, although it is reported to occur uniquely when there is direct release of ethanol into the systemic veins. Collapse can occur after release of tourniquets in extremities that have been injected with ethanol. It is critical that the radiologist communicate with the anesthesiologist whenever ethanol is being injected as well as before the deflation of the tourniquet. Similarly, the anesthesiologist must alert the radiologist immediately if there is any acute change in the patient's vital signs. It has been recommended that any child at significant risk of systemic ethanol egress should have a pulmonary artery catheter placed before the procedure to identify changes in pulmonary artery pressure that might herald electromechanical dissociation. Significant elevations in pulmonary artery pressure due to pulmonary vasoconstriction necessitate interruption of ethanol administration until the pressure normalizes. Significant fluctuations in vital signs include an elevation in pulmonary artery pressure, a decrease in systemic blood pressure, decrease in end-tidal CO_2, or oxygen saturation, cardiac arrhythmias, or full cardiac arrest. Complete cardiovascular collapse is rare but has resulted in patient deaths and cerebral injury (personal correspondence). In our practice, sudden desaturation without arrhythmia or hypotension has occurred with ethanol administration. Massive pulmonary embolism caused by thrombus dislodgement from the vascular malformation has also occurred, and some children have demonstrated mild (mid 80%-low 90% oxygen saturation) but prolonged (24 to 48 hours) hypoxemia that is probably caused by microthromboembolism (personal experience). Such children have been successfully managed by systemic anticoagulation without long-term sequelae.

Ethanol can produce a state of intoxication. The ethanol used for embolization and sclerotherapy is 95% to 98% pure. Children who receive greater than 0.75 mL/kg can be clinically intoxicated. Blood levels correlate with the volume of ethanol administered, regardless of the location or type of vascular malformation (Fig. 46-11).[84] On extubation, these children display either significant agitation or excessive sedation and analgesia. Narcotics should be administered to these children with caution because our experience has shown that children who receive significant ethanol (maximum dosage at our institution is 1 mL/kg) are slow to emerge from anesthesia and may have a strong odor of alcohol on their breath. Increased serum levels of ethanol can be analgesic. Opioids have a synergistic effect with ethanol and potentially cause unwanted respiratory depression. Modest doses of opioids should be administered until the child is extubated and confirms the presence of pain. Ketorolac may be administered intravenously after the invasive catheters are removed and hemostasis ensured.

Children with vascular malformations, especially venous malformations, can have preexisting coagulation disturbances that resemble disseminated intravascular coagulation.[111-115] Children with laboratory values indicative of a preexisting consumptive coagulopathy should have a hematology consultation and, if possible, receive heparin for 2 weeks before the procedure to replenish their fibrinogen levels. The anesthesiologist frequently will be requested to administer cryoprecipitate or platelets during the procedure to promote clotting and successful sclerosis. The use of ethanol for sclerosis or embolization can elicit a coagulation disturbance that resembles disseminated intravascular coagulation. There is a statistical relationship between the amount (mL/kg) of ethanol administered and the degree of coagulation disturbance elicited.[116] Additional cryoprecipitate or fresh frozen plasma transfusions are given only in severe cases because the coagulopathy is generally not symptomatic and resolves in about 5 days. However, major surgery should be deferred until the coagulation parameters have normalized.

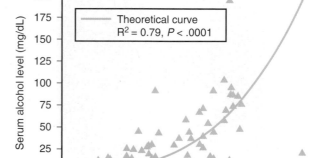

Figure 46-11. Positive relationship between serum ethanol level and amount of ethanol administered. (From Mason KP, Michna E, Zurakowski D, et al: Serum ethanol levels in children and adults after ethanol embolization or sclerotherapy for vascular anomalies. Radiology 2000; 217:127-132.)

It is important to be aware of the potential morbidity associated with embolizations. Arteriovenous malformations involving the head and neck frequently require cannulation of the external carotid artery branches and the thyrocervical trunk. All children scheduled for embolization should be typed and crossmatched for blood in anticipation of possible major hemorrhage. Those children who undergo embolizations of arteriovenous malformations of the head and neck are at risk for stroke, cranial nerve palsies, skin necrosis, blindness, infection, and pulmonary embolism.[117] It is important to document full return of neurologic status after the child is extubated. Vascular malformations involving the airway are particularly challenging (Fig. 46-12). The anesthesiologist and radiologist should review the imaging studies (usually MRI) before the procedure. The scans should be evaluated for patency of the nares, nasopharynx, hypopharynx, and oropharynx—as well as for an uncompromised trachea, carina, and bronchi. MRI will also confirm that there is no malformation in the nares or nasopharynx, which could be damaged or bleed during intubation. Most interventional radiology suites are not situated in the operating room. If there is any potential for airway compromise, difficulty in attaining a mask airway, or failure to intubate, the airway is secured in the main operating room and then the child is transported to interventional radiology. Generally, an otolaryngologist or another specialist skilled in bronchoscopy and tracheotomy remains in the operating room suite prepared to perform bronchoscopy (fiberoptic or rigid) or tracheostomy should the airway be lost.

If post-sclerotherapy edema and vascular congestion involving the airway structures is anticipated, the child is intubated nasally, remains intubated after the procedure, and usually remains intubated for 48 hours or longer until the swelling is reduced. Nasal intubation is preferred to minimize the risk of endotracheal tube dislodgement or premature extubation. The decision for postoperative intubation and ventilation is usually made before the start of the procedure, after the anesthesiologist

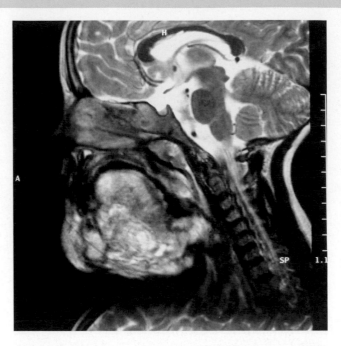

Figure 46-13. MR image showing airway involvement of lymphatic malformations.

and radiologist together review the MR images (Fig. 46-13). Usually, the child is extubated while in the ICU after confirmation of an air leak around the endotracheal tube or a flexible nasal fiberoptic view of the airway that can be performed at the bedside. If there is any doubt regarding the patency of the airway, these children are transferred to the operating room for extubation in a controlled setting with an otolaryngologist present. Despite the best attempts to minimize airway calamity, these patients are challenging. Alternative airway devices (e.g., oral airway, nasal trumpet, LMA) should be readily accessible in any area where these patients are managed (operating room, interventional suite, intensive care unit).

Venous malformations involving the head, neck, or airway structures typically swell with dependency or Valsalva maneuver (e.g., crying) (Fig. 46-14). Before extubation, these children should be positioned in a head-up position to promote venous drainage and minimize swelling. Efforts should be made to minimize coughing and bucking before extubation. In the event of respiratory compromise, venous malformations can enlarge when the child coughs, increases intrathoracic pressure, or utilizes accessory muscles. Attempts at re-intubation, cricoid pressure, head extension, and mask ventilation can further enlarge the malformation. Mask ventilation can be challenging, sometimes impossible, if the malformation is swollen and firm. Achieving an occlusive mask seal is particularly difficult when there is swelling of the cheek, tongue, lip, chin, or nares. Venous malformations of the lips and tongue, because of their blue color, can make it difficult to assess the patient for hypoxemia in the event of respiratory distress. Re-intubation can become impossible in these situations because all maneuvers to achieve a mask seal are increasing venous pressure and swelling. When attempting to re-intubate the trachea of a child with intraoral or pharyngeal malformations, special care should be taken to avoid damaging the integrity of the malformation: even a small nick can create significant bleeding. In the event of

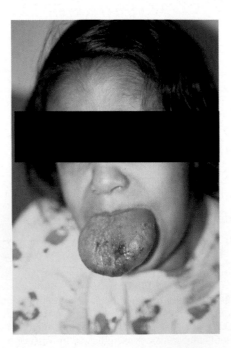

Figure 46-12. Vascular malformation of the tongue.

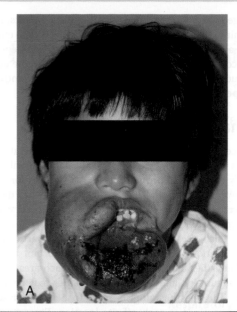

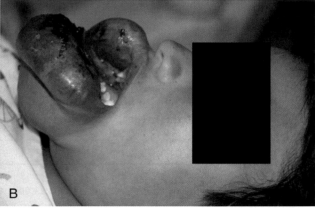

Figure 46-14. Venous malformation of face with patient sitting upright (**A**) and supine (**B**).

oropharyngeal bleeding and inability to mask ventilate and/or intubate, it is critical to have alternate airway devices immediately available. LMAs in particular can be lifesaving. Proper insertion and inflation of the LMA can secure an airway and, more importantly, tamponade bleeding. Because the LMA rests above the vocal cords, it does not protect the airway from pulmonary aspiration.

Risks Associated with Intravascular Contrast Media

All intravascular studies require contrast. It is important that the anesthesiologist be aware of the risks and potential side effects of contrast media. It is estimated that approximately 500 fatalities occur annually in the United States as a direct result of having received intravascular contrast media.[118,119] Almost all life-threatening reactions occur immediately or within 20 minutes of contrast agent administration. Low-osmolality ionic and nonionic contrast media are associated with a lower incidence of adverse events, especially non–life-threatening events, as compared with high-osmolality contrast media. Serious contrast reactions are estimated at 1 to 2 per 1,000 studies using high-osmolality contrast media versus 1 to 2 per 10,000 studies with low osmolality contrast media.[120-122] Adverse reactions can range from nausea, vomiting, hypotension, urticaria, bronchospasm, anxiety, chills, fever, and facial flushing to seizures, pulmonary edema, and cardiovascular collapse. Mortalities have been heralded by hypotension, cardiac dysrhythmia, and symptoms of respiratory distress.[123-125] Anaphylactoid shock is the most worrisome of all contrast reactions and may occur as early as 1 minute after administration of the contrast material and as late as several hours later. Although the occurrence of an adverse reaction to intravascular contrast media cannot be predicted, there are some identifiable risk factors. Those who suffer from allergies or an atopic disease, children with asthma, significant cardiovascular disease, or paraproteinemia, and children with prior contrast reactions have an increased incidence of adverse reactions.[126] Children who have been identified as being at increased risk of a contrast reaction should be premedicated with corticosteroids and antihistamines. The American College of Radiology suggests that corticosteroid premedication, along with low osmolality contrast media, should be used for those at risk.[126-129]

Because the contrast agent is hypertonic relative to plasma, attention needs to be paid to the risk of an initial hypertensive response followed by a hyperosmotic diuresis with the potential for hypotension. Equilibration with the extracellular fluid compartment occurs within 10 minutes, heralded by the onset of diuresis. For this reason, special attention should be paid when administering iodine contrast to any patient with a history of congestive heart failure. The initial increase in blood volume may precipitate cardiovascular compromise. Renal failure from contrast media can occur with high and low osmolality contrast media. Although the etiology of the acute renal failure is not known, risk factors include preexisting renal insufficiency (serum creatine $\geq$1.5 mg/dL), diabetes mellitus, dehydration, cardiovascular disease, age 70 years or older, myeloma, hypertension, and hyperuricemia. For these at-risk patients, good hydration must be maintained along with careful follow-up of renal function (following serum creatine levels as compared with baseline) and, possibly, the use of an antioxidant such as N-acetylcysteine.[130-133] Children with paraproteinemias (multiple myeloma, Waldenström macroglobulinemia) are predisposed to irreversible renal failure from protein precipitation in renal tubules, which is preventable with proper hydration.[134]

Endoscopic Procedures

Gastrointestinal endoscopy has become increasingly common practice for the pediatric gastroenterologist. Because of the potential for airway compromise together with the difficulty to achieve a motionless condition using deep sedation during an upper endoscopy, general anesthesia is rapidly becoming a standard for children. The choice of deep sedation versus general anesthesia with or without an endotracheal tube depends on the medical condition, the risks associated with the procedure, and the anticipated duration. Upper esophagogastroduodenoscopy in infants (<10 kg) generally requires an endotracheal tube so as to avoid airway compromise by the scope. Although all anesthesia-delivery areas must meet the requisite ASA standard, there may not always be effective scavenging and ventilation in these suites to enable inhalation anesthetics to be used. In these cases, total intravenous anesthetics should be substituted for the inhalation agents.

There are many techniques that may be employed successfully to maintain adequate conditions for upper and lower gas-

Table 47-1. Suggested Essential Bedside Equipment

- Oxygen supply with regulated flows
- Oxygen face masks and face tents for spontaneous ventilation (various sizes)
- Stethoscope
- Resuscitation bags: self-inflating (Ambu) and Mapleson type
- Anesthesia face masks for positive-pressure ventilation (pediatric sizes 0, 1, 2, 3, adult, small, medium, large)
- Oral airways (sizes 00, 0, 1 to 5)
- Nasal airways (sizes 12 Fr to 36 Fr)
- Suction and appropriate suction catheters (sizes $6\frac{1}{2}$ to 14 Fr); tonsil-type (Yankauer) attachment
- Needles, syringes, alcohol wipes, Betadine solution, gauze pads
- Arterial blood gas kit
- Gloves (preferably non-latex)
- Pulse oximeter and sensors (size appropriate, stick-on type preferred to clip on type)
- ECG monitor and pads
- Manual and automated blood pressure device
- All sizes of blood pressure cuffs

postoperative care, similar to a typical Pediatric Intensive Care Unit (PICU). Equipment (Table 47-1) and available medications (Tables 47-2 and 47-3) should be standardized throughout the unit and, if possible, match and be compatible with transport monitors as well as devices used in other pediatric care units.

Personnel working in the perioperative area should be trained in child-specific care and be familiar with neonatal and pediatric advanced life support. This includes nurses, residents, fellows, as well as attending physicians. Ideally, the team should participate in mock codes and simulations to train for an emergency. Patient sign outs should be standardized, include checklists, and follow an institutional specific protocol. All personnel also should be familiar with the equipment and be able to use it instantaneously (mobile crash carts). We recommend instituting equipment and policies according to the guidelines published by the American Academy of Pediatrics "Pediatric Postoperative Environment."[1]

The Transport

Transport from the operating room to the PACU should be carried out under the direct supervision of a trained expert. A check of the security and patency of the endotracheal tube (if a child is to remain intubated) or laryngeal mask airway, all intravenous lines, the arterial line, chest tubes, drains, and the urinary catheter should be made before transport. Children should be in presentable condition (e.g., removal of blood, secretion) before transport to the PACU or PICU. Children should be kept warm throughout transport to avoid hypothermia. Unless children are wide awake, with protective airway reflexes intact, or unless there is a specific contraindication, it is sensible to transport extubated children in the lateral position (tonsil) so that the tongue and secretions and possible vomitus are less likely to be aspirated or cause airway obstruction. A hand holding the chin up helps maintain a child's airway and serves as a breath monitor; the exhaled breath can be felt on the hand. For sleepy children, continued use of the precordial stethoscope

or a portable oxygen saturation device serves as a monitor of respiration and circulation. Oxygen delivery via face mask or nasal cannula may be indicated. We recommend that children in a potentially unstable condition be transported with a battery-powered pulse oximeter, an electrocardiographic (ECG) monitor, and a blood pressure cuff or a transduced arterial line. The monitoring lines, intravenous drips, infusion pumps, and other equipment should be clearly labeled and simplified before transport. For sick patients, intubated children, and children with potential airway difficulties, an appropriate resuscitation bag, face mask, oral airway, oxygen tanks (oxygen levels should be checked), functioning laryngoscopes, endotracheal tube, and medications (including atropine and succinylcholine) should be carried en route to the PACU or PICU. A tackle box containing all of this equipment is helpful, especially when children are transported to the PICU in an elevator. Children receiving vasopressors or vasodilators require battery-powered infusion pumps so that these agents can be continuously administered at precise titrated levels.

Transport to the PACU or PICU is a time of potential danger. Distance and duration of travel should be minimized. When designing pediatric perioperative areas or reallocating space, strong emphasis should be put on ergonomics.

Table 47-2. Suggested Emergency Supplies for "Crash Cart" or Central Location

- Laryngoscopes with blades: Miller 0, 1, 2, 3; Macintosh 2, 3, 4; extra laryngoscope bulbs, batteries
- Endotracheal tubes, sizes 2.0 mm ID through 8 mm ID (cuffed and uncuffed tubes for all sizes when available)
- Laryngeal mask airways: sizes 1, 1.5, 2, 2.5, 3, 4, and 5
- ProSeal laryngeal mask airway sizes 1.5, 2, 2.5, 3, 3.5, 4 and 5
- Fast-Track laryngeal mask airway
- Stylet appropriate for each endotracheal tube size
- Syringe for endotracheal cuff inflation
- Tape and liquid adhesive for endotracheal tube fixation
- 14-gauge IV catheter with 3-mm ID endotracheal tube adapter for emergency cricothyroidotomy (see also Fig. 12-27)
- Cricothyrotomy kits appropriate for age (see Figs. 12-27 and 12-28)
- Back-up resuscitation bags and masks and oral airways for each bedside
- Nasogastric tubes
- Intravenous infusion solutions, tubing, drip chambers
- Supplies for intravenous cannulation, catheter sizes 24 to 14 gauge
- Cutdown tray, tracheostomy, and suture sets
- Central venous catheter insertion sets (3 to 7 Fr single and multiple lumen)
- Tube thoracotomy set and system for suction and underwater seal
- Defibrillator (adult, child paddles)
- Electrocardiogram
- Pressure transducer system and oscilloscope monitor
- Sterile gowns, gloves, masks, towels, drapes
- Urinary catheters of appropriate pediatric size
- Bedboard for cardiopulmonary resuscitation

Table 47-3. Suggested Recovery Room Medications*

Suggested Emergency Medications on "Crash Cart"

Atropine

Epinephrine

Sodium bicarbonate

Dextrose

Calcium chloride or gluconate

Lidocaine (intravenous and topical)

Succinylcholine and rocuronium

Thiopental and propofol

Etomidate

Ketamine

Diphenhydramine

Hydrocortisone, dexamethasone, methylprednisolone

Neostigmine

Physostigmine

Naloxone

Flumazenil

Furosemide

Dopamine

Norepinephrine

Sodium nitroprusside

Heparin

Verapamil

Amiodarone

Propranolol, atenolol, esmolol, labetalol

Phenytoin or phosphenytoin

Mannitol

Racemic epinephrine (for inhalation)

Medications to Be Kept Under Lock

Fentanyl

Morphine

Meperidine

Ketamine

Midazolam (IV and PO)

Diazepam

Phenobarbital

Potassium chloride

Other Medications for Central Location

Antibiotics

Acetaminophen (PO and PR)

Dantrolene

Digoxin

Pancuronium, rocuronium, vecuronium

Antiemetics (e.g., $5HT_3$ antagonist, promethazine, metoclopramide)

Protamine

Insulin

Potassium chloride

*Alternate or additional medications may be needed because this is merely a list of proposed medications.

A child often appears awake after the stimulation of extubation and transfer to the stretcher but may subsequently become more obtunded, and obstruction of the airway may occur during transit. Just as frequently, children may become restless during transit. Guard rails may be helpful, but most important is the anesthesiologist's constant observation of the child. As always, the cause of restlessness must be sought.

The Arrival

Attention is first directed to airway patency, the color of the lips and mucous membranes, oxygen saturation, and adequacy of ventilation, perfusion, and central nervous system function. Heart rate, blood pressure, oxygen saturation, respiratory rate, and temperature are recorded. The nurse-to-patient ratio should be 1:1 for sick children and 1:2 or 1:3 for routine cases. Supplemental oxygen is administered as indicated. Many children object to placement of an oxygen mask, and a funnel-type mask or open hose with large flow rates may be less objectionable (although less optimal). Thereafter, a report should be given to the nurses and physicians in attendance. Ideally, the nurses taking care of the child postoperatively will already be familiar with the child and family from the preoperative setting (see Perioperative Environment). The transfer of care protocol should be standardized. This report should include, at a minimum, patient identification, age, preoperative vital signs, and specific circumstances, such as language barrier or developmental delay. The size and location of catheters, a description of the child's current problem, past medical history, medications and allergies, operative procedure, and pertinent surgical problems should be outlined. The following should be described to the PACU team: the premedication and anesthetic agents used at induction and for maintenance, techniques used, reversal of neuromuscular blockade (adequacy of the train-of-four response), estimated blood loss, fluid replacement (including amount and type of solution), urine output, and vasoactive drugs, bronchodilators, and intraoperative medications (e.g., antibiotics) used. Regional anesthesia issues, such as epidural, location, drug, drug concentration and contents, effective level of analgesia, and infusion rate should be clearly transmitted. The administration of analgesics (time and dose, such as rectal acetaminophen), local blocks and wound infiltration with local anesthetics, problems with either surgery or anesthesia (difficult intravenous access, difficult intubation, intraoperative hemodynamic instability or cardiac changes), and potential problems in the PACU should be listed. Finally, the anesthesia team must remain with the child until the patient is stable and the PACU team is comfortable and ready to assume the care of the child.

Central Nervous System

The Pharmacodynamics of Emergence

Emergence from anesthesia is faster after a relatively insoluble inhaled anesthetic agent such as sevoflurane or desflurane than it is after a more soluble agent such as halothane. However, the clinical importance of these differences may be minimal and vary with the duration of anesthesia and the medications co-administered (see later). Differences in the times to discharge from the PACU and the hospital are even harder to detect when specific comparisons are made between inhalation agents

Table 47-4. Pediatric Anesthesia Emergence Delirium (PAED) Scale

	0	1	2	3	4
Child makes eye contact with caregiver	Extremely	Very much	Quite a bit	Just a little	Not at all
Child's actions are purposeful	Extremely	Very much	Quite a bit	Just a little	Not at all
Child is aware of his/her surroundings	Extremely	Very much	Quite a bit	Just a little	Not at all
Child is restless	Not at all	Just a little	Quite a bit	Very much	Extremely
Child is inconsolable	Not at all	Just a little	Quite a bit	Very much	Extremely
Total Score					

Modified from Sikich N, Lerman J: Development and psychometric evaluation of the pediatric anesthesia emergence delirium scale. Anesthesiology 2004; 100:1138-1145.

because so many other factors such as pain management, agitation, availability of hospital beds, and family circumstances affect discharge readiness.

Patient age generally exerts a minimal influence on the washout of inhaled anesthetic agents and thus has little impact on the rapidity of emergence. The one age group in which age might be a factor is in infants younger than 1 year of age,[2] but the overall clinical implications of age-related differences in emergence are virtually undetectable.[3]

The rate of emergence correlates more closely with the duration of anesthesia. The greater the duration of anesthesia, the more saturated the tissue compartments and thus the more time is required to eliminate these agents. For example, emergence from 30 minutes of sevoflurane anesthesia will be significantly faster than it is after 2 hours of anesthesia, which in turn is more rapid than after 8 hours of anesthesia.[4] This relationship, between emergence time and the duration of anesthesia, is even more marked for agents that are more soluble (e.g., halothane).

Emergence from intravenous agents can vary significantly from that of inhaled agents. Several studies have evaluated the quality and rapidity of emergence after intravenous anesthetic agents compared with that after inhaled agents. For outpatient surgery, emergence after propofol anesthesia is as rapid as that after sevoflurane but may have the advantage of a reduced incidence of agitation and fewer pain behaviors than after sevoflurane anesthesia.[5,6] The recovery characteristics of propofol with remifentanil total intravenous anesthesia have been compared with those after desflurane inhaled anesthesia. Recovery appears to be as rapid as that after inhaled agents but with less agitation and no difference in the rates of nausea and vomiting.[7]

Midazolam is rarely used for maintenance of anesthesia but is often used for oral or intravenous premedication, anxiolysis, or amnesia in preparation for anesthesia. Several studies have shown that the early emergence after a brief anesthetic is prolonged by adding midazolam to inhaled agents or propofol. However, with cases of greater duration or when considering late emergence, this effect is minimal[8]; midazolam does not appear to affect postoperative agitation.[9,10]

Emergence Agitation/Delirium—Excitement

Emergence agitation (also referred to as emergence delirium [Video Clip 47-1, see website]) is a well-known entity that was first described in a large cohort of postsurgical patients nearly 40 years ago.[11] From a clinical perspective, it is often impossible to differentiate pure "agitation" from "delirium," the latter implying a specific set of thought disorders and hallucinations based on the American Psychiatric Association's *Diagnostic and Sta-tistical Manual of Mental Disorders,* 4th edition (DSM-IV). Despite numerous investigations, differentiating emergence delirium from postoperative pain has also proven to be difficult. Emergence delirium is usually manifest by the child who is thrashing, disoriented, crying, screaming, unable to recognize parents or surroundings, inconsolable, and talking irrationally during early emergence from anesthesia. It occurs more often in children (at a rate of 10%-20%) than in adults, and particularly in those younger than 6 years of age.[12,13] The etiology of emergence delirium is not clear but may in part reflect pharmacodynamic differences in clearance of insoluble inhalation agents from the central nervous system. Recently, an emergence delirium scale has been developed and validated that may provide both clinicians and investigators with a tool to differentiate emergence delirium from pain.[14] See Tables 47-4 and 47-5 for two scoring systems used to evaluate emergence behaviors in children.

Table 47-5. Postanesthesia Behavior Assessment (PABA) Scale*

Perceptual disturbances (maximal score 3)
- 0 None evident
- 1 Feelings of depersonalization (verbalizes situation is not real, comments on "out of body" feelings)
- 2 Visual illusions or misperceptions (misidentifies objects such as urinates in trash can)
- 3 Markedly confused about external reality (misidentifies self or surroundings such as being at school)

Hallucination type (maximal score 6)
- 0 None evident
- 1 Auditory hallucinations only (responds to questions not asked)
- 2 Visual hallucinations or misperceptions (responds to things only the child can see)
- 3 Tactile, olfactory (responds to sensations not obvious to others, e.g., there is a bug crawling on the leg)

Psychomotor behavior (maximal score 3)
- 0 No significant agitation
- 1 Mild restlessness, tremulousness, or anxiety
- 2 Moderate agitation with pulling at IV lines
- 3 Severe agitation, needs to be restrained, combative

*A higher PABA score is associated with a greater degree of postanesthetic distress.

Reproduced with permission from Przybylo HJ, Martini DR, Mazurek AJ, et al: Assessing behavior in children emerging form anaesthesia: can we apply psychiatric diagnostic techniques? Pediatr Anesth 2003; 13:609-616.

Whereas our understanding of emergence delirium/agitation continues to evolve, it is clear that it occurs both after surgical procedures and after procedures that are free from pain, such as magnetic resonance imaging.[12,15,16] For reasons that remain unexplained, emergence delirium appears to occur more frequently after less-soluble inhaled anesthetics such as sevoflurane and desflurane than after more-soluble inhaled anesthetics such as halothane and isoflurane[17,18]; there may be a greater incidence of emergence delirium after painful procedures, thereby emphasizing the difficulty of separating agitation due to pain and agitation due to the direct effects of the inhalation agents on the sensorium.[19] In addition, emergence delirium occurs more commonly in children 2 to 5 years of age than in older children, generally lasts 5 to 15 minutes, and resolves spontaneously if the children are left undisturbed or they are held by their parents.[12]

Several strategies have been used to decrease the duration and intensity of emergence delirium. Opioids appear to be the most effective agents in this regard. Low-dose fentanyl (intranasal [2 µg/kg] or intravenous [1.0-2.5 µg/kg]) has been shown to decrease the duration and intensity of emergence delirium,[20] even in the absence of significant painful stimuli.[15] Other adjunctive agents used to treat this phenomenon include ketorolac and acetaminophen in the setting of ear tube placement and midazolam; the effectiveness of midazolam, however, has been mixed.[21,22] More recently, dexmedetomidine has been shown to decrease the incidence of emergence delirium, but the cost-effectiveness of this treatment compared with others remains to be evaluated.[23] Regional analgesia in the form of caudal blocks has also been shown to reduce the incidence of emergence delirium, although this is probably related to improved pain control, which eliminates pain as a source of agitation.[24]

Although there is no evidence of long-term consequences, in the current era of fast-tracking anesthesia, emergence delirium can represent a significant time expenditure for nurses in the PACU. Discharge from the PACU may be delayed in part while waiting for the delirium to wane or for the effects of the interventional drugs to dissipate. Injury to the child who is extremely agitated is a theoretical concern. In addition, parental satisfaction decreases when severe emergence delirium occurs. Finally, although the impact of extreme delirium on the child is not fully known, evidence suggests that the incidence of postoperative maladaptive behaviors increases in children who experience marked emergence delirium.[25]

Respiratory System

Criteria for Extubation

In most cases, extubation may be safely performed in the operating room. However, a child's condition may necessitate delayed extubation at an appropriate time in the PACU or PICU. There is widespread agreement that children who have been anesthetized with a full stomach, children at risk for airway obstruction (including those whose jaws are wired shut and those with Pierre Robin syndrome, Treacher-Collins syndrome, hemifacial microsomia, or other syndromes associated with difficult airway maintenance, e.g., obstructive sleep apnea), premature infants, and other infants predisposed to apnea should be awake before extubation is attempted. Beyond this, the timing of extubation is a matter of individual judgment. For example, the practice at some institutions is to extubate when a child is awake and demonstrating eye opening and other purposeful movement; the practice at others is to extubate while the child is under a deep plane of inhalation anesthesia. Clinicians report only rare problems with either approach. Most clinicians would agree (expert opinion rather than conclusive data with a high level of evidence) that either approach is preferable to extubation in a very light plane of anesthesia, when laryngospasm may be more likely and vomiting may occur while protective reflexes are impaired.

Procedure for Extubation in the Operating Room or in the PACU

Immediately after extubation, oxygen should be administered and the child should be observed for adequate ventilation, satisfactory oxygen saturation, color of the mucous membranes, and the presence of laryngospasm or vomiting. Transport of children should not be undertaken until the patency of the airway and the adequacy of oxygenation and ventilation have been confirmed, meaning stable, satisfactory oxygen saturation in room air. Our criteria for transporting the child from the operating room to the PACU without oxygen is a stable oxygen saturation of 95% or greater in room air. If the child cannot sustain this level of oxygen saturation, then either more time for recovery in the operating room is taken or the child is transported with oxygen with a means for providing positive-pressure ventilation.

For children whose tracheas are extubated in the PACU, respiratory insufficiency is the most worrisome and most frequent complication; when associated with emergence from anesthesia in children, this comprises approximately two thirds of critical perioperative events.[26] Respiratory insufficiency may manifest as obvious signs of difficulty breathing, or it may occur more subtly, as anxiety, unresponsiveness, tachycardia, bradycardia, hypertension, arrhythmia, seizures, or even cardiac arrest. When any of these conditions are present, respiratory insufficiency must be considered as the root cause. Hypoxemia, hypoventilation, and upper airway obstruction are the three most common respiratory events that occur in children in the PACU; this is particularly true of children after tonsillectomy with associated obesity and possible obstructive sleep apnea as well as in children who have undergone diagnostic bronchoscopy.

Hypoxemia

Hypoxemia in children may result from hypoventilation, diffusion hypoxia, upper airway obstruction, bronchospasm, aspiration of gastric contents, pulmonary edema, pneumothorax, atelectasis or, rarely, postobstructive pulmonary edema or pulmonary embolism. Hypoxia occurs more rapidly and may be more profound during emergence from general anesthesia because general anesthesia inhibits the hypoxic and hypercapnic ventilatory drive, reduces functional residual capacity, and alters hypoxic pulmonary vasoconstriction. In addition, shivering will further increase oxygen consumption and exacerbate hemoglobin desaturation.

Postoperative hemoglobin desaturation is more common in children with, or in those recovering from, an active upper respiratory tract infection, probably owing to increased reactivity of upper and lower airways as well as pulmonary atelectasis and secretions than in children without a history of upper tract infection.[27,28] In neonates, hypoxia will result in an *increase* in ventilation for approximately 1 minute and then it will *depress* respiratory drive (respiratory rate and tidal volume).[29] Infants such as former preterm infants with severe bronchopulmonary dysplasia who have sustained an hypoxic injury have delayed development of a normal ventilatory response to hypoxia for several months, thereby placing them at particular risk.[30]

Hypoventilation

Minute ventilation is the product of tidal volume and respiratory rate. It decreases when tidal volume, respiratory rate, or both, decrease. Hypoventilation leads to hypercarbia and promotes alveolar collapse. Severe hypoventilation results in respiratory acidosis, hypoxemia, carbon dioxide narcosis, and apnea. The ventilatory response to carbon dioxide is age dependent. In infants who breathe spontaneously under halothane anesthesia, 3.7% inspired CO_2 triggers no ventilatory response, whereas in children older than 6 months of age, this concentration of CO_2 increases minute ventilation by 34%.[31,32]

Hypoventilation results from a decrease in ventilatory drive, insufficiency of the muscular system, or mechanical reasons. Ventilatory drive is decreased in all children by volatile agents, opioids, benzodiazepines, and other sedating medications. At particular risk for hypoventilation in the PACU, and for some time thereafter, are children with underlying disturbances in respiration, such as infants with apnea of prematurity; former preterm infants of less than 60 weeks' postconceptual age; those with central nervous system injury such as head injury, strokes, and intracranial surgery; and obese children, especially those with obstructive sleep apnea. Some of these special children require prolonged observation in the PACU or postoperative care in an ICU or a special, monitored bed.

Muscular weakness may also contribute to respiratory insufficiency. It may be the result of preexistent muscular disease (e.g., the various muscular dystrophies) and inadequate reversal of neuromuscular blockade (with special considerations to myasthenia gravis, myasthenic syndrome, pseudocholinesterase deficiency, succinylcholine-induced phase II block, and anticholinesterase overdose).

Respiratory insufficiency may also result from upper airway obstruction. Airway obstruction is a feature in children with known airway problems due to unusual facies (particularly those with midfacial hypoplasia) and obese children with a history of obstructive sleep apnea. Finally, inadequate analgesia can lead to splinting and hypoventilation, which in turn may depress oxygen saturation.

Airway Obstruction

Among the most common and serious problems in the PACU is an extrathoracic airway obstruction. Clinical hallmarks include oxygen desaturation with inspiratory stridor, inspiratory retraction, and paradoxical chest wall motion. Initial intervention requires common measured maneuvers to improve airway patency, such as stimulating the child, repositioning (sitting up, roll of towels under the shoulders), suction of secretions, performing a jaw thrust, insertion of an oral or nasal airway, and application of positive end-expiratory pressure (see Fig. 12-10). In children who remain drowsy, respiration improves with these measures alone. However, if these measures fail, one must consider the patency of both the upper and the lower airway, that is, whether gas exchange is being compromised by laryngospasm, subglottic narrowing as the result of edema, bronchospasm, atelectasis, or tracheal secretions. Incomplete recovery from general anesthesia or neuromuscular blockade, wound hematoma, and vocal cord paralysis may also lead to upper airway obstruction.

If the airway is not cleared by any of the above maneuvers, then placement of a tracheal tube preceded by administration of oxygen by mask with continuous positive airway pressure and atropine (0.02 mg/kg IV) and succinylcholine (0.5 to 1 mg/kg IV or 5 mg/kg IM) may be necessary. Postobstructive pulmonary edema is a complication of acute upper airway obstruction and the relief of chronic airway obstruction after tonsillectomy. The mechanism appears to be the generation of extreme negative intrathoracic pressure against a closed glottis or obstructed airway and its sudden release, resulting in a dramatic increase in pulmonary blood flow, thereby causing noncardiogenic or neurogenic pulmonary edema. This complication should be suspected when significant hypoxia, persistent tachypnea, or tachycardia follow a prolonged episode of laryngospasm, airway obstruction, or tonsillectomy and the child has pink frothy secretions.[33-35]

Postintubation croup or subglottic edema has been associated with a number of factors, including traumatic intubation, tight-fitting endotracheal tubes, coughing while the tracheal tube is in situ, a change in the child's position during surgery, prolonged duration of intubation, surgery of the head and neck, and in children with a history of croup.[36] Treatment should be initiated with the inhalation of cool mist. If the symptoms do not abate, inhalation of nebulized epinephrine (0.5 mL in 3 mL of normal saline over 10 minutes) should be administered, although its effects are temporary and its use may be followed by rebound edema. In general, the use of nebulized epinephrine implies that a period of prolonged observation will occur. For outpatients, this implies that the child may have to be admitted to the hospital overnight or observed for an extended period.

Respiratory Effort

If the airway is patent, attention turns to the adequacy of ventilatory effort. Residual neuromuscular blockade can be diagnosed by observation (the patient's ability to lift extremities against gravity, perform a sustained head lift, breathing pattern [paradoxical chest movement]) and quantitatively by assessment with a peripheral nerve stimulator. Depending on the severity and the clinical situation, this condition may be treated with either supplemental doses of reversal agents or ventilatory assistance. If the respiratory rate is slow, suggestive of opioid-induced respiratory depression, then titrated doses of naloxone should be administered. Administration of naloxone in small incremental doses (0.5-1.0 µg/kg) (if the situation permits) will reverse the respiratory depression without precipitating acute anxiety, pain, or pulmonary edema. If naloxone is effective, then measures for continuous or repeated doses should be taken because the effects of intravenous naloxone are likely to wane before the respiratory depressant effects of the opioid. Residual sedation from benzodiazepines may similarly be antagonized with flumazenil.

Children who have an adequate airway and adequate muscular strength may experience difficulty breathing because of pain, restriction from bandages or casts, abdominal distention, pneumothorax, atelectasis, aspiration pneumonitis, or cardiogenic or postobstructive pulmonary edema. In most cases, the history and physical examination will focus the differential diagnosis, and, when necessary, investigations including a chest radiograph, blood gas analysis, and possibly invasive hemodynamic monitoring will identify the underlying etiology and determine an effective treatment.

Preterm Infants and Discharge from PACU

Preterm infants (≤36 weeks' gestation at birth) are at risk for apnea after sedation and general anesthesia.[37,38] As the postconceptual age (PCA, the sum of the gestational and postnatal ages) increases, the risk for apnea decreases.[39] Given the fact that there are inadequate randomized controlled trials and underpowered individual institutional studies, and the fact that apnea has been reported even after more modern anesthetic agents (desflurane and sevoflurane), it is recommended that former preterm infants who are 55 to 60 weeks' PCA who are not anemic and not experiencing apnea be observed for an extended period of time and, if stable, later discharged. However, infants younger than 55 weeks' PCA, those who are anemic (hematocrit <30%), and those with ongoing apnea should be admitted for monitoring.[39-45] Prophylactic administration of caffeine (10 mg/kg) may be administered to reduce the risk of apnea after general anesthesia in infants at high risk,[46,47] although it should not supplant postoperative admission and monitoring. Preterm infants younger than 55 weeks' PCA, particularly those with anemia, or those with major cardiorespiratory or neurologic disorders, should be admitted and monitored for at least 12 apnea-free hours after general or regional anesthesia (see Chapter 4).[39]

Although preterm infants who undergo surgery under spinal anesthesia have fewer respiratory and cardiovascular complications compared with general anesthesia,[39,40,45,48] these infants remain at risk for apnea. It is unknown if this risk is greater after a spinal anesthetic (with nothing administered to the child but the local anesthetic for the spinal) than the preexisting baseline risk. Infants who have received a spinal anesthetic supplemented with ketamine or midazolam are at greater risk for apnea[45] than those who have not. Despite evidence of a reduced risk of apnea after regional anesthesia,[48,49] and the discharge of former premature infants on the day of surgery after uncomplicated spinal anesthetics in some institutions,[49,50] there is currently insufficient evidence to make general recommendations regarding this practice. Our recommendation is to admit and monitor them.

Full-term neonates and infants with no history of apnea and bradycardia have a reduced risk of apnea and bradycardia after general anesthesia. Opinions vary on the minimum PCA for ambulatory surgery in this age group, varying between 44 and 50 weeks PCA; many children's hospitals admit all full-term neonates (<30 days of age) for overnight monitoring after general anesthesia, although this is not evidence based. All full-term infants with a history of apnea and bradycardia or those who have siblings who have had sudden infant death syndrome should be observed for an extended period if not admitted for overnight monitoring after general anesthesia.

Cardiovascular System

Bradycardia

Bradycardia is the most common dysrhythmia in the pediatric patient and requires immediate attention because of its association with a decrease in cardiac output. *The most common cause of bradycardia in infants and children is hypoxemia until proven otherwise.* Other possible causes for the bradycardia include vagal responses (i.e., passage of a nasogastric tube), medications (i.e., neostigmine, β-adrenergic blockade and opioids such as fentanyl), increased intracranial pressure, and high neuraxial anesthetic block. Treatment is directed at correcting the underlying cause, including the administration of oxygen and ensuring a patent airway. Bradycardia should be immediately treated with oxygen and, if necessary, with ventilation. If this "first line" intervention with oxygen does not immediately result in restoring the heart rate, then atropine (0.02 mg/kg) is administered; and if no response is found within 30 seconds, then administration of epinephrine (2-10 µg/kg) is indicated. If there is no response to epinephrine, then chest compressions are instituted and standard cardiopulmonary resuscitation algorithms followed (see Chapter 40). Bradycardia associated with hypotension must be treated immediately with epinephrine and cardiopulmonary resuscitation.

Tachycardia

Tachycardia is an important postoperative sign signifying an attempt by the body's compensatory mechanisms to maintain adequate cardiac output or oxygen delivery or a response of the body to reflex stimuli (pain) or drugs (epinephrine, atropine). In addition, tachycardia may be due to hypoxemia, hypercarbia, hypovolemia, emergence delirium, anxiety, sepsis (fever), hypervolemia, a full bladder, a previously unrecognized conduction abnormality (particularly in children with congenital heart disease [see Chapter 21]), or heart failure. Treatment is directed to correct the underlying cause. Occasionally, children present with a sustained tachycardia that is refractory to the usual therapy. A cardiac consultation will be required to investigate and identify rarer causes, such as an aberrant conduction system or ectopic foci.

Other Arrhythmias

Postoperative arrhythmias are relatively rare in children except for bradycardia and tachycardia. Development of premature ventricular beats or premature atrial beats may first occur in the PACU. Multifocal premature ventricular beats are not common in children. They may occur as a result of inadequately treated pain, cardiac conduction defect, or, in rare instances, may be a harbinger of malignant hyperthermia (see Chapter 41), acute rhabdomyolysis with hyperkalemia, inadequately treated pain, a congenital conduction defect, or the presence of a structural cardiac defect. Children with known congenital heart disease should have continuous ECG monitoring in the PACU, because ectopic foci commonly occur in this population (see Chapter 21).

Blood Pressure Control

Hypotension

The anesthesiologist should be familiar with the normal blood pressure ranges of infants and children (see Chapter 2). The measurement should be obtained with an appropriately sized blood pressure cuff (two-thirds the length of the upper arm). An improperly sized cuff will give spurious readings. Small cuffs may yield a false high reading, whereas a large cuff may yield a false low reading. Proper placement of the cuff is essential if errors in interpretation are to be avoided.

The most common cause of hypotension in children is hypovolemia from inadequate replacement of blood and fluids lost during the surgical procedure or ongoing blood loss. Clinical hallmarks of hypovolemia are tachycardia, urine output of less than 1 mL/kg/hr, slow capillary refill (>3 seconds), and narrowing of the pulse pressure. If the hematocrit is adequate, hypovolemia may be treated with isotonic crystalloids and albumin. An initial fluid bolus of 10 mL/kg should be given and then repeated until the blood pressure is age appropriate. If the hematocrit is inadequate, packed red blood cells (PRBCs) or whole blood should be administered. In this case, a rough guide for the volume of blood required is 4 mL/kg packed cells or 6 mL/kg whole blood to raise the hemoglobin 1 g/dL in children and adults (see Chapter 10). If a more accurate restoration of the hematocrit is preferred, then the volume of PRBCs required may be estimated to be

$$\frac{(Desired\ hematocrit - present\ hematocrit) \times EBV}{The\ hematocrit\ in\ the\ PRBCs.}$$

If the child does not respond to volume expansion, then other causes for the hypotension need to be considered, especially ongoing but not clinically evident blood loss (e.g., intra-abdominal, retroperitoneal, intrathoracic [blocked chest tube] or cardiac tamponade). Any factor that interferes with venous return can result in hypotension; such factors include positive-pressure ventilation, auto-positive end-expiratory pressure, tension pneumothorax, pericardial tamponade, and compression of the inferior vena cava.

High-dose inhalation agents, local anesthetic agents, opioids, as well as interactions between benzodiazepines and opioids may produce hypotension through vasodilation (relative hypovolemia) and direct myocardial depression. However, these factors rarely make significant contributions in the PACU. Other rare causes may include anaphylaxis (e.g., latex allergy, antibiotics), transfusion reaction, adrenal insufficiency, systemic inflammation, infection, severe liver failure, and the administration of antihypertensive, antidysrhythmic, and anticonvulsant medications. Increased body temperature may cause vasodilation and a relative hypovolemia. In addition, the increased metabolic demands of fever may compromise an already stressed myocardium. If a child arrives in the PACU requiring vasopressors and subsequently develops hypotension, then a cause for the hypotension including pump failure, a disconnect or kink in the vasopressor infusion, disruption of the intravenous access, or a disconnect from the pump must be considered and corrected.

Vasodilation caused by sympathetic blockade associated with regional anesthesia occasionally will cause hypotension, especially with a high blockade and restricted fluid intake. This is generally only a problem in children older than 6 years of age. Owing to the developmental changes in the sympathetic nervous system, most children younger than age 6 are normally peripherally vasodilated and therefore have little response to further vasodilation with a regional block.[51]

Decreased inotropy (caused by myocardial ischemia), dysrhythmia, calcium-channel blockers, sepsis, hypothyroidism, negative inotropic agents, and congestive heart failure are other rare causes of hypotension in children. Treatment is directed at the underlying cause, such as correcting hypovolemia with volume loading, treating the allergic reaction, or treating the sepsis. Decreased cardiac contractility may be treated by diuresis and the administration of inotropic agents, that also decrease the afterload.

Hypertension

Postoperative hypertension in children is less common than hypotension and most often is due to incorrect measurement or to pain. A blood pressure cuff that is too small may yield a spuriously high blood pressure reading and should be one of the first considerations in the differential diagnosis, especially if the child is not manifesting other symptoms consistent with pain. Causative factors besides pain include hypervolemia, preexisting hypertension (renal disease with inadequate continuity of antihypertensive medications), distended bladder, hypercarbia, hypoxemia, agitation and delirium, increased intracranial pressure, and exogenous vasoactive drugs (e.g., epinephrine). Pheochromocytoma and other vasoactive secreting tumors may rarely occur as a cause of hypertension in the PACU. A previously unrecognized coarctation of the aorta may be ruled out by comparing upper and lower extremity blood pressures and palpation of the quality of femoral and brachial pulses. Therapy for hypertension includes but is not limited to treatment of pain, drainage of the bladder, a review of current and intraoperative medications (vasopressor pump malfunction), and treatment of intracranial pressure. In unusual clinical situations, antihypertensive medications such as β-adrenergic blockers, calcium-channel blockers, hydralazine, nitrates, and α-adrenergic blockers, may be required.

Renal System

Complications related to the renal system are rare in the postoperative period. The most likely cause of low urine output (<1 mL/kg/hr) is hypovolemia as discussed previously (e.g., postoperative hypotension). Mechanical obstruction downstream from the kidneys could be due to either direct surgical interference or a misplaced or dysfunctional urinary catheter (blood clot or kink). If the child has a regional (spinal or epidural) anesthetic that includes an opioid, and there is no urinary catheter in place, then placement of a Foley or straight catheter may be indicated. Renal failure is a rare possibility in children who have had major operations or have systemic inflammatory disease. If screening tests such as blood urea nitrogen, creatinine elevations, and abnormal urine analysis (abnormal or inappropriate osmolality and sodium excretion) are suggestive, then a pediatric nephrologist should be consulted.

Gastrointestinal System

Postoperative Nausea and Vomiting

Postoperative nausea and vomiting (PONV) is one of the most bothersome side effects of anesthesia and surgery. Unlike adults, most children are unfamiliar with and have never experienced nausea. It is unlikely that they will warn the PACU personnel that they are nauseated. In children, vomiting and/or complaining of a "sore tummy" are likely the first and only manifestations of gastrointestinal upset. Another distinguishing feature of PONV in children is that age seems to be a factor, that is, PONV is inversely related to age.[52] The incidence of PONV is small in very young children, increases throughout childhood, reaching a zenith in adolescents, in whom the incidence exceeds that in adults.[52]

The type of surgery also influences the incidence of PONV.[52] The incidence of PONV in children is greatest after tonsillectomy, strabismus repair, hernia repair, orchiopexy, microtia, and middle ear procedures.[53] Before puberty there are no gender-related differences in PONV. The medical complications of PONV include pulmonary aspiration, dehydration, electrolyte imbalance, fatigue, wound disruption, and esophageal tears. Aside from the medical complications, PONV can produce psychological effects that may produce anxiety in both the children and parents and lead them to avoid further surgery. The cost implications of PONV can be major because of delayed recovery and discharge, increased medical care, and occasionally reoperation. Although these problems are seldom life-threatening, the cumulative costs in terms of prolonged PACU stays, unplanned admissions, and patient dissatisfaction are serious.[54]

Evidence-Based Consensus Management of PONV

The management of PONV is complex, and a very large number of treatment strategies have been formulated (Fig. 47-1). Almost all have been shown to be effective in one study or another. However, the superiority of some treatments over others may not have been established, in part because of study design flaws such as inadequate dosing, small sample sizes, or variable periods of observations and data collection (some studies monitored PONV only during the first few hours after surgery whereas others monitored the children for 24 to 48 hours after surgery). To make sense of the conflicting data that exist, a consensus-based management strategy for the prevention and management of PONV has been devised.[55] These guidelines advise first identifying patients at significant risk for PONV as outlined earlier; prophylaxis for PONV is recommended for children in high-risk groups.

The consensus guidelines also recognize that the choice of anesthetic can influence the incidence of PONV in children. Propofol-based anesthesia when used in procedures with a high incidence of PONV has been shown to have a much smaller rate of PONV than isoflurane-based anesthesia, even when both groups are given prophylactic 5-HT$_3$ inhibitors.[56] Similarly, multimodal therapy that is a combination of PONV treatment strategies has been shown to be more effective than single treatment strategy. For instance, the combination of propofol anesthesia plus ondansetron has been shown to significantly reduce the incidence of PONV when compared with the use of propofol alone (7% vs. 22%).[57] The combination of dexamethasone and ondansetron is more effective than either intervention in isolation but also permits the dose of ondansetron to be reduced by 50%.[58] A slightly more contentious effect has been the elimination of nitrous oxide, which has been shown to decrease the incidence of PONV in patients undergoing highly emetogenic surgery with a number needed to treat of only five patients. However, that same meta-analysis also revealed a disturbing incidence of awareness if nitrous oxide was omitted.[59]

Other strategies recommended to decrease the rate of PONV include the use of the smallest dose of opioids that still provides adequate pain control and the use of regional anesthesia where possible. In addition, the use of nonopioids such as acetaminophen and ketorolac should also be considered. Adequate parenteral hydration and avoidance of early postoperative fluid ingestion has also been shown to improve PONV status (see Chapter 4).

Prophylactic Therapy for PONV in Children

Ondansetron has been studied extensively in children and has been shown to decrease both early and late PONV at doses of 50 to 100 µg/kg.[60] Because the 5-HT$_3$ antagonists as a group have greater efficacy in the prevention of vomiting versus nausea, they are the drugs of first choice for prophylaxis in children. Dexamethasone has also been shown to be effective in decreasing PONV.[61] Administration of dexamethasone either alone or in combination with other antiemetics has been shown to extend the period of effective treatment up to 24 hours. In a

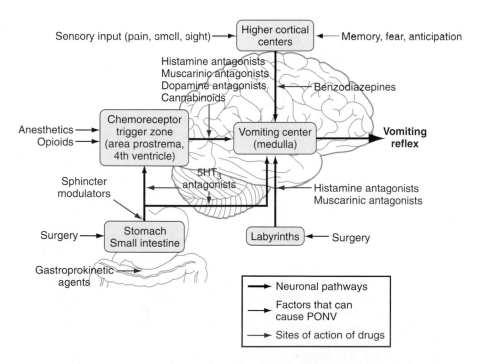

Figure 47-1. Treatment strategies for postoperative nausea and vomiting. PONV, postoperative nausea and vomiting.

systematic review, Steward and associates demonstrated that children who received a single dose of dexamethasone (0.15 to 1 mg/kg) were two times less likely to vomit after tonsillectomy and adenoidectomy than those who did not receive dexamethasone.[62,63] A randomized prospective dose finding study of dexamethasone administered to children undergoing tonsillectomy found no difference between 0.0625 mg/kg compared with 1.0 mg/kg, suggesting that very low doses of dexamethasone are equally effective as very high doses (see Fig. 31-6)[64]; a similar trial has not been carried out in the PACU for children who are already experiencing PONV. Prior to the black box warning for droperidol, it was also recommended for prophylaxis of PONV,[65] but only as a last resort because of the issues of extrapyramidal effects and significant sedation.

The most effective prophylaxis strategy in children at moderate or high risk for PONV is to utilize combination therapy that includes a 5-HT$_3$ antagonist and a second drug such as low dose dexamethasone. Antiemetic rescue therapy should be administered to children who vomit after surgery. An emetic episode more than 6 hours postoperatively can be treated with any of the drugs used for prophylaxis except dexamethasone and transdermal scopolamine.[66]

Rescue Therapy

The consensus panel recommends that children who did not receive intraoperative prophylaxis or those who fail prophylaxis should receive a 5-HT$_3$ receptor antagonist at the first signs of PONV.[39] The consensus guideline—recommended dose should be one fourth of that used for prophylaxis—for all other therapies the data on efficacy for rescue are sparse and doses are not known. One study found that promethazine and droperidol were as effective as ondansetron in a general surgical population of adults, but similar studies have not been conducted in children.[59]

Alternative Treatments

Alternative methods for nausea and vomiting prophylaxis deserve consideration. In a prospective randomized study, isopropyl alcohol significantly reduced postoperative vomiting, although the effect was transient.[67] In a meta-analysis that evaluated 24 randomized studies on the alternative anti-nausea and vomiting techniques, the authors concluded that acupuncture, electro-acupuncture, transcutaneous electrical nerve stimulation, acupoint stimulation, and acupressure each have a significant effect when compared with placebo in preventing early postoperative nausea and vomiting in adults, but not in children.[68]

Pain Management in the PACU

Acute postoperative pain management strategies are discussed in detail in Chapter 44. In this section, the discussion is limited to the management of pain in the PACU. More than in any other unit of the hospital, a given child's level of pain (or the perception of pain) changes rapidly in the PACU. Frequent and consistent use of pain scores for children of all ages, including those with developmental disabilities, is critical. A large number of pain scales have been validated for use in children (see Chapter 44). More important than the specific scale that is employed is that the scale be used consistently and follow simple principles. For instance, children who are verbal and developmentally appropriate should be encouraged to report their pain using a self-report scale (e.g., the Oucher scale). Young children or those without verbal skills should be assessed using an objective pain behavior scale (e.g., the FLACC scale).[69,70] Just as important is the consistent application of protocols to treat pain, that is, the treatment of a given pain level should not vary from shift to shift or from one nurse to another.[71]

As with other areas of pediatric pain control, a multimodal approach to postoperative pain is recommended. A plan for pain management should be discussed among the family, surgical team, and anesthesia team before surgery.[72] Depending on the surgery, such a plan may include any or all of the following: acetaminophen, nonsteroidal agents, local anesthesia, nerve blocks, regional anesthesia, clonidine, opiates, patient-controlled analgesia (PCA), and patient-controlled epidural analgesia (PCEA). Acetaminophen and nonsteroidal drugs act through inhibition of prostaglandins and their metabolites. Most of these drugs are given orally and should be given preoperatively or intraoperatively to be effective in the PACU. Occasionally, they may be indicated in the PACU if they were not administered before arrival. Oral acetaminophen (15 mg/kg) or ibuprofen (10 mg/kg) have been shown to decrease opioid requirements by 20% to 30% after a variety of surgical procedures.[73,74] Acetaminophen can also be given rectally in doses of 35 to 45 mg/kg; however, because absorption is variable and delayed (peak level 60 to 180 minutes after rectal administration), this route is not recommended for use in the PACU.[75] The pharmacokinetics of the rectal route are such that a greater interval between doses is recommended (6 hours) and that subsequent doses are reduced (20 mg/kg) so that the total dose per 24 hours does not exceed 100 mg/kg.[76] There are no data to provide guidance for rectal acetaminophen beyond 24 hours. If a child has received rectal acetaminophen, then the first oral dose should be delayed until 6 hours after the rectal dose. The nonsteroidal anti-inflammatory drug ketorolac can decrease opioid requirements by approximately 30%. The recommended dosage is 0.2 to 0.5 mg/kg given intravenously every 6 hours.[77] Caution is warranted in postoperative children when bleeding is a significant problem or when any history of renal insufficiency is present.[78] The manufacturer recommends limiting doses to 15 mg total for patients weighing less than 50 kg and 30 mg total for heavier patients.

Opioids are indicated during the immediate postoperative period for any surgery or procedure in which moderate or severe pain is not being managed by other means. Morphine, hydromorphone, and fentanyl are all effective and have a long history of safe use for pediatric patients. Repeated doses of meperidine are generally not recommended in children because of the potential for seizures from epileptogenic metabolites (normeperidine).[79] Opioid dosing should be initiated according to body weight, physiologic development, underlying medical/surgical conditions, co-administered medications, and the severity of the pain. The goal should be effective and rapid pain relief. Subsequent dosing of the medications should be titrated based on response to the initial dose. Administration of multiple, small, ineffective doses results in prolongation of pain, stress, and anxiety without improving the safety of care provided. With this caveat in mind, patient-controlled analgesia (PCA) and patient-controlled epidural analgesia (PCEA) (see Chapter 44) may be used in the PACU environment; however, this intervention should be started only after acute pain has been adequately treated. The small doses administered by PCA are generally not adequate to completely treat acute postoperative pain and may add to a sense that the PCA is not "working" for a given child.[80]

Regional analgesia using caudal or epidural blocks is a common mode of intraoperative pain control in the child that extends into the PACU (see Chapter 42). The most important question for the PACU personnel is "how do we know it is working?" This question needs to be approached in a systematic manner.

The regional block should be placed in a manner that provides analgesia for the surgical incision site and visceral pain. Evidence that the regional block is effective should first be detected during surgery. In the presence of an effective regional block, the anesthetic requirements are usually reduced. For instance, a caudal block will generally not be effective for a midabdominal incision. The addition of hydrophilic opioids or clonidine may extend the level of analgesia to some extent over the course of several hours; however, a block that is many dermatome segments away from the site of the surgical incision will likely not be adequate. Furthermore, the addition of opioids to an epidural or spinal block increases the risk of pruritus, urinary retention, and emesis. Similarly, visceral pain such as bladder spasms (which have thoracic innervation) or the sore throat after intubation are not attenuated by a lumbar epidural catheter and must be managed by other measures (belladonna alkaloids, benzodiazepines, opioids, or ketorolac).[81]

Verification needs to be obtained that the catheter is in the epidural space. Several methods exist to answer this question. Older children can be questioned about their sensation level using ice or other cold sensation to determine the level of sympathectomy. Preverbal or developmentally disabled patients require some other objective form of confirmation. Previous reports have focused on electrical stimulation via the epidural catheter at the time of catheter placement to determine the level of insertion.[82] More recently ultrasound methods for detecting epidural catheter placement have been described.[83] Perhaps most practical in the PACU may be the use of radiographic confirmation of dermatome level of the tip of the catheter and to ensure appropriate placement in the epidural space.[84] A small amount (<1 mL) of contrast (e.g., Omnipaque 180 or 240) can be infused into the catheter with one radiograph taken to confirm placement.

Temperature Management

Intraoperative normothermia is key to maintaining a normal temperature postoperatively. Hypothermia (see Chapter 25) is associated with discomfort, bleeding, infections, altered metabolism of drugs, delayed return of cognitive functions, and prolonged recovery.[85-89] Because most heat loss (about 90%) occurs via the skin, only heat exchange via the skin provides an adequate way of warming children. Intraoperatively, this method of warming is enhanced by the vasodilation properties of most anesthetic agents. Forced-air warming blankets are currently the most effective way of maintaining body temperature in children.[90] Given the vasoconstriction that occurs after anesthesia, attempts at warming are less effective postoperatively than intraoperatively and most of the detrimental physiologic changes have already taken place. Given the growing body of literature documenting the detrimental effects of hypothermia and the availability of effective warming devices, children should arrive in the PACU with a normal body temperature.

Table 47-6. Discharge Criteria (Inpatients)

1. Recovery of airway and respiratory reflexes adequate to support gas exchange and to protect against aspiration of secretions, vomitus, or blood
2. Stability of circulation and control of any surgical bleeding
3. Absence of anticipated instability in categories 1 and 2
4. Reasonable control of pain and vomiting
5. Appropriate duration of observation after narcotic or naloxone flumazenil administration (a minimum of 60 minutes after intravenous naloxone and up to 2 hours after flumazenil)
6. Return to baseline level of consciousness unless transfer is to an ICU environment

Infants and children may suffer burns from overly aggressive rewarming measures. This is particularly true for nonverbal children, children who are somnolent, and children who have decreased sensation due to disease or use of regional anesthesia techniques. Recommendations from the device manufacturer and recent literature should be carefully reviewed before instituting routine use of warming devices.

Discharge Criteria (Fast Track)

The recovery process and discharge criteria vary from institution to institution. Various criteria are used for readiness for discharge from the PACU. The modified Aldrete score is the most common system used to assess discharge readiness, but specific criteria are actually dependent on the particular situation or environment to which the child will be discharged. For example, a child with a slight degree of postextubation croup or stridor may be discharged for monitoring on a pediatric floor or ICU but the same child would not be discharged to parental care and a 2-hour drive home. The criteria for discharge of children to a general inpatient setting are summarized in Table 47-6; for outpatients, these criteria hold and the additional criteria outlined in Table 47-7 must generally be met before

Table 47-7. Discharge Criteria (Outpatients)

All criteria in Table 47-6, plus:

1. Cardiovascular function and airway patency are satisfactory and stable.
2. The child is easily arousable, and protective reflexes are intact.
3. The child can talk (if age appropriate).
4. The child can sit up unaided (if age appropriate).
5. For a very young or handicapped child, incapable of the usually expected responses, the preanesthetic level of responsiveness or a level as close as possible to the normal level for that child should be achieved unless the child is to be transferred to another monitored location.
6. The state of hydration is adequate.
7. It may be permissible for parents to carry their children without full recovery of gait (parents must be advised that the child is at risk of injury if improperly supervised).
8. Control of pain should be achieved to permit adequate analgesia via the oral route thereafter.
9. Control of nausea and vomiting should be achieved to allow for oral hydration (see "Discharge Criteria" in text).

discharge. Traditionally, pediatric patients have been allowed to recover in a "first-stage" recovery unit until the airway was considered stable, consciousness is regained, baseline motor activity is confirmed, vital signs are stable, and oxygen saturations are stable (or at baseline) without respiratory support (unless needed at baseline). In addition, pain should generally be well controlled. Often children can then be transferred to a second-stage recovery unit where more complete recovery would take place with a reduced nurse-to-child ratio until children have met criteria for adequate hydration, minimal emesis, appropriate wound status, good vital signs, and appropriate ambulation and mental status. In general, requirements for children to eat/drink and void before leaving the secondary recovery area have been shown to significantly delay discharge. Efforts should be made to ensure fluid replacement and adequate hydration, thus negating any physiologic imperative for oral intake in the immediate postoperative time frame. Other than children who are at particularly high risk for urinary retention (e.g., those with a history of urinary retention or urethral surgery), there is little evidence that discharge before voiding results in readmission for voiding problems and, therefore, this requirement is no longer part of standard discharge criteria.[91] Children who have received a caudal block for surgery are likewise at low risk for urinary retention as long as opioids have not been added to the caudal medication.[92]

Although there are few data on the current status of recovery processes across the country, there appears to be a trend toward one-stage (fast track) recovery for pediatric outpatients.[93,94] This process allows selected children to bypass the first-stage recovery and go directly to the second-stage unit based on appropriate level of consciousness, physical activity, vital signs, respiratory status, and pain control (Table 47-8). Such systems have proven successful and quite safe, although appropriate attention to issues such as pain control must be addressed when initiating such a program.

Acknowledgment

The authors wish to thank Alberto J. de Armendi, MD, and I. D. Todres, MD, for their prior contributions to this chapter.

Table 47-8. Discharge Criteria for Fast-Tracking

	Score
Level of Consciousness	
Aware and oriented	2
Arousable with minimal stimulation	1
Responsive only to tactile stimulation	0
Physical Activity	
Able to move all extremities on command	2
Some weakness in movement of extremities	1
Unable to voluntarily move extremities	0
Hemodynamic Stability	
Blood pressure <15% of baseline MAP value	2
Blood pressure 15% to 30% of baseline MAP value	1
Blood pressure >30% of baseline MAP value	0
Respiratory Stability	
Able to breathe deeply	2
Tachypneic with good cough	1
Dyspneic with weak cough	0
Oxygen Saturation Status	
Maintains value >95% on room air	2
Requires supplemental oxygen (nasal prongs)	1
Saturation <90% with supplemental oxygen	0
Postoperative Pain Assessment	
None, or mild discomfort	2
Moderate to severe pain controlled with intravenous analgesics	1
Persistent, severe pain	0
Postoperative Emetic Symptoms	
None, or mild nausea with no active vomiting	2
Transient vomiting or retching	1
Persistent moderate to severe nausea and vomiting	0
Total*	14

MAP, mean arterial pressure.
*Pediatric patients must score 14 to bypass the phase 1 (PACU) recovery unit to be admitted to the "step-down" unit.
From White PF, Song D: New criteria for fast-tracking after outpatient anesthesia: a comparison with the modified Aldrete's scoring system. Anesth Analg 1998; 88:1069-1072.

Annotated References

Birmingham PK, Tobin MJ, Henthorn TK, et al: Twenty-four-hour pharmacokinetics of rectal acetaminophen in children: an old drug with new recommendations. Anesthesiology 1997; 87:244-252
This study was one of the first to shed light on the need to use relatively large doses of acetaminophen when it was administered rectally as opposed to orally. They concluded that the oral dosing regimen of 10 to 15 mg/kg is inadequate and that the initial dose of rectal acetaminophen should be approximately 40 mg/kg.

Cravero JP, Beach M, Thyr B, Whalen K: The effect of small dose fentanyl on the emergence characteristics of pediatric patients after sevoflurane anesthesia without surgery. Anesth Analg 2003; 97:364-367
The authors performed a prospective, randomized, blinded trial in which they studied patients undergoing MRI with general inhaled sevoflurane anesthesia via a laryngeal mask airway. The authors concluded that small doses of opiates decrease emergence agitation without increasing unwanted side effects.

Gan TJ, Meyer T, Apfel CC, Chung F, et al: Consensus guidelines for managing postoperative nausea and vomiting. Anesth Analg 2003; 97:62-71

The authors present a review of the available literature concerning postoperative nausea and vomiting. They use "strength of evidence" criteria where possible and expert opinion where data are lacking.

Hackel A, Badgwell JM, Binding RR, et al: Guidelines for the pediatric perioperative anesthesia environment. American Academy of Pediatrics, Section on Anesthesiology. Pediatrics 1999; 103:512-515

The American Academy of Pediatrics Guideline for the pediatric perioperative anesthesia environment addresses the facility- and personnel-based components of the postoperative care setting for children.

Kain ZN, Caldwell-Andrews AA, Maranets I, et al: Preoperative anxiety and emergence delirium and postoperative maladaptive behaviors. Anesth Analg 2004; 99:1648-1654

This study is extremely unusual in its ability to relate perioperative anxiety with the incidence of emergence agitation. Preoperative anxiety is significantly related to the incidence of emergence agitation and, even more importantly, the incidence of agitation is related to the rate of postoperative maladaptive behaviors. This study argues strongly for identifying children at risk for emergence agitation and gives some evidence for why it is worth effort to prevent or ameliorate this phenomenon.

References

Please see www.expertconsult.com

Sedation for Diagnostic and Therapeutic Procedures Outside the Operating Room

CHAPTER 48

Richard F. Kaplan, Joseph P. Cravero, Myron Yaster, and Charles J. Coté

Definition of Levels of Sedation	**Specific Sedation Techniques**
Goals of Sedation	Local Anesthetics
Risks and Complications Associated with Sedation	Anxiolytics/Sedatives
Guidelines	Barbiturates
Implementation of Sedation Guidelines	Opioids
Documentation	Systemic Anesthetics

THE USE OF SEDATION and analgesia for diagnostic and thera- peutic procedures performed by anesthesiologists and non- anesthesiologists outside the operating room has dramatically increased. It is estimated that millions of such procedures are performed each year throughout the world. Great progress has been made in the understanding of sedation and analgesia within and outside the operating room. The mere restraint of a child of any age for a frightening and/or painful procedure is completely unjustified.[1-4] Procedures performed outside the operating room require the same attention to anxiolysis, analgesia, and sedation as procedures performed in the operating room. Painful proce- dures that frequently are performed outside the operating room (e.g., bone marrow aspiration, lumbar puncture, repair of minor surgical wounds, insertion of arterial or venous catheters, burn dressing changes, fracture reduction, bronchoscopy, endoscopy) require analgesia and often sedation that may reach levels of deep sedation/general anesthesia, particularly in children age 6 years and younger. Nonpainful procedures require sedation and immobility. Children undergoing diagnostic studies (e.g., com- puted tomography [CT], magnetic resonance imaging [MRI], positron emission tomography, electroencephalography [EEG], electromyography) or who require high doses of ionizing radia- tion also require deep levels of sedation and anesthesia because as part of the procedure they must remain absolutely motionless and be immobile for 10 to 90 minutes or longer.[5] Given these requirements, a team approach is required to provide adequate care to the child and conditions for the planned procedure.

Young children, as well as developmentally and medically handicapped children, are often unable to remain motionless for even short periods of time. Many older children and adults are unable to enter the confined space and often frightening envi- ronment of a diagnostic imaging scanner. The fear and anxiety associated with procedures are difficult to control and may be exacerbated by parental anxiety, separation from parents, and the pain or anticipation of pain from the procedure. Although distraction, guided imagery, and the use of videos and music have clear and documented benefit, they are often not enough to efficiently and successfully complete procedures.[6-10]

The pharmacologic armamentarium for sedation has greatly expanded to include drugs classified as sedatives as well as those classified as anesthetics. Who uses these drugs and what quali- fications are needed to provide sedation is controversial. Anes- thetic agents used by anesthesiologists outside the operating room for sedation and analgesia have provided conditions that are much improved compared with older traditional sedation agents used by non-anesthesiologists.

The demand for safe efficient sedation and analgesia outside the operating room has outstripped the available supply of anesthesiologists. The lack of sufficient anesthesiology care pro- viders has lead to the demand to create sedation services led by non-anesthesiologists (i.e., nurse practitioners, pediatricians, emergency department physicians, intensivists, and dentists) who often use sedative agents including anesthetics. The devel- opment of pediatric sedation services has taken many direc- tions. In a recent survey of pediatric sedation practice in 116 children's hospitals in the United States and Canada,[11] only 50% of the hospitals had a formal pediatric sedation service. Fifty- four percent utilized a "mobile" provider model. Hospital cre- dentialing for non-anesthesiology providers varied between 66% and 76% for "deep" and "conscious" sedation (now classified as moderate sedation), respectively. A nurse-physician provider combination was the most common and was utilized in 59% of hospitals. Anesthesiologists were the sole sedation providers in only 26% of institutions. Anesthetic agents such as propofol were used regularly by non-anesthesiologists for sedation of nonintubated (42%) and intubated (63%) children. Eighty-seven percent of institutions reported barriers to development of pediatric sedation services. The most common barrier was a shortage of providers, particularly anesthesiologists. In this chapter we focus on the definition of sedation and the goals, risks, and guidelines for creation of safe conditions for the care of children who are scheduled for diagnostic and therapeutic procedures outside the operating room.

Definition of Levels of Sedation

Several organizations have created guidelines and definitions of sedation for use in children. The most frequently used and agreed upon are the definitions of the American Academy of Pediatrics (AAP), the American Society of Anesthesiologists (ASA), and the Joint Commission on Accreditation of Healthcare Organizations (JCAHO).[12-15] These organizations defined sedation and analgesia for procedures as a continuum of consciousness to unconsciousness with four levels previously described as "anxiolysis," "conscious sedation," "deep sedation," and "general anesthesia." In 2002, the AAP changed the terminology of "conscious sedation" to "moderate sedation" because "conscious sedation" was too confusing. The present continuum of sedation ranges from minimal sedation (anxiolysis) to moderate sedation (previously conscious sedation) to deep sedation and general anesthesia. Note that a child may easily pass from a light level of sedation to general anesthesia (Fig. 48-1).

A clear understanding of the definition of sedation is mandatory to recognize when the child has progressed to a deeper level of sedation than anticipated and is at increased risk (i.e., from moderate sedation to deep sedation or from deep sedation to general anesthesia). Recognition of this transition allows escalation of monitoring and care to avoid complications. The AAP, ASA, and the JCAHO formalized and defined the concepts of minimal sedation, moderate sedation, deep sedation, and general anesthesia. The definitions that follow are taken from the JCAHO manual (2006)[15] and are in agreement with AAP and ASA definitions:

- *Minimal sedation (anxiolysis):* A drug-induced state during which patients respond normally to verbal commands. Although cognitive function and coordination may be impaired, ventilatory and cardiovascular functions are unaffected (Video Clip 48-1).
- *Moderate sedation* (previously called conscious sedation or sedation/analgesia): A drug-induced depression of consciousness during which patients respond purposefully to verbal commands either alone or accompanied by light tactile stimulation. No interventions are required to maintain a patent airway, and spontaneous ventilation is adequate. Cardiovascular function is usually maintained (Video Clip 48-2).
- *Deep sedation:* A drug-induced depression of consciousness during which patients cannot be easily aroused but respond purposefully after repeated or painful stimulation (*note:* reflex withdrawal from a painful stimulus is not considered a purposeful response). The ability to independently maintain ventilatory function may be impaired. Patients may require assistance in maintaining a patent airway and spontaneous ventilation may be inadequate. Cardiovascular function is usually maintained (Video Clip 48-3).
- *General anesthesia:* A drug-induced loss of consciousness during which patients are not arousable, even to painful stimulation. The ability to independently maintain ventilatory function is often impaired. Patients often require assistance in maintaining a patent airway, and positive-pressure ventilation may be required because of depressed spontaneous ventilation or drug-induced depression of neuromuscular function. Cardiovascular function may be impaired (Video Clip 48-4).

The assessment of the depth of sedation based on response to stimulation is illustrated in Figure 48-2. The assessment of response to stimulation is difficult in children and depends on their verbal abilities, age, level of maturity, and underlying condition. Most nonpainful procedures in children are performed with the child either moderately or deeply sedated. Almost all painful procedures are done with children deeply sedated. A common problem with the classification of a child as either moderately or deeply sedated is to misinterpret any movement in response to touch as "purposeful" and therefore a sign of "moderate sedation." A child who is moderately sedated should respond to touch or firm rubbing by saying "ouch," pushing your hand away, and pulling up the covers. *No response or nonpurposeful movement is a sign that the child has progressed to a level of deep sedation and should lead to escalation of care of the patient because respiratory depression may occur.*[16-19] Similarly, children who are deeply sedated should respond purposefully to painful stimulation. *Reflex withdrawal or a nonpurposeful response to painful stimulation is a sign that the child has progressed to a level of anesthesia and should be cared for using guidelines and personnel for general anesthesia.*

ASA AND JCAHO DEFINITION OF SEDATION

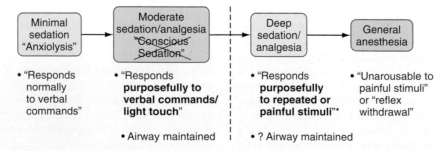

Figure 48-1. The sedation continuum. A patient may readily pass from a light level of sedation to deep sedation or general anesthesia. Health care providers must be prepared to increase vigilance and intensity of monitoring consistent with the depth of sedation. One should consider all children younger than the age of 6 years as deeply sedated because "conscious sedation" in this age group for most children is an oxymoron. (ASA, American Society of Anesthesiologists; JCAHO, Joint Commission on Accreditation of Healthcare Organizations.)

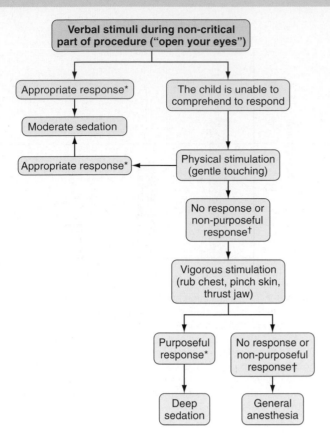

* Purposeful: opens eyes, talks back, pushes you out of the way
† Nonpurposeful: winces, shrugs shoulders, nonspecific
  withdrawal to pain

Figure 48-2. Sedated children must be continuously evaluated for depth of sedation and appropriateness of response. As diagrammed here, sedation is a continuum. Note that a purposeful response to voice or light touch is consistent with moderate sedation. A purposeful response to pain is consistent with deep sedation. A nonpurposeful response to pain is consistent with general anesthesia.

Children may quickly move from one level of sedation to another. A study in a large pediatric hospital showed that the goal of either moderate or deep sedation was only attained in 50% to 75% of patients. An awake state was noted in 12% to 28% of children, and a level consistent with general anesthesia was observed in up to 35% of children.[20] The need for accurate assessment of the sedated child has brought about several scoring systems.

The Ramsay scale was described by Ramsay and colleagues[21] in 1974 for the purpose of monitoring sedation with alphaxa-

Table 48-2. Modified Ramsay Sedation Scale

Score	Characteristics
1	Awake and alert, minimal or no cognitive impairment
2*	Awake but tranquil, purposeful responses to verbal commands at conversation level
3*	Appears asleep, purposeful responses to verbal commands at conversation level
4†	Appears asleep, purposeful responses to verbal commands but at louder than usual conversation level or requiring light glabellar tap
5†	Asleep, sluggish purposeful responses only to loud verbal commands or strong glabellar tap
6‡	Asleep, sluggish purposeful responses only to painful stimuli
7§	Asleep, reflex withdrawal to painful stimuli only (no purposeful responses)
8§	Unresponsive to external stimuli, including pain

*Minimal
†Moderate
‡Deep
§GA
GA, general anesthesia

lone/alphadolone (Table 48-1). It continues to be the most widely used scale for assessing and monitoring sedation in daily practice, as well as in clinical research. It spans the continuum of sedation but does not clearly separate purposeful from nonpurposeful responses. The Ramsey scale has been modified to more clearly coincide with the AAP and JCAHO guidelines (Table 48-2).[22] A score of 2 to 3 is anxiolysis, 4 to 5 is moderate sedation, 6 is deep sedation, and 7 to 8 is general anesthesia.

The Observer's Assessment of Alertness/Sedation scale (OAA/S)[23] is often cited as a scale for sedation. It is scored as follows: 1, no response to shaking; 2, responds to mild prodding; 3, responds to name called loudly; 4, lethargic response to name; and 5, readily responds to name. However, its inability to clearly categorize deep levels of sedation and lack of a clear differentiation between purposeful and nonpurposeful responses limit its usefulness. The University of Michigan Sedation Scale (UMSS)[24] is an assessment tool that has been shown to be valid when compared to the OAA/S scale and other scales of sedation (Table 48-3). It readily separates patients into the sedation categories defined by the AAP, ASA, and JCAHO.

These assessment tools all have the disadvantage of intermittently stimulating the child during the procedure and thereby undoing the very reason that sedation was given in the first

Table 48-1. Ramsay Scale

Level	Characteristics
1	Patient awake, anxious, agitated, or restless
2	Patient awake, cooperative, orientated, and tranquil
3	Patient drowsy, with response to commands
4	Patient asleep, brisk response to glabella tap or loud auditory stimulus
5	Patient asleep, sluggish response to stimulus
6	Patient has no response to firm nail-bed pressure or other noxious stimuli

Table 48-3. University of Michigan Sedation Scale (UMSS)

Score	Characteristics
0	Awake and alert
1	Minimally sedated: tired/sleepy, appropriate response to verbal conversation and/or sound
2	Moderately sedated: somnolent/sleeping, easily aroused with light tactile stimulation or a simple verbal command
3	Deeply sedated: deep sleep, arousable only with significant physical stimulation
4	Unarousable

place! Furthermore, assessing the child after stimulation may arouse the child to a lighter level of sedation than he or she was at before the stimulus and therefore inappropriately categorizes the child into a lighter level of sedation. A nonstimulating continuous assessment tool using processed EEG and particularly the bispectral index (BIS) monitor has been extensively explored. The BIS was derived from empirically estimating processed EEG parameters that best predicted OAA/S levels in adult volunteers receiving a wide variety of anesthetics, analgesics, and sedatives.[25] BIS values in adults range from 100 to 95, awake; 95 to 70, light to moderate sedation; 70 to 60, deep sedation with low probability of explicit recall; and 60 to 40, general anesthesia.[26] The EEGs in children vary markedly with age and therefore may render processed EEG measures unreliable.[27,28] Multiple studies have attempted to correlate BIS values with depth of sedation in children with varying success. One study involved 96 healthy children between 1 and 12 years of age sedated with chloral hydrate, meperidine and promethazine, midazolam, fentanyl, or pentobarbital and showed a good correlation between BIS and UMSS scores.[29] Another study examined 327 observations on 39 children aged birth to 18 years and compared levels of sedation to BIS after volatile anesthetic, chloral hydrate, midazolam, and fentanyl.[30] There was overall validity between the BIS and sedation scores, but this study also revealed ongoing limitations when attempting to distinguish moderate from deep sedation. For example, the researchers concluded that a BIS of 80 is the best cutoff for determining deep sedation; this value is inconsistent with that found in the adult literature. The overlap between different levels of sedation, relatively few large well-controlled studies in children, and overall quality of BIS data in some studies, as well as a lack of information for different ages and specific drugs, makes validation of the BIS for use in sedated children premature.[31]

All the definitions and tools just discussed attempt to assess sedation and thereby decrease risk by quantitating the response to stimulation or EEG activity. These tools, however, do not directly measure the risk of loss of the airway, which is the primary cause of death and injury during sedation.[32] The implication is that there is a direct quantifiable correlation between response to touch or painful stimulation and ability to control the airway. Thus, a moderately sedated child who can respond to light touch can protect his or her airway and a deeply sedated child who can respond appropriately only to pain may not be able to control the airway. *The important assessment of the child is not response to stimulation but the ability to protect the airway.* Furthermore, different sedative drugs have differing effects on analgesia versus airway obtundation. Propofol is not a profound analgesic but has profound effects on the airway.[33] Conversely, the sedative drug dexmedetomidine may provide profound sedation with little depression of respiratory function. Ketamine produces intense analgesia and most children maintain a patent airway and adequate respiratory effort.[34] Until recently, a quantifiable assessment of control of the airway in sedated children was not available.[35] Studies on the changes of airway dimensions under different anesthetic and sedative agents, the effect of different positions of the upper airway,[36-38] and upper airway collapsibility with different concentrations of sedative drugs are starting to emerge and will give us a more meaningful assessment of airway risk and protection using different sedative drugs and allow us to more carefully care for sedated children.

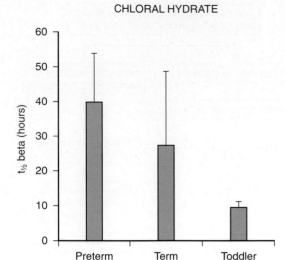

CHLORAL HYDRATE

Figure 48-3. Beta-elimination half-life of the active metabolite of chloral hydrate, trichloroethanol, in preterm infants, term infants, and toddlers. Note the extremely prolonged half-lives and the large standard deviations in all age groups. Although often thought of as a short-acting sedative, chloral hydrate can have profoundly long sedative effects with a real possibility of re-sedation after a procedure when the child is left undisturbed. It is for this reason that we recommend a longer period of observation in a step-down area before discharge.

Assessment of sedation must also focus on appropriate discharge readiness. Adverse effects including death have occurred after premature discharge following sedation for a procedure.[32] These events have mostly occurred when a long lasting (long half-life) sedative such as chloral hydrate has been given (Fig. 48-3). This can result in the child being unable to spontaneously unobstruct his or her airway.[39] A simple Modified Maintenance of Wakefulness score (infants had to stay awake for at least 20 minutes in a quiet environment before discharge) ensured that more then 90% of children had returned to baseline, compared with only 55% of children assessed as "street ready" according to usual hospital discharge criteria.[40]

Goals of Sedation

The goals of pediatric sedation can be summarized as follows[19,41]:

- Guard the child's safety and welfare.
- Minimize physical discomfort and pain.
- Control anxiety, minimize psychological trauma, and maximize the potential for amnesia.
- Control behavior and/or movement to allow the safe completion of the procedure.
- Return the child to a state in which safe discharge from medical supervision, as determined by recognized criteria, is possible.

Risks and Complications Associated with Sedation

The foremost goal is to optimize patient safety and thereby decrease the risk and associated complications. The assessment of risk for pediatric sedation must include age, type of procedure, underlying medical conditions, and how these might influence the response to sedating medications, intended level of sedation, the pharmacology and pharmacodynamics of the medications used, guidelines (i.e., training, equipment, personnel, monitoring), and discharge criteria. Complications and risk assessment must also include whether the procedure was successfully and efficiently completed, stress and pain of the subject, and postdischarge return to baseline activity, as well as the full range of complications from mild to moderate to life-threatening and death. There are numerous case reports and anecdotes describing pediatric sedation complications but few large sufficiently powered multicenter trials to evaluate safety. As importantly, the lack of sedation failures or complications ignores the fact that many children who need sedation are not getting sedation at all or in sufficient amounts. Sedation centers in the United States were much less likely to offer sedation for painful procedures than similar centers in Europe. Thirty percent of U.S. respondents to a mail survey reported performing bone marrow biopsies in children without significant sedation more than 50% of the time as compared with 0% of European centers![42]

The psychological consequences of no or insufficient sedation have not been specifically studied but can be inferred from other stressful situations. Inadequate preoperative sedation is clearly linked to increased anxiety in children and their families. Fifty-four percent of children undergoing stressful anesthesia induction have postoperative maladaptive behaviors.[43] The incidence of these behaviors is decreased through the use of appropriate preoperative sedation. Similar severe effects have been shown in pediatric intensive care units when Rennick and associates documented post-traumatic stress syndrome in children after repeated invasive procedures.[44] Although the number of children having adverse psychologic outcomes due to no or less than optimal sedation during diagnostic and therapeutic procedures is not known, one can assume that it would be similar to that in these situations.

There are many reports of relatively few patients (<200) receiving a variety of sedative medications in a variety of settings with successful completion of the procedure and no fatality.[45-55] A typical example is that of Vardi and colleagues[55] who in 105 procedures performed by intensivists compared propofol 200 μg/kg/min to a combination of ketamine/fentanyl/midazolam. Ten percent in the ketamine group had emergence delirium and one needed intubation; 20% of the propofol group required airway support and positive-pressure ventilation. Despite these complications, the conclusion reached was that propofol administered by pediatric intensivists is safe but must be used with "vigilance." Another study prospectively followed 1140 children (mean age 2.96 ± 3.7 years) sedated for procedures by non-anesthesiologists following AAP guidelines and using a quality assurance tool.[56] Approximately 13% of the children received inadequate sedation. There were no deaths or sedation-induced crises, but they reported a 5.3% incidence of respiratory events, including one in which a child stopped breathing. Given that the expected incidence of a sedation-induced crisis should be on the order of one in tens of thousands, it is not surprising that these studies rarely uncover a critical event.[57] If a study were designed to detect a difference between one sedation method with a fatality rate of 1 in 5,000 compared with another method with a fatality rate of 1 in 20,000, the study would require more than 50,000 children in each group!

Other research techniques have been used to identify common causes associated with sedation complications. In 2000, a retrospective review was undertaken of 95 cases of sedation-related deaths and critical incidents derived from the U.S. Food and Drug Administration's (FDA) adverse drug event reporting system, the U.S. Pharmacopeia, and a survey of pediatric specialists.[39] This analysis revealed that (rather than being related to a specific medication) the overwhelming majority of critical events were preventable and caused by operator error or lack of robust rescue systems when incidents occurred. Whereas a number of the incidents cited in this study occurred over 20 years, the findings are still applicable today. Drug interactions were the most common associated factor, followed by drug overdose, inadequate monitoring, inadequate cardiopulmonary resuscitation skills, inadequate evaluation before sedation, and premature discharge from medical supervision. The report emphasizes the fact that most sedation complications are related to the inability of the child to control or protect the airway; 80% of children with critical events presented with respiratory compromise. A high percentage progressed to cardiac arrest, indicating a lack of rescue skills of the practitioners. A disproportionately large number of severe complications and deaths occurred when sedation was performed in offices outside of hospitals, indicating a lack of personnel and training to provide rescue.

Another approach to the assessment of safety is to carefully observe relatively small groups of children and track minute-to-minute changes in their level of sedation. This has been accomplished by the creation of the Dartmouth Operative Conditions Scale.[58] This scale was derived from observing 110 videos of pediatric sedation outside the operating room and is a scale that allows quantification of children based on observable behavior. Continuously applying this scale allows for careful tracking of state of sedation, effectiveness of sedation, uncontrolled side effects, and the timing of induction of sedation and recovery. These data can be helpful in quantifying the quality of sedation and best practices.

Simulations have been used to carefully examine rare adverse effects in pediatric sedation and ability to rescue.[59,60] A simulated scenario of a sedation complication consisted of a standard reproducible event in which physiologic variables degraded with inappropriate interventions and improved when treated effectively. The simulation was brought to actual sedation settings throughout the hospital and used on various sedation provider teams (postanesthesia care unit, emergency department, radiology, sedation unit). The event was videotaped and scored based on deviations from best practice and quantifies episodes of hypoventilation, apnea, hypoxia, and cardiovascular collapse. Hypoxia and hypotension lasted 90 seconds in the pediatric sedation unit but on average were four times longer (360 seconds) in the emergency and radiology settings.[61] Such studies demonstrate that simulation of rare events in sedation can identify areas in need of improvement and have a positive impact on patient safety.

There has been a recent effort to carefully capture large numbers of patient sedation information to understand the nature and frequency of adverse reactions to sedation. The Pediatric Sedation Research Consortium comprises a group of over 30 institutions in the United States and North America who share prospective data on pediatric sedation.[62] Over 50,000 sedation encounters delivered by anesthesiologists and non-anesthesiologists have been entered into the data bank at this time. Preliminary analysis of the first 30,000 records identified demographics, procedures, sedation techniques, outcomes, and adverse events: (1) there were no deaths and only one cardiac arrest reported; (2) unanticipated admission occurred once in every 1500 sedations; (3) vomiting occurred once in every 200 sedations including one aspiration; (4) 1 in 400 procedures were associated with stridor, laryngospasm, wheezing, or apnea; and (5) 1 in 200 sedations required airway or ventilatory manipulations.[61] Risk factors included age younger than 3 months, ASA Physical Status greater than or equal to 3, type of provider, and different drugs used for sedation. Initial review of the data identifies particular areas of sedation adverse events. As this large database grows and is carefully examined, it will give us the correct numerator and denominator to assess adverse sedation events and their causes.

Guidelines

The first guidelines for sedation were published in 1985 from the Committee on Drugs, Section on Anesthesiology, American Academy of Pediatrics.[63] The guidelines provided the first framework to improve safety for children requiring sedation for a procedure. The guidelines emphasized systems issues, such as the need for informed consent, appropriate fasting before sedation, frequent measurement and charting of vital signs, the availability of age and size-appropriate equipment, the use of physiologic monitoring, the need for basic life support skills, as well as proper recovery and discharge procedures. The guidelines were the first to state that an independent observer whose only responsibility was to monitor the patient was required for deep sedation. Advanced airway and resuscitation skills were encouraged but not required. In 1992, the guidelines were revised.[12] These guidelines emphasized that a child could readily progress from one level of sedation to another and that the practitioner should be prepared to increase vigilance and monitoring as indicated. Pulse oximetry was recommended for all patients undergoing sedation. In 2002, the same Committee on Drugs of the AAP updated and amended the guidelines.[13] It eliminated the use of the confusing term *conscious sedation* and replaced it with the term *moderate sedation*. It also emphasized the application of these guidelines outside the hospital in recognition of the relatively high complication rate in non–hospital-based settings. In 1996, the ASA adopted guidelines for sedation and analgesia by non-anesthesiologists.[64] They were in agreement and reinforced the AAP guidelines, but they did not address the issue of deep sedation. The ASA guidelines were reviewed and updated in 2002 to include deep sedation.[65] The 2002 practice guidelines were systematically developed by a task force of 10 members who reviewed published evidence, obtained opinions from a panel of experts, and built a consensus within the community of practitioners likely to be affected by the guidelines. The task force reviewed the strength of evidence and made recommendations that include the following:

- *Patient Evaluation:* Clinicians should be familiar with the sedation-related aspects of the patient's medical history. These include (1) abnormalities of major organ systems, (2) previous adverse effects with sedation and general anesthesia, (3) drug allergies, current medications, and drug interactions, (4) time and nature of oral intake, and (5) history of tobacco, alcohol, or substance abuse. A focused physical examination including vital signs, auscultation of the heart and lungs, and evaluation of the airway is recommended.

- *Preprocedural Preparation:* Patients should be informed of and agree to sedation, including its risks, benefits, limitations, and alternatives. Sufficient time should elapse before a procedure to allow gastric emptying in elective patients. Minimum fasting periods of 2 hours (clear liquids), 4 hours (breast milk), and 6 hours (infant formula, nonhuman milk, and light meal), are recommended for healthy patients. If urgent, emergent, or other situations impair gastric emptying, the potential for pulmonary aspiration of gastric contents must be considered in determining the target level of sedation, delay, or intubation.

- *Monitoring Level of Consciousness:* Monitoring of verbal commands should be routine during moderate sedation, with the exception of young children and mentally impaired, uncooperative patients or when the response would be detrimental. During deep sedation the response to a more profound stimulus should be sought to be sure the patient has not drifted into general anesthesia.

- *Physiologic Monitoring:* All patients undergoing sedation/analgesia should be monitored by pulse oximetry with appropriate alarms. In addition, ventilatory function should be continually monitored by observation or auscultation. Monitoring of end-tidal carbon dioxide ($ETCO_2$) should be considered for all patients receiving deep sedation and for patients whose ventilation cannot be directly observed during moderate sedation. (Of note is a recent study verifying the usefulness of CO_2 sampling other than via an endotracheal tube. A nasal cannula designed to obtain gas sampling simultaneously from the nose and mouth was used in deeply sedated children for cardiac catheterization [ages 4 days to 18 years]. $ETCO_2$ provided a reasonable reflection of blood CO_2 when a good waveform was present.) When possible, blood pressure should be determined before sedation/analgesia is initiated. Once sedation/analgesia is established, blood pressure should be measured at regular intervals during the procedure, unless such monitoring interferes with the procedure (e.g., pediatric MRI, in which stimulation from the blood pressure cuff could arouse an appropriately sedated child). Electrocardiographic (ECG) monitoring should be used in all patients undergoing deep sedation. It should also be used during moderate sedation in patients with significant cardiovascular disease or those who are undergoing procedures in which dysrhythmias are anticipated.

- *Recording of Monitored Parameters:* For both moderate and deep sedation, the patients' level of consciousness, ventilatory and oxygenation status, and hemodynamic variables should be assessed and recorded at a frequency that depends on the type and amount of medication administered, the length of the procedure, and the general condition of the patient. At a minimum, this should be (1) before the beginning of the procedure; (2) after administration of sedative-analgesic agents; (3) at regular intervals during the procedure; (4) during initial recovery; and (5) just before discharge. If recording is performed automatically, device alarms should be set to alert the care team to critical changes in patient status.

- *Availability of an Individual Responsible for Patient Monitoring:* A designated individual, other than the practitioner performing the procedure should be present to monitor the patient throughout procedures performed with sedation/analgesia. During deep sedation, this individual should have no other responsibilities. However, during moderate sedation, this individual may assist with minor, interruptible tasks once the patient's level of sedation/analgesia and vital signs have stabilized, provided that adequate monitoring for the patient's level of sedation is maintained.

- *Training of Personnel:* Individuals responsible for patients receiving sedation/analgesia should understand the pharmacology of the agents that are administered, as well as the role of pharmacologic antagonists for opioids and benzodiazepines. Individuals monitoring patients receiving sedation/analgesia should be able to recognize the associated complications. At least one individual capable of establishing a patent airway and positive-pressure ventilation, as well as a means for summoning additional assistance, should be present whenever sedation/analgesia is administered. It is recommended that an individual with advanced life support skills be immediately available (within 5 minutes) for moderate sedation and within the procedure room for deep sedation.
- *Availability of Emergency Equipment:* Pharmacologic antagonists as well as appropriately sized equipment for establishing a patent airway and providing positive-pressure ventilation with supplemental oxygen should be present whenever sedation/analgesia is administered. Suction, advanced airway equipment, and resuscitation medications should be immediately available and in good working order. A functional defibrillator should be immediately available whenever deep sedation is administered and when moderate sedation is administered to patients with mild or severe cardiovascular disease.
- *Use of Supplemental Oxygen:* Equipment to administer supplemental oxygen should be present when sedation/analgesia is administered. Supplemental oxygen should be considered for moderate sedation and should be administered during deep sedation unless specifically contraindicated for a particular patient or procedure. If hypoxemia is anticipated or develops during sedation/analgesia, supplemental oxygen should be administered.
- *Combinations of Sedative/Analgesic Agents:* Combinations of sedative and analgesic agents may be administered as appropriate for the procedure being performed and the condition of the patient. Ideally, each component should be administered individually to achieve the desired effect (e.g., additional analgesic medication to relieve pain; additional sedative medication to decrease awareness or anxiety). The propensity for combinations of sedative and analgesic agents to cause respiratory depression and airway obstruction emphasizes the need to appropriately reduce the dose of each component as well as the need to continually monitor respiratory function.
- *Titration of Intravenous Sedative/Analgesic Medications:* Intravenous sedative/analgesic drugs should be given in small, incremental doses that are titrated to the desired end points of analgesia and sedation. Sufficient time must elapse between doses to allow the effect of each dose to be assessed before subsequent drug administration. When drugs are administered by nonintravenous routes (e.g., oral, rectal, intramuscular, transmucosal), allowance should be made for the time required for drug absorption before supplementation is considered. Because absorption may be unpredictable, administration of repeat doses of oral medications to supplement sedation/analgesia is not recommended.
- *Anesthetic Induction Agents Used for Sedation/Analgesia (Propofol, Methohexital, Ketamine):* Even if moderate sedation is intended, patients receiving propofol or methohexital by any route should receive care consistent with that required for deep sedation. Accordingly, practitioners administering these drugs should be qualified to rescue patients from any level of sedation, including general anesthesia. Patients receiving ketamine should be cared for in a manner consistent with the level of sedation that is achieved.
- *Recovery Care:* After sedation/analgesia, patients should be observed in an appropriately staffed and equipped area until they are near their baseline level of consciousness and are no longer at increased risk for cardiorespiratory depression. Oxygenation should be monitored periodically until patients are no longer at risk for hypoxemia. Ventilation and circulation should be monitored at regular intervals until patients are suitable for discharge. Discharge criteria should be designed to minimize the risk of central nervous system (CNS) or cardiorespiratory depression after discharge from observation by trained personnel.
- *Consultation and Availability of an Anesthesiologist:* Whenever possible, appropriate medical specialists should be consulted before administration of sedation to patients with significant underlying conditions. The choice of specialists depends on the nature of the underlying condition and the urgency of the situation. For severely compromised or medically unstable patients (e.g., anticipated difficult airway, severe obstructive pulmonary disease, coronary artery disease, or congestive heart failure), or if it is likely that sedation to the point of unresponsiveness will be necessary to obtain adequate conditions, practitioners who are not trained in the administration of general anesthesia should consult an anesthesiologist.

At the same time as the guideline development described earlier, other organizations including the American College of Emergency Physicians wrote their own guidelines for sedation.[66-70] This guideline has important variations to the AAP and ASA guidelines, particularly in the definition of the continuum of sedation. This guideline does not use moderate or deep sedation but rather the term *procedural sedation.* It is defined "as a technique of administering sedatives, analgesics, dissociative agents, or in some combination to induce a state that allows the patient to tolerate unpleasant procedures while maintaining cardiopulmonary function." It is intended to result in a depressed level of consciousness but one that allows the patient to "independently and continuously" maintain airway control. The lack of uniform agreement on definitions of sedation has lead to considerable confusion among practitioners and regulatory bodies. The situation will not be resolved quickly.

The AAP in 2006 has again updated their guidelines.[71] In general, these guidelines reinforce the ASA guidelines mentioned earlier. The recent revision retains the same definitions of the continuum of sedation that are identical to the ASA and JCAHO definitions. The new AAP guidelines emphasize a systematic approach to sedation.

These new guidelines include the following:

- *No administration of sedative medications without the safety net of medical supervision* (i.e., no sedative medications given at home)
- *Careful pre-sedation evaluation* to include review of pertinent medical and surgical conditions
- *Careful history for ingestion of neutraceuticals and other medications that may alter drug metabolism and prolong sedation*
- *A "time out" should be performed before sedation*
- *Appropriate fasting guidelines* for elective and urgent procedures. There should be a balance between the depth of sedation and the risk for those who are unable to fast because of the urgent nature of the procedure
- *Focused airway examination* with particular attention to anatomic airway abnormalities and enlarged tonsils
- *Understanding of the pharmacologic and pharmacodynamic effects of sedation medications and drug interactions*
- *Appropriate training and skills in airway management to allow for rescue.* Deep sedation requires training in pediatric advanced life support
- *Immediate availability of size and age appropriate airway, monitoring, and resuscitation equipment*
- *Appropriate medications and reversal agents*
- *Sufficient numbers of sedation providers* to carry out the procedure and monitor the child
- *Appropriate physiologic monitoring* during and after the procedure; use of capnography is encouraged
- *Appropriate recovery personnel, monitoring, and discharge criteria* with return to baseline condition before discharge
- *Prolonged observation of children in a step-down unit* who have been sedated with drugs known to have a long half-life (e.g., chloral hydrate, DPT [see later])
- *Continuous quality improvement to track common markers of potential safety issues such as desaturation events, airway obstructions, laryngospasm, unplanned hospital admission, unsatisfactory sedation, and medication errors*
- *Use of simulators to practice how to manage rare adverse events*
- *Assume all children younger than age 6 years to be deeply sedated from the beginning of the sedation process*

In addition to recommendations from clinical organizations it is mandatory that sedation policies used in hospitals conform to JCAHO standards. Hospitals risk loss of federal funding without compliance. In 2004, 18% of hospitals were found non-compliant in planning the administration of moderate or deep sedation.[72] The most recent JCAHO regulations are from 2006[73]; guidelines for sedation are mentioned in Provision of Care, Treatment and Services (PC13.20, 13.30, 13.40), Improving Organization Performance (PI 2.20), and Management of Information (MI 6.30). These standards address both moderate and deep sedation and anesthesia. The standards require that each hospital develop specific appropriate protocols for patients receiving sedation. These protocols must be consistent with professional standards and address the following:

1. Qualified individuals in sufficient numbers to perform and monitor patients during and after the procedure. A registered nurse must supervise perioperative nursing care.
2. Competency-based education, training, and experience in evaluating patients. These must include the following:

   a. Evaluating patients before the sedation
   b. Performing moderate and deep sedation, including rescuing patients who slip into a deeper than desired level of sedation. These include the following:
      i. Moderate sedation—are qualified to rescue patients from deep sedation and are competent to manage a compromised airway and to provide adequate oxygenation and ventilation.
      ii. Deep sedation—are qualified to rescue patients from general anesthesia and are competent to manage an unstable cardiovascular system as well as a compromised airway and inadequate oxygenation and ventilation.
3. Appropriate equipment for care and resuscitation
4. The following must occur before moderate or deep sedation:

   a. Appropriate needs of the patient are assessed
   b. Preprocedural education is provided according to a plan of care
   c. A "time out" is conducted immediately before starting as described in universal protocol
   d. A licensed independent practitioner plans or concurs with the planned procedure
5. Appropriate monitoring of vital signs during and after the procedure including, but not limited to, heart rate and oxygenation using pulse oximetry, respiratory frequency and adequacy of pulmonary ventilation, monitoring of blood pressure at regular levels, and cardiac monitoring (by ECG or use of a continuous cardiac monitoring device) in patients with significant cardiovascular disease or when dysrhythmias are anticipated or detected
6. Documentation of care before, during, and after the procedure
7. Monitoring of outcomes. In particular, analysis of data is performed on adverse events or patterns of adverse events during moderate or deep sedation.

Implementation of Sedation Guidelines

Different institutions may choose to implement various sedation services to meet their particular needs. Large institutions where sedation is performed in many areas at all hours may choose a decentralized approach where individual departments have practitioners who perform sedation under strict guidelines and oversight. This is the approach that is used at the Children's National Medical Center in Washington, DC. Other institutions may be able to have one area where most children who require sedation are brought and a small team of sedation providers to care for them. This is the organization model at Dartmouth Medical Center in New Hampshire. Anesthesiologists, intensivists, or radiologists may supervise this area. Other institutions may have teams of sedation nurses or hospitalists who go where sedation is required. Other institutions may use a combination of these practices. In all cases, institutional oversight is required for a successful service.

The implementation of a successful institution-wide policy involves organization, education, record keeping, enforcement, and continuing quality improvement.[74] A sedation committee must be carefully organized and involves many departments, practitioners, and geographic areas within the institution. The goal of the committee must be to create a sedation policy that can facilitate patient care without placing undue burden on practitioners. Ideally, the committee should be composed of representatives from at least one and preferably two to three sedation practitioner services (e.g., an endoscopist, intensivist, dentist, surgeon, or emergency medicine), anesthesiology, nursing, pharmacy, hospital administration, and risk management. The responsibilities of the sedation committee include the creation of hospital (institution)-wide sedation policies, determination of hospital (institution)-wide personnel and equipment needs, creation of educational programs, monitoring of sedation problems, and modification of policies as needed. Involving risk management is also advised.

The Department of Anesthesiology (chairman or designate) plays a pivotal if not central role. Because JCAHO combines anesthesia and sedation regulations the Department of Anesthesiology is instrumental in formulating policy, educating non-anesthesiology sedation practitioners, acting as consultants on difficult patients, and determining when sedation by a non-anesthesiologist is inappropriate. The Department of Anesthesiology should approve sedation flow sheets and records and be involved, along with the committee and the institution's risk management department in periodic review of the records and compliance with documentation and institutional policies and procedures. A member of the Department of Anesthesiology should also serve in the process of continuous quality improvement. Continuous quality improvement is needed to review complications, incident reports, and sedation flow sheets to ensure compliance with policy and recommend changes to the sedation committee. Finally, sedation and analgesia require a treatment plan. The Department of Anesthesiology must play a decisive role in determining which sedatives, hypnotics, general anesthetics, and analgesics can be safely used alone and in combination in each institution. Several drugs in particular can easily produce deep sedation/general anesthesia, airway obstruction, an unprotected airway, and cardiorespiratory collapse, namely, methohexital, thiopental, nitrous oxide (when combined with other sedating medications), ketamine, propofol, and remifentanil. Whether these drugs can or should be administered by non-anesthesiologists and, if so, under what conditions must be determined on an institution-by-institution basis. Education is vital to maintain safety. An ongoing educational institution-wide program on sedation emphasizing physician (dentist) responsibility, nursing responsibility, guidelines, and the pharmacology of drugs should be given frequently enough to train the staff and to accommodate staff turnover (usually one to two times a year). Teaching modules, videos, and handouts, simulations, and hands-on supervision have been used to supplement this program.[57] Our institution (Children's National Medical Center, Washington, DC) uses a computerized teaching module that includes a review of hospital policy, equipment, personnel, pharmacology of drugs used, and rescue from deeper levels of sedation. A quiz must be successfully completed at the end of the computerized teaching module. The module is part of each physicians' and nurses' orientation and hospital privileging procedure and must be complete before they can administer sedation. The module must be reviewed and successfully completed every 2 years. Staff privileges also require Basic Life Support or equivalent for those giving moderate sedation and Pediatric Advanced Life Support or equivalent for those giving deep sedation. Each chief or supervisor must attest to the practitioner's competency to provide the desired level of sedation.

Education must also emphasize the limits of sedation by the non-anesthesiologist and criteria for a sedation consultation and/or sedation by an anesthesiologist. Of particular concern is upper airway obstruction that would likely become worse with the administration of sedatives.[39] Tonsil and adenoid hypertrophy is common in children aged 2-12 years, and is associated with loud snoring or obstructive sleep apnea. Parents will frequently tell the practitioner that their child snores loudly and then "stops breathing." These children are at increased risk for airway obstruction and should be referred to an airway specialist (anesthesiologist, pediatric intensivist, pediatric emergency medicine specialist) for procedures requiring any sedation.[75,76] Problems for which consultation with an anesthesiologist is suggested are listed below:

1. Medical Problems
   - ASA Physical Status III or IV
   - Pulmonary: airway obstruction (tonsils/adenoids)
     Loud snoring, obstructive sleep apnea
     Poorly controlled asthma
   - Morbid obesity ($\geq$2 times ideal body weight)
   - Cardiovascular: cyanosis, congestive heart failure
   - Prematurity: less than 60 weeks postconceptual age
   - Residual pulmonary, cardiovascular, gastrointestinal, neurologic problems
   - Neurologic:
     Poorly controlled seizures
     Central apnea
   - Gastrointestinal: uncontrolled gastroesophageal reflux
2. Procedures requiring deep sedation in patients with a full stomach
3. Management problems
   - Severe developmental delay
   - Patients who are difficult to control
   - History of failed sedation
   - Oversedation
   - Hyperactive (paradoxical) response to sedatives

The role of nursing cannot be overemphasized. Nurses are the "front line" in sedation and frequently the part of the sedation team that identifies variation in policy compliance. Their support and education is mandatory. In addition, state nursing regulations must be considered because many states restrict the administration of certain drugs such as propofol and ketamine by registered nurses.

The performance improvement administrative part of sedation implementation is the final piece of the puzzle. Compliance can be monitored by the Medical and Dental Staff Office, the Department of Nursing, as well as a committee charged with the responsibility of continuing quality improvement. *This committee should fall under the purview of risk management.* Nursing and medical staff offices should monitor compliance with educational certification for appropriate credentialing. Every 6 months, the Medical Staff Office should report to the department chairman and nursing office a list of individuals who need to be recertified in sedation. It is the responsibility of the department chairman and nursing supervisors to secure individual staff compliance. Finally, variance reports should be reported and generated when sedation policy is not followed or when a critical incident occurs. The appropriate institutional review committee reviews the incident and reports to the sedation committee. Educational and corrective action should take place as quickly as possible. This committee should not be viewed as

INPATIENT / OUTPATIENT
MODERATE/DEEP SEDATION
FLOWSHEET
Page 2 of 4

Children's National Medical Center.

Label or Addressograph

ASSESSMENT KEY

STIMULATION RESPONSE Identify the lightest stimulation needed to elicit a response to:
V = Voice   T = Touch   P = Pain: appropriate response   U = Unarousable or inappropriate response to pain   N = Not done 2nd procedure

Mod Sedation: HR, RR, SaO2, Vent., Stim. Response & BP (May defer Stim Resp. & BP if interferes with procedure). **Record q 15 min.**
Deep Sedation & ASA-PS III or IV: HR, RR, SaO2, Vent., Stim Response & B/P. (EKG if indicated). **Record q 5 min.**
Default Monitor Alarm Limits: Pulse Oximeter: High SA02 = 100; Low SA02 = 94

Mode * (Age)	Low heart rate	High heart rate	Apnea delay	Low RR	High RR
Neonatal (0-2 yrs)	80	180	20 sec	20	60
Pediatric (2 yr-10 yr)	60	150	20 sec	18	40
Adult (>10 yr)	50	100	20 sec	12	30

ASSESSMENT/MONITORING: SEDATION & RECOVERY

Time & Initials	HR	RR	BP	SaO₂	FiO₂	Vent Adequate Yes/No	End Tidal CO₂	Stimulation Response	Cardiac Monitoring	Maintains Own Airway	COMMENT
/											*Pre-sedation Assessment (HR, RR, BP, SaO₂, Stimulation Response)*
/						☐ Yes ☐ No				☐ Yes ☐ No	
/						☐ Yes ☐ No				☐ Yes ☐ No	
/						☐ Yes ☐ No				☐ Yes ☐ No	
/						☐ Yes ☐ No				☐ Yes ☐ No	
/						☐ Yes ☐ No				☐ Yes ☐ No	
/						☐ Yes ☐ No				☐ Yes ☐ No	
/						☐ Yes ☐ No				☐ Yes ☐ No	
/						☐ Yes ☐ No				☐ Yes ☐ No	
/						☐ Yes ☐ No				☐ Yes ☐ No	
/						☐ Yes ☐ No				☐ Yes ☐ No	
/						☐ Yes ☐ No				☐ Yes ☐ No	
/						☐ Yes ☐ No				☐ Yes ☐ No	
/						☐ Yes ☐ No				☐ Yes ☐ No	
/						☐ Yes ☐ No				☐ Yes ☐ No	
/						☐ Yes ☐ No				☐ Yes ☐ No	
/						☐ Yes ☐ No				☐ Yes ☐ No	
/						☐ Yes ☐ No				☐ Yes ☐ No	
/						☐ Yes ☐ No				☐ Yes ☐ No	
/						☐ Yes ☐ No				☐ Yes ☐ No	
/						☐ Yes ☐ No				☐ Yes ☐ No	
/						☐ Yes ☐ No				☐ Yes ☐ No	
/						☐ Yes ☐ No				☐ Yes ☐ No	
/						☐ Yes ☐ No				☐ Yes ☐ No	
/						☐ Yes ☐ No				☐ Yes ☐ No	
/						☐ Yes ☐ No				☐ Yes ☐ No	
/						☐ Yes ☐ No				☐ Yes ☐ No	
/						☐ Yes ☐ No				☐ Yes ☐ No	
/						☐ Yes ☐ No				☐ Yes ☐ No	

Signature/Title/Initials	Signature/Title/Initials	Signature/Title/Initials

18407 (Rev. 11/04)

* 18407 *

Figure 48-5 (continued)

DO NOT WRITE IN THIS SPACE

INPATIENT / OUTPATIENT MODERATE/DEEP SEDATION FLOWSHEET
Page 3 of 4

Children's National Medical Center.

Label or Addressograph

Time/Initial	DISCHARGE FROM SEDATION CRITERIA	Criteria Met *(If "no", please explain)*
/	Vital signs WNL for age	☐ Yes ☐ No
/	Absence of respiratory distress	☐ Yes ☐ No
/	Supplemental O$_2$ ≤ pre-sedation level	☐ Yes ☐ No
/	Awake & responsive to commands	☐ Yes ☐ No
/	Speaks/communicates *(age appropriate)*	☐ Yes ☐ No
/	Sits, stands/walks *(minimal assistance)*	☐ Yes ☐ No
/	Tolerating clear liquids	☐ Yes ☐ No
/	Absence of nausea & vomiting	☐ Yes ☐ No
/	Pain score:_____. Score is ≤ pre-sedation score	☐ Yes ☐ No

/	**DISPOSITION:** ☐ Discharged home ☐ Remained on unit ☐ Transferred to CNMC ☐ *Inpt Unit* ☐ *ETU* ☐ *Clinic* ☐ _____ ☐ Transferred To Other Facility_____ **ACCOMPANIED BY:**_____ *(RESPONSIBLE ADULT)* **TRANSPORT MODE:** ☐ Stretcher ☐ Bed ☐ WC ☐ Crib ☐ Stroller/Carriage ☐ Carried by Parent ☐ Walked ☐ _____
/	**Sedation Discharge Teaching** ☐ Done ☐ States Understanding ☐ Instructions Reviewed & Given to Parent/Guardian

Date of Discharge: **Time of Discharge:**

LIP Discharge patient for sedation *(Signature/Title/Initials)*	Nurse Discharging Patient From Sedation *(Signature/Title/Initials)*	Instructions Received By *(Name of Guardian)*

Time/Initials	ADDITIONAL DOCUMENTATION / MEDICATIONS *(Optional, use as needed)*
/	
/	
/	
/	
/	
/	
/	
/	
/	
/	
/	
/	
/	

Signature/Title/Initials	Signature/Title/Initials	Signature/Title/Initials

MEDICATION SECTION IS FOR OUTPATIENT & EMTC USE ONLY. INPATIENT MEDICATION ADMINISTRATION IS DOCUMENTED ON THE MAR.

Order Time / Init	MD Dose Time / Init	RN Dose Time / Init	Given Time / Init	MEDICATION NAME	Milligram or microgram/kg *(Specify)*	Times pt wt in kgs = dose in milligram or microgram	Route	Concentration per ml	Volume
/	/	/	/		/kg	X kgs=		/ml	ml
Dose Verification	/				/kg	X kgs=		/ml	ml
/	/	/	/		/kg	X kgs=		/ml	ml
Dose Verification	/				/kg	X kgs=		/ml	ml
/	/	/	/		/kg	X kgs=		/ml	ml
Dose Verification	/				/kg	X kgs=		/ml	ml
/	/	/	/		/kg	X kgs=		/ml	ml
Dose Verification	/				/kg	X kgs=		/ml	ml

18407 (Rev. 11/04)

* 18407 *

Figure 48-5 (continued)

OPS: OBJECTIVE PAIN SCALE - Operational Definitions - For a score ≥ 6, patient receives a narcotic analgesic

BEHAVIOR		SCORE	DEFINITION
Blood Pressure (Systolic)	= 10% preop	0	
	>10 - 20% preop	1	
	>20% preop	2	
Crying	Not crying	0	Awake and not crying or asleep.
	Crying but responds to TLC	1	Crying is controlled by being touched, reassured or held by nurse/parent.
	Crying does not respond to TLC	2	Crying uncontrollably. Measures to comfort child are unsuccessful.
Movement	None	0	Asleep or if patient is awake, lying or playing quietly.
	Restless	1	Child unable to sit or lie still. Frequent position changes. No threat of self harm.
	Thrashing	2	Child kicking and/or squirming. Has to be protected or restrained for safety.
Agitation	Asleep or calm	0	Asleep or awake and calm.
	Mild	1	Tense, voice quivering. Responds rationally to questions and/or responds to attempt to console.
	Hysterical	2	Does not appear rational, eyes wide. May be clinging to nurse/parent. Does not respond to attempts to console.
Verbal Evaluation or Body Language			
Asleep or states no pain (Preverbal child-No special posture)		0	
Mild pain or cannot localize (Preverbal child-Flexing extremities)		1	Complains of general feeling of discomfort, but unable to describe location of pain or states pain is mild in nature. Legs drawn up. Arms may be folded across body.
Moderate pain and can localize (Preverbal child-Holding location of pain)		2	Complains of pain that is bothersome and is able to point to or describe location of pain. Holding, guarding, or touching location of pain. Infants with legs drawn up, fists clenched.

WONG-BAKER FACES PAIN RATING SCALE
(recommended for persons age 3 years and older)

0   2   4   6   8   10

10 9 8 7 6 5 4 3 2 1 0
Most Pain   NUMERIC PAIN RATING SCALE: No Pain
(for older children and adolescents)

Explain to the person that each face is for a person who feels happy because he has no pain (hurt) or sad because he has some or a lot of pain.

Face 0 is very happy because he doesn't hurt at all.
Face 2 hurts just a little bit.
Face 4 hurts a little more.
Face 6 hurts even more.
Face 8 hurts a whole lot.
Face 10 hurts worst.

Ask the person to choose the face that best describes how he is feeling.

PAIN CHARACTER:
S = Sharp
T = Throbbing
D = Dull

FREQUENCY:
C - Constant
I - Intermittent
O - Occasional

INTERVENTIONS:
PCA = Pump
POS = Position change
COM = Comfort Measure
MED = Medication

TREATMENT OUTCOMES:
N = No Relief
MI = Minimal Relief (Relief for < 1hr)
MO = Moderate Relief (Relief for 1-2 hrs)
MA = Maximum Relief (Relief for 3-4 hrs)

INPATIENT / OUTPATIENT MODERATE SEDATION — FLOWSHEET INSTRUCTIONS

- The department performing the procedure initiates the Sedation Flowsheet.
- All required sections must be completed, including the signature, title and initials of those who provide documentation.
  NPO guidelines: If NPO guidelines cannot be met, the benefit of proceeding must be weighed against the risk of harm.
- The LIP must reassess the patient immediately prior to the administration of the sedation medications.
- All entries for medications and assessments must be timed and initialed with signature/title/initials written in the appropriate boxes below the "Medication" and "Assessment" sections.
- **Medication orders for Inpatients** are written on an inpatient order sheet, transcribed onto the MAR and sent to the Pharmacy.
- **Medication orders for Outpatient & EMTC patients** are written on the Sedation Flowsheet.
- **Narcotic Medication orders:** LIP must write order per hospital policy. Before administration 2 RN's or an RN/LIP must separately verify patient weight, calculate dose in writing, and document amount/administration volume.
- **Presedation Procedural Pause: Verify informed consent, ASA-PS classification, assessment & reassessment has been completed prior to the administration of the sedating agent(s).**
- The patient must receive continuous heart rate and SaO2 monitoring until recovered and returned to pre-sedation level. Continuous respiratory rate and cardiac monitoring is required if deep sedation occurs.
- Each assessment box must be completed at the appropriate timed intervals *(see table below)*.
- PCT's and Technicians may obtain and document vital signs per RN direction.
- The timed interval assessments *(see table below)* will continue until the patient is fully recovered from the sedation medication and has returned to the pre-sedation level.
- Assessments that cannot be obtained due to a need for the patient to remain undisturbed during the procedure will be documented as such *(see "N" in the item keys)*.
- **IF THE PATIENT ASSESSMENT INDICATES THAT DEEP SEDATION HAS OCCURRED, THE FOLLOWING MUST BE DONE:**
  One care provider must remain at bedside to continuously monitor patient as their sole responsibility. Appropriate interventions will be provided as needed (e.g., position airway, Administer oxygen if needed, etc.). Patient assessments must be performed and documented Q 5 minutes until patient transitions to the moderate sedation level, at which time the assessments may return to Q 15 minutes (see also table below).

SEDATION LEVEL	CHARACTERISTICS OF THE DRUG-INDUCED SEDATION LEVEL	REQUIRED CONTINUOUS MONITORING	REQUIRED FREQUENCY OF FULL ASSESSMENT
Minimal (Anxiolysis)	• State when pain & anxiety is diminished / eliminated • Cognitive function and coordination may be impaired • Ventilatory and cardiovascular functions unaffected • No significant risk of losing protective reflexes	Patients who are not undergoing a diagnostic or therapeutic procedure & are receiving narcotics, sedatives or other medications that place them at risk for cardio/respiratory depression will be placed on cardiac/resp and/or pulse ox monitor	(see CH PC#: TM:#: "Cardiac/Respiratory and Pulse Oximetry Monitoring on Acute Care Units)
Moderate (Conscious) Chloral Hydrate > or equal to 50 mg/kg is considered moderate sedation	• Depression of consciousness • Responds purposefully to verbal commands, either alone or accompanied by light tactile stimulation • Able to maintain patient airway without interventions • Spontaneous ventilation is adequate • Cardiovascular function is usually maintained	Heart rate, SaO2 and ventilation monitored via direct visualization or capnography; Needs cardiac monitor if significant cardiovascular disease or when dysrhythmia anticipated or detected	**ASA I & II:** Q 15 minutes *(or more frequently if indicated)* until returned to pre-sedation level **ASA III, IV:** Q 5 minutes until returned to pre-sedation level
Deep	• Depression of consciousness • Patient cannot be easily aroused • Responds only to repeated painful stimuli • May require assistance in maintaining patient airway • Spontaneous ventilation may be inadequate • Cardiovascular function is usually maintained	H R, RR, SaO2 & Vent. Monitored via direct visualization or capnography; Cardiac Monitor if significant CV disease or when dysrhythmia anticipated or detected. Deep sedation is performed in cardiac cath, upper endoscopy, bronchoscopy, & anesthesia sed. service.	Q 5 minutes until returned to moderate sedation level
Anesthesia	• Loss of consciousness • Not arousable, even by painful stimulation • Often require assistance in maintaining patient airway • Often has impaired ability to independently maintain ventilatory function due to depression of spontaneous ventilation or neuromuscular function • May require positive pressure ventilation • Cardiovascular function may be impaired	Page anesthesia. (pager 6001)	As per anesthesia protocols.

- The patient must meet ALL "Discharge from Sedation Criteria" before monitoring/vital sign assessments cease.
- At the discretion of the LIP/RN, the sedated patient may be transferred to a patient care area within the Hospital. Appropriate monitoring and assessment will continue during and after transport until "Discharge from Sedation Criteria" is met. *The RN or Physician will continue appropriate monitoring & assessment during the transfer process.*
- The nurse/physician discharging the patient from sedation must sign the discharge section.
- The parent/legal guardian must sign the discharge section to indicate that instructions were received and understood.

18407 (Rev. 11/04)

Figure 48-5 (continued)

Table 48-4. Recommended Intensity of Monitoring, Documentation, Personnel, and Equipment for Different Levels of Sedation

	Moderate Sedation	Deep Sedation
Monitoring	Pulse oximetry continuous Heart rate continuous Respiratory rate every 15 min Level of consciousness every 15 min (if possible)	Pulse oximetry continuous Heart rate continuous Respiratory rate every 5 min Level of consciousness every 5 min (if possible)
Documentation	Pulse oximetry every 15 min Heart rate every 15 min Respiratory rate every 15 min Level of consciousness every 15 min, if possible	Pulse oximetry every 5 min Heart rate every 5 min Respiratory rate every 5 min Level of consciousness every 5 min, if possible
Personnel	The same individual may observe the child and assist with procedure.	Dedicated independent observer—may not assist with procedure
Equipment	Pulse oximeter Blood pressure device Stethoscope Resuscitation equipment immediately available	Pulse oximeter Blood pressure device Stethoscope EKG monitor Resuscitation equipment immediately available
Airway Equipment	Age and size appropriate	Age and size appropriate (including a defibrillator)

DEPARTMENT OF PEDIATRIC RADIOLOGY PRESEDATION PHONE CALL AND ASSESSMENT

**Department of Radiology/Nursing Database
Patient Sedation Phone Call Form**

Pre-sedation Screen Calls Attempted: 72 hours_____ **48 hours**_____ **24 hours**_____
(RN's Initials)　　　　　(RN's Initials)　　　　(RN's Initials)

PATIENT Name: _____ Age: _____ Date of Exam:_____
Diagnosis: _____ Respondent _____
Relationship: _____ Language Services needed: ☐ _____ ☐ Language Services contacted
Home Phone # _____ Work Phone # _____ Cell Phone #_____

Type of Exam: _____ ☐ Single Study ☐ Double Study
Patient Arrival Time: _____ **Scheduled Exam Time:** _____
(**1½** hours early for MRI, **1** hour for CT-sedation and **2** hours early for CT Abdomen)
(0830 sedation slot on Thursday should arrive at 0730, if no sedation required then ½ hour before scan)

- **Pre-op instructions:** No solid foods and milk products after: _____. (**8 hours prior to exam time.**)
- Clear liquids (water, pedialyte, and clear juices) and breastmilk up until _____. (**4 hours prior to exam time.**)
- We require the presence and signature of a parent or legal guardian.
- You will need to arrange to be with your child for the testing and recovery phase. **A minimum of 3 to 4 hours.**
  Please note that other children are not permitted in the testing area for safety reasons.

- **Please remember to bring your Insurance Card, referral and/or authorization #.**

INPATIENTS Only: Working PIV _____ Precautions/Isolation _____ How will the patient travel? _____.
We need a parent present and/or a phone number where they can be reached for consent _____.

☐ **You must confirm your child's exam by calling 000-000-0000.**
☐ If you have any questions please call us at 000-000-0000.
☐ If you need to reschedule this exam please call 000-000-0000.

Form completed by _____. Date: _____.

Form completed by _____. Date: _____.

NPO INSTRUCTION TIMES FOR ALL SEDATION PATIENTS

1. NPO for **solids, formula and milk products** eight **(8) hours** prior to **exam time**.
2. NPO for **clear liquids and breast milk** four **(4) hours** prior to **exam time**. (Per anesthesia discretion clears may be moved up to 2 hours prior to exam time for o/w healthy patients)
3. **Arrival time 1½ hours** prior to **exam time** for **MRI** and **1 hour** for **CT**.
** **Encourage the parents to give clear liquids 4 hours prior to exam time, especially for infants and small children** **

Figure 48-6. Sample Department of Radiology/Nursing database patient sedation phone call and assessment form (see website for downloadable figure). (Courtesy of Children's National Medical Center, Washington, DC.)

CURRENT HEALTH HISTORY

Cold symptoms fever or rash _____ Chronic pain _____
History of reflux, snoring and/or apnea _____.
Prior sedation _____ When? _____ Medication used?_____.
Any complications with sedation? _____.
Any history of difficult IV starts? _____.
History of developmental delay, behavior problems and/or autism? _____.
Allergies: **NKDA** _____ Latex _____ Environmental _____ Food_____
Identify allergies to Medicines _____ Describe Reaction _____.
Current Medications? _____.
(May take meds with sip of water) (Use PRN Nebulizer prior to arrival)

PAST MEDICAL HISTORY

PREMATURITY (Inquire if patient is <1 year)

Weeks Gestation _____ Length of Hospital stay _____ Intubated _____ Oxygen Requirement _____
Apnea monitor? _____ Hx. BPD _____

CARDIAC

Heart Murmur _____ Congenital Heart Defect _____
Hypertension _____ Currently seeing a Cardiologist _____ MD's Name _____ Date Last Seen _____
(Please bring in last clinic letter if available.)

RESPIRATORY

Asthma _____ URI _____ Pneumonia _____ TB _____ Chicken Pox Exposure _____ If yes when _____.

HEMATOLOGY/ONCOLOGY

Sickle Cell Disease (Inform parent to increase fluids prior to informed NPO instructions)
Trait _____ Last Crisis? _____ Type _____ Severity? _____ Treatment? _____
Last Transfusion _____ Last Hgb _____ Cancer _____ HIV _____ Hepatitis/Bleeding Disorders? _____
Who is the MD following your child? _____ Last seen by MD on _____
(Please bring in last clinic letter if available.)

NEUROMUSCULAR

Spina Bifida _____ Cerebral Palsy _____ Hypotonia _____ Muscle disease _____
Seizures _____ Development Delays _____ Speech _____ Motor _____

Liver Disease _____ Kidney Disease _____ GI/GU _____ Overweight_____ Diabetes _____

If there are significant problems; CV, PULM, HEM/ONC, go to EPRS and find last clinic information.
Show to Anesthesiologist.
☐ **EPRS Checked/Reviewed** _____.

POST-EXAM CALL

Sedation type _____ Call made to/or message _____ Date: _____
Completed by: _____ RN.

This is a follow-up phone call. Do you feel your child experienced any unexpected reaction following his/her exam?
Do you have any questions or concerns we could help you with?

Please call us at 000-000-0000 and speak with a Radiology Nurse.
Thank you for choosing Children's National Medical Center.

Figure 48-6 (continued)

Specific Sedation Techniques

A *sedation treatment plan* analyzing the requirements for analgesics, anxiolytics, or both is necessary for each child and will vary depending on the procedure and the anxiety of the child and family. Psychological techniques to allay anxiety (cuddling, parental support, warm blankets, a gentle reassuring voice, and hypnosis) are extraordinarily useful adjuncts to the sedation plan.[6-10]

Although the FDA is responsible for approval of the use of drugs, for a variety of reasons many of the drugs used for sedation and analgesia in children are not approved by the FDA for use in young children (e.g., fentanyl < 2 years; morphine < 12 years, bupivacaine < 12 years, and propofol < 2 months). Although midazolam is approved even in preterm infants, the reversal agent flumazenil is not approved in children younger than 1 year of age! The lack of "approval" by the FDA does not imply that a drug should not be used; rather, it only means that

⊙Children's
National Medical Center©   *Serving Children and Their Families Since 1870*

111 Michigan Avenue, N.W.
Washington, D.C. 20010-2970
(202) 884-5000

DIAGNOSTIC IMAGING & RADIOLOGY

DISCHARGE TEACHING INFORMATION SHEET

The following medications were given to your child for sedation:

Chloral Hydrate_____   Benadryl_____   Nembutal_____

Versed_____   Fentanyl_____   Propofol by Anesthesia MD

Please review the following instructions with your nurse prior to discharge:

1)   Your child will need assistance to walk, sit or crawl until the medication is worn off. Please hold onto your child's hand or carry your child at all times until the medication is worn off.

2)   DO NOT allow your child to walk, sit, or crawl alone until your child is steady. Limit activity for the remainder of the day. Encourage quiet play. No toys with wheels, no swimming, no playing outside for the remainder of the day.

3)   Please keep your child away from unsafe objects or areas of your home such as stairs, furniture, corners, bath tubs.

4)   Increase your child's diet slowly from clear liquids to semi-solids to solids.

5)   Do not feed unless child is fully awake.

6)   If your child falls asleep on the way home be sure to position your child's head tilted back or to the side while sitting up in the car. Do not allow your child's head to fall forward while sleeping. If your child feels sick to his stomach at any time, place him on his side.

CONTACT CHILDREN'S HOSPITAL IF ANY OF THE FOLLOWING OCCUR:

difficulty swallowing   dizziness   excessive vomiting

**Radiology Nurses are available from 7am – 7pm at 000-000-0000
After 7pm you may call 000-000-0000 for assistance.**

Thank you for choosing Children's National Medical Center. Please expect a follow-up call from our Nursing Staff during the next business day.

Figure 48-7. Sample Diagnostic Imaging and Radiology discharge teaching information sheet (see website for downloadable figure). (Courtesy of Children's National Medical Center, Washington, DC.)

the manufacturer never carried out the appropriate studies to gain FDA approval.[16,80-83] A number of legislative changes are intended to improve drug research in children and improve drug labeling; however, some of the drugs are no longer under patent and there is no motivation for drug companies to study their use in children.[84-86] It is hoped that the newer legislative efforts will improve drug labeling for children; see Chapter 6 for a more complete discussion of this issue.

It is important to review the child's pre-sedation medications. Particular note of the use of protease inhibitors used by many patients with human immunodeficiency virus infection must be sought. These protease inhibitors (e.g., nelfinavir, ritonavir, saquinavir) are potent inhibitors of the cytochrome P-450 CYP3A metabolic pathway. This pathway is responsible the metabolism of many sedatives, including midazolam, and may markedly prolong its duration of action and may lead to life-threatening respiratory depression. Erythromycin and some calcium channel blockers may also inhibit the cytochrome system and delay metabolism of midazolam.[87-89] A new concern for the practitioner is the widespread use of herbal medicines that can enhance or shorten sedative medication activity.[90-94] Herbal medicines (e.g., St. John's wort or echinacea) may alter drug pharmacokinetics through inhibition of the cytochrome P450 system, resulting in prolonged drug effect and altered (increased or decreased) blood drug concentrations. Kava may increase the effects of sedatives, and valerian may itself produce sedation (see also Table 4-6).[95]

maximum of approximately 100 cm² surface area; for those 10 to 20 kg, apply to a maximum of approximately 600 cm² surface area; and for those more than 20 kg, apply to a maximum of approximately 2000 cm² surface area). The duration of action is 1 to 2 hours after the cream is removed. Adverse reactions include erythema, itching, rash, and methemoglobinemia. It also causes blanching of the skin, which can make intravenous access difficult. It is contraindicated in children younger than 1 month of age, in children with congenital or idiopathic methemoglobinemia, or in infants receiving methemoglobinemia-inducing drugs (e.g., phenytoin, phenobarbital, acetaminophen, and sulfonamides).

ELA-Max and L-M-X 4 (Ferndale Laboratories, Inc., Ferndale, MI) is a topical 4% liposomal lidocaine solution whose effect occurs in 30 minutes.[101] The S-Caine patch (ZARS, Inc., Salt Lake City, UT) is a eutectic mixture of 70 mg of lidocaine and 70 mg tetracaine in a bioadhesive layer that contains a heating element. The 20-minute application is effective in lessening pain from venipuncture procedures.[102]

Anxiolytics/Sedatives

The most commonly used anxiolytics/sedatives in pediatric sedation are chloral hydrate, diazepam, and midazolam.

Chloral hydrate is one of the most widely used sedatives in neonates and children younger than 3 years of age (Table 48-6).[103-106] It is widely used as a sedative to facilitate nonpainful diagnostic procedures such as EEG and CT or MRI.[105] It is rapidly and completely absorbed when given orally. Rectal administration is erratically absorbed and therefore not recommended. Onset of sedation is 30 to 60 minutes, and the usual clinical duration is 1 hour. Although it has a long safety record, it can cause respiratory depression due to airway obstruction, and deaths have been associated with its use alone and when combined with other sedating medications.[39,76,107-110] One large series showed a 0.6% incidence of respiratory depression especially at larger doses (75-100-mg/kg).[111] Its effect is primarily mediated by the active metabolite trichloroethanol (TCE), which is formed by the liver and erythrocytes.[112] TCE has a half-life of 10 hours in toddlers, 18 hours in term infants, and 40 hours in preterm infants (Fig. 48-10).[113] The prolonged effects of chloral hydrate warrant a longer period of post-sedation observation; chloral hydrate can also cause side effects after discharge, which include motor imbalance (31%), gastrointestinal effects (23%), agitation (19%), and restlessness (14%). Agitation and restlessness lasted more than 6 hours in more than one third of children who experienced these effects, 5% of whom did not return to baseline activity for 2 days after the procedure.[40,114] The unpredictable onset and active metabolites dictate that this drug (as well as all sedatives for sedation) is given only in facilities capable of resuscitation (AAP guidelines) and that discharge occurs when sedation is clearly lessening and the child meets discharge criteria. Airway obstruction and death has occurred after chloral hydrate sedation in a child who was in a child's car seat in the back of a car while going home after procedural sedation.[39] Despite being restricted in some countries as a result of potential carcinogenicity, in the United States the AAP states that there is insufficient evidence to avoid single doses of chloral hydrate.[115]

The *benzodiazepines* are commonly used in pediatric sedation. They are anxiolytic, amnestic, sedative hypnotics with anticonvulsant activities but no analgesic properties. Their high

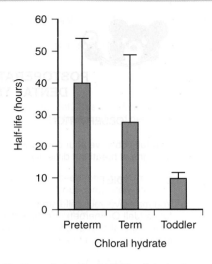

Figure 48-10. Beta elimination half-life of the active metabolite of chloral hydrate, trichloroethanol, in preterm infants, term infants, and toddlers. Note the extremely long half-lives in all age groups and the large standard deviation. Although often thought of as a short-acting sedative, chloral hydrate can have profoundly long effects. (Data abstracted from Mayers DJ, Hindmarsh KW, Sankaran K, et al: Chloral hydrate disposition following single-dose administration to critically ill neonates and children. Dev Pharm Ther 1991; 16:71-77.)

lipid solubility at physiologic pH accounts for the rapid CNS effects. As opposed to diazepam, midazolam is delivered in a water-soluble form (pH 3.5), which markedly decreases the incidence of pain on injection and thrombophlebitis.[112] However, the resulting decrease in fat solubility markedly delays transport into the CNS (peak EEG effect 4.8 minutes for midazolam versus 1.6 minutes for diazepam (Fig. 48-11).[116,117] The benzodiazepines exert their effects by occupying the benzodiazepine receptor that modulates γ-aminobutyric acid (GABA), the major inhibitory neurotransmitter in the brain. The clearance of benzodiazepines is decreased by liver enzyme inhibition that occurs during concomitant use of erythromycin and cimetidine and protease inhibitors.[88]

The sedated child usually becomes compliant but does not lose consciousness. Children frequently move, and another agent, such as an opioid, may be necessary if the child must not move to successfully accomplish the procedure. Although many children initially act disinhibited and "drunk" after small doses of benzodiazepines, some children have a true paradoxical response.[118] One to 15% of children may show paradoxical responses such as combativeness, disorientation, hyperexcitability, and agitation.[119] It is wiser to switch to a different sedative drug in these children because increasing the dose of benzodiazepines may lead to severe agitation followed by unconsciousness and respiratory compromise. The benzodiazepines have the advantage of antegrade amnesia in a significant number of patients.[120,121] The markedly prolonged and variable elimination half-life and active metabolite of diazepam (desmethyldiazepam) make midazolam a superior sedative drug in children, particularly infants.[122-127] Time to peak effect after intravenous administration of midazolam is 2 to 4 minutes, and duration is 45 to 60 minutes. Midazolam can be given intravenously, intranasally, sublingually, orally, or rectally (see Table 48-6). It is the

Table 48-6. Sedation Regimens for Children

Drug Regimen	Dose/Route	Onset (minutes)	Duration (minutes)	Comments
Pentobarbital	4-6 mg/kg IV or PO	IV: 2-5 PO: 20-60	IV: 15-45 PO: 60-240	Long history of safety. Slow onset. Prolonged emergence. May have paradoxical excitement. Half-life increased by valproic acid and MAO inhibitors. Contraindicated in porphyria.
Midazolam	0.5-0.75 mg/kg PO 0.025-0.5 mg/kg IV 0.2 mg/kg intranasal 0.1-0.15 mg/kg IM	15-30 1-3 10-15 10-15	60-90 45-60 60 60-90	Paradoxical response not infrequent. Intranasal route very irritating and should be avoided. Increased respiratory depression when used with opioids; reduce midazolam dose by 25%. Prolonged duration with protease inhibitors. Antagonist: flumazenil.
Chloral hydrate	50-100 mg/kg PO (Max not to exceed 2 grams)	30-60	60-120	Very popular for nonpainful radiologic procedures in small children when IV not available. Effects unreliable over age 1-2. Prolonged sedation and paradoxical responses noted. Respiratory depression and obstruction reported with tonsil hypertrophy and anatomic abnormalities. Moderate sedation guidelines required. Markedly prolonged half-life in neonates. Contraindicated in porphyria.
Etomidate	0.1-0.4 mg/kg IV	<1	5-15	No analgesic effect. Higher doses cause general anesthesia, respiratory depression, and loss of airway. Stable cardiovascular profile. Little data in children. Must be credentialed for deep sedation/anesthesia. No reversal drug. Causes adrenal suppression ~12 hours.
Methohexital	0.25-0.50 mg/kg IV 20-25 mg/kg rectal 10 mg/kg IM	<1 10-15 10-15	10-20 30-60 30-60	Avoid if temporal lobe epilepsy or porphyria. IV doses quickly lead to general anesthesia. Rectal doses cause high frequency of apnea and should be avoided. Deep sedation/anesthesia credentialing. Contraindicated in children younger than age 3 months, psychosis, stimulation of oropharynx, increased intracranial pressure, head injury, glaucoma.
Fentanyl with propoful	Fentanyl 1-2 µg/kg IV with propofol 50-150 mg/kg/min infusion IV	1-2	30-60	Child may rapidly become anesthetized with loss of airway. Advanced airway management skills required with appropriate credentialing.
Midazolam with fentanyl	Midazolam 0.020 mg/kg IV with fentanyl 1-2 µg/kg IV	2-3	45-60	Commonly used for painful procedures. Careful titration needed to avoid deep sedation/anesthesia with apnea and hypoxia. Reduce dose of fentanyl when combined with benzodiazepine. Reduce dose with protease inhibitors.
Ketamine	3-4 mg/kg IM 1-2 mg/kg IV 4-6 mg/kg PO	5 1 10-20	30-60 30-60 30-90	Nausea and vomiting common after procedure. Laryngospasm, apnea, agitation, hallucinations reported but uncommon. Midazolam may not help emergence delirium. Anticholinergic to control secretions. Larger doses can produce state of general anesthesia. Usually causes tachycardia, hypertension, and bronchodilatation. Paradoxical hypotension in critically ill patients. No antagonist available.
Remifentanil	0.1-0.25 µg/kg/min	1	10-15	Difficulty in titration frequently leads to apnea and general anesthesia. Few studies in children. Exclusively used by anesthesiologists.
Nitrous oxide	50% in 50% oxygen for "minimal sedation," up to 70% used by some for moderate sedation	<5	On discontinuing	Requires specialized equipment for delivery, monitoring, and scavenging. When used alone or with local anesthesia is considered "minimal sedation." Higher doses or addition of other sedatives/analgesics requires a minimum of "moderate sedation" guidelines. Contraindications include respiratory failure, altered mental status, otitis media, bowel obstruction, and pneumothorax. No antagonist available.

used for intraoperative sedation by anesthesiologists and in intubated children in the ICU.[163-166] It has recently been suggested that children may develop opioid tolerance to this drug after several hours of infusion.[167] Remifentanil is associated with a high incidence of apnea and chest wall rigidity and should not be used by the non-anesthesiologist for pediatric sedation (see Table 48-6).[168]

Opioid antagonists specifically reverse the respiratory and analgesic effects of opioids and should be readily available when opioids are used (see Table 48-6). Naloxone (Narcan) is the most commonly used antagonist.[169] Opioid antagonists should not be used for routine reversal of the sedative effects of opioids but reserved for reversal of respiratory depression/respiratory arrest. Naloxone may be given intravenously, intramuscularly, or subcutaneously.[170] The initial dose for respiratory depression is 0.01 mg/kg titrated to effect every 2 to 3 minutes. Ten to 100 µg/kg up to 2 mg may be required for respiratory arrest. Adverse reactions from reversal of analgesia include nausea, vomiting, tachycardia, hypertension, delirium, and pulmonary edema.[171-173] Children on long-term opioid therapy should be given opioid reversal agents in low doses and with extreme caution because withdrawal seizures and delirium may occur. Children given naloxone may again have opioid effects after 1 hour. *If naloxone is used, then the child should be observed for a minimum of 2 hours.* Repeat naloxone may be necessary. Nalmefene (Revex) has a longer half-life (~10 hours) than naloxone.[174] Although experience in children is limited it has been shown to accelerate recovery from sedation.[175] Its half-life outlasts the effects of fentanyl and negates the treatment of pain with opioids for several hours.

Systemic Anesthetics

Systemic anesthetics traditionally have been used in the operating room by anesthesiologists to produce a state of deep sedation (i.e., monitored anesthesia care) or general anesthesia. With appropriate monitoring and skilled personnel, these agents can be safely used outside the operating room for diagnostic and therapeutic procedures. These drugs are extremely difficult if not impossible to titrate in children. The child may quickly become deeply sedated and develop airway compromise such that a level of deep sedation and/or anesthesia must be assumed. *These drugs should be used only by anesthesiologists or other practitioners who have specific training in their use and have advanced airway management skills because airway obstruction, apnea, and cardiovascular instability may quickly and unpredictably occur.* The use of these agents in the operating room for monitored anesthesia care/general anesthesia by anesthesiologists is discussed elsewhere. In the following discussion we will emphasize the use of these drugs for sedation outside the operating room when an anesthesiologist may not be directly involved.

Ketamine has been available since the 1960s. It is one of the few sedatives that produce both amnesia and analgesia. It is structurally similar to phencyclidine and exerts its dissociative properties by interacting with the limbic/thalamic systems. Additional mechanisms postulated are antagonism of *N*-methyl-D-aspartate (NMDA) receptors and agonism of opioid subgroups.[112] The clinical appearance is that of a child who has opened eyes (usually with horizontal nystagmus) but does not respond to pain. Ketamine has been shown to preserve cardiovascular function in most cases and to have limited effects on respiratory mechanics and allows for spontaneous respirations.[176] Although it is certainly not a new drug, ketamine has recently experienced resurgence in popularity, particularly in the emergency department. Some emergency medicine physicians suggest that ketamine not be considered an anesthetic but a "dissociative sedation" drug with unique properties that warrant their own separate monitoring guidelines.[177] Intramuscular and intravenous ketamine (with and without midazolam) is frequently used for closed fracture reductions and other painful minor procedures in the emergency department (see Table 48-6).[178-180] In an emergency department series of 1022 patients, the following adverse airway events were noted: airway malalignment (0.7%), transient laryngospasm (0.4%), and transient apnea or respiratory depression (0.3%). All were quickly identified and treated with no sequelae.[181]

Ketamine has also been investigated in children for gastroendoscopic procedures: 636 children were given ketamine (1.0 to 1.3 mg/kg IV) for upper gastrointestinal endoscopy. Adverse effects included transient laryngospasm (8.2%), emesis (4.1%), recovery agitation (2.4%), partial airway obstruction (1.3%), apnea and respiratory depression (0.5%), and excessive salivation (0.3%).[52] The analgesic effects of ketamine make it very useful for sedation for burn dressing changes. Under strict supervision the outcomes of 522 sedation events were studied: 4.9% of procedures had potential adverse outcomes, of which 2.9% required intervention. Eight events were related to the airway.[182] Certainly, ketamine sedation/analgesia is very safe, perhaps having advantage over other sedation regimens, but these studies clearly indicate that potentially life-threatening events can and do occur with ketamine sedation, thus negating the concept that this drug is "different" from other sedative/analgesic regimens. Ketamine is also associated with nonpurposeful motion, which limits its usefulness when immobility is necessary (e.g., use during CT). Ketamine can markedly increase cerebral blood flow and is contraindicated in children with increased intracranial pressure. Other contraindications include those with head injury, open globe injury, hypertension, and psychosis. Ketamine can decrease the response to hypercarbia, as well as cause laryngospasm, coughing, and apnea. No antagonist is available.

Typical starting doses[183] are 1 to 2 mg/kg intramuscularly, 0.25 to 1.0 mg/kg intravenously, or 4 to 6 mg/kg orally.[184-186] The onset after intramuscular injection is 2 to 5 minutes, with a peak of 20 minutes; duration can be 30 to 120 minutes. Onset after intravenous administration occurs in less than 1 minute, with a peak effect in several minutes and duration of action of approximately 15 minutes. Oral doses of 4 to 6 mg/kg are usually combined with atropine and have an effect in 30 minutes and last up to 120 minutes.[19] Larger doses or supplementation with other sedatives or opioids may produce deep sedation/general anesthesia. Ketamine should be administered with an antisialagogue (atropine, 0.02 mg/kg, or glycopyrrolate, 0.01 mg/kg) because copious secretions from ketamine alone may induce laryngospasm.[187] Although initially thought to maintain airway reflexes, this is not always the case; ketamine may not protect against aspiration.[188] However, aspiration is extremely rare. One author states that in 30 years of regular use for sedation there have been no documented cases of clinically significant aspiration.[69] Unpleasant dysphoric reactions (so-called emergence reactions) (up to 12%) can be severe but are usually mild.[189]

The prophylactic use of midazolam does not decrease this incidence.[190]

Etomidate is a carboxylated imidazole that is primarily used as an induction agent for anesthesia. Its mechanism is thought to be due to potentiation of GABA inhibitory neurotransmission via alteration of chloride conductance. Loss of consciousness occurs in 15 to 20 seconds, and recovery is due to redistribution and occurs in 5 to 10 minutes. It is hydrolyzed in the liver to inactive metabolites and excreted (90%) in the urine.[112] Etomidate produces sedation/anesthesia, anxiolysis, and amnesia similar to the barbiturates and propofol. Its major advantage is its lack of adverse cardiovascular effects. Etomidate has been used in adults and children for procedural sedation, although the end point of sedation is not well described and often is general anesthesia. In one study of 53 children having fracture reductions in the emergency department, success was reported with a mean dose of 0.2 mg/kg in combination with fentanyl or morphine for pain relief.[48] Although the drug is associated with myoclonus this did not occur in this study; one patient developed hypotension and tachycardia. Transient adrenal suppression can occur after multiple doses and after single dose administration.[191] Because of its limited use in pediatric sedation and the ease with which it may cause general anesthesia with loss of the airway, etomidate is not recommended for sedation use in children.

Propofol is an anesthetic that is widely used for pediatric sedation and anesthesia. It is an isopropyl phenol derivative whose mechanism of action appears to be activation of the sodium channel of the β_1 subunit of GABA, thereby enhancing inhibitory transmission.[192] Its onset is within 30 seconds. It is highly lipid soluble and is provided in a lipid solution that is the same as the lipid component in total parenteral solutions. The lipid solubility makes the drug effect diminish extremely quickly (5-15 minutes).[193] It has no analgesic properties, but it does have antiemetic and antipruritic properties. Although small doses of propofol (25-50 µg/kg/min) can provide moderate sedation in adults, deep sedation and airway obstruction quickly occur in children. Dosing in adults for sedation is recommended at 25 to 200 µg/kg/min, whereas many children require considerably higher doses. Propofol is a profound respiratory depressant and can lead to rapid airway obstruction and apnea. Reported rates of respiratory complications range from 8% to 30%.[194] It is generally best administered by titration with an infusion pump. Other adverse reactions include increased salivary and tracheobronchial secretions, myoclonic movements, anaphylactic reactions, and bacterial contamination. Pain on injection can be lessened by the addition of lidocaine to the solution. Hypotension is mild and usually not clinically significant. Cases of fatal metabolic acidosis, myocardial failure, and lipemic serum have been reported in children who received prolonged propofol treatment.[195-198] Durations of propofol for more than 5 hours have been associated with propofol infusion syndrome but not during shorter procedures for sedation. Children should be assumed to be deeply sedated or anesthetized when using this drug, and it should be administered only by practitioners with advanced airway skills.

Propofol "procedural sedation" delivered by non-anesthesiologists is growing rapidly in intensive care units, emergency departments, dentistry, oral surgery, and gastroenterology suites (see Table 48-6).[55,199-203] The dosing recommendations for use in "procedural sedation" in these areas frequently do not cause sedation but rather anesthesia as defined by the JCAHO.[194] In particular, doses, airway maintenance, and response to stimulation frequently go beyond the classification of "procedural sedation" and into "anesthesia." "Procedural sedation" is defined as a depressed level of consciousness but one that allows the patient to maintain airway control "independently and continuously."[70] However, multiple studies show that propofol procedural sedation frequently causes anesthesia with inability to maintain the airway. In one study of propofol administration in 105 painful procedures in the pediatric intensive care unit, 21% of children required airway repositioning, 17% had apnea, 5% had hypotension, and 45% had events that required intervention. The doses of propofol used were 2.5 to 3 mg/kg, with infusions of 200 µg/kg/min.[55] In a study in the emergency department, propofol was administered to 113 children such that they were motionless during the reduction of fractures. Propofol caused desaturation in 21%, laryngospasm in one child, and an oxygen requirement in 25%. Doses of propofol totaled 4.5 mg/kg in addition to fentanyl (1 to 2 µg/kg).[204] A study of sedation by non-anesthesiologists for bone marrow procedures, lumbar punctures, and esophagoscopies titrated propofol to a target of "not arousable"; 21 children age 27 weeks to 18 years were studied. One hundred percent adequate sedation was accomplished only after a BIS score of 45 or less. Propofol total doses were 520 µg/kg/min for these short procedures.[205] Clearly, these responses to stimulation, effect on the airway, doses of propofol, and BIS levels fall outside the range of procedural sedation and into the definition of general anesthesia.

As the studies just outlined clearly indicate, the field of "pediatric sedation" or "procedural sedation" has evolved to a point at which providers who are not trained in anesthesiology regularly deliver deep sedation and anesthesia. This insight is further confirmed by the fact that many of these practitioners have been credentialed in their hospitals to deliver this care and bill under anesthesia codes. The American Medical Association recently released its annual refinement of the Current Procedural Terminology (CPT) codes and descriptions for moderate sedation, including pediatric qualifiers.[206] Codes now exist for moderate sedation provided by a practitioner while performing a procedure, and additional codes exist for providing sedation (only) while another practitioner performs a procedure. Unfortunately, because the sedation provided for children is much deeper than "moderate," these codes are often ignored in preference of anesthesia-based codes.* Over the past 5 years, this issue has been become particularly contentious surrounding the use of propofol. Just as propofol is debated today, dexmedetomidine, remifentanil, and other drugs will be debated in the future. Regardless of the shape these future discussions take, anesthesiologists will have a key role in demanding the same high monitoring and competency standards that have led to marked improvement in operative and nonoperative care in our field. The controversy over whom and under what conditions propofol (or other potent sedatives) should be administered for pediatric sedation needs to be addressed and agreed upon on a national level.

Methohexital is a short-acting oxybarbiturate that is rapidly metabolized and redistributed and has a rapid recovery (see

---

*Personal communication from Shani Freilich, MD, director of Sedation Service at Scottish Rite Children's Hospital, Atlanta, GA.

Complications

Hematoma is usually of no serious consequence.

Infection/thrombosis may be limited by aseptic technique.[25-27] One study of 642 Teflon catheters in 525 patients showed that the risk of catheter complications in children was extremely low and would not be reduced significantly by routine replacement.[28] Catheter life span has been found to be unrelated to insertion site, cannula size, or brand in infants younger than 12 months of age.[29]

Skin sloughing is usually caused by subcutaneous infiltration of calcium, potassium, or hypertonic solutions; it may be avoided by frequent inspection, such as checking IV function before injecting medications.[30] The risk of subcutaneous infiltration is increased with the administration of medications and parenteral nutrition solutions compared with the use of 10% dextrose compared with 5% dextrose solutions, but it is not increased with the use of potassium solutions ($\leq$20 mEq/L vs. >20 mEq/L); there is apparently no difference between gravity-controlled versus infusion delivery devices.[31]

There are insufficient data to support the use of heparin for prolonging patency of peripheral IV catheters in neonates and children.[32]

Central Venous Pressure Measurement

There are a number of studies in children and adults that have described a reasonable correlation between peripheral intravenous catheters and central venous catheters even in critically ill children. Hypothermia (peripheral vasoconstriction) decreases the accuracy of such measurements, but it is useful to understand that transducing the pressure of a peripheral vein may provide valuable information regarding right-sided cardiac filling pressures.[9,10,33-36]

Establishing a Large Intravenous Catheter in Small Patients

Indications

This procedure is used for any child in whom there is the potential for massive, rapid hemorrhage.

1. Prepare and drape the appropriate area using standard sterile techniques.
2. Perform a standard intravenous cannulation of an antecubital, saphenous, or external jugular vein with a small (22- or 20-gauge) intravenous catheter.
3. Pass a small, flexible guidewire (0.18 mm) through the intravenous catheter, remove the catheter, and with a No. 11 blade make a small incision at the entry point of the wire at the skin.
4. Pass the next larger size intravenous catheter over the wire to dilate the vein and leave in place; stiff intravenous catheters are more effective than soft ones. An alternative is to use a small dilator from a pulmonary artery catheter introducer and leave the introducer in place. The wire is removed, and the next larger size wire is inserted (0.25 mm). The catheter (or introducer) is removed, leaving this larger wire within the vein.
5. Pass the next larger size intravenous catheter over the wire (usually 18 gauge) several times and then pass the next larger size catheter (usually 16 gauge); remove the guidewire, leaving the intravenous catheter within the vein.
6. Pass the next larger flexible guidewire (0.35 mm) into the vein, remove the 16-gauge intravenous catheter, and insert a 14-gauge catheter. An alternative is to leave progressively larger pulmonary artery introducers in the vein; both techniques provide a reasonably rapid method of establishing a large-bore intravenous infusion site (see Table 49-1 for wire sizes that will pass through each IV catheter size).

Rapid Infusion Catheters and Introducer Sheaths

Special rapid volume catheters (6F and larger, Arrow International, Reading, PA) allow venipuncture with a needle or small IV catheter, passage of a guide wire, then introduction of a dilator and sheath with fewer steps required (see Fig. 10-10).

Intravenous Cutdown

Indications

- Percutaneous cannulation is unsuccessful.
- Percutaneous cannulation is tenuous.
- The catheter in place is inadequate for the planned surgical procedure.

The most common sites for insertion are the saphenous vein at the ankle (medial malleolus) and the brachiocephalic vein in the arm (antecubital fossa). This procedure may require a significant period of time to perform and has limited utility for emergent venous access.[37]

Complications

Intravenous cutdown has a high incidence of infection and therefore should be used only on a short-term basis.

Saphenous Vein Cannulation

The saphenous vein is often a reliable point for intravenous access in infants and children that may be directly visualized or

Table 49-1. Comparison of IV Safety Mechanisms

Safety Mechanism	Operator Activation Required	Syringe Attachment	Rapid Flash	Bulky	Advantages	Disadvantages	Devices (Manufacturers)
Retractable needle	Yes	No	Yes	Yes	Unobstructed and rapid blood flash Similarity in use to non-safety devices	Bulky Requires operator activation No syringe attachment	Angiocath Autoguard (BD Medical, Franklin Lakes, NJ) Secure IV (SpanAmerica Medical Systems, Inc., Greenville, SC)
Blunted needle	No	Yes	No	No	Passive action requiring no operator activation Syringe attachment possible	Slow blood flash if needle has been partially withdrawn	Introcan Safety IV (B. Braun, Bethlehem, PA) Protectiv Acuvance (Ethicon Endo-Surgery, Inc., Somerville, NJ)

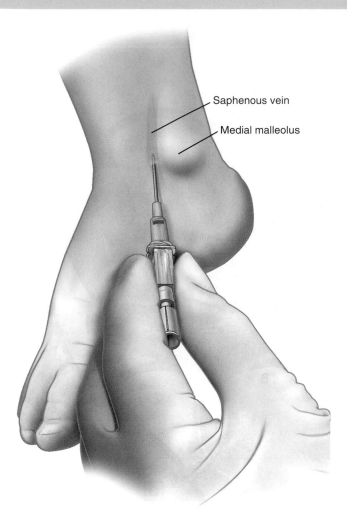

Saphenous vein

Medial malleolus

Figure 49-1. Saphenous vein cannulation.

cannulated with a "blind" technique (Fig. 49-1). It is consistently found lateral to the medial malleolus of the foot one-half to one fingerbreadth over the anterior quadrant.

1. The area should be cleansed in the standard fashion after a tourniquet is applied to the lower extremity below the knee.
2. The saphenous vein may or may not be palpated and visualization may not be possible.
3. Enter the skin at a 30-degree angle at the expected site of the saphenous vein at the level of the medial malleolus with the tip of the needle directed toward the upper two thirds of the calf. If there is not evidence of venipuncture on insertion, the needle should be slowly withdrawn because the flash of blood may occur while exiting the vein.
4. If unsuccessful on the first attempt, fan medially then laterally from the same insertion point slowly advancing and withdrawing the catheter until blood return is obtained.

Safety IV Catheters

In the United States it is now federally mandated that retractable or sheathed needles designed to reduce the potential for needlestick injury are available to health care personnel (see Table 49-

1).[38] A study comparing traditional IV catheters to safety devices found that a larger proportion of children younger than 3 years old required more than one catheter to successfully gain IV access. The retractable IV catheter compared with traditional catheters was associated with a nearly fourfold increase in the splattering and spilling of blood.[39] It should be understood that the U.S. federal legislation requires that these devices are available but the ultimate decision to use them rests with the physician in his or her patient's best interest. *Therefore, the type of catheter should not be dictated by the hospital but rather by the individuals who place the catheters.*

Central Venous Catheterization

Indications

- Provision of a secure means for administration of fluid and blood when major shifts in intravascular volume are anticipated (e.g., multiple trauma, intestinal obstruction, burns)
- Monitoring of cardiac filling pressures
- Infusion of drugs and fluids that are sclerosing to peripheral veins (e.g., antibiotics, vasopressors, and hyperalimentation fluids)
- Need for blood sampling
- Measurement of mixed venous acid-base balance or estimation of cardiac output (Fick principle) or measurement of cardiac output (dye dilution)
- Route for aspiration of air emboli

The common sites for central venous cannulation are the external and internal jugular veins, the subclavian and brachiocephalic veins, the femoral vein, and the umbilical vein in neonates. Invasive approaches such as via the internal jugular and subclavian veins should be used with extreme caution in the presence of a bleeding diathesis. The percutaneous approach to central venous cannulation is often successful using a modified Seldinger technique (Fig. 49-2).[40,41] The advantages of this technique are that it avoids the need for a cutdown, only one venipuncture is made with a thin-walled small gauge needle, a guidewire directs the catheter within the blood vessel, introducing a large catheter through the small venipuncture site minimizes the chances of significant hematoma formation even after systemic heparinization, and the procedure can often be accomplished when access is required emergently. Alternative techniques include locating the vein with a small gauge needle, followed by venipuncture with a large needle (Intracath, Deseret, Sandy, UT) through which the catheter is threaded. This technique is successful in the hands of experienced operators but has the disadvantage of requiring several venipunctures, and the larger needle may cause hematoma formation or may damage surrounding tissues and nerves (Horner syndrome)[42] and may make carotid artery puncture more likely.[43] Whenever a central line is inserted, care must be taken to ensure that the catheter tip is not inserted against the wall of a major blood vessel, deep in the right atrium, or in a ventricular position, because these positions have been associated with perforation of large vessels and the myocardium (Fig. 49-3) as well as a source of ventricular arrhythmias.[44]

Ultrasound guidance or pressure waveform analysis may help to prevent complications related to central catheter placement.[45,46] Ultrasound-guided access has been demonstrated to be successful for cannulation of the internal jugular vein[45] and infraclavicular axillary vein[46] specifically. A meta-analysis of 18 trials with 1646 participants, including

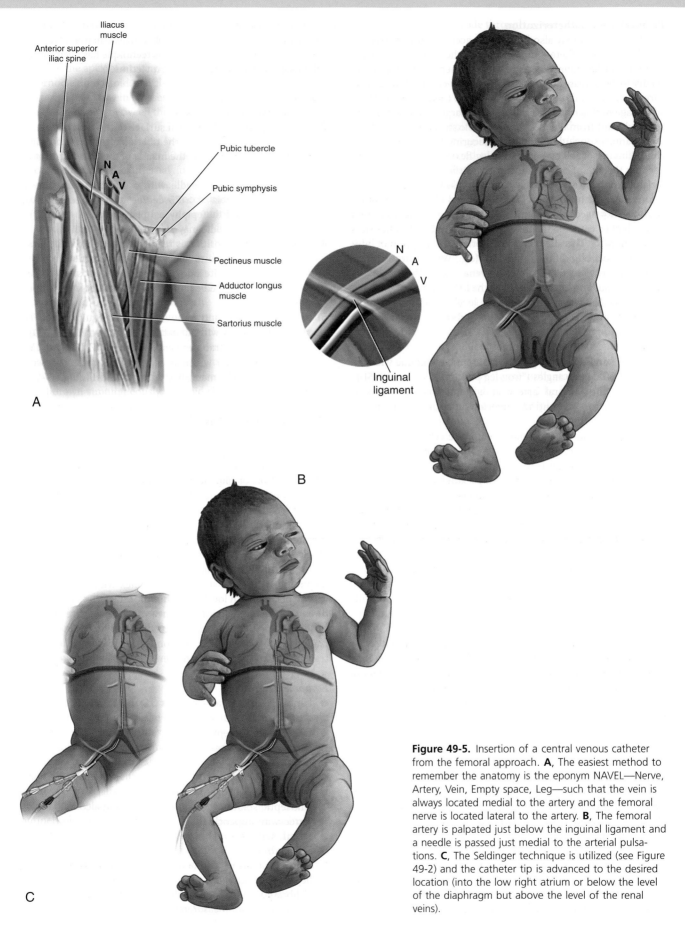

Figure 49-5. Insertion of a central venous catheter from the femoral approach. **A,** The easiest method to remember the anatomy is the eponym NAVEL—Nerve, Artery, Vein, Empty space, Leg—such that the vein is always located medial to the artery and the femoral nerve is located lateral to the artery. **B,** The femoral artery is palpated just below the inguinal ligament and a needle is passed just medial to the arterial pulsations. **C,** The Seldinger technique is utilized (see Figure 49-2) and the catheter tip is advanced to the desired location (into the low right atrium or below the level of the diaphragm but above the level of the renal veins).

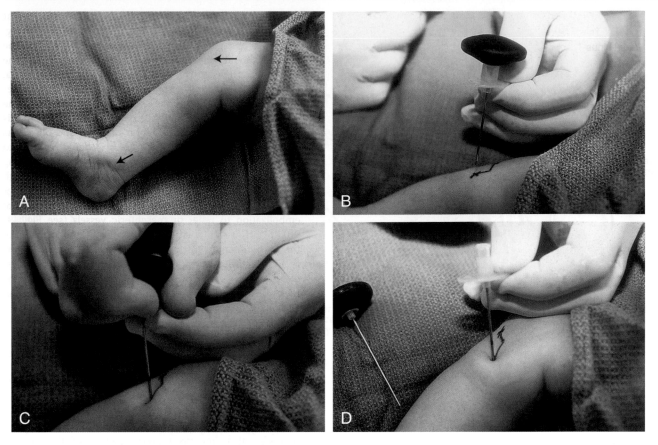

Figure 49-6. A, The intraosseous needle may be inserted in either of two locations: at a point 1 to 2 cm below and medial to the tibial tuberosity or at the medial malleolus (*arrows*). **B** and **C**, The leg is prepared, and the intraosseous needle punctures the skin (note the two X marks connecting the tibial tuberosity with the point of needle insertion); the needle is advanced with a twisting motion in a caudal direction. **D**, The stylet is removed, and the selected solution is infused.

Technique

1. Prepare and drape the umbilicus with sterile technique; cut the cord approximately 1 cm above the umbilicus. The umbilical vein orifice is more patulous and thin walled than the two umbilical arteries (Fig. 49-8).

2. Holding the catheter filled with heparinized solution 2 cm from the tip, gently introduce it into the vein. In some situations, forceps can aid in directing the catheter. Traction of the umbilical stump *caudad* may facilitate the catheter's advancement (see Fig. 49-8). The catheter is passed a distance that approximates the length between the umbilical stump and the right atrium. Blood should freely aspirate into a syringe. Inability to withdraw blood may occur if the tip of the catheter is resting against a vessel wall or if a clot is present within the catheter lumen. *It is important that the tip of the catheter be placed in the proper position, that is, at the junction of the inferior vena cava and right atrium.* A radiograph confirms proper catheter position. Monitoring changes in the configuration of the electrocardiogram during insertion may allow for a more accurate placement within the right atrium but is limited to neonates with a normal tracing.[101] At times, the catheter may fail to traverse the ductus venosus and may become wedged in the liver. This position is potentially dangerous because portal necrosis and subsequent cirrhosis may result should hyperosmolar or sclerosing solutions be injected (calcium, sodium bicarbonate, 25% to 50% glucose).[105,106] A low position might be acceptable for short-term use if one is unable to pass the catheter centrally, but the distance of insertion should be no more than 3 to 4 cm or just until blood is freely aspirated.

3. Suture the catheter in place, cover the insertion site with antibiotic ointment, and tape it to the abdominal wall. The catheter is then connected to a constant-infusion system and should be removed as soon as the indications for its insertion have passed. Complications appear to relate in part to the duration of insertion.[103,105,107]

Complications

- Thrombosis of portal or mesenteric veins[105,108]
- Infection (septicemia)[103]
- Endocarditis
- Pulmonary infarction (misplacement of the catheter into the pulmonary vein through a patent foramen ovale)
- Portal cirrhosis and esophageal varices later in life[109-112]
- Cardiac tamponade[113]
- Liver abscess and subcapsular hematoma[102,106]

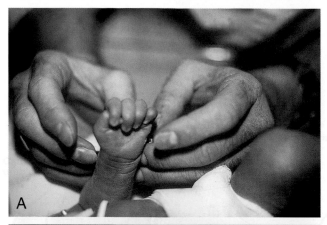

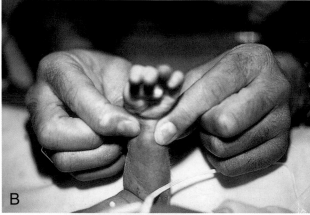

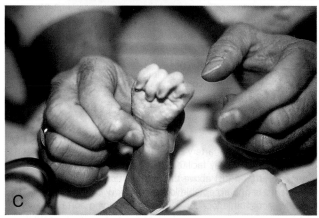

Figure 49-10. Modified Allen test. **A**, Color and perfusion of the hand are noted. **B**, The hand is first passively clenched, and then both radial and ulnar vessels are occluded. **C**, The ulnar artery is released while the radial artery remains occluded. If flow through the ulnar artery is adequate, then the color and perfusion should rapidly return.

noted. The hand is passively clenched, and the radial and ulnar arteries are simultaneously compressed at the wrist (see Fig. 49-10B). The ulnar artery is then released, and flushing (reperfusion) of the blanched hand is noted (see Fig. 49-10C). If the entire hand is well perfused while the radial artery remains occluded, indicating adequate collateral flow, catheterization of the radial artery is performed.

2. Secure the hand on an armboard with slight extension of the wrist to avoid excessive median nerve stretching. The finger-

tips should be left exposed when the hand is taped down so that any peripheral ischemic changes due to spasm, clot, or air can be observed.

3. Observe the course of the radial artery in a neonate with the aid of a fiberoptic light source directed toward the lateral side or dorsal aspect of the wrist. Use of a Doppler device may also be of some value.[141,142]

4. Use a 20-gauge needle to make a small skin puncture over the maximal pulsation of the radial artery, usually at the second proximal wrist crease. This step eases passage of the cannula by reducing resistance offered by the skin. A method to avoid accidental puncture of the artery is to pull the overlying skin laterally to make the skin nick.

5. Perform cannulation with a 24-gauge or 22-gauge catheter either on direct entry of the artery at an angle of 15 to 20 degrees or on withdrawing the cannula after transfixion of the artery (Fig. 49-11A-C). A wire (0.018 inch) may be used as an aid in advancement for 22-gauge and nontapered 24-gauge catheters.

6. Attach the catheter firmly to a T-connector to permit continuous infusion of isotonic saline (1 U/mL) at the rate of 1 to 2 mL/hr via a constant-infusion pump (see Fig. 49-10D). The catheter is securely taped in place. A pressure transducer is connected to allow continuous arterial pressure monitoring. To ensure accurate blood pressure measurement, it is essential that the transducer be calibrated to the neonate's/child's heart level, that all air bubbles be removed from the system, and that no more than 3 feet of tubing be used between the neonate/child and the transducer to minimize artifacts caused by the monitoring tubing.[143]

7. Obtain blood samples by clamping off the distal end of the T-connector, cleaning the injection port of the T-connector with povidone-iodine, introducing a 22-gauge needle, and allowing three to four drops of blood to flow out. A sample of blood is obtained by use of a heparinized syringe, with minimal blood loss and minimal manipulation of the system.[132,144] An alternative is the use of a 3-mL syringe on a 3-way stopcock: aspirate 2 to 3 mL, clamp the system, and then take the sample of blood from the T-connector as just described. After sampling, the clamp is released and continuous infusion is resumed or flush is run into the 3-mL syringe and then the system is gently manually flushed intermittently with the syringe but the flush syringe is changed just once per 24 hours. This method of sampling maintains a closed system with reduced potential for sources of infection. Bolus flushes are avoided, which is an important consideration because bolus flushing has been associated with retrograde blood flow to the brain. Disastrous results may occur if an air bubble or blood clot should accompany a bolus flush.[145] *All arterial lines must be clearly identified (red tape) to avoid accidental infusion of hypertonic solutions and sclerosing medications.*

Complications
- Infection at the site of the catheter insertion, with possible septicemia
- Arterial thrombus formation. This is dependent on the size of catheter inserted, the material of which it is constructed, the technique of insertion, and the duration of cannulation.
- Emboli. A blood clot or air may embolize to the digits, resulting in arteriolar spasm or more serious ischemic necrosis.

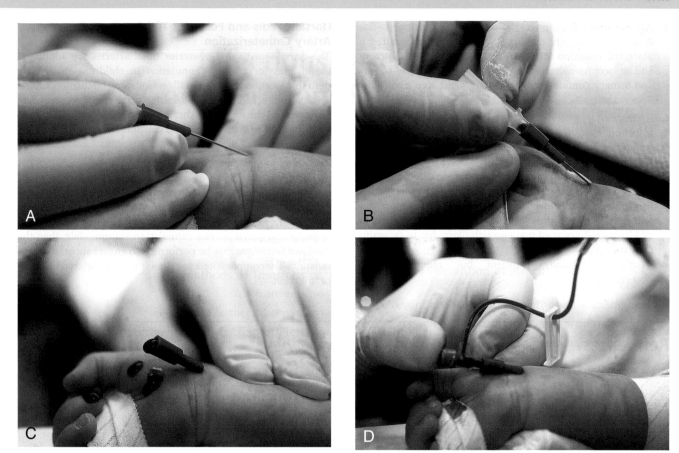

Figure 49-11. A, After adequate collateral circulation has been ensured, the radial artery is palpated and the appropriate catheter is advanced into the vessel. **B**, After blood return is noted, the catheter is threaded over the needle and into the artery. **C**, Pulsatile back-bleeding confirms intra-arterial position. **D**, A T-connector with appropriate flush solution is connected; the catheter is aspirated to clear air bubbles and then gently flushed. Antibiotic ointment and benzoin are applied. The injection port should be clearly marked as "arterial" so as to minimize accidental drug administration into the artery. A Luer-lock connection is preferred to prevent accidental disconnection.

- Disconnection of the catheter from the infusion system. Blood loss may be life-threatening, especially in an infant.
- Ischemia. The radial artery cannula should be withdrawn if ischemic changes develop.
- Vasospasm. Usually transient but requires careful observation.

The method just described is the traditional percutaneous radial artery cannulation at the ventral aspect of the wrist. The radial artery on the dorsal aspect of the wrist within the anatomic snuff box may be used as an alternative site.[146] Once an attempt at cannulation of the radial artery is made, the ipsilateral ulnar artery should not be instrumented to ensure adequate perfusion of the entire hand. Strict indications for inserting radial artery catheters are necessary, and their removal must be considered at the earliest possible time.[147-150]

Temporal Artery Catheterization

When the radial artery has been previously cannulated or is inaccessible, the temporal artery may be used.[151] The complication of cerebral infarction has been described with this technique. The infarction appears to be related to retrograde embolization of air or a blood clot.[152]

An advantage of this sampling site is that it provides preductal blood gas values. However, in our experience, the tortuous course of the artery and the resultant apposition of the distal tip of the catheter and the arterial wall have caused difficulties in freely drawing blood samples.

Femoral Artery Catheterization

Femoral catheterization in infants and children includes a greater risk of vascular injury or thrombosis resulting in ischemia[153] and is not recommended if other peripheral sites are available. In situations in which peripheral arterial cannulation is impossible (e.g., in burned patients or children with poor peripheral perfusion), the femoral artery should be used rather than not having any invasive arterial monitoring: one has to balance the remote possibility of a line complication versus a greater likelihood of life-threatening complications owing to less than ideal monitoring.[154]

Technique
1. Locate the femoral artery by palpation at the groin; this can be confirmed with ultrasonic guidance. Anatomically, it is situated midway between the anterior superior iliac spine and the pubic tubercle.
2. After sterile preparation of the skin, insert a catheter of appropriate size into the femoral artery using the Seldinger technique. The artery is entered at the point of maximal pulsation, approximately 1 cm below the line joining the anterior superior iliac spine and the pubic tubercle.

Table 50-11. Suggested Initial Dose and Time to Redosing for Antimicrobials Commonly Used for Surgical Prophylaxis

Antimicrobial	Half-Life Normal Renal Function (hr)	Half-Life End-Stage Renal Disease (hr)	Recommended Infusion Time (min)	Standard Intravenous Dose (g)	Weight-Based Dose Recommendation* (mg)	Recommended Dosing Interval[†] (hr)
Aztreonam	1.5-2	6	3-5[‡]	1-2	Max 2 g (adults)	3-5
Ciprofloxacin	3.5-5	5-9	60	400 mg	400 mg	4-10
Cefazolin	1.2-2.5	40-70	3-5[‡] 15-60[§]	1-2	20-30 mg/kg 1 g < 80 kg 2 g ≥ 80 kg	2-5
Cefuroxime	1-2	15-22	3-5[‡] 15-60[§]	1.5	50 mg/kg	3-4
Cefamandole	0.5-2.1	12.3-18[‖]	3-5[‡] 15-60[§]	1	20-40 mg/kg	3-4
Cefoxitin	0.5-1.1	6.5-23	3-5[‡] 15-60[§]	1-2	20-40 mg/kg	2-3
Cefotetan	2.8-4.6	13-25	3-5[‡] 20-60[§]	1-2	20-40 mg/kg	3-6
Clindamycin	2-5.1	3.5-5.0[¶]	10-60 (Do not exceed 30 mg/min)	600-900	<10 kg: at least 37.5 mg ≥10 kg: 3-6 mg/kg	3-6
Erythromycin base	0.8-3	5-6	NA	1 g orally 19, 18, 9 hr before surgery	9-13 mg/kg	NA
Gentamicin	2-3	50-70		1.5 mg/kg**	See footnote**	3-6
Neomycin	2-3 hours (3% absorbed under normal GI conditions)	12-≥24	NA	1 g orally 19, 18, 9 hr before surgery	20 mg/kg	NA
Metronidazole	6-14	7-21 no change	30-60	0.5-1	15 mg/kg (adult) 7.5 mg/kg on subsequent doses	6-8
Vancomycin	4-6	44.1-406.4 (Cl$_{cr}$ <10 mL/ min)	1 g ≥ 60 min (use longer infusion time if dose < 1 g)	1.0	10-15 mg/kg (adult)	6-12

*Weight-based doses are primarily from published pediatric recommendations.

[†]For procedures of long duration, antimicrobials should be redosed at intervals of 1 to 2 times the half-life of the drug. The intervals in the table were calculated for patients with normal renal function.

[‡]Dose injected directly into vein or running intravenous fluids.

[§]Intermittent intravenous infusion.

[‖]In patients with a serum creatinine value of 5 to 9 mg/dL.

[¶]The half-life of clindamycin is the same or slightly increased in patients with end-stage renal disease compared with patients with normal renal function.

**If the patient's weight is 30% above the ideal body weight, dosing weight can be determined as follows: DW = IBW + 0.4 (total body weight − IBW).

DW, dosing weight; IBW, ideal body weight; NA, not applicable.

incision, it is important to administer the antibiotics as soon as possible after intravenous access is established. If vancomycin must be used for prophylaxis, it should be infused slowly over 60 minutes (to minimize the risk of severe hypotension) beginning within 2 hours of skin incision. If a tourniquet is required, the full antibiotic dose should be administered before the tourniquet is pressurized.[126] Postsurgical prophylactic antibiotics are not necessary for most procedures and should generally be stopped within 24 hours after the surgical procedure.[126]

Allergy to β-Lactams

Several studies have shown that the true incidence of allergy is less than that reflected in medical charts.[127] For surgical procedures where cephalosporins are the prophylaxis of choice, alternative antibiotics should be administered to those children at high risk for serious adverse reactions or allergy, based on their history or diagnostic tests (e.g., skin testing). However, the incidence of adverse reactions to cephalosporins in children with reported allergy to penicillin is rare; further-more, skin testing does not reliably predict the likelihood of adverse reactions to cephalosporins in those with reported allergy to penicillin.[128-130] For the most part, "allergies" to oral antibiotics that appear on children's charts (rash, vomiting, gastrointestinal disturbances) are reactions to the additives in the antibiotic formulation including food dyes, fillers, and other compounds. Intravenous administration of small test doses of the pure

Table 50-12. Wound Classification System

Wound Category	Description
Class I/clean	Uninfected wound with no inflammation and the respiratory, alimentary, genital, or uninfected urinary tract is not entered. Clean wounds primarily are closed and drained, when necessary, with closed drainage. Operative wounds after blunt trauma may be included in this category if they meet criteria.
Class II/clean contaminated	Operative wound in which the respiratory, alimentary, genital, or urinary tract is entered under controlled conditions and without unusual contamination. Specifically, operations involving the biliary tract, appendix, vagina, and oropharynx are included in the category, provided no evidence of infection or major break in technique is encountered.
Class III/contaminated	Open, fresh, accidental wounds; operations with major breaks in sterile technique (e.g., open cardiac massage) or gross spillage from the gastrointestinal tract; and incisions in which acute, nonpurulent inflammation is encountered
Class IV/dirty-infected	Old traumatic wounds with retained devitalized tissue and those that involve existing clinical infection or perforated viscera, suggesting that the organisms causing postoperative infection were present in the operative field before operation.

From Neville HL, Lally KP: Pediatric surgical wound infections. Semin Pediatr Infect Dis 2001; 12:124-129.

antibiotics in a fully monitored (and anesthetized) child with a so-called allergy may be used to establish the child's susceptibility to an allergic reaction to the antibiotic.

In the case of surgical procedures where antibiotic prophylaxis is mainly directed at gram-positive cocci, children who are truly allergic to β-lactams (cephalosporins) should receive either vancomycin or clindamycin.[122]

Indications for Prophylactic Antibiotics

Surgical wounds are classified in four categories (Table 50-12). The use of antibiotic prophylaxis for postoperative infections is well established for clean-contaminated procedures. Within the clean category, prophylaxis has been traditionally reserved for surgical procedures involving a foreign body implantation or for any surgical procedure where a surgical site infection would be catastrophic (e.g., cardiac surgery or neurosurgical procedures). However, there is evidence to demonstrate that postoperative infections resulting from procedures not involving prosthetic elements are underreported; estimates show that over 50% of all complications occur after the patient is discharged from hospital and are unrecognized by the surgical team. Therefore, antibiotic prophylaxis is also recommended for certain procedures such as herniorrhaphy.[131,132] The direct and indirect costs of these complications will not affect the hospital budget; however, they represent a high cost for the community at large. In the case of contaminated or dirty procedures, bacterial contamination or infection is established before the procedure begins. Accordingly, the perioperative administration of antibiotics is a therapeutic, not a prophylactic, measure. The use of antibiotics in children has implications not only for the response to the current treatment but also to future treatments. Thus, all medical professionals are jointly responsible for the rational use of antibiotics.

Protocols, although effective, require continuous feedback on their acceptance and surgical site infection results. No surgical protocol can replace the judgment of the medical professional; clinical reasoning must be tailored to the individual circumstances. Finally, children with congenital heart disease and many of those with repaired congenital heart disease will require subacute bacterial endocarditis prophylaxis (see also Tables 14-1 and 14-2).[133]

Annotated References

Hota B: Contamination, disinfection, and cross-colonization: are hospital surfaces reservoirs for nosocomial infection? Clin Infect Dis 2004; 39:1182-1189

Although much about the spread of nosocomial infection remains unknown, several facts have been established by existing data: (1) inanimate environmental surfaces can become durably contaminated after exposure to colonized patients; (2) although an organism may be endemic within an institution, specific isolates may predominate in the inanimate environment (e.g., vancomycin-resistant enterococci); and (3) contaminated rooms may be a risk factor for the acquisition of nosocomial pathogens by unaffected patients. This author elaborates on the need for improved infection control measures for preventing nosocomial infections.

Rizzo M: Striving to eliminate catheter-related bloodstream infections: a literature review of evidence-based strategies. Semin Anesth Perioper Med Pain 2005; 24:214-225

This paper reviews and emphasizes the need for preventive measures that could help to avoid or reduce most nosocomial catheter-related infections. The use of protocol evidence-based standardized protocols will result in "best practices" and markedly reduce such infections.

Sagoe-Moses CH, Pearson R, Perry J, Jagger J: Risks to health care workers in developing countries. N Engl J Med 2001; 345:538-541

Protecting health care workers in developing countries from exposure to blood-borne pathogens will involve some cost. Health care workers are a crucial resource in the health care systems of developing nations. In many countries, including those in sub-Saharan Africa, workers are at high risk for preventable, life-threatening occupational infections. This paper expands on the need for improved support of health care workers throughout the world with appropriate supplies of gloves, barriers, sharps disposal, and the need for educational accident programs.

References

Please see www.expertconsult.com

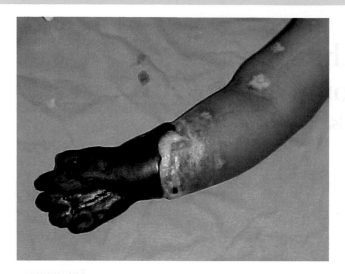

Figure 51-1. Peripheral gangrene of the hand. Severe dehydration in this infant was caused by severe gastroenteritis. Dehydration in association with delayed presentation, hypernatremia, herbal medications, and pneumonia are common contributors to this disastrous outcome.

Superstition may also play a role in compounding the anesthetic risk. For example, rural Vietnamese believe that it is not good to die with an empty stomach; parents consider surgery an enormous risk so they feed their children beforehand. Passage of a nasogastric tube before induction of anesthesia is routine, although it is quite likely that the stomach will not be completely emptied of solids despite the tube.[24]

Perinatal mortality in some parts of the developing world is ten times greater than those in developed countries.[25] The common denominators are early childbearing, poor maternal health, and, above all, the lack of appropriate and quality medical services. Although lifesaving practices for most infants have been known for decades, currently one third of pregnant women still have no access to medical services during pregnancy, and almost 50% do not have access to medical services for childbirth.[15,19,26] The majority of parturients give birth at home or in rural health centers,[19] where basic neonatal resuscitation equipment is often deficient or nonexistent.[15] Those who require surgery may need to be transferred, but specialized transport teams rarely exist.

In some hospitals, neonates are not candidates for surgery because "they always die,"[27] whereas in others they undergo surgery without anesthesia[8] because "it's safer" and because some still believe that neonates do not feel pain. When surgery is performed in neonates, there are additional challenges, particularly in emergency situations.[8] Not only is there a lack of appropriately sized equipment,[21] but it may be extremely difficult to maintain normothermia even in relatively warm climates without improvisation. Regional anesthesia can play a significant role in neonatal anesthesia[15,21,28] and in some centers may be the only choice for anesthesia.[19,29] Apart from providing analgesia without respiratory depression, the need for postoperative ventilatory support for conditions such as esophageal atresia,[30] congenital diaphragmatic hernia,[31] and abdominal wall defects are reduced by continuous epidural analgesia (Fig. 51-2).

Regrettably, even neonates who have skillful anesthesia and surgery may die because of inadequate postoperative care.[29]

Overwhelming infection, sepsis, respiratory insufficiency, and surgical complications are the main causes of morbidity and mortality.[15,19] The development of highly specialized neonatal anesthetic and surgical services,[25,27] essential for a good outcome after neonatal surgery,[15,19,21] is a low priority.

While the burden of diseases is dominated by infections and malnutrition; pediatric trauma has low advocacy and as such is given scant attention.[15,21,32] Socioeconomic advances in some countries have introduced a new danger in the form of faster more powerful vehicles without the necessary maintenance culture or road discipline. Road traffic accidents are inevitable and effective systems to handle the polytrauma victims that result are hard to find.[21]

Even simple bone fractures may have disastrous outcomes. Inappropriate management by traditional bonesetters may frequently result in compartment syndromes or even gangrene.[32] Road traffic accidents are common and injuries are highly preventable. Trauma prevention strategies are given low priority despite the acknowledged impact it has on the economy of any country. Additionally, many developing countries are at war and this has led to massive trauma and injuries to children who may be participants in the fighting or innocent bystanders.

Children and War

Children may be victims of all aspects of violence; they face an intense struggle for survival as a consequence of displacement, separation from or loss of parents, poverty, hunger, and disease. They are vulnerable to the abuse of abandonment, abduction, rape, and forced soldiering. An estimated 300,000 children are currently used as child soldiers in over 30 countries.[33] Many

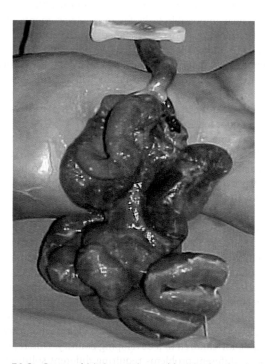

Figure 51-2. Gastroschisis is a major problem in the developing world. The outcome is poor because of a paucity of facilities for neonates. This defect was not diagnosed antenatally and presented late for closure, which proved difficult. Ventilatory support was not available, and a silo thus was fashioned. Unfortunately the child died of overwhelming sepsis a week later.

sustain physical injuries and permanent disabilities, whereas a large number acquire sexually transmitted diseases, including HIV/AIDS. These HIV-positive child soldiers then become vectors in communities where they are deployed.[34]

For many of these children acts of violence become the only form of normality: the former victims become the perpetrators.[17] Survivors are subjected to the total collapse of economic, health, social, and educational infrastructures. Lost and abandoned children sleep on the streets and are forced to beg for

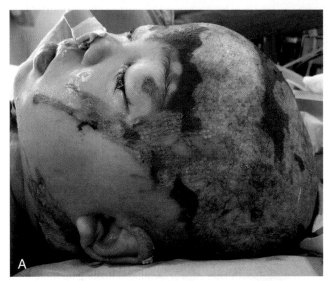

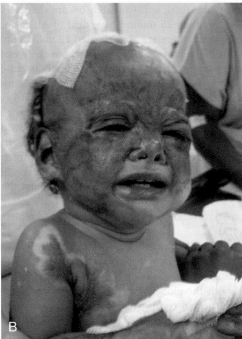

Figure 51-3. Facial burns. Burn injuries are common in the developing world, and these children may require multiple anesthetic procedures. **A,** Flame burns of the face are invariably associated with inhalation injuries that may necessitate ventilatory support in intensive care units, which are often not readily available; **B,** Pain management and pain assessment are challenging. The pained expression on this child's face is one of fear (and possibly the indignity of having the photograph taken!) rather than actual pain.

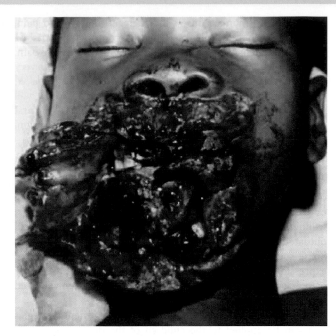

Figure 51-4. Children and war. This 8-year-boy bit a detonator he found while playing. Endotracheal intubation proved a major challenge without a fiberoptic laryngoscope, a luxury in the developing world.

food while trying to find their families. Many become child laborers or turn to crime or prostitution for survival.[35]

Children in war-torn areas sustain bullet, machete, or shrapnel wounds, whereas others are burned; these mutilating injuries (Figs. 51-3 and 51-4) are not commonly seen in civilians.[36] Land mines are responsible for killing or maiming an estimated 12,000 civilians per year. In Angola, a country with the highest rate of amputees in the world, there were an estimated 5.5 land mines for every child. Continuing land mine explosions remain a chronic legacy of this conflict.[36] These blast injuries leave children without feet or lower limbs, with genital injuries, blindness, and deafness—a pattern of injury that has become a post–civil war syndrome encountered by surgeons worldwide.[36] Although the war in Angola is essentially over, the cost of land mine removal is beyond the means of local governments. Ironically, artificial limb manufacture has become a developing industry.[36]

The terrible psychologic effects of war persist even though the armed conflict may be over. Mental and psychiatric disorders with all the ramifications of post-traumatic stress disorder are common among child survivors.

Pain
Unfortunately, pain management modalities for children in developed countries are vastly different from those available to practitioners working with limited resources and inadequately trained personnel in the developing world. Attempting to apply similar standards is fraught with difficulty. Illiteracy, malnutrition, poor cognitive development, differing coping strategies, pharmacogenetic, cultural, and language differences all contribute to the complexity of the problem.

Children of the developing world cope with vastly different problems. They may be victims of poverty, malnutrition, or

perinatal transmission by more than 90% compared with the 1993 rate.[51]

Differentiating those infants who are infected by vertical transmission from those who are not infected presents a difficult dilemma because one cannot easily differentiate between actively or passively acquired antibodies. All children born to HIV-positive mothers will have acquired HIV antibody in the first 6 to 18 months. Only 30% to 40% of those infants who are actually infected may go on to develop AIDS. The presence of HIV antibody is, therefore, not a reliable indicator of infection. More sophisticated expensive tests have been developed but are not yet widely available. All children born to HIV-positive mothers, therefore, should be considered potentially infected; if antibody persists beyond 15 months, infection should be assumed.

Progression of the disease depends on the mode of transmission; vertically acquired infection is more aggressive. Twenty to 30 percent of HIV-infected children will develop profound immune deficiency and AIDS-defining illnesses within a year, whereas two thirds will have a slowly progressive disease. The course of the disease depends on a variety of factors including the timing of infection in utero, viral load, and mother's stage of the disease.

The clinical manifestations of HIV infection in infants and children vary. The majority may have asymptomatic infections, and the presentation may be subtle, such as failure to thrive, lymphadenopathy, hepatosplenomegaly, interstitial pneumonia, chronic diarrhea, or persistent oral thrush. Some present for the first time with severe life-threatening disease. Chronic diarrhea, wasting, and severe malnutrition predominate in Africa, whereas systemic and pulmonary pathologic processes are more common in the United States and Europe. Recurrent bacterial infections, chronic parotid swelling, lymphocytic interstitial pneumonitis, and early onset of progressive neurologic deterioration are characteristic of children with AIDS.

Pulmonary disease is the leading cause of morbidity and mortality.[52,53] Bacterial pneumonia, viral pneumonia, and pulmonary tuberculosis (TB) are common in children throughout the developing world. The course of these infections is more fulminant when associated with HIV infection. Acute opportunistic infections occur when the CD4 T-cell count falls; these include *Pneumocystis carinii* pneumonia (PCP), *P. jirovecii* pneumonia (PJP), cytomegalovirus, as well as the more typical *Haemophilus influenzae*, *Streptococcus pneumoniae*, and respiratory syncytial virus infections.[52,53] The classic presentation of PCP is fever, tachypnea, dyspnea, and marked hypoxemia, but in some children the presentation is more indolent, with hypoxemia preceding clinical or radiologic changes.

A slowly progressive chronic form of lung disease, lymphocytic interstitial pneumonitis or pulmonary lymphoid hyperplasia, occurs in older children and can lead to an insidious onset of dyspnea, cough, and chronic hypoxia with normal auscultatory findings. In contrast to adults, lymphocytic interstitial pneumonitis may cause acute respiratory failure in children and is treated with corticosteroids and bronchodilators. Management of the upper airway may be difficult in the presence of stomatitis and gingival disease. Intubation may be difficult in the presence of acute (candidal) or chronic epiglottitis (lymphoid hyperplasia), necrotizing laryngotracheitis, Kaposi sarcoma (Fig. 51-6), or laryngeal papillomas (Fig. 51-7). These comorbid respiratory disorders will challenge even the most experienced pediatric anesthesiologist (Fig. 51-8).

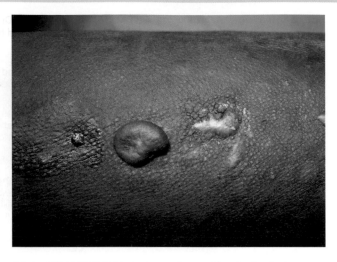

Figure 51-6. HIV/AIDS is an increasing problem in developing countries, particularly in sub-Saharan Africa. Skin manifestations of Kaposi sarcoma seen here in an 8-year-old boy indicate an AIDS-defining tumor.

Cardiac disease is being recognized with increasing frequency in HIV-infected children. The pathogenesis of the cardiomyopathy is multifactorial and includes pulmonary insufficiency, anemia, nutritional deficiencies, specific viral infections, and drug therapy. Left and right ventricular dysfunction, arrhythmias, and pericardial effusions are seen. HIV may directly infect the myocardium itself, leading to early electrocardiographic changes: abnormal echocardiograms show either hyperdynamic left ventricular dysfunction or evidence of diminished contractility.

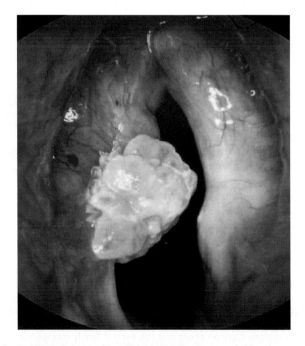

Figure 51-7. Laryngeal papilloma. Papillomas, caused by the human papillomavirus, are prevalent in low socioeconomic groups, with the highest incidence in the 2- to 5-year age group. This age distribution is changing in the HIV-exposed population. Even in well-equipped institutions, anesthesia for these children can be challenging.

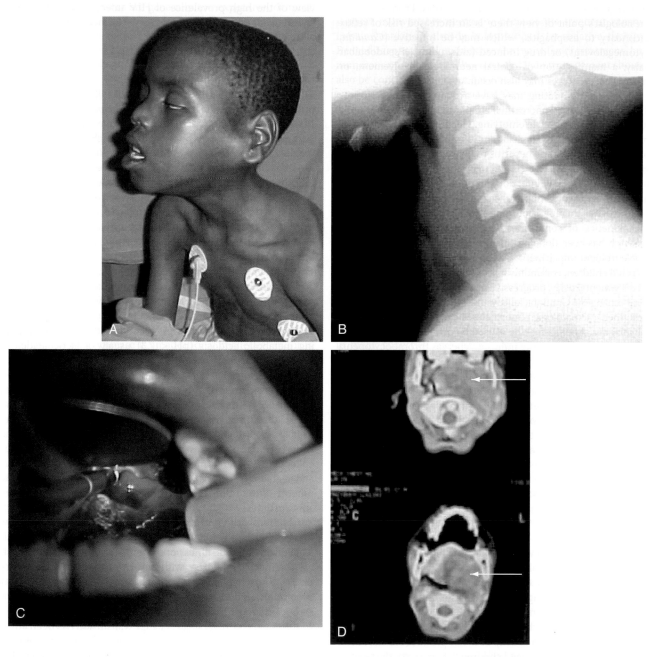

Figure 51-8. Kaposi sarcoma is a marker for AIDS. It was previously considered to be rare in children but may even affect the airway at different levels, as shown in this child. **A,** This 12-year-old girl is clearly fatigued from the respiratory distress caused by Kaposi sarcoma at three levels: base of the tongue, tonsil, and trachea. In addition, she has an underlying pneumonia. Significant supraclavicular recession suggesting upper airway obstruction is evident. **B,** A Kaposi sarcoma of the base of the tongue, tonsil, and trachea is shown on this poor-quality lateral neck radiograph that is illustrative of one of the many difficulties faced in remote areas. **C,** Laryngoscopic view of the Kaposi sarcoma at the base of tongue and tonsil. **D,** CT scan showing a large retropharyngeal Kaposi sarcoma (*arrows*) obstructing the upper airway. The poor quality of the CT image is typical of scans performed by inexperienced radiographers using poor quality equipment commonly found in developing countries.

considered dangerous in an environment where the oxygen supply is erratic[66] and agent monitors are not available.[10] The erratic supply of soda lime and compressed gas cylinders further limits it use. Consequently, the potential benefits and cost savings of low-flow anesthesia are lost.[66]

Regional anesthesia has many benefits, in terms of safety, cost savings, and immediate postoperative analgesia.[1,8,15,19,21,28,67,68] Generally, children in developing countries are very accepting of this form of analgesia. However, there seems to be a general reluctance to perform regional anesthesia in children[14,21] even in some institutions in the developed world. Possible reasons include lack of training or expertise, fear of failure, and the unavailability of drugs and disposable and other ancillary equipment.

Improvisation may be the key. Access to the epidural space can be obtained if the appropriate equipment is not available by using a technique first described before the introduction of pediatric epidural needles into clinical practice. A catheter can be threaded well into the epidural space through an intravenous cannula inserted into the caudal space via the sacral hiatus in neonates and small infants.[69] Furthermore, inexpensive noninsulated needles can be used for peripheral nerve blocks when more expensive insulated needles are not available.[70]

Blood Safety

An estimated 70% of all blood transfusions in Africa are given to children with severe anemia caused by malaria. Blood transfusion services, if they exist, aim to provide a lifesaving service by ensuring an adequate supply of safe blood.[71] Patients, particularly children, in developing countries face the greatest risks from unsafe blood and blood products.[72]

Fewer than 30% of developing countries have a nationally coordinated blood transfusion service. Many of these do not even perform the most rudimentary tests for diseases such as HIV infection or hepatitis B and C because of economic constraints. Even limited testing doubles the basic cost of a unit of blood. It is estimated that some 6 million tests that should be done globally to check for infections are not done annually.

Many countries still rely on paid donors or family members to donate blood before surgery. In Argentina, for example, up to 92% of the blood supply is derived from family members. Although voluntary unpaid blood donation has increased to 20% in the past 5 years in Pakistan, family donors constitute 70% and paid donors 10% of the blood donors in 2004.[72] Over the past decade, through concerted efforts by the World Health Organization to improve blood safety worldwide, the number of voluntary unpaid donors has increased considerably. For example, voluntary blood donation in China increased from 45% of donations in 2000 to 90% in 2004. Similarly, the rate of voluntary, unpaid donations in Bolivia increased from 10% in 2002 to 50% in 2005. Malaysia, China, and India reached 100% screening of donated blood for HIV infection by the year 2000.[73]

There are risks in any system. Family and paid donors may hide aspects of their health and lifestyle that could make the blood unsafe for different reasons. Family members may feel pressured to donate, whereas paid donors are driven by need and avoid important details about their health status. The commercial plasma industry and blood trade can fuel the transmission of HIV. In 1999, 26 million liters of plasma were fractionated for global use;[74] the major source was paid donors from developing countries. Voluntary unpaid donors have a greater sense of responsibility toward their community and keep themselves healthy so as to be able to keep giving safe blood. South Africa has had 100% voluntary, unpaid donation since it established a national blood service. With HIV prevalence approaching 30% in the adult population Africa, only 0.02% of its regular blood donors in South Africa have contracted HIV infection.

Storage of blood is difficult considering the unreliable and unpredictable electricity supply in many of the developing countries. To obviate the risk of transmission of malaria, HIV, and other infectious diseases, blood should be transfused only when absolutely necessary. In sophisticated blood transfusion units, the use of predonated autologous blood is an option.[75] In poorer countries this is not practical because malnutrition and chronic anemia are common. There is often a lack of appropriate equipment, and cost is also prohibitive. Similarly, intraoperative blood salvage, let alone cell savers appropriate for use in children, are simply not available. Recombinant factor VII, which is being used more and more frequently to reduce blood usage by those who can afford it,[75] is beyond the scope (and cost) of practice in many countries.

Equipment

Electrical supplies are unreliable in many hospitals in the developing world. In some, particularly in rural areas, neither main electricity nor a reliable functional generator are available.[2] General facilities for infection control, such as running water, disinfectants, or gloves, are not always available and the reuse of disposable equipment such as endotracheal tubes is normal practice in many countries.[2]

Essential equipment to provide safe anesthesia for children and particularly neonates is lacking.[2,10,15,21] Neonatal or pediatric ventilators are virtually nonexistent outside the main centers.[15] Small intravenous cannulas are a precious commodity, and butterfly needles are still used (and in some cases reused!). Syringe pumps and other control devices are impractical in environments that have an erratic electricity supply. Laryngoscopes, both metal and plastic, are usually available but generally not well maintained. Batteries may be in short supply and light bulbs unreliable. Endotracheal tubes in the full pediatric range are rarely found and are invariably recycled because there is no alternative. Laryngeal mask airways in pediatric sizes are less freely available. Intravenous fluids are very expensive if not manufactured locally, and many developing countries do not have any local production facilities.[3] The choice of intravenous fluid is, therefore, limited and in short supply.

Monitoring is very basic and done with a precordial stethoscope and a finger on the pulse.[1] Electrocardiographic monitoring is used when available but is dependent on a constant electricity supply and proper maintenance. Appropriately sized blood pressure cuffs are scarce. Pulse oximetry has been shown to be the most useful monitor and should be available in all centers where pediatric surgery is performed.[1,10] Unfortunately, this ideal is far from reality.

Anesthetic machines in developing countries fall into two categories: modern sophisticated machines or simple low maintenance equipment. Modern electronic machines, provided by well-meaning donors, have a poor track record in austere environments. Sophisticated equipment needs to be understood, but this is not aided by operating manuals that are printed in a foreign language. Sophisticated machines require maintenance, and individuals trained to repair equipment are seldom available. Service contracts are not considered viable. Unfortunately these machines are invariably discarded when the first fault occurs because guarantees are unlikely to be honored and faults are considered too expensive to repair. Poorly maintained equipment becomes hazardous and even life-threatening in untrained hands.

Simplicity and safety have long been the keys to anesthetic equipment in developing countries.[1-3,76] Ideally, a suitable anesthetic machine should be inexpensive, versatile, robust, and able to withstand extreme climatic conditions, able to function even if the supply of cylinders or electricity is interrupted, easy to understand and operate by those with limited training, economical to use, and easily maintained by locally available

skills.[77,78] The least expensive, most practical, and most widely used anesthetic is inhalational anesthesia administered through an EMO (Epstein Macintosh Oxford) or OMV (Oxford Miniature Vaporizer) draw-over vaporizer. Oxygen concentrators supplement oxygen delivery and eliminate the need for expensive oxygen cylinders whose reducing valves are often faulty or destroyed in these austere environments. The most appropriate ventilator is the Manley Multivent Ventilator, which essentially functions like a mechanical version of the OIB (Oxford Inflating Bellows) and can be used with a draw-over system.[78]

A general scheme for inhalation anesthesia in developing countries is shown in Figure 51-9,[79] which was first proposed by Ezi Ashi and associates in 1983.[66] By applying this scheme, four different modes can used and modified according to the available supplies and services. The basic mode A is for use when there is no electricity and no supply of compressed gases. The

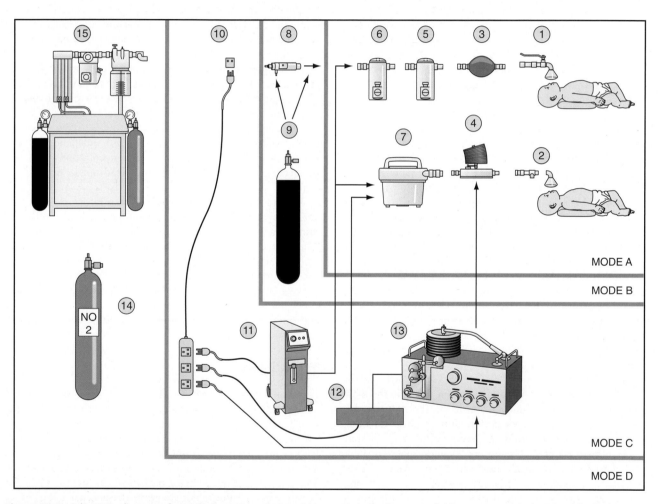

Figure 51-9. Schematic diagram of anesthetic systems that could be used depending on available resources. Mode **A** provides basic inhalation anesthesia with air, spontaneous ventilation, or self-inflating bags. Draw-over vaporizers are required. Mode **B** provides oxygen enrichment but requires the availability of oxygen cylinders. Plenum vaporizers can be used. Mode **C** requires electricity to power the oxygen concentrator, air compressor, and/or ventilator. A mechanical ventilator (e.g., Manley) does not require electrical power. Mode **D** requires a Boyles machine and nitrous oxide cylinders. (1), T-piece with reservoir tube and face mask; (2), Ambu Paedi valve; (3), self-inflating bag (Ambu); (4), Oxford inflating bellows (OIB); (5), Oxford miniature vaporizer (OMV) with halothane; (6), OMV with trichloroethylene; (7), EMO vaporizer with ether. These circuits and manual ventilators are interchangeable and ether, halothane, and trichloroethylene can be used on their own or in series. (8), Farman's entrainer with an oxygen cylinder (9) can be used to supplement oxygen; or an electrical power source (10) is available with an oxygen concentrator (11), air compressor (12), or Manley ventilator (13). Nitrous oxide (14) and Boyles apparatus (15) allow anesthesia practice equivalent to that of developed countries.

apparatus consists of a low-resistance vaporizer linked by valves to the patient to act as a draw-over system with room air as the carrier gas. The self-inflating bag or hand bellows makes it possible to provide artificial ventilation while the vaporizer remains as a draw-over. The addition of low flow oxygen to the inspired gas in mode B depends on the availability of an oxygen cylinder. The addition of a length of reservoir tubing to the circuit enables oxygen to be stored on expiration, to be used on the next inspiration, substantially improving its economy.[80]

When electricity is available (mode C), the operation of the anesthetic apparatus can be extended by permitting the use of (1) an air compressor to provide continuous gas flow (which in turn would allow the use of a Boyles apparatus and plenum vaporizer); (2) oxygen concentrator; and (3) ventilators. When nitrous oxide is available (mode D) all types of inhalation anesthesia currently available in developed countries can be practiced. In situations where services and supplies are interrupted even acutely, it is possible to change from one mode to another without requiring other anesthetic apparatus.

These techniques may be of little interest to the anesthesiologist working comfortably in the well-maintained sophisticated environment of developed nations. Their role, however, is considerable in the field situations (war, natural disasters), and today's anesthesiologist should be acquainted with their functioning in this unpredictable world.

Draw-Over Anesthesia

Draw-over anesthesia enables inhalation anesthesia to be administered using atmospheric air as the carrier gas. The essential features of this system consist of a calibrated vaporizer with sufficiently low resistance (EMO and OMV) to allow the negative pressure created by the child's inspiratory effort to draw room air through the vaporizer during spontaneous ventilation. Positive-pressure ventilation can be provided by means of a self-inflating bag or bellows (OIB), with a valve to prevent the gas mixture reentering the vaporizer, as well as a unidirectional valve at the child's airway to direct expired gases to the atmosphere, preventing rebreathing (see mode A, Fig. 51-6). In this way, an anesthetic can be administered in the absence of compressed gases. The vaporizer has an inlet for supplementary oxygen that can be attached to the oxygen output tube of an oxygen concentrator or oxygen cylinder when available (see modes B and C, Fig. 51-6).

The EMO (Epstein, Macintosh, Oxford: Penlon, Ltd.) and the OMV (Oxford Miniature Vaporiser: Penlon, Ltd.) are the more commonly used low resistance vaporizers. The EMO is calibrated only for ether, but its performance is linear for other agents. The OMV is calibrated for a variety of agents;[27,78] despite the lack of temperature compensation its performance is stable under most conditions. Both these vaporizers have been used successfully in pediatric anesthetic practice,[18] but it is recommended that they be converted to form a T-piece for greater safety.

The OMV has been evaluated as a simple draw-over system for pediatric anesthesia. Wilson and associates[27] showed that when a self-inflation bag is used in a draw-over mode, more efficient vaporization occurs despite vaporizer cooling. However, the respiratory efforts of neonates or weak infants are insufficient to operate the valve mechanisms of the self-inflating bag (e.g., Ambu bag), necessitating continuous assisted ventilation even in the presence of ether, which stimulates ventilation.

Oxygen Concentrators

Improved oxygen availability, independent of compressed gas and electrical power supply, can be provided by linking oxygen concentrators to a draw-over anesthetic apparatus as first described by Fenton.[65] Maintenance requirements are low, and servicing is recommended only after approximately 10,000 hours of usage. The benefits are enormous, but a reliable electricity supply is critical.

The concentrator functions by using a compressor to pump ambient air alternately through one of two canisters containing a molecular sieve of zeolite granules that reversibly absorbs nitrogen from compressed air.[63,78] The controls are simple and comprise an on/off switch for the compressor and a flow-control knob to deliver 0 to 5 L/min. Flow of oxygen continues uninterrupted as the canisters are alternated automatically so that oxygen from one canister is available while the other regenerates. A warning light on a built-in oxygen analyzer illuminates if the oxygen concentration is less than 85% and the concentrator switches off automatically when the oxygen concentration is less than 70%. This is heralded by visual and audible alarms. Air is then delivered as the effluent gas. Modern machines are relatively silent.

The oxygen output of the concentrator depends on the size of the unit, the inflow of oxygen, the minute volume, and pattern of ventilation. The addition of dead space (or oxygen economizer tube) at the outlet improves the performance, and predictable concentrations of more than 90% oxygen can be obtained with flows between 1 and 5 L/min independent of the pattern of ventilation. Much lower concentrations and less predictability was noted when the dead space tubing was omitted.[80]

The possible hazards of oxygen concentrators are few, provided they are positioned in the operating room so that the indraw area is free from pollutants. Failure of power supply or failure of the zeolite canisters will result in the delivery of ambient air. A bacterial filter at the outlet combined with the use of dust-free zeolite should prevent contamination of the delivered gas. Dirty internal air filters may produce lower oxygen concentrations and must be checked. An oxygen storage tank and booster pumps afford protection against the vagaries in electrical supply.

The Visitor

Personality traits compatible with survival have been suggested as a prerequisite for working in the austere environments of the developing world. These personality traits include an almost pathologic desire for hard work, a willingness to merge or at least sympathize with a different culture, patience to relate to and teach people sometimes far removed educationally, the ability to withstand prolonged periods of cultural isolation, but mostly, a never failing ability to improvise and make the best of a bad situation.[79,81] There is no place for risk taking.[81]

International travel, particularly visits to many parts of the developing world, needs careful preparation and planning whether the anesthetist is part of a volunteer organization[18,82,83] or traveling as an individual. Detailed advice[82,83] is beyond the scope of this chapter, but some generalizations are made based on personal experience and those of colleagues. Changing political climates and international health guidelines dictate visa and vaccinations requirements. Expert advice should be sought to tailor the traveler's needs according to the individual's medical and immunization history, the duration of stay, and the proposed itinerary.

Physical acclimatization (ranging from jet lag to altitude sickness, heat, or sunburn) will be necessary, as well as an adjustment to the local culture and cuisine. Social graces acceptable in a western culture may be deemed offensive in some other cultures. An interpreter is an important ally. However, the inability to understand a language or the local dialect places a visiting anesthesiologist at a serious disadvantage, particularly when dealing with children. Children often use subtle ways to describe their feelings that even a skilled interpreter may fail to convey.

The hospital environment may be disconcerting for some. In contrast to the familiar comforts of a clean child-friendly hospital, the visitor may be struck by the relatively shabby, bland appearance of many hospitals in developing countries. The buildings may not have received a coat of paint since they were originally built, and broken windowpanes provide the only air conditioning. Children are usually cared for in adult wards.

In the operating room the visitor may be faced with anesthetic equipment barely recognizable from its original manufacture or in a state of disrepair with nonstandard improvisations in attempts to make it functional. The choice of drugs may be limited, and the names of locally manufactured generic drugs and the presentation of intravenous solutions may add to the confusion. Surgical safety may be the next issue. Informed consent, as we know it, and patient identification in the absence of parents may not be obvious to the newcomer. A local or itinerant surgeon may suggest an extensive procedure on a malnourished child without consideration for monitoring, blood transfusion, or availability of intensive care or postoperative analgesia in an unmonitored environment. The anesthesiologist is obliged to carefully consider the risks and benefits in such circumstances.

Summary

The practice of anesthesia in an austere environment in a developing country will always be challenging, particularly for those who provide anesthesia for children. The challenges vary from country to country and even within a given country. Expect the unexpected, and have the flexibility to improvise in the face of an ever-changing world racked by famine, violence, natural disasters, and political unrest. The nuances of practice in different communities will inevitably vary and may even challenge some fondly held beliefs in pediatric anesthesia.

Different standards may emerge from different parts of the world. Such standards need not necessarily be considered inferior but may well open the way for the assimilation of new ideas.[84] A safe anesthetic is not necessarily the most expensive one. After all, it is generally not the agents that we use but the skill with which we use them that determines outcome. It should never be necessary to depart from the dictum *primum non nocere*. Simplicity may be the key, but there is no place for double standards. Guidelines, evolved over time in the United Kingdom, United States, and Australia may be untenable in many parts of the world,[84] but every attempt should be made to exercise the same standard of care as expected in the developed countries. Our children deserve no less!

Acknowledgments

One author (ATB) acknowledges the input provided by Haydn Perndt (Ethiopia), Anneke Meursing (Malawi), Carol Parrot (Vietnam), Annette Davis (Mocambique), Richard Ing (South Africa, Ethiopia, Nicaragua,), Jeff Morray (Khazakstan), David Baines (East Timor), Narko Tuotuo (Solomon Islands), Zippy Gathuya (Kenya), Felix Namboya (Malawi), and Sats Bhagwanjee, Dave Muckart, Larry Hadley (South Africa), all of whom have worked or are working in a developing country. All tried, as I did, to ensure that important points were not omitted. The author would also like to thank my hosts Philemon Amambo (Namibia), Eric Borgstein (Malawi), Ali Salaama (Sudan), Carlos Parsloe (Brazil), Dr. Gunnesar (Mauritius), the Indian Society of Paediatric Critical Care, the Malaysian Society of Anaesthetists, the Zimbabwean Society of Anaesthetists, and Operation Smile, Inc., who afforded me the opportunity to visit their respective countries and gain a glimpse of anesthetic practice in those parts of the world.

References

Please see www.expertconsult.com

litigation process. This involves your family and colleagues and, occasionally, psychiatric assistance. The most difficult emotion to deal with is anger when you realize the system may not be about the truth but rather how the lawyers can persuade and sway the jury. Another source of emotional stress is the qualifications (or lack of qualifications) of plaintiff's experts, which will at times surprise you with distortions or exaggerations of fact.[21]

Summary

The manner in which physicians interface with the law in their daily practice of medicine varies greatly. The need for a pediatric anesthesia caregiver to be informed of legal issues arising from his or her practice has become essential. It has also meant that the breadth of knowledge that those who support care in your practice must acquire has increased significantly. This requires that educational materials to keep you and your staff up to date with pertinent legal issues is a necessary part of your practice. In addition, you may want to have access to a health care lawyer who can provide advice and counsel on a periodic basis. Your facility may have such a lawyer on staff or your practice may have an attorney to whom you can turn when the need arises.

This chapter provides a framework for some of the common issues that you may encounter in your daily practice. There are many more legal issues such as billing regulations and regulations that govern your practices' interactions with a hospital or other health care facility that have not been addressed here.

Annotated References

Davidson AJ, Huang GH, Czarnecki C, et al: Awareness in children: a prospective cohort study. Anesth Analg 2005; 100:653-661

This paper defines the incidence of awareness under anesthesia in children, which may be higher than in adults, but further study is needed.

Eichhorn JH: Organized response to major anesthesia accident will help limit damage: update of "Adverse Event Protocol" provides valuable plan. APSF Newsletter, Spring 2006. Available at http://www.apsf.org/assets/Documents/SUMMER_06.pdf

This is a select article from an entire issue of the Anesthesia Patient Safety Foundation regarding the management of an adverse event; in particular, an organized "adverse event protocol" is described.

Feldman JM: Do anesthesia information systems increase malpractice exposure? Results of a Survey. Anesth Analg 2004; 99:840-843

This paper demonstrates with a small cohort that an automated record in general is more helpful in defending an anesthesiologist should an adverse event occur primarily because there is more precise recording of the event at the time of occurrence rather than a record being filled in hours later after the event has occurred.

Gross JB, Bachenberg KL, Benumof JL, et al: Practice guidelines for the perioperative management of patients with obstructive sleep apnea: a report by the American Society of Anesthesiologists Task Force on Perioperative Management of patients with obstructive sleep apnea. Anesthesiology 2006; 104:1081-1093

This guideline has made significant changes in the management of all patients with obstructive sleep apnea, including children. Close attention will indicate particular recommendations regarding children in selecting those who are and are not appropriate candidates for same-day surgery.

Sebel PS, Bowdle TA, Ghoneim MM, et al: The incidence of awareness during anesthesia: a multicenter United States study. Anesth Analg 2004; 99:833-839

This article is important because it defines the incidence of awareness under anesthesia in adults.

References

Please see www.expertconsult.com

Pediatric Equipment

Richard H. Blum and Charles J. Coté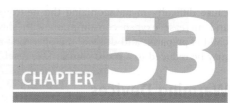

CHAPTER 53

Heating and Cooling Systems

The operating room, which is comparable to a large infant incubator, provides the physical environment for the conduct of anesthesia. Readily controlled heating and cooling systems are crucial for thermal stability of the child, that is, control of the external environment. The neonate or small infant requires a warmer room temperature than an adult and should be considered poikilothermic particularly if preterm, critically ill, or stressed. With approximately 40% of heat loss by radiation and 35% by convection, increasing the operating room temperature warms the walls, which decreases radiation heat loss, and warms the air, which decreases convection heat loss (see Chapters 25, 35, and 36). Exposure to a cool room temperature during induction of anesthesia and surgical preparation may cause significant thermal stress, particularly in the preterm neonate and young infant. Mild to moderate hypothermia may cause acidosis and apnea in infants, alter the pharmacokinetics of medications,

oximeter senses the motion of the pulse but light is transmitted around the finger or toe, thus providing a falsely high hemoglobin saturation. Only size-appropriate oximeter probes should be used in infants and children. In critically ill children and those with thermal injuries, problems with finding a suitable site to apply the probe can be overcome by using a modified oximeter probe applied to the tongue (see Fig. 34-13A-D).[262,263] The tongue provides a rich blood supply unaffected by vasoconstriction, and electrocautery interference is less. If the tongue moves, the sensor may dislodge or record a false heart rate. Thermal injury secondary to the interface of incompatible sensor probes and cables (i.e., equipment from more than one manufacturer) has been reported, as has pressure necrosis resulting from too tight an application.[264,265]

Newer-Generation Pulse Oximeters

Recent advances in pulse oximetry technology have attempted to make several major improvements, including (1) software that provides motion artifact compensation; (2) software that allows uninterrupted readings even in low-flow states; (3) software that provides more accurate assessment of oxygenation in cyanotic children; and (4) software that allows measurement of methemoglobin and carboxyhemoglobin levels.[155] Conventional pulse oximetry time-averages a signal over 5 to 10 seconds, depending on the default settings of the oximeter. This signal represents the ratio of transmitted red and infrared light, and the instrument uses this to determine the child's hemoglobin saturation. This averaging smooths over motion-induced artifacts but may ultimately lessen the sensitivity and response time of a conventional oximeter in situations of hypoxemia or even delay the recognition of asystole or severe bradycardia by several seconds. More recent models are designed to recognize motion artifact and discard signal aberrations secondary to motion using proprietary signal filtering techniques. Some devices combine two different approaches to signal processing to arbitrate the correct saturation based on dual signal filtration techniques using both "pattern matching" and "adaptive comb filtering." This technique is designed to detect motion and reject analysis of data generated during motion. Other oximeter manufacturers take a different approach using spectrophotometer principles to generate a saturation signal. That saturation signal may contain several component saturations corresponding to different absorption artifacts of blood and other tissues, including venous blood. The signal is then processed using a discrete saturation transform (DST) algorithm that then extracts the highest and presumably the arterial component saturation and then reports this value as the hemoglobin oxygen saturation.[266-269] Conventional pulse oximeters can either overestimate or underestimate the degree of desaturation and therefore may have less accuracy and greater signal dropout rate (i.e., no reading or poor quality signal associated with an alarm) especially in children with hypoxemia. These deviations may be improved with the newer generation pulse oximeters, but this has yet to be definitively demonstrated.[270] The newer-generation pulse oximeters perform better than conventional pulse oximetry in hypothermic low flow states during cardiopulmonary bypass.[271] Movement artifact is the main cause of false alarms in sedated or awake children who require oximetry monitoring. This artifact is significantly reduced with the current generation of pulse oximeters in both adult and pediatric patient populations.[272-276] It is hoped this improvement will result in greater utilization in non–operating room and non–critical care venues where children are not under the effects of muscle relaxants (e.g., the emergency department, the recovery room, children receiving opioids on patient wards, and in the ICU).

Reflectance Oximetry

Reflectance pulse oximetry has been available for many years, but with recent technologic improvements several devices have achieved FDA approval and are currently marketed. The technology behind reflectance oximetry involves the emission of multiple wavelengths of red and infrared light that are sensed in two or more photo detectors located a distance away from the diodes on the same probe sensor (Fig. 53-15). These devices measure reflected rather than transmitted light. The technology used to create these oximeter probes permit usage on the forehead, in the esophagus, and on the fetal scalp. The forehead devices have had the largest use among pediatric anesthesiologists. Studies of reflectance oximeters in general demonstrated that these devices are more susceptible to erratic measurements when the probe is placed directly over an artery[277] and vein.[278] The oximetry measurements can be significantly decreased when compared with traditional pulse oximetry. Some potential advantages to using reflectance oximetry on the forehead include better signals during conditions of poor perfusion, lack of motion, and faster response time than conventional peripheral oximeter probes. However, possible disadvantages include a potentially high signal dropout rate and poor accuracy.[279] Several studies report good correlation between concurrent measurements of oxygen saturation comparing reflectance oximetry on the forehead,[280] esophagus,[281] and around the chest of preterm infants,[282] compared with extremity pulse oximetry and arterial co-oximetry measurements but also report a clear dropout rate.

Near-Infrared Spectroscopy

Near-infrared spectroscopy (NIRS) is a noninvasive, optical technology that bears similarities to pulse oximetry in that it uses the relative absorption of near-infrared light, 700 to 900 nm, through biologic tissues to determine tissue oxygenation.[283] Oxyhemoglobin and deoxyhemoglobin absorb light at different frequencies, and the use of a probe that emits and detects different frequencies of near-infrared light can be used to estimate tissue oxygenation. This device has been most widely used to measure "regional" cerebral oxygen saturation (rSO_2).[284-287] Pulse oximetry requires the measurement of the pulsatile (arterial) component of the total light transmitted by the biologic tissue. Because NIRS does not require the subtraction of the pulsatile component, the signal is more than 100 times stronger and unaffected by poor perfusion compared with pulse oximetry. It is, however, susceptible to motion artifact and ambient light noise. A probe placed on the child's forehead measures the concentration of oxyhemoglobin and deoxyhemoglobin in the tissue underlying the probe. The device functionally measures the oxygenation of blood in the underlying tissues, including blood in the arterioles, capillaries, and venules. The majority (approximately 85%) of the signal originates from the venules; skin and bone and extracranial blood absorb only limited amounts of light that is subtracted from the signal and does not have significant impact of the measurement in infants and children.[288,289] NIRS thus measures the oxygen saturation in venous, as well as arterial, blood and, as such, represents an average saturation across blood vessels and tissue. In cerebral oximetry, the oxygen saturation of the blood in the tissue (i.e., between

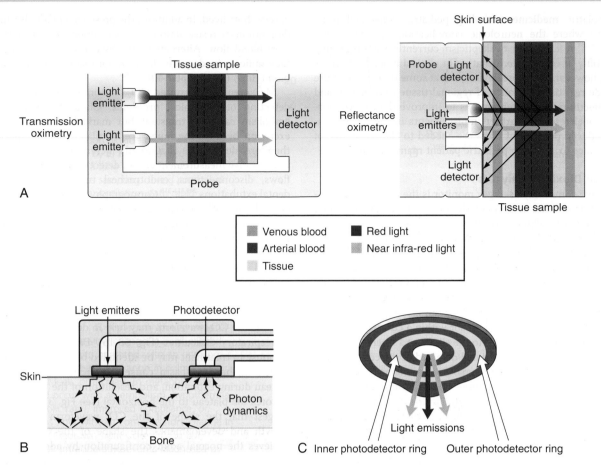

Figure 53-15. A, Comparison of conventional transmission pulse oximetry with reflectance oximetry. Note that with conventional oximetry that the light detector is located directly opposite on the other side of a digit and detects light transmitted through the digit; with reflectance oximetry the light detector is located next to the light emitters and detects the light reflected back through and from the tissues. **B,** Typical configuration of a reflectance oximeter. **C,** Another configuration where several light detectors are located at different distances from the light emitters. In addition, reflectance oximeters may emit light in more than just 2 wavelengths, which is typical of conventional transmission pulse oximeters. (Redrawn with permission from Kugelman A, Wasserman Y, Mor F, et al: Reflectance pulse oximetry from core body in neonates and infants: comparison to arterial blood oxygen saturation and to transmission pulse oximetry. J Perinatol 2004; 24:366-371, and Keogh BF, Kopotic RJ: Recent findings in the use of reflectance oximetry: a critical review. Cur Opin Anesth 2005; 18:649-654.)

the sending and emitting probe) depends on factors that affect oxygen transport, including cerebral blood flow, hemoglobin saturation, hemoglobin-oxygen binding affinity, and oxygenation saturation in the arterial blood. Therapies aimed at improving oxygen delivery or decreasing oxygenation consumption to the brain will potentially increase cerebral oxygenation (rSO_2).[290,291] This technology is not new; however, only one device is currently FDA approved for commercial use to measure cerebral oxygenation (INVOS Cerebral Oximeter, Somanetics Corporation, Troy, MI). The absolute accuracy of the current Somanetics device is plus or minus 10% to 15%, making the measurement of absolute oxygenation unreliable, although it is reasonably accurate for changes in oxygenation (±5%), making this device useful only for following trends in cerebral oxygenation.[292-295] Other devices are more accurate and capable of measuring oxygenation in other tissues but are not currently FDA approved.

Studies of healthy children and animals using devices that have been shown to have greater accuracy than the Somanetics Cerebral Oximeter demonstrate that normal regional cerebral oxygen saturation (rSO_2) is 60% to 80%.[296,297] In controlled hypoxic-ischemic states in animals, electroencephalographic slowing and increased tissue lactic acid levels occur at rSO_2 between 40% and 45%. The EEG becomes flat at rSO_2 between 30% and 35%, and if the cerebral ischemia is protracted, it may be associated with tissue infarction.[297]

There are many important limitations to this technology, including the lack of accuracy of the actual measurements. Currently, this device is used only to follow the trends of each child. The relationship between the amount of tissue damage and clinical outcome depends on the site of the tissue damage. This monitor measures only the saturation in tissue below the probe and reflects more accurately on focal tissue oxygenation and/or damage. If the probe is placed on the forehead, it will reflect the state of the tissue in the frontal cortex and may not reflect other areas of the brain.

Although there are no studies that have as yet demonstrated that cerebral oximetry improved outcomes, published data do support the potential efficacy of this technology in many areas